Handbook of Medical Psychiatry

D0543804

SECOND EDITION

Handbook of Medical Psychiatry

David P. Moore, M.D.
Associate Clinical Professor of Psychiatry,
University of Louisville School of Medicine;
Frazier Rehab Institute,
Louisville, Kentucky

James W. Jefferson, M.D.
Distinguished Senior Scientist,
Madison Institute of Medicine, Inc.;
Clinical Professor of Psychiatry,
University of Wisconsin Medical School,
Madison

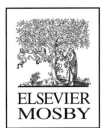

ELSEVIER
MOSBY

ELSEVIER
MOSBY
An Affiliate of Elsevier

170 S. Independence Mall W.
300 E.
Philadelphia, PA 19106-3399

HANDBOOK OF MEDICAL PSYCHIATRY, 2nd Edition   ISBN 0-323-02911-6

NOTICE

Medicine is an ever-changing field. Standard safety precautions must be followed, but as new research and clinical experience broaden our knowledge, changes in treatment and drug therapy may become necessary or appropriate. Readers are advised to check the most current product information provided by the manufacturer of each drug to be administered to verify the recommended dose, the method and duration of administration, and contraindications. It is the responsibility of the licensed physician, relying on experience and knowledge of the patient, to determine dosages and the best treatment for each individual patient. Neither the publisher nor the editor assumes any liability for any injury and/or damage to persons or property arising from this publication.

Previous edition copyrighted 1996.

Library of Congress Cataloging-in-Publication Data

Moore, David P.
Handbook of medical psychiatry/David P. Moore, James W. Jefferson.—2nd ed.
   p. ; cm.
  Includes bibliographical references and index.
  ISBN 0-323-02911-6
  1. Biological psychiatry—Handbooks, manuals, etc. I. Title: Medical psychiatry.
II. Jefferson, James W. III. Title.
  [DNLM: 1. Mental Disorders—Handbooks. WM 34 M821h 2004]
RC455.4.B5M64 2004
616.89—dc22   2004044821

Acquisitions Editor: Susan F. Pioli
Editorial Assistant: Joan Ryan
Publishing Services Manager: Joan Sinclair
Project Manager: Mary Stermel

Printed in the United States of America

Last digit is the print number: 10   9   8   7   6   5   4   3   2   1

Scribere actum fidei est.

To my wife
Nancy G. Moore, Ph.D.
my children,
Ethan, Nathaniel and **Joshua**
and to my editor
Susan Pioli
who has been, and remains, a godsend

DPM

◆

Cui dono lepidum novum libellum
arido modo pumice expolitum?
Catullus c.84–c.54 BC

To
Susan Mary Cole
my wife of many years,
Lara, Shawn and **James,**
my children of quite a few years,
and **Cole** and **Dean,**
my grandchildren

JWJ

Preface to the Second Edition

In the preface to the first edition of the *Handbook of Medical Psychiatry* we stated that it was our intention to write a comprehensive, thorough and practical textbook of psychiatry, presented firmly within the medical model. We are happy to say, judging by the reviews the *Handbook* received in many journals, that it appears we succeeded.

This second edition builds on the strengths of the first. The *Handbook* continues to cover almost every psychiatric, neurologic and general medical condition capable of causing disturbances in thought, feeling or behavior, together with almost every psychopharmacologic agent currently available in America. Further, it continues to provide sufficient detail such that the reader will be better equipped to assess, diagnose and treat whatever case may be encountered in the clinic, on the ward or during consultations.

Finally, at its heart, it remains extremely practical – the sort of text that the student and resident will keep on the ward (and next to the phone at night), and to which the practitioner may refer when in need of a refresher or when confronted with a rare or unusual condition.

The pace of research in psychiatry has quickened since the first edition, and we have aimed to keep the *Handbook* current. To that end, the entire text has been revised and updated, and 26 new chapters have been added.

We trust, as we did before, that the reader will find this text useful, and we hope that it will further solidify psychiatry's place as a medical specialty.

David P. Moore
James W. Jefferson

Contents

SECTION IV
Schizophrenia and Other Psychotic Disorders

SECTION V
Mood Disorders

SECTION VI
Anxiety Disorders

SECTION VII
Somatoform Disorders

SECTION VIII
Dissociative Disorders

SECTION XXX
Electroconvulsive Treatment

GENERAL SYMPTOMATOLOGY

1 General Symptomatology

As is the case with all medical specialty areas, the symptoms described in this chapter are of varying specificity and sensitivity. In some cases specificity is fairly high; for example, Schneiderian delusions, although not specific for schizophrenia, are strongly suggestive of this disorder. Unfortunately, this degree of specificity is rare for most symptoms in psychiatry; rather, most symptoms, such as depressed mood, may be found in a host of disorders.

Given the relative nonspecificity of most of the symptoms described below, becoming familiar with, at the least, the most common disorders described in this book is necessary. The importance of the overall clinical picture cannot be overstressed; in most cases one cannot rely on any one or two symptoms. The box on p. 2 lists the signs and symptoms covered in this chapter.

A. APPEARANCE

The overall appearance of the patient may offer valuable diagnostic clues. Dress, grooming, and demeanor may be an integral part of the symptomatology of an illness.

Some patients may appear bizarre, unkempt or disheveled. The hair may be uncut, dirty, and uncombed; the fingernails long and likewise dirty. The clothing may be torn, mismatched for color and pattern, and is often layered with redundant shirts, sweaters, and socks. Ornaments and bits of jewelry may be oddly placed; some patients may wear tin foil to keep off noxious influences, or have their ears plugged with cotton to keep away the voices. Such an overall appearance may be seen in schizophrenia.

Depression, when severe, may render certain aspects of dress and grooming such an effort that they are left undone. The hair, though perhaps clean, may only be halfheartedly combed; women may omit their makeup. When less severe, patients may be able to keep up appearances, but their overall demeanor may indicate their illness. The shoulders sag, the posture is slumped, the head may be hung, and the over-all impression is of a body drained of life. In some cases this drained appearance can be truly remarkable. During depression the skin may become deeply lined and lack turgor, the hair appear lifeless and dull, and the eyes lack any vibrancy. Upon recovery the change may be startling. Patients may appear to have become 10 years younger; the eyes may sparkle, the hair appear almost lustrous, and the skin appear smooth and vital.

In contrast with depressed patients, manic patients may appear overvitalized. Dress is often overly colorful, at times clashing. Jewelry may be in abundance and overly gaudy; at times patients may be absolutely festooned with jewelry. Veritable headdresses may be worn, and women may plait their hair, often intertwining it with flowers or colorful ribbons. Colorful appearance may also be seen in patients with a histrionic personality disorder. The dress of histrionic patients, however, though perhaps tastefully colorful, rarely becomes as garish as that sported by the manic.

Some patients with anorexia nervosa attempt to hide their emaciation with long hair, bulky sweaters, and long heavy skirts. The drawn, sunken face, however, belies the robust impression offered by the dress.

B. DISTURBANCES OF ACTIVITY

B1. Inactivity

Inactivity may stem from a variety of causes including psychomotor retardation and lack of interest (or anhedonia), as seen in depression, a general slowing of all processes as may be seen in hypothyroidism, ambivalence and "annihilation of the will" as in schizophrenia, abulia of the frontal lobe syndrome, and the peculiar combination of paralyzing ambivalence and tension seen in catatonic stupor.

In depression patients lose their hedonic capacity: they take no pleasure in things; nothing excites or motivates them; and they lose interest in former pleasures. For them, all the color seems drained away from life, leaving it stale and tasteless, a wearisome burden. Coupled with this lack of interest, there is typically a more or less profound anergia, or lack of energy. Patients complain of feeling fatigued, drained, and exhausted. Some also experience an oppressive heaviness and a sense of painful inhibition of all processes. At times the oppressive fatigue may be so severe as to make simple actions, such as picking up a fork, impossible.

Thus fatigued and unexcited by life, depressed patients may sit motionless for hours; simple tasks are accomplished only with the greatest of effort. They may speak little, and, when they do, it may be but a whisper, soon to trail off again into silence.

The slowing seen in hypothyroidism primarily consists of fatigue and lack of energy. In contrast to depressed patients, hypothyroid patients often retain some interest, and rarely complain of a sense of oppressive inhibition.

The ambivalence seen in schizophrenia may paralyze the patient into inaction. Here it is not so much a case of an inability to exert the will, but rather the simultaneous appearance of two opposite but equally strong inclinations. When faced with a choice, the patient may thus be unable to commit to one or another course of action. In one case, a patient, though hungry, sat through a meal without eating, being unable to decide whether to use a fork or a spoon.

In other cases of schizophrenia, an actual annihilation of the will may be seen: the capacity to act volitionally, to conceive of a purpose and follow it, may be lost. Such patients are unable to summon themselves to purposeful activity and may spend their

Signs and Symptoms

■

A. Appearance	F7. Delusions of reference
B. Disturbances of activity	F8. Schneiderian delusions
B1. Inactivity	F9. Bizarre delusions
B2. Agitation and hyperactivity	F10. Erotomanic delusions
B3. Impulsivity	F11. Pseudomemories
B4. Bizarre behavior	G. Hallucinations
C. Abnormal movements	G1. Auditory hallucination
C1. Tics, chorea, and tremors	G2. Visual hallucination
C2. Stereotypies	G3. Tactile hallucination
C3. Mannerisms	G4. Olfactory hallucination
C4. Catatonic symptoms	G5. Gustatory hallucination
D. Relationship to the examiner	H. Disturbances of thought
E. Disturbances of mood and	H1. Loosening of associations
affects	H2. Poverty of thought and
E1. Depressive symptoms	speech
E2. Manic symptoms	H3. Thought blocking
E3. Irritability	H4. Mutism
E4. Anxiety	I. Cognitive defects
E5. Labile affect	I1. Confusion
E6. Inappropriate affect	I2. Disorientation
E7. Flat affect	I3. Decreased memory
F. Delusions	I4. Calculations
F1. Somatic delusions	I5. Abstractions
F2. Delusions of poverty	I6. Judgment and insight
F3. Nihilistic delusions	J. Other symptoms
F4. Delusions of sin	J1. Obsessions and
F5. Delusions of persecution	compulsions
F6. Delusions of grandeur	J2. Phobias

hours in meaningless tasks, such as gathering up bits of dust, or doing nothing except sitting still or lying in bed.

Abulia, as seen in the frontal lobe syndrome, shares certain characteristics with annihilation of the will seen in schizophrenia. The abulic patient, though neither depressed, slowed down, nor fatigued, appears apathetic and lacking in motivation. With their mental horizons undisturbed by any impulses or strivings, such patients may sit quietly for long periods.

In stuporous catatonia patients may lie motionless for hours, days, weeks, or even longer. Saliva may drool from their mouths, and the contents of bowel and bladder may be loosed into their clothing. Yet no matter how profound the stupor, such patients never appear quite dead inside, and at times, as proof of this, they may suddenly erupt into a frenzy of catatonic excitement.

B2. Agitation and Hyperactivity

Depressed patients may at times exhibit an extraordinary degree of psychomotor agitation. They may wail loudly, plead for relief, or even for death. They may pace agitatedly about their room or up and down the hall, and classically one sees prominent and unceasing hand-wringing.

Excited catatonia presents a different picture. Here patients are neither despairing nor pleading for help; rather their hyperactivity seems senseless and bizarre. One patient may stand in a corner, bellowing in a declamatory voice; another may pace about the ward from one door to another always touching the doorknobs twice; another may simply march frantically in place, first in one spot, then another. In extreme catatonic excitation patients may jump up, scooch across the floor, turn somersaults, tear up the bed linen, and eventually require restraint.

Manic excitation differs from the psychomotor agitation seen in depression by virtue of the abundance of energy seen in mania, and differs from catatonic excitement by the presence of purpose in the manic behavior. Exalted and energized, patients may rush from one person to another to loudly proclaim their news. They may bang on the doors, jump to the tabletop to give a speech, pour everyone water and insist it be drunk "now," and in general, in their overbusyness, inflict themselves on any who come into view. In acute mania and certainly in delirious mania, discerning the purpose behind a patient's hyperactivity may be difficult. Distractibility becomes so severe that patients no sooner embark on one purposed activity before another commands their attention and resources. Eventually their behavior becomes characterized by competing and ever-changing fragments of purpose. Hundreds of things may be started, some simultaneously, yet none are completed.

B3. Impulsivity

Although isolated impulsive acts may occur in a large number of disorders, impulsivity per se is less common. Of the various disorders characterized, at least in part, by impulsivity, mania and excited catatonia are the two most important.

The behavior of a manic patient is almost a veritable blossoming of impulsivity: one after another impulse overrides whatever steadying forces still exist in the patient. No interference is tolerated, and no obstacle is too great as the patient gives free rein to whatever at the moment he wants to do. Indeed, should anyone attempt to block the patient's impulse, such a person may be met with a torrent of irritable abuse.

The impulsivity of a patient with excited catatonic schizophrenia (and, to a lesser degree, the other subtypes of schizophrenia) is less constant and free flowing than that seen in mania. Indeed, between impulsive acts, catatonic patients may be withdrawn and even mute. Suddenly, however, with no warning or provocation, a catatonic patient may leap up, smash furniture, scream a song, assault a passerby, or rip off clothing; then, just as suddenly, the patient may again break off all contact and withdraw, perhaps to a corner, or into bed.

Attention-deficit/hyperactivity disorder in children or adolescents may be marked by impulsivity, and such youngsters may blurt out whatever comes to mind or act on whatever impulse arises.

Active alcoholics may display considerable impulsivity, not only when intoxicated, but also when more or less sober. The irritability and often fierce resentments harbored by the alcoholic easily overwhelm whatever restraint and good judgment are left. Those addicted to cocaine, stimulants, or opioids may become very impulsive indeed when their supply is cut off and the craving is strong. In such situations impulsive acts of violence are not uncommon. Patients with a histrionic personality disorder display almost a caricature of impulsivity. Good drama requires impulsive deeds, and these patients, to keep the limelight trained on themselves, may go so far as to feign impulsivity. A different picture obtains for patients with borderline personality disorder: here patients lack reliable internal controls; under stress, the patients' restraint and good judgment become brittle and frail, leaving them prey to their own self-destructive impulses.

Patients with dementia (especially those with the frontal lobe syndrome) or with mental retardation either lose or, in the case of mental retardation, never fully acquire self-restraint. Thus when they see something they want, little or nothing internal impedes them from trying to get it. In this sense they are like normal 2-year-olds, who seem to act as if they believed that everything in view belongs, or perhaps should belong, to them.

B4. Bizarre Behavior

Bizarre or grossly disorganized behavior should always raise the question of schizophrenia. Under the influence of delusions patients may heap rotting fruits in a corner, paper their room with tinfoil to ward off noxious rays, paint windows black to thwart those spying on them, or take an ad in the paper announcing their plans for world peace through strict vegetarianism. At times, however, the bizarre behavior is apparently without motivation: bits of paper may be zealously stuffed into pockets; patients may march in place, walk backward, declaim to a wall, or turn their furniture upside down.

Mania, especially in the delirious stage, may produce a similar and at times almost indistinguishable picture of bizarre behavior. Here, as pointed out in the chapter on bipolar disorder, the differential rests on demonstrating the existence of more typical signs of mania before the patient's behavior became bizarre and disorganized.

Some patients with autism may be particularly bizarre. During an interview such patients may exhibit gaze avoidance, looking anywhere but at the person interviewing them. They may demonstrate a peculiar flapping tremor when stressed, skitter into a corner, squat, defecate, and crawl under a chair, all the while chattering away. The sometimes difficult differential between autism and schizophrenia of childhood onset is discussed in the chapter on autism.

Bizarre behavior may also be seen in metachromatic leukodystrophy, hepatic porphyria, interictal psychoses, and drug intoxication with phencyclidine.

C. ABNORMAL MOVEMENTS
C1. Tics, Chorea, and Tremors

Abnormal movements, such as tics, chorea, and peculiar tremors, are strongly suggestive of certain specific disorders. They must, however, be distinguished from stereotypies and mannerisms, which are discussed later.

Tics are repetitive rapid involuntary movements that bear a greater or lesser degree of similarity to purposeful behavior. Simple tics may consist of things such as eye blinking or grimacing; complex tics much more resemble purposeful behavior and may even consist of vocalizations. Coprolalia, or the involuntary utterance of obscenities, is a classic, albeit not common, example of a complex vocal tic. Tics should always raise the suspicion of Tourette's syndrome, but may be seen also as side-effects of various medications (e.g., stimulants, carbamazepine or lamotrigine), as part of tardive dyskinesia, and, rarely, in Huntington's disease, neuroacanthocytosis and Sydenham's chorea.

Chorea consists of rapid purposeless movements occurring randomly both in time and in spatial location on the body. Indeed, choreiform movements may seem to dart from one part of the body to another like summer lightning. Common causes of chorea include Huntington's disease, tardive dyskinesia and Sydenham's chorea; other causes include medications (e.g., phenytoin, oral contraceptives and stimulants), hyperthyroidism and lupus.

Tremor is generally postural, rest or intention in type. Postural tremor may be seen in essential tremor, anxiety, hyperthyroidism, hypoglycemia, as a side-effect to numerous medications, during delirium of various causes, and, above all, during alcohol withdrawal. Rest tremor is found in parkinsonism, whether due to Parkinson's disease or some other cause, as for example as a side-effect of an antipsychotic. Intention tremor is seen with cerebellar lesions or during intoxication with alcohol or sedative-hypnotics, such as benzodiazepines.

A peculiar flapping tremor may be seen both in autism and in Wilson's disease.

C2. Stereotypies

Stereotypy represents a kind of perseveration, which may be found in schizophrenia and in some cases of intoxication with cocaine or stimulants. In schizophrenia, stereotypies are often bizarre. One patient read a page, turned it, read the other side, then turned back to the original side, and repeated this over and over again in a stilted, ritualized way until the page disintegrated. Another sang the same fragment of a song recurrently through the morning, in a screeching, halting voice. Still another, shuffling along the hallway, all the while facing the wall, would lay one curiously bent finger on the wall every few feet, going thus up and down the hall for hours. Some patients exhibit stereotyped speech, repeating the same, often nonsensical, phrase again and again. Such verbal stereotypy, when fairly rapid and enduring, is known as verbigeration.

In those instances of intoxication with cocaine or stimulants that are characterized by stereotyped behavior, the resultant stereotypies, at least initially, tend to be more purposeful than the stereotypies seen in schizophrenia. Typically, machines are involved: one patient repetitively took apart then put back together a radio, while another attempted the same maneuver with a watch. In severe intoxication, however, purpose may be lost: one patient simply rapidly and repetitively struck his forehead with his hand.

C3. Mannerisms

Manneristic behaviors are characterized by affectation, stiltedness, or bizarre ritualization. Normal activity thus loses its grace, fluidity, and easy purpose and is transformed into an almost alien caricature of normal behavior. Rather than break into a smile, the face may contort into a bizarre, lopsided grin; a patient's hand, extended to shake the physician's hand, may be offered with the fingers spread and arched back. Gestures are particularly prone to manneristic transformations. At times the fingers and hands seem to have a life of their own, alien and strange to whatever the patient is otherwise saying or doing. The fingers may writhe or perhaps assume positions that seem totally unnatural and divorced from any possible gestural communication. Facial expression may also display mannerisms. In particular one may see repetitive bizarre grimacing.

Mannerisms may be seen in mental retardation and in a variety of deliria and dementias. Thus in the presence of confusion or of defects in memory, orientation, or abstracting ability, mannerisms are diagnostically nonspecific. However, in the presence of a clear sensorium and intact memory, orientation and abstracting ability, mannerisms are strongly suggestive of schizophrenia.

C4. Catatonic Symptoms

Traditionally the following symptoms have been considered catatonic: catalepsy and waxy flexibility, posturing, negativism, and automatic obedience (including echopraxia and echolalia).

Although most typically seen in catatonic schizophrenia or in a depressive or manic episode, these symptoms are at times seen with lesions of the frontal lobes, in epilepsy-related psychoses and as a side-effect to certain medications, most notably disulfiram.

In catalepsy, patients maintain whatever position they are placed into by the examiner, no matter how awkward. Indeed the limbs and torso may be molded into the most unnatural position, and patients stay that way perhaps for hours with no sign of fatigue until, over a brief period of time, a normal position is again assumed. Often, catalepsy is accompanied by waxy flexibility (also known as flexibilitas cerea). Here the examiner meets with a peculiar stiffness upon attempting to move the patient's limbs, as if bending a soft waxen rod, or perhaps one made of solder.

In catatonic posturing, patients spontaneously, without any recognizable motivation, assume bizarre postures and then maintain them for varying periods of time. One patient stood with one leg raised, like a stork; another sat with head hung and arms outstretched in front, as if attempting to catch something.

Negativism, or the tendency to do or say the opposite of what is asked or what is appropriate to the situation, is often confused with simple stubbornness or oppositionalism. The difference between negativism and stubbornness is qualitative: in stubbornness a patient's behavior is purposeful and is to some degree modifiable by argument or persuasion. By contrast, negativism has an instinctual quality to it, as if the patient has no choice but to do the opposite. This difference between stubbornness and negativism is most apparent when the negativism is severe. Examples include refusing to dress, drawing the hand away when the physician offers to shake hands, and resolving into a cramped grimace and remaining mute when asked a question.

Automatic obedience is almost the exact opposite of negativism. Here patients do or say whatever is asked of them, regardless of consequences. This is not mere agreeableness, for the patients act in a wooden, mechanical way, almost like robots, and seem heedless of any danger. For example, in the nineteenth century, patients, upon request, would hold the tongue protruded despite knowing that the examiner intended to pierce it with a pin, and neither flinch nor attempt to withdraw as the piercing occurred. In some cases of automatic obedience one may see echolalia or echopraxia. Here, without being asked, the patient's behavior mirrors whatever is said or done by the interviewer. If the examiner speaks, the patient repeats the words, often in a monotonous voice. If the examiner raises an arm the patient does likewise.

D. RELATIONSHIP TO THE EXAMINER

Defining the quality of the relationship between a patient and physician is sufficiently difficult such that few diagnostic schemes use it as one of their diagnostic criteria. Nevertheless, the feeling that the examiner has during the interview can offer important diagnostic clues. This is particularly the case with the "praecox feeling" related to schizophrenia and the "infectious good humor" of mania.

The term "praecox feeling" is derived from the older name for schizophrenia, dementia praecox. In the course of interviews with some patients with schizophrenia, interviewers may find themselves possessed of an eerie feeling as if they were speaking to someone alien, to someone who, in certain fundamental ways, is not reacting normally. With patients with other disorders, a certain affective harmony occurs between physician and patient, and the physician's reactions, whether sympathy, anger, or pity, clearly interlock with the patient's own emotional state. With some

patients with schizophrenia, however, the affective bond does not form: there seems no way to connect with the patient, as if one were speaking with an automaton.

The infectious good humor of mania is often welcomed by the physician. Manic patients, when euphoric, are in such high spirits and are possessed of such good and high humor, that the physician can scarcely keep from laughing with the patient. Thus when a physician feels unaccountably energized and almost recklessly cheerful during an interview, mania should be at the top of the differential diagnosis.

A similar sympathetic response may leave the physician morose, despondent, and pessimistic after interviewing a depressed patient.

E. DISTURBANCES OF MOOD AND AFFECT

In speaking of mood one is referring to a patient's sustained, relatively long-lasting emotional tone. Thus moods may be depressed, manic (either euphoric or irritable), or anxious. In contrast, affect refers to the emotional "look" of the patient: facial expression, gestures, and postures, all of which convey a certain emotion. Whereas mood is fairly constant, affect may change from one minute to the next in the context of a patient's ongoing reaction to events and other people. Indeed, in certain cases, affect may change so rapidly as to merit the term "labile." To use an analogy, mood is to affect as climate is to weather.

Distinguishing an abnormal mood from a normal one may at times be difficult, as all persons at times experience depression, irritability, elation, and anxiety. The key differential point is the presence or absence of autonomy, or independence, of the patients' moods, not only from their own attempts at control, but also from the events of their lives. In normal life, moods gradually come and go, are understandable in light of the events of the patients' lives, and, to a considerable extent, are subject to some degree of control: most persons are able to "shake off" a bad mood and get on with life. Pathologic moods, however, are autonomous and have a life of their own. They are out of proportion to the patients' lives; they are simply too profound or too long-lasting in light of any supposed precipitating event. Furthermore, in cases where the presumed precipitating stress is resolved, the mood in question persists, rather than gradually clearing, again for no apparent reason. The autonomy of a pathologic mood is also evident in its persistence despite all reasonable attempts by patients to "shake it off" or "pull themselves out of it."

E1. Depressive Symptoms

Pathologically depressed mood is often accompanied by a characteristic depressive "cognitive set" and by symptoms such as decreased energy, decreased interest, and difficulty with concentration and memory. Other depressive symptoms are described in the chapter on major depression.

A depressed mood may be described in a variety of ways. Patients may speak of being "down," "blue," unhappy, or simply sad. In some cases patients may speak more of being drained and empty, whereas in others there may be a sense of heaviness and oppression. In severe cases patients may deny having any feelings at all: some say they are simply "dead inside."

In depression, thinking may become distorted by a pervasive pessimism: thoughts and perceptions that fail to resonate with the depression either simply fail to register or are discarded. In reviewing the past, patients think only of misfortune and misdeeds: if someone else reminds the patient of past successes or accomplishments, they are either belittled and undercut, or simply dismissed as not important. In looking to the future the patient sees only futility and failure. Hopelessness may be so profound as to inhibit the patient from venturing anything. In looking at themselves patients see only that they do not measure up and are burdened with guilt, shame, and a sense of utter helplessness. In severe cases patients may come to "ruminate." Here the same damning and depressive thoughts come again and yet again, as a burdensome chain that the patient cannot throw off.

Anergia may manifest as either a sense of being drained and lifeless, or a sensation of heaviness and leaden fatigue. Everything becomes an effort, and when anergia is severe even the smallest obstacles may become insurmountable. One patient simply could not summon the energy to get dressed for work and sat motionless in a bedroom chair for hours.

The loss of interest in formerly pleasurable activities is perhaps more properly construed as anhedonia, or an inability to experience pleasure. For anhedonic patients the world seems to have lost its color and appeal. Food may taste like cardboard, and things may actually come to appear in shades of gray, as if all the color had drained out from them. Libido is lost, and sexually provocative situations, which in the past would leave patients excited, now leave them cold and unmoved.

Memory and the ability to concentrate may be lost. Patients cannot remember names or where they put things; they may lose their train of thought in the middle of a sentence. Thinking becomes slow and effortful, and patients have great difficulty in attending to what others say or to what they are reading. They may ask others to repeat themselves, or they may read a paragraph again and again and still not comprehend it. Some describe a sense of being "wooden headed," as if nothing can get in, nothing can be grasped. Some may lose track of the date. One patient was absolutely unable to comprehend how it was possible to get through morning chores and, thus perplexed, remained in bed. In such cases patients may complain that it is as if a fog lay over everything. Indeed one of the first signs of recovery may be the sense that the "fog" is lifting.

E2. Manic Symptoms

Heightened mood (either euphoric or irritable), increased energy, flight of ideas and pressured speech, and hyperactivity constitute the cardinal manic symptoms and are a mirror image of the depressive symptoms. They may be seen in bipolar disorder, cyclothymia, hyperthymia, and secondary mania.

Euphoric patients may burst with amusement and good cheer. Everything appears to them wonderful, satisfying, and beyond contentment. They may positively beam with confidence and good will, and no task seems insurmountable to them. Their enthusiasm and good humor, as noted earlier, are often "infectious," and indeed only the dour physician can avoid being swept up in their mirth.

Irritability may be extreme and can eventuate in violence. Some manic patients are predominantly irritable, whereas others may tend toward euphoria and only flash into irritability when one of their many designs are thwarted. Irritable patients tend to be overbearing, insistent, quick to take offense, and are constantly pressing their own opinions and plans. As they seek to control all around them they inevitably come into conflict with others, whereupon they often become threatening and may flash into violence.

The energy level, like mood, is heightened in mania, at times to an almost boundless degree. These patients seem inexhaustible,

attack each new project with unflagging enthusiasm, and often find that they need little or no sleep. Fatigue has become a stranger to them. Some may work for days on end, without a break, leaving their exhausted coworkers far behind. In severe mania the energy level may surpass that which the patient is able to channel, and like a locomotive at full throttle the patient may find himself out of any possible control.

In almost all cases hyperactivity, as might be expected, accompanies this increased level of energy. These patients seem always on the go, restless, and unable to sit down and be still. In mild forms of mania the activity is often channeled and clearly purposeful, however misguided. One patient began three new businesses, bought a house, married, and visited every single relative throughout the state, all in a few days time. When hyperactivity becomes more severe, however, the patient's behavior begins to disintegrate into multiple and at times conflicting fragments of purpose. Too many projects are begun and few, if any, are brought even close to completion.

In flight of ideas, patients find their thoughts passing in a rapid, uncontrollable, and at times disorganized progression. Some complain that they have "too many thoughts," that their thoughts "race"; others speak of "jumbled" thoughts that cannot be grasped.

Pressured speech is almost unmistakable. Patients pour forth a veritable torrent of words, inundating anyone close enough to hear. Speech is rapid, often loud, and typically laced with rhymes, puns, and clang associations. Others can "barely get a word in edgewise."

E3. Irritability

The quality of irritability is strongly influenced by the disorder in which it appears. Patients with paranoia tend to be querulous; those with mania tend to be more actively and constantly argumentative and threatening. In patients with paranoid schizophrenia the irritability, though ever-present, is held in check, almost like a constant veiled threat.

E4. Anxiety

Anxiety may be either chronic or come in attacks, often referred to as "panic attacks," that may or may not have precipitants. It is generally accompanied by autonomic symptoms such as tremulousness, palpitations, and diaphoresis.

The most common causes of chronic anxiety are dysthymia, a depressive episode, generalized anxiety disorder, substance use (e.g., caffeine), and importantly, alcohol or sedative-hypnotic withdrawal.

Precipitated anxiety attacks (also known as "situationally bound or predisposed attacks") may occur in the phobias (simple, social, and agoraphobia), panic disorder, post-traumatic stress disorder, separation anxiety disorder, and in patients with obsessive-compulsive disorder when they are unable to follow through on their compulsions.

Unprecipitated anxiety attacks are seen in panic disorder, during depressive episodes, and in various other conditions, as for example hypoglycemia.

E5. Labile Affect

In normal adults affects tend to be slowly aroused, endure for some time, and clear slowly. By contrast, in lability of affect the affects may come and go like brief summer storms. Such lability is normal in children, and a good example of lability may be found in almost any 3- or 4-year-old child.

Among adults lability may be found in mania, histrionic personality disorder, delirium, and dementia. Among those in acute or delirious mania affect may be extremely mercurial, with changes occurring for no apparent reason every few seconds. By contrast, in histrionic personality disorder, usually a precipitant for the affective change is seen, but in most cases the precipitant is relatively minor, and the resultant affect tends to be dramatic and disproportionately extreme. Likewise, demented patients may weep or laugh whereas others might feel only slight sorrow or mirth.

Pathological laughing and crying, as described in the chapter on pseudobulbar palsy, represents a peculiar form of lability. Here patients may laugh or cry for no apparent reason; in addition they may honestly deny feeling happy or sad. A divorce occurs between felt emotion and the facial expression of emotion.

E6. Inappropriate Affect

Inappropriate affect, as seen in schizophrenia, often has a bizarre tinge to it, as the patients' affective expressions, in part or in whole, become inappropriate to what they claim to be feeling. For example, one patient spoke of grief over a parent's death; yet even while speaking of the grief, a grin appeared on the left side of the face. Another example is a patient who, though recounting horrible tortures endured every day, had a beatific facial expression.

The term "inappropriate affect" has also been used in situations where emotion and affect correspond, but those listening to the patient find the emotional display offensive or inappropriate to the occasion. For example, though it is inappropriate for someone to laugh at a parent's funeral, and certainly shocking to other mourners, such an emotional display might not indicate pathology. If the parent had been abusive and the person was seething with triumphant hatred, then the laughter in this light would be "appropriate" to the emotion that the person had. To avoid confusion one may best reserve the term "inappropriate affect" only to those situations where a discordance exists between what the patient feels and what shows on the face.

E7. Flat Affect

In flattened affect patients become devoid of all feeling and of all emotional expression. This symptom is almost specific for schizophrenia and is often accompanied by a remarkable degree of indifference. Though not depressed, these patients are unmoved by events around them and display no emotion. Lighter degrees of this symptom are often termed "blunting" of affect.

The masked or flattened facies of parkinsonism may be distinguished from flattened affect by virtue of the fact that these patients still have feelings but simply cannot express them by facial movement.

Expressive aprosodia likewise differs from flattened affect in that these patients still experience feelings. A global aprosodia may be quite difficult to distinguish from flattened affect. The absence, however, of any other signs or symptoms typical for schizophrenia should prompt a thorough search for a lesion affecting the right parietotemporal cortex.

F. DELUSIONS

A delusion is a false belief that cannot be accounted for on the basis of a patient's culture, upbringing, or religion. For example, to a Confucian the belief in the resurrection of the dead would be considered a delusion, whereas to a Christian it would not. Some beliefs, of course, are never normal regardless of background and may be assumed to be delusions: an example might be the belief that one's hairs have been transformed into myriad antennae designed to pick up electronic signals from alien beings.

In some cases delusions develop gradually and mature slowly into unshakable beliefs. In others they appear suddenly, as if by revelation. Once established, delusions may be either systematized or unsystematized. When they are systematized, delusions often form an elaborate, more or less internally logical view of the world. Such systematization is common in delusional disorder, but somewhat less so in paranoid schizophrenia. By contrast unsystematized delusions are often fragmentary and may be mutually contradictory—a fact that often fails to trouble the patient holding them.

Perhaps the most important clinical distinction among delusions is whether they are mood-congruent or mood-incongruent. In the middle half of the twentieth century, at least in America, it was often erroneously thought that the presence of delusions almost certainly indicated a diagnosis of schizophrenia. We now know that delusions are fairly common in mania and in depression, and that in these cases they are usually congruent with the patient's mood. For example, when depressed patients full of self-loathing and guilt develop the belief that they had committed unpardonable sins, this seems logical and understandable in light of their mood. Likewise, one would not be surprised to find manic patients believing that they had inherited millions of dollars. A not uncommon corollary to such a grandiose delusion is the belief that the patient is being persecuted by those who wish to steal the fortune.

Certain delusions, however, are almost never mood-congruent. For example, the belief that one's thoughts are extracted or withdrawn and sucked into telephone wires bears no relationship to any conceivable mood. Although such non-mood-congruent delusions are more likely in schizophrenia, exceptions do occur, especially in delirious mania. What follows is a compilation of relatively common delusions.

F1. Somatic Delusions

Patients may come to believe themselves to be afflicted in all manner of ways. Rumblings in the belly indicate a tumor, headache a stroke, and cough a cancer. They are convinced they are ill, no matter what the physicians say. The bones are becoming brittle, the skin dry and about to fall off. The intestines have turned to concrete, the brain to dust, and all the internal organs are shriveled and dry. In the most extreme cases patients may come to believe that they are already dead.

Such somatic delusions, however, must be distinguished from hypochondriacal concerns, wherein patients merely suspect that they have a serious illness.

F2. Delusions of Poverty

Patients are convinced that their resources are depleted, that they have lost all. The situation is hopeless; creditors will take the house and all possessions; the family will starve. Displaying a healthy bank statement to such patients is of no avail; they dismiss it; they claim the bank is in error or their recent withdrawals have not as yet been tabulated. Destitution awaits them, they will sleep in the gutter, die unknown, and be buried in a pauper's grave.

F3. Nihilistic Delusions

Here the patient believes that everything has become dead, lifeless, and inanimate. Figures may walk around, but they are not people; rather they are automatons. Trees and animals slowly turn to ashes. Some patients believe that a part of them has died: though an arm may yet still move, the patient knows that it is dead, useless, and fit only for amputation.

F4. Delusions of Sin

As guilt-ridden patients survey their lives they may begin to see many sins, some of them appearing monstrous. They cheated in school, they stole from neighbors, and they treated younger siblings roughly. They have committed adultery in their hearts, embezzled funds, and squandered the rent money. In severe cases these delusions may become quite fantastic. Patients may believe they have threatened the President, poisoned the reservoir, or betrayed their country. Some may present themselves to the authorities, demanding arrest and the ultimate punishment.

F5. Delusions of Persecution

Persecutory beliefs may leave patients feeling hemmed in, hounded, and attacked from all sides. They are followed, tailed, and the phone is tapped. Large organizations may be involved, such as the CIA, the FBI, or the mafia. Carloads of agents cruise the street in front of the house; patients find evidence that someone has broken in. At times these delusions may become bizarre. Patients report that they are attacked at night, cut with knives, subjected to electric shocks, or burned with scalding water. Others are convinced that torture, even execution, is imminent. They hear the chains, smell the burning flesh, see lumber hauled away to make the gallows.

F6. Delusions of Grandeur

Delusions of grandeur may occur alone; however, often they are accompanied by delusions of persecution. In their milder form certain grandiose delusions may be hard to identify as such. For example, paupers may insist that their parents were in fact millionaires and that they had fallen on hard times. Typically, however, grandiose delusions fly in the face of reality. Patients declare that they have billions, that they have invented a perpetual motion machine, or that the President has sought their opinion. They may reveal themselves as heirs to the throne, the elect of God, or the bearer of peace and salvation. Superhuman powers may be asserted: the patient could break down the walls, break the restraints, or lift cars high in the air.

Such delusions, though typical of mania, may also be seen in schizophrenia and in delusional disorder.

F7. Delusions of Reference

Here patients come to believe that chance events and encounters in some way or other refer or pertain to them. Typically these delusions of reference serve to bolster other delusions, such as delusions of sin, grandeur, or persecution.

Patients convinced they have sinned may note the peculiar way a police officer stands: a sign that apprehension is near. The pealing of church bells stops as patients pass by: an indication that their souls are lost, that no prayers will be offered for them. Someone across the room laughs, and patients are convinced that their shameful deeds have become known and have made them a laughing stock.

For grandiose patients a stroll down the street may be an occasion for exaltation. Horns honk to signal their coming; passersby cross the street to get a better view; the clouds part to bestow the radiance of angels upon them.

Delusions of reference are perhaps most common in those patients who believe themselves persecuted. Conversation stops when they enter the room, and patients are convinced that others were talking about them. The lights blink when they enter a building, a sign to their pursuers that their quarry has entered. Patients find indirect allusions to themselves in the newspaper, hear them on the radio, or see them on television. Attempts to convince patients that these are mere coincidences are doomed to failure. To the patients simply too many coincidences have occurred. Everything has meaning, and they are skilled at reading the signs. They are perhaps cleverer than those who torment them.

F8. Schneiderian Delusions

Kurt Schneider, a German psychiatrist, described a number of delusions that he believed to be of the "first rank" and more common in schizophrenia than in other disorders, including delusions of influence, thought broadcasting, thought insertion and thought withdrawal.

Patients with a delusion of influence, or control, believe that their thoughts, feelings, or actions are no longer under their own control but are in fact influenced and directed by some outside force or agency. Patients may believe that their thoughts are orchestrated by radio waves directed at them from a distant computer. Others may experience themselves as automatons or marionettes. Though their legs move in walking and their lips in speech, these are not their movements but are rather under the direct control of aliens who beam radar onto them.

In the delusion of thought broadcasting, patients believe that their thoughts literally leave their heads whereupon they are picked up or read by others. Some patients speak of telepathy, others of thoughts radiating out like radio waves. One patient sensed that thoughts were drawn out by magnets, then transmitted across telephone wires to waiting machines.

The delusion of thought insertion involves the belief that thoughts, which are not the patients' own, are placed or somehow inserted directly into their heads. One patient, a physician, compared the inserted thought to a "foreign body in the mind"; though clearly it was the physician thinking the thought, clearly also it was alien, and not the physician's own.

The delusion of thought withdrawal is in a sense the opposite of thought insertion. In thought withdrawal patients experience one or more of their thoughts being sucked out or somehow withdrawn from them by an outside force. A train of thought may suddenly be cut off, with all the succeeding thoughts withdrawn. The patient has no idea how to carry on with the previous thought. When thought withdrawal occurs while the patient is speaking, the observed sign is called thought blocking, as described below.

F9. Bizarre Delusions

Especially from disorganized patients, one may hear at times any number of fantastic beliefs that resist any clear classification except that of being bizarre. Ants crawl out the pupils; hair is electrified; light shines forth from the fingernails; dwarfs come out at night and mess the sheets.

F10. Erotomanic Delusions

Here patients come to believe that someone else, often someone of much higher social stature, has fallen in love with them, but for one compelling reason or another is unable to openly profess that love. Such a delusion is not uncommon in delusional disorder or in paranoid schizophrenia.

F11. Pseudomemories

More often than is appreciated, patients will report as memories events and experiences that either did not or could not have occurred. In some cases what the patient believes happened represents a twist or modification of actual events, and at other times the belief has no basis in fact. Such pseudomemories can make the history of the present illness that is obtained from patients unreliable.

One patient with paranoid schizophrenia reported that the persecution had begun only after graduating with a doctorate several months earlier. Upon questioning relatives, it was discovered that the patient had dropped out of undergraduate school.

Another less organized patient related with simple honesty being born into a royal family, kidnapped by gypsies, and sent to live in an orphanage. Confronted with the certificate of an otherwise prosaic birth, the patient dismissed the paper as a "forgery."

Such pseudomemories should be distinguished from simple lies on the basis of the fact that the patient has believed them since they first came to mind; they were not suggested by someone else, nor did they begin as a lie, only to become gradually accepted as the truth.

G. HALLUCINATIONS

Hallucinations may occur in each of the five sensory modalities: patients may hear, see, feel, smell, or taste things that are not in fact there.

Patients react differently to these experiences. Occasionally patients have insight about these and recognize that although these experiences appear as vivid and clear as things that other people hear and see, they are not in fact real. More often, however, patients insist these experiences are real, and when the physician denies hearing or seeing the same things, the patients may assume that the physician is lying or is perhaps part of the plot against them. In such cases trying to convince patients that they are wrong is useless. One patient hallucinated the devil sitting in another chair in the room; the physician, trying to convince the patient otherwise, got up and sat in the chair the devil was supposed to be in. The patient was unimpressed and commented that "everyone knows the devil is a spirit."

Hallucinations, like delusions, may or may not be mood-congruent. For example, a voice announcing a guilty verdict and a death sentence would be quite congruent with the mood of a profoundly depressed patient who had a delusion of sin. Or an exalted manic patient might well see angels descending and hear a chorus of heavenly voices from the clouds. An example of a mood-incongruent hallucination, however, is found in a depressed patient who heard giggling voices uttering obscenities. Although exceptions do exist, in general the finding of mood incongruent hallucinations argues strongly against the diagnosis of a mood disorder, suggesting rather a diagnosis of schizophrenia, schizoaffective disorder, or some other similar condition.

Hallucinations may also be seen in dementia, delirium, secondary psychosis, alcohol hallucinosis, various intoxications, and in some withdrawal states.

G1. Auditory Hallucinations

At times only simple sounds are heard: bells, cracklings, "the voice of chewing," or the roar of animals. Music may be heard. When voices occur they may be only in a whisper or mumbled indistinctly. At other times they may be distinct, even overpowering. Short phrases or just single words may be heard: "whore," "murderer," "guilty," "look-out." At other times patients hear long sentences, even conversations.

For the most part what the voices say is unpleasant, even frightening. Sometimes, however, patients hear soothing voices, even congratulatory ones.

At times patients hear "command hallucinations," or voices that direct them to do specific things. They may be innocuous: a voice commanding them to get dressed or to not eat certain foods. At other times, however, patients may be commanded to do dangerous things: the voices may even tell them to kill themselves or someone else. Most often patients are able to resist such command hallucinations, but not always.

Most patients have a sense of where the voices come from. They may be "in the air," in walls or furniture, or emanating from television, radios, or electrical appliances. Not uncommonly they are heard in the midst of music, in what is said on the radio, in rushing water, or from the wind as it rustles the leaves of trees. At times they are located in the body, perhaps the spleen, or some other organ.

Kurt Schneider identified three types of auditory hallucinations that he believed were of the "first rank" and found more commonly in schizophrenia than in other conditions. These three hallucinations consist of the following: voices talking to each other, voices commenting on what the patient is doing, and voices that repeat or speak out loud the patient's thoughts. This last hallucination, often known as "audible thoughts," is perhaps the most suggestive of schizophrenia. Patients hear their own thoughts spoken out loud, as if they were echoed, and they often believe that others can hear them also and thus know what the patients are thinking. Sometimes, indeed, they feel as if the thoughts were spoken from a loudspeaker.

G2. Visual Hallucinations

Visual hallucinations may range in complexity from simple flashes of light to the most detailed scenes. Sometimes shadows are seen "out of the corner of the eye." At other times fleeting shapes are seen in the darkness of the night, "as if someone were there." Colored shapes may float in the air. The faces of others may become disfigured, grotesque, or even melt. Bodies may float through the air; a skeleton is seen outside the window. The heavenly host appears on the horizon; the jurors march in to render their verdict.

Visual hallucinations that accompany auditory ones have no special diagnostic significance and may be seen in schizophrenia, mania, depression, dementia, delirium, and in other disorders. However, when visual hallucinations occur in the complete absence of auditory ones, then one is most likely dealing with a dementia, delirium, or secondary psychosis.

G3. Tactile, or Haptic, Hallucinations

Any imaginable tactile sensation may be hallucinated. In formication, bugs may be felt crawling over the face or swarming over the body. Internal stirrings or electric sensations deep in the bowels may be felt. Burns or prickings of hundreds of needles are felt on the skin. Less commonly, tactile hallucinations may be pleasant, often sexual in nature: a feeling as of soft velvet drawn across the skin, ineffable pleasures are felt, and at times orgasm may occur.

Tactile hallucinations may occur in schizophrenia, mania, depression, intoxications (especially with cocaine), and withdrawal from alcohol or sedative-hypnotics.

G4. Olfactory Hallucinations

Patients may speak of a foul stench, "as if death." Poisonous gas may be smelled, or sulfurous fumes "from hell." Occasionally there may be pleasant odors, as of perfume. Such hallucinations may be seen in schizophrenia and also in simple or complex partial seizures, so-called "uncinate fits."

G5. Gustatory Hallucinations

Hallucinated tastes are almost always disagreeable. Food may taste rotten or putrid. Patients may experience a taste of feces.

Metallic tastes may be found in simple or complex partial seizures and may also occur in some poisonings with heavy metals.

H. DISTURBANCES OF THOUGHT

H1. Loosening of Associations

Loosening of associations, called "formal thought disorder," may be seen in schizophrenia, schizoaffective disorder, or delirious mania, and as such is a symptom of great diagnostic import.

When loosening of associations occurs, the interviewer can often make little or no sense of what the patient is saying. Thoughts seem to lack goal-directedness; they appear to be joined together as if by accident, almost at random, as if fragments of disparate thoughts had all been haphazardly mixed. An example may help to clarify this. Upon being asked by the physician what had occasioned this admission to the hospital, a patient with schizophrenia replied: "Oh, but doctor, the trams, the cars and stars, I wrote my mother a letter, the dog, I see was blue, if only once, twice, nice day to you too!" At its most severe, loosening of associations is characterized by a "word salad" wherein the various words spoken by the patient have no relation with each other at all, much as if they had been tossed together in a linguistic salad.

Typically if the physician confesses to some difficulty in understanding what patients say and asks for an explanation, patients show little or no concern and generally make no effort to clarify what they meant.

Neologisms often accompany loosening of associations. Here the patient uses a totally private and invented word as readily as any word in common usage. For example, when asked to describe a favorite activity, one patient responded "birkenstunning." When asked what this meant, the patient simply repeated the word.

Given the diagnostic import of a finding of loosening of associations, differentiating it from other symptoms, namely flight of ideas and aphasia, is critical.

Flight of ideas, as may be seen in mania, is characterized by abrupt jumps from one thought to another, with each thought being left behind before it can be fully developed. Although this is often a rapid process, exceptions do occur and at times the flight may be quite slow. The key to differentiating flight from loosening of associations lies in the presence or absence of coherence. In flight of ideas, although thoughts are not fully developed, they are nevertheless coherent, as far as they go, in contrast with loosening of associations, wherein coherence is lost.

Expressive aphasia is distinguished from loosening of associations by virtue of the fact that the aphasic patient is still able to communicate in modalities other than speech. The aphasic patient may write, use sign language, or "body language." The patient with loosened associations, however, makes no attempt to communicate ideas more clearly in other modalities. Receptive, or Wernicke's, aphasia may be very difficult to differentiate from loosening of associations. Like patients with loosening of associations, these aphasics do not understand well what is said to them, and often their incoherent speech is impossible to understand. Furthermore, like patients with loosened associations, they may at times show no concern over their incoherence and the inability of others to understand them. Preserved facial and gestural displays of emotion may be a clue. Patients with Wernicke's aphasia often still respond to emotional displays and may make appropriate emotional displays in return. By contrast, loosening of associations is almost always accompanied by an abnormal affect, whether it be flattened, manneristic, or blunted.

H2. Poverty of Thought and of Speech

In poverty of thought, as the name implies, patients simply have few if any thoughts. Consequently they may say little or nothing spontaneously. This is different from the psychomotor retardation seen in depression, as these patients are not depressed. It is also different from mutism, as these patients respond to questions, albeit laconically.

In poverty of speech the patient may talk a normal amount, even at length, and yet "say" little. With an abundance of words, but a dearth of content and meaning, sentences tend to be full of stock phrases, repetitions, and vague or even bizarre references.

Poverty of thought and poverty of speech may be seen in schizophrenia and in some cases of dementia.

H3. Thought Blocking

Thought blocking may be suspected when patients suddenly cease to talk in the middle of a sentence or even of a word and look as if their minds just went blank. If the physician asks what happened, patients may respond that their minds did indeed go blank. If pressed as to how that happened patients often express the delusion of thought withdrawal, discussed above under Schneiderian delusions. The thoughts were taken away, patients were "deprived" of them; "the voices took them."

Thought blocking differs from the sparse, halting speech seen in the psychomotor retardation of depression. In depression all speech is slow, and when it stops its cessation appears a natural consequence of the slow grinding down that characterized what the patient was saying previously. By contrast, just before thought blocking occurs, a patient may talk at a quite normal, even lively, rate.

H4. Mutism

Mutism, or the absence of any verbal production, may occur in a number of conditions. Depressive stupor is suggested by the depressive affect, slumped posture, and similar signs. In catatonic stupor one typically sees other catatonic symptoms, such as rigidity or waxy flexibility. In selective mutism patients are typically children or young teenagers who otherwise appear normal. Patients with a severe global or Broca's aphasia may not speak, but may make efforts to communicate in some other way. Akinetic mutism, as may occur with mesial frontal lesions, is suggested when a global akinesia is seen in addition to mutism without any accompanying depressive or catatonic symptoms.

I. COGNITIVE DEFECTS

Traditionally the cognitive symptoms have included the following: confusion, disorientation, decreased memory, deficient calculating ability, deficient abstracting ability, and poor judgment and poor insight. Their diagnostic significance is greatly heightened by attention to their course and to any associated features. For example, the failure of these abilities to develop at the expected age in childhood generally indicates either mental retardation or a specific developmental disability, such as developmental dyscalculia. "Acquired" deficiencies may be seen in delirium, dementia, depression, delirious mania, and schizophrenia. Associated vegetative symptoms might suggest depression, whereas mannerisms might suggest schizophrenia.

I1. Confusion

Confused patients fail to apprehend clearly both their own thoughts and feelings and events around them. Attention wanders, and the patient has difficulty grasping what is going on. "It was all like a dream," said one patient.

Synonyms for confusion include "clouding of the sensorium" and "clouding of consciousness."

I2. Disorientation

Patients are assessed for orientation in three spheres: person, place, and time. Orientation to time is assessed by asking patients to give the date: the month, the day, and the year. Orientation to place is assessed by simply asking patients to name the building they are in and the city in which the building is found. Orientation to person is almost never lost. Exceptions occur in cases of profound dementia, dissociative amnesia, and fugue.

When assessing psychotic patients, one must beware of misinterpreting delusional disorientation as true disorientation. Patients with schizophrenia may say they are in a castle in the year 1584. When carefully pressed, however, these patients admit the correct date.

I3. Decreased Memory

From a clinical point of view it is most useful to conceive of three forms of memory: immediate, short-term, and long-term. Immediate memory is assessed by giving patients ever longer series of random digits to remember, noting the maximum. Most normal persons can recall seven digits forward and five or six in reverse. Short-term memory is assessed by giving patients the names of three unrelated things and asking them to memorize them. Five minutes later they are asked to recall them: care must be taken not to introduce disturbing or distracting material in the intervening five minutes. Normal persons can recall all three words. Long-term memory is assessed by asking patients about historical facts they would be likely to recall, such as where they went to school, the names of their children, and what they were doing before they were admitted to the hospital. Testing for long-term memory is typically done informally, during the course of the general interview, and always with reference to events that the examiner can verify.

I4. Calculations

Calculating ability may be assessed by asking patients to do simple addition or subtraction, e.g., subtracting 3 from 9. If successful one might move to two-digit subtraction, asking the patient what remains after 4 is taken away from 13. If the patient is successful in this the interviewer may proceed to serial sevens, asking the patient to subtract 7 from 100, then 7 from that answer, and so on. Serial sevens requires considerable concentration and thus, in patients having difficulty with concentration, serial sevens may not be a valid indicator of calculating ability. Although found in mental retardation, dementia, and various deliria, deficient calculating ability by itself does not necessarily imply pathology, as it may be seen in someone who has had little formal education.

I5. Abstractions

The ability to think abstractly may be gauged by asking patients to say in their own words what certain proverbs mean. A typical proverb is, "People who live in glass houses should not throw stones." An abstract answer might be something along the lines of, "Everyone has his faults." On the other hand a concrete answer might be, "Because the glass will break."

This inability to abstract is often called concreteness, or concrete thinking. Hints of concrete thinking can often be found in the general interview. A classic example of this is when the physician asks patients what brought them to the hospital and receives a reply such as "a car." Concrete thinking may be found in mental retardation, dementia, and delirium. It may also be seen in schizophrenia; here one may also hear bizarre answers to questions concerning proverbs. For example, to the "glass houses" proverb, such a bizarre reply might be, "The transparency of glass and opaqueness of stone stand in juxtaposition to the yin and yang of life force."

I6. Judgment and Insight

Judgment, or the ability to adequately assess new situations and to chart appropriate responses to them, may suffer in various disorders, most notably schizophrenia, dementia, and delirium. Judgment may be assessed in two ways: with specific test questions and with more individually tailored questions. A test question might be: "What would you do if you were in a theater and smelled smoke?" Tailored questions take account of the patient's current position: for example, a police officer might be asked how to respond if a suspect resisted arrest.

Poor judgment is certainly not specific for disease: many normal persons exercise poor judgment at times. If, however, poor judgment is present, the examiner must inquire further to see whether it stems from a symptom, such as concrete thinking (which might impair assessment of the situation), or delusions or hallucinations or other symptoms. When poor judgment does arise secondary to such a symptom, the deficiency in judgment may itself be considered part of the pathologic picture.

The term "insight," as used here, refers simply to a recognition, or appreciation, by patients that parts of their experiences of life are not normal. Some patients with hallucinations have no insight at all, and perhaps wonder why the physician denies hearing the voices. On the other hand some patients recognize that, though they hear the voices, these voices are not in fact real and are not heard by others. This insight that a symptom is just that—a symptom of an illness and not real—is much to be desired, as it may motivate a patient to seek and accept treatment. Patients who realize that they are "sick" are more likely to take their medicine than those who believe that "nothing is wrong."

J. OTHER SYMPTOMS
J1. Obsessions and Compulsions

Obsessions are thoughts that are unwarranted, involuntary, occur repetitively, and persist despite a patient's effort to think of something else (examples may be found in the chapter on obsessive-compulsive disorder). Obsessions typically have an intrusive quality and often strike the patient as absurd. Defined thus in a medical sense, they must be distinguished from what lay people often refer to as an obsession. For example, although someone who thought of little else than work might be styled as "obsessed" by lay people, such a person would not be considered to have an obsession as defined in the medical sense. The difference is that the person obsessed with work wants it that way, works hard to keep it that way, and resists any counsels to slow down and enjoy life.

A compulsion is a more or less irresistible urge to repetitively do something, usually in response to an obsessive fear that something bad will happen should the compulsive act not be undertaken. The patient recognizes that the fear is irrational yet is nevertheless unable to dispel the fear or quiet the urge. Indeed, attempts to resist the urge are met initially with ever-increasing anxiety. Common compulsions include the urge to wash the hands for fear of contamination, the urge to check and recheck the stove for fear it may not have been turned off, and the urge to go back again and again to check on the door for fear it may not have been locked. Characteristically, when a patient gives in to the compulsion and carries out the compulsive act, the anxiety lessens, and for a moment the urge wanes. Soon thereafter, however, doubts recur: perhaps the hands were not thoroughly washed; perhaps, in checking to see if the door was locked, it was inadvertently reopened. Thus the urge to go back mounts as the anxiety grows.

Obsessions and compulsions may be seen in obsessive-compulsive disorder, a depressive episode, schizophrenia, Tourette's syndrome, Sydenham's chorea, or as a side-effect to certain antipsychotics, such as clozapine, olanzapine and risperidone.

J2. Phobias

Phobias are fears of specific things or situations that the patient recognizes as unreasonable. For example, a patient phobic of moths may readily admit that "there is nothing to be scared of," yet if closed in a room with a moth may nonetheless rapidly develop a panicky fear.

From a clinical point of view, phobias are usually subdivided into the following: simple (or "specific") phobia, social phobia, agoraphobia, and "school" phobia. In a simple phobia the patient is fearful of specific things such as spiders, snakes, heights, closed spaces, and so forth. In a social phobia the patient fears being humiliated or embarrassed in a specific situation. Examples include fear of public speaking, fear of eating in public, fear of urinating in a public rest room, and the like.

In agoraphobia the patient is fearful of being in a situation where help is not immediately available or from which immediate escape is not possible should a situation arise in which the patient needed help. The agoraphobic thus might fear being alone in crowds, or stuck in a traffic jam on a bridge, or going on a long trip to an unknown destination. In extreme cases patients may be so fearful that they become housebound and refuse to leave the safety of home.

"School phobia," more properly known as "separation anxiety disorder," is similar to agoraphobia in that the child, anxiously fearful of leaving the safety of mother and home, refuses to go to school.

Each one of the foregoing phobias is more thoroughly described in its respective chapter.

BIBLIOGRAPHY

Bleuler E. *Dementia praecox or the group of schizophrenias,* translated by Zinken J, New York, 1950, International Universities Press.

Bleuler E. *Textbook of psychiatry,* translated by Brill AA, New York, 1976, Arno Press.

Hamilton M, editor. *Fish's clinical psychopathology,* ed 2, Bristol, England, 1975, John Wright & Sons.

Kraepelin E. *Dementia praecox and paraphrenia,* translated by Barclay RM, Huntington, NY, 1971, Robert E. Krieger.

Kraepelin E. *Manic-depressive insanity and paranoia,* translated by Barclay RM, New York, 1976, Arno Press.

Kraepelin E. *Clinical psychiatry: a textbook for students and physicians,* translated by Diefendorf AR, Delmar, NY, 1981, Scholars' Facsimiles and Reprints.

Moore DP. *Textbook of Clinical Neuropsychiatry,* London, 2001, Arnold.

Schneider K. *Clinical Psychopathology,* New York, 1959, Grune & Stratton.

DISORDERS USUALLY FIRST DIAGNOSED IN INFANCY, CHILDHOOD, OR ADOLESCENCE

2 Mental Retardation (DSM-IV-TR #317–319)

In mental retardation a patient's development fails to progress beyond a certain point in both an intellectual and social sense despite adequate opportunity. By convention mental retardation is divided into four grades as outlined in Table 2-1, which roughly correspond to various levels of development seen during infancy and childhood.

Mental retardation is a syndrome secondary to any of multiple different causes, as discussed under Etiology. The prevalence of any degree of mental retardation is about 1% of the general population. The lighter grades of mental retardation are more common: 80% to 85% of all cases are mild; 10% to 12% are moderate; 3% to 7% severe; and perhaps only 1% are profoundly retarded. Among the mildly retarded, males are more common; however, the sex ratio gradually approaches equality in the more severe grades.

ONSET

In most cases mental retardation is congenital. Exceptions would include postnatal etiologies, such as severe malnutrition, phenylketonuria, or erythroblastosis fetalis. The age at which the mental retardation becomes clinically apparent, however, varies with its severity, ranging anywhere from infancy for the profoundly retarded up to, perhaps, the end of elementary school for those with quite mild mental retardation.

CLINICAL FEATURES

Mild mental retardation may not become apparent until the child is in elementary school. These children have difficulty learning to read, write, and do arithmetic, and at best these patients may eventually progress academically to a fourth, fifth, or perhaps sixth grade level. Thinking is more or less concrete, and seeing things from another person's point of view or appreciating the importance of anything that lies outside of their immediate concerns is difficult. These patients fail to grasp social nuances and typically appear "immature." Affects tend to be exaggerated with little shading: a patient may slip from joyful exuberance to profound, seemingly inconsolable despair within moments. Judgment tends to be poor, and a certain degree of gullibility is often displayed. Sudden changes or new situations often catch these patients helpless and render them in need of direct, one-on-one supervision if they are to make it successfully through the transition. In tranquil circumstances, however, many of these patients are able to work simple jobs and to live independently or with minimal supervision.

Moderate mental retardation is apparent during preschool years. These children are often able to talk but have great difficulty in learning to read, write, or do arithmetic and at best may eventually progress academically to a second grade level. Thinking is sparse, very concrete, and limited to immediate needs. These patients fail to understand elementary social conventions and have great difficulty in getting along with others. With close supervision they may be able to perform simple work and live outside of an institution, perhaps in a group home.

Severe mental retardation is generally apparent during the first several years of life. Malformations may be apparent at birth, and seizures are not uncommon. These infants are slow to laugh, have difficulty in imitating others, and at best acquire limited speech. They do not learn to write or do any arithmetic beyond simple counting, and at best may be able to recognize certain simple words. Some are able to live with the family or in tightly organized group homes, whereas others are unable to survive outside of an institution. Regardless of where they live, however, close or relatively constant supervision is required.

Profound mental retardation is usually apparent during the first year of life. Malformations are common, as are seizures. These infants are generally unable to walk, and some may be unable to stand or even sit. Speech is generally not acquired, and vocalizations are generally limited to grunts, cries, or some expression of pleasure. Constant close supervision is required to maintain adequate nutrition and personal hygiene. Institutional care is often required.

In addition to the specific deficits just described, patients with mental retardation are apt to display a number of associated features. Aggression, impulsivity, and a low frustration tolerance may be seen in all degrees of mental retardation. An insistence on following routines is also commonly seen. Among those with moderate and higher degrees of retardation, stereotypies may be seen, as may self-injurious behavior. Among the severely and profoundly retarded, rectal digging and coprophagia may occur.

The ability to delay gratification and to endure frustration, like social nuances, are rarely attained by retarded patients, and when they do not "get their way," temper tantrums or aggressive behavior may appear.

A fondness for routine is seen in most retarded patients. In extreme cases the entire day may become ritualized, and the patient may become enraged if the rituals are broken. For such patients moving from one family or institution to another may be catastrophic.

Common stereotypies include repetitive rocking, head-rolling, waving or hand-flapping, finger-sucking, or repeated meaningless

■**TABLE 2-1.** Grades of Mental Retardation

Grade	Age Level (years)	IQ
Profound	<1	<20-25
Severe	1-3	20-25 to 35-40
Moderate ("trainable")	3-7	35-40 to 50-55
Mild ("educable")	7-11	50-55 to 65-75

utterances. Repetitive self-injurious behaviors include slapping, scratching, head-banging, hair pulling, biting hands or arms, and eye-gouging. Lip biting suggests a diagnosis of the Lesch-Nyhan syndrome.

Rectal digging is generally seen only among the severely or profoundly retarded who live in institutions. At times it may be secondary to some irritating condition, such as hemorrhoids; however, often it simply appears to be intrinsic to the retardation. Feces may also be smeared, and at times coprophagia may occur.

Pica, ruminative vomiting, and refusal of solid food may occur and may endanger the patient. Occasionally the vomiting or refusal of solid food may be secondary to some other condition, such as a cleft palate, pharyngeal spasticity, or esophageal dysmotility; however, often, as with rectal digging, no cause other than the mental retardation itself can be found.

Patients with mental retardation are several times more likely than the general population to experience other psychiatric disorders, such as hyperactivity, autism, developmental disabilities, depression, and bipolar disorder. In instances where another disorder does occur the mental retardation itself modifies the clinical presentation of the second disorder, occasionally making it almost unrecognizable. Depression may present merely as insomnia, weight loss, and psychomotor change. Mania may present as agitation, increased irritability, and an absence of sleep. Should schizophrenia occur, its presence may be betrayed only by mannerisms or bizarre affect. Because mental retardation impairs the reporting of symptoms, one should rely much more on signs in approaching the diagnosis of these concurrent conditions.

COURSE

With few exceptions (such as in certain storage diseases), mental retardation, though chronic and lifelong, is not progressive.

COMPLICATIONS

As children and adolescents these patients are often subject to teasing and ridicule by their peers. Puberty is an exceptionally difficult transition. Those with mild mental retardation may be able to work independently and raise a family, albeit with greater difficulty than those of normal intelligence. Higher degrees of mental retardation are generally disabling and render the patient dependent on others for survival.

ETIOLOGY

Overall, the etiology may be determined in from 50% to 80% of all cases of mental retardation. In mild mental retardation, a specific etiology may be determined in about 50% of cases, with the remainder either being idiopathic or presumably due to polygenic, familial causes. As one proceeds to the higher grades of mental retardation, the likelihood of determining an etiology rises to the point where in cases of profound retardation a cause may be found in over 90%.

Currently, over 1000 etiologies have been discovered; importantly, however, most of these are quite rare and in practice only several dozen etiologies account for the vast majority of cases. Etiologies may be divided into several groups: genetic or chromosomal (e.g., Down's syndrome, Fragile X syndrome), accounting for roughly one-half of all the known causes; intrauterine insults (e.g., the fetal alcohol syndrome), accounting for perhaps one-fifth; and perinatal or postnatal factors (e.g., erythroblastosis fetalis), accounting roughly for one-third. Examples of etiologies for each group are found in the box on this page. By far, the most common causes of mental retardation in America are Down's syndrome, Fragile X syndrome, and the fetal alcohol syndrome.

In working up a patient with mental retardation, if one cannot confidently make an etiologic diagnosis, it is appropriate to seek consultation with a specialist.

DIFFERENTIAL DIAGNOSIS

Certain developmental disabilities, such as developmental dysphasia, may preclude academic advancement; however, here one does not see the generalized deficit present in mental retardation. For example, a child with a severe developmental dysphasia may yet show by his behavior a keen and subtle awareness of social nuances.

Severe autism, especially if accompanied by mutism, may mimic mental retardation. Here, however, one sees a definite avoidance of human contact, in sharp contrast to the childlike, at times clinging, behavior of the mentally retarded. However, as noted in the section on autism, mental retardation may often accompany the syndrome of autism.

Childhood-onset schizophrenia may preclude academic progress and thus mimic mental retardation. However, here one sees not only bizarreness but also often a fluctuating course, features that are not seen in mental retardation.

Profound deprivation, as may be seen in some orphanages or in cases of severe abuse, may leave a child appearing almost indistinguishable from one with mental retardation. Here the differential may be in doubt until one places the child in a more nurturing

Some Etiologic Factors in Mental Retardaton ■

GENETIC AND CHROMOSOMAL DEFECTS
Tuberous sclerosis*
Von Recklinghausen's disease*
Lesch-Nyhan syndrome*
Prader-Willi syndrome*
Bardet-Biedl Syndrome*
Aminoacidurias, e.g., phenylketonuria
Storage disease, e.g., Tay-Sachs disease
Down's Syndrome*
Fragile X syndrome*
Klinefelter's syndrome*

INTRAUTERINE INSULTS
Radiation
Alcohol *(fetal alcohol syndrome*)* or other drugs, e.g., phenytoin
Infections, e.g., rubella, toxoplasmosis, cytomegalovirus, HIV
Hypothyroidism*
Hyperparathyroidism

PERINATAL AND POSTNATAL FACTORS
Severe malnutrition
Erythroblastosis fetalis
Prematurity
Birth trauma
Perinatal anoxia

*See the respective chapter.

environment. In a similar vein patients from other cultures or those deprived of education may have difficulty adapting to complex social situations and may test falsely low on standard IQ tests. Deaf persons lacking appropriate educational resources may likewise do very poorly on IQ tests.

Dementia may produce a clinical picture similar to mental retardation. Here, however, the course is fundamentally different, in that dementia represents a retrogression from a previously attained level. In mental retardation not so much a retrogression is seen, as a failure of further progression. In a sense the intellectual and social development of the patient with mental retardation seems to stall out and plateau at some point in childhood. The situation, of course, may be complicated in some disorders, such as Down's syndrome, which produce not only mental retardation but also eventually a dementia in many patients.

TREATMENT

Appropriately geared education and training generally serve to increase patients' abilities either to care for themselves or to assist or cooperate with others in their care.

Family counseling is generally helpful in enabling family members to adjust to the special needs of the mentally retarded child. In hereditary cases genetic counseling should be offered.

Although no specific treatment for mental retardation per se exists, certain associated features may respond to specific treatments. Aggressivity and impulsivity may respond to behavior modification; aggressivity and impulsivity and overall disruptive behaviors may also respond to antipsychotics, especially risperidone in doses of from 0.02 to 0.06 mg/kg/d. Lithium may also be effective for impulsivity. Troublesome stereotypies may likewise respond to behavior modification or antipsychotics. Self-injurious behaviors appear resistant to antipsychotics, but may respond to clomipramine; behavior modification may also be helpful; however, helmets, mittens, or restraints may be required. Other associated features, such as rectal digging, fecal smearing or coprophagia, and feeding problems, may respond to behavior modification.

Concurrent disorders, such as hyperactivity, autism, or mood disorders may generally be treated in their customary fashion. An exception would be hyperactivity occurring in a mentally retarded child with stereotypies. Here, because stimulants may increase stereotypies, alternatives, as discussed in the chapter on attention-deficit/hyperactivty disorder, may be preferred. Furthermore, should a mentally retarded patient have both seizures and a mood disorder, one may consider using an antiepileptic drug which may be effective for both conditions, e.g. carbamazepine for either depression or mania, lamotrigine for depression as part of bipolar disorder, or divalproex for mania.

BIBLIOGRAPHY

Aman MG, Collier-Crespin A, Lindsay RL. Pharmacotherapy of disorders seen in mental retardation. *European Child & Adolescent Psychiatry* 2000;9(Suppl1):98-107.

Cherry KE, Penn D, Matson JL, et al. Characteristics of schizophrenia among persons with severe or profound mental retardation. *Psychiatric Services* 2000;51:922-924.

King BH, State MW, Shah B, et al. Mental retardation: a review of the past 10 years. Part I. *Journal of the American Academy of Child and Adolescent Psychiatry* 1997;36:1656-1663.

Lewis BH, Bodfish JW, Powell SB, et al. Clomipramine treatment for self-injurious behavior of individuals with mental retardation: a double-blind comparison with placebo. *American Journal of Mental Retardation* 1996;100:654-665.

State MW, King BH, Dykens E. Mental retardation: a review of the past 10 years. Part II. *Journal of the American Academy of Child and Adolescent Psychiatry* 1997;36:1664-1671.

Stromme P. Aetiology in severe and mild mental retardation: a population-based study of Norwegian children. *Developmental Medicine and Child Neurology* 2000;42:76-86.

Stromme P, Valvatne K. Mental retardation in Norway: prevalence and sub-classification in a cohort of 30037 children born between 1980 and 1985. *Acta Paediatrica* 1998;87:291-296.

Szymanski L, King BH. Summary of practice parameters for the assessment and treatment of children, adolescents, and adults with mental retardation and comorbid disorders. *Journal of the American Academy of Child and Adolescent Psychiatry* 1999;38:606-610.

3   Fetal Alcohol Syndrome

The fetal alcohol syndrome, caused by *in utero* exposure to alcohol, is characterized by a distinctive facial dysmorphism, varying degrees of intellectual deficits, and behavioral problems, most notably hyperactivity. This is a not uncommon disorder, occurring with a frequency of 1 in 1000 live births or more, and appears equally common in males and females. Patients with mild forms of the syndrome are generally said to have "fetal alcohol effect."

ONSET

Although this is a congenital disorder, mild forms, especially those lacking prominent facial dysmorphism, may not become evident until school years when intellectual deficits or behavioral problems become evident.

CLINICAL FEATURES

In its fully developed form the facial dysmorphism is characterized by microcephaly, shortened palpebral fissures, epicanthal folds, microphthalmia, maxillary hypoplasia, a thin upper lip and absence of the philtrum, and a degree of micrognathia.

Intellectual deficits range in severity from mental retardation to specific learning disabilities.

Behavioral problems, in addition to hyperactivity, include distractibility and irritability.

Cardiac abnormalities may also be found, including atrial or ventricular septal defects.

MRI scanning may be normal in mild cases; however, in severe cases one may find cortical atrophy, ventriculomegaly, hypoplasia or absence of the corpus callosum, cavum septi pellucidi or cavum vergae.

COURSE

Although some improvement occurs during adolescence, especially with regard to dysmorphic facial features, the overall course is one of chronicity.

COMPLICATIONS

The complications of mental retardation are as described in that chapter; the complications of the behavioral problems are similar to those described in the chapter on attention-deficit/hyperactivity disorder.

ETIOLOGY

Although the syndrome is clearly related to maternal ingestion of alcohol during pregnancy, it is not clear whether it is alcohol itself which is the main toxin or alcohol's metabolite, acetaldehyde, nor is it clear what the mechanism is underlying the toxicity: one theory suggests that alcohol or acetaldehyde triggers apoptosis in developing neurons; another that neuronal migration is disturbed. Further, it is also not known whether there is a "threshold" of alcohol consumption, below which there is no risk, nor is it clear when, during pregnancy, the greatest risk is: some authors believe it is in the first trimester, whereas others point to animal data suggesting that third trimester exposure is most important.

Macroscopically, in severe cases, there is cortical atrophy, lissencephaly, ventriculomegaly, agenesis of the corpus callosum and cerebellar hypoplasia. Microscopically, neuronal heterotopias are found in the periventricular white matter and in the leptomeninges.

DIFFERENTIAL DIAGNOSIS

The characteristic facial dysmorphism, coupled with a history of maternal alcohol use, strongly suggests the diagnosis. In partial syndromes, or in older children or adults in whom there has been substantial regression of the dysmorphic features, differentiating the fetal alcohol syndrome from other causes of mental retardation, learning disabilities or attention-deficit/hyperactivity syndrome may be difficult: in these cases, obtaining early childhood photographs may be helpful.

TREATMENT

The treatment of mental retardation and learning disabilities is as discussed in those chapters. Although there are no controlled studies, it appears that the hyperactivity of the fetal alcohol syndrome responds to the treatments described in the chapter on attention-deficit/hyperactivity disorder.

BIBLIOGRAPHY

Jones KL, Smith DW. Recognition of fetal alcohol syndrome in early infancy. *Lancet* 1973;2:999-1001.

Larsson G, Bohlin A-B, Tunell R. Prospective study of children exposed to variable amounts of alcohol in utero. *Archives of Disease in Childhood* 1985;60:316-321.

Olney JW, Wozniak DF, Farber NB, et al. The enigma of fetal alcohol neurotoxicity. *Annals of Medicine* 2002;34:109-119.

Roebuck TM, Mattson SN, Riely EP. A review of the neuroanatomical findings in children with fetal alcohol syndrome or prenatal exposure to alcohol. *Alcoholism, Clinical and Experimental Research* 1998;22: 339-344.

Steinhausen HC, Spohr HL. Long-term outcome of children with fetal alcohol syndrome: psychopathology, behavior, and intelligence. *Alcoholism, Clinical and Experimental Research* 1998;22:334-338.

Swayze VW, Johnson VP, Hanson JW, et al. Magnetic resonance imaging of brain anomalies in fetal alcohol syndrome. *Pediatrics* 1997;99:232-240.

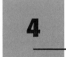

4   Fragile X Syndrome

Fragile X syndrome, which may occur in both males and females, is a variably penetrant disorder associated with a fragile site on the long arm of the X chromosome, which in turn is caused by an expanded trinucleotide repeat at the fragile site. Patients may or may not be retarded and may or may not display a characteristic facial dysmorphism. Almost all postpubertal males will have macroorchidism. A minority of male patients also display autistic features or have the full syndrome of autism.

Fuller penetrance is seen more often among males than females, with about 80% of males being affected and only about one third of females. The prevalence of fragile X syndrome among the general male population is about 0.08%; among females it is about 0.04%. Discovered in 1969, this syndrome is now known to be the second most common known cause of mental retardation of genetic or chromosomal origin, ranking just behind Down's syndrome.

ONSET

Facial dysmorphism, if present, is evident in infancy. The age at which mental retardation or autism is recognized is a function of severity and is discussed in the respective chapters. Macroorchidism may or may not be evident in childhood, but is almost always in evidence after puberty.

CLINICAL FEATURES

The clinical picture is extremely variable, and it is not at all uncommon for patients to display only a part of the syndrome.

Most clinical studies have utilized male patients, and in this population the clinical picture has been well characterized. Although most patients have some degree of mental retardation, ranging from mild to severe, a minority may be of average intelligence; in such cases, however, one almost always finds some

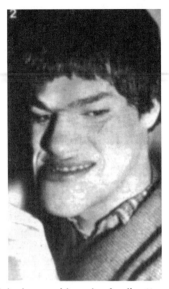

FIG. 4-1. Facial dysmorphism in fragile X syndrome. (From Wiedemann HR, Kunze J, Dibbern H. *Atlas of clinical syndromes: a visual aid to diagnosis*, ed 2, London, 1992, Wolfe.)

(FMRP). The gene itself contains a sequence of CGG trinucloetide repeats, and in normal individuals one finds anywhere from 5 to 50 of these triplets. An expansion of this sequence to from 50 to 200 repeats is known as a "premutation," whereas an expansion to over 200 repeats represents a full mutation. Patients with a premutation are asymptomatic and considered carriers. In cases with a full mutation, transcription of the gene does not occur, levels of the FMRP protein are very low or undetectable, and symptoms result.

The relatively minor symptomatology seen in females with the full mutation is due to random inactivation of the X chromosome, which allows for the presence of some normal X chromosomes and the consequent production of a clinically significant, albeit reduced, amount of the FMRP protein.

Interestingly, although the carrier status may be seen in both females and males, it is only from female carriers that individuals may inherit the full mutation and thus have symptoms. The reason for this is that although expansion can and does occur during oogenesis, it is very unlikely to occur during spermatogenesis.

MRI studies have demonstrated hypertrophy of the hippocampi and atrophy of both the superior temporal gyrus and the cerebellar vermis; an autopsy study revealed widespread abnormalities of dendritic spines.

DIFFERENTIAL DIAGNOSIS

Macroorchidism is an important diagnostic clue; the presence of other features is helpful; however, their absence, given the variability of the clinical picture, does not argue against the diagnosis. Testing all males with mental retardation or autism may be prudent, and any females with characteristic dysmorphic facies.

TREATMENT

The treatment for mental retardation, autism and hyperactivity are as described in those chapters; importantly, hyperactivity in these patients responds well to methylphenidate. Prior reports of beneficial effects of folic acid treatment have not been borne out. Genetic testing and counseling should be available to the patient and all first-degree relatives.

linguisitic deficits, with both receptive and expressive elements. Facial dysmorphism, illustrated in Figure 4-1, is present to some degree in the majority and may include any or all of the following: prognathism; a high, broad forehead; a long, thin face; and variously malformed ears. Macroorchidism, as noted earlier, is found in almost all postpubertal male patients; however, hypogonadism does not appear to occur. The vast majority of patients also display one or more autistic traits, such as gaze avoidance, stereotypies (such as hand flapping), or inappropriate verbal behavior (such as echolalia), but only a small minority will have the full syndrome. Other associated features include hyperactivity, mitral valve prolapse, pectus excavatum, and a high arched palate. Either grand mal or partial complex seizures may occur in a minority of patients.

Females with the fragile X syndrome are less severely affected than males: only about one-half will have a degree of mental retardation, and facial dysmorphism is seen in only a small minority. Schizotypal features, such as social isolation, mannerisms, and odd communications, may also be seen in a minority of these female patients.

Diagnosis is by genetic testing for the expanded trinucleotide repeat with either polymerase chain reaction (PCR) assay or with Southern blot analysis.

COURSE

Although in most cases the cognitive deficit, if one is present, remains stable, in a minority, and generally only in males, one may see a progressive deterioration in intellectual ability.

COMPLICATIONS

The complications are as discussed in the chapters on mental retardation and autism.

ETIOLOGY

The responsible gene, located on the long arm of the X chromosome, is known as the fragile X mental retardation-1 gene (FMR-1), and codes for the fragile X mental retardation-1 protein

BIBLIOGRAPHY

de Vries BB, Halley DJ, Oostra BA, et al. The fragile X syndrome. *Journal of Medical Genetics* 1998;35:579-589.

de Vries BB, Mohkamsing S, van den Ouweland AM, et al. Screening for the fragile X syndrome among the mentally retarded: a clinical study. *Journal of Medical Genetics* 1999;36:467-470.

Enfiled SL, Tonge BJ, Florio T. Behavioral and emotional disturbance in fragile X syndrome. *American Journal of Medical Genetics* 1994; 51:386-391.

Freund LS, Reiss AL, Hagerman R, et al. Chromosome fragility and psychopathology in obligate female carriers of the fragile X chromosome. *Archives of General Psychiatry* 1992;49:54-60.

Hagerman RJ, Murphy MA, Wittenberger MD. A controlled trial of stimulant medication in children with the fragile X syndrome. *American Journal of Medical Genetics* 1988;30:377-392.

Mostofsky SH, Mazzocco MM, Aakalu G, et al. Decreased cerebellar posterior vermis size in fragile X syndrome: correlation with neurocognitive performance. *Neurology* 1998;50:121-130.

Musumeci SA, Hagerman RJ, Ferri R, et al. Epilepsy and EEG findings in males with fragile X syndrome. *Epilepsia* 1999;40:1092-1099.

Reisss AL, Lee J, Freund L. Neuroanatomy of fragile X syndrome: the temporal lobe. *Neurology* 1994;44:1317-1324.

Rogers SJ, Wehner DE, Hagerman R. The behavioral phenotype in fragile X: symptoms of autism in very young children with fragile X syndrome, idiopathic autism, and other developmental disorders. *Journal of Developmental and Behavioral Pediatrics* 2001;22:409-417.

Rousseau F, Heitz D, Biancalana S, et al. Direct diagnosis of the fragile X syndrome of mental retardation. *The New England Journal of Medicine* 1991;325:1673-1681.

Rudelli RD, Brown WT, Wisniewski K, et al. Adult fragile X syndrome: clinico-neuropathologic findings. *Acta Neuropathologica* 1985;67: 289-295.

Sabaratnam M, Vroegop PG, Gangadharan SK. Epilepsy and EEG findings in 18 males with fragile X syndrome. *Seizure* 2001;10:60-63.

5 Klinefelter's Syndrome

Klinefelter's syndrome occurs only in males and is caused by the presence of one or more extra X chromosomes. It is relatively common, being present in about 0.02% of males.

A patient with classical Klinefelter's syndrome is tall, eunuchoid, and infertile. Although Klinefelter's syndrome is an important cause of mental retardation, most patients are in fact not retarded; however, they may experience linguistic delay, and they may have considerable difficulty in negotiating the developmental tasks of adolescence and early adulthood. This classical picture, however, is by no means universal. Some patients have no obvious signs or symptoms and come to medical attention only during an infertility workup. Others, especially those with two, three, or more extra X chromosomes, may have a high degree of mental retardation and readily recognizable malformations.

ONSET

Mental retardation, when present, is usually mild and may not be apparent until later childhood. Other features of Klinefelter's syndrome gradually appear after puberty.

CLINICAL FEATURES

The patient is often tall, with disproportionately long legs. Obesity is not uncommon, and the beard is sparse or nonexistent. Most patients have a heterosexual orientation; however, libido may be low, and impotence may occur. History may reveal a tumultuous adolescence, and a certain degree of psychosocial immaturity is generally present. Academic performance may have been poor, and patients may have had elements of developmental dysphasia or developmental dyslexia.

Although Klinefelter's syndrome is a relatively common cause of mental retardation, accounting for perhaps 2% of all retarded patients, most patients with Klinefelter's syndrome have a Full Scale IQ within the normal range.

Gynecomastia, which ranges in severity from being barely palpable to embarrassingly noticeable, is present in a majority of patients. Axillary hair may be sparse or absent, and a female escutcheon is often present. An 18-year-old man with Klinefelter's syndrome is shown in Figure 5-1. The testicles are almost invariably small and firm, and the penis may be small.

Azoospermia and infertility are present in almost all patients. Testosterone levels may be normal, especially in early adolescence; however, by early adult years most patients tend to have low levels of testosterone. Luteinizing hormone and, more constantly,

follicle-stimulating hormone levels tend to be elevated. Estradiol levels tend to rise above normal as the patient passes through adolescence.

Diagnosis depends on demonstrating one or more extra X chromosomes and may be accomplished via a buccal smear, or, more accurately, by karyotyping.

A minority of patients also display thyroid dysfunction. The TSH response to TRH may be blunted, and, likewise, the thyroid may be insensitive to TSH. Other associated disorders found in a minority of patients include bipolar disorder, grand mal seizures, chronic obstructive pulmonary disease, systemic lupus erythematosus,

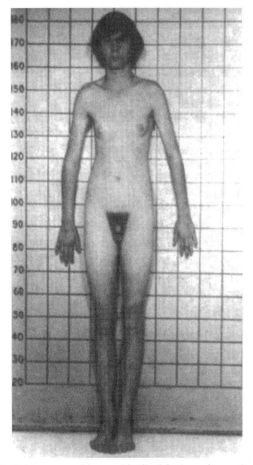

FIG. 5-1. Eighteen-year-old man with Klinefelter's syndrome. (From Kelly TE. *Clinical genetics and genetic counseling*, ed 2, Chicago, 1986, Mosby.)

leukemia, and diabetes mellitus, which is usually mild. Breast cancer, though uncommon, is yet 20 times more frequent among those with Klinefelter's syndrome than among the general male population.

COURSE

The evolution of symptoms is usually completed by early adult years, and the clinical picture tends to remain stable for the rest of the patient's life.

COMPLICATIONS

The complications of mental retardation are as described in that chapter. For those who are not retarded, relatively poor verbal skills may limit occupational achievement.

ETIOLOGY

Patients may have one or more extra X chromosomes and some 10% will display a mosaic pattern. The classic karyotype is 47XXY, and this pattern is secondary to nondisjunction during meiosis in either the mother or the father.

Hyalinization and fibrosis of the testes generally begin during puberty and progressively worsen throughout adolescence, with progressively decreasing testosterone production.

DIFFERENTIAL DIAGNOSIS

The classical presentation is fairly distinctive; diagnostic difficulties generally arise, however, in milder cases, and the diagnosis may only be made during a workup for impotence, infertility, or gynecomastia.

TREATMENT

Psychotherapy may better enable these patients to master the developmental tasks of adolescence. If speech or reading difficulties are present, special education may help, and mental retardation is treated as outlined in that section. If testosterone levels are low, testosterone may be given as testosterone enanthate, testosterone cypionate, or via a transdermal patch, with gradual improvement of libido and potency, mood and energy, and the appearance of facial hair. Infertility, however, will persist.

Gynecomastia does not regress with testosterone replacement treatment and may indeed worsen. If embarrassing, reduction mammoplasty may be indicated.

BIBLIOGRAPHY

Barker TE, Black FW. Klinefelter syndrome in a military population. Electroencephalographic, endocrine, and psychiatric status. *Archives of General Psychiatry* 1976;33:607-610.

Everman DB, Stoudemire A. Bipolar disorder associated with Klinefelter's syndrome and other chromosomal abnormalities. *Psychosomatics* 1994;35:35-40.

Khalifa MM, Struthers JL. Klinefelter syndrome is a common cause for mental retardation of unknown etiology among prepubertal males. *Clinical Genetics* 2002;61:49-53.

Manning MA, Hoyme HE. Diagnosis and management of the adolescent boy with Klinefelter syndrome. *Adolescent Medicine* 2002;13:367-374.

Nielsen J, Pelsen B, Sorensen K. Follow-up of 30 Klinefelter males treated with testosterone. *Clinical Genetics* 1988;33:262-269.

Smyth CM, Bremmer WJ. Klinefelter syndrome. *Archives of Internal Medicine* 1998;158:1309-1314.

Tatum WO, Passaro EA, Elia M, et al. Seizures in Klinefelter's syndrome. *Pediatric Neurology* 1998;19:275-278.

6   Down's Syndrome

Down's syndrome, first described by John Langdon Down in 1866, is one of the most common causes of mental retardation, accounting for anywhere from 10% to 16% of all retarded patients. It occurs in 1 in 600 to 1 in 1000 live births and is almost always secondary to trisomy 21, with less than 5% of cases secondary to a translocation. It appears to be equally common among males and females. Although almost half of these patients die in childhood, a significant percentage survive into teenage and adult years. Perhaps half of those who live beyond the age of 40 will develop clinical evidence of Alzheimer's disease.

ONSET

The diagnosis is usually made at birth on the basis of some of the characteristic signs noted below.

CLINICAL FEATURES

The head is generally small, with a flattened occiput. The palpebral fissures show a characteristic oblique slant, and epicanthal folds are present. The bridge of the nose is usually broad, and the mouth may be small with a protruding tongue. A 15-year-old girl with Down's syndrome is shown in Figure 6-1.

The patients tend to be of short stature. The hands tend to be broad and foreshortened, with a characteristic "simian crease." The fifth finger tends to be shorter than normal and to curve inward. The first and second toes are often separated by a wide gap. The muscles are often hypotonic. The external genitalia are often small, puberty may be delayed, and fertility is reduced, more so in the male.

The mental retardation may range from mild to severe. These patients tend to be placid, easy-going, and often cheerful and affectionate. However, in a minority a significant degree of disruptiveness is seen.

Congenital heart disease is found in up to 40% of patients. Ventriculoseptal defects and patent ductus arteriosus are common. At times these defects may give rise to cerebral emboli (some of which may be septic), and multiple cerebral infarctions, which, in turn, may give rise to a multi-infarct dementia.

Hypothyroidism may occur in from 20% to 30% of patients, and in the majority of these, anti-thyroid antibodies are present.

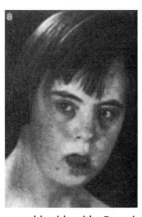

FIG. 6-1. Fifteen-year-old girl with Down's syndrome. (From Wiedeman HR, Kunze J, Dibben H. *Atlas of clinical syndromes: a visual aid to diagnosis*, ed 2, London, 1992, Wolfe.)

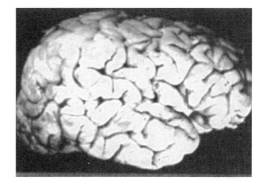

FIG. 6-2. Typical brain in Down's syndrome. (From Parisi JE, Schochet SS. *Principles and practice of neuropathology*, St. Louis, 1993, Mosby.)

Duodenal obstruction, intestinal stenosis, or megacolon may occur. Seizures may occur in a minority of patients, and the risk of leukemia is 10 to 20 times greater than in the general population. Atlanto-axial instability occurs in about one-fifth of patients and may lead to compression or transection of the cervical spinal cord. A small minority have obstructive sleep apnea, with daytime fatigue and irritability, and in a very small minority autism may occur.

Among patients who survive into adulthood, precocious aging is common with baldness, graying, and cataracts; a minority also develop depressive symptoms, which at times may be so severe as to cause the dementia syndrome of depression.

Of great interest is the fact that Alzheimer's disease occurs with ever-increasing frequency as these patients pass the age of 20, with almost half of all the patients showing definite evidence of dementia during the fifth and sixth decades.

Although the diagnosis may be made reliably on clinical grounds, karyotyping is indicated, not only to make the diagnosis conclusive, but also to determine whether the syndrome is secondary to trisomy 21 or to a translocation.

COURSE

The average age of death is 12 years; most who do die before adult years succumb to infection or to congenital heart disease. Those who survive into adult years eventually succumb in the midst of precocious aging or Alzheimer's disease. Those developing Alzheimer's disease generally survive for only about 5 more years.

COMPLICATIONS

These are as described in the chapters on mental retardation and on Alzheimer's disease.

ETIOLOGY

Approximately 95% of all cases of Down's syndrome are secondary to trisomy 21 occurring due to non-disjunction during meiosis, with this non-disjunction occurring in the mother in almost all cases. The risk of non-disjunction in the mother rises dramatically with age, from about 1 in 1000 in the early 20's to close to 1 in 100 at the age of 40 and almost 1 in 50 at the age of 45. In a very small proportion of cases mosaicism occurs and such patients generally have much milder symptomatology. In the other 5% of cases of Down's syndrome, one finds a translocation, generally from

chromosome 21 to chromosome 14, with such translocations either occurring sporadically or being inherited from an asymptomatic carrier parent.

The brain is small and rounded, often with a blunted occiput; the sulcal pattern may be poorly developed, and the superior temporal gyrus is often abnormally small. A typical brain in Down's syndrome is shown in Figure 6-2. The cerebellum and brainstem are likewise hypoplastic. Microscopically, one finds a reduced number of cortical neurons, and those pyramidal neurons which are present typically demonstrate a reduced number of dendritic spines with fewer than normal synapses. With age, neurofibrillary tangles and senile plaques appear, and indeed in those over 40, they are found in almost all patients. Although these pathologic changes are not identical to those seen in Alzheimer's disease, they are extraordinarily similar, and in this regard, it is of interest that chromosome 21 contains the gene for the amyloid precursor protein, a major consituent of senile plaques.

DIFFERENTIAL DIAGNOSIS

The diagnosis of Down's syndrome itself is straightforward, as the signs are almost pathognomonic. Should a dementia supervene, consideration is given not only to Alzheimer's disease, but also to hypothyroidism and, rarely, a multiinfarct dementia.

TREATMENT

If karyotyping reveals a translocation, all first-degree relatives should be offered karyotyping to determine their carrier status.

The general treatment of mental retardation is outlined in that chapter. All patients should have a CT scan of the cervical spine and if there is evidence of atlanto-axial instability, sports should be forbidden. Given the relatively high incidence of hypothyroidism, it is prudent to perform yearly screening with TSH and free T4 levels. Should Alzheimer's disease develop, it is appropriate to consider treatment with a cholinesterase inhibitor such as donepezil; however, it must be borne in mind that these agents have not as yet been conclusively shown effective in these patients.

BIBLIOGRAPHY

Collacott RA, Cooper SA, Branford D, et al. Behavior phenotype for Down's syndrome. *The British Journal of Psychiatry* 1998;172: 85-89.

Cooper SA, Collacot RA. Clinical features and diagnostic criteria of depression in Down's syndrome. *The British Journal of Psychiatry* 1994;165:399-403.

Down JLH. Observation on an ethnic classification of idiots. *Clinical Letters and Reports of the London Hospital* 1866;3:259-262.

Holland AJ, Hon J, Huppert FA, et al. Population-based study of the prevalence and presentation of dementia in adults with Down's syndrome. *The British Journal of Psychiatry* 1998;172:493-498.

Hyman BT, West HL, Rebeck GW, et al. Neuropathological changes in Down's syndrome hippocampal formation. Effect of age and apolipoprotein E genotype. *Archives of Neurology* 1995;52:373-378.

Kallen B, Mastroiacovo P, Robert E. Major congenital malformations in Down syndrome. *American Journal of Medical Genetics* 1996;16:160-166.

Karlsson B, Gustafson J, Hedov G, et al. Thyroid dysfunction in Down's syndrome: relation to age and thyroid autoimmunity. *Archives of Disease in Childhood* 1998;79:242-245.

Kent L, Evans J, Paul M, et al. Comorbidity of autistic spectrum disorders in children with Down syndrome. *Developmental Medicine and Child Neurology* 1999;41:153-158.

Levanon A, Tarasiuk A, Tal A. Sleep characteristics in children with Down syndrome. *The Journal of Pediatrics* 1999;134:755-760.

Lund J, Munk-Jorgensen P. Psychiatric aspects of Down's syndrome. *Acta Psychiatrica Scandinavica* 1988;78:369-374.

Pearson E, Lenn NJ, Cail WS. Moyamoya and other causes of stroke in patients with Down's syndrome. *Pediatric Neurology* 1985;1:174-179.

Prasher VP. Epilepsy and associated effects on adaptive behavior in adults with Down syndrome. *Seizure* 1995;4:53-56.

Prasher VP, Huxley A, Haque MS, et al. A 24-week, double-blind, placebo-controlled trial of donepezil in patients with Down syndrome and Alzheimer's disease—pilot study. *International Journal of Geriatric Psychiatry* 2002;17:270-278.

Rasmussen P, Borjesson O, Wentz E, et al. Autistic disorders in Down syndrome: background factors and clinical correlates. *Developmental Medicine and Child Neurology* 2001;43:750-754.

Stoll C, Alembik Y, Dott B, et al. Study of Down syndrome in 238,942 consecutive births. *Annales de Genetique* 1998;41:44-51.

Warren AC, Holroyd S, Folstein MF. Major depression in Down's syndrome. *The British Journal of Psychiatry* 1989;155:202-205.

7   Sturge-Weber Syndrome

Sturge-Weber syndrome (also known as Sturge-Weber-Dimitri syndrome and encephalotrigeminal angiomatosis), first described by William Allen Sturge in 1879, is a rare disorder characterized by a facial port-wine stain, seizures, and mental retardation. Cortical calcification may be imaged ipsilateral to the port-wine stain.

ONSET

The port-wine stain is typically present at birth; other symptoms often begin within the first year or two, and calcification becomes apparent on neuroimaging in early childhood.

CLINICAL FEATURES

The facial port-wine stain, or nevus flammeus, covers minimally the area of distribution of the first division of the trigeminal nerve, and may also cover the area of the second and third division, sometimes even down the side of the neck: Figure 7-1 illustrates a port-wine stain in an adult. In almost all cases the stain is unilateral. The great majority of patients will also have seizures, often beginning in the first year of life. Partial seizures, which may undergo secondary generalization, are most common, and if motor or sensory in type, the manifestations, such as clonic movements, appear contralateral to the side with the port-wine stain. Hemiplegia, hemiatrophy and hemianopia may develop, again contralateral to the port-wine stain, and mental retardation is seen in about one-half of patients. It is apparent also that most patients will experience stroke-like episodes or transient ischemic attacks.

An enlarged eye (also known as bupthalmos, or "ox-eye") may be seen in some patients at birth, and glaucoma becomes increasingly common with age, eventually occurring in from one-third to one-half of patients.

Cerebral cortical calcification ipsilateral to the port-wine stain may be seen on plain films or CT or MRI scanning. Serpiginous calcifications involving the cortex of the left occipito-parietal area are displayed in Figure 7-2. The latter two modalities also reveal a degree of ipsilateral cortical atrophy. Although calcification is most common in the occipito-parietal area, it may involve the entire hemisphere, and rarely may be bilateral.

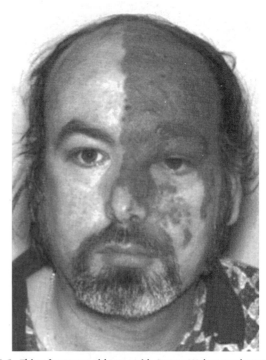

FIG. 7-1. Thirty-four-year-old man with Sturge-Weber syndrome. (From Parsons M. *Color atlas of clinical neurology*, ed 2, London, 1993, Wolfe.)

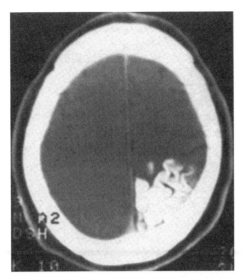

FIG. 7-2. Serpiginous cortical calcifications in Sturge-Weber syndrome. (From Haaga JR, Alfidi RJ, eds. *Computed tomography of the whole body*, vol 1, ed 2, St. Louis, 1988, Mosby.)

COURSE

Though in most patients the degree of intellectual impairment remains static after early childhood, in some cases a progressive decline may be seen, which in turn appears to be associated with persistent uncontrolled seizure activity. In such cases it may be more proper to speak of a dementia rather than mental retardation.

COMPLICATIONS

The complications of mental retardation are as described in that chapter.

ETIOLOGY

The hallmark of this disorder is a leptomeningeal angiomatosis, which, though generally confined to the occipito-parietal area, may extend forward to the frontal lobe or even occur bilaterally. Vessels of the subjacent cortex are thickened and eventually undergo calcification, and free calcium deposits may also be seen in the brain parenchyma. Gliosis and neuronal loss occur, accounting for the atrophy seen on neuroimaging.

In some cases venous stasis may occur in the leptomenigeal angiomatous malformations, with subsequent venous infarction of the underlying cortex.

Almost all cases of Sturge-Weber syndrome are sporadic; in the few familial cases recorded, inheritance seems to follow an autosomal recessive pattern.

DIFFERENTIAL DIAGNOSIS

Port-wine stains are not uncommon, but in the vast majority of cases they are not indicative of Sturge-Weber syndrome: a port-wine stain on the forehead in combination with seizures and mental retardation, however, is almost pathognomonic for this disorder. Very rarely, the port-wine stain may be absent, and in such cases the differential expands to include celiac disease which may be associated with seizures and occipital calcification.

TREATMENT

Given that recurrent seizures may lead to a progressive intellectual impairment, aggressive anti-epileptic drug treatment is essential, and carbamzepine is recommended: in treatment-resistant cases, surgery may be considered. Intraocular pressure should be monitored, generally on an annual basis, and glaucoma should be aggressively treated. Some authorities recommend low-dose aspirin for patients with stroke-like episodes or transient ischemic attacks; however, in children one must carefully balance the potential benefit against the risk of Reye's syndrome. The port-wine stain may be subjected to laser treatments. The overall treatment of mental retardation is as described in that chapter.

BIBLIOGRAPHY

Arzimanoglou AA, Andermann F, Aicardi J, et al. Sturge-Weber syndrome: indications and results of surgery in 20 patients. *Neurology* 2000;55: 1472-1479.

Benedikt RA, Brown DC, Walker R, et al. Sturge-Weber syndrome: cranial MR imaging with Gd-DTPA. *American Journal of Neuroradiology* 1993;14:409-415.

Chapieski L, Friedman A, Lachar D. Psychological functioning in children and adolescents with Sturge-Weber syndrome. *Journal of Child Neurology* 2000;15:660-665.

Maria BL, Neufeld JA, Rosainz LC, et al. High prevalence of bihemispheric structural and functional defects in Sturge-Weber syndrome. *Journal of Child Neurology* 1998;13:595-605.

Maria BL, Neufeld JA, Rosainz LC, et al. Central nervous system structure and function in Sturge-Weber syndrome: evidence of neurologic and radiologic progression. *Journal of Child Neurology* 1998;13: 606-618.

Pascual-Castroviejo I, Diaz-Gonzalez C, Garcia-Melian RM, et al. Sturge-Weber syndrome: study of 40 patients. *Pediatric Neurology* 1993;4: 283-288.

Sturge WA. A case of partial epilepsy, apparently due to a lesion of one of the vaso-motor centres of the brain. *Transactions of the Clinical Society of London* 1879;121:162-167.

Sujansky E, Conradi S. Sturge-Weber syndrome: age of onset of seizures and glaucoma and the prognosis for affected children. *Journal of Child Neurology* 1995;10:49-58.

Sujansky E, Conradi S. Outcome of Sturge-Weber syndrome in 52 adults. *American Journal of Medical Genetics* 1995;57:35-45.

Taly AB, Magaraja D, Das S, et al. Sturge-Weber-Dimitri disease without facial nevus. *Neurology* 1987;37:1063-1064.

Ville D, Enjolras O, Chiron C, et al. Prophylacticantiepileptic treatment in Sturge-Weber disease. *Seizure* 2002;11:145-150.

8 Tuberous Sclerosis

Tuberous sclerosis, also known as epiloia and Bourneville's disease, is a systemic disorder affecting not only the brain but also the skin, retina, kidneys, lungs, and other organs. Although classically this disease presents in childhood with the triad of mental retardation, seizures, and adenoma sebaceum, the presentation may be delayed until early adult years, in which case it may present as a dementia. This is a rare disorder, with a prevalence of perhaps 1 in 10,000. It may be more frequent among males than females.

ONSET

Although symptoms referable to the central nervous system typically do not appear until early childhood and indeed, as noted above, occasionally may not present until early adult years, cutaneous manifestations are present from birth. Almost 100% of patients have scattered, small, leaf-shaped areas of depigmentation at birth, some of which may be visible only with Wood's light. By the age of 4, approximately 90% display adenoma sebaceum.

CLINICAL FEATURES

In childhood-onset tuberous sclerosis mental retardation is seen in about two-thirds of patients and autism may be seen in up to one-quarter of all patients, with many others displaying isolated autistic features. Seizures occur in about three-quarters: initially they tend to manifest as infantile spasms (or "salaam" seizures); however, with age, focal, myoclonic, or typical generalized tonic-clonic convulsions tend to appear. Adenoma sebaceum, when fully mature, presents as multiple minute nodules, often distributed in a butterfly pattern on the face, typically sparing the upper lip, as shown in Figure 8-1. Other cutaneous manifestations include subungual fibromas and "shagreen" patches, which are circumscribed leathery areas of skin often found on the lower back.

Rarely, tuberous sclerosis may remain latent until adult years, wherein it may present as a progressive dementia or occasionally as a new onset seizure disorder.

Retinal phakomas, which are small, flat, rounded tumors, are often found; other common manifestations include renal cysts or angiomyolipomata, cardiac rhabdomyomata, and, somewhat less commonly, pulmonary cysts.

In perhaps 10% of cases a tuber may undergo malignant transformation, generally to a giant cell astrocytoma. Furthermore, should a tuber or astrocytoma obstruct the foramen of Monro, hydrocephalus may occur with headache, nausea, gait deterioration and cognitive deterioration.

The electroencephalogram is often abnormal, with generalized slowing and epileptiform activity.

Skull x-rays may show multiple calcified tubers. CT scanning likewise shows many calcified tubers, which tend to be subependymal in location, often close to the foramen of Monro. Uncalcified tubers may escape detection on CT scanning but are reliably picked up on MRI scanning; Figure 8-2 demonstrates noncalcified subependymal tubers.

COURSE

Children with severe disease rarely live more than 15 years; cognitive functioning gradually declines, and seizures frequently increase. Death may occur secondary to status epilepticus, or cardiac or renal disease. On the other hand, those with adult-onset disease may experience only a slowly progressive dementia and may not die of the disease unless an astrocytoma or other tumor should occur.

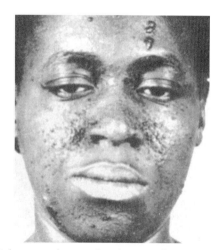

FIG. 8-1. Adenoma sebaceum in tuberous sclerosis. (From Goodman RM, Gorlin RJ. *Atlas of the face in genetic disorders*, St. Louis, 1977, Mosby.)

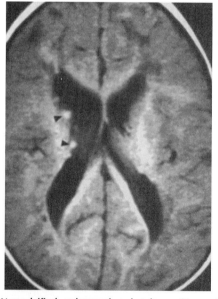

FIG. 8-2. Noncalcified subependymal tubers. (From Osborn AG. *Diagnostic neuroradiology*, St. Louis, 1994, Mosby.)

COMPLICATIONS

These are as described in the chapters on dementia and on mental retardation.

ETIOLOGY

At autopsy, numerous sclerotic tumors, known as tubers, are found, many of which are calcified. These may be found on the surface of the cortex, in the white matter, and, most typically, subependymally. These subependymal tumors project into the ventricle and at times are so numerous as to give the ventricular surface the classic "candle guttering" appearance. Less commonly, tubers are found in the cerebellum or the brain stem. The tubers themselves are composed of a combination of enlarged, atypical glial cells and neuronal elements which are often extraordinarily large and vacuolated.

Tuberous sclerosis is a genetic disorder: in about one-third of cases, the disease is inherited in an autosomal dominant pattern with the rest of the cases representing spontaneous mutations. Mutations may be seen in one of two genes: TSC1 is located on chromosome 9 and codes for a protein known as hamartin whereas TSC2 is located on chromosome 16 and codes for tuberin. Both TSC1 and TSC2 function as "tumor suppressor genes," and it is presumably the lack of a normal amount of "suppression" which allows for the development of tubers and other manifestations of the disease.

DIFFERENTIAL DIAGNOSIS

When the classic triad is present in childhood, the diagnosis is difficult to miss. In adults who present with dementia, cutaneous manifestations may suggest the diagnosis. If these are missed, the finding of multiple tumors, many calcified, on CT or MRI scanning suggests the correct diagnosis.

TREATMENT

Aggressive antiepileptic treatment is imperative, and in treatment-resistant cases surgery may be considered when there is a single, well-localized epileptogenic zone; surgery may also be considered in cases of obstructive hydrocephalus. Mental retardation, autism and dementia are treated as outlined in the respective chapters; importantly, however, potentially cardiotoxic drugs should probably be avoided given the frequency with which cardiac rhabdomyomata occur. Genetic counseling should be offered to patients. Apparently unaffected parents of patients should be carefully examined (with consideration given to MRI scanning of the head, echocardiography, renal ultrasound and chest x-ray) before assuming that the patient's disease represents a spontaneous mutation.

BIBLIOGRAPHY

Baker P, Piven J, Sato Y. Autism and tuberous sclerosis complex: prevalence and clinical features. *Journal of Autism and Developmental Disorders* 1998;28:279-285.

Franz DN, Tudor C, Leonard J, et al. Lamotrigene therapy of epilepsy in tuberous sclerosis. *Epilepsia* 2001;42:935-940.

Guerreiro MM, Andermann F, Andermann E, et al. Surgical treatment of epilepsy in tuberous sclerosis: strategies and results in 18 patients. *Neurology* 1998;51:1263-1269.

Gutierrez GC, Smalley SL, Tanguey PE. Autism in tuberous sclerosis complex. *Journal of Autism and Developmental Disorders* 1998;28:97-103.

Gutowski NJ, Murphy RP. Late onset epilepsy in undiagnosed tuberous sclerosis. *Postgraduate Medical Journal* 1992;68:970-971.

Hunt A. Tuberous sclerosis: a survey of 97 cases. I: Seizures, pertussis immunization and handicap. *Developmental Medicine and Child Neurology* 1983;25:346-349.

Hunt A. Tuberous sclerosis: a survey of 97 cases. II: Physical findings. *Developmental Medicine and Child Neurology* 1983;25:350-352.

Langkau N, Martin N, Brandt R, et al. TSC1 and TSC2 mutations in tuberous sclerosis, the associated phenotypes and a model to explain observed TSC1/TSC2 frequency ratios. *European Journal of Pediatrics* 2002;161:393-402.

Pampiglione G, Moynahan EJ. The tuberous sclerosis syndrome: clinical and EEG studies in 100 children. *Journal of Neurology, Neurosurgery, and Psychiatry* 1976;39:663-673.

Weig SG, Pollack P. Carbamazepine-induced heart block in a child with tuberous sclerosis and cardiac rhabdomyoma: implications for evaluation and follow-up. *Annals of Neurology* 1993;34:617-619.

9 Bardet-Biedl Syndrome

The Bardet-Biedl syndrome is a rare genetic disorder characterized by obesity, retinal dystrophy, polydactyly and, in about one-half of patients, mental retardation. Although this syndrome is well-characterized, there is some inconsistency in the literature regarding its name: originally called the "Laurence-Moon-Biedl syndrome," the currently preferred name is Bardet-Biedl syndrome.

ONSET

Obesity and mental retardation are generally apparent in infancy or early childhood.

CLINICAL FEATURES

Obesity is generally truncal, and patients may be of short stature; a typical patient is seen in Figure 9-1. Polydactyly is present in about two-thirds, with the remainder having either syndactyly or brachydactyly. Mental retardation, when present, ranges from mild to severe. Most males have hypogenitalism, with small testes and penis, and almost all females have significant menstrual irregularities. Diabetes mellitus, cardiac and renal disease are commonly seen. Retinal dystrophy with a gradual loss of central vision may not be apparent for many years, and blindness is generally delayed until middle years.

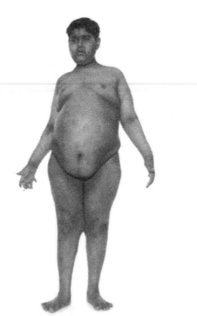

FIG. 9-1. Typical male with Bardet-Biedl syndrome. (From Hall R, Evered DC. *Color atlas of endocrinology*, ed 2, London, 1990, Wolfe.)

COURSE

As noted, retinal dystrophy is gradually progressive; of those with renal disease, progression may also occur and in a small minority renal failure may supervene.

COMPLICATIONS

These are as described in the chapters on mental retardation and on obesity.

ETIOLOGY

Six loci (BBS1 through BBS6) have been identified and, in most cases, an autosomal recessive mode of inheritance is present. As yet no characteristic pathology of the central nervous system has been delineated.

DIFFERENTIAL DIAGNOSIS

Both the Prader-Willi and Alstrom-Hallgren syndromes are characterized by obesity and an autosomal recessive mode of inheritance; neither of these syndromes, however, are characterized by polydactyly. Further differentiating factors include a ravenous appetite in the Prader-Willi syndrome and sensorineuronal deafness in the Alstrom-Hallgren syndrome.

TREATMENT

Treatment is as outlined in the chapters on mental retardation and on obesity. Testosterone does not appear to be helpful.

BIBLIOGRAPHY

Beales BL, Warner AM, Hitman GA, et al. Bardet-Biedl syndrome: a molecular and phenotypic study of 18 families. *Journal of Medical Genetics* 1997;34:92-98.

Green GS, Parfrey PS, Harnett JD, et al. The cardinal manifestations of Bardet-Biedl syndrome, a form of Laurence-Moon-Biedl syndrome. *The New England Journal of Medicine* 1989;321:1002-1009.

Katsanis N, Lupski JR, Beales PL. Exploring the molecular basis of Bardet-Biedl syndrome. *Human Molecular Genetics* 2001;10: 2293-2299.

Mykytyn K, Braun T, Carmi R, et al. Identification of the gene that, when mutated, causes the human obesity syndrome BBS4. *Nature Genetics* 2001;28:188-191.

Mykytyn K, Nishimura DY, Searby CC, et al. Identification of the gene (BBS1) most commonly involved in Bardet-Biedl syndrome, a complex human obesity syndrome. *Nature Genetics* 2002;31:435-438.

Ozer G, Yuksel B, Suleymanova D, et al. Clinical features of Bardet-Biedl syndrome. *Acta Paediatrica Japonica* 1995;37:233-236.

Riise R, Tornqvist K, Wright AF, et al. The phenotype in Norwegian patients with Bardet-Biedl syndrome with mutations in the BBS4 gene. *Archives of Ophthalmology* 2002;120:1364-1367.

10 Velocardiofacial Syndrome

The velocardiofacial syndrome is a genetic disorder occurring secondary to a deletion on chromosome 22 which manifests with a distinctive facial dysmorphism, intellectual deficits, and, of great interest to psychiatry, a psychosis which closely resembles schizophrenia. This is not an uncommon disorder, being found in approximately 1 in 4000 live births.

ONSET

Although the facial dysmorphism and intellectual deficits are apparent in childhood, the psychosis, which occurs in about one-third of all patients, generally is delayed until late adolescence or early adult years.

CLINICAL FEATURES

The facial dysmorphism is characterized by a large, often bulbous, nose with a "squared-off" nasal root, a degree of micrognathia, and a flattening of affect. A high, nasal voice is often present, and this may or may not be accompanied by a submucosal cleft palate.

A little less than one-half of patients will have mental retardation, which, in most cases, is of mild degree.

Although not without controversy, it appears that up to one-third of patients will, as adolescents or adults, develop a psychosis phenotypically very similar to that seen in schizophrenia.

Other clinical findings include congenital heart defects (most commonly ventricular septal defects) and hypoparathyroidism.

COURSE

The course is chronic; although some die of complications of heart defects, most survive and live a normal life span.

COMPLICATIONS

The complications of mental retardation and of secondary psychosis are as described in those chapters.

ETIOLOGY

The velocardiofacial syndrome occurs secondary to a microdeletion on the long arm of chromosome 22. Although in most cases this is inherited in an autosomal dominant pattern, de novo cases may also occur.

DIFFERENTIAL DIAGNOSIS

The diagnosis is suggested by the facial dysmorphism and the nasal voice.

TREATMENT

There is no specific treatment for the syndrome; mental retardation and psychosis may be treated as outlined in those chapters.

BIBLIOGRAPHY

Bartsch O, Nemeckova M, Kocarek E, et al. DiGeorge/velocardiofacial syndrome: FISH studies of chromosomes 22q11 and 10p14 and clinical reports on the proximal 22q11 deletion. *American Journal of Medical Genetics* 2003;117:1-5.

Eliez S, Schmitt JE, White CD, et al. Children and adolescents with velocardiofacial syndrome: a volumetric MRI study. *The American Journal of Psychiatry* 2000;157:409-415.

Eliez S, Antonarakis SE, Morris MA, et al. Parental origin of the deletion 22q11.2 and brain development in velocardiofacial syndrome: a preliminary report. *Archives of General Psychiatry* 2001;58:64-68.

Pike AC, Super M. Velocardiofacial syndrome. *Postgraduate Medical Journal* 1997;73:771-775.

Swillen A, Devriendt K, Legius E, et al. Intelligence and psychosocial adjustment in velocardiofacial syndrome: a study of 37 children and adolescents with VCFS. *Journal of Medical Genetics* 1997;34:453-458.

11 Prader-Willi Syndrome

Prader-Willi syndrome is a congenital disorder characterized by short stature, micromelia, mild mental retardation, hypogonadism, and obesity secondary to a remarkable hyperphagia. It occurs in both males and females and affects up to 0.01% of the population.

ONSET

During the first 6 to 24 months of life these infants tend to be somnolent and hypotonic and to eat very little. Indeed some may require tube feeding. This phase is then replaced by alertness and the characteristic hyperphagia.

CLINICAL FEATURES

These patients have a ravenous appetite and go to great lengths to satisfy it. They often steal food and may eat almost anything, including pet food. Parents typically end up locking cabinets and refrigerators, but even that may not be sufficient, as some patients may eat the garbage. Almost inevitably, morbid obesity eventually develops.

Mental retardation may be present in from one-half to three-quarters of these patients; however, it is typically mild. Emotional lability, stubbornness, and temper tantrums are common, as is skin-picking, which at times may be quite severe. Many patients also engage in ritualistic behaviors, and a minority may develop depression. Hypersomnolence is common and appears to be multifactorial in origin with contributions from sleep apnea, the Pickwickian syndrome and as yet unidentified hypothalamic mechanisms. Typically the head is narrow, the eyes almond shaped, and the upper lip narrow; these patients may also display micromelia, with thin arms and legs and small hands and feet. A teenage boy with this syndrome is shown in Figure 11-1.

In males hypogonadism manifests with micropenis and cryptorchidism. In females the hypogonadism manifests with a lack of breast development and pubic hair, hypoplastic labia, and varying degrees of amenorrhea.

The diagnosis may be confirmed by DNA methylation analysis, as discussed below.

COURSE

These patients generally die of one of the complications of obesity.

COMPLICATIONS

Complications are as described in the chapters on mental retardation and obesity. The massive obesity seen in this condition may lead to diabetes mellitus, hypertension, and, as noted above, sleep apnea and the Pickwickian syndrome.

ETIOLOGY

The Prader-Willi syndrome occurs in individuals who lack a critical portion of paternally derived chromosome 15. Such a deficit can occur in one of three ways: first, and most commonly, there is a microdeletion on the paternal chromosome; second, there may be "uniparental disomy" wherein both chromosomes are derived from the mother; third, and rarely, there may be a mutation in that critical portion of the paternally derived chromosome. Determining whether or not a given patient's chromosome 15 is paternally derived is facilitated by the fact that the methylation pattern of paternally derived chromosome 15 is different from the methylation pattern of the maternally derived chromosome; consequently,

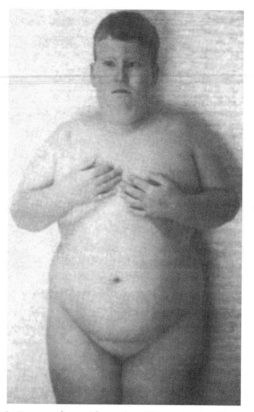

FIG. 11-1. Teenage boy with Prader-Willi syndrome. (From Kelly TE. *Clinical genetics and genetic counseling*, ed 2, Chicago, 1986, Mosby.)

if DNA methylation analysis indicates a lack of paternally derived material, then one may be confident that the diagnosis is correct.

Little is known regarding the neuropathology of this syndrome: one study found a reduced number of neurons in the paraventricular and supraoptic nuclei of the hypothalamus.

DIFFERENTIAL DIAGNOSIS

The differential diagnosis for obesity is as discussed in that chapter, and for the mental retardation as discussed in that chapter.

TREATMENT

Early dietary management is essential; in some cases institutionalization may be required to restrict the patient from food.

Growth hormone injections may induce increased activity and an increase in lean body mass. Fenfluramine, in a double-blinded study, reduced hyperphagia and aggressiveness, and, in an open study, risperidone (in a mean dose of approximately 1.5 mg/d) had the same effects.

The vast majority of cases are sporadic: as noted earlier most cases are secondary to microdeletions in the paternal chromosome or to maternal uniparental disomy, and neither of these phenomena is heritable.

BIBLIOGRAPHY

Boer H, Holland A, Whittington J, et al. Psychotic illness in people with Prader-Willi syndrome due to chromosome 15 maternal uniparental disomy. *Lancet* 2002;359:135-136.

Butler JV, Whittington JE, Holland AJ, et al. Prevalence of, and risk factors for, physical ill-health in people with Prader-Willi syndrome: a population-based study. *Developmental Medicine and Child Neurology* 2002;44:248-255.

Bye AM, Vines R, Fronzek K. The obesity hypoventilation syndrome and the Prader-Willi syndrome. *Australian Paediatric Journal* 1983;19:251-255.

Carrel AL, Myers SE, Whitman BY, et al. Benefits of long-term GH therapy in Prader-Willi syndrome: a 4-year study. *The Journal of Clinical Endocrinology and Metabolism* 2002;87:1581-1585.

Clarke DJ, Boer H, Whittington J, et al. Prader-Willi syndrome, compulsive and ritualistic behaviors: the first population-based survey. *The British Journal of Psychiatry* 2002;180:358-362.

Clift S, Dahlitz M, Parkes JD. Sleep apnoea in the Prader-Willi syndrome. *Journal of Sleep Research* 1994;3:121-126.

Durst R, Rubin-Jabotinsky K, Raskin S, et al. Risperidone in treating behavioral disturbances of Prader-Willi syndrome. *Acta Psychiatrica Scandinavica* 2000;102:461-465.

Fridman C, Varela MC, Kod F, et al. Prader-Willi syndrome: genetic tests and clinical findings. *Genetic Testing* 2000;4:387-392.

Greenswag LR. Adults with Prader-Willi syndrome: a survey of 232 cases. *Developmental Medicine and Child Neurology* 1987;29:145-152.

Hellings JA, Warnock JK. Self-injurious behavior and serotonin in Prader-Willi syndrome. *Psychopharmacology Bulletin* 1994;30:245-250.

Manni R, Politini L, Nobili L, et al. Hypersomnia in the Prader-Willi syndrome: clinical-electrophysiological features and underlying factors. *Clinical Neurophysiology* 2001;112:800-805.

Selikowitz M, Sunman J, Pendergast A, et al. Fenfluramine in Prader-Willi syndrome: a double blind, placebo controlled trial. *Archives of Disease in Childhood* 1990;65:112-114.

Symons FJ, Butler MG, Sanders MD, et al. Self-injurious behavior and Prader-Willi syndrome: behavioral forms and body locations. *American Journal of Mental Retardation* 1999;104:260-269.

Lesch-Nyhan syndrome is a very rare X-linked recessively inherited disease associated with an almost complete deficiency of hypoxanthine-guanine phosphoribosyltransferase. Clinically, patients present with choreoathetosis, spasticity, striking self-mutilation, and varying degrees of mental retardation.

ONSET

Abnormal involuntary movements are generally apparent within the first year of life.

CLINICAL FEATURES

Although mental retardation was once assumed to be at least of mild or moderate degree, IQ scores are in some cases falsely low secondary to the severe movement disorder, and some of these children may be of almost normal intelligence and be quite aware of their plight.

Toward the end of the first year of life choreoathetosis becomes evident. Dysarthria and dystonia may also be evident. Some children also display spasticity, with a scissoring gait and hyperreflexia. A minority have seizures, and in a smaller minority a megaloblastic anemia occurs.

The characteristic self-mutilation usually appears in childhood after the third year of life. Despite being normally sensitive to pain these patients repeatedly bite at their lips, tongue, buccal mucosa, and fingers. In extreme cases the fingers and lips are literally chewed off by the patient's teeth; two such patients are shown in Figure 12-1.

Serum uric acid is almost always elevated, and tophaceous gout and gouty nephropathy may occur in adolescence.

The diagnosis is confirmed either by finding a grossly decreased level of hypoxanthine-guanine phosphoribosyltransferase activity in erythrocytes, hair roots, or cultured skin fibroblasts, or by PCR analysis.

COURSE

Most patients die of infection or of renal failure in their teenage or early adult years.

COMPLICATIONS

Institutionalization is required in almost all cases.

ETIOLOGY

The almost complete absence of hypoxanthine-guanine phosphoribosyltransferase (HPRT) activity occurs secondary to any one of over 100 known mutations in the gene for HPRT, which is located on the X chromosome. Although the resultant disturbance in purine metabolism leads to excessive uric acid production, the resultant hyperuricemia is apparently epiphenomenal and not causally related to the central nervous system dysfunction.

PET studies have demonstrated reduced dopaminergic activity in the frontal cortex, striatum and midbrain tegmentum, and MRI has revealed atrophy of the caudate nucleus. Further evidence of disturbed dopaminergic activity comes from CSF studies which

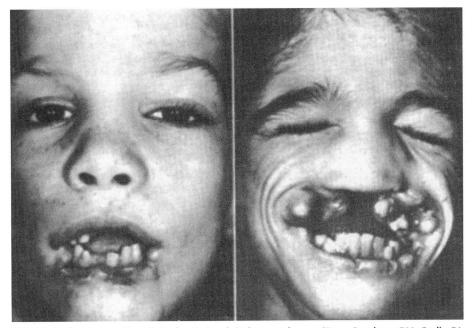

FIG. 12-1. Self-amputation of the lips in Lesch-Nyhan syndrome. (From Goodman RM, Gorlin RJ. *Atlas of the face in genetic disorders*, St. Louis, 1977, Mosby.)

reveal decreased HVA levels, and from a post-mortem study which indicated a reduced concentration of dopamine in the caudate.

DIFFERENTIAL DIAGNOSIS

Many patients with other forms of mental retardation bite themselves, as noted in that chapter. However, the degree of self-mutilation seen in other cases of mental retardation rarely even approaches that seen in the Lesch-Nyhan syndrome.

TREATMENT

Allopurinol, by forestalling gouty nephropathy, may prolong life but has no effect on the central nervous system symptoms.

Restraints are often required to protect the fingers. Interestingly these patients often appear quite relieved when restraints are applied, as if, although wishing to stop biting, they were yet unable to do so. Mouth or lip guards or face masks, may reduce lip injury, but in some cases teeth may have to be extracted to protect the lips. Antipsychotics, such as fluphenazine, haloperidol, or risperidone may reduce choreoathetosis and self-mutilation; there are also reports of reduced self-mutilation with carbamazepine and with gabapentin. Oral 5-hydroxytryptophan does reduce choreoathetosis but is ineffective against self-mutilation.

Current research focuses on gene replacement therapy. Antenatal diagnosis by amniocentesis and assay of cultured fibroblasts is currently available.

BIBLIOGRAPHY

Allen SM, Rice SN. Risperidone antagonism of self-mutilation in a Lesch-Nyhan patient. *Progress in Neuro-psychopharmacology & Biological Psychiatry* 1996;20:793-800.

Christie R, Bay C, Kaufman IA. Lesch-Nyhan disease: clinical experience with nineteen patients. *Developmental Medicine and Child Neurology* 1982;24:293-306.

Ernst M, Zametkin AJ, Matochik JA, et al. Presynaptic dopaminergic deficits in Lesch-Nyhan disease. *The New England Journal of Medicine* 1996;334:1568-1572.

Frith CD, Johnston EC, Joseph MH, et al. Double-blind trial of 5-hydroxytryptophan in a case of Lesch-Nyhan syndrome. *Journal of Neurology, Neurosurgery, and Psychiatry* 1976;39:656-662.

Harris JC, Lee RR, Jinnah HA, et al. Craniocerebral magnetic resonance imaging measurement and findings in Lesch-Nyhan syndrome. *Archives of Neurology* 1998;55:547-553.

Jankovic J, Caskey TC, Stout JT, et al. Lesch-Nyhan syndrome: a study of motor behavior and cerebrospinal fluid neurotransmitters. *Annals of Neurology* 1988;23:466-469.

Lesch M, Nyhan WL. A familial disorder of uric acid metabolism and central nervous system function. *The American Journal of Medicine* 1964;36:561-570.

McManaman J, Tam DA. Gabapentin for self-injurious behavior in Lesch-Nyhan syndrome. *Pediatric Neurology* 1999;20:381-382.

Mizuno T. Long-term follow-up of ten patients with Lesch-Nyhan syndrome. *Neuropediatrics* 1986;17:158-161.

Roach ES, Delgado M, Anderson L, et al. Carbamazepine trial for Lesch-Nyhan self-mutilation. *Journal of Child Neurology* 1996;11:476-478.

Saito Y, Ito M, Hanaoka S, et al. Dopamine receptor up-regulation in Lesch-Nyhan syndrome: a post-mortem study. *Neuropediatrics* 1999;30:66-71.

Wong DF, Harris JC, Naidu S, et al. Dopamine transporters are markedly reduced in Lesch-Nyhan disease in vivo. *Proceedings of the National Academy of Sciences of the United States of America* 1996;93:5539-5543.

13 Introduction to the Developmental Disabilities (communication, learning, and motor skills disorders)

In the course of normal development, children, in a more or less sequential fashion, come to be able to do the following: put their thoughts into spoken words and understand what is said to them, articulate clearly, read, do arithmetic, write, and do things in a dexterous, coordinated fashion. Children who fail to develop these abilities at the expected time in the absence of any other apparent cause are said to have a developmental disability. These disabilities have been given specific names in DSM-IV; however, they are also often referred to by the names given to their adult onset "equivalents" that occur secondary to acquired lesions such as strokes, tumors, and the like. For example, children who have trouble learning to write are said by DSM-IV to have "Disorder of Written Expression," but are often simply characterized as having developmental dysgraphia. Table 13-1 lists the various developmental disabilities, with both DSM-IV and equivalent terminology. In general this text refers to these disabilities by the names derived from their adult "equivalents."

Each of these disabilities is considered individually in the following chapters. The features they have in common are discussed here.

These disabilities are very common. Though precise estimates are not available, up to 15% of the elementary school age population suffers from one or more of them. For the most part they are far more common in boys than in girls, by a ratio of anywhere from 2:1 to 4:1.

ONSET

These disabilities first become apparent when the child fails to keep developmental pace with his peers. Thus, in general, developmental or receptive dysphasia has the earliest age of onset, at times being

■**TABLE 13-1.** Developmental Disabilities

DSM-IV	Equivalent Terms
Communication Disorders	
Expressive language disorder	Developmental dysphasia
Mixed expressive-receptive language disorder	Developmental dysphasia
Language Disorder	
Phonologic disorder	Developmental dysarticulation
Learning Disorders	
Reading disorder	Developmental dyslexia
Mathematics disorder	Developmental dyscalculia
Disorder of written expression	Developmental dysgraphia
Motor Skills Disorder	
Developmental coordination disorder	Developmental clumsiness

apparent at the age of 2 years. On the other extreme, developmental dysgraphia generally has the latest onset, sometimes not being apparent until the age of 10, by which time most children, at least in our culture, have come to be able to write reasonably well.

CLINICAL FEATURES

Individual descriptions of each disability are provided in the respective chapters; importantly, although a developmental disability may occur in isolation, it is more often the case that any given patient will have a mixed condition, with two or more concurrent disabilities. In particular, dyslexia is often accompanied by dysgraphia and dyscalculia, and it is unusual to find either dysgraphia or dyscalculia in isolation. Furthermore, although clumsiness often does occur in isolation, it may also be seen in conjunction with dysarticulation or dysphasia.

Hyperactivity may be associated with developmental disabilities, especially developmental dyslexia, dysphasia, dyscalculia and clumsiness.

COURSE

In the natural course of events most affected children experience at least partial remission of their symptoms. The degree and timing of remission varies. On the one hand most children with developmental dysarticulation substantially improve before early teenage years; on the other hand developmental dysphasia tends to be a lifelong problem.

COMPLICATIONS

In addition to their own sense of embarrassment and shame these children are often subject to ridicule and humiliation. School failure is common. Debate is ongoing as to whether the presence of developmental disability predisposes to the development of a conduct disorder, and eventually to an antisocial personality disorder.

ETIOLOGY

With the exception of clumsiness, all of these developmental disabilities are known to run in families. In the case of developmental dysphasia and developmental dyslexia, neuropathologic changes have been found that are highly suggestive of maturational dysgenesis of the cortex.

In cases where a child has more than one developmental disability, either he has two independent disabilities or one of the disabilities is secondary to the other. This secondary phenomenon is perhaps most clearly seen in a child with developmental receptive dysphasia and dyslexia or dysgraphia. A child who lacks the ability to understand what is said to him is disabled from learning to read or write.

DIFFERENTIAL DIAGNOSIS

Congenital or early-onset blindness or deafness often disables a child; however, these are easily checked for.

In mental retardation the child's abilities are far below his peers across the board. Occasionally, however, one ability may be far below the others possessed by the retarded child. In such a case then a diagnosis of both mental retardation and developmental disability should be made.

Children with autism, whether retarded or not, show very uneven development. In contrast to mental retardation, however, such unevenness, being universally present in autism, does not indicate the presence of a separate developmental disability. Overall the autistic child is distinguished from the developmentally disabled child by his indifference to or active avoidance of human contact.

In the rare instance of early childhood onset schizophrenia certain abilities do not develop. Here, however, one finds peculiarities and bizarreness not present in children with developmental disabilities.

Deprivation or educational lack may leave a child unable to read, write, or do arithmetic and, in extreme cases of deprivation, unable to speak or understand what is said. Here, however, given the opportunity to learn and a certain amount of trust in the teacher, these children rapidly gain these abilities, in contrast to the slow acquisition demonstrated by developmentally disabled children.

Children with hyperactivity often fail to make satisfactory progress in learning to read, write, or do arithmetic. Here, however, the poor performance is secondary to the child's inability to sit still and pay attention in class. Once the hyperactivity is successfully treated these children generally make rapid progress.

Acquired defects should never be mistaken for a developmental disability. Any child who loses an ability already mastered, as, for example, reading, must be carefully evaluated for disorders such as depression, schizophrenia, or a dementing illness such as adrenoleukodystrophy, metachromatic leukodystrophy, and subacute sclerosing panencephalitis.

The foregoing differential diagnostic considerations apply to all of the developmental disabilities. Additional considerations are presented in the respective chapters.

TREATMENT

Remedial education is essential and successful. With the exception of piracetam (not available in the United States) for developmental dyslexia, medications do not appear to be helpful.

Parents may benefit from education regarding these disabilities; many may see their child as willful, lazy, or stubborn, and their approach to the child may become far more constructive when they realize the nature of the disability.

If to avoid shame or humiliation the child withdraws or rebels from schoolwork or play with friends, individual psychotherapy may be helpful.

When the entire family has been affected by the disability, family counseling may likewise be beneficial.

Early school screening and timely remedial intervention may prevent many of the complications of these developmental disabilities.

BIBLIOGRAPHY

Anonymous. Practice parameters for the assessment and treatment of children and adolescents with language and learning disorders. *Journal of the American Academy of Child and Adolescent Psychiatry* 1998;37(Suppl 10):46-62.

Beitchman JH, Young AR. Learning disorders with a special emphasis on reading disorders: a review of the past 10 years. *Journal of the American Academy of Child and Adolescent Psychiatry* 1997;36: 1020-1032.

Sonnander K. Early identification of children with developmental disabilities. *Acta Paediatrica Scandinavica* 2000;89(Suppl):17-23.

14 Developmental Dysphasia (expressive language disorder and mixed receptive-expressive language disorder, DSM-IV-TR #315.31, 315.32)

Children with developmental dysphasia typically have deficits in both receptive and expressive language. Rarely one may see an isolated developmental expressive dysphasia; isolated developmental receptive dysphasia probably does not occur in pure form. Children with a receptive deficit fail to understand what is said to them, as if they are not listening. Those with an expressive deficit are able to grasp the meaning of what is said to them, yet are unable to express their own thoughts. The expressive form of developmental dysphasia is also called "expressive language disorder," and the mixed expressive-receptive type of developmental dysphasia is also called "mixed receptive-expressive language disorder."

The prevalence of developmental dysphasia among school-age children is not known with certainty. Estimates range from less than 1% to up to 15% depending on the criteria used. Conservative estimates place the prevalence at about 6%. Developmental dysphasia is more common in boys than girls.

ONSET

Depending on its severity developmental dysphasia may first become apparent anywhere from the age of 2 up to late childhood. As children normally come to understand what is said long before they can adequately express themselves, a pure expressive deficit tends to appear later than a mixed receptive-expressive one.

CLINICAL FEATURES

In the interest of clarity, receptive and expressive deficits are described separately. However, as noted earlier, though an expressive deficit can and does at times appear in isolation, typically the child has elements of both.

In the most severe cases of receptive dysphasia children do not seem to be affected at all by the content of what is said to them. Their attention may be captured by tone of voice, but the words themselves, spoken in a monotone and stripped of prosody, seem to fall on deaf ears. They may hum a tune they have heard or imitate a dog barking, yet they cannot understand the words that are spoken to them. In less severe cases, the child may come to grasp simple words, such as "cat" or "candy," and at times even simple sentences such as "sit down." More complex words and sentences, however, leave them baffled. Milder cases may not come to light until early school years, when the child shows difficulty in understanding difficult sentences or paragraphs. Conditional and concessive statements may have to be broken down into simple declarative sentences before the patient can grasp what is being said.

Children with isolated developmental expressive dysphasia can follow directions, even complex ones, yet have extraordinary difficulty in speaking or in putting their thoughts into spoken words. The vocabulary is limited to simpler words. At times lacking a complex vocabulary item for a complex thought, the patient may engage in circumlocution, using his simple vocabulary in an attempt to express his complicated thought. At other times he may have difficulty finding simple words. In milder cases where the child is able to speak in sentences, the sentences themselves tend to be short, incomplete, and at times telegraphic. Words, such as verbs, are often omitted. Complex sentence construction, as, for example, those with dependent clauses, are often not used at all.

Children with severe cases of the mixed receptive-expressive form of developmental dysphasia may not speak at all, perhaps for years. In such cases, when speech is acquired it tends to be idiosyncratic and almost inaccessible except to those who know the patient well.

Other disorders commonly found in patients with developmental dysphasia include developmental clumsiness, enuresis, and attention-deficit/hyperactivity disorder.

COURSE

Although improvement tends to occur over the years, developmental dysphasia is in general a chronic disorder.

Children with mixed receptive-expressive dysphasia tend, in the natural course of events, to have a poor prognosis. Although those with a mild case may eventually come to understand enough of what is said to them to get by reasonably well, those severely afflicted may never understand what is said and may never speak.

The outlook for children with isolated expressive dysphasia is better. Many acquire serviceable speech by early school years, and most have generally normal speech by early adolescence.

COMPLICATIONS

Developmental dysphasia may be extremely disabling. Unable to adequately communicate, these children are less able to progress either socially or academically.

ETIOLOGY

Developmental dysphasia tends to be familial. Furthermore among the first-degree relatives of developmentally dysphasic children, one also finds a higher than expected incidence of dyslexia, dysgraphia, and dysarticulation.

At autopsy, one patient displayed asymmetry of the plana temporalia and focal cortical dysplasia of the inferior surface of the left frontal gyrus, suggesting a disorder of neuronal migration. Sleep EEG studies have demonstrated a greater than normal amount of paroxysmal activity, again consistent with the presence of cortical dysplasia.

DIFFERENTIAL DIAGNOSIS

Deafness, of course, can simulate developmental dysphasia; however, here the deaf child, unlike the dysphasic child, fails to respond to tone of voice.

Selective mutism is distinguished by its later age of onset and by the ability of the child to communicate with selected others.

Severe deprivation may leave the child unexposed to speech and thus unable to understand or speak. Such children, however, once able to trust others generally show rapid strides in speech. In a somewhat similar vein, youngest children whose older siblings "do all the talking for them" may likewise appear dysphasic, yet here these children likewise rapidly come to speak when they are chronically kept in a situation where no one else can speak for them and their wants are not met unless they engage in conversation.

Autistic children often appear inaccessible to those speaking to them. Furthermore their own speech is often idiosyncratic, and some may be mute. In contrast to dysphasic children, however, autistic children are emotionally aloof. The dysphasic child shows relatively normal affection; the autistic child remains distant.

Mental retardation always includes deficits in language; however, here one sees an inability to learn by any means. In contrast the dysphasic child may grasp complex visual or spatial concepts.

In the exceedingly rare instance of early childhood onset schizophrenia, language is disordered. Here, however, in contrast to dysphasia one finds bizarre speech and bizarre behavior.

Children with severe developmental dysarticulation may be almost unintelligible and appear to have developmental expressive dysphasia. Careful examination, however, discloses a normal syntax, which is not found in severe cases of expressive dysphasia.

Tumors, encephalitides, and trauma may cause dysphasia but may be distinguished either by their acquired, rather than developmental, aspect or by associated focal signs or seizures: a very important cause of acquired aphasia in children is the Landau-Kleffner syndrome, characterized by progressively worsening seizures and aphasia.

TREATMENT

Remedial education is critical and often very helpful. Children with receptive dysphasia may be taught to lip-read.

Some authors advocate the use of antiepileptic drugs, such as divalproex, in cases associated with paroxysmal electroencephalographic activity; however, this has not as yet been clearly demonstrated to be beneficial.

BIBLIOGRAPHY

Bartak L, Rutter M, Cox A. A comparative study of infantile autism and specific developmental receptive language disorder: I. the children. *The British Journal of Psychiatry* 1975;126:127-145.

Beitchman JH, Wilson B, Johnson CJ, et al. Fourteen-year follow-up of speech/language impaired and control children: psychiatric outcome. *Journal of the American Academy of Child and Adolescent Psychiatry* 2001;40:75-82.

Billard C, Toutain A, Loisel ML, et al. Genetic basis of developmental dysphasia. Report of eleven familial cases in six families. *Genetic Counseling* 1994;5:23-33.

Caulfield MB, Fischel JE, DeBaryshe BD, et al. Behavioral correlates of developmental language disorder. *Journal of Abnormal Child Psychology* 1989;17:187-201.

Cohen D, Caparulo B, Shaywitz B. Primary childhood aphasia and childhood autism: clinical, biological, and conceptual observations. *Journal of the American Academy of Child and Adolescent Psychiatry* 1976;4: 604-645.

Cohen D, Campbell R, Yaghmai F. Neuropathological abnormalities in developmental dysphasia. *Annals of Neurology* 1984;25:567-570.

Duvelleroy-Hommet C, Billard C, Lucas B, et al. Sleep EEG and developmental dysphasia: lack of a consistent relationship with paroxysmal EEG activity during sleep. *Neuropediatrics* 1995;26:14-18.

Karlin IW. Congenital verbal auditory agnosia. *Pediatrics* 1951;7:60-68.

Paul R, Cohen DJ, Caparulo BK. A longitudinal study of patients with severe developmental disorders of language learning. *Journal of the American Academy of Child and Adolescent Psychiatry* 1983;22:525-534.

Picard A, Cheliout Heraut F, Bouskraoui M, et al. Sleep EEG and developmental dysphasia. *Developmental Medicine and Child Neurology* 1998;40:595-599.

15 Developmental Articulation Disorder (phonological disorder, DSM-IV-TR #315.39)

Developmental articulation disorder, also known as developmental dysarticulation or, most recently, phonological disorder, is characterized by a difficulty in pronunciation. The child may lisp, or at times the child's speech may resemble "baby talk."

Up to 3% of children below the age of 8 have some degree of developmental dysarticulation. Although the sex ratio has not been clearly defined, the clinical impression is that it is more common in boys.

ONSET

Developmental dysarticulation usually becomes evident between the ages of 3 and 6, as the difference between the child's speech and the progressively better articulated speech of peers becomes more and more apparent.

CLINICAL FEATURES

These children often have difficulty pronouncing consonants. Rather than saying "with me" they may say "wif me"; other examples include "tak" for "talk," "wim" for "swim," or "ollipop" for "lollipop." At times there may be a distinct lisp. Speech may be slow and at times almost effortful. The child knows exactly what he wants to say, and when others don't grasp his meaning he may become frustrated or, perhaps just as frequently, angry at his listeners for not understanding.

Mild cases may almost escape detection. The child may only be reproached for talking "baby talk." In more severe cases, however, speech may be almost unintelligible except to those who have lived with the child.

Developmental dysarticulation may be seen in association with developmental clumsiness.

COURSE

In the majority of cases developmental dysarticulation goes into remission before the age of eight; patients who remain symptomatic much beyond that may experience some gradual improvement over many years but overall the course tends to be chronic.

COMPLICATIONS

These children may suffer ridicule from their peers and reprimands from uninformed parents. When dysarticulation is so severe as to render speech unintelligible, academic and social progress may be very difficult.

ETIOLOGY

Developmental dysarticulation appears more frequently than expected by chance among the first-degree biologic relatives of affected children.

DIFFERENTIAL DIAGNOSIS

Deaf children, unable to monitor their articulation, may make numerous articulatory errors.

Certain dialects may favor what to the general culture appears to be an articulatory defect. Here, however, children raised to speak such a dialect may readily learn the common tongue, unlike the child with developmental dysarticulation, who, despite effort, experiences only slow improvement.

Dental malocclusion or cleft palate may produce dysarticulation. Such anatomic defects are generally readily apparent.

Children with cerebral palsy may also have dysarticulated speech. The typical signs and symptoms of cerebral palsy, whether hemiplegic or dystonic, serve to make the diagnosis.

Children with mental retardation may have dysarticulate speech, yet in contrast to developmental dysarticulation, one finds a global decrement in abilities.

Autistic children may also have dysarticulate speech. Here, in contrast to developmental dysarticulation, one sees a typical indifference or aversion to people.

In severe cases of developmental dysarticulation one may have some difficulty in differentiating this from developmental expressive dysphasia. In both instances speech may be almost unintelligible. As noted in the section on dysphasia, however, the differential point is the presence or absence of syntax. Dysarticulate speech evidences syntax, whereas in expressive dysphasia the syntax is deficient.

TREATMENT

Speech therapy appears quite effective. Parents, by persistently modeling proper pronunciation and gently calling attention to errors, may be especially helpful.

BIBLIOGRAPHY

Almost D, Rosenbaum P. Effectiveness of speech intervention for phonological disorders: a randomized controlled trial. *Developmental Medicine and Child Neurology* 1998;40:319-325.

Berthal J, Bankson N. *Articulation and phonological disorders,* ed 4. Englewood Cliffs, 1998, Prentice Hall.

Felsenfeld S, Broen PA, McGue M. A 28-year follow-up of adults with a history of moderate phonological disorder: linguistic and personality results. *Journal of Speech and Hearing Research* 1992;35:1114-1125.

Felsenfeld S, Broen PA, McGue M. A 28-year follow-up of adults with a history of moderate phonological disorder: educational and occupational results. *Journal of Speech and Hearing Research* 1994;37:1341-1353.

Mowrer DE, Wahl P, Doolan SJ. Effect of lisping on audience evaluation of male speakers. *Journal of Speech and Hearing Disorders* 1978;43: 140-148.

16 Developmental Dyslexia (reading disorder, DSM-IV-TR #315.00)

Children with developmental dyslexia, though able to understand spoken language, have undue difficulty in learning how to read. Learning to spell and write is also often unduly difficult. The ability to speak, however, is generally unimpaired. Synonyms for this disorder include congenital word blindness and reading disorder.

The prevalence of all degrees of developmental dyslexia in elementary school children is about 4%. Although earlier studies indicated that it was some four times more common in boys than girls, more recent epidemiologic studies suggest only a slightly greater prevalence in males.

ONSET

The difficulty in learning to read generally first comes to light when the child would normally be expected to acquire this skill, anywhere between the ages of 6 and 9, or from the first through the fourth grades. The more severe the case, the earlier it is recognized.

CLINICAL FEATURES

In attempting to read out loud, these children seem to stumble over certain words. They may skip over a word and try the next, or at times they may misread it and say a different word than the one on the page. The error thus produced often seems "understandable" in a way; certain letters in the word or on the page may have been omitted, or misrecognized as a different yet similar letter. On closer inspection certain letters are reversed, such as "d" for "b," or at times the whole word may be reversed such as "top" for "pot." Reading comprehension is also often limited; after haltingly completing the reading of a paragraph, the child may not be able to put it into her own words. In contrast if the paragraph is read to her out loud, she may be able to paraphrase it herself with no difficulty.

These peculiar difficulties in reading are often also seen in writing, whether spontaneous or to dictation. "Pat" may be written when "tap" was meant; letters are reversed; at times whole sentences may be reversed, with the patient writing from right to left. Interestingly even with such a large error, if the child is asked if anything is amiss with what was written, the reply is often "no."

In attempting to read, these children often become very frustrated, even irritable. Some may refuse to try. Others may develop strategies to disguise their inability to read, such as memorizing what has to be read before class.

Developmental dyslexia is often associated with hyperactivity, developmental dysgraphia, and developmental dyscalculia.

COURSE

Most patients continue to experience some difficulty reading all their lives. However, with time and practice, most come to read reasonably well. Those with a higher IQ tend to do best.

COMPLICATIONS

Embarrassed over their difficulty these patients may seek to escape humiliation by refusing to read in class or by refusing to attend class at all. Thus withdrawn from the academic environment, they may fail at other subjects also.

A debate continues as to whether dyslexic children are more likely to develop a conduct disorder. Undoubtedly in some cases repeated school failure may lead to unapproved behavior, yet it appears that when these children grow up they are no more likely to engage in criminal behavior than anyone else.

ETIOLOGY

Developmental dyslexia appears to be inherited. Almost half of the first-degree relatives of dyslexic children have dyslexia themselves. Furthermore, whereas the concordance rate for dyslexia is about 25% for dizygotic twins, it is almost 75% for monozygotic twins. Linkage studies have provided evidence for loci on chromosomes 1, 2, 3, 6 and 15.

Some MRI studies have suggested that patients with developmental dyslexia have an abnormal symmetry of the plana temporalia, in contrast to the normal asymmetric enlargement of the left planum temporale compared with the right; however, this finding has not been consistently replicated. PET scanning suggests decreased metabolic activity in the left parietotemporal area. Limited autopsy samples have shown neuronal ectopia and dysplasias. These, however, are not confined to the left parietotemporal area, but appear to be scattered throughout the cortex. Further autopsy work has also demonstrated abnormalities in the magnocellular layers of the lateral geniculate nuclei.

DIFFERENTIAL DIAGNOSIS

Difficulty in learning to read may be secondary to partial blindness or to an undue amount of anxiety about learning of any sort.

Childhood dementing diseases, should their onset coincide with the early elementary school years, may present with reading difficulty. Here, however, the subsequent evolution of other symptoms rules out developmental dyslexia.

TREATMENT

Remedial education strictly focused on reading is often dramatically effective. Mild cases may improve to the point where reading appears completely normal. Piracetam, unavailable in the United States, also improves reading and comprehension.

Antivertigo agents, elimination and other diets, and megavitamin therapy have all been tried, but none help consistently.

BIBLIOGRAPHY

Galaburda AM, Sherman GF, Rosen GD, et al. Developmental dyslexia: four consecutive patients with cortical abnormalities. *Annals of Neurology* 1985;18:222-233.

Grigorenko EL, Wood FB, Meyer MS, et al. Linkage studies suggest a possible locus for developmental dyslexia on chromosome 1p. *American Journal of Medical Genetics* 2001;105:120-129.

Habib M. The neurological basis of developmental dyslexia: an overview and working hypothesis. *Brain* 2000;123:2372-2399.

Humphreys P, Kaufmann WE, Galaburda AM. Developmental dyslexia in women: neuropathological findings in three patients. *Annals of Neurology* 1990;28:727-738.

Hynd GW, Semrud-Clikeman M, Lorys AR, et al. Brain morphology in developmental dyslexia and attention deficit/hyperactivity. *Archives of Neurology* 1990;47:919-926.

Livingstone MS, Rosen GD, Drislane FW, et al. Physiological and anatomical evidence for a magnocellular defect in developmental dyslexia. *Proceedings of the National Academy of Sciences of the United States of America* 1991;88:7943-7947.

Nodola-Hemmi J, Myllyluoma B, Haltia T, et al. A dominant gene for developmental dyslexia on chromosome 3. *Journal of Medical Genetics* 2001;38:658-664.

Orton ST. Word blindness in school children. *Archives of Neurology and Psychiatry* 1925;14:581-615.

Rumsey JM, Donohue BC, Brady DR, et al. A magnetic resonance imaging study of planum temporale asymmetry in men with developmental dyslexia. *Brain and Language* 1999;70:187-204.

Wilsher CR, Bennett D, Chase CH, et al. Piracetam and dyslexia: effects on reading tests. *Journal of Clinical Psychopharmacology* 1987;7:230-237.

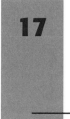

17 Developmental Dysgraphia (disorder of written expression, DSM-IV-TR #315.2)

Children with developmental dysgraphia, also known as disorder of written expression, though able to understand what is said, speak clearly and read, yet have undue difficulty in learning to write. The defect is not one of handwriting or penmanship but rather of punctuation, spelling, and the overall construction of the sentences and paragraphs.

Although the prevalence of developmental dysgraphia is not known, the clinical impression is that it is uncommon. Likewise, though the sex ratio is also not known, the impression is that it is more common in boys.

ONSET

The difficulty in learning to write usually comes to light between the ages of 7 and 10, perhaps in the third or fourth grade, when most students are normally able to master this skill.

CLINICAL FEATURES

Children with developmental dysgraphia often misspell words; however, as the written word is often spelled in a phonetic way, the reader can usually guess what the child meant to write. Written sentences tend to be short and lacking in grammar and syntax; whole words may be omitted. Paragraphs are short and poorly organized; sentences tend to be of the run-on variety. Often there is a "telegraphic" aspect to their composition.

Although these children, by what they say, are clearly capable of complex and at times sophisticated thinking, what they write often fails to reflect that.

Developmental dyslexia is often seen in association with developmental dysgraphia. Deficient penmanship may or may not occur; often the handwriting itself far outshines what is actually written.

COURSE

The course of developmental dysgraphia is not known. The clinical impression is that, though waning in severity over the years, it tends to be chronic.

COMPLICATIONS

Once apprised of their deficiencies by parents, teachers, or other peers, these children may become apprehensive about writing. Indeed, to avoid reprimand or ridicule, they may refuse to write at all.

ETIOLOGY

Dysgraphia appears to be more common among the first-degree biologic relatives of these children. Additionally, a greater frequency of dyslexia, dyscalculia, and developmental dysphasia exists among these relatives.

DIFFERENTIAL DIAGNOSIS

Children with developmental clumsiness or simply with poor handwriting may produce difficult-to-read compositions. However, on inspection, it is clear that with these children paragraph and sentence construction, punctuation, and spelling are all correct, merely being masked by the deficient handwriting.

TREATMENT

Remedial education focused specifically on writing is often effective in ameliorating the dysgraphia.

BIBLIOGRAPHY

Deuel RK. Developmental dysgraphia and motor skills disorders. *Journal of Child Neurology* 1995;10(Suppl 1):6-8.

Gubbay SS, de Klerk NH. A study and review of developmental dysgraphia in relation to acquired dysgraphia. *Brain & Development* 1995;17:1-8.

Houck C, Billingsley B. Written expression of students with and without learning disabilities: differences across the grades. *Journal of Learning Disabilities* 1989;22:561-567.

Myklebust H. *Developmental Disorders of Written Language.* New York, 1973, Grune and Stratton.

Newcomer PL, Barenbaum EM. The written composing ability of children with learning disabilities: a review of the literature from 1980 to 1990. *Journal of Learning Disabilities* 1991;24:578-593.

Temple CM. Developmental dysgraphias. *The Quarterly Journal of Experimental Psychology* 1986;38:77-110.

18 Developmental Dyscalculia (mathematics disorder, DSM-IV-TR #315.1)

■

Children with developmental dyscalculia experience an undue difficulty in learning arithmetic. Although their ability to communicate orally and to read and write may develop normally, they have trouble with numbers and the manipulation of numbers. Developmental dyscalculia has also been called acalculia, developmental arithmetic disorder, anarithmia, and mathematics disorder.

The prevalence of isolated developmental dyscalculia is not known with certainty; estimates range from 1% to 6% of the school-age population.

ONSET

Difficulty with arithmetic usually comes to light at some point during elementary school, usually between the ages of 6 and 10. In most cases the difficulty is obvious by the third grade.

CLINICAL FEATURES

Children with developmental dyscalculia may experience a range of difficulties with arithmetic. Some are unable to recognize numerals or write them; some may have trouble counting to 10. Children may have difficulty in understanding what adding, subtracting, multiplying, or dividing means, and show an inability to perform these tasks. Some may be able to perform simple operations, such as adding single-digit numbers, but more complex operations, such as adding double-digit numbers, seem to leave them baffled. The concept of "carrying" may be impossible for them to grasp.

Although developmental dyscalculia may appear in isolation, these children often also experience developmental dyslexia, developmental dysgraphia and attention-deficit/hyperactivity disorder.

COURSE

The course of developmental dyscalculia has not been adequately well studied; perhaps half these children will experience significant improvement by teenage years.

COMPLICATIONS

Many children with developmental dyscalculia may "get by" in school by depending on their intact abilities to read and write. Without remedial education, however, these children are limited in their occupational choices.

ETIOLOGY

Developmental dyscalculia is clearly familial in about one-half of cases, and the association with developmental dyslexia appears to be genetically mediated. In a small minority of cases, dyscalculia appears to occur as part of either the Fragile X syndrome or petit mal epilepsy.

DIFFERENTIAL DIAGNOSIS

Mental retardation is distinguished by an overall intellectual impairment, and acquired dyscalculia, as may be seen with lesions of the left parietal lobe, is distinguished by a loss of a previously acquired calculating ability, in contrast with developmental dyscalculia where such ability is never fully acquired.

TREATMENT

Remedial education is effective in helping these children learn how to do arithmetic.

BIBLIOGRAPHY

Knopik VS, Alarcon M, DeFries JC. Comorbidity of mathematics and reading deficits: evidence for a genetic etiology. *Behavior Genetics* 1997;27:447-453.

Rourke BP, Conway JP. Disabilities of arithmetic and mathematical reasoning: perspectives from neurology and neuropsychology. *Journal of Learning Disabilities* 1997;30:34-46.

Shalev RS, Gross-Tsur V. Developmental dyscalculia and medical assessment. *Journal of Learning Disabilities* 1993;26:134-137.

Shalev RS, Gross-Tsur V. Developmental dyscalculia. *Pediatric Neurology* 2001;24:337-342.

Shalev RS, Weirtman R, Amir N. Developmental dyscalculia. *Cortex* 1988;24:555-561.

Shalev RS, Manor O, Auerbach J, et al. Persistence of developmental dyscalculia: what counts? Results from a 3-year prospective follow-up study. *The Journal of Pediatrics* 1998;133:358-362.

Shalev RS, Auerbach J, Manor O, et al. Developmental dyscalculia: prevalence and prognosis. *European Child & Adolescent Psychiatry* 2000;9(Suppl 2):58-64.

19 Developmental Clumsiness (developmental coordination disorder, DSM-IV-TR #315.4)

Developmental clumsiness renders the child incapable of coming to move with precision, adroitness, and grace. Ridiculed and humiliated by their more motorically adept peers, these children may tend to restrict their activities to imagination and talk. Numerous synonyms for developmental clumsiness are in use: congenital maladroitness, developmental apraxia, developmental coordination disorder, clumsy child syndrome, and congenital clumsiness.

Developmental clumsiness may exist in as many as 6% of all elementary school-age children; although most studies indicate a higher prevalence in males, recent work suggests that this might be due to referral bias and that the actual sex ratio may be close to 1.

ONSET

In severe cases this clumsiness may be apparent in a 2- or 3-year-old who repeatedly stumbles as he tries to run. In less severe cases it may not be apparent until the age of 5 or 6, when the child repeatedly fumbles as he attempts to dress himself or button his shirt.

CLINICAL FEATURES

As the child grows and his interests and abilities evolve, the clumsiness becomes apparent in different ways. Infants may have trouble sitting up or crawling; toddlers stumble often, especially if they attempt to run. Preschoolers trip and fall, often splayed out, as they attempt to skip or play hopscotch. Early school-age children fumble at tying shoelaces, zipping up pants, or brushing their teeth. Playing with blocks and Lincoln Logs may be particularly frustrating. Older elementary school-age children are unable to put together the intricate small pieces of model airplanes or battleships; they may abandon such projects or they may smash the models in frustration. Sports are seen as an arena for failure: shooting baskets, catching footballs, or pitching a baseball are simply beyond their ability. The clumsiness may also extend to such activities as penmanship and drawing.

Some children, in addition to clumsiness, may also display mild abnormal movements, which are variously described as choreiform, mirror, and adventitious or "overflow."

Although developmental clumsiness may occur in isolation, these children often also have developmental dysphasia or dysarticulation and close to one-half will also have attention-deficit/hyperactivity disorder.

COURSE

Developmental clumsiness appears to be chronic. Even though over the years the clumsiness may become less noticeable, perhaps due to compensation or spontaneous partial remission, as adults the residual aspects of childhood clumsiness are still apparent.

COMPLICATIONS

These children tend to avoid activities in which their clumsiness is apparent. They may refuse to participate in gym class or after-school games in the neighborhood. Some, embarrassed by their handwriting, may refuse to do assignments. Academic and social progress may be stunted.

ETIOLOGY

Little is known about the etiology of developmental clumsiness.

DIFFERENTIAL DIAGNOSIS

Mentally retarded children are often clumsy and motorically awkward, yet here one also finds a proportionate decrement in all other skills.

Cerebral palsy may present with poor coordination. Here, however, additional motor defects are evident, such as hemiplegia or dystonia.

Acute cerebellar ataxia, Friedreich's ataxia, cerebellar tumors, and ataxia telangiectasia may occasionally enter into the differential diagnosis, but may be distinguished either by the age or mode of onset or by associated features.

Hyperactive children may appear clumsy; however, on close inspection the bumps and falls suffered by these children are caused by their overall hyperactivity and impulsiveness rather than by clumsiness per se.

TREATMENT

Remedial physical education is generally offered; other approaches are at times advocated, but there is little empirical support for them.

BIBLIOGRAPHY

Fox AM, Lent B. Clumsy children. Primer on developmental coordination disorder. *Canadian Family Physician* 1996;42:1965-1971.

Gordon N, McKinley I. *Helping Clumsy Children.* London, 1980, Churchill Livingstone.

Gubbay SS, Ellis E, Walton JN, et al. Clumsy children. A study of apraxic and agnosic defects in 221 children. *Brain* 1965;88: 295-312.

Kadesjo B, Gillberg C. Developmental coordination disorder in Swedish 7-year-old children. *Journal of the American Academy of Child and Adolescent Psychiatry* 1999;38:820-828.

Pless M, Carlsson M, Sundelin C, et al. Preschool children with developmental coordination disorder: a short-term follow-up of motor status at seven to eight years of age. *Acta Paediatrica* 2002;91: 521-528.

Rasmussen P, Gillberg C. Natural outcome of ADHD with developmental coordination disorder at age 22 years: a controlled, longitudinal, community-based study. *Journal of the American Academy of Child and Adolescent Psychiatry* 2000;39:1424-1431.

Shaw L, Levine MD, Belfer M. Developmental double jeopardy: a study of clumsiness and self esteem in children with learning problems. *Journal of Developmental and Behavioral Pediatrics* 1982;3:191-196.

20 Developmental Stuttering (stuttering, DSM-IV-TR #307.0)

Developmental stuttering, or stammering, occurs in about 1% of elementary school-age children. It is three to four times more common in boys than girls.

ONSET

Stuttering generally appears insidiously sometime between the ages of 2 and 10; most often it first appears at about 5 years of age.

CLINICAL FEATURES

Stuttering may occur with nearly every word, or only at certain sounds. B's, D's, K's, P's, and T's are common precipitants. In attempting to say the word the patient often feels "blocked" and may appear to stumble over it, repeating the first letter or syllable again and again, sometimes with explosive force. Often these attempts are accompanied by repetitive grimacing, blinking, hissing, or forceful thrusting of the head, arm, or trunk. After the sound is finally enunciated there may be a veritable cascade of words, all correctly pronounced, until the next stumbling block is reached.

Stuttering is generally worse when the patient feels rushed, under pressure, or has to speak in front of a group. Interestingly, even in severe cases, patients may be able to sing or read aloud without difficulty. Furthermore, spontaneous speech may likewise become free of stuttering if the patient is extremely angry or if he is by himself.

Occasionally, stuttering may be seen in children with developmental dysphasia or developmental dysarticulation.

COURSE

Spontaneous remission is seen in about three-quarters of patients by early teenage years, and this is more likely in girls and in those with mild cases; among the rest, although some improvement may be seen the disorder nevertheless remains chronic. Interestingly, in patients who do experience a full remission, the onset of Parkinson's disease in later years may be associated with a relapse of the stuttering.

COMPLICATIONS

Embarrassment, shame, ridicule, and humiliation await most patients. To escape these affects, some withdraw from any spoken involvement with others.

ETIOLOGY

Stuttering is clearly familial: the incidence among first-degree relatives is higher than in the general population, and the concordance rate for monozygotic twins is higher than that for dizygotic twins. Left-handedness is more common in stutterers than in the general population, and PET studies have demonstrated underactivation of the left temporal area.

DIFFERENTIAL DIAGNOSIS

Acquired stuttering is distinguished from developmental stuttering on two counts. First, in acquired stuttering, the "block" may appear on any syllable, rather than primarily the first one as in developmental stuttering. Second, although patients with acquired stuttering may express frustration upon being "blocked," one rarely sees the forceful efforts to overcome the block that is characteristic of patients with developmental stuttering.

Acquired stuttering may occur with lesions, such as infarctions, affecting the dominant frontal or parietal cortices, the subjacent white matter or the basal ganglia. Various drugs may also have stuttering as a side-effect including antipsychotics, tricyclics, SSRIs, benzodiazepines, methylphenidate, phenytoin and theophylline.

TREATMENT

Speech therapy may be dramatically effective. In treatment-resistant cases one may consider clomipramine in doses, for adults, of 150 mg/d, or either haloperidol or risperidone. Although haloperidol, in doses of about 3 mg, is often effective, side-effects are often limiting. Risperidone is generally better tolerated, and at a dose of 0.5 mg/d is effective; interestingly, with higher doses of risperidone the beneficial effect may be lost.

BIBLIOGRAPHY

Brady JP. Drug-induced stuttering: a review of the literature. *Journal of Clinical Psychopharmacology* 1998;18:50-54.

Costa D, Kroll R. Stuttering: an update for physicians. *Canadian Medical Association Journal* 2000;167:1849-1855.

Gordon CT, Cotelingam GM, Stager S, et al. A double-blind comparison of clomipramine and desipramine in the treatment of developmental stuttering. *The Journal of Clinical Psychiatry* 1995;56:238-242.

Helm NA, Butler RB, Benson DF. Acquired stuttering. *Neurology* 1978;28:1159-1165.

Ingham RJ. Brain imaging studies of developmental stuttering. *Journal of Communication Disorders* 2001;34:493-516.

Kidd KK, Heimbuch RC, Records MA. Vertical transmission of susceptibility to stuttering with sex-modified expression. *Proceedings of the National Academy of Sciences of the United States of America* 1981;78:606-610.

Maguire GA, Riley GD, Franklin DL, et al. Risperidone for the treatment of stuttering. *Journal of Clinical Psychopharmacology* 2000;20:479-482.

Murray TJ, Kelly P, Campbell L, et al. Haloperidol in the treatment of stuttering. *The British Journal of Psychiatry* 1977;130:370-373.

Shahed J, Jankovic J. Re-emergence of stuttering in parkinson's disease: a hypothesis. *Movement Disorders* 2001;16:114-118.

21 Autism (autistic disorder, DSM-IV-TR #299.00)

Autism is a chronic lifelong disorder that is characterized by an inability on the patient's part to form normal relationships with others. Patients with autism often form peculiarly disturbed relationships with others, often acting toward them as if they were inanimate objects. A peculiarly machine-like quality is evident in their relationships, as if they fail to sense the difference between the animate and the inanimate. At its most severe, patients may be almost totally inaccessible; in very mild cases an observer may note only a peculiar awkwardness and stiltedness around others.

Classic autism was first described by Kanner in 1943 and is still at times referred to as Kanner's syndrome. Another synonym is early infantile autism. Classic autism generally presents with symptoms in infancy; indeed in some cases symptoms may be apparent in the first few months of life. By contrast, in some mild cases, especially those with normal intelligence and relatively unimpaired language, symptoms may not become apparent until the child enters elementary school. There is debate as to whether such cases represent a discrete, separate disorder or are simply just mild cases of autism. Some authors claim that a separate disorder does exist, namely Asperger's syndrome (or, Asperger's disorder), whereas others, as in this text, conceive of such patients as merely constituting the very "high-functioning" end of the spectrum of autism.

Another controversial diagnosis is Heller's syndrome, also referred to as childhood disintegrative disorder. Here, patients are said to develop normally up until the age of two or three, after which there is a cataclysmic regression into an autistic state. Although there is no debate that such cataclysmic regressions, though rare, do occur, it is unclear whether they represent a discrete distinct disorder, namely Heller's syndrome, or whether the "disintegration" is due to some well-characterized disorder such as the Landau-Kleffner syndrome.

Autism is a relatively rare disorder, with a lifetime prevalence of about 0.05%; the sex ratio of males to females is roughly 3-4:1. Although recent studies have demonstrated an increase in the diagnosis of autism it is unclear whether this represents merely a broadening of diagnostic criteria or whether there is a true increase in the prevalence of this disorder.

ONSET

As noted, classic autism presents in infancy, typically in an insidious fashion. Affected infants may cry infrequently and do not seek to be held. Typically the full clinical picture is evident before the age of 3 years. In mild cases, however, the symptoms may be so mild that they escape notice until the patient enters elementary school and becomes compared with his normal classmates. Occasionally parents date the onset to a specific event, such as the birth of a sibling. However, with careful retrospective study, one usually sees that the symptoms long predated the supposedly "precipitating" event.

CLINICAL FEATURES

The various symptoms of autism are perhaps best illustrated by describing the clinical picture as it may be seen in middle childhood.

For the most part these children prefer solitary activities; they tend to not play with others and, when they do, tend to use others as "mechanical props" in their play. One gets the impression that a mannequin would be as satisfactory a playmate for these children as would another child. In their play they rarely imitate grownups; one rarely finds them playing "house" or "cops and robbers."

At times the activity of these children may seem bizarre. They may have what are known as "fascinations." Here the child appears quite fascinated with certain objects, such as a piece of cloth, jewelry, or, classically, with something spinning, such as a top. Occasionally the child himself starts to spin. At other times the child may repetitively touch or tap things; the page of a book may be turned again and again, with no attempt to see what is on the page. Even more unusual behavior may be seen: repetitious arm or hand flapping, persistent finger flicking, posturing, or classically, toe-walking. Head-banging may occur; the child may also repeatedly bite himself.

When the child is involved with others, this involvement has a distinctive, unusual, mechanical quality to it. Eye contact is unusual; indeed, often gaze avoidance is evident. The child may stare fixedly past one or seem to be looking through the other person. If one attempts to hug an autistic child, the child stiffens up; if an autistic child is hurt, he will not accept comfort. Speech, at best, is used to arrange others; rarely does he seem to have an interest in communicating on a "feeling" level. Rather than having a conversation, these patients seem to be having more of a monologue. The speech itself is often dysprosodic. It may be monotone or curiously inflected, at times in a "sing-song" fashion. Pronomial reversals occur, with the patient saying "you" when he clearly means "I." Echolalia may occur. At times one may also see a private language; for example, a child may say "cloud, cloud, cloud" when he wants a favorite fork. In severe cases the child may be mute.

A classic symptom of autism is the "insistence on sameness." The aisles in the grocery store must be traversed in the same direction and sequence as always; while watching television others must sit in the same places; place settings at the table must never vary. When routines are changed, the child's reaction may be truly catastrophic.

Autistic children may display an indifference to pain. Paradoxically, however, their reaction to certain innocuous stimuli may be extreme. A scratching or ringing may induce terrifying anxiety.

In addition to these autistic symptoms per se, about three quarters of children with autism also have mental retardation, and from one quarter to one third of autistic children also have seizures. Furthermore in almost all cases, regardless of the total IQ, cognitive development tends to be uneven. One may see otherwise normal "islets" of functioning in an otherwise retarded, autistic child.

When present, mental retardation ranges from mild to profound; most patients fall within the moderate range. Regardless of the degree of mental retardation, however, these doubly afflicted children still bear the unmistakable stamp of autism.

Seizures are not more common in those with mental retardation than in those with normal IQs. Seizure onset shows two peaks, the first in early childhood and the second in adolescence. In children one may see infantile spasms, whereas in adolescents or adults grand mal or complex partial seizures are most common.

The "islets" of better functioning within an otherwise retarded autistic child may be quite striking. Such children, for example, though unable to think abstractly, may be capable of prodigious feats of memory. Entire airline schedules may be memorized; large portions of the telephone book may be recited. Another common islet is musical ability. One child, though unable to speak, played a symphony on the piano before he was 3. In the past such children were described as "idiot savants," and though this is an unfortunate term, it does convey forcefully the impression one is left with after seeing such children.

Such islets of superior functioning, however, are the exception. For the most part, the unevenness of cognitive development is less dramatic. The child who is unable to add or subtract may read reasonably well; the child who cannot speak may be able to repair small appliances. Typically, on formal IQ testing, a scattering of scores is seen on the various scales.

Although the foregoing discussion of clinical features as seen in middle childhood is applicable in most cases, some further discussion is in order regarding patients with very mild cases, that is to say those with "Asperger's syndrome." These mildly affected patients are of normal intelligence, but display the typical "machine-like" qualities noted earlier. In conversation they seem oblivious to social cues and often evidence a pedantic and formalized speech. Overall their behavior is eccentric, and their interests, though often vigorously pursued, are narrow.

COURSE

As noted earlier, autism is a chronic, lifelong disorder. The clinical expression, however, changes over time as the child passes through normal developmental stages. From a prognostic point of view, the age of 5 or 6 is a critical point in autism. Improvement in linguistic and social skills at that time suggest strongly that the outcome will be better than what might have been expected. Puberty, a difficult time for any adolescent, is apt to be particularly stormy for the autistic teenager. Patients may display pervasive stubborn rebelliousness; violent confrontations may occur. With adult years comes a general diminution of symptoms, which then tend to remain static for the remainder of a patient's life.

The eventual outcome in adulthood is quite variable, but generally predictable on the basis of the individual history. In rare instances patients may graduate from college or even graduate school and achieve some occupational standing. Rarely, however, do these patients marry, and often they have few if any friends. Work that requires social interaction is avoided; solitary work with machines, particularly computers, is preferred. Furthermore, regardless of how good the outcome is, residual symptoms always exist. Speech may be stilted or dysprosodic; often it has a curious lilt to it. Behavior with others is stiff and awkward, with little awareness of social conventions. On the other extreme, the outcome may be quite poor, and the patient may require lifelong institutional care. For the most part, however, patients may be maintained in the community, provided that others give substantial structure for them.

COMPLICATIONS

The complications of autism are predictable on the basis of the individual patient's symptoms. Success in the community often depends on social skills, and to the extent that these are disturbed in autism, so too will the individual's chances of making his way in the world be reduced. Should mental retardation be present, the outcome, as in any child with mental retardation, varies with the degree of retardation.

ETIOLOGY

Etiologic theories about autism have changed radically over the past few decades. This disorder was once thought to be the result of faulty child-rearing, that the parents were cold and distant, and that under this influence the child developed the typical symptoms of autism. This theory has been soundly discredited. Clearly parents of autistic children are no different from the parents of other seriously ill children. The abnormalities noted in parents of autistic children were themselves the result of trying to raise an autistic child and not the cause itself of the autism. Current research focuses on genetics and neuropathology.

Family studies strongly suggest genetic factors. As noted earlier the incidence of autism in the general population is about 0.05%; among siblings, however, it rises to about 5%, and among monozygotic twins the concordance rate ranges from 60% to 90%. Genetic studies strongly suggest a complex mode of inheritance, with linkage studies suggesting loci on chromosomes 2, 3, 7, 15, 19 and X.

Electroencephalographic examination of these patients yields a variety of abnormalities; however, these do not appear to be consistent, and they do not correlate well with the actual symptoms.

MRI studies have been inconclusive: both failures of replication and contradictory results have been obtained. Perhaps the most promising findings include megalencephaly (particularly affecting the occipital, parietal and temporal lobes) and vermal hypoplasia, but clearly more research is needed.

Autopsy studies have likewise been inconclusive; however, here too, there have been some promising findings including a reduction in the number of cerebellar Purkinje cells and the presence of microdysgenetic changes in the cerebral cortex.

Although in the vast majority of cases the etiology remains thus unclear, there is a small minority of cases, perhaps 10%, where the autism is clearly part of another condition. Such cases are often

Some Causes of "Secondary" Autism

Tuberous sclerosis*	Down's syndrome*
Fragile X syndrome*	CMV encephalitis
von Recklinghausen's disease*	Congenital rubella
Rett's syndrome*	Phenylketonuria

*See the respective chapter.

referred to as "secondary" autism, and the various responsible conditions are listed in the box above: of these, by far the most common are tuberous sclerosis and the fragile X syndrome. Given the existence of such secondary cases, considerations should be given to appropriate genetic and karyotypic studies when working up patients.

DIFFERENTIAL DIAGNOSIS

The key points that differentiate autism from other disorders are its age of onset and the peculiar lack of social relatedness. Keeping these points in mind allows one to differentiate autism from the following: mental retardation of other causes, childhood-onset schizophrenia, developmental dysphasia, and certain other disorders that occasionally present some diagnostic difficulty.

Patients with mental retardation of other causes may at times engage in stereotyped repetitive behaviors and thus appear similar to an autistic child who also happens to have mental retardation. However, the desire for social contact is preserved in otherwise straightforward mental retardation. Upon approaching the child with uncomplicated mental retardation, one may be greeted with a smile and an expectant posture. In contrast, the child with autism may show no more interest in the approaching physician than he might if a machine entered the room.

In differentiating schizophrenia from autism, one finds the age of onset often quite helpful. As noted earlier, in almost all cases autism begins before the age of 5 years. In contrast, finding schizophrenia beginning before the age of 8 is very rare. The presence of hallucinations and delusions and of inappropriate affect also point to a diagnosis of schizophrenia.

Children with developmental dysphasia may at times appear autistic, especially if they have elements of both an expressive and a receptive dysphasia, as is generally the case. However, here, in contrast to autism, the desire for social contact is preserved. Though unable to communicate verbally, the child with developmental dysphasia makes it clear by her looks and gestures that she wishes for human contact.

Selective mutism is usually easily differentiated from autism. Here, the failure to speak is generally evident only in certain situations, such as at school. At home or perhaps in the neighborhood the child may speak. Furthermore, the selectively mute child may communicate by gestures or facial expression in contrast to the mute autistic child.

Congenital deafness or blindness may at times occasion diagnostic confusion with autism, yet, as in mental retardation, so also in deafness or blindness, the desire for social contact remains intact.

A child who has suffered extreme neglect or abuse, as may be seen in reactive attachment disorder, may become listless and apathetic and fail to make any effort at social contact. Thus he may appear to have autism. In contrast to the autistic child, these children eventually respond to consistent nurturance. Their capacity for social relatedness, though dormant, yet survives.

Tourette's syndrome and obsessive-compulsive disorder may present with repetitive or stereotyped behaviors, similar to those seen in autism. However, in both of these the desire for social contact is preserved. Furthermore, in obsessive-compulsive disorder one usually sees an attempt on the patient's part to resist engaging in the behavior; in autism the patient almost seems to enjoy what he is doing.

A host of other rare disorders may present with a disintegration of behavior in a previously healthy child, thus mimicking Heller's syndrome. These include the Landau-Kleffner syndrome, metachromatic leukodystrophy, subacute sclerosing panencephalitis, progressive rubella panencephalitis, Canavan's disease, Alexander's disease, the aminoacidurias, Lesch-Nyhan syndrome, and Tay-Sachs disease. One of these may be suspected if the child presents with symptoms atypical for autism (such as ataxia, blindness, myoclonus, and others) or with a course that is persistently downhill.

TREATMENT

Treatment of autism often involves behavior modification, family counseling, special education, and medication. All components are important, and most children benefit from a combination of all of these.

Behavior modification programs that target specific symptoms, such as head-banging or aggressive behavior, are often very effective. Unfortunately, however, there is often very little generalization. The learning of autistic children is often quite state specific: whereas a behavior program may eliminate head-banging at school, the same program must also be physically instituted at home. Consequently, parents or other caretakers should become in a quite real sense behavioral cotherapists.

Family counseling is aimed at helping parents adjust to their ill child and to continuing or implementing appropriate behavior programs at home. Given that some parents may still feel at fault for the illness, one must outline what is known about the etiology of the disease to dispel any guilt they may have.

Special education classes are almost always indicated. A class that is highly structured is more effective in fostering better classroom behavior and better grades than is a more permissive or "open" classroom. In some areas special schools for autistic children may be found.

A number of different medications have proved superior to placebo in autism. Antipsychotics are perhaps most commonly used, and include haloperidol and risperidone, both in doses of $\frac{1}{2}$ to 3 mg/d. Clomipramine, in doses of ~150 mg/d for adults, is an alternative to antipsychotics, but is not as well tolerated as is haloperidol. Fluvoxamine, in doses of 250 to 300 mg/d in adults, may be an alternative to clomipramine. Clonidine, in weekly patches delivering about 0.005mg/kg/d, is modestly effective, but sedation and fatigue are often limiting. Both naltrexone (in doses of 0.3 mg/kg/d) and methylphenidate reduce hyperactivity, but either may increase irritability and social withdrawal.

In planning pharmacologic treatment of autism it is important to adopt a methodical approach, using one agent at a time, and giving each successive agent a "good" trial, not only in terms of dosage but also duration, keeping in mind that weeks or months may be required to see the full effect at any given dose. Often, an antipsychotic is used first, and given the higher risk of tardive dyskinesia with haloperidol, it is reasonable to try risperidone first. Given, however, this risk of tardive dyskinesia, many prefer to start with clomipramine or fluvoxamine. Clonidine, naltrexone and methylphenidate are generally second choices, given their at best modest effectiveness, and, in the cases of naltrexone and methylphenidate, the risk of increasing irritability and withdrawal.

BIBLIOGRAPHY

Bailey A, Luthert P, Dean A, et al. A clinicopathological study of autism. *Brain* 1998;121:889-905.

Courchesne E, Karns CM, Davis HR, et al. Unusual brain growth patterns in early life in patients with autistic disorder: an MRI study. *Neurology* 2001;57:245-254.

Croen LA, Grether JK, Hoogstrate J, et al. The changing prevalence of autism in California. *Journal of Autism and Developmental Disorders* 2002;32:207-215.

Fankhauser MP, Karumanchi VC, German ML, et al. A double-blind, placebo-controlled study of the efficacy of transdermal clonidine in autism. *The Journal of Clinical Psychiatry* 1992;53:77-82.

Feldman HM, Kolman BK, Gonzaga AM. Naltrexone and communication skills in young children with autism. *Journal of the American Academy of Child and Adolescent Psychiatry* 1999;38:587-593.

Handen BL, Johnson CR, Lubetsky M. Efficacy of methylphenidate among children with autism and symptoms of attention-deficit hyperactivity disorder. *Journal of Autism and Developmental Disorders* 2000;30: 245-255.

Kanner L. Autistic disturbances of affective content. *Nervous Child* 1943;2:217-250.

McCracken JT, McGough J, Shah R, et al. Risperidone in children with autism and serious behavioral problems. *The New England Journal of Medicine* 2002;347:314-321.

McDougle CJ, Naylor ST, Cohen DJ, et al. A double-blind, placebo-controlled study of fluvoxamine in adults with autistic disorder. *Archives of General Psychiatry* 1996;53:1001-1008.

Malhotra S, Gupta N. Childhood disintegrative disorder. Re-examination of the current concept. *European Child & Adolescent Psychiatry* 2002; 11:108-114.

Prater CD, Zylstra RG. Autism: a medical primer. *American Family Physician* 2002;61:1667-1674.

Remington G, Sloman L, Konstantareas M, et al. Clomipramine versus haloperidol in the treatment of autistic disorder: a double-blind, placebo-controlled, crossover study. *Journal of Clinical Psychopharmacology* 2001;21:440-444.

Rinehart NJ, Bradshaw JL, Brereton AV, et al. A clinical and neuro-behavioral review of high-functioning autism and Asperger's disorder. *The Australian and New Zealand Journal of Psychiatry* 2002;36: 762-770.

Ritvo ER, Mason-Brothers A, Freeman BJ, et al. The UCLA-University of Utah epidemiologic survey of autism: the etiologic role of rare diseases. *The American Journal of Psychiatry* 1990;147:1614-1621.

Shao Y, Wopert CM, Raiford KL, et al. Genomic screen and follow-up analysis for autistic disorder. *American Journal of Medical Genetics* 2002;114:99-105.

Treffert DA. The idiot savant: a review of the syndrome. *The American Journal of Psychiatry* 1988;145:563-572.

Volkmar FR, Nelson DS. Seizure disorders in autism. *Journal of the American Academy of Child and Adolescent Psychiatry* 1990;29: 127-129.

---

22 Rett's Syndrome (Rett's disorder, DSM-IV-TR #299.80)

◾

Rett's syndrome, first described by Andreas Rett in 1966, is characterized by mental retardation, microcephaly, autistic features, and peculiar stereotypic hand movements. This is a rare disorder, with a prevalence of from 1 in 10,000 to 1 in 15,000. The overwhelming majority of cases occur in females: cases in males are very, very rare.

ONSET

Infants with Rett's syndrome are apparently normal until close to the end of the first year of life. In retrospect, however, some parents will report that these infants tended to be unusually placid and to display a tremor of the neck.

CLINICAL FEATURES

The clinical features of Rett's syndrome may be roughly divided into four stages, as outlined in Table 22-1.

These stages are described in more detail below. These are rough divisions only, and considerable overlap may occur among the various features particular to each stage.

Stage I is characterized by a stagnation or generalized slowing of normal development and generally becomes apparent at about 10 months of age. One may see a failure to make expected weight gain and to progress to normal crawling; many infants will display a persistent "bottom shuffling." Patients may persist in this stage for anywhere from a month up to a year and a half.

Stage II is characterized by a regression, typically occurring at about the age of 18 months: although this regression is typically gradual, occurring over weeks or months, it may, occasionally, occur precipitously over days. Patients withdraw from contact with their surroundings and their parents and begin to display the characteristic hand stereotypies of Rett's syndrome. Initially patients may suck their hands or grasp their tongues; however, with time, the more characteristic hand-wringing, hand-clasping, or washing movements appear. A 12-year-old with Rett's syndrome with microcephaly and hand-wringing movements is shown in Figure 22-1. There may also be attacks of violent screaming, teeth gnashing, and nocturnal awakenings accompanied by peculiar laughter. Most patients also display episodes of irregular respiration while awake, with periods of hyperventilation followed by apneic periods that are often characterized by a Valsalva maneuver. During stage II head growth also decelerates, and patients with previously normal head size may eventually become microcephalic. A more or less generalized growth failure also eventually appears, which is often most apparent in the feet. Stage II generally lasts about a year and a half.

Stage III, or the "pseudostationary" stage, typically begins at about 3 years of age. Early on in this stage, communicative abilities lost during stage II may be partially restituted, but for the most

■**TABLE 22-1.** Stages of Rett's Syndrome

Stage	Stage Name	Age at Onset	Characteristics
I	Stagnation	10 months	Slowing of normal development
II	Regression	18 months	Loss of previously acquired abilities and appearance of mental retardation, autistic features, and hand stereotypies
III	Pseudostationary	3 years	Partial remission of signs seen in stage II
IV	Late motor deterioration	End of childhood or later	Gradual appearance of scoliosis and dystonia

part this stage is one of relative stability, with persistence of most of the symptoms apparent during stage II. Most patients are severely retarded, with the intellectual capacity generally not progressing beyond that of a normal 2-year-old. Ambulation may or may not occur. Seizures, if not already evident in stage II, typically appear in stage III, and may be either complex partial or grand mal in type. The EEG is almost always abnormal, with epileptiform spikes and widespread delta slowing. Most girls remain in stage III for many years, occasionally into young adulthood or even middle years.

Stage IV, or the stage of late motor deterioration, is characterized by scoliosis, which may be particularly severe; dystonia, which often affects most prominently the lower extremities; and a lower motor neuron type of wasting, often most apparent in the lower extremities.

Although the clinical stages just described are the rule, one occasionally sees mild (or "variant") cases with relatively preserved speech. Such "formes frustes" may be understood on the basis of the complex genetics of Rett's syndrome, as described below.

COURSE

Stage IV may persist for decades, and some patients may live into their sixties. Early deaths, however, may occur secondary to respiratory infections or postoperative complications.

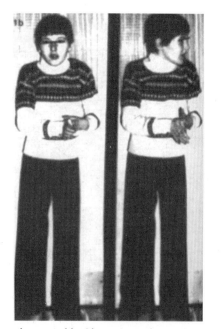

FIG. 22-1. Twelve-year-old with Rett's syndrome. (From Wiedemann HR, Kunze J, Dibbern H. *Atlas of clinical syndromes: a visual aid to diagnosis*, ed 2, London, 1992, Wolfe.)

COMPLICATIONS

Complications are similar to those described for mental retardation and for autism, as described in those chapters. In addition, the motor deterioration of stage IV often leaves these patients wheelchair-bound.

ETIOLOGY

Rett's syndrome is caused by a mutation in the gene for methyl-CpG-binding protein 2 (MECP2) located on the X chromosome. Over 70 different mutations have been identified and it appears that variations in the severity of the phenotype are related not only to non-random X-inactivation in females but also to the particular mutation present. Almost all cases represent sporadic mutations: in the rare familial cases, it appears that the mother was a "carrier" with a very mild phenotype. The extreme rarity of the syndrome in males is probably best explained by the lethality of most of the mutations: females with these lethal mutations escape death by virtue of a non-mutated MECP2 on the normal X-chromosome, whereas most males, lacking the buffer of a normal X-chromosome, die. Males with Rett's syndrome who do survive owe their survival to the presence of a non-lethal mutation.

At autopsy, the brain is small. In the cortex, pyramidal neurons exhibit small dendritic trees; the pars compacta of the substantia nigra, though of normal size, is severely depleted of melanin. Interestingly, although gliosis is absent in the brains of children with Rett's syndrome, it is present in adults.

DIFFERENTIAL DIAGNOSIS

The combination of mental retardation, microcephaly, autistic features, and hand stereotypies is highly suggestive. The overall evolution of symptoms as patients pass from normalcy into stage I, II, and III, however, may be more distinctive, for here unlike the other childhood encephalopathies a partial restitution of abilities occurs, rather than a steady progression.

Rarely, a similar picture may be seen with ornithine transcarbamylase deficiency or with a pontine tumor.

TREATMENT

Habilitative efforts similar to those discussed in the chapter on mental retardation are indicated.

Seizures may be difficult to control: carbamazepine, lamotrigene or valproate are recommended.

Bromocriptine may reduce agitation and autistic withdrawal in a small minority of patients; however, this effect may not be sustained.

Naltrexone may hasten progression of the disease and should not be used.

BIBLIOGRAPHY

Amir RE, Van den Vyver IB, Schultz R, et al. Influence of mutation type and X chromosome inactivation on Rett syndrome phenotype. *Annals of Neurology* 2000;47:670-679.

Armstrong DD. Neuropathology of Rett syndrome. *Mental Retardation and Developmental Disabilities Research Reviews* 2002;8:72-76.

Bienvenu T, Villard L, De Roux N, et al. Spectrum of MECP2 mutations in Rett syndrome. *Genetic Testing* 2002;6:1-6.

Dotti MT, Orrico A, De Stefano N, et al. A Rett syndrome MECP2 mutation that causes mental retardation in men. *Neurology* 2002; 58:226-230.

Hagberg B, Aicardi J, Dias K, et al. A progressive syndrome of autism, dementia, ataxia, and loss of purposeful hand movement in girls: Rett's syndrome: report of 35 cases. *Annals of Neurology* 1983;14:471-479.

Hyman SL, Batshaw ML. A case of ornithine transcarbamylase deficiency with Rett's syndrome manifestations. *American Journal of Medical Genetics* 1986;1(Suppl)339-343.

23 | Attention-Deficit/Hyperactivity Disorder (DSM-IV-TR #314.00-314.01)

Attention-deficit/hyperactivity disorder, often referred to as "ADHD," is a common disorder, occurring in from 3% to 7% of school age children: it is more common in boys, with sex ratios varying from 2:1 to 10:1 depending on the diagnostic criteria used. Synonyms for ADHD include minimal brain dysfunction, hyperkinesis, hyperkinetic syndrome or simply hyperactivity.

ONSET

In retrospect, the age at which symptoms first become apparent varies widely, from infancy up to the age of 7. Infants may have experienced sleeplessness and an unusual degree of fussiness or colic. Parents may recall that during toddler years the child seemed to skip learning to walk, literally "took off running," was always "on the go," and uncontrollably "into" everything, as if the "motor" never stopped. The preschooler may be impatient and impulsive and indeed may be ungovernable in the household. The actual diagnosis, however, is often delayed until the first or second grade, when symptoms bring the patient into direct conflict with the rules and expectations of the classroom.

CLINICAL FEATURES

Clinically, ADHD may present with hyperactivity and impulsivity or with inattention. When the clinical picture is dominated by hyperactivity and impulsivity, one speaks of attention-deficit/hyperactivity disorder, predominantly hyperactive-impulsive type, and when it is dominated by inattention, one speaks of attention-deficit/hyperactivity disorder, predominantly inattentive type. In cases where all symptoms are present to a more or less equal degree, then as one might expect, one speaks of attention-deficit/hyperactivity disorder, combined type.

In children, of all these symptoms, hyperactivity is often most prominent. These children are always on the move. In the classroom they may be unable to remain in their seat, or they may fidget and squirm uncomfortably. They may be incessant talkers; other children are bothered, and teachers often find themselves expending an inordinate amount of effort simply to keep the child seated. At home the child may be unable to sit through story time or stay in front of the television long enough to watch a favorite program. Trips to the store may be a nightmare for the parent as the child restlessly roams and disappears among the maze of aisles. In severe cases the hyperactivity may be evident in all situations; however, in most instances the symptoms may not be apparent in certain situations, such as a one-to-one interview with a physician.

The impulsivity of such children often prompts adults to say the child "doesn't think first" but always acts first, seemingly without any sense of the consequences of such "thoughtless" behavior. In class the child may blurt out an answer before finishing the problem, or perhaps even before the teacher has finished asking the question. In the lunch line the child may barge ahead to get a favorite dessert, and at recess may grab the ball out of turn, or may rush uninvited into the midst of other children who are playing their own game. At home the child may incessantly come into conflict with siblings or neighborhood children or may commandeer their toys. Thrust headlong by uncontrollable impulses, the child may run into the street, climb a roof, or race a bicycle down a dangerously steep hill.

Inattentiveness in these children is most apparent in the classroom. They fail to pay attention to what the teacher is saying and to the schoolwork at hand, and this is especially the case whenever attention to detail is required. In many cases this inattentiveness appears to represent an easy distractibility. In the midst of an assigned task, the child may suddenly be attracted to something outside the window, or to a disturbance in the hallway, or perhaps simply to an item on another pupil's desk. If called back to task by the teacher, the patient may indeed pay attention to the academic matter at hand, yet often within moments is once again no longer attending to it. The attention of these children seems attracted to almost everything, as if nothing were more important than anything else. At home parents may complain that the only way to get these children's attention is to literally hold their heads in their hands and make them look them straight in the eye, and even then the message may not get through.

The hyperactivity, inattentiveness and impulsivity of these children make it very difficult for adults to discipline them and keep them at task and out of trouble. Neighbors may complain, and repeated trips to the principal's office are more the rule than the exception. They fall behind in school and eventually may become demoralized and simply stop trying altogether. Rejected by siblings and neighborhood children, they may become vengeful and aggressive. Temper tantrums are not uncommon. Frequently the behavior of these children becomes so untoward that a diagnosis of conduct disorder is merited.

In adolescents, the syndrome is marked by a partial remission of all symptoms, most particularly hyperactivity: the grosser elements of hyperactivity clear up and the patient is left with such relatively subtle manifestations as foot tapping and fidgeting. Persistent impulsiveness, however, often brings these adolescents to clinical attention. At a minimum their impulsivity may result merely in a few too many "larks" and an excessive number of confrontations with those in authority when their impulses leave them breaking through the rules. At worse they may be in fights as others retaliate or stand their ground; thoughtless use of alcohol may be followed by car wrecks. Often these adolescents are seen as irritable and unstable. Inattentiveness abetted by the normal adolescent restlessness continues to mar schoolroom performance and derail solitary attempts at homework.

Amongst adults with ADHD, a further general partial remission of symptoms is seen, most notably in hyperactivity and impulsivity. Hyperactivity may now manifest only as a certain unsettled restlessness, and impulsivity as a tendency to flightiness. Inattentiveness, however, often remains very significant, and may severely limit the patient's ability to advance at work.

A number of other disorders are associated with hyperactivity. Developmental disabilities, especially developmental dyslexia, are not uncommon. Developmental clumsiness may also be seen, as may right/left confusion. In the clinic one may see a higher than expected prevalence of Tourette's syndrome in children with hyperactivity. Whether this represents a true association or the effect of a biased sample is not as yet known.

COURSE

ADHD, in most cases, gradually undergoes a spontaneous remission. By late adolescence, only about one-half still evidence the full syndrome, and the figure falls to about one-third in the early twenties; by the late twenties only about a tenth are still fully affected. These reassuring figures, however, are tempered by the fact that residual symptoms are seen in a greater proportion of patients, which, though of much less severity, may still cause some impairment.

COMPLICATIONS

As noted earlier, academic failure and truancy are not uncommon and the misconduct that ADHD impels children into may be so severe and pervasive as to occasion a diagnosis of conduct disorder. Furthermore, in adult years these patients are more likely to have antisocial personality disorder and to engage in the abuse of various substances, notably alcohol.

ETIOLOGY

The concordance of ADHD rises dramatically from siblings to dizygotic and finally monozygotic twins, where it is above 50%. Linkage studies have suggested loci on several chromosomes and some, but not all, studies have supported a connection with certain polymorphisms at the DRD4 gene. MRI studies have at times been contradictory; however, certain findings appear promising, notably an overall reduction in cerebral and cerebellar volumes and a disproportionately greater reduction in the volume of the posterior-inferior cerebellar vermis.

Although the vast majority of cases of ADHD are idiopathic, a small number may be directly traced to a lead encephalopathy or to a rare, inherited resistance to thyroid hormones.

DIFFERENTIAL DIAGNOSIS

A chaotic upbringing may leave a child restless, impulsive, and distractible; however, these children rarely have hyperactivity per se. In doubtful cases prolonged observation of the child in a more benevolent and structured environment may be required to make the diagnosis.

The fetal alcohol syndrome, which may also cause hyperactivity, is suggested by a characteristic facial dysmorphism, as described in that chapter.

Mentally retarded children may appear more hyperactive and impulsive than normal children of the same age; however, when compared with children of the same developmental age, the hyperactivity of these mentally retarded patients appears normal.

Autistic children may be extremely hyperactive and distractible and may be very impulsive. These symptoms, however, occur in the setting of typical symptoms of autism and do not indicate the presence of an additional disorder such as ADHD. Indeed these hyperactive autistic children may get worse if treated with stimulants.

Phenobarbital, as may be prescribed for epilepsy, may cause hyperactivity in children as a side effect.

Children with mania may appear quite similar to children with ADHD; however, in mania one sees an exuberance of energy and a pressure to complete tasks, in contrast to the purposelessness and restlessness of a hyperactive child.

Children with an agitated depression may likewise at first glance appear to have ADHD; however, here one sees despair and fatigue, symptoms not typical of ADHD.

Children with schizophrenia, especially the catatonic type, may be quite active and impulsive; however, the presence of delusions and bizarre behavior rules out ADHD.

The diagnosis of ADHD in adults is particularly difficult. Restlessness, distractibility, and impulsivity are associated with many disorders, including the affective disorders, schizophrenia, antisocial personality disorder, Briquet's syndrome, substance use disorder, and borderline personality disorder, and may not indicate the presence of a concurrent ADHD. With the aid of a history obtained from parents and teachers, establishing a continuity of symptoms back to childhood is perhaps the only currently reliable way to make the diagnosis in an adult. The "detective work" involved in such a diagnostic endeavor is often prodigious.

TREATMENT

A large number of medications are useful in ADHD, including stimulants (or stimulant-like medications), antidepressants, lithium, and alpha-2 autoreceptor blocking agents. As a group, the stimulants are most effective.

Stimulant and stimulant-like medications include methylphenidate, mixed amphetamine salts (marketed under the trade name "Adderall"), dextroamphetamine, atomoxetine, modafinil and pemoline. Methylphenidate and mixed amphetamine salts are generally equal in effectiveness, and methylphenidate is probably superior to dextroamphetamine. Although atomoxetine and modafinil are both superior to placebo, their effectiveness relative to methylphenidate is not clear. Pemoline is generally held in reserve, given its potential hepatotoxicity.

Antidepressants effective in ADHD include bupropion, the tricyclics nortriptyline and desipramine, and the MAOI tranylcypromine. Bupropion is roughly equivalent in efficacy to methylphenidate and is the preferred antidepressant. Of the two tricyclics, desipramine is generally not used in children, given concerns over possible cardiotoxicity. The MAOI tranylcypromine is generally a last choice given the wide range of restricted foods and possible drug-drug interactions.

Lithium, in one preliminary, double-blinded study in adults, was equivalent to methylphenidate.

The alpha-2 autoreceptor blockers guanfacine and clonidine are more effective than placebo, but overall their effect is relatively modest, and side-effects such as sedation are often limiting: of these two, guanfacine is better tolerated. Clonidine may be initiated in a total daily dose of 0.1 mg, increasing in similar increments every week until a satisfactory response or unacceptable side-effects occur. This total daily dose should be divided into 3 or 4 doses; most patients respond to a total daily dose of 0.5 mg or less.

Barring the existence of certain complicating conditions, noted below, it is reasonable to start with either methylphenidate or mixed amphetamine salts. Both agents are available in immediate and time-release preparations and it is customary to begin with an immediate release preparation, dividing the total daily dose generally into two doses, with the first falling in the very early morning and the second around mid-day: in some cases an early evening dose may be required but dosing this late in the day risks causing insomnia. Methylphenidate is begun in a total daily dose of 10 mg and increased in 10 mg increments every 4 to 7 days to a maximum of 60 mg. Mixed amphetamine salts are begun in total doses of from 5 to 10 mg, with incremental increases of from 5 to 10 mg every 7 days to a maximum of 40 mg. Once an optimum dose has been established with either agent, an attempt may be made to switch to the time-release preparation, giving the entire total daily dose in the early morning. Although most patients do well with this (and indeed, in many cases it may be practical to initiate treatment with the time-release preparation), in a minority the immediate release preparations are clearly more effective.

In cases where stimulants offer little benefit or are poorly tolerated, bupropion is a reasonable next step. Treatment may be initiated with the sustained release preparation at a dose of 150 mg in the morning, and then, after four to seven days, increased to 150 mg in the morning and 150 mg in the early afternoon.

Certain complicating conditions may dictate a change in strategy, and these include substance abuse, depression, tic disorders, schizophrenia and bipolar disorder. Substance abusers should generally not be given stimulants, and here bupropion is a reasonable alternative to start with. In the case of depression, it makes sense to kill two birds with one stone by using one medication for both the depression and the ADHD, and here again, bupropion is a reasonable first choice. Tic disorders used to be thought to constitute a contraindication to stimulants, given that, albeit in a minority, stimulants may exacerbate tics. Recent research, however, has shown that most patients with tics can, and do, take stimulants without experiencing a significant increase in the severity of their tics, thus clearing the way for treatment with stimulants. In the minority of cases where tics do worsen, or when one wishes to kill two birds with one stone and treat both the tic disorder and the ADHD with one medication, then consideration may be given to an alpha-2 autoreceptor blocker or, in adults, desipramine. Schizophrenia constitutes a relative contraindication to stimulants,

which can exacerbate psychosis, and here either an antidepressant or lithium are reasonable alternatives. Finally, bipolar patients are at risk of mania if given stimulants or antidepressants, and here lithium is the obvious first choice.

Regardless of which medication is used, it is reasonable, given the course of ADHD, to occasionally give "drug holidays" (as for example during the summer school break for children) to see if treatment is still required. For children, this is especially important in the case of stimulants, for it is during such "holidays" that "catch-up" growth may occur.

In most cases, parent-training classes and classroom-based behavior modification programs are also helpful; however, it must be emphasized that, as a rule, medications, in particular stimulants, are more effective. Indeed, in some cases, medications are required before hyperactivity and impulsivity subside to the point where behavioral treatment is even possible.

BIBLIOGRAPHY

Anonymous. Clinical practice guidelines: diagnosis and evaluation of the child with attention-deficit/hyperactivity disorder. *Pediatrics* 2000;105: 1158-1170.

Berquin PC, Giedd JN, Jacobson LK, et al. Cerebellum in attention-deficit/hyperactivity disorder: a morphometric MRI study. *Neurology* 1998;50:1087-1093.

Castellanos FX, Lee PP, Sharp W, et al. Developmental trajectories of brain volume abnormalities in children and adolescents with attention-deficit/hyperactivity disorder. *The Journal of the American Medical Association* 2002;288:1740-1748.

Dorrego MF, Canevaro L, Kuzis G, et al. A randomized, double-blind, crossover study of methylphenidate and lithium in adults with attention-deficit/hyperactivity disorder: preliminary findings. *The Journal of Neuropsychiatry and Clinical Neurosciences* 2002;14:289-295.

Fisher SE, Francks C, McCracken JT, et al. A genomewide scan for loci involved in attention-deficit/hyperactivity disorder. *American Journal of Human Genetics* 2002;70:1183-1196.

Hauser P, Zametkin AJ, Martinez P, et al. Attention-deficit/hyperactivity disorder in people with generalized resistance to thyroid hormone. *The New England Journal of Medicine* 1993;328:997-1001.

Kuperman S, Perry PJ, Gaffney GR, et al. Bupropion SR vs. methylphenidate vs. placebo for attention-deficit/hyperactivity disorder in adults. *Annals of Clinical Psychiatry* 2001;13:129-134.

Mannuzza S, Klein RG, Bessler A, et al. Adult outcome of hyperactive boys. Educational achievement, occupational rank, and psychiatric status. *Archives of General Psychiatry* 1993;50:565-576.

Mannuzza S, Klein RG, Klein DF, et al. Accuracy of recall of childhood attention-deficit/hyperactivity disorder. *The American Journal of Psychiatry* 2002;159:1882-1888.

Michelson D, Allen AJ, Busner J, et al. Once-daily atomoxetine treatment for children and adolescents with attention-deficit/hyperactivity disorder: a randomized, placebo-controlled study. *The American Journal of Psychiatry* 2002;159:1896-1901.

Pelham WE, Gnagy EM, Chronis AM, et al. A comparison on morning-only and morning/late afternoon Adderall to morning-only, twice-daily, and three times-daily methylphenidate in children with attention-deficit/hyperactivity disorder. *Pediatrics* 1999;104:1300-1311.

Prince JB, Wilens TE, Biederman J, et al. A controlled study of nortriptyline in children and adolescents with attention deficit hyperactivity disorder. *Journal of Child and Adolescent Psychopharmacology* 2000;10:193-204.

Scahill L, Chappell PB, Kim YS, et al. A placebo-controlled study of guanfacine in the treatment of children with tic disorders and attention-deficit/hyperactivity disorder. *The American Journal of Psychiatry* 2001;158:1067-1074.

Spencer T, Biederman J, Coffey B, et al. A double-blind comparison of desipramine and placebo in children and adolescents with chronic tic disorder and comorbid attention-deficit/hyperactivity disorder. *Archives of General Psychiatry* 2002;59:649-656.

Taylor FB, Russo J. Efficacy of modafinil compared to dextroamphetamine for the treatment of attention-deficit/hyperactivity disorder in adults. *Journal of Child and Adolescent Psychopharmacology* 2000;10: 311-320.

Taylor FB, Russo J. Comparing guanfacine and dextroamphetamine for the treatment of adult attention-deficit/hyperactivity disorder. *Journal of Clinical Psychopharmacology* 2001;21:223-228.

Zametkin A, Rapoport JL, Murphy DL, et al. Treatment of hyperactive children with monoamine oxidase inhibitors. I. Clinical efficacy. *Archives of General Psychiatry* 1985;42:962-966.

24   Conduct Disorder (DSM-IV-TR #312.8)

■

Of children and adolescents, anywhere from 1% to 10% repetitively and persistently break important rules, destroy property, and harm others, and this is much more common in males than females by a ratio of from 3:1 to 5:1.

About half of all these individuals eventually evidence an antisocial personality disorder as adults; the rest are generally able to conduct themselves into reasonably satisfactory compliance with societal norms and laws.

ONSET

In boys conduct disorder tends to begin before the age of 8, whereas in girls onset may be delayed until puberty or shortly thereafter.

CLINICAL FEATURES

Preschoolers may be defiant and oppositional. Temper tantrums are common, and aggressiveness may earn the child a "reputation." Other children, especially younger ones, whether at home, school, or in the neighborhood, may be bullied or beaten, sometimes unmercifully so. Toys and clothing may be stolen, as may some of the parents' belongings. Toward the end of elementary school years many of these children have either gravitated into gang membership or have established themselves as "loners." The loner tends to be more aggressive and seems to lack any concept of loyalty or friendship. Group members, on the other hand, may be quite "tight" with each other and display a considerable degree of loyalty. Lying, "conning," stealing, destruction of property, and fire setting may occur. Cruelty to animals or other children may occur and in the loner may be extreme. When caught these children neither appear contrite nor are they prone to confess. Rather they almost invariably blame others. Remorse is lacking, and although they attempt to avoid punishment they have no true sense of guilt. Classroom disruptiveness is the rule, and grades are uniformly low. Truancy, though more common in adolescence, may begin in elementary school.

The adolescent with conduct disorder, though he may engage in less frequent misconduct, often shows evidence of planning when he does, and the misconduct itself tends to be much more severe. Picking fights and using weapons during them may become commonplace. Theft, often surreptitious in childhood, now becomes more blatant, with breaking and entering, purse-snatching, or even threats with a weapon. Vandalism and wanton destruction of property may occur. Truancy becomes common, and these teenagers often run away from home, staying away for several days or longer. Drinking and smoking begin at an early age, as does sexual activity. Rape may occur. Girls may become promiscuous and have unwanted pregnancies.

Attention-deficit/hyperactivity disorder is very commonly present, especially in those with an early age at onset.

COURSE

As noted earlier about one half of patients with conduct disorder eventually display an antisocial personality disorder. Indicators of such a poor prognosis include childhood onset under the age of 10, greater severity and frequency of antisocial behaviors, especially aggressive behavior, and being a loner. By contrast, those with an adolescent onset—over the age of 10, less severe misconduct, and some evidence of group loyalty—tend to have a better prognosis and often grow up to be responsible and law-abiding adults.

COMPLICATIONS

Academic failure is common, and these patients may be incarcerated or institutionalized.

ETIOLOGY

Both hereditary and environmental influences are important, and when both are present an additive effect occurs.

Antisocial personality disorder, especially in the father, and alcoholism are more common among the biologic parents of conduct-disordered children than in the general population.

Typically in the family of origin, discipline is harsh, inconsistent, and at times capricious. Conflict between the parents is often severe, and supervision may be minimal or entirely lacking. In some cases abandonment may occur, with a legacy of foster homes or orphanages.

As noted earlier, attention-deficit/hyperactivity disorder appears more commonly among these children than in others and if severe may make it impossible for the child to learn discipline.

EEG abnormalities and "soft" findings on a neurologic examination are not uncommon; one study found that indicators of autonomic hypoarousal, such as low heart rate and decreased skin conductance in adolescence, reliably predicted criminal activity in early adulthood.

DIFFERENTIAL DIAGNOSIS

Misconduct may occur as part of simple adolescent rebelliousness or may be secondary to specific disorders, such as attention-deficit/hyperactivity disorder (ADHD), depression, mania, schizophrenia or mental retardation.

Adolescent rebelliousness may manifest as misconduct but here the onset is in the early teens and the history prior to that is generally unremarkable, in contrast to conduct disorder which usually has an onset in childhood and indeed may not have been preceded by a period of normal functioning.

ADHD, as noted earlier, is often present in patients with conduct disorder, and in these cases it may merely be a concurrent disorder or it may have played an etiologic role. ADHD occurring in isolation may lead to misconduct; however, here one finds that the misconduct is more "accidental" and a by-product of generally impulsive and hyperactive behavior, rather than being the result of planning, as is often seen in conduct disorder. Furthermore, with treatment of "isolated" ADHD the misconduct generally clears, whereas in the case of concurrent ADHD and conduct disorder, although there may be some lessening of misconduct with treatment of the ADHD, the overall pattern of misbehavior persists.

From a clinical point of view, depression (or dysthymia) remains one of the most important and at times most difficult differentials for conduct disorder. The depressed child or adolescent, lacking interest, energy, and the ability to think clearly, falls behind in school, out of favor at home, and becomes "easy prey" for those with a conduct disorder who are looking to recruit someone into their group. The more chronic the depression, the more ingrained the group's antisocial "values" become until the depressed youngster's behavior eventually becomes almost indistinguishable from that seen in conduct disorder, and indeed may continue that way even if the depression goes into remission. Diagnostic clues include the following: a history from teachers or parents of a relatively rapid fall in grades followed by "hanging around with the wrong crowd," and on the mental status examination a certain sullen and psychomotorically retarded attitude that stands in contrast to the nimble animation of the youngster with a conduct disorder. When in doubt, a trial of an antidepressant is generally in order.

Mania, as may be seen in bipolar disorder, typically propels patients into impulsive and injudicious endeavors that often burst the bounds of legality and propriety. Here, however, the heightened mood, pressured speech and increased energy with decreased need for sleep stand in contrast with the sullen impulsivity of the conduct-disordered youth who, though perhaps energetic, still requires sleep.

Schizophrenia may present with misconduct; however, here one finds delusions, hallucinations or bizarre behavior, features lacking in conduct disorder.

Mentally retarded patients may engage in much misconduct; however, here the misconduct stems from an inability to understand rules coupled with an overall inability to exercise self-control.

TREATMENT

Neither group therapy, dynamically oriented individual psychotherapy, nor family therapy has been shown effective for conduct disorder. Highly structured residential programs, though capable of improving behavior during the period of incarceration, are not associated with long-term improvement after discharge.

In contrast, parent training has been found effective and is followed by an improvement in the youngster's behavior. Furthermore, social skills training may serve as a useful adjunct, enhancing the results of parent training.

ADHD, if present, should be aggressively treated, and although stimulants are generally preferred, the presence of substance abuse, common in conduct disorder, should prompt consideration of an alternative, such as bupropion or atomoxetine.

Pharmacologic treatment of conduct disorder per se plays a relatively minor role. However, for aggressive youths, lithium, haloperidol and risperidone have each been shown to be superior to placebo; lithium and haloperidol have also been compared to each other, and it appears that lithium is superior.

BIBLIOGRAPHY

Bassarath L. Conduct disorder: a biopsychosocial review. *Canadian Journal of Psychiatry* 2001;46:609-616.

Campbell M, Small AM, Green WH, et al. Behavioral efficacy of haloperidol and lithium carbonate. A comparison in hospitalized aggressive children with conduct disorder. *Archives of General Psychiatry* 1984;41:650-656.

Findling RL, McNamara NK, Branicky LA, et al. A double-blind pilot study of risperidone in the treatment of conduct disorder. *Journal of the American Academy of Child and Adolescent Psychiatry* 2000;39:509-516.

Lahey BB, Loeber R, Burke J, et al. Adolescent outcomes of childhood conduct disorder among clinic-referred boys: predictors of improvement. *Journal of Abnormal Child Psychology* 2002;30:333-348.

Robins L. Deviant Children Grown Up. Boston, 1966, Williams and Wilkins.

Storm-Mathisen A, Vaglum P. Conduct disorder patients 20 years later: a personal follow-up study. *Acta Psychiatrica Scandinavica* 1994;89:416-420.

Wolfenden SR, Williams K, Peat JK. Family and parenting interventions for conduct disorder and delinquency: a meta-analysis of randomized clinical trials. *Archives of Disease in Childhood* 2002;86:251-256.

Tourette's Syndrome (Tourette's disorder, DSM-IV-TR #307.23)

Tourette's syndrome is a chronic disorder characterized by multiple tics, both motor and vocal, that vary over time in location, intensity, and character. It is at least three times more common in males than females, and the lifetime prevalence is about 0.05%.

This syndrome was first described by Georges Gilles de la Tourette in 1885 and is often referred to as Gilles de la Tourette's syndrome. Other synonyms include tic convulsif and maladie des tics.

ONSET

Tourette's syndrome may first appear anywhere between the ages of 2 to 18 years; the average age of onset is about 7 years, and the vast majority of patients manifest symptoms before the age of 15. The onset is generally heralded by a simple tic, more often motor than vocal, and more often on the head or face than elsewhere.

CLINICAL FEATURES

Both motor and vocal tics are present, and these may be either simple or complex; sensory tics, previously thought to be relatively rare, are now known to occur in almost all patients. The tics themselves are experienced as involuntary; although patients may be able to suppress them for a time, the tics inevitably appear. Simple tics appear purposeless; complex tics present fragments of otherwise purposeful-appearing behavior. Anxiety or tension often increases the tics; however, at times tics may decrease in these conditions. The tics may appear during sleep, particularly REM sleep, although they are much less frequent than during wakefulness.

Motor tics generally appear first in the head or face, and if progression occurs, as is often the case, it is seen in a rostral-caudal sequence.

Simple motor tics include blinking, brow wrinkling, grimacing, and shoulder shrugging. Complex motor tics include touching, smelling, hopping, throwing, clapping, bending over, or squatting. In more complex tics patients may hit or bite themselves, twist about, engage in echopraxia, or repetitively make obscene gestures.

Simple vocal tics include snorting, hissing, coughing, sniffing, throat clearing, shouting, or, classically, barking. In complex vocal tics patients may suddenly utter words, phrases, or at times entire sentences. Echolalia may occur, as may pallilalia, the perseverative repetitive utterance of what the patient has already said. Only a minority of patients, perhaps 10%, display the classic coprolalia, involuntarily giving voice to obscenities.

Sensory tics come in one of two forms. In one, there is merely the experience of an itch or a tickle, and this occurs in up to one-quarter of all patients. The other form is also known as a "premonitory urge" and this is seen in almost all patients. This "urge to tic" is experienced just before a motor or verbal tic, and in some cases may be resisted, thus quashing the tic.

About one-half of all patients with Tourette's syndrome also experience obsessions and/or compulsions, which typically have an onset about five years after the appearance of tics. Compulsions often later become associated with a powerful sense of having to get things "just right."

About one-half of children who are seen by physicians also have attention-deficit/hyperactivity disorder (ADHD), and display the restlessness, impulsiveness, and inattentiveness characteristic of that disorder. It appears, however, that this may represent not a true association of the two disorders but rather the fact that these doubly affected children are more likely to be seen in consultation.

The tics seen in Tourette's syndrome change remarkably, sometimes from moment to moment, and certainly over days or weeks. In a dramatic example a patient, in scarcely a minute or two, may bark, grimace, shout, snort, jump up from the chair, bark an obscenity, scratch at an ear and sniff the palms, with these tics appearing and disappearing with a lightning-like rapidity.

COURSE

In those with childhood-onset cases, symptoms tend to gradually worsen to a peak around the age of ten; subsequently there is a very gradual remission lasting into early adult years whereupon about one half of patients are left with chronically persistent, clinically significant symptoms while the other half are either in full remission or left with trivial, insignificant tics.

COMPLICATIONS

The most common complications ensue from shame and embarrassment at having tics and from the social ostracism that may follow. In extreme cases relationships with others are virtually impossible to sustain. Friendships are lost, and attendance in the classroom or work place may become impossible to sustain.

In rare instances patients with severe tics have injured their eyes or sustained articular damage. Sensory tics rarely have led to excoriation.

ETIOLOGY

Tourette's syndrome is clearly familial, with concordance rates rising from 5% in siblings to about 10% in dizygotic twins to over 50% in monozygotic twins. Indeed, if one accepts the presence of simple tics in relatives as evidence of the disorder, then the concordance rate in monozygotic twins rises to over 90%. Although linkage studies have indicated multiple loci on various chromosomes (including 2, 7, 8 and 11), the mode of inheritance is not clear. Whereas earlier studies had supported a autosomal dominant mode with sex-mediated penetrance, more recent work has implicated the involvement of multiple genes.

MRI studies, though at times contradictory or suffering from a failure of replication, do, however, provide some support for the notion of a reduction in the size of the basal ganglia, and the limited number of autopsy studies also suggest abnormalities in the same area. In this regard, it is of great interest that serum anti-putaminal antibodies are present in many patients.

Overall, the evidence is consistent with the notion that Tourette's syndrome occurs secondary to a disturbance in the cortico-striatal-pallido-thalamo-cortical circuit which, at least in some cases, may be related to an autoimmune assault upon the putamen. The inherited nature of the disorder is consistent with this speculation, as what may be inherited is a susceptibility to such an autoimmune disturbance.

In a small minority of cases, Tourette's syndrome occurs secondary to an autoimmune disturbance triggered by a preceding group A beta-hemolytic streptococcal pharyngitis. Such cases are said to belong to the PANDAS syndrome (Pediatric Autoimmune Neuropsychiatric Disorders Associated with Streptococcal infections), which also includes a subset of patients with obsessive-compulsive disorder. In this syndrome, the preceding streptococcal infection triggers an immune response which cross-reacts with neurons in the basal ganglia. Clues to this diagnosis include not only the presence of a preceding streptococcal pharyngitis but also the presence of elevated titers of anti-streptolysin O, anti-DNAase B or anti-hyalouronidase.

DIFFERENTIAL DIAGNOSIS

Tourette's syndrome is basically a movement disorder, and thus the first step in differential diagnosis is to determine whether the patient indeed has tics, rather than another abnormal movement, such as chorea, dystonia, athetosis, ballism, myokymia, hemifacial spasm, or myoclonus.

Tics are sudden, brief, repetitive, often stereotyped involuntary movements or vocalizations that at times may appear purposeful. In chorea the jerks and twitches dance from one part of the body to another in a lightning-like nonrepetitive fashion. Often the patient attempts to elaborate on the choreic movement to make it look purposeful, but persistent observation reveals their utterly purposeless nature. Both dystonic and athetoid movements are of slower onset and longer duration; in addition the athetoid movements have a peculiar writhing quality to them. Ballism is violent and continuous. Myokymia displays the characteristic continuous "live flesh" appearance. Hemifacial spasm, as the name implies, is a repetitive spasm, quite unlike the grimacing one may see in Tourette's syndrome. Myoclonus, when well localized, may be difficult to distinguish from a tic; one clue is the absence of any semblance of purpose.

Stereotypies, as may be found in schizophrenia, may appear to have some purpose; however, the overall appearance is one of bizarreness.

Compulsions, as may be seen in obsessive-compulsive disorder, appear similar to complex tics; however, here the movements are intentional. They are in the service of a definite purpose, rather than merely seeming purposeful, as is the case with complex tics.

Assuming that the foregoing disorders have been ruled out and that the patient does have tics and not some other kind of abnormal movement, the next step is to search out those disorders that may secondarily produce tics.

Autism may present with tics, but the invariable defect in social relationships distinguishes this disorder. Intoxication with amphetamines and related dopamine agonists may cause tics; in such cases the history of antecedent use facilitates the diagnosis. Tardive dyskinesia rarely may present primarily with tics, resulting in "tardive Tourette's." In tardive Tourette's, however, one generally also sees choreiform movements and the invariable history of prolonged antipsychotic use. Occasionally a patient with Tourette's syndrome who has been treated with antipsychotics may have both Tourette's

syndrome and tardive Tourette's. Sydenham's chorea may also occasionally present with tics; however, here choreiform movements are also present, and one may usually be able to elicit a history of antecedent rheumatic fever. Neuroacanthocytosis may present with simple tics and with lip biting; however, here usually chorea is also seen; if doubt persists a peripheral smear shows acanthyocytes. Postviral encephalitides may include tics (von Economo's encephalitis being the most famous); the antecedent history of an encephalitis, however, makes the diagnosis. Intoxication with either carbon monoxide or gasoline may leave tics as sequelae; however, here the history of antecedent exposure makes the diagnosis. Hallervorden-Spatz disease, rarely, may present with motor or vocal tics, and there is also a case report of motor and vocal tics occurring as a side effect of lamotrigene.

Assuming that the foregoing disorders, which may secondarily produce tics, have been ruled out, the final task is to distinguish Tourette's syndrome from the other two idiopathic tic disorders, namely transient tic disorder and chronic motor or vocal tic disorder. As will be pointed out in the chapter on other tic disorders, this may be something of an academic distinction, as current research suggests strongly that these disorders actually lie on a continuum.

Patients with motor or vocal tics lasting less than a year are said to have transient tic disorder. When tics last longer than a year, the patient is said to have either chronic motor or vocal tic disorder or Tourette's syndrome. The distinction between these two rests on whether both motor and vocal tics are present. If both are present, the diagnosis is Tourette's syndrome. If, however, only motor or vocal tics are present for over a year, the diagnosis is chronic motor or vocal tic disorder.

TREATMENT

Various medications are effective in Tourette's syndrome, including antipsychotics (olanzapine, risperidone, ziprasidone, haloperidol and pimozide), the alpha-2 autoreceptor blockers clonidine and guanfacine, the tricyclic antidepressant desipramine, and a benzodiazepine, clonazepam.

Of the antipsychotics, olanzapine may be started at a dose of 5 mg, and then increased, if necessary, to a maximum of 10 mg two weeks later. The starting dose for risperidone is 0.5 mg, for ziprasidone 5 mg, for haloperidol 0.25 to 0.5 mg, and for pimozide 1 mg, and each agent may be increased in similar increments every seven days until a satisfactory response, limiting side-effects or a maximum dose. Maximum doses (and average effective doses) for these agents are: for risperidone 6 mg (2-4 mg), for ziprasidone 40 mg (20-30 mg), for haloperidol 10 mg (3-4 mg), and for pimozide 10 mg (3-4 mg). Choosing among the various antipsychotics is not entirely straightforward. The second-generation antipsychotics olanzapine and risperidone are overall better tolerated in terms of extrapyramidal side effects (e.g., akathisia) but may be associated with hyperlipidemia, diabetes or weight gain; furthermore, use of risperidone in Tourette's syndrome is fairly strongly associated with dysphoria and depression. Haloperidol is perhaps the best studied agent, but both it and pimozide are prone to cause extrapyramidal side effects; furthermore, both these agents may also, in children, induce a syndrome almost identical with school phobia (also known as separation anxiety disorder). Finally, pimozide carries the unfortunate liability of prolonging the corrected QT interval, thereby increasing the risk of a fatal arrhythmia. Bearing in mind all these considerations, it may be reasonable to begin with a second-generation agent such as olanzapine. Should this prove unsuccessful, then consideration may be given to either risperidone or haloperidol. Pimozide is definitely a third choice, given its cardiac profile.

Of the alpha-2 autoreceptor blockers, clonidine is most widely used, and is given in two divided doses, initially at a total daily dose of 0.1 mg, with increases in similar increments every seven days until one begins to see a response, limiting side effects occur, or a maximum dose of 1.0 mg is reached. Importantly, whereas the response to an antipsychotic is fairly prompt, the full response to clonidine may not occur for weeks or months; hence it is reasonable, in titrating the dose, to pause when one first begins to see a response and then wait until that response plateaus before considering another dose increase: most patients respond to about 0.5 mg.

The tricyclic desipramine may be started at a dose of 25 mg and increased every few days to a dose of about 100 mg, after which the patient should be observed for weeks to assess the response. Importantly, although desipramine may be used safely in adults, it should generally be avoided in children, given its potential cardiotoxicity in this age group.

The benzodiazepine clonazepam should be given in two divided doses, beginning with a total daily dose of 0.5 mg and increasing in similar increments every week until one sees a satisfactory response, limiting side effects occur, or a maximum dose of 4 mg is reached: most patients respond to a dose of about 2 mg.

Clearly, there is a formidable number of different agents available for the treatment of Tourette's syndrome, and, unfortunately, there is no hard and fast rule to guide one in choosing among them. Although the antipsychotics, by and large, produce the most robust response, concerns about tardive dyskinesia and akathisia temper one's enthusiasm. Should an antipsychotic be selected, keep in mind that an akathisia may manifest as an exacerbation of tics, rather than with any motor restlessness. The alpha-2 autoreceptor blocker clonidine, although perhaps not as effective as an antipsychotic, is often preferred in order to avoid incurring the risk of tardive dyskinesia. Furthermore, clonidine is also effective for ADHD, a definite advantage given how many clinic patients with Tourette's syndrome also have ADHD. Importantly, if clonidine is used, caution must be exercised in the event it is discontinued because an abrupt discontinuation may be followed by a severe "rebound" exacerbation of tics which may persist for weeks or months: clearly, a gradual tapering is appropriate. Desipramine, like clonidine, is also effective against both Tourette's syndrome and ADHD, and thus may be attractive when treating adults with both disorders. Clonazepam is less effective than antipsychotics and clonidine, and is often used adjunctively.

In summary, then, for uncomplicated Tourette's syndrome, it appears reasonable to begin with either an antipsychotic (e.g., olanzapine) or the alpha-2 autoreceptor blocker clonidine. In cases, however, where ADHD is also present, clonidine may be the preferred agent, with consideration also given, in adults, to desipramine. When concurrent obsessions or compulsions require treatment, one may add an SSRI such as fluoxetine, or one may consider using risperidone, as this agent may, in addition to reducing tics, also be effective for obsessions and compulsions. It must be emphasized, however, that these are suggestions only: there simply are not enough comparative studies available to allow for definitive recommendations. In many cases, a methodical approach, giving one agent a good trial, both in terms of dose and duration, and then another, is required to find the best agent and dose for any given patient.

Finally, in those cases where the Tourette's syndrome is occurring as part of PANDAS, consideration may be given to plasma exchange to remove the offending anti-basal ganglia antibodies. Furthermore, a good case may be made for prophylactic treatment with penicillin in these patients in order to prevent another streptococcal pharyngitis.

BIBLIOGRAPHY

Bruun RD. Subtle and underrecognized side effects of neuroleptic treatment in children with Tourette's disorder. *The American Journal of Psychiatry* 1988;145:621-624.

de la Tourette G. Étude sur une affection nerveuse, caractérisée par de l'incoordination motrice, accompagnée d'écholalie et de coprolalie. *Archives of Neurology* (Paris) 1995;9:158-200.

Gaffney CR, Perry PJ, Lund BC, et al. Risperidone versus clonidine in the treatment of children and adolescents with Tourette's syndrome. *Journal of the American Academy of Child and Adolescent Psychiatry* 2002;41:330-336.

Haber SN, Kowall NW, Vonsattel JP, et al. Gilles de la Tourette's syndrome. A postmortem neuropathological and immunohistochemical study. *Journal of the Neurological Sciences* 1986;75:225-241.

Jankovic J. Tourette's syndrome. *The New England Journal of Medicine* 2001;345:1184-1192.

Klawans HL, Falk DK, Nausieda PA, et al. Gilles de la Tourette syndrome after long-term chlorpromazine therapy. *Neurology* 1978;28:1064-1066.

Leckman JF. Tourette's syndrome. *Lancet* 2002;360:1577-1586.

Leckman JF, Ort S, Caruso KA, et al. Rebound phenomena in Tourette's syndrome after abrupt withdrawal of clonidine. Behavioral, cardiovascular, and neurochemical effects. *Archives of General Psychiatry* 1986;43:1168-1176.

Leckman JF, Walker DE, Cohen DJ. Premonitory urges in Tourette's syndrome. *The American Journal of Psychiatry* 1993;150:98-102.

Leckman JF, Walker DE, Goodman WK, et al. "Just right" perceptions associated with compulsive behavior in Tourette's syndrome. *The American Journal of Psychiatry* 1994;151:675-680.

Leckman JF, Zhang H, Vitale A, et al. Course of tic severity in Tourette syndrome: the first two decades. *Pediatrics* 1998;102:14-19.

Margolese HC, Annable L, Dion Y. Depression and dysphoria in adult and adolescent patients with Tourette's syndrome treated with risperidone. *The Journal of Clinical Psychiatry* 2002;63:1030-1034.

Mikkelsen EJ, Detlor J, Cohen DJ. School avoidance and social phobia triggered by haloperidol in patients with Tourette's syndrome. *The American Journal of Psychiatry* 1981;138:1572-1576.

Northam RS, Singer HS. Postencephalitic acquired Tourette-like syndrome in a child. *Neurology* 1991;41:592-593.

Onofrj M, Paci C, D'Andreamatteo G, et al. Olanzapine in severe Gilles de la Tourette syndrome: a 52-week double-blind cross-over study vs. low-dose pimozide. *Journal of Neurology* 2000;247:443-446.

Perlmutter SJ, Leitman SF, Garvey MA, et al. Therapeutic plasma exchange and intravenous immunoglobulin for obsessive-compulsive disorder and tic disorders in childhood. *Lancet* 1999;354:1153-1158.

Pulst SM, Walshe TM, Romero JA. Carbon monoxide poisoning with features of Gilles de la Tourette's syndrome. *Archives of Neurology* 1983;40:443-444.

Sallee FR, Nesbitt L, Jackson C, et al. Relative efficacy of haloperidol and pimozide in children and adolescents with Tourette's disorder. *The American Journal of Psychiatry* 1997;154:1057-1062.

Sallee FR, Kurlan R, Goetz CG, et al. Ziprasidone treatment of children and adolescents with Tourette's syndrome: a pilot study. *Journal of the American Academy of Child and Adolescent Psychiatry* 2000;39:292-299.

Scarano V, Pellecchia MT, Filia A, et al. Hallervorden-Spatz syndrome resembling a typical Tourette syndrome. *Movement Disorders* 2002;17:618-620.

Simonic I, Nyholt DR, Gericke GS, et al. Further evidence for linkage of Gilles de la Tourette syndrome (GTS) susceptibility loci on chromosome 2p11, 8q22 and 11q23-24 in South African Afrikaners. *American Journal of Medical Genetics* 2001;105:163-167.

Singer HS, Brown J, Quaskey S, et al. The treatment of attention-deficit/hyperactivity disorder in Tourette's syndrome: a double-blind placebo-controlled study with clonidine and desipramine. *Pediatrics* 1995;95:74-81.

Singer HS, Giuliano JD, Hansen BH, et al. Antibodies against human putamen in children with Tourette syndrome. *Neurology* 1998;50:1618-1624.

Swedo SE, Leonard HL, Garvey M, et al. Pediatric autoimmune neuropsychiatric disorders associated with streptococcal infections: clinical descriptions of the first 50 cases. *The American Journal of Psychiatry* 1998;155:264-271.

26 Other Tic Disorders (transient tic disorder and chronic motor or vocal tic disorder, DSM-IV-TR #307.21, 307.22)

Much evidence supports the notion that transient tic disorder and chronic motor or vocal tic disorder lie on a continuum with Tourette's syndrome. By convention if the patient has motor or vocal tics lasting less than a year, a diagnosis of transient tic disorder is made. If the tics last longer than a year, then the diagnosis is changed to either Tourette's syndrome or chronic motor or vocal tic disorder. In patients who have had tics for more than a year, a diagnosis of Tourette's syndrome is given if both motor and vocal tics have been present at some point, whereas if the illness is characterized by only motor or only vocal tics, then the diagnosis of chronic motor or vocal tic disorder is made.

Whereas Tourette's syndrome is relatively rare, up to 15% of children at some point have tics. Furthermore, in contrast to Tourette's syndrome, the sex ratio for other tic disorders is less heavily weighted toward males.

ONSET AND CLINICAL FEATURES

These are similar to those described for Tourette's syndrome, with the exception that vocal tics are less commonly seen than are motor ones.

COURSE

When evaluating a child whose tics have lasted less than a year, currently no means are available for predicting whether these tics will remit in less than a year or become chronic. In those cases wherein they do remit within a year—that is to say, those with transient tic disorder—repeat episodes of tics may appear later either in adolescent or adult years. In cases where tics persist chronically for over a year, remission occurs in adolescence in about two-thirds with the rest pursuing a chronic course.

COMPLICATIONS

Complications are the same as those discussed in the section on Tourette's syndrome but are less severe.

ETIOLOGY

The etiology is probably the same as that for Tourette's syndrome.

DIFFERENTIAL DIAGNOSIS

The differential diagnostic scheme outlined in the section on Tourette's syndrome may also be applied here. As noted earlier if the tics last longer than a year, the diagnosis must be revised to either Tourette's syndrome or chronic motor or vocal tic disorder, depending on whether one sees a combination of motor and vocal tics, or only motor or only vocal tics present.

TREATMENT

Treatment may be pursued generally as outlined for Tourette's syndrome; however, given the relative mildness of symptoms, antipsychotics are generally not the first choice.

BIBLIOGRAPHY

Corbett JA, Mathews AM, Connell PH, et al. Tics and Gilles de la Tourette's syndrome: a follow-up study and clinical review. *The British Journal of Psychiatry* 1969;115:1229-1241.

Evidente VG. Is it a tic or Tourette's? Clues for differentiating simple from more complex tic disorders. *Postgraduate Medicine* 2000;108: 179-182.

Golden GS. Tics and Tourette's: a continuum of symptoms? *Annals of Neurology* 1978;4:145-148.

Kurland R, Behr J, Medved L, et al. Transient tic disorder and the spectrum of Tourette's syndrome. *Archives of Neurology* 1988;45: 1200-1201.

Spencer T, Biederman J, Harding M, et al. The relationship between tic disorders and Tourette's syndrome revisited. *Journal of the American Academy of Child and Adolescent Psychiatry* 1995;34: 1133-1139.

27 Separation Anxiety Disorder (DSM-IV-TR #309.21)

Separation anxiety disorder is a fairly common disorder of childhood with a prevalence in school age children of from 2% to 5%. Affected children demonstrate extreme anxiety upon actual, or at times only threatened, separation from their parents. Thus these children avoid any activity that might effect such a separation, including going to school, camp, or a friend's home for an overnight stay, or perhaps even going to bed in their own room. This disorder appears to be equally common in boys and girls.

Separation anxiety disorder has also been referred to as "school phobia." However, this term is somewhat misleading because the child is not afraid of, or phobic about, approaching school; rather it is the separation from parents which evokes anxiety.

ONSET

Onset is generally at the age of 6 or 7; it may be as early as the preschool years, only very rarely does it begin in teenage years. No consistent premorbid findings are apparent, nor has a prodrome been identified. Occasionally a precipitating event may be seen, and it is usually one that involves loss or separation. It may follow a death of a relative, another child, or perhaps a pet, or it may follow a move to a new and strange neighborhood.

CLINICAL FEATURES

Characteristically, at the threat of separation these children become very anxious. If it is time to go to school they may complain of headaches or stomachaches, and may even vomit. If allowed to stay home with a parent, however, these symptoms generally rapidly remit. If the parents attempt to go out for a night, the child may throw a temper tantrum or may cling to the parents and plead with them not to go. Bedtime may be particularly difficult. These children may refuse to go to sleep in their own rooms. They may sneak into their parents' bed or, if the door is locked, sleep in the hallway just outside their parents' bedroom.

These children often worry something awful might befall them or perhaps befall their parents. They may worry that an accident or an illness might occur or that they might be lost or even kidnapped. Often there are nightmares, in which the parents come to harm or death. They may be afraid of the dark or believe monsters might be in the closet or under the bed.

In some children the fear of separation becomes so pervasive that they become clinging and never want the parent out of sight. Some may become quite controlling, insisting on either having a parent at home or knowing exactly where they are at all times.

Occasionally some of these children experience some depressive symptoms; at times an actual depressive episode may occur.

COURSE

Symptoms tend to slowly wax and wane for months or years. The overall outlook, however, is good. It is very rare for symptoms to persist into college years.

COMPLICATIONS

Family discord is an almost inevitable complication of the disorder, especially when one of the parents tends at all toward overprotectiveness. If too much school is missed, grades may fall.

ETIOLOGY

Separation anxiety disorder is clearly familial, and, although controversial, there is some evidence that it represents an "equivalent" of panic disorder with agoraphobia.

DIFFERENTIAL DIAGNOSIS

Separation anxiety is a normal part of the developmental phase of separation and individuation that occurs generally between the ages of 8 and 24 months. All children experience this to a certain degree, and it should not be confused with separation anxiety disorder, which, as noted earlier, often comes at 6 or 7 years of age. Another normal part of growing up is homesickness as may be seen when a child goes to summer camp. The fact that children "get over" homesickness in a week or two clearly distinguishes this from separation anxiety disorder wherein the anxiety persists.

At times, under the influence of an overprotective mother or father, a child may become timid, fearful, and reluctant to do anything new, such as go to school. Two features often allow a differential diagnosis to be made. First, in these cases parental overprotectiveness preceded the onset of the child's timidity; second, the child will go to school if he believes that it makes mother pleased.

Separation anxiety may be seen in autism, schizophrenia, and depression. The other symptoms associated with these illnesses indicate the correct diagnosis. Separation anxiety disorder may also occur as a side-effect to treatment with haloperidol, risperidone or pimozide.

In some instances the child may get anxious at the prospect of going to school, not out of fear of separation from a parent, but out of fear of what will happen to him at school. The prospect of having to face a critical teacher or a bullying classmate has made many a child nauseated on a school morning.

TREATMENT

Parents must be educated about the disorder. Overprotectiveness must be discouraged; however, on the other hand, a demanding critical approach must also be avoided. A behavior program is set up in conjunction with parents whereby the child is reinforced for enduring progressively longer separations from his parents. Family and individual therapy are often utilized, but the evidence for their superiority over routine supportive therapy is not conclusive.

If the child has missed a lot of school, remedial work at home and a prompt return to school should be primary goals.

In cases where psychosocial approaches are unsatisfactory, medication may be considered. Although the initial positive double-blinded study of imipramine was not replicated in a subsequent smaller study, this agent still has the most empirical support: treatment is initiated at 10 to 25 mg hs and increased in similar increments every week until limiting side effects or a maximum dose of 100 mg is reached; full effects may not be seen for six to eight weeks. Benzodiazepines such as clonazepam (up to 1 mg/d) or alprazolam (up to 2 mg/d) are used, but lack any double-blinded support. Open studies and case reports also support the use of SSRIs (e.g., fluoxetine) or buspirone.

Which medication constitutes an optimum first choice is a matter of great debate. Imipramine, though possessed of the most support, is often poorly tolerated. Benzodiazepines, though well tolerated, lack good empirical support and carry the risk of neuroadaptation and withdrawal. Both an SSRI and buspirone, like the benzodiazepines, are generally well supported; they do not, however, carry the risk of neuroadaptation. For these reasons, and despite the lack of double-blinded support, one of these agents is often tried first. If pharmacologic treatment is successful it should be continued until the child is symptom-free for at least two months, after which the dose may be gradually tapered.

BIBLIOGRAPHY

Battaglia M, Bertella S, Politi E, et al. Age at onset of panic disorder: influence of family liability to the disease and of childhood separation anxiety disorder. *The American Journal of Psychiatry* 1995;152:1362-1364.

Bernstein GA, Garfinkel BD, Borchardt CM. Comparative studies of pharmacotherapy for school refusal. *Journal of the American Academy of Child and Adolescent Psychiatry* 1990;29:773-781.

Gittelman-Klein R, Klein DF. School phobia: diagnostic considerations in the light of imipramine effects. *The Journal of Nervous and Mental Disease* 1973;156:199-215.

Graae F, Milner J, Rizzotto L, et al. Clonazepam in childhood anxiety disorders. *Journal of the American Academy of Child and Adolescent Psychiatry* 1994;33:372-376.

Hanna GL, Fluent TL, Fischer DJ. Separation anxiety disorder in children and adolescents treated with risperidone. *Journal of Child and Adolescent Psychopharmacology* 1999;9:277-283.

Klein RG, Koplewicz HS, Kanner A. Imipramine treatment of children with separation anxiety disorder. *Journal of the American Academy of Child and Adolescent Psychiatry* 1992;31:21-28.

Last CG, Hansen C, Franco N. Cognitive-behavioral treatment of social phobia. *Journal of the American Academy of Child and Adolescent Psychiatry* 1998;37:404-411.

Linet LS. Tourette syndrome, pimozide, and school phobia: the neuroleptic separation anxiety syndrome. *The American Journal of Psychiatry* 1985;142:613-615.

Manicavasagar V, Silove D, Rapee R, et al. Parent-child concordance for separation anxiety: a clinical study. *Journal of Affective Disorders* 2001;65:81-84.

Mikkelsen EJ, Detlor J, Cohen DJ. School avoidance and social phobia triggered by haloperidol in patients with Tourette's disorder. *The American Journal of Psychiatry* 1981;138:1572-1576.

28 Encopresis (DSM-IV 787.6, 307.7)

Encopresis is a form of childhood-onset fecal incontinence characterized by repeated soiling of clothing or, less commonly, bedding, which cannot be explained by the direct effects of such general medical conditions as rectal stenosis.

Encopresis is present in from 1 to 1.5% of children aged 5 through 8 years, and is far more common in boys than girls, by a ratio of up to 4:1.

ONSET

Onset may be anywhere from ages 4 through 8 years, and may or may not have been preceded by the establishment of fecal continence. Most children attain fecal continence by the age of 4: in cases where continence was never fully established one speaks of "primary" encopresis, whereas in cases where the encopresis was preceded by a year or more of continence, the encopresis is said to be "secondary."

CLINICAL FEATURES

In both primary and secondary encopresis soiling occurs repeatedly, at a minimum at least monthly for three months.

The primary and secondary forms of encopresis, besides being distinguished by their onset, are also distinguished by the absence or presence of constipation. In primary encopresis, constipation is generally absent. By contrast, in secondary encopresis, constipation is generally severe, and the fecal incontinence is of the "overflow" type, with the passage of soft or liquid stool around the hard mass of retained feces. In these cases characterized by overflow of stool, the incontinence may be frequent, sometimes several times a day, with the passage of small amounts of stool onto underwear, or, less commonly, sheets.

COURSE

In the natural course of events most cases of encopresis gradually resolve by adolescence.

COMPLICATIONS

Encopresis makes parents angry and leaves children ashamed and humiliated. There may be unpleasant confrontations between parents and children, and the children themselves may become withdrawn and unwilling to spend time with friends, or even go to school, for fear of soiling. In some cases the conflict between parents and children may become profound, and assume a life of its own, persisting far past the resolution of the encopresis.

ETIOLOGY

Primary encopresis appears to represent a developmental delay of sphincter control. Secondary encopresis develops in the setting of severe constipation, which, itself, may occur for a variety of reasons. In many cases, children with secondary encopresis were subject to harsh or inconsistent toilet training and here the anxiety over possibly making a "mess" impels children to retain their stool, which then becomes hardened and impacted. At this point, a vicious cycle may begin, wherein any attempt to pass the impaction incites pain, which in turn only increases the anxiety associated with defecation, leading to further retention of stool. Eventually, overflow incontinence occurs. In other cases, the constipation may begin in the midst of dehydration associated with a febrile illness, the administration of constipating medications (e.g., certain antihistamines) or a significant change in daily routine, as may occur during trips: regardless of the cause, the resulting constipation, if associated with painful defecation, may lead to retention and overflow incontinence.

DIFFERENTIAL DIAGNOSIS

Various general medical illnesses must be ruled out, including spina bifida, rectal stenosis, hypothyroidism and Hirschsprung's disease.

Many authorities include the voluntary passage of stool in inappropriate places under the rubric of encopresis; however, this pattern is so radically different in terms of etiology and treatment from encopresis as described above that such "lumping" may not be useful. Children who intentionally defecate on the floor or on others' beds are generally defiant and vindictive, and such behavior often forms but a part of an overall pattern of misconduct: they generally do not benefit from the treatment programs described below, and indeed will continue to "send a message" with their inappropriate defecation until the overall pattern of misconduct itself is successfully addressed. Given that such children are, however, often diagnosed with "encopresis" it is very important, in making clinical reports or writing papers, that one specify whether the fecal incontinence is "involuntary" or "voluntary."

TREATMENT

For both primary and secondary encopresis, it is critical to explain to both parents and children the nature of the problem and to defuse the conflict between parents and children and relieve the children's shame and embarrassment.

In primary encopresis, it is appropriate to continue non-punitive toilet training, emphasizing regular toilet times, which should generally fall some 10 to 20 minutes after a meal to take advantage of the gastrocolic reflex. Here, "tincture of time" is essential as one waits for a full developmental "catch-up." In some cases, adding a reward system, as described for secondary encopresis below, may be helpful.

In secondary encopresis, it is essential to free the bowel of any hard or impacted stool. In some cases, digital disimpaction or an enema may be required, whereas in others laxatives will be sufficient. Once this has been accomplished it is appropriate to put measures in place to prevent, as much as possible, constipation from recurring, including adequate hydration, a high fiber diet (accomplished either with a daily helping of bran cereal or daily administration of a bulk-forming agent, such as psyllium), and a daily dose of a stool softener, in either a capsule or liquid form, whichever is better tolerated. A system should also be devised that, while not punishing children for "mistakes," does reward them for defecation in the toilet. In some cases a simple "star chart" suffices; however, in many this must be combined with rewards, such as small toys, for every defecation in the toilet. As for primary encopresis, it is also helpful to establish regular twice daily toilet times, generally 10 to 20 minutes after a meal. When children do make a "mistake" they should clean themselves but should not be required to clean the clothing or bedding; this often backfires as the incredibly anxious child makes a further mess in the attempt at cleaning: in such cases, the soiled clothing may simply be placed in a hamper by the child, and any soiled bedding should be left to the parent to take care of. Most children with secondary encopresis respond well to such a program, usually within a matter of weeks. Once continence has been maintained for a month or more, the star chart and rewards may be phased out, but it is probably prudent to continue adequate hydration, high fiber and stool softeners for some time thereafter. Biofeedback training does not appear any more effective than this approach.

BIBLIOGRAPHY

Borowitz SM, Cox DJ, Sutphen JL, et al. Treatment of childhood encopresis: a randomized trial comparing three treatment protocols. *Journal of Pediatric Gastroenterology and Nutrition* 2002;34:378-384.

Foreman DM, Thambirajah MS. Conduct disorder, enuresis and specific developmental delays in two types of encopresis: a case-note study of 63 boys. *European Child & Adolescent Psychiatry* 1996;5: 33-37.

Kuhn BR, Marcus BA, Pitner SL. Treatment guidelines for primary nonretentive encopresis and stool toileting refusal. *American Family Physician* 1999;59:2171-2178, 2184-2186.

Nolan T, Catto-Smith T, Coffey C, et al. Randomized controlled trial of biofeedback training in persistent encopresis with anismus. *Archives of Disease in Childhood* 1998;79:131-135.

29 Selective Mutism (DSM-IV-TR #313.23)

In selective, or, as it was formerly called, elective mutism, children, while yet capable of speech, become more or less mute in specific social situations that typically lie outside their family or customary circle of friends.

Selective mutism is probably more common in girls than boys. It is an uncommon disorder, with a prevalence among early elementary school age children of from 0.06% to 0.7%.

ONSET

The onset is generally gradual, occurring sometime between the ages of 3 and 6. Most cases, however, do not come to clinical attention until the child enters school.

CLINICAL FEATURES

These children are often shy and withdrawn. They may talk with their siblings, parents, or with a few close friends, but outside of this circle they become mute. At school or with strangers they may follow directions and even answer questions by nodding their heads, but when called upon to speak, they do not. There may be clinging or sulkiness; at times negative and oppositional behavior may be seen.

COURSE

Remission occurs in from one-third to one-half of patients in from months to five or ten years; in the remainder, considerable improvement is the rule.

COMPLICATIONS

These children fail to make satisfactory academic progress; they may be unmercifully ridiculed by their schoolmates.

ETIOLOGY

Selective mutism is probably a syndrome with multiple different etiologies. In some, mutism appears to be but one more expression of shyness and sensitiveness present since infancy, and in such cases it is felt that selective mutism may constitute a variant form of social phobia of the generalized type. In others maternal overprotectiveness appears to be a factor. Developmental dysphasia or dysarticulation is more common in these children than controls and is evident before the onset of the mutism. Recently immigrated children, who have not as yet mastered the language, are likewise more likely to become electively mute.

DIFFERENTIAL DIAGNOSIS

Many young children may evidence shyness and a reticence to speak upon beginning school. This reticence, however, is not abnormal and tends to clear within a few days and certainly within a month.

Some younger immigrants may simply be unwilling to speak their new language. In contrast to the elective mute, however, they may be quite vocal if placed in a school that uses their native tongue.

A number of other conditions exist wherein a child may be mute; however, in each of these the mutism is not elective, but occurs in all settings, including home. These include developmental dysphasia, acquired dysphasia secondary to a tumor or some other lesion, "cerebellar mutism" (as may be seen following removal of a posterior fossa tumor), deafness, autism, major depression, schizophrenia, mental retardation, and conversion disorder.

TREATMENT

Behavior therapy appears effective, and treatment with fluoxetine, in doses of approximately 0.6 mg/kg/d, is modestly effective.

BIBLIOGRAPHY

Bergman RL, Piacentini J, McCracken JT. Prevalence and description of selective mutism in a school-based sample. *Journal of the American Academy of Child and Adolescent Psychiatry* 2002;41: 938-946.

Black B, Uhde TW. Treatment of elective mutism with fluoxetine: a double-blind, placebo-controlled study. *Journal of the American Academy of Child and Adolescent Psychiatry* 1994;33:701-703.

Remschmidt H, Poller M, Herpetz-Dahlmann B, et al. A follow-up study of 45 patients with elective mutism. *European Archives of Psychiatry and Clinical Neuroscience* 2001;251:284-296.

Steinhausen HC, Juzi C. Elective mutism: an analysis of 100 cases. *Journal of the American Academy of Child and Adolescent Psychiatry* 1996;35:606-614.

30 Reactive Attachment Disorder (reactive attachment disorder of infancy or early childhood, DSM-IV-TR #313.89)

Infants subjected to severe and persistent neglect or abuse or deprived of the opportunity to attach themselves to an adult, as may happen in an institution, may develop a syndrome characterized by apathy, withdrawal, and a degree of emotional inaccessibility. In addition, some of these children may evidence failure to thrive, and in severe cases marasmus, with growth retardation and wasting of the extremities, may develop.

This is a very uncommon syndrome, about which little is known with certainty. In the past it was known as "hospitalism" or the "maternal deprivation syndrome."

ONSET

Symptoms typically appear within the first few years of life, generally before the age of 5.

CLINICAL FEATURES

Younger infants with this syndrome appear withdrawn, sad, and listless. They do not smile, and the normal tendency to follow others about the room with the eyes is lost. If these children are picked up they fail to reach out; they seem dead to the opportunity for affection and human contact.

Older infants are apathetic and uninterested in their surroundings. They take no interest in playing "peek-a-boo" and may show little distress if left alone. Toys are left alone, and the infant may present an overall picture of placid misery.

Older children with this disorder tend to evidence either of two types of disturbed relations. In the inhibited type the patient remains generally withdrawn and watchful and very ambivalent about forming any social relationships. By contrast in the disinhibited type the child may indiscriminantly form relationships, even with complete strangers.

Some infants with this syndrome may also display rumination, head banging, or stereotyped rocking, and some may also evidence failure to thrive, with a progressively lower than expected weight for age in the face of a relatively more normal height. In severe cases marasmus may occur, with emaciation, hypotension, and bradycardia. In such cases the growth hormone level is either elevated or within normal limits.

COURSE

Untreated, this is a chronic disorder; at times death from starvation or intercurrent illness may occur.

COMPLICATIONS

Regardless of whether the inhibited or disinhibited pattern emerges, these patients remain incapable of forming normal personal relations.

ETIOLOGY

Any factor that consistently frustrates the development of a normal bond between the infant and parent or parent substitute may cause this syndrome. Thus neglect, abuse, being moved multiple times from one caretaker to another, or an emotionally sterile atmosphere have all been cited as etiologic.

DIFFERENTIAL DIAGNOSIS

In autism the infant fails to attach to his parents; however, this is not due to the generalized sort of apathy seen in reactive attachment disorder. To the contrary, the autistic infant may be quite interested in things, provided that they are inanimate.

Severe grades of mental retardation may be difficult to distinguish from reactive attachment disorder. Here, however, one generally does not see a generalized listlessness nor a dramatic improvement with adequate care, as is typically seen with reactive attachment disorder.

Infants with the diencephalic syndrome may become emaciated; however, in contrast to those with a reactive attachment disorder, these infants often remain quite active and may at times appear happy.

The Cockayne syndrome is distinguished by a progressive decrease in relative head circumference and by a peculiar facial appearance.

When failure to thrive or marasmus occurs, other causes of these conditions, such as congenital heart disease or chronic renal disease, must be sought.

TREATMENT

Improvement gradually ensues upon the institution of adequate parenting. In some cases parental counseling may be adequate. In others the infant may have to be hospitalized and perhaps permanently placed in another home.

BIBLIOGRAPHY

Barbero GJ, Shaheen E. Emotional failure to thrive: a clinical view. *The Journal of Pediatrics* 1967;71:639-641.

Casey PH, Bradley R, Wortham B. Social and nonsocial home environments of infants with nonorganic failure-to-thrive. *Pediatrics* 1984;73:348-353.

Evans SL, Reinhart JB, Succop RA. Failure to thrive. A study of 45 children and their families. *Journal of the American Academy of Child and Adolescent Psychiatry* 1972;11:440-457.

Provence S, Lipton RC. *Infants and Institutions.* New York, 1962, International Universities Press.

Richters MM, Volkmar FR. Reactive attachment disorder of infancy or early childhood. *Journal of the American Academy of Child and Adolescent Psychiatry* 1994;33:328-332.

Tibbits-Kleber AL, Howell RJ. Reactive attachment disorder of infancy (RAD). *Journal of Clinical Child Psychology* 1985;14:304-310.

Zeanah CH. Disturbances of attachment in young children adopted from institutions. *Journal of Developmental and Behavioral Pediatrics* 2000;21:230-236.

31 Psychosocial Dwarfism

Psychosocial dwarfism, also known as deprivation dwarfism, represents a distinctive form of pituitary dwarfism. Under the influence of persistent and severe abuse or neglect, these children, though not malnourished, slowly stop gaining in stature. Concurrently they may also evidence apathy or other symptoms, such as bizarre eating habits.

Reliable data are not available regarding either the sex ratio or prevalence of psychosocial dwarfism.

ONSET

Onset is generally between the ages of 2 and 4, after a period of relatively normal growth.

CLINICAL FEATURES

These children are quite short, often below the third percentile for their age; however, they are not malnourished. Indeed some may be somewhat overweight. Otherwise their habitus is unremarkable.

Apathy and depression are not uncommon; one may, however, see irritability, temper tantrums, cruelty, and hostility. Few of these children can sustain friendships with other children, and some may appear mildly retarded. The most striking abnormality, however, consists of their bizarre eating habits. Some may eat or drink almost anything: dog food, garbage, toilet water, or water from rain puddles. Insomnia may occur, and these children may roam the house at night, secretly eating their unpalatable foods. Older children may experience delayed puberty.

Growth hormone and insulin-like growth factor I (IGF-I, formerly called somatomedin-C) levels are generally decreased, and the majority will show a deficient growth hormone response to provocative tests such as insulin-induced hypoglycemia, levodopa, arginine or clonidine.

COURSE

The long-term course untreated is not known.

COMPLICATIONS

Deficient academic and social development may significantly impair the child's adjustment to the demands of adolescence and adulthood.

ETIOLOGY

Presumably, this disorder results from a predisposition for a specific hypothalamic dysfunction in the face of abuse or neglect, leading to reduced growth hormone-releasing factor secretion or perhaps increased somatostatin production and subsequently low growth hormone level and growth failure.

DIFFERENTIAL DIAGNOSIS

The first step in the differential diagnosis of dwarfism is to determine whether skeletal or facial abnormalities are present; if so then one looks for further evidence of such disorders as the osteochondrodysplasias or the mucopolysaccharidoses. If not, that is to say if the child is otherwise of normal appearance and proportion, the next step is to undertake provocative tests to determine if there is a deficiency of growth hormone.

If there is a deficiency of growth hormone, one looks first for lesions of the hypothalamus or pituitary (e.g., inflammation or a tumor, especially a craniopharyngioma). In the absence of an identifiable lesion, one may be dealing with a genetic disorder (e.g., a mutation in the gene for the GHRH receptor in the pituitary) or psychosocial dwarfism. The differential at this point rests on the response to adequate care: as noted below, in psychosocial dwarfism growth hormone secretion promptly normalizes whereas in other disorders it remains depressed.

In cases where there is not a deficiency of growth hormone, consideration may be given to hypothyroidism, Cushing's syndrome or certain chronic disease (e.g., chronic renal failure, congenital heart disease, inflammatory bowel disease). In cases where the workup still remains unrewarding, one may be dealing with "constitutional short stature" and in such cases one finds that the parents were quite short in their own childhoods.

TREATMENT

With hospitalization and adequate care, growth hormone levels generally normalize within a few days, and within weeks the child may begin to grow and to behave more normally. Placement in a foster home is often required, as a return to the previous home is often followed by relapse. It is not clear whether, even with the best of foster parenting, all the signs and symptoms will eventually remit.

BIBLIOGRAPHY

Albanese A, Hamill G, Jones J, et al. Reversibility of physiological growth hormone secretion in children with psychosocial dwarfism. *Clinical Endocrinology* 1994;40:687-692.

Green WH, Campbell M, David R. Psychosocial dwarfism: a critical review of the evidence. *Journal of the American Academy of Child and Adolescent Psychiatry* 1984;23:39-48.

Money J. The syndrome of abuse dwarfism (psychosocial dwarfism or reversible hyposomatotropism). *American Journal of Diseases of Children* 1977;131:508-513.

Powell GF, Brasel JA, Blizzard RM. Emotional deprivation and growth retardation simulating idiopathic hypopituitarism. I. Clinical evaluation of the syndrome. *The New England Journal of Medicine* 1967;276: 1271-1278.

Powell GF, Brasel JA, Raiti S, et al. Emotional deprivation and growth retardation simulating idiopathic hypopituitarism. II. Endocrinologic evaluation of the syndrome. *The New England Journal of Medicine* 1967;276:1279-1283.

Silver HK, Finkelstein M. Deprivation dwarfism. *The Journal of Pediatrics* 1967;70:317-324.

Sydenham's chorea, also known as Saint Vitus' dance, rheumatic chorea, or chorea minor, is one of the manifestations of rheumatic fever, occurring in a minority of cases, and more frequently in girls than boys. In addition to chorea these patients typically also experience obsessions and compulsions, restlessness, delirium, or at times an excited psychosis, known as "maniacal chorea."

ONSET

Most cases occur between the ages of 10 and 15, and typically a latent period is evident between the more typical manifestations of rheumatic fever and the onset of Sydenham's chorea, averaging about 2 or 3 months and ranging from 1 week to 7 months.

The onset itself is generally subacute, spanning several weeks, during which there may be "fidgetiness," restlessness, irritability, mood lability and obsessions or compulsions.

CLINICAL FEATURES

The chorea is typically generalized, affecting the extremities and the face, and is often accompanied by dysarthria. In a minority of cases hemichorea may occur, and in a small percentage an almost flaccid paralysis occurs rather than chorea.

Mild symptoms such as irritability, emotional lability, emotional instability, crying spells, and difficulty with concentration and memory are common, occurring in the vast majority of patients. Obsessions and compulsions are also seen in the majority of patients, and these may be severe. Occasionally, tics are seen. Rarely, the chorea may be accompanied by delirium, mania, depression or a psychosis with delusions and hallucinations.

In a majority of cases, other evidence of rheumatic fever may be found; carditis and arthritis are most frequent. It must be kept in mind, however, that in a small minority of cases all other symptoms of rheumatic fever may have gone into remission before the onset of the chorea, leaving a case of "pure" Sydenham's chorea. A small minority of patients will also have seizures, which may be either grand mal or complex partial.

Routine "rheumatic" laboratory studies such as throat culture, ESR, ASO and anti-DNAase B may or may not be abnormal, depending on how much time has passed since the fateful streptococcal pharyngitis; of all these, anti-DNAase B levels tend to remain elevated the longest, in some cases for up to six months. CT scanning is generally normal; however, MRI scanning may reveal enlargement and increased signal intensity on T-2 weighted scans of the basal ganglia; in some cases, foci of increased signal intensity may also be seen in the thalamus, centrum semiovale and cerebral cortex.

COURSE

The overall duration of an episode of Sydenham's chorea ranges from as little as a week to over two years, averaging from four to six months; very rarely the chorea may persist in a chronic, life-long fashion. Recurrences may appear if the patient again develops a streptococcal pharyngitis.

COMPLICATIONS

Although most patients appear to recover completely, many will re-experience mild and transient choreiform movements with stress or fatigue, or upon taking certain medications, such as stimulants. Furthermore, in a significant minority of women who had Sydenham's chorea in childhood there will be a major recurrence of chorea with pregnancy, whereupon one speaks of "chorea gravidarum," or upon taking an oral contraceptive. In addition, some patients, both male and female, may be left with a degree of clumsiness or emotional lability.

It also appears that some patients, after recovering from Sydenham's chorea, will, as adolescents or adults, develop obsessive-compulsive disorder or Tourette's syndrome. Whether such cases should be subsumed under the new rubric of PANDAS (Pediatric Autoimmune Neuropsychiatric Disorders Associated with Streptococcal infections) is not clear.

ETIOLOGY

Sydenham's chorea results from a streptococcal-induced autoimmune process directed at small vessels, astrocytes, and neurons throughout the central nervous system, with the basal ganglia, cerebral cortex, and cerebral white matter suffering the brunt of the damage, and anti-basal ganglia serum antibodies may be found in almost all patients.

DIFFERENTIAL DIAGNOSIS

Few other conditions are capable of producing a clinical condition similar to this in children or young adolescents. Consideration may be given to systemic lupus erythematosus, the primary anti-phospholipid syndrome, hyperthyroidism, Wilson's disease, treatment with phenytoin or levodopa, intoxication with cocaine and tardive dyskinesia.

TREATMENT

Regardless of the severity of the chorea, all patients should receive penicillin VK 500 mg bid (or, if allergic, erythromycin 250 mg qid) for ten days: antibiotics should be given whether there is any clinical evidence of pharyngitis or not, as it is critical to eradicate all vestiges of the streptococcal infection. Subsequently, most patients should be treated prophylactically with benzathine penicillin G, 1.2 million U every four weeks until they finish High School.

A variety of medications show promise for the symptomatic treatment of Sydenham's chorea, including divalproex, carbamazepine and haloperidol. Divalproex may be given in a dose of 10 to 25 mg/kg/d. Carbamazepine is initiated at 10 mg/kg/d and increased gradually to a dose of from 600 to 800 mg/d. Haloperidol may be given in doses of from 1 to 4 mg/d. Overall, although there are no blinded studies of any of these agents, the impression is that divalproex is most effective. Some authors also advocate use of corticosteroids (e.g., prednisolone in doses of 2 mg/kg/d) on the not unreasonable supposition that aborting the underlying autoimmune process may not only be effective in limiting the current attack but also in reducing the chances of complications. In the case of divalproex, carbamazepine or haloperidol, treatment should generally be continued until the patient has been symptom-free for several weeks after which the dose is tapered: a re-emergence of symptoms indicates a need for further treatment. The optimum length of treatment for corticosteroids is not clear.

BIBLIOGRAPHY

Cardosos F, Eduardo C, Silva AP, et al. Chorea in fifty consecutive patients with rheumatic fever. *Movement Disorders* 1997;12:701.

Ch'ien LT, Economides AN, Lemmi H. Sydenham's chorea and seizures. Clinical and electroencephalographic studies. *Archives of Neurology* 1978;35:382-385.

Church AJ, Cardoso F, Dale RC, et al. Anti-basal ganglia antibodies in acute and persistent Sydenham's chorea. *Neurology* 2002;59:227-231.

Giedd JN, Rapoport JL, Kruesi MJ, et al. Sydenham's chorea: magnetic resonance imaging of the basal ganglia. *Neurology* 1995;45:2199-2202.

Green LN. Corticosteroids in the treatment of Sydenham's chorea. *Archives of Neurology* 1978;35:53-54.

Groothuis JR, Groothuis DR, Mukhopadhyay D, et al. Lupus-associated chorea in childhood. *American Journal of Diseases of Children* 1977; 131:1131-1134.

Moore DP. Neuropsychiatric aspects of Sydenham's chorea: a comprehensive review. *The Journal of Clinical Psychiatry* 1996;57:407-414.

Pena J, Mora E, Cardozo J, et al. Comparison of the efficacy of carbamazepine, haloperidol and valproic acid in the treatment of children with Sydenham's chorea: clinical follow-up of 18 patients. *Arquivos de Neuro-Psiquiatria* 2002;60:374-377.

Swedo SE, Leonard LH, Schapiro MB, et al. Sydenham's chorea: physical and psychological symptoms of St Vitus dance. *Pediatrics* 1993;91:706-713.

Van Horn G, Arnett FC, Dimachkie MM. Reversible dementia and chorea in a young woman with the lupus anticoagulant. *Neurology* 1996; 46:1599-1603.

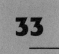

33 Kleine-Levin Syndrome

The Kleine-Levin syndrome is characterized by episodes of hypersomnolence accompanied by hyperphagia and, in most cases, altered sexual behavior. This is a rare disorder, seen most commonly in adolescent males.

ONSET

The first episode usually occurs sometime in adolescence or late childhood.

CLINICAL FEATURES

Episodes may be ushered in by a prodrome, lasting one to three days, of malaise, headache and lethargy. During the episode proper hypersomnia is prominent, with patients sleeping 18 or more hours per day. When not sleeping, most patients experience a ravenous appetite and display hyperphagia; many also display an unusual hypersexuality, with exhibitionism, unwelcome sexual advances, and excessive and sometimes public masturbation. Affective lability is common, and although depression may occur, a kind of euphoria appears more prominent. Humming, singing, and restlessness may be seen. Delusions, often persecutory, may occur, as may hallucinations, which tend to be visual. In a minority of cases there may be a degree of confusion.

The duration of an episode ranges from a few days up to a month; most seem to last a week or two. Upon recovery most patients are at least partially amnestic for the events occurring during the episode.

Although most patients are normal in the interval between episodes, some may demonstrate minor mood changes, such as irritability or forgetfulness and a decreased academic ability.

Polysomnography performed during the episode typically reveals decreased slow-wave sleep and multiple awakenings from stage 2 sleep. The multiple sleep latency test (MSLT) may demonstrate sleep-onset REM.

COURSE

The duration of the symptom-free intervals between episodes varies from as little as a few days to as much as a year. Early in the course, episodes tend to occur every 3 to 6 months. Over the ensuing years, however, episodes tend to become less severe and to be more widely spaced. In most patients, episodes spontaneously cease in the twenties or, occasionally, as late as the thirties.

COMPLICATIONS

Episodes derail the patient's academic and occupational progress and are extremely disruptive of family and social life.

ETIOLOGY

Most, but certainly not all, cases are preceded by a viral illness, such as an upper respiratory infection, and there is a long-standing suspicion that the Kleine-Levin syndrome represents an autoimmune disorder triggered by such a disorder. Although MRI studies have been unrevealing, there have been three autopsy studies with findings suggestive of diencephalic or brainstem involvement, and two of these studies documented gliosis. The alterations in sleep, appetite and sexuality have all suggested hypothalamic involvement, but efforts to find endocrinologic changes in the syndrome have not been consistently successful.

DIFFERENTIAL DIAGNOSIS

The Kleine-Levin syndrome is almost unique in its ability to produce episodes, lasting from days to months, of hypersomnia. Narcolepsy may come to mind, but here the episodes are quite brief, lasting no more than a half hour. Other disorders capable of producing hypersomnia, such as sleep apnea, are not episodic but are characterized by chronic sleepiness.

TREATMENT

There are no controlled studies here. Chronic treatment with lithium is often recommended, and during episodes themselves stimulants or stimulant-like medications, such as methylphenidate or modafinil, may be given.

BIBLIOGRAPHY

Carpenter S, Yassa R, Ochs R. A pathologic basis for Kleine-Levin syndrome. *Archives of Neurology* 1982;39:25-28.

Critchley M. Periodic hypersomnia and megaphagia in adolescent males. *Brain* 1962;85:627-656.

Dauvilliers Y, Mayer G, Lecendreux M, et al. Kleine-Levin syndrome: an autoimmune hypothesis based on clinical and genetic analyses. *Neurology* 2002;59:1739-1745.

Fenzi F, Simonati A, Crosato F, et al. Clinical features of Kleine-Levin syndrome with localized encephalitis. *Neuropediatrics* 1993;24:292-295.

Gadoth N, Kesler A, Vainstein G, et al. Clinical and polysomnographic characteristics of 34 patients with Kleine-Levin syndrome. *Journal of Sleep Research* 2001;10:337-341.

Koerber RK, Torkelson R, Haven G, et al. Increased cerebrospinal fluid 5-hydroxytryptamine and 5-hydroxyindoleacetic acid in Kleine-Levin syndrome. *Neurology* 1984;34:1597-1600.

Levin M. Periodic somnolence and morbid hunger: a new syndrome. *Brain* 1936;59:494-504.

Mayer G, Leonhard E, Krieg J, et al. Endocrinological and polysomnographic findings in Kleine-Levin syndrome: no evidence for hypothalamic and circadian dysfunction. *Sleep* 1998;21:278-284.

Muratori F, Bertini N, Masi G. Efficacy of lithium treatment in Kleine-Levin syndrome. *European Psychiatry* 2002;17:232-233.

Sagar RS, Khandelwal SK, Gupta S. Interepisodic morbidity in Kleine-Levin syndrome. *The British Journal of Psychiatry* 1990;157:139-141.

SUBSTANCE USE AND RELATED DISORDERS

34 Introduction to Substance Use Disorders

People take various substances because they like the effects. In some, such use stays at a "recreational" or "social" level; in others, abusive use occurs; and in still others, addiction, or compulsive use, occurs. Differentiating among these three forms of use is important not only with regard to prognosis but also with regard to treatment.

Most of these substances have the capacity to produce tolerance and withdrawal, whereas others generally do not. Those that routinely produce tolerance and withdrawal include the following: caffeine, cannabis, inhalants, nicotine, amphetamines, cocaine, opioids, sedative-hypnotics, and alcohol. Those that lack substantial capacity to produce tolerance and withdrawal include hallucinogens and phencyclidine.

The transition from recreational use to abusive use can occur in anyone and is probably heavily influenced by peer pressure and personal stresses from which the user seeks escape. The transition from abusive use to addiction, however, appears to occur only in those predisposed to develop a compulsive craving for the substance. In the case of some substances, for example alcohol, the presence or absence of this predisposition appears to be genetically determined. In the case of other substances, such as cocaine, the genesis of a craving for these substances is not clearly understood. Craving seems to develop only for those substances capable of producing tolerance and withdrawal. For example, the craving of an alcoholic for alcohol is a familiar phenomenon. On the other hand, even the most inveterate user of hallucinogens does not speak of a craving. Though he may want to "trip out," he does not experience a compulsion to use the hallucinogens; indeed he can stop if he wants to.

Tolerance and withdrawal, however, must not be equated with addiction. For example, a burn patient treated with an opioid may experience withdrawal when the opioid is finally stopped, yet in the vast majority of cases such patients experience no craving for the drug. They may have liked the way it made them feel, but they do not go out of their way to get more. Or a long-distance truck driver may take amphetamines for days in a row while on the road and then experience a significant withdrawal "crash" after getting home and stopping the amphetamine; glad that it is not needed anymore, the driver may not resume use until the next long-distance job.

TOLERANCE AND WITHDRAWAL

Tolerance is said to occur when the patient has to take ever-increasing amounts of the substance to get the desired effect. Tolerance may also be inferred when, over time, even though the

patient continues to use the same amount, the effect becomes progressively less.

Withdrawal symptoms occurring after use is discontinued often constitute a "rebound" from the effects of intoxication. For example, the placid alcohol-intoxicated patient may become tremulous, or the patient stimulated during cocaine intoxication may undergo a dysphoric, depressive "crash." During withdrawal many patients resort to "relief" use of the substance to quell the withdrawal symptoms, such as the "relief drinking" of an alcoholic who takes the "morning drink" to "steady the nerves" and "stop the shakes." Such a need for relief, however, must not be equated with a craving for the substance. Consider, for example, a patient who had taken a benzodiazepine exactly as prescribed for years, without ever exceeding the dose but who accidentally left the medicine at home while going on vacation. After a sleepless night and experiencing tremulousness the next day, the patient calls the physician who explains to the patient that these constitute withdrawal symptoms. Such a patient, though desperate for relief, may nevertheless decide that "it isn't worth it," and because she has no craving may simply not take anymore, "tough out" the withdrawal, and then get on with life.

In the past these phenomena of tolerance and withdrawal have been termed "physiologic dependence." However, because the word "dependence" often conjures up the image of addiction, another term, "neuroadaptation," has been coined. Neuroadaptation is clearly the preferred term for two reasons: first, it speaks to the underlying neuronal mechanism; and second, it is neutral with respect to addiction, thus emphasizing that tolerance and withdrawal, though ubiquitous in addiction, can also occur with abusive use, occasionally with recreational use, and also during appropriate medical treatment.

RECREATIONAL USE

Most Americans, at some point or other, "experiment" with substances, such as caffeine, nicotine, alcohol, cannabis, and, with ever-increasing frequency, cocaine. A morning cup of coffee and social drinking are typical examples. In some cases the substance produces some sort of dysphoria, and the person never uses it again. An example would be the teenager who gets "paranoid" the first time he smokes marijuana. In other cases peer pressure or a certain appreciation for the effects of the substance may prompt the patient to use the substance occasionally. Here the person is in the "take it or leave it alone" mode, and going to get the substance is no more important than, say, going to a good movie. He can "walk away from it" without a second thought.

In the case of caffeine, alcohol, cannabis, and perhaps also hallucinogens and phencyclidine, substance use for many appears to stay at a "recreational" level. Although a progression to abusive use may occur with any of these, a progression from recreational to abusive use appears more common for tobacco, stimulants, and especially cocaine and opioids. The likelihood of this progression is increased with intravenous use or with smoking "crack" cocaine.

ABUSIVE USE

In a minority of those who engage in recreational use, an abusive pattern of use will emerge. In some cases this progression is due to peer pressure, in others because neuroadaptation has occurred and "relief" use seems highly desirable, and in yet a third group abusive use may occur either because the person gets substantial enjoyment from the substance or because it helps the patient "cope" with life's problems.

Peer pressure is particularly important among teenagers and young adults. Since "everybody" is using, say, cannabis or alcohol to be "one of the crowd," these patients go along and use more than might be the case if left to their own devices.

The need for "relief" use may occasionally prompt use beyond that which the patient wishes. A salesperson, for example, may find daily drinking "necessary" for work as customers are entertained. Eventually, though, morning shakiness starts to occur, and though not welcoming the idea, such an individual finds it very difficult to hold off until a drink can be had with lunch.

For those whose lives are far from what they want, substance use may appear the only way to gain solace and peace, no matter how temporary, and if their lives continue in disarray, they may continue to use far more than is "normal" for them. Depressed patients are particularly prone to this genesis of substance abuse.

Regardless of what prompts them to go beyond recreational use, the results are the same: patients continue to use the substance despite suffering consequences directly attributable to that use. Thus an alcohol abuser may continue to drink despite the fact that spouse and friends say they do not like it. Or a cannabis abuser may continue to smoke marijuana even though a cough has developed and school grades have started to fall.

At some point substance abusers weigh the consequences against what they get out of the substance use. When the consequences are relatively mild the patient may consider them to be acceptable losses and continue to use. In cases where the consequences become severe, however, most patients, at the least, attempt to stop or moderate their use.

At this point, if not before, "denial" becomes apparent as patients minimize or simply pay no attention to the consequences of abusive use. If pressed they may become irritable and insist that they can "handle it."

In many cases, however, the consequences eventually outweigh any satisfaction from substance use, and the patient either substantially moderates his use back to a recreational level or stops altogether. Some who attempt to stop may do it on their own; others, especially those with significant withdrawal symptoms or those whose lives seem intolerable without substance use, may require treatment. Though such patients may miss the intoxication and find it hard to imagine going on without it, they as yet do not experience a craving for it. "Walking away from it" may be more difficult than it is for the recreational user, but fundamentally it is still a matter of choice. Once the patient has made a choice and put his heart into abstinence, success usually follows.

ADDICTION

In a minority of those who abuse substances, addiction may occur. This transition is marked by the appearance of a craving for the substance.

The significance of craving cannot be overstated. These patients experience an overpowering compulsion to use the substance and are driven by that compulsion to repeated use despite the most disastrous consequences. Despite repeated attempts to control their use, by either moderating it or stopping it altogether, addicts find themselves again and again intoxicated.

The appearance of craving may be gradual and insidious or at times acute. But in the history of every addict is a time when she "crosses the line" and is no longer able to stop.

Once craving develops, denial becomes severe. Cocaine addicts driven to theft and robbery to support their "habit" may insist that they are "in charge." Or alcoholics literally living in the gutter may blame all their problems on everyone and everything else except, of course, the bottle. At times denial may be so severe that the patients themselves have no awareness of the problem. For example, an alcoholic recently discharged from the hospital after experiencing delirium tremens (DTs) and seizures simply walked into a bar without any compunction or reservation whatsoever, experiencing no more concern than a drinker who has a drink perhaps only twice a year.

Most of the time, however, addicts are aware of the consequences, yet continue to use. They may miss work, fail to keep social engagements, or neglect spouse and children. Health may fail; the alcoholic may develop cirrhosis; the cocaine addict, a perforated nasal septum; the tobacco addict, emphysema, even lung cancer; and yet they continue to use.

Eventually, substance use becomes the primary, if not the sole, motivating factor in the patient's life. Family, friends, and work pale by importance, and all the patient's efforts become directed to one thing: ensuring an unbroken supply of the substance.

Although most addicts at times attempt to moderate or stop altogether, in some cases no such attempt occurs. In these cases denial is so strong that the only things that reliably stop use are incarceration or death. Those who do try and stop on their own generally fail in the attempt, and after numerous attempts may eventually give up trying.

SUMMARY

At the risk of oversimplification, these three forms of substance use may be epitomized as follows. Recreational users can "take it or leave it" and suffer few, if any, consequences from their use. Abusive users, however, find themselves continuing to use despite significant consequences. Although they can still "take it or leave it," the leaving of it may require considerable effort. Finally, addicts, or compulsive users, have lost the power of choice due to their craving. They must continue taking the substance and, despite the greatest exertion of individual will, find it impossible to leave it alone despite the most disastrous consequences.

As noted earlier, neuroadaptation, or the development of tolerance and withdrawal, may or may not develop during abusive use. However, neuroadaptation appears to occur in almost all cases of addiction.

In the following chapters some of the more important substances are discussed. Those for which significant craving does not occur and for which addiction does not occur include the following: caffeine, hallucinogens and phencyclidine. Those that may become craved and to which addiction may occur include the following: cannabis, inhalants, nicotine, stimulants, cocaine, opioids, sedative-hypnotics, and alcohol. (Following the chapter on alcoholism are a series of chapters on the many alcohol-related disorders.)

Before closing this introductory section, some comments are appropriate about the word "addiction." Many would prefer that it be expunged from the language, as it conjures up the most sordid of images. They wish instead to use the word "dependence." Unfortunately, as noted earlier, "dependence" has at least two meanings, and the employment of such a word invites misunderstanding. On the other hand, the word "addiction" is well understood, and, as for its negative connotations, perhaps we should welcome them. Addiction should not be sanitized. It is a sordid affair, and drags patients into undreamt of degradation. Sugarcoating this decline by calling it dependence may only serve the patient's denial.

BIBLIOGRAPHY

Koob GF, Nestler EJ. The neurobiology of drug addiction. *The Journal of Neuropsychiatry and Clinical Neurosciences* 1997;9:482-497.

Lyvers M. Drug addiction as a physical disease: the role of physical dependence and other chronic drug-induced neurophysiological changes in compulsive drug self-administration. *Experimental and Clinical Psychopharmacology* 1998;6:107-125.

McLellan AT, Lewis DC, O'Brien CP, et al. Drug dependence, a chronic mental illness: implications for treatment, insurance, and outcomes evaluation. *The Journal of the American Medical Association* 2000;284:1689-1695.

Tomkins DM, Sellers EM. Addiction and the brain: the role of neurotransmitters in the cause and treatment of drug dependence. *Canadian Medical Association Journal* 2001;164:817-821.

Weiss F, Porrino LJ. Behavioral neurobiology of alcohol addiction: recent advances and challenges. *The Journal of Neuroscience* 2002;22:3332-3337.

35 Caffeine Related Disorders (DSM-IV-TR #305.90, 292.89)

A majority of Americans use caffeine on a daily basis for its mild stimulant effect without any untoward effects. A minority, however, develop a pattern of abusive use wherein they continue to use caffeine despite recurrent episodes of caffeine intoxication or the development of other consequences, such as exacerbation of peptic ulcer disease secondary to coffee. Tolerance and withdrawal may also occur.

A cup of coffee contains about 100 mg of caffeine, tea about 50 mg, and caffeinated soft drinks anywhere from 25 to 200 mg. Over-the-counter analgesic and "cold" preparations, "stimulants," anorectics, herbal products and health food products may contain anywhere from 25 to 200 mg. Caffeine is almost completely absorbed, reaching peak blood levels in from 30 to 60 minutes. Metabolism is via the cytochrome P450 1A2 hepatic enzyme system, with a half-life ranging from three to five hours.

ONSET

Caffeine abuse tends to occur in early or middle adult years.

CLINICAL FEATURES

In caffeine-naive patients, about 100 mg of caffeine produces an increased sense of alertness and decreased fatigue. At doses between 200 and 500 mg, however, caffeine intoxication begins. Patients feel apprehensive, restless, and even agitated, and complain of headache and insomnia. Tremor and tachycardia may appear. At doses of about 1 g, intense anxiety to the point of panic occurs. Agitation may be extreme, and tremor and tachycardia are now quite prominent. Premature beats and muscle twitches may occur. Significantly higher doses (e.g., 10 gm) may produce serious arrhythmias, such as ventricular fibrillation, grand mal seizures, respiratory depression and death.

Provided that no further caffeine is ingested, symptoms of intoxication tend to clear in a matter of hours, and recovery is generally complete within 6 to 12 hours. Neuroadaptation may develop after daily use of only 500 mg of caffeine over a couple of weeks time. Tolerance is manifest by the ability of the patient to consume, without ill effect, doses of caffeine that would cause intoxication in caffeine-naive individuals. Withdrawal tends to occur in 12 to 24 hours after the last dose and is characterized by headache, poor concentration, fatigue, anxiety, irritability, and depressed mood, all gradually clearing in from 2 days up to a week.

COURSE

The course of caffeine abuse is not known.

COMPLICATIONS

The agitation and irritability seen in intoxication may strain the patient's relations at work and at home. Long-term coffee use may aggravate peptic ulcers, gastroesophageal reflux, fibrocystic disease and hypertension.

DIFFERENTIAL DIAGNOSIS

Panic attacks may be confused with caffeine intoxication; however, attacks tend to be of much more acute onset and to remit in 15 minutes or so rather than lasting for hours. Of course, as noted in the chapter on panic disorder, panic attacks in patients with panic disorder may at times be precipitated by caffeine.

Chronic caffeine intoxication may very closely mimic generalized anxiety disorder; indeed abstinence from caffeine may be required to make the diagnosis.

Chronic intoxication in a patient taking an antipsychotic may resemble akathisia; however, in akathisia tremor and tachycardia generally are not seen. In doubtful cases prohibiting caffeine or using a test dose of benztropine may resolve the issue.

TREATMENT

Caffeine intoxication itself generally requires no specific treatment, and the same is generally true of caffeine withdrawal.

In most cases, with education about the consequences of caffeine abuse, most caffeine abusers are able to either moderate their use or to stop altogether without undue difficulty. In some cases it may be helpful to keep a "caffeine diary" to establish the daily dosage, and then to gradually withdraw the caffeine at a rate of about 10% of the total daily dose per day.

BIBLIOGRAPHY

Brice CF, Smith AP. Effects of caffeine on mood and performance: a study of realistic consumption. *Psychopharmacology* 2002;164:188-192.

Bruce M, Scott N, Shine P, et al. Anxiogenic effects of caffeine in patients with anxiety disorders. *Archives of General Psychiatry* 1992;49:867-869.

Cannon ME, Cooke CT, McCarthy JS. Caffeine-induced cardiac arrythmia: an unrecognized danger of healthfood products. *The Medical Journal of Australia* 2001;174:520-521.

Donovan JL, DeVane CL. A primer on caffeine pharmacology and its drug interactions in clinical psychopharmacology. *Psychopharmacology Bulletin* 2001;35:30-48.

Griffiths RR, Bigelow GE, Liebson IA. Human coffee drinking: reinforcing and physical dependence producing effects of caffeine. *The Journal of Pharmacology and Experimental Therapeutics* 1986;239:416-425.

Hughes JR, Higgins SD, Bickel WK, et al. Caffeine self-administration, withdrawal, and adverse effects among coffee drinkers. *Archives of General Psychiatry* 1991;48:611-617.

36 | Cannabis Related Disorders (DSM-IV-TR #305.20, 305.30, 292.89, 292.11, 292.12, 292.81)

■

Although occasional use of cannabis is as common as that of alcohol, cannabis abuse or dependence occurs in only a small minority of adolescents or young adults, perhaps 5% or less.

"Cannabis" comes from the Greek word for hemp and refers to the flowering tops of the hemp plant, Cannabis sativa. In the United States the two most commonly available preparations of cannabis are marijuana and hashish. Marijuana (also known as "grass," "pot," "reefer," "weed," or "Mary Jane") is simply a dried collection of the flowers and nearby leaves and sprouts of the hemp plant and is usually rolled into a cigarette. Hashish, on the other hand, is more potent and is the resin that is scraped from the leaves and flowers of the plant.

The principal intoxicant in cannabis is the delta-9 isomer of tetrahydrocannabinol, or THC. Marijuana contains anywhere from 1% to 15% THC, whereas hashish contains at a minimum 10%, with the concentrated hashish oil containing up to 60%.

THC is highly lipid soluble and readily crosses the blood-brain barrier. Two endogenous cannabinoid receptors have been identified in the central nervous system, namely CB1 and CB2; the CB1 receptors appear responsible for the euphoriant effects of THC, and are concentrated in the basal ganglia, hippocampus, cerebral cortex and cerebellum. After either marijuana or hashish is smoked, central nervous system effects begin to appear within minutes and reach their peak within a half hour. Although the intoxication lasts for only 3 or 4 hours, the half-life of THC is much longer, up to three or four days, owing in large part to its storage in, and slow release from, lipocytes. THC or its metabolites may be detected in the urine for anywhere from 2 to 6 days in infrequent users and up to several weeks in chronic users.

Marijuana is occasionally taken orally, often mixed in brownies or cookies. After oral use, CNS effects begin to appear in about one half hour; peak effects coincide with peak blood levels and occur at about 2 or 3 hours.

In a minority of users marijuana intoxication may be complicated by a variety of symptoms including the following: anxiety, which may be extreme to the point of panic; psychosis; and delirium.

ONSET

Cannabis abuse generally begins in adolescence. Moderate or "social" users tend to reduce their use or stop altogether as they enter into adult years and assume more responsibilities. The adolescent who used cannabis heavily, however, is likely to persist in that use into early adult years.

CLINICAL FEATURES

Cannabis intoxication is characterized for most individuals by a dreamy sense of well-being. The senses feel heightened; color and sounds appear unusually sharp and clear. Time seems to slow down, and minutes may seem like hours. Thinking becomes less logical, and everyday things may come to seem ridiculous and amusing. Laughter and giggling may occur, and although this may leave the unintoxicated unmoved, it often is infectious to others who are intoxicated.

While intoxicated, most individuals have difficulty remembering things and paying attention. The mouth is dry, and most experience increased hunger, often for cookies or brownies. The conjunctivae are reddened, sometimes markedly so. A mild degree of ataxia may be seen. The heart rate is generally elevated, and although the supine blood pressure is often elevated, orthostatic hypotension may occur upon standing.

In a minority of cases the intoxication may be complicated by any of a number of events. Perhaps the most common complication is anxiety, which at times may be as severe as that seen in a panic attack. This cannabis-induced anxiety generally passes as the intoxication does. Depersonalization or derealization may also occur during intoxication.

A less common complication is the development of a psychosis. This "cannabis-induced psychotic disorder," as it is sometimes called, is characterized by the fairly abrupt appearance during intoxication of compelling delusions of persecution, which may be accompanied by auditory or visual hallucinations. Extreme anxiety is commonly associated with this, and although patients rarely attack their "persecutors," many will flee or seek safety in some other way. The psychosis generally outlasts the intoxication per se, and indeed may persist for 1 to 3 days.

These two complications, anxiety and psychosis, may occur after smoking only a relatively small amount of marijuana. When much higher doses are taken, a delirium may occur. This cannabis intoxication delirium is characterized by confusion and, often, agitation. Thinking is quite illogical, and delusions and hallucinations often appear. This delirium may clear as the intoxication does or it may last for up to a few days.

The pattern of recurrent intoxication is quite different between the "social user" and the patient with cannabis abuse or dependence. Social use is often confined to weekends and generally occurs with friends. Cannabis abusers typically smoke marijuana or hashish on a daily basis, and often do so alone. The pattern is similar for cannabis addicts, whose entire lives often center on getting and staying intoxicated and who also develop either tolerance or withdrawal.

Tolerance is manifested by a decreased euphoria and a diminution in the tachycardia and blood pressure changes. If withdrawal occurs it tends to be mild and to appear anywhere from 3 to 12 hours after the cannabis was last used. Patients are anxious, irritable, and restless and almost always complain of some insomnia. Anorexia and increased sweating are seen, and some patients may develop a fine tremor. Symptoms generally peak in 1 to 2 days and resolve spontaneously within 4 to 5 days.

Most patients with cannabis abuse also use other substances to excess. Alcohol and cocaine use are perhaps the most common associated substances; however, use of opioids, hallucinogens, or phencyclidine may also occur. Occasionally, phencyclidine or an hallucinogen may be mixed into the cannabis and taken simultaneously.

Before ending this discussion on symptomatology, one controversial area must be touched on, namely whether or not heavy chronic cannabis use may cause a chronic psychotic condition. Some patients in the midst of active cannabis use clearly may develop an illness very similar to paranoid or undifferentiated schizophrenia that may persist for months or years after cessation of cannabis use. What is not clear is whether this represents merely a coincidence of two independent illnesses, cannabis abuse and schizophrenia, or a "triggering" of a latent schizophrenia by cannabis. Most clinicians doubt that chronic cannabis use per se can cause such a condition directly.

COURSE

The long-term course of cannabis abuse and dependence is not known.

COMPLICATIONS

Impaired performance may lead to automobile or airplane crashes or accidents with hazardous machinery.

The symptoms of schizophrenia may be exacerbated by cannabis.

Flashbacks, similar to those seen with hallucinogens, may occur in a minority of cases.

Chronic marijuana or hashish smoking may result in bronchitis. Whether the risk of cancer is increased is not clear. Cannabis-induced tachycardia may aggravate classic angina.

THC is excreted in the breast milk, and infants may become intoxicated. Babies born of women who abuse cannabis during pregnancy may be underweight at birth.

DIFFERENTIAL DIAGNOSIS

Cannabis intoxication at times may be mimicked by alcohol or hallucinogen intoxication. More to the point, since multiple substance use is common among cannabis users, the diagnostician may be faced with a mixed intoxication. The mere finding of cannabinoids in the urine does not necessarily indicate that the patient used cannabis himself. Those who spend a considerable amount of time in an enclosed space with people using cannabis may inhale enough secondary smoke to produce a false positive urine test.

Delusions occurring during amphetamine or cocaine intoxication may be similar to those occasionally seen in cannabis intoxication; however, here the patient is often more agitated than the cannabis-intoxicated patient.

Delirium appearing in cannabis intoxication apparently has no distinctive features, and if the history of cannabis use is not available, the differential becomes similar to that described in the chapter on delirium.

TREATMENT

Uncomplicated intoxication rarely requires any treatment. An exception may be a patient who was intent on using potentially hazardous machinery who might have to be detained until the intoxication clears.

Patients who have become panic stricken during an intoxication can often be "talked down"; occasionally a benzodiazepine with a long half-life, such as diazepam 10 mg, may be required.

Psychosis, if persistent and troubling, may be treated either with an anxiolytic or an antipsychotic. Haloperidol, 5 to 10 mg, is often given; although a second generation antipsychotic, such as olanzapine, is better tolerated, it does not appear to be more effective. Given the natural course of the delusions, prolonged treatment is not required.

Delirious patients may require admission for their own protection; treatment is as outlined in the chapter on delirium.

Cannabis withdrawal is generally mild and specific treatment is not required.

Treatment aimed at abstinence is both difficult and frustrating. Many patients see no need for treatment, and many adolescents rebelliously refuse to cooperate. Group therapy with other cannabis abusers may hold some promise; most of these patients do not feel "at home" in Alcoholics Anonymous or Narcotics Anonymous and generally do not follow through with these referrals. When patients live at home with their parents, as is often the case, family therapy may be helpful. Inpatient care is rarely required; however, it may be useful for patients who cannot avoid intoxication long enough to engage in outpatient treatment.

BIBLIOGRAPHY

Ashton CH. Pharmacology and effects of cannabis: a brief review. *The British Journal of Psychiatry* 2001;178:101-106.

Berk M, Brook S, Trandafir AI. A comparison of olanzapine with haloperidol in cannabis-induced psychotic disorder: a double-blind randomized controlled trial. *International Clinical Psychopharmacology* 1999;14:177-180.

Duffy A, Millin R. Case study: withdrawal syndrome in adolescent chronic cannabis users. *Journal of the American Academy of Child and Adolescent Psychiatry* 1996;35:1618-1621.

Hall W, Degenhardt L. Cannabis use and psychosis: a review of clinical and epidemiological evidence. *The Australian and New Zealand Journal of Psychiatry* 2000;34:26-34.

Hall W, Solowij N. Adverse effects of cannabis. *Lancet* 1998;352: 1611-1616.

Haney M, Ward AS, Comer SD, et al. Abstinence symptoms following oral THC administration to humans. *Psychopharmacology* 1999;141: 385-394.

Keeler MH, Reifler CB, Liptzin MB. Spontaneous recurrence of marijuana effect. *The American Journal of Psychiatry* 1968;125:384-386.

Pope HG, Gruber AJ, Hudson JI, et al. Neuropsychological performance in long-term cannabis users. *Archives of General Psychiatry* 2001;58: 909-915.

37 Hallucinogen Related Disorders (DSM-IV-TR #305.30, 292.89, 292.11, 292.12, 292.84)

The hallucinogens, also known as psychedelics or psychotomimetics, may be roughly divided into two groups: the indolealkylamines, such as LSD, and the phenylalkylamines, such as mescaline (Table 37-1). Although each drug differs somewhat in its effects, the drugs' similarities are sufficient to permit them to be considered as a group.

With the exception of dimethyltryptamine (DMT), which must be smoked, insufflated, or injected, all of the hallucinogens are generally taken orally. The hallucinatory intoxication is the desired effect; however, unwanted effects are not uncommon. The intoxication itself may be complicated by extreme dysphoria and panic and turn into a "bad trip." In some the intoxication may be followed by sustained depression and anxiety. A more serious sequela, however, is a prolonged psychosis that in some may be very similar to schizophrenia. Finally a substantial minority of patients may experience recurrent "flashbacks."

Although occasional use of an hallucinogen is not uncommon, occurring in from 10 to 20% of all adolescents and adults, abuse of hallucinogens is apparently relatively uncommon, appearing in less than 0.5% of adolescents and young adults. Interestingly one of the earliest descriptions of personal experience of mescaline intoxication in the medical literature comes to us from the eminent nineteenth and early twentieth century physician, S. Weir Mitchell.

ONSET

Hallucinogen abuse typically begins in adolescence.

CLINICAL FEATURES

After oral use of most hallucinogens, intoxication begins gradually within 20 minutes to 1 hour. A certain tension or apprehension may occur, soon followed by an alteration in the state of consciousness that is difficult to describe. Although fully alert and oriented, patients describe a "cosmic" sense of unity with those around them. Heretofore trivial, mundane phenomena become imbued with deep meaning. A sense of the profound surrounds thoughts, and memories may rush to mind as if they were present, palpable realities. Visual illusions and hallucinations are common, and patients often relate to them as they would to a movie. Patients acknowledge that they are not real, yet they are captivated by them. Rippling colors and geometric forms may occur; bodies may appear distorted, and at times complex visual hallucinations of people or things may occur. After-images may occur, and a previous perception may be superimposed as in a double exposure on the current percept. Auditory hallucinations may also occur but are far less common and tend to be noncomplex. Occasionally synesthesiae may occur: colors may be heard, or a touch may be experienced as a color.

Intoxication with MDMA ("Ecstasy") is somewhat different than that seen with other hallucinogens, being characterized by an initial "rush," followed by a heightened sense of empathy or connectedness with others.

Not uncommonly the intoxication may become extremely dysphoric as it evolves into a "bad trip." Anxiety sets in as the patient vainly attempts to control his thoughts and perceptions. Some fear dissolution; others are in terror that they are losing their minds and that the trip will never end. Delusions of reference and persecution may occur, and the patient, panic-stricken, may be brought to the hospital.

On examination of the intoxicated patient one finds mild degrees of tachycardia, hypertension, mydriasis, fine tremor, poor coordination, and generalized hyperreflexia: in the case of MDMA, bruxism may also be seen. The temperature may be elevated.

Regardless of whether the intoxication is pleasant or not, patients generally recover within 6 to 24 hours after most hallucinogens with the exceptions of psilocybin and DMT, which produce shorter intoxications of only 2 to 6 hours.

■ TABLE 37-1. Hallucinogens

Name	Source
Indolealkylamines	
Lysergic acid diethylamide (LSD)	Synthetic
Psilocybin	Psilocybe mushroom
Dimethyltryptamine (DMT)	Synthetic
Phenylalkylamines	
Mescaline	Peyote cactus or synthetic
Dimethoxymethylamphetamine (DOM)	Synthetic
Dimethoxyamphetamine (DMA)	Synthetic
Methylenedioxyamphetamine (MDA)	Synthetic
3,4-methylenedioxymethamphetamine (MDMA or "Ecstasy")	Synthetic
3,4-methylenedioxy-N-ethylamphetamine (MDEA, or "Eve")	Synthetic

Tolerance to the euphoriant effect occurs rapidly, within days, to all hallucinogens, with the sole exception of DMT. Importantly, however, tolerance does not develop to the autonomic effects of hallucinogens, such as tachycardia, hypertension, and tremor. Interestingly, despite the development of tolerance, there are no withdrawal symptoms.

As noted earlier several sequelae may be seen after the intoxication has resolved: various mood changes, a psychosis that may be prolonged, and flashbacks. A minority of patients develop an hallucinogen-induced mood disorder shortly after the intoxication resolves, usually within days. Most commonly, depression is seen with anxiety, insomnia, and an unrelenting fear that the drug has caused permanent damage. At times, patients are severely agitated, and suicide attempts have occurred. Less commonly, manic symptoms may occur, and one may see a heightened mood, hyperactivity, pressured speech, and a decreased need for sleep. These mood changes tend to be relatively brief, lasting only a few days; rarely, however, they may persist for much longer, up to weeks.

Also in a small minority of patients, an hallucinogen-induced psychotic disorder may emerge shortly after the intoxication resolves. This may be characterized by any of the symptoms seen during the intoxication with one critical difference: here the patient believes that they are real. Although generally lasting only a few days, some cases have been reported with durations running to weeks, months, or longer, and in such cases the clinical picture is very similar to that seen in schizophrenia.

Flashbacks (also known as "hallucinogen persisting perception disorder") may occur in up to a quarter of all patients. Here, while not intoxicated, the patient experiences one or more of the symptoms seen in the intoxication. Generally the flashback itself is quite brief, sometimes lasting only seconds. Patients may experience complex visual hallucinations, or only shapes, color, or "trailing" of after-images. Auditory and tactile hallucinations may also be seen. Flashbacks may occur spontaneously or may be precipitated by moving into a darkened area, or by the use of alcohol, marijuana, or an antipsychotic. They may be infrequent or occur multiple times every day. In the majority, flashbacks cease to occur within weeks or months; however, in some they may become chronic, lasting years.

"Social" use of hallucinogens is generally fairly limited. Most people who take hallucinogens do so only a few times and then stop. Some find the first intoxication so dysphoric that they never take one again. A minority of those who use hallucinogens recreationally may enjoy the experience and may continue to use the drug intermittently; this is particularly the case with MDMA, which is often repeatedly used by young people at all-night parties known as "raves." Given the tolerance that rapidly develops, frequent daily use almost never occurs as patients must wait at least a few days before intoxication is again possible. In the meantime, other drugs, such as marijuana, alcohol, or phencyclidine, are often used. Hallucinogen abuse is relatively rare and is generally accompanied by a concurrent disorder such as a borderline personality disorder or an antisocial personality disorder.

COURSE

Although the long-term course of hallucinogen abuse is not known with certainty, many patients stop or moderate their use by middle adult years.

COMPLICATIONS

The ability to work and sustain normal relationships is generally seriously impaired during intoxication or a subsequent disorder of mood or a subsequent psychosis.

Overdosage with hallucinogens is generally not fatal; exceptions, however, occur, with DMA, MDA and, especially, MDMA ("Ecstasy"). In the case of MDMA, overdose may result in hyperpyrexia, cardiac arrhythmia, seizures, rhabdomyolysis with renal failure, disseminated intravascular coagulation and hepatic necrosis.

MDMA causes destruction of serotoninergic neurons in non-human primates, and there is suggestive evidence for the same effect in humans. Furthermore, there is good evidence for mild cognitive impairment, even in recreational users, which persists into abstinence for years.

Although LSD use is associated with an increased rate of spontaneous abortion and fetal malformations, whether this is directly related to LSD or to contaminates is not clear. LSD does not appear to cause chromosomal abnormalities.

ETIOLOGY

All the hallucinogens have complex agonist/antagonist activity at either presynaptic or postsynaptic serotonin receptors.

The mechanism underlying postintoxication mood changes or flashbacks is not known. In cases where a postintoxication psychosis becomes prolonged, it is speculated that the patient had a preexisting diathesis for schizophrenia.

DIFFERENTIAL DIAGNOSIS

Intoxications with other substances are generally readily distinguished by the appearance of drowsiness, sedation, or disorientation—effects not typically caused by hallucinogens. Phencyclidine may produce a picture similar to an hallucinogen; however, here one finds nystagmus, which is not seen with hallucinogens.

Should a postintoxication mood change be prolonged, one might consider an affective disorder. The history of hallucinogen use and the presence of any other sequelae, such as flashbacks, would suggest the correct diagnosis.

A prolonged psychotic sequela, as noted earlier, may appear very similar to schizophrenia. As noted in the subsection on etiology, however, some believe that the differential question here is moot, as it appears that the hallucinogen may have precipitated schizophrenia in a patient so predisposed.

Flashbacks, especially visual ones, may be mimicked by partial sensory seizures, peduncular hallucinations, migrainous auras, and local ocular disturbances.

TREATMENT

Dysphoric intoxication may usually be managed by supportively "talking the patient down." Occasionally a short-acting benzodiazepine, such as lorazepam, may be helpful. Antipsychotics have also been used, but paradoxic reactions have been seen. Theoretically the serotonin blocker cyproheptadine should be helpful.

Postintoxication mood changes are generally best managed with supportive care. Hospitalization may be required if the risk of suicide is significant. Given the short course of the disorder, antidepressants are generally not indicated.

Likewise postintoxication psychoses are generally best approached initially with supportive watchful waiting. Antipsychotics may be used if symptoms are severe or prolonged; although the first-generation agent haloperidol has been most widely used, consideration may be given to a second-generation agent such as risperidone.

Flashbacks generally require no treatment except reassurance. Clonidine and clonazepam have each, anecdotally, been effective; antipsychotics are generally not effective, and, indeed, risperidone may exacerbate flashbacks.

Treatment of hallucinogen abuse per se is very difficult. Concurrent disorders, such as borderline or antisocial personality disorder, must be taken into account.

BIBLIOGRAPHY

Abraham HD, Mamen A. LSD-like panic from risperidone in post-LSD visual disorder. *Journal of Clinical Psychopharmacology* 1996;16: 238-241.

Henry JA. Ecstasy and the dance of death: sèvere reactions are unpredictable. *British Medical Journal* 1992;305:5-6.

Kalant H. The pharmacology and toxicology of "ecstasy" (MDMA) and related drugs. *Canadian Medical Association Journal* 2001;165: 917-928.

Lerner AG, Gelkopf M, Skladman I, et al. Flashback and hallucinogen persisting perception disorder: clinical aspects and pharmacological treatment approach. *The Israel Journal of Psychiatry and Related Sciences* 2002;39:92-99.

Morgan MJ, McFie L, Fleetwood H, et al. Ecstasy (MDMA): are the psychological problems associated with its use reversed by prolonged abstinence? *Psychopharmacology* 2002;159:294-303.

Peroutka SJ, Newman H, Harris H. Subjective effects of 3,4 methyldioxymethamphetamine in recreational abusers. *Neuropsychopharmacology* 1988;1:273-277.

Reneman L, Lavalaye J, Schmand B, et al. Cortical serotonin transporter density and verbal memory in individuals who stopped using 3,4-methylenedioxymethamphetamine (MDMA or "ecstasy"): preliminary findings. *Archives of General Psychiatry* 2001;58:901-906.

38 Phencyclidine (or Phencyclidine-Like) Related Disorders (DSM-IV-TR #292.89, 292.81, 292.11, 292.12, 292.84, 304.60, 305.90)

Phencyclidine and its closely related derivative ketamine are arylcyclohexylamines developed as "dissociative" anesthetics: the frequent occurrence of a post-operative psychosis with phencyclidine led to its abandonment as an anesthetic; however, ketamine, as it is less problematic in this regard, is still used in anesthetic practice. Both these drugs are used also as intoxicants, and the popularity of ketamine as a "club" drug appears on the rise. Phencyclidine is also known as "PCP," "angel dust," "Hog," and "peace pill"; ketamine may be referred to as "K," "Special K," "Vitamin K," "Cat Valium," "Kat" or "Kit-Kat."

The intoxication produced by phencyclidine has similarities to that produced by amphetamines and by hallucinogens such as LSD. Sufficient differences exist, however, for phencyclidine and related compounds such as ketamine to be considered in a class by themselves. Presuming that users have found the optimum intoxicating dose for themselves, these drugs may produce a euphoric state in which users feel at a distance, or are dissociated, from their environment. Unfortunately, however, the intoxicating dose is very close to the toxic dose, and serious toxic effects have been common.

Delusions, hallucinations, and bizarre and at times violent behavior may occur; at higher doses, stupor, coma, and respiratory depression may also be seen.

The prevalence of recreational use is not known with certainty, but it appears that at least several percent of adolescents and young adults use one of these drugs at least occasionally. Abuse is less common, and whether or not addiction occurs is not clear—if it does, it is rare. Exclusive use of these drugs is rare; most users also avail themselves of alcohol or marijuana.

Phencyclidine and ketamine may be taken orally, by intranasal "snorting," intravenously, or by smoking. Blood levels rise slowly after oral or intranasal administration; rapid rises are seen after intravenous or pulmonary administration. Both drugs undergo extensive hepatic metabolism.

Phencyclidine is both a weak base and lipophilic, and these two characteristics have significant clinical consequences. As a weak base phencyclidine is secreted into and sequestered in the acid gastric fluids, and considerable gastroenteric recirculation occurs. Being lipophilic it is also sequestered in adipose tissue. Thus protected from hepatic metabolism by sequestration in the stomach or adipocytes, the parent compound may be detectable in the blood for weeks, and occasionally longer.

It is doubtful whether tolerance or withdrawal occurs with phencyclidine or ketamine. Some patients may describe depressive symptoms after cessation of long-term use, but such complaints are not common and not impressive. Whether or not craving per se develops is controversial.

Both phencyclidine and ketamine act as non-competitive antagonists at cation channels within the NMDA receptor complex, and although numerous other receptors are also affected, it is this action at the NMDA receptor which appears responsible for the intoxicant and psychotogenic effects of these drugs.

ONSET

Phencyclidine and ketamine use usually begin in teenage years. Initial exposure may be accidental, with phencyclidine being present as a contaminant of marijuana, stimulants, or hallucinogens.

CLINICAL FEATURES

Intoxication with phencyclidine or ketamine may, as noted below, be roughly characterized as mild, moderate or severe: ketamine is less potent than phencyclidine and only rarely produces the severe, and potentially life-threatening, intoxication not uncommonly seen with phencyclidine. Intravenous use is rare, and oral use, given its slow onset and often unpredictable results, is uncommon: "snorting" or smoking is preferred, with, in the case of smoking, an onset of intoxication in minutes or less.

Mild intoxication is characterized by euphoria and a peculiar sense of detachment. Users may feel as if they are floating; the body often appears misshapen. Agitation and labile affect may occur; at times users may appear lethargic. Bizarre, unpredictable behavior may occur, and violent aggressive behavior appears to occur more frequently during intoxication with phencyclidine than with other substances. Users often complain of vertigo, and nausea and vomiting are experienced by some. Characteristic signs often accompany the intoxication. Users are often dysarthric and ataxic. Nystagmus is particularly characteristic and may be rotatory, horizontal, or vertical. Increased salivation, diaphoresis, and flushing may occur. Myoclonus and tremor may also be observed. Tachycardia, increased blood pressure, an increased respiratory rate, and an elevated temperature may be seen. Miosis may be present; the corneal and gag reflexes may be depressed or absent. Sensation is generally reduced in the extremities. The deep tendon reflexes are often increased.

A moderate degree of intoxication is characterized by delirium, which may be accompanied by persecutory delusions and also by hallucinations that tend to be visual. Catatonic posturing, bizarre repetitive stereotyped movements, and facial grimacing may be seen. Muscular rigidity, opisthotonotic posturing, and dystonia along with convulsions may be seen. Agitation may be extreme and rhabdomyolysis may occur with possible acute renal failure.

In severe intoxication stupor or coma may be seen. In stupor, users may show random purposeless movements or may lie still; painful stimuli, however, still elicit a response. Myoclonus is frequent, and the deep tendon reflexes may be greatly exaggerated. With even higher doses coma may supervene. Typically users evidence a sort of "coma vigil": the eyes are open and the patient appears vigilant, yet there is no response to pain or to nearby events. The EEG may show profound slowing. The temperature is elevated, as is the blood pressure, and a hypertensive encephalopathy may occur. Respiratory depression may also occur. As users emerge from stupor or coma they again display the previously described signs of moderate and then mild intoxication; indeed, the clinical picture may fluctuate between stupor and lesser degrees of intoxication for days.

The duration of the intoxication varies directly with its severity, but tends to be shorter with ketamine, which has a half-life of about three hours compared to seven to 20 hours for phencyclidine. Other factors which prolong the intoxication seen with phencyclidine are its sequestration in the acidic gastric contents and its retention within lipocytes. Overall, intoxication with ketamine is generally resolved within four to six hours, whereas with phencyclidine the duration ranges from hours up to several days.

After all signs of intoxication have finally remitted, many users experience dysphoria, irritability, and insomnia, and this "letdown" may last for a day or more.

Most users recover completely from intoxication. In occasional users, however, certain residual symptoms may persist. Although certain syndromes of such persistent symptoms do in fact occur in "pure culture," in many users the persistent phenomena are characterized by a mixture of symptoms. The syndromes that have been characterized include the following: first, delusions and hallucinations; second, delirium; and third, mood changes that may be either manic or depressed.

Persistent delusions are generally persecutory; any accompanying hallucinations are often visual. When such symptoms do appear in pure culture, without any confusion, the clinical picture resembles that seen in paranoid schizophrenia. This syndrome generally lasts for days, or a week or more.

When a persistent delirium occurs, users remain confused; they may tend to wander and are generally not capable of caring for themselves. This syndrome likewise tends to last for days or a week or so.

Manic symptoms, such as euphoria, grandiosity, pressured speech, hyperactivity, and the like, may last for over a week. A depressive syndrome, however, tends to last much longer, often for several weeks. In general the postintoxication depressive syndrome tends to occur only in those who have engaged in long-term heavy use of phencyclidine.

In rare instances, and generally after only severe prolonged use of phencyclidine, a dementia may occur, which may persist for months or a year or more, long after phencyclidine has been eliminated. Memory loss, diminished abstracting ability, and aphasia of the expressive type are generally seen. Although generally mild, such symptoms nonetheless may be socially incapacitating. A personality change may also occur with dysphoria, irritability, and impulsivity. In addition scattered case reports of a prolonged illness symptomatically similar to schizophrenia have occurred after severe, prolonged abuse.

The overall pattern of phencyclidine or ketamine abuse may be either episodic or continuous. In the episodic pattern, users engage in "binges" lasting for several days, during which they stay more or less intoxicated. Such binges usually terminate when users become exhausted, run out of the drug, or, if moderately or severely intoxicated, are forcibly separated from the drug by friends or the authorities. The interval between binges varies usually from only a few days up to a week or more. In the continuous pattern users take the drug generally in small doses on an almost daily basis. Regardless of whether the pattern is episodic or continuous the majority of users do not confine themselves to phencyclidine or ketamine alone. Marijuana, alcohol, cocaine, and occasionally stimulants are also used.

COURSE

Few data are available regarding the long-term use of either phencyclidine or ketamine: it does appear, however, that abusers tend to moderate or stop by their late 20s.

COMPLICATIONS

Repeated intoxications generally render users incapable of obtaining or maintaining stable relationships or jobs. Violent behavior may result in incarceration. Suicide may occur, particularly during moderate intoxication or during a postintoxication depressive syndrome. Users with preexisting schizophrenia may experience a severe exacerbation of the schizophrenia if they use phencyclidine or ketamine.

Phencyclidine is neurotoxic in fetuses, and children born of phencyclidine-abusing mothers are often underweight.

ETIOLOGY

Why some users of phencyclidine eventually come to abuse the drug, while others remain "social" users or relinquish its use entirely, is not clear.

DIFFERENTIAL DIAGNOSIS

Differentiating mild or moderate degrees of phencyclidine or ketamine intoxication from intoxication with other substances is often relatively straightforward. Alcohol intoxication may present with euphoria, dysarthria, ataxia, and nystagmus. Generally, however, alcohol-intoxicated individuals do not perceive their bodies as distorted, as occurs in phencyclidine or ketamine intoxication. Furthermore they do not display the catatonic or bizarre behavior seen in moderate intoxication. Intoxication with hallucinogens, such as LSD, may produce a euphoria along with vivid hallucinations; however, these users generally evidence mydriasis, not the miosis seen with phencyclidine and ketamine. Furthermore hallucinogens fail to produce the nystagmus, ataxia, and dysarthria so common with phencyclidine and ketamine. Similarly, stimulants and cocaine also generally produce mydriasis rather than miosis, and likewise do not cause the cerebellar signs seen with phencyclidine and ketamine. In most cases a urine sample for toxicology may be useful; this may remain positive for several days after phencyclidine use. In doubtful cases a fat biopsy may reveal phencyclidine sequestered within the adipocytes.

Differentiating a severe case of phencyclidine or ketamine intoxication from other causes of stupor or coma may be difficult. If the patient has a reliable history of recent use and of antecedent good health, and if the toxicology screen is confirmatory, then one may be fairly confident. Often, however, these stuporous or comatose users are presented at the emergency room with no history, and in such cases the multiple other possible causes of stupor or coma must be ruled out.

Differentiating the postintoxication syndromes from schizophrenia or from an affective disorder often rests on demonstrating whether these symptoms antedated the recent use. If they did, then one may be seeing merely an exacerbation of a preexisting disorder. If they did not then in all likelihood one is seeing a postintoxication syndrome. In instances where a reliable history is unobtainable

or in cases where the use has been chronic and severe, such a differential point may not be ascertainable. In such cases, observation over time aids in the diagnosis. Symptoms that persist beyond a few weeks, presuming abstinence, or which progressively worsen over that time, are probably caused by a disorder other than intoxication.

Differentiating a postintoxication delirium from delirium of other causes requires the same approach used for stupor and coma.

TREATMENT

The goals of treatment are to ensure complete abstinence from future use of phencyclidine and ketamine, and other substances, and to reduce the symptoms of intoxication and the postintoxication syndromes.

Given the lethality of severe intoxication, all patients in stupor or coma should be hospitalized. Patients with moderate degrees of intoxication also often require admission for their own and often others' protection. Patients with mild degrees of intoxication, provided that no risk of progression to a higher degree of intoxication exists, may be seen as outpatients but only with careful outpatient supervision. The postintoxication syndromes are often sufficiently disabling to likewise require admission.

Treatment of intoxication may be either directed at the symptoms themselves or, in the case of phencyclidine, at hastening the elimination of the drug and thus shortening the course of the symptoms.

Haloperidol in doses used as described in the chapter on Rapid Pharmacologic Treatment of Agitation is effective in reducing delusions, hallucinations, confusion and agitation. Hyperthermia may be treated with a cooling blanket; hydralazine or nitroprusside may be used for hypertension. Opisthotonotic posturing and severe dystonia may be treated with intravenous (IV) lorazepam. Isolated seizures may not require treatment; repetitive seizures may be terminated with IV lorazepam. If that fails, IV fosphenytoin may be useful. Increased salivation may require suctioning; intubation may be required for respiratory depression.

Successful use of ECT has been reported for moderate degrees of intoxication; lacking formal studies, however, one should hold such an approach in reserve pending the failure of other approaches.

Awake patients should be protected from any unnecessary stimulation. Isolation in a dimly lit, quiet, well-protected room with close monitoring is often best. In contrast to patients intoxicated with hallucinogens, these patients cannot be "talked down." Indeed such efforts often make phencyclidine intoxicated patients worse. Restraints may be required; however, given the possibility that their use may increase muscle breakdown, thus increasing the risk of renal failure due to myoglobinuria, their use is to be avoided if possible.

Three methods are available whereby the elimination of phencyclidine may be hastened. Activated charcoal binds the drug, and, when aspiration is not a risk, is recommended. Further, in light of phencyclidine's sequestration in the acidic gastric contents, some authorities recommend continuous nasogastric suctioning. Finally, and controversially, some recommend acidification of the urine with oral or intravenous ascorbic acid to "trap" phencyclidine in the urine, followed by administration of furosemide. As such acidification, however, may increase the risk of renal failure, it is not currently recommended.

Post-intoxication psychosis and post-intoxication delirium may be treated symptomatically with low-dose haloperidol. The optimum treatment for post-intoxication mood disorders is not clear; in the case of depression symptoms generally remit before an antidepressant could take effect.

Upon resolution of the intoxication or of any post-intoxication syndrome, efforts are directed at engendering abstinence. Patients with phencyclidine abuse generally do not tolerate the confrontation and emotional turmoil present in most currently available inpatient programs. They tend to become overstimulated. Long-term outpatient programs, such as Narcotics Anonymous, appear to offer some hope.

BIBLIOGRAPHY

Anis NA, Berry SC, Burton NR, et al. The dissociative anesthetics ketamine and phencyclidine selectively reduce excitation of central mammalian neurons by N-methyl aspartate. *British Journal of Pharmacology* 1983;79:565-575.

Delgarno PJ, Shewan D. Illicit use of ketamine in Scotland. *Journal of Psychoactive Drugs* 1996;28:191-199.

Giannini AJ, Eighan MS, Loiselle RH, et al. Comparison of haloperidol and chlorpromazine in the treatment of phencyclidine psychosis. *Journal of Clinical Pharmacology* 1984;24:202-204.

Giannini AJ, Underwood NA, Condon M. Acute ketamine intoxication treated by haloperidol: a preliminary study. *American Journal of Therapeutics* 2000;7:389-391.

Grover D, Yeragani VK, Keshavan MS. Improvement of phencyclidine-associated psychosis with ECT. *The Journal of Clinical Psychiatry* 1986;47:477-478.

Hansen G, Jensen SB, Chandresh L, et al. The psychotropic effects of ketamine. *Journal of Psychoactive Drugs* 1988;20:419-425.

Lahti AC, Weiler MA, Tamara Michaelidis BA, et al. Effects of ketamine in normal and schizophrenic volunteers. *Neuropsychopharmacology* 2001;25:455-467.

McCarron MM, Schulze BW, Thompson GA, et al. Acute phencyclidine intoxication: clinical patterns, complications and treatment. *Annals of Emergency Medicine* 1981;10:290-297.

Mattson MP, Rychlik B, Cheng B. Degenerative and axon outgrowth-altering effects of phencyclidine in human fetal cerebral cortical cells. *Neuropharmacology* 1992;31:279-291.

Rosen AM, Mukherjee S, Shimbach K. The efficacy of ECT in phencyclidine-induced psychosis. *The Journal of Clinical Psychiatry* 1984;45: 220-222.

Weiner AL, Vieira L, Mckay CA, et al. Ketamine abusers presenting to the emergency department: a case series. *The Journal of Emergency Medicine* 2000;18:447-451.

39 Inhalant Related Disorders (DSM-IV-TR #292.89, 305.90, 304.60, 292.82)

The volatile ingredients of many readily available products are often inhaled for intoxication. These include airplane or model glue, paint thinner, kerosene and gasoline, various cleaners and industrial solvents, the propellants in aerosol sprays and spray paints, fingernail polish or polish remover, and typewriter correction fluid. Each of these products contains various mixtures of aliphatic or aromatic hydrocarbons, some of which may be halogenated. Of all these intoxicating hydrocarbons, toluene appears to be most significant for inhalant abuse.

Inhalant abuse is sometimes also known as solvent abuse or, more loosely, "glue sniffing." The actual prevalence of inhalant abuse is not known; however, over 10% of all high school seniors have at least "experimented" with inhalants. Inhalant abuse is more common among males than females.

ONSET

Inhalant abuse generally begins in late childhood or early adolescence.

CLINICAL FEATURES

The volatile substances may be soaked in a rag and held to the face, or placed in a plastic or paper bag; a tell-tale rash may indicate where the bag was positioned. Intoxication usually begins within minutes. Users often describe a euphoric dreamy "high." Often some drowsiness, dizziness, dysarthria, diplopia, nystagmus, and ataxia occur. Hallucinations, generally visual, and confusion may occur, and some may experience delusions. Some users become agitated, irritable, and impulsive. In severe intoxication stupor or

coma may occur. Symptoms of intoxication subside gradually after about an hour or so.

In most instances, at least initially, "sniffing" is done in groups of youngsters. Often alcohol and marijuana are also taken. Most abusers and addicts seek intoxication frequently, often daily. In some instances a user may "titrate" his inhalation and stay intoxicated the entire day.

Tolerance may develop; withdrawal has also been reported and is characterized by nausea, tremulousness, diaphoresis, irritability and insomnia.

COURSE

The long-term course of inhalant abuse and addiction is not known with certainty: some appear to stop by their late 20's; some "graduate" to dependence on other substances, such as opioids; and some, often those with a concurrent antisocial personality disorder, live out an isolated existence that centers on chronic intoxication with inhalants.

COMPLICATIONS

Several complications may occur during intoxication. These include bronchospasm, seizures, ventricular arrhythmias (e.g., ventricular fibrillation), respiratory arrest, acute renal failure, vomiting with aspiration pneumonia and suffocation in plastic bags.

School failure, truancy, and delinquency are common. Other complications may appear after years of use, among which an inhalant-induced persisting dementia is the most serious.

This dementia generally presents with concreteness, forgetfulness, apathy, and emotional dullness; typically these demented patients also have cerebellar ataxia and some degree of generalized hyperreflexia. CT scanning shows cerebral atrophy; MRI scanning, in addition to the atrophy, shows increased signal intensity in the cerebral white matter, consistent with patchy or widespread, confluent, areas of demyelinization.

N-hexane, a common contaminant, may cause a chronic, primarily motor polyneuropathy that, unfortunately, may continue to progress after cessation of use. Other hydrocarbons can cause aplastic anemia, nephrotoxicity, or hepatotoxicity.

A fetal alcohol-like syndrome may occur in children born of women who use inhalants during pregnancy.

ETIOLOGY

Although clearly the intoxicating hydrocarbons have a direct effect on lipid membranes, the precise mechanism whereby the clinical features of intoxication are produced is not known.

Likewise the factors that determine which young "experimenter" goes on to abuse or addiction, and which does not, are not clear. Although most inhalant abusers are found among impoverished minority groups, privileged youngsters may also be affected.

DIFFERENTFIAL DIAGNOSIS

Intoxication with alcohol, benzodiazepines, or other sedative-hypnotics may resemble that seen with inhalants. A "solvent odor" on the breath or clothing, though not always present, is a clue. A blood alcohol level and urine or serum toxicology may be helpful, but it must be kept in mind that inhalant users often consume multiple different substances.

TREATMENT

Inhalant abusers rarely seek treatment; almost universally they are sent by family members, the schools, or the courts. They are generally unmoved by the available treatment approaches and tend to drop out as soon as they can.

BIBLIOGRAPHY

Altenkirch H, Mager J, Stoltenburg G, et al. Toxic polyneuropathies after sniffing a glue thinner. *Journal of Neurology* 1977;214:137-152.

Aydin K, Sencer S, Demir T, et al. Cranial MR findings in chronic toluene abuse by inhalation. *American Journal of Neuroradiology* 2002;23: 1173-1179.

Caldemeyre KS, Armstrong SW, George KK, et al. The spectrum of neuroimaging abnormalities in solvent abuse and their clinical correlation. *Journal of Neuroimaging* 1996;6:167-173.

Evans AC, Raistrick D. Phenomenology of intoxication with toluene-based adhesives and butane gas. *The British Journal of Psychiatry* 1987;150: 769-773.

Filley CN, Heaton RK, Rosenberg NL. White matter dementia in chronic toluene abuse. *Neurology* 1990;40:532-534.

Hormes JT, Filley CM, Rosenberg NL. Neurologic sequelae of chronic solvent abuse. *Neurology* 1986;36:698-702.

King GS, Smialek JE, Trouthman WG. Sudden death in adolescents resulting from inhalation of typewriter correction fluid. *The Journal of the American Medical Association* 1985;253:1604-1609.

King MD, Day RE, Oliver JS, et al. Solvent encephalopathy. *British Medical Journal* 1981;283:663-665.

King PJ, Morris JG, Pollard JD. Glue sniffing neuropathy. *The Australian & New Zealand Journal of Medicine* 1985;15:293-299.

Rosenberg ML, Kleinschmidt-Demasters BK, Davis KA, et al. Toluene abuse causes diffuse central nervous system white matter changes. *Annals of Neurology* 1988;23:611-614.

Watson JM. Glue sniffing: two case reports. *Practitioner* 1979;222:845-847.

40 Nicotine Related Disorders (DSM-IV-TR #305.10, 292.0)

Although nicotine is the substance in question, the term "tobacco addiction" may be more clinically useful, as tobacco is the only "vehicle" whereby nicotine addiction occurs. Of the various ways in which tobacco is used, cigarette smoking is by far the most clinically important. Although oral cancer and tobacco addiction may occur with chewing tobacco and pipe or cigar smoking, the numbers pale in comparison with cigarette smoking.

In the United States alone some 45 million or more regularly smoke cigarettes, and this accounts for over 400,000 premature deaths every year. When a cigarette is smoked, over 4000 different compounds are produced, which may exist in either gaseous or particulate form. Important gaseous components include carbon monoxide and hydrogen cyanide. In the particulate phase one finds nicotine and a substance known as "tar," which contains for the most part polycyclic aromated hydrocarbons. Nicotine is the active habituating substance in tobacco; among the polycyclic hydrocarbons are found the carcinogens.

Inhaled nicotine is rapidly absorbed across the alveoli and reaches the brain in seconds, where, given its highly lipophilic nature, it rapidly crosses the blood-brain barrier. The half-life of nicotine is about 2 hours. None of its metabolites possess any substantial pharmacologic activity. A major metabolite, cotinine, has a half-life of about 20 hours and is often sought in urine drug screens.

Despite the well-publicized hazards of smoking, new smokers continually appear, and among them are more and more females. Among older smokers men far outnumber women, but among teenagers and young adults the sex ratio is approximately equal.

ONSET

In almost all cases tobacco dependence begins in adolescence. Extensive, seductive advertising by tobacco companies, simple curiosity, and peer pressure are among the factors that prompt the first experimentation. Then follows a transition period of more or less irregular smoking until the use of cigarettes and the craving for their effect have become established. For most this transition to addiction takes from 1 to 3 years; however, in some cases the transition may occur within months, or, exceptionally, only weeks.

CLINICAL FEATURES

Especially with the first cigarette of the day, the smoker experiences a sense of euphoria, which, although mild and lasting only minutes, is most desired. Memory improves, any irritability wanes, and an overall sense of satisfaction is felt. Nicotine also causes a degree of tachycardia, increased blood pressure, and increased peristaltic activity. Palpitations may occur as well as nausea and vomiting in those not tolerant to the effects of nicotine. Appetite decreases, and frequent smokers may lose a modest amount of weight, perhaps 5 or 10 pounds.

Over time most regular smokers develop some degree of tolerance to the effects of nicotine. Thus by the end of a day of heavy smoking, little is gained from a cigarette. This tolerance, however, is generally short-lived, and after a night's sleep most smokers once again find smoking pleasurable. Similarly the number of cigarettes that can be smoked without nausea or vomiting increases dramatically over weeks of daily smoking, from perhaps only one cigarette in a tobacco-naive subject up to dozens for a chronic smoker.

Among those addicted to tobacco, the number of cigarettes smoked per day averages perhaps 20 and ranges from 5 or less up to 100 or more. A cigarette may be sought immediately upon awakening, and cigarettes are often carried wherever the smoker goes. Desperate smokers may "light up" even in nonsmoking areas and may continue to smoke even when they have respiratory complaints and each inhalation triggers another retching paroxysm of coughing. Over the years facial skin becomes coarse and leathery, and tobacco stains may be seen on the fingers and teeth.

In some, withdrawal symptoms play a prominent part in the perpetuation of smoking. For most, nicotine withdrawal occurs within 24 hours of the last cigarette; however, in heavy smokers symptoms may appear within as little as 2 hours. A restless craving for a cigarette occurs. The smoker often becomes tense and irritable. The smoker may have headaches and may have difficulty in concentrating. Insomnia commonly occurs, as does an increase in appetite. In most smokers, the desire for a cigarette peaks within a day or two and then along with most other symptoms declines gradually over a matter of weeks. In a minority of smokers, however, withdrawal symptoms may persist for months, during which time some gain considerable weight. The actual craving for a cigarette may intermittently recur for years, especially in times of stress.

The denial seen in some tobacco addicts may be profound. Those rendered emphysematous may still smoke, even though they have become oxygen dependent. Some who have had a laryngectomy for cancer continue to smoke through their tracheostomies. Most smokers, however, eventually try to stop. Sadly, though, most of these will fail in their attempt.

COURSE

In the vast majority of cases, tobacco addiction, in the natural course of events, is lifelong: some will continue to smoke on their deathbeds as they lie dying of lung cancer.

COMPLICATIONS

The complications of cigarette smoking include the following: gingivitis; esophageal reflux; peptic ulcer disease; cancer of the mouth, larynx, or lung; cancer of the esophagus, bladder, and pancreas; chronic obstructive pulmonary disease (COPD); coronary artery disease and myocardial infarction; subarachnoid hemorrhage and ischemic cerebral infarction; peripheral vascular disease; and exacerbation of Raynaud's phenomenon. Of all these complications, cancer, COPD, and heart disease cause the greatest morbidity and mortality. Smoking during pregnancy may cause spontaneous abortion, abruptio placentae, low birth weight, and increased perinatal mortality.

Polycyclic hydrocarbons also cause liver enzyme induction, which may reduce levels of various antidepressants (clomipramine, imipramine, desipramine, nortriptyline, doxepin and fluvoxamine), antipsychotics (haloperidol, fluphenazine, olanzapine and clozapine), propranolol and theophylline. Importantly, patients who stop smoking (as may happen upon hospital admission) will experience blood level elevations of these agents, with increased side effects.

"Passive" smoking by nonsmokers increases the risk of cancer and of respiratory disease, particularly in children.

ETIOLOGY

Among adolescents who experiment with smoking, some go on to develop tobacco addiction and others do not. The reason for this is not entirely clear. Adoption and twin studies indicate a genetic factor; however, environmental factors, such as peer pressure, are undoubtedly involved.

DIFFERENTIAL DIAGNOSIS

Very few who smoke cigarettes do so casually. Although a minority can quit whenever they want, most American adults who continue to smoke today despite the ubiquitous warnings against the dangers of smoking are addicted.

TREATMENT

The physician should tell the patient in a nonjudgmental yet forceful way to stop smoking. For those in whom denial is still strong, videotapes of those with cancer or COPD may be helpful. A personal visit with such patients in the hospital may be even more effective. For patients who are unable to stop on their own, various treatments are available.

Patients should choose a reasonable "quit date" which, ideally, should fall during a relatively stress-free period in the not too distant future. Patients should generally be instructed to stop smoking completely on that day and to avoid, if possible, situations or gatherings where smoking is likely to occur. Various smoking "triggers" or "cues" (e.g., after meals, while driving) should be anticipated and alternative strategies developed. Although some patients may be able to quit on these bases alone, the vast majority will not, and it is thus appropriate to offer psychotherapeutic support, medications, or both, to all patients.

"Stop-smoking" groups, many using a cognitive-behavioral approach, are generally helpful and should be offered to all patients. Medications may include either nicotine replacement products or either bupropion or nortriptyline, and it appears that a combination of nicotine replacement and bupropion is better than bupropion alone. Nicotine replacement is available in 16- or 24-hour transdermal patches (available in various strengths, e.g., 7, 14 or 21 mg), gum tablets (available in 2 and 4 mg sizes), lozenges (also available in 2 and 4 mg sizes), inhaler canisters (delivering about 2 mg) and nasal spray (delivering about 0.5 mg per spray). Given that the average cigarette delivers, depending on how avidly it is smoked, anywhere from 1 to 3 mg, the average daily dose of cigarette-derived nicotine may be roughly estimated based on the number of cigarettes smoked per day. A nicotine replacement dose may then be calculated which generally should be somewhat less than the average daily cigarette-derived dose. Most patients appear to prefer the patches; if another vehicle is used it is important to roughly schedule the dosing in such a way as to avoid any significant withdrawal symptoms. Some patients who use the 24-hour patch may experience insomnia and in such cases the patch should be removed before bedtime. The optimum tapering schedule for replacement nicotine has not been determined: recommendations range anywhere from six to twenty weeks, and considerable clinical judgment may be required. For otherwise healthy patients who cannot remain abstinent from cigarettes without nicotine replacement, a strong case may be made for indefinite treatment.

Both bupropion and nortriptyline are effective in increasing cessation rates, regardless of whether patients are or ever have been depressed. Both appear equally effective: bupropion, though perhaps the better tolerated overall of the two, is contraindicated in patients with a history of seizures or bulimia; nortriptyline should be used with caution in patients with cardiac disease. Bupropion may be initiated at 150 mg and increased after several days to 150 mg bid; nortriptyline is begun at 25 mg and increased in 25 mg increments every three or four days to 75 mg, if tolerated. Both of these medications should be started at least two weeks before the "quit date," and continued until the patient has been continuously abstinent for at least several months.

Although the above treatment recommendations are generally applicable, there are two disorders which, if present, may alter treatment strategy. The first is alcoholism. Most alcoholics smoke, and given the stresses of early sobriety it is generally appropriate to forestall efforts to stop smoking until sobriety is well-established, lest the stress of stopping smoking tips patients back into drinking, whereupon almost all will once again pick up smoking again. The second disorder is major depression. For reasons not yet clear, patients with major depression, even though not currently in the midst of an episode of depression, are at high risk for a recurrence of depression during the first year of abstinence from smoking, and for such patients antidepressant medication (which, all other things

being equal, should be either bupropion or nortriptyline) should be started on a preventive basis and continued for at least a year.

Regardless of what approach is used, during the first year relapses are the rule rather than the exception, and such "slips" should not be seen as failures. Since weight gain is so common and may not be prevented by nicotine replacement, patients should be warned about this and instructed that a weight loss program may be required once they are reasonably comfortable in their abstinence. Those who remain continuously abstinent from tobacco for a year or more generally have a very favorable prognosis.

BIBLIOGRAPHY

Benowitz NL, Henningfield JF. Establishing a nicotine threshold for addiction. The implications for tobacco regulation. *The New England Journal of Medicine* 1994;331:123-125.

Breslau N, Johnson EO, Hiripi E, et al. Nicotine dependence in the United States: prevalence, trends and smoking persistence. *Archives of General Psychiatry* 2001;58:810-816.

da Costa CL, Younes RN, Laurenco MT. Stopping smoking: a prospective, randomized, double-blind study comparing nortriptyline to placebo. *Chest* 2002;122:403-408.

Froom P, Melamed S, Benbasel J. Smoking cessation and weight gain. *The Journal of Family Practice* 1998;46:460-464.

Glassman AH, Covey LS, Stetner F, et al. Smoking cessation and the course of major depression: a follow-up study. *Lancet* 2001;357:1929-1932.

Hall SM, Humfleet GL, Reus VI, et al. Psychological intervention and antidepressant treatment in smoking cessation. *Archives of General Psychiatry* 2002;59:930-936.

Hughes JR, Hatsukami D. Signs and symptoms of smoking withdrawal. *Archives of General Psychiatry* 1986;43:289-294.

Hurt RD, Sachs DPL, Glover ED, et al. A comparison of sustained-release bupropion and placebo for smoking cessation. *The New England Journal of Medicine* 1997;337:1195-1202.

Jorenby DE, Leischow SS, Nides MA, et al. A controlled trial of sustained-release bupropion, a nicotine patch, or both for smoking cessation. *The New England Journal of Medicine* 1999;340:685-691.

Karnath B. Smoking cessation. *The American Journal of Medicine* 2002;112:399-405.

Kendler KS, Neale MC, Sullivan P, et al. A population-based twin study in women of smoking initiation and nicotine dependence. *Psychological Medicine* 1999;29:299-308.

Prochazka AV, Waver MJ, Keller RT, et al. A randomized trial of nortriptyline for smoking cessation. *Archives of Internal Medicine* 1998;158:2035-2039.

Shiffman S, Dresler CM, Hajek P, et al. Efficacy of a nicotine lozenge for smoking cessation. *Archives of Internal Medicine* 2002;162:1267-1276.

41 Amphetamine (or Amphetamine-Like) Related Disorders (DSM-IV-TR #304.40, 305.70, 292.89, 292.0, 292.81, 292.11, 292.12)

Of the many stimulants that have been abused, amphetamine, dextroamphetamine and methamphetamine are the worst offenders; methylphenidate has also been abused as have some of the "diet" drugs, such as diethylpropion, benzphetamine and phenteramine. Of all these, amphetamine and methamphetamine are the most important clinically.

These drugs may be taken orally or crushed, dissolved, and taken intravenously. Occasionally they are also "snorted." Highly purified methamphetamine ("ice") may also be smoked. Within the central nervous system the stimulants act primarily as indirect, but also possibly as direct, sympathomimetics, releasing both norepinephrine and dopamine; the amphetamines are predominantly noradrenergic and methylphenidate predominantly dopaminergic.

The lifetime prevalence of stimulant abuse or dependence has been estimated at 1.7% in the United States.

ONSET

Abuse of stimulants generally begins in teenage or early adult years, and in some cases has its genesis in medically supervised use for the treatment of attention-deficit/hyperactivity disorder, narcolepsy or obesity. The time required for the appearance of craving and neuroadaptation varies from months in the case of oral use to only weeks with intravenous use or with inhalation of methamphetamine.

CLINICAL FEATURES

Stimulant intoxication may begin almost immediately with inhalation or intravenous use, producing an intensely pleasurable "rush," whereas an hour or more may pass after oral use before the user experiences a somewhat less profound elation or sense of intense well-being. Typically, the user feels more confident, energetic, and active. The user is disposed to talk; there may be some grandiosity, and often a degree of vigilant watchfulness with some suspiciousness is seen. The pupils are dilated, the blood pressure, both systolic and diastolic, is increased, and the heart rate may be either increased or reflexively slowed. The deep tendon reflexes are symmetrically brisk. Such a degree of intoxication rarely brings the user to medical attention.

A severe degree of intoxication, one seen not uncommonly in the emergency room, is characterized by agitation and at times bizarre behavior. Often a peculiar interest in things mechanical is observed, and users may spend hours taking apart and then attempting to put back together clocks, radios, televisions, and the like. Fleeting delusions of persecution and auditory hallucinations

may arise, and formication may occur. Bruxism and choreoathetotic movements may be seen, and in severe cases generalized dystonia. The temperature is raised, and extreme diaphoresis may occur. The user may experience nausea, vomiting, abdominal cramping, and diarrhea. Occasionally, in even higher degrees of intoxication, a stimulant-intoxication delirium may occur with confusion, extreme apprehension, incoherence, and at times violent assaultive behavior. Seizures, hypertensive encephalopathy, and various arrhythmias may also occur.

Regardless of the degree of intoxication most users recover a few hours later or perhaps in a day or more.

In some users a stimulant-induced psychotic disorder may occur, and although this is typically restricted to chronic IV users, it has been reported in normal volunteers given very high oral doses. The user becomes intensely suspicious, guarded, and watchful. Delusions of persecution develop, as may both auditory and visual hallucinations; formication is not uncommon. Typically these users remain free of confusion and incoherence. In extreme cases the user may attack the "persecutors." With abstinence the symptoms of the psychosis gradually fade, generally over anywhere from days to weeks. Exceptionally, however, the psychosis may persist for anywhere from months to a year or more. Those who resume daily use may display sensitization wherein over time recurrent paranoid psychoses occur at ever lower doses. Tolerance to the effects of stimulants, including euphoria, develops with continued use, and especially in IV users a progressive escalation in dose is common. At times this may be extreme: some have been known to take several grams a day, with little effect.

Withdrawal symptoms typically occur after extended use of stimulants. As the intoxication clears, users become dysphoric and fatigued. They may be irritable, and some users become agitated. Suicidal ideation, which may be intense, is not uncommon. Some users experience a dreadful insomnia, whereas others sleep excessively, at least initially. This acute withdrawal syndrome, or "crash," as it is often called, may undergo considerable clearing within days or a week or more; however, dysphoria and sleep disturbance may linger for weeks or months.

For the stimulant addict the need for the drug becomes paramount. Some seem able to confine themselves to moderate daily use, somehow getting by, whereas many others become binge users. Over one or several days the stimulant is taken again and again, often intravenously, until either the money runs out or the addict becomes debilitated and unable to go on. Several days or more of withdrawal then ensue, until the next binge begins. Regardless of whether the addict develops daily or binge use, sedative or alcohol use is very common, both for their own effect and to modulate the intoxication and "smooth it out."

COURSE

The long-term course of stimulant addiction is not known with certainty; it appears that in some cases a spontaneous partial or complete remission may occur after a decade of use.

COMPLICATIONS

The user neglects family, friends, and work, and indeed these may be lost or swept aside in favor of the drug. Craving at times may be desperately strong, and some may kill to obtain a fresh supply.

Both intracerebral hemorrhage and ischemic cerebral infarction may occur, and these seem related not only to hypertension but also to a stimulant-induced vasculopathy. Rare complications include myocardial infarction, cardiomyopathy, rhabdomyolysis and shock. In addition, IV users are at risk for AIDS and hepatitis.

Those who develop a stimulant-induced psychotic disorder may become aggressive and commit crimes.

The withdrawal syndrome, as noted earlier, may be accomplished by suicidal ideation, and completed suicides have occurred.

Methamphetamine, alone among the stimulants, also appears to be neurotoxic to both dopaminergic and serotoninergic neurons. Specifically, even after a year of abstinence, methamphetamine addicts demonstrate mild memory impairment and motor slowing, both of which have been related to a reduction of dopamine transporters in the striatum.

ETIOLOGY

The euphoriant effect of stimulants appears to be mediated via dopamine release in the nucleus accumbens; however, why craving develops in some users and not others is unclear.

DIFFERENTIAL DIAGNOSIS

Cocaine intoxication may be clinically indistinguishable from stimulant intoxication.

Occasionally the increased activity and talkativeness seen during intoxication may suggest a manic episode. The history of antecedent use or a positive toxicology are of course helpful; however, one may also rely on mydriasis and bradycardia, a combination that is rare in mania. In doubtful cases abstention on a secure drug-free ward for a day or two will resolve the diagnostic question.

When the stimulant-induced psychosis follows a typical short course, one can rule out paranoid schizophrenia. In cases, however, where it is prolonged for months or more, only very long-term observation may suffice. Indeed some believe that in these cases the stimulant use merely precipitated a paranoid schizophrenia in an individual so predisposed.

The withdrawal syndrome may suggest a depressive episode; however, the brevity of the severe symptoms indicates the correct diagnosis.

TREATMENT

Mild degrees of intoxication require only observation and general support. If agitation is severe or if delirium occurs, antipsychotics, such as haloperidol or chlorpromazine, may be used, as described in the chapter on rapid treatment. Acidification of the urine with ammonium chloride, in a dose of 500 mg q 4h, hastens excretion of amphetamines. Severe hypertension may be treated with nitroprusside, seizures with intravenous lorazepam, and arrhythmias with propranolol.

The psychosis may be treated with antipsychotics, such as haloperidol, keeping in mind that the natural course of this disorder is such as to dictate relatively brief use of these agents.

Treatment of the withdrawal syndrome involves observation and support. Hospitalization may be indicated if significant suicidal ideation is present.

The overall treatment of stimulant addiction has as its goal abstinence. Hospitalization is often indicated to break the pattern of use. Support groups, such as Cocaine Anonymous or Narcotics Anonymous, may be very helpful; in any case, patients must avoid contact with "using" friends and with situations that might prompt use. Regular urine sampling may be a potent motivator for abstinence, especially when patients have contracted ahead of time that a positive urine test automatically triggers notification of their employer.

BIBLIOGRAPHY

Angrist B, Lee HK, Gershon S. The antagonism of amphetamine-induced symptomatology by a neuroleptic. *The American Journal of Psychiatry* 1974;131:817-819.

Derlet RW, Rice P, Horowitz BZ, et al. Amphetamine toxicity: experience with 127 cases. *The Journal of Emergency Medicine* 1989;7:157-161.

Drevets WC, Gautier C, Price JC, et al. Amphetamine-induced dopamine release in human ventral striatum correlates with euphoria. *Biological Psychiatry* 2001;49:81-96.

Iwanami A, Sugiyama A, Kuroki N, et al. Patients with methamphetamine psychosis admitted to a psychiatric hospital in Japan. A preliminary report. *Acta Psychiatrica Scandinavica* 1994;89:428-432.

Janowsky DS, Risch C. Amphetamine psychosis and psychotic symptoms. *Psychopharmacology* 1979;65:73-77.

Parran TV, Jasinski Dr. Intravenous methylphenidate abuse. Prototype for prescription drug abuse. *Archives of Internal Medicine* 1991;151:781-783.

Volkow ND, Chang L, Wang GJ, et al. Association of dopamine transporter reduction with psychomotor impairment in methamphetamine abusers. *The American Journal of Psychiatry* 2001;158:377-382.

Yen DJ, Wang SJ, Ju TH, et al. Stroke associated with methamphetamine inhalation. *European Neurology* 1994;34:16-22.

42 Cocaine Related Disorders (DSM-IV-TR #304.20, 305.60, 292.89, 292.0, 292.81, 292.11, 292.12)

Several different preparations of cocaine are available illegally. Cocaine hydrochloride is a white powder that may be "snorted" into the nasal passages where it is absorbed through the nasal mucosa; cocaine hydrochloride is also water soluble and may be injected intravenously. Cocaine hydrochloride is destroyed by heat, and is thus not suitable for smoking; however, it may be treated with sodium bicarbonate and then either extracted with ether to yield a "free base" preparation, or warmed to create a "rock" of cocaine. Both the free base and crack preparations evaporate with heating and thus may be smoked.

After snorting, peak blood levels are reached within 30 to 60 minutes, and the total duration of intoxication is about a half hour. By contrast, when cocaine is taken intravenously or by smoking, peak levels occur within seconds and the intoxication, though briefer, lasting only 5 to 20 minutes, is far more intense.

Within the central nervous system cocaine both inhibits the reuptake and enhances the release of monoamines by presynaptic neurons. Although the reuptake of norepinephrine and serotonin are both inhibited, it appears that the euphoriant effects of cocaine are for the most part mediated by blockade of reuptake of dopamine in the dopaminergic mesocortical and mesolimbic pathways.

Cocaine is rapidly hydrolyzed by plasma and hepatic esterases to relatively inactive metabolites, such as benzoylecgonine and ecgonine methylester. Although the plasma half-life for cocaine is short, ranging from 30 to 90 minutes, its metabolites may be detected in the urine for up to 2 to 3 days after only one dose, and up to a week and a half with chronic use. In some cases, perhaps due to a release of stored cocaine from adipocytes, a "negative" urine may be followed by a "positive" one without any intervening cocaine use.

Cocaine, in certain forms, is the most addicting substance known. Craving may develop within days with the smoking of free base cocaine or intravenous injection of cocaine hydrochloride. Laboratory animals, if given free access to cocaine, ignore sex, food, even water, and repeatedly administer cocaine until they die.

The lifetime prevalence of cocaine abuse and dependence in the United States is roughly 2%. It appears that many are able to "snort" cocaine hydrochloride "recreationally" and not become addicted. With graduation to injection or smoking, however, abuse or addiction becomes very likely; indeed with crack cocaine the transition from "recreational" use to addiction may take place within days.

ONSET

Although cocaine addiction may develop at any age, most patients develop a pattern of regular use in adolescence or occasionally in early adult years. The rapidity with which addiction occurs depends in part on the preparation and routes of administration. As just described regular usage of IV cocaine hydrochloride or inhaled crack cocaine may eventuate in addiction within days. Intranasal snorting of cocaine hydrochloride, however, may be practiced regularly for months or even years before addiction occurs. Often addiction is ushered in by the development of "binging" wherein the patient continuously uses cocaine for a day or more, sometimes up to a week.

CLINICAL FEATURES

During intoxication users becomes euphoric, hyperalert, talkative, and grandiose. Hyperactivity is common, and with higher doses agitation may occur; some patients may also experience visual hallucinations, often consisting of insects, the notorious "cocaine bugs"; some of these patients may also experience tactile hallucinations, typically of formication, and in such cases patients may excoriate themselves in an attempt to get rid of the "bugs." The appetite for food and sleep is routinely lost, and with mild intoxication sexual desire increases, accompanied by delayed ejaculation. With greater intoxication, however, partial or complete impotence may occur. Users may experience tachycardia or palpitations; headache, nausea, and vomiting may also occur. Rarely choreoathetosis ("crack dancing") may occur. Mydriasis and increased blood pressure are routinely found; occasionally the user may have fever and chills. Users often take sedatives, alcohol, or opioids to enhance the intoxication or dampen the unwanted effects; a favored combination is the "speedball," a mixture of cocaine and heroin. The duration of the intoxication, as noted earlier, varies with the preparation. Regardless, however, of the route of administration, the autonomic and cardiovascular effects tend to persist for 20 to 60 minutes.

Most users experience a "crash" shortly after using cocaine and this tends to be more severe after taking cocaine intravenously or smoking it. During the "crash," users experience fatigue, depression, irritability, and anxiety; the overall dysphoria may be intense. The crash may come within 15 minutes after IV use or smoking; after snorting, the crash may not appear for 30 to 60 minutes. Generally this crash resolves within hours, or a day at the most.

After 2 years or so of cocaine use, a cocaine-induced psychotic disorder may occur during intoxication, characterized by delusions of persecution and reference, which may at times be accompanied by auditory hallucinations. Of note, one may, in these patients, see evidence of "sensitization" wherein with repeated intoxication the psychosis appears more regularly and at progressively lower doses. Although in most cases this psychosis clears shortly after the intoxication does, in some cases it may persist into abstinence for days, weeks, or, rarely, months.

During severe intoxication after intravenous use or smoking, some users may develop a cocaine-induced delirium. Confusion, apprehension, and incoherence may be seen. The mood is often labile, and delusions and hallucinations, as just described, are common. Users in the midst of such a delirium are prone to aggression and violence. In general the delirium clears within hours; afterward the user may be amnestic for the event.

The pattern of cocaine use may be one of either continuous, often daily, use or of episodic use in "binges," also known as cocaine "runs." Users who display a continuous pattern for the most part confine their usage to snorting. Binges may be as short as a few hours but generally last a day; in exceptional cases they may persist for up to a week. During the binge, IV cocaine or smoking free base cocaine is preferred, and doses may be repeated as often as every 10 or 15 minutes. Most users find that with repeated doses, the euphoriant effects wane, whereas the "crashes" and craving become more intense. Eventually either exhaustion or an inability to get more cocaine will terminate the binge. The interval between binges is quite variable; at times only a few days separate the binges; conversely weeks or months may pass before another "run" occurs.

In addition to craving, cocaine addiction is universally characterized by the phenomena of tolerance and withdrawal. The craving for cocaine may be particularly intense. It may occur concurrent with the crash and may last much longer. Some users may resort to the most extreme measures to ensure an unbroken supply of cocaine. Some may sell their children; others may prostitute themselves, rob, or kill.

Tolerance appears to occur much more rapidly with IV use or smoking than if cocaine is snorted. Indeed during a "run" of IV use, tolerance may appear within a day. Unfortunately such tolerance develops only to the euphoriant effect of cocaine and not to its cardiovascular effects. Thus the progressively higher doses required to achieve the euphoria may eventually cause a lethal event, such as an arrhythmia, before the euphoria can be reached.

Withdrawal symptoms seem in some sense to be an extension and elaboration of the frequently occurring post-intoxication "crash," described earlier. Withdrawal tends to occur only after a minimum of several days of heavy use; the withdrawal symptoms themselves tend to reach a maximum in several days and then remit gradually over days or weeks. Typically a user in withdrawal experiences depression, irritability, fatigue, anhedonia, a tense craving for more cocaine, insomnia, and occasionally hyperphagia. Suicidal ideation is not uncommon and suicide attempts may occur.

When evaluating a patient with cocaine addiction, one should inquire after the symptoms of certain other disorders that commonly are associated with it. Abuse or addiction to alcohol or opioids is often seen. Furthermore most patients with cocaine addiction also have a personality disorder; antisocial, narcissistic, or borderline types being most common.

COURSE

The natural course of cocaine addiction is not known with certainty.

COMPLICATIONS

Cardiovascular and cerebrovascular complications during intoxication are not rare. Cardiac complications include arrhythmias (e.g., ventricular tachycardia), severe hypertension, angina or myocardial infarction. Cerebral infarction may also occur; however, it appears that subarachnoid or intracerebral hemorrhages are more common. Seizures may also occur and these may be either grand mal or partial in type. Other organ systems may also be affected, and one may see bowel infarction, renal infarction, rhabdomyolysis, hyperpyrexia or shock.

In addition to complications occurring during intoxication, one may also see complications that progress beyond the dissipation of the intoxication, including myocarditis, a dilated cardiomyopathy or a cerebral vasculitis.

Although any of the foregoing complications may occur with any preparation of cocaine, one complication, namely perforation of the nasal septum, is peculiar to "snorting" cocaine. Here, locally induced vasospasm eventually causes necrosis and destruction of the septum.

Cocaine use by pregnant women may be followed by fetal death, miscarriage, or abruptio placentae, and infants may go through cocaine withdrawal in the first days of life if the mother was using just before delivery. Intrauterine growth retardation may also occur, and some infants are born microcephalic.

Intravenous users who share needles are at risk for AIDS and hepatitis; prostitution and hypersexuality put the user at risk for syphilis, AIDS and other sexually transmitted diseases.

ETIOLOGY

The etiology of cocaine addiction is not clearly delineated. Whether inherited abnormalities of the central nervous system exist that predispose a "recreational" or "social" user to progress to addiction is not known.

DIFFERENTIAL DIAGNOSIS

Because at times intoxication with stimulants or with phencyclidine may be quite similar to cocaine intoxication, obtaining a urine sample for toxicologic analysis is often quite useful.

In those rare instances where a manic episode has a hyperacute onset, one may initially diagnose cocaine intoxication. The persistence of manic hyperactivity, euphoria, and grandiosity long past the half-life of cocaine, however, serves to indicate the correct diagnosis.

Cocaine withdrawal may be mistaken for depression. However, in contrast to depression, the withdrawal symptoms clear within days or weeks. Thus the persistence of depressive symptoms and certainly their worsening beyond 2 weeks should suggest the diagnosis of a depressive illness.

TREATMENT

Neither uncomplicated cocaine intoxication, nor the post-intoxication "crash," given their brevity, require anything other than supportive care. Cocaine-induced psychosis and cocaine-induced delirium may or may not require symptomatic treatment, depending on their severity and duration: where appropriate, haloperidol, used as described in the chapter on Rapid Pharmacologic Treatment of Agitation, may be utilized.

Cocaine withdrawal, if severe, may be partially relieved by amantadine in doses of 100 mg bid.

Arrhythmias may be treated with labetolol, hypertension with sodium nitroprusside, and seizures with intravenous lorazepam.

The overall goal in the treatment of cocaine addiction is complete abstinence, not only from cocaine but also from alcohol and other substances, with the possible exceptions of caffeine and tobacco. Some might include these latter two substances; however, the continued use of caffeine and tobacco does not in fact appear to make relapse more likely, whereas alcohol and other substances do.

Depending on the severity of the withdrawal and craving, inpatient care may or may not be required for detoxification.

Narcotics Anonymous and Cocaine Anonymous, organizations modeled after Alcoholics Anonymous, are useful in maintaining abstinence. Family therapy has not been found helpful. In combination with behavioral contracting, group or individual therapy may be helpful. In these cases random urine screenings are obtained, and, according to a contract, should one be positive, notification is given to the patient's employer or licensure board. Such contracts, however, by commingling the role of therapist and police officer, create tension within the therapeutic relationship. Overall a prudent approach is to refer the patient to a support group and to provide supportive psychotherapy and overall medical management.

Overall, pharmacologic treatment plays no role in the treatment of cocaine addiction per se, with one possible exception: it appears that in those cocaine addicts who also suffer from depression that treatment with desipramine may facilitate abstinence.

BIBLIOGRAPHY

Bartlett E, Hallin A, Chapman B, et al. Selective sensitization to the psychosis-inducing effects of cocaine: a possible marker for addiction relapse vulnerability? *Neuropsychopharmacology* 1997;16:77-82.

Brady KT, Lydlard RB, Malcom B, et al. Cocaine-induced psychosis. *The Journal of Clinical Psychiatry* 1991;52:509-512.

Burke WM, Ravi NV, Dhopesh V, et al. Prolonged presence of metabolite in urine after compulsive cocaine use. *The Journal of Clinical Psychiatry* 1990;51:145-148.

Daras M, Koppel BS, Atos-Radzion E. Cocaine-induced choreathetoid movements ("crack dancing"). *Neurology* 1994;44:751-752.

Kampman KM, Volpicelli JR, Alterman AI, et al. Amantadine in the treatment of cocaine-dependent patients with severe withdrawal symptoms. *The American Journal of Psychiatry* 2000;157:2052-2054.

Klonoff DC, Andrews BT, Obana WG. Stroke associated with cocaine use. *Archives of Neurology* 1989;46:989-993.

Krendel DA, Ditter SM, Frankel MR, et al. Biopsy-proven cerebral vasculitis associated with cocaine use. *Neurology* 1990;40:1092-1094.

Rose RB, Collins JP, Fay-McCarthy M, et al. Phenomenologic comparison of idiopathic psychosis of schizophrenia and drug-induced cocaine and phencyclidine psychoses: a retrospective study. *Clinical Neuropharmacology* 1994;17:359-369.

Roth D, Alarcon FJ, Fernandez JA, et al. Acute rhabdomyolysis associated with cocaine intoxication. *The New England Journal of Medicine* 1988;319:673-677.

Satel SL, Southwick SM, Gawin FH. Clinical features of cocaine-induced psychosis. *The American Journal of Psychiatry* 1991;148:495-498.

Siegel RK. Cocaine hallucinations. *The American Journal of Psychiatry* 1978;135:309-314.

Withers NW, Pulvirenti L, Koob GF, et al. Cocaine abuse and dependence. *Journal of Clinical Psychopharmacology* 1995;15:63-78.

43 Opioid Related Disorders (DSM-IV-TR #304.00, 305.50, 292.89, 292.0)

An opiate is any intoxicant naturally found in opium. The term "opioid" is more general and refers to any substance, either synthetic or naturally occurring, that has morphine-like effects.

Opium is obtained from the juice of the poppy plant, and within opium are found two opiates, namely morphine and codeine. Synthetic and semi-synthetic derivatives include heroin, hydromorphone, merperidine, hydrocodone, oxycodone and pentazocine. Methadone and buprenorphine are derivatives used, as noted below, in the treatment of opioid addiction, but these may also be abused. Of all the opioids, heroin is by far the most commonly abused.

The intoxicant effects of the opioids are mediated by their binding to mu and, to a lesser extent, kappa receptors within the central nervous system. Most opioids, such as morphine, heroin, and hydromorphone, are pure agonists and act primarily at the mu receptor; pentazocine and buprenorphine, however, are mixed agonist-antagonist agents which affect both mu and kappa receptors.

Although some of the opioids, such as morphine, heroin, pentazocine, and methadone, may be used orally, in most instances a parenteral route is preferred, as the effect is more immediate and intense. Thus illicit heroin, or tablets or capsules of licit drugs, are crushed, dissolved and filtered (often through cigarette filters) to yield a more or less adulterated or contaminated liquid for injection. Most addicts progress from "skin popping," or subcutaneous injection, to "mainlining" the drug intravenously. Occasionally heroin may be snorted or smoked or, in the practice known as

"chasing the dragon," heated, with subsequent inhalation of the heroin vapor.

The lifetime prevalence of opioid addiction is probably about 0.4% in the United States, and, particularly in the case of heroin addiction, males far outnumber females. Among professional groups, opioid dependence, as might be expected given their availability, is more common in physicians and nurses than in lawyers, accountants or teachers.

ONSET

Most patients begin using opioids with their friends during adolescence or early adult years. Typically use escalates within a year or so until addiction has set in.

Less commonly, the initial exposure is by prescription of an opioid for its analgesic or antitussive effect to a patient predisposed to addiction. Soon thereafter the patient seeks the drug for its intoxicating effect and may begin a career of "doctor shopping" to maintain the supply. For physicians, pharmacists, and nurses opioids are generally easily obtained by diverting hospital supplies or through mail order catalogs.

CLINICAL FEATURES

The intoxication produced by opioids is intensely seductive. Within minutes after the intravenous injection of heroin, morphine, or hydromorphone the user may be rewarded by an intense rush. The body is suffused with warmth, and orgasmic sensations may be felt. In less than a minute the rush tends to pass, to be replaced by a drowsy, vaguely euphoric feeling that may last for hours. Dysarthria and difficulty with concentration may occur. The pupils are constricted, peristalsis is slowed, and constipation ensues; urinary hesitancy or retention may occur. Some experience generalized pruritus. During the intoxication most users are slowed down, and some may "nod off." Aggressiveness and sexual desire are blunted, and an opioid-intoxicated user rarely harms others during the actual intoxication.

Meperidine intoxication may have distinctive clinical features. Meperidine is metabolized to normeperidine, and this metabolite may cause agitation, tremor, dilated pupils, increased deep tendon reflexes, and occasionally myoclonus or seizures.

Pentazocine intoxication may also possess distinctive features. Especially with higher doses dysphoria, anxiety, hallucinations, and bizarre thoughts may occur. Diaphoresis and dizziness are common. Some addicts combine pentazocine with an antihistamine called tripelennamine, also known as a "T and B" (the "T" from "Talwin" and the "B" from the blue color of the tripelennamine tablet). This combination, when taken intravenously, is said by some to produce a better "rush" than heroin.

Opioid overdose is not uncommon. The purity of "street" heroin varies widely. A "100 mg" packet may in fact contain only 5 or 10 mg of pure heroin, the rest being adulterants and additives. The unsuspecting acquisition of purer grades may lead to overdose. Overdose also occurs when opioid addicts resume use after a period of abstinence. Having lost their tolerance they may find themselves overdosed on an amount that heretofore had only minimal effect.

In an overdose the user is stuporous or comatose. Initially the pupils are pinpoint; however, with respiratory depression and cerebral anoxia pupillary dilatation may occur. Temperature falls, and the skin is often cold and clammy. Respirations decrease not uncommonly to less than five breaths/minute. Pulmonary edema is not uncommon. Intracranial pressure may rise, and seizures may occur. Death is usually caused by respiratory arrest.

With frequent, repeated use tolerance develops to almost all of the effects of the opioids, with the notable exception of miosis and constipation. Ever higher doses must be used to obtain the rush and euphoria; some addicts may eventually take astounding doses, sometimes over a gram of morphine at a time, and not experience any respiratory depression.

Concurrent with the development of tolerance, users also begin to experience withdrawal symptoms. Although subtle withdrawal symptoms may appear after a relatively brief period of sustained use, in some cases of after only a few days, most patients remain untroubled by them for longer periods of time. Eventually, however, significant withdrawal symptoms occur, and when they do the addict may continue using opioids as much to prevent withdrawal as to achieve euphoria.

In those addicted to heroin or morphine, withdrawal symptoms gradually emerge anywhere from 6 to 12 hours after the last dose. The user becomes uneasy and experiences a craving for the drug. Yawning, lacrimation, and rhinorrhea appear; diaphoresis is also seen. Several hours later the user may fall into a restless sleep, known as "yen" sleep. Upon awakening, the earlier symptoms intensify, and the user soon thereafter becomes irritable, demanding, and intensely dysphoric. Insomnia may be extreme. Nausea, vomiting, intestinal cramping, and diarrhea occur, and the user begins to experience waves of goose flesh that may be so severe as to make flesh resemble that of a plucked turkey, an appearance that prompted the phrase "cold turkey." Intense bone and muscle pain in the back, arms, and legs occurs. Often, seemingly involuntary kicking movements occur, a phenomenon that prompted another proverbial phrase "kicking the habit." The pupils are dilated, and the temperature, pulse, and blood pressure are all increased. Leukocytosis may be present. Fluid loss secondary to vomiting and diarrhea may lead to dehydration and rarely circulatory collapse.

The withdrawal syndrome from heroin or morphine usually peaks in 2 to 3 days. Although it is generally not life threatening, in contrast, say, to delirium tremens, most addicts find it so intensely noxious that they go to almost any length to avoid it. After peaking, symptoms gradually subside over the following week or week and a half.

The symptoms of withdrawal from other opioids, such as meperidine, pentazocine, and methadone, are in general similar to those just described for heroin or morphine; however, the course is somewhat different. Meperidine withdrawal tends to appear in only a few hours, peaks in 8 to 12 hours, and tends to clear in 4 to 5 days. The course of pentazocine withdrawal is even more rapid. By contrast, withdrawal symptoms from methadone are generally delayed for 1 to 4 days, peak in about 1 week, and may take 2 weeks or more to subside completely.

Subsequent to the resolution of the classic withdrawal symptoms described above, patients may display a less clearly defined protracted withdrawal syndrome that may last from several weeks up to a half a year. Addicts complain of dysphoria, irritability, anhedonia, insomnia and drug craving.

The life of the opioid addict often becomes centered on only one thing: obtaining the drug. The restless anticipation of the rush, the deep craving for the drug, and the intense fear of withdrawal symptoms combine to irresistibly drive the addict to do whatever is necessary to maintain the supply. Prostitution and murder may occur; some may sell children.

Most opioid addicts use other substances, including cocaine, amphetamines, alcohol, benzodiazepines and marijuana. At times these may be used primarily as adjuncts to the opioid (cocaine to reduce sedation and alcohol or a benzodiazepine to ease withdrawal); however, many opioid addicts also become addicted to these. Indeed cocaine addiction and alcoholism are not uncommonly found concurrent with opioid addiction.

Opioid addiction is also strongly associated with antisocial personality disorder, major depression, and various phobias.

COURSE

The overall long-term prognosis is poor. By their early 40s no more than one-third of addicts have become abstinent, and the rest are either still using, or incarcerated, or dead from suicide, homicide or one of the many complications of opioid dependence, most notably AIDS or an overdose.

COMPLICATIONS

Those who become involved in the drug "subculture" are liable to violent death at the hands of others. Suicide attempts are not at all uncommon. Those who survive may end up losing all in their pursuit of the drug.

Overdose may be followed by pulmonary edema, aspiration pneumonia, respiratory depression or death. Those who survive a significant period of cerebral hypoxia may be left with a post-anoxic dementia and are at risk for a delayed post-anoxic leukoencephalopathy.

Intravenous use brings the risk of bacteremia with pulmonary abscess, endocarditis, cerebral abscess, cerebral mycotic aneurysm, meningitis, osteomyelitis (with a predelection for the lumbar vertebral bodies) and tetanus: in the case of tetanus, the rigidity and spasm seen here may be mistaken for the "kicking" seen in withdrawal. Parenteral users also often share needles and thus are at risk for AIDS, hepatitis and syphilis. Furthermore, the presence of particulates in the injected fluid (as may occur when cigarette filters are used to filter the dissolved opioid) may lead to pulmonary fibrosis, pulmonary hypertension and right ventricular failure. Particulates also collect in regional lymph nodes causing a chronic lymphadenopathy with edema, especially of the hands.

"Skin popping" may be followed by a cellulitis or ulceration, and those who repeatedly inject heroin intramuscularly may develop a myositis which may lead to ossification.

Patients who "chase the dragon" and inhale heroin are at risk for a progressive leukoencephalopathy.

Illegally manufactured "street" meperidine may be contaminated with a byproduct of its synthesis, namely methyl-phenyl-tetrahydropyridine (MPTP), which may cause an irreversible parkinsonism.

Other complications include progressive renal failure, rhabdomyolysis, transverse myelitis, plexopathies and peripheral neuropathies. The cause of these complications is unclear, but the effect of contaminants is suspected. Finally, opioid addicts are at increased risk for tuberculosis.

ETIOLOGY

Recent work suggests that, in the presence of certain environmental factors, as noted below, genetic factors may increase the risk of developing opioid addiction.

The families of origin of opioid addicts tend to be severely disturbed; alcoholism, opioid addiction, or other substance use disorders are common among the parents.

Opioid addicts often have a history of antisocial behavior before ever using opioids, and, as noted earlier, antisocial personality disorder is common among opioid addicts. Criminal activity accelerates during addiction and tends to persist into abstinence, albeit to a lesser degree.

DIFFERENTIAL DIAGNOSIS

Other intoxications, especially those from alcohol or sedative hypnotics, may present a clinical picture somewhat similar to opioid intoxication. In these cases, however, one fails to see the striking miosis that characterizes opioid intoxication. In doubtful cases a urine toxicologic screen is helpful; heroin is metabolized to morphine and thus may be detected in the urine for up to a day or two after heroin use. The possibility of a mixed intoxication secondary to multiple substances must also be kept in mind.

TREATMENT

In a patient comatose from opioid overdose, naloxone may be given as described in that chapter. The goal of treatment with naloxone is to restore the respiratory rate, gag reflex, and consciousness. Care must be taken not to "overshoot" and precipitate a hyperacute opioid withdrawal syndrome. This is particularly important to prevent in pregnant patients, as withdrawal may be associated with fetal death. Since agitation may occur as the patient emerges from the coma, one should prepare for instant application of restraints. As noted in the chapter on naloxone repeated doses are generally necessary, since the half-life of naloxone is considerably shorter than that of any of the opioids. As noted earlier, convulsions may occur during overdose. With certain exceptions, such as meperidine, naloxone is quite effective in controlling these, whereas anticonvulsants appear of limited value.

Patients wishing to be withdrawn from opioids should generally be admitted to a secure inpatient unit. Given the intense dysphoria and drug craving that often occurs, one may decide to keep some patients confined to the ward and to prohibit all but fully supervised visits until the withdrawal syndrome has run its course. Currently three treatment approaches to withdrawal are available: "cold turkey," methadone withdrawal, and clonidine treatment. Which one has the best success rate in terms of eventual abstinence is not clear.

Very few patients opt to go "cold turkey." However, as withdrawal is generally not life threatening, this may be appropriate for some. It is generally contraindicated if the patient is pregnant. Prochloperazine may be used for vomiting, diphenoxylate for diarrhea.

Oral methadone may be substituted for the patient's opioid and then gradually tapered. When withdrawal symptoms appear, a starting dose of 10 to 20 mg may be given orally, with repeat doses of from 5 to 10 mg every four hours as needed to suppress withdrawal symptoms. Most patients may be stabilized on from 20 to 40 mg daily, after which the dose may be tapered in decrements of from 5 to 10 mg daily.

Clonidine is not as effective in suppressing withdrawal symptoms as is methadone, but in instances where methadone is not available, or if in the interest of long-term abstinence it appears prudent not to use any opioids, including methadone, then clonidine represents a viable alternative. This approach, however, as is the case with "cold turkey," is generally contraindicated in pregnant patients. Clonidine appears most effective against nausea and diarrhea, less effective against insomnia, and has little effect on drug craving, restlessness, and "kicking." Once withdrawal begins, an initial dose of 0.1 to 0.3 mg is given. Repeated doses may then be given every 2 or 3 hours until the desired clinical effect is seen. Based on the initial dose required, a regular dosage given four times daily is then established. However, as withdrawal symptoms may not peak for several days, provision for p.r.n. doses should be made and the regular dose accordingly adjusted upward until no further p.r.n. doses are required. In most instances a final total daily dosage ranges from 0.6 to 2.4 mg. Before each dose patients should be checked for sedation and postural hypotension. The patient is generally "covered" with clonidine for about 7 to 10 days, that is to say for the natural course of the withdrawal. During this time, dosage reduction may be required to prevent sedation and constipation. Once the withdrawal has run its course, clonidine is tapered over 3 or 4 days and then discontinued.

There is one additional mode of withdrawal that deserves mention, known as "rapid" or "ultra-rapid" detoxification. Although details differ among programs, in most cases patients are first "covered" with clonidine and an anti-emetic and then either sedated with a benzodiazepine or anesthetized with propofol or midazolam. Naloxone and naltrexone are given and the potentially extremely dysphoric withdrawal is thus precipitated while the patient is more or less unconscious. Consciousness is then allowed to return and patients are continued on naltrexone and, temporarily, also on clonidine and an anti-emetic. It is not at all clear whether these techniques increase the chance of abstinence, nor whether any purported successes outweigh the risks of general anesthesia.

With regard to long-term treatment, an ongoing debate exists about the relative merits of methadone or buprenorphine maintenance versus abstinence. Most patients in maintenance programs evidence a clinically significant reduction in criminal behavior and in the use of other opioids, along with increased employment. On the other hand, both these agents are clearly capable of causing euphoria, and patients in maintenance programs often continue to use other substances, especially alcohol and benzodiazepines. Abstinence, clearly, is a preferable goal. Unfortunately, however, given the status quo few patients are able to achieve this goal.

Methadone maintenance is conducted only in clinics that have secured necessary federal, state, and local approval. In some methadone clinics chronic indefinite treatment is presumed, and doses range anywhere from 80 to 120 mg of methadone a day. By contrast, at other clinics eventual abstinence is the goal, and patients are initially stabilized on lower doses of anywhere from 20 to 60 mg a day. When patients have consistently tested free of other opioids or any other intoxicants for about a year, the dose of methadone is tapered on a weekly basis in decrements ranging anywhere from 5% to 10% and eventually discontinued. Despite extensive counseling during methadone maintenance the majority of patients relapse, usually within several months after discontinuation of methadone.

Buprenorphine maintenance may be conducted on an outpatient basis by any physician in the United States who has satisfied certain Federal criteria, and most patients may be managed at doses of from 16 to 32 mg sublingually given three times weekly.

Regardless of whether methadone or buprenorphine are used, it must be borne in mind that both drugs are metabolized by cytochrome P450 3A4, hence dosage adjustments will be required if an inducer (e.g., rifampin, carbamazepine or phenytoin) or inhibitor (e.g., ketoconazole, ritonavir, indinavir, saquinavir, erythromycin or cimetidine) is added.

Treatment approaches that have as their goal abstinence and that do not use methadone maintenance include Narcotics Anonymous and the various therapeutic communities. Narcotics Anonymous, modeled after Alcoholics Anonymous, is perhaps the most viable nonresidential treatment approach. A number of residential therapeutic communities exist, each with a somewhat different approach. All, however, strongly emphasize confrontation, and most encourage a stay of a year or more.

In patients who are highly motivated toward abstinence, naltrexone may be a valuable adjunct to outpatient treatment during the first few months to a half a year after discharge. Naltrexone effectively prevents opioid-induced euphoria and thus, if the patient does "slip," prevents the incredibly reinforcing "rush." Use of naltrexone is as described in that chapter. Those who lack commitment to abstinence rarely agree to take naltrexone, or if they do, drop out within a few weeks. In some cases, however, particularly among physicians, nurses, and others who still maintain and value social connections outside the drug subculture, naltrexone may play a critical role during the first all-important few months of abstinence, especially if used in a "contingency" program wherein the occurrence of a positive urinary drug screen is followed by notification of the appropriate authorities.

Should a concurrent major depression or phobia require pharmacologic treatment, the monoamine oxidase inhibitors are generally contraindicated because the combination of an MAOI and meperidine may cause delirium, coma, convulsions and death. Other antidepressants, however, appear quite safe, as do lithium, valproate, and carbamazepine.

BIBLIOGRAPHY

Bell JR, Young MR, Masterman SC, et al. A pilot study of naltrexone-accelerated detoxification in opioid dependence. *The Medical Journal of Australia* 1999;171:26-30.

Carroll KM, Ball SA, Nich C, et al. Targeting behavioral therapies to enhance naltrexone treatment of opioid dependence: efficacy of contingency management and significant other involvement. *Archives of General Psychiatry* 2001;58:755-761.

Challoner KR, McCarron MM, Newton EJ. Pentazocine (Talwin) injection: report of 57 cases. *The Journal of Emergency Medicine* 1990;8:67-74.

de Gans J, Stam J, van Wijugaarden GK. Rhabdomyolysis and concurrent neurological lesions after intravenous heroin abuse. *Journal of Neurology, Neurosurgery, and Psychiatry* 1985;48:1057-1059.

Haastrup S, Jepsen PW. Eleven year follow-up of 300 young opioid addicts. *Acta Psychiatrica Scandinavica* 1988;77:22-26.

Hser YI, Anglin D, Powers K. A 24-year follow-up of California narcotics addicts. *Archives of General Psychiatry* 1993;50:577-584.

Jasinski JR, Johnson RE, Kocher TR. Clonidine in morphine withdrawal. Differential effects on signs and symptoms. *Archives of General Psychiatry* 1985;42:1063-1066.

Johnson RE, Chutuape MA, Strain EC, et al. A comparison of levomethadyl acetate, buprenorphine, and methadone for opioid dependence. *The New England Journal of Medicine* 2000;343:1290-1297.

Kriegstein AR, Shungu DC, Miller WS, et al. Leukoencephalopathy and raised brain lactate from heroin vapor inhalation ("chasing the dragon"). *Neurology* 1999;53:1765-1773.

McGregor C, Ali R, White JM, et al. A comparison of antagonist-precipitated withdrawal under anesthesia to standard inpatient withdrawal as a precursor to maintenance naltrexone treatment in heroin users: outcomes at 6 and 12 months. *Drug and Alcohol Dependence* 2002;68:5-14.

Torrens M, San L, Cami J. Buprenorphine versus heroin dependence: comparison of toxicologic and psychopathologic characteristics. *The American Journal of Psychiatry* 1993;150:822-824.

44 Sedative, Hypnotic, or Anxiolytic Related Disorders (DSM-IV-TR #304.10, 305.40, 292.89, 292.0, 292.81)

The sedatives, hypnotics, and anxiolytics, including the benzodiazepines, barbiturates, and related drugs, comprise a large group of agents often referred to as "sedative-hypnotics," all of which have an effect that is more or less similar to that of alcohol. Although most commonly used in combination with alcohol or other substances, they are at times used in isolation, and for clarity of exposition they shall for the most part be treated that way in this chapter.

Classifying the sedative-hypnotics according to the duration of their effect is clinically useful, as this allows one to make a rough prediction as to when withdrawal, seizures, or delirium is likely to occur (see the box on this page).

The popularity of each of these various agents has changed over time. The barbiturates, chloral hydrate, and paraldehyde, once commonly abused, have generally been supplanted by the benzodiazepines. Among the benzodiazepines, diazepam, lorazepam, and alprazolam are currently the most popular among abusers, with diazepam heading the list. Reliable estimates of current prevalence are not available. Clinically, isolated addiction to sedative-hypnotics appears uncommon; however, addiction to one of them in conjunction with alcohol, opioids, cocaine or amphetamines appears to be quite common.

ONSET

When sedative-hypnotics are used in isolation, the onset of their addiction appears to occur in late teenage or early adult years; however, one to two decades may be required before the full picture of addiction is established. But if these drugs are used in conjunction with alcohol or other drugs, the onset generally parallels that of the other agent.

CLINICAL FEATURES

Descriptions of sedative-hypnotic intoxication, withdrawal, withdrawal seizures and withdrawal delirium are provided below, followed by a discussion of the overall form that sedative-hypnotic addiction may take.

In intoxication the user, though often euphoric, may at times display some emotional lability. Judgment is impaired, and sexual or aggressive urges that are normally inhibited may be acted upon. With somewhat more severe intoxication, reaction time is markedly slowed, and the user may appear drowsy or lethargic. Dysarthria, poor coordination, ataxia, and nystagmus are common at this point. Blackouts similar to those described in the chapter on alcoholic blackouts may occur. Severe intoxication may produce stupor, coma, respiratory depression and death.

The onset of withdrawal symptoms varies according to the duration of the agent's effect. Roughly speaking, withdrawal may be expected in less than 1 day for short-acting agents, 2 to 3 days for intermediate-acting agents, and 2 to 6 days for longer-acting agents. For certain very-long-acting agents, such as diazepam or phenobarbital, a "self-tapering" process may occur as the blood level falls very slowly, so withdrawal symptoms may be relatively mild compared with other agents. The patient in withdrawal is anxious and irritable and generally craves the drug. Autonomic signs, such as tremor, tachycardia, and diaphoresis, are common, and muscle weakness is a typical complaint. Nausea and vomiting may occur, as may postural hypotension. Insomnia is common and may be quite severe. For short- and intermediate-acting agents withdrawal symptoms tend to peak at 1 to 3 days and persist for 1 to 2 weeks; for longer-acting agents, the peak may not occur for 5 to 7 days, and the syndrome may persist for 2 to 3 weeks. Insomnia is usually the last symptom to clear, and sleep may not normalize for a month or more.

If seizures occur they generally do so in the context of the withdrawal syndrome. They are more common in barbiturate than benzodiazepine withdrawal, and when secondary to barbiturate withdrawal they tend to be much more severe than those seen in alcohol withdrawal. Multiple seizures are not uncommon, and status epilepticus may occur.

Withdrawal delirium is generally seen only in those users who have been addicted to sedative-hypnotics for many years and who have experienced multiple episodes of withdrawal. Typically the delirium arises out of the withdrawal syndrome. Insomnia and autonomic symptoms become markedly heightened, and fever may appear. Confusion and disorientation occur, and the user experiences visual, tactile, or less frequently auditory hallucinations. Persecutory delusions may appear, as may catatonia, and one commonly sees agitation that may be extraordinarily severe. The

Duration of Effect of Certain Sedative-Hypnotics

SHORT-ACTING AGENTS (DURATION GENERALLY LESS THAN 6 HOURS)	LONG-ACTING AGENTS (DURATION GENERALLY LONGER THAN 24 HOURS)
Triazolam	Quazepam
Alprazolam	Prazepam
Zolpidem	Halazepam
Zaleplon	Flurazepam
	Clorazepam
INTERMEDIATE-ACTING AGENTS (DURATION GENERALLY FROM 6 TO 18 HOURS)	Diazepam
	Amobarbital
Oxazepam	Secobarbital
Temazepam	Pentobarbital
Lorazepam	Phenobarbital
Chlordiazepoxide	Butalbital
Meprobamate	
Chloral hydrate	

delirium tends to persist for days or a week or two, then gradually clears.

Users who become addicted to sedative-hypnotics generally are introduced to the drug in one of two ways: either the user received the drug illicitly from a dealer or friend, or the drug was initially prescribed for anxiety, insomnia, depression or headache. In most cases use escalates over time. In some a binge pattern develops, whereas in others daily use becomes the rule. Regardless of the pattern of use, sedative-hypnotic addicts come to experience a craving for the substance. It must be borne in mind, however, that the mere fact that benzodiazepines are subject to abuse should not unduly discourage their use, as the vast majority of patients who receive such prescriptions do not in fact end up abusing the drug.

Daily users may develop a remarkable degree of tolerance: some may end up taking the equivalent of hundreds of milligrams of diazepam a day, with little or no evidence of sedation. Concurrent use of alcohol or other substances is not uncommon.

COURSE

Sedative-hypnotic addiction tends to be chronic, especially when occurring in combination with alcohol. Only a minority of patients become abstinent in the natural course of events.

COMPLICATIONS

Intoxicated patients may fall and suffer fractures or head trauma; motor vehicle accidents may also occur. Furthermore, those who display a daily pattern of use often become depressed and irritable, and some may attempt suicide. Accidental overdose is not rare and is particularly injurious when combined with alcohol; fatalities have occurred.

ETIOLOGY

As noted earlier, sedative-hypnotic addiction often arises in the context of other addictions: opioid addicts may use these drugs to relieve opioid withdrawal, stimulant addicts may use them to "modulate" the "high," and alcoholics may use them to dampen the withdrawal "shakes." The reason why some of these users develop dependence on sedative-hypnotics, or why such a dependence develops in the person who uses sedative-hypnotics in an "isolated" fashion is not clear.

DIFFERENTIAL DIAGNOSIS

Sedative-hypnotic addiction must be distinguished from appropriate, medically supervised use that has become complicated by neuroadaptation. An example would be an elderly patient who has taken 5 or 10 mg of diazepam nightly for 10 years to ease the transition to sleep. Leaving the medicine at home on vacation, the patient notes several days later anxiety and worsening insomnia. These complaints are related to the physician, who calls in a prescription for a small supply to tide the patient over until returning home. The difference here is that this patient, in contrast to the sedative-hypnotic addict, neither craves the drug nor escalates the use of it.

TREATMENT

Blacked-out or intoxicated patients may simply be observed in a safe environment until the intoxication has passed. In cases of profound intoxication with benzodiazepines where respiratory depression occurs, flumazenil, as described in that chapter, may obviate the need for intubation. Flumazenil is not effective for barbiturates or other sedative-hypnotics. In the case of barbiturate overdose, gastric lavage, followed by repeated doses of activated charcoal, all in the setting of intensive support, are useful: when these measures fail, hemodialysis should be considered.

Withdrawal from sedative-hypnotics should generally be treated be re-instituting the offending agent at a dose sufficient to abolish the withdrawal symptoms, and then gradually tapering the dose by roughly 10% per day. Some authors recommend the use of diazepam or clonazepam rather than the abused drug; however, there is no compelling evidence for the superiority of this approach, and, in the case of barbiturates, it may be dangerous. It appears that cross-tolerance between benzodiazepines and barbiturates may be far less than complete, and consequently, only barbiturates will suffice to treat barbiturate withdrawal. In cases of barbiturate dependence where the average daily dose of the barbiturate is not known, one may give phenobarbital at a dose of 90 to 120 mg every one to two hours until the withdrawal is suppressed.

In the case of benzodiazepine withdrawal, another option is carbamazepine. After the benzodiazepine withdrawal has been brought under control by a benzodiazepine, carbamazepine, in a dose of 400 to 800 mg daily, may be added, after which the benzodiazepine may be rapidly tapered over two or three days. Subsequently, the carbamazepine is continued for the anticipated duration of the withdrawal, after which it is tapered over two or three days and then discontinued. Importantly, it must be stressed that carbamazepine is not effective in barbiturate withdrawal, and may not be as effective in alprazolam withdrawal as it is for other benzodiazepines.

Propranolol, in total daily doses of from 60 to 120 mg, may be used adjunctively to suppress tremor; however, it must be borne in mind that propranolol does not prevent either withdrawal seizures or withdrawal delirium.

The best treatment for withdrawal delirium is prevention, and withdrawal symptoms should be promptly brought under control. Should a withdrawal delirium occur, aggressive treatment with the appropriate sedative-hypnotic is pursued in the setting of general supportive measures, as outlined in the chapter on delirium.

The overall goal of treatment is abstinence. Those addicted to sedative-hypnotics alone or to a combination of sedative-hypnotics and alcohol may do well in Alcoholics Anonymous and may be approached as described in the chapter on alcoholism. However, in those who use sedative-hypnotics in combination with opioids, cocaine, or stimulants, a judgment call is required as to whether the sedative-hypnotic or the other agent is the "drug of choice." Treatment then is focused on this "drug of choice" with the expectation that once controlled the concurrent drug use will either come under control or represent a relatively minor problem.

BIBLIOGRAPHY

Allgulander C, Borg S, Vikander B. A 4-6-year follow-up of 50 patients with primary dependence on sedative and hypnotic drugs. *The American Journal of Psychiatry* 1984;141:1580-1582.

Anonymous. Treatment of benzodiazepine overdose with flumazenil. The Flumazenil in Benzodiazepine Intoxication Multicenter Study Group. *Clinical Therapeutics* 1992;14:978-995.

Aragona M. Abuse, dependence, and epileptic seizures after zolpidem withdrawal: review and case report. *Clinical Neuropharmacology* 2000;23:281-283.

Busto UE, Sellers EM. Anxiolytics and sedative-hypnotics dependence. *British Journal of Addictions* 1991;86:1647-1652.

Chern CH, Chern TL, Wang LM, et al. Continuous flumazenil infusion in preventing complications arising from severe benzodiazepine intoxication. *The American Journal of Emergency Medicine* 1998;16:238-241.

Janecek E, Kapur BM, Devenyi P. Oral phenobarbital loading: a safe method of barbiturate and nonbarbiturate hypnosedative withdrawal. *Canadian Medical Association Journal* 1987;137:410-412.

Martinez-Cano H, Vela-Bueno A, de Iceta M, et al. Benzodiazepine withdrawal seizures. *Pharmacopsychiatry* 1995;28:257-262.

Raja M, Altavista MC, Azzoni A, et al. Severe barbiturate withdrawal syndrome in migrainous patients. *Headache* 1996;36:119-121.

Rosebush PI, Mazurek MF. Catatonia after benzodiazepine withdrawal. *Journal of Clinical Pharmacology* 1996;16:315-319.

Schweizer E, Rickels K, Case WG, et al. Carbamazepine treatment in patients discontinuing long-term benzodiazepine therapy. Effects on withdrawal severity and outcome. *Archives of General Psychiatry* 1991;48:448-452.

45 Alcoholism and Alcohol Abuse (alcohol dependence, DSM-IV 303.90; alcohol abuse, DSM-IV 305.00)

Alcoholism, also known as alcohol dependence, is a common disorder. Lifetime prevalence rates vary widely according to the methodology used, but probably close to 10% of the U.S. population is affected. Asians, however, particularly those from China, Korea, and Japan, appear to have much lower rates. At all ages alcoholism is more common among males than females; however, given the somewhat later age of onset in females, the ratio tends to decrease in higher age groups. Overall the ratio is probably 3:1.

Alcoholics and alcohol abusers are recurrently and persistently beset with an urge to drink, an urge that is of sufficient compellingness for them to continue to drink despite the fact that because of their drinking they sustain substantial damage to their health and personal or business affairs. Amongst alcoholics, but not in alcohol abusers, one also sees the development of both craving and of neuroadaptation, with either tolerance or withdrawal.

This chapter deals with alcoholism and alcohol abuse in an overall sense. The following chapters cover alcohol intoxication, alcohol withdrawal, delirium tremens, and other alcohol-related disorders.

ONSET

The onset of alcoholism or alcohol abuse is generally insidious and spans many years. For men, onset is generally dated to the late teens or the early twenties; however, most alcoholics are not recognized as such until their late twenties or early thirties, and many more years may pass before the alcoholic or someone else recognizes the need for treatment. Although some otherwise typical onsets have been described in patients over 60, it is rare for the onset to occur past the age of 45.

The onset in women tends to be later than that in men.

Alcoholics who concurrently have an antisocial personality disorder seem to have an earlier onset, generally in the teenage years.

Although precisely dating the onset is very difficult, many alcoholics, in retrospect, can point to a period in their lives when they "crossed the line," after which their efforts to control their drinking became futile.

CLINICAL FEATURES

In a full-blown case of alcoholism, drinking has become the primary need in an alcoholic's life, to the detriment or neglect of almost all other activities. The urge to drink may be experienced as a craving, an imperious need, or a compulsion; at times, however, when the alcoholic is off guard it may merely sneak up insidiously, and the alcoholic may begin drinking without knowing why.

Denial is ubiquitous in alcoholism. Almost all alcoholics deny they have a problem with drinking or rationalize it one way or another. They are often quick to lay blame for their drinking on situations or other people. Upon close inquiry, however, one often sees that drinking is in large part autonomous. Although stressful events may be followed by increased alcohol consumption, the alcoholic is also intoxicated during the good times, or simply the neutral times of life.

Most alcoholics make attempts to control their drinking, and although they may have some successes, these are generally short-lived. This "loss of control" was at one point considered the hallmark of the alcoholic. However, it may be just as fair to say that the hallmark is rather a sense of a need to control. Normal people do not experience a need to control their drinking; they simply stop, without giving it a second thought.

When alcoholics do drink, most eventually become intoxicated, and it is this recurrent intoxication that eventually brings their lives down in ruins. Friends are lost, health deteriorates, marriages are broken, children are abused, and jobs terminated. Yet despite these consequences the alcoholic continues to drink. Many undergo a "change in personality." Previously upstanding individuals may find themselves lying, cheating, stealing, and engaging in all manner of deceit to protect or cover up their drinking. Shame and remorse the morning after may be intense; many alcoholics progressively isolate themselves to drink undisturbed. An alcoholic may hole up in a motel for days or a week, drinking continuously. Most alcoholics become more irritable; they have a heightened sensitivity to anything vaguely critical. Many alcoholics appear quite grandiose, yet on closer inspection one sees that their self-esteem has slipped away from them.

Most alcoholics also display an alcohol withdrawal syndrome when they either reduce or temporarily cease consumption. Awakening with the "shakes" and with the strong urge for relief drinking is a common occurrence; many alcoholics eventually succumb to the "morning drink" to reduce their withdrawal symptoms.

Some degree of tolerance occurs in all alcoholics. Here the alcoholic finds that progressively larger amounts must be consumed to get the desired degree of intoxication; if the amount is not increased, the alcoholic finds that the degree of intoxication becomes less and less. Some alcoholics, however, late in the course of the disorder may experience a relatively abrupt loss of tolerance that can be profound. The alcoholic who routinely drank a quart of bourbon a day now finds that a couple of shots of bourbon leads to hopeless intoxication.

Excessive use of other intoxicants is common among alcoholics. Benzodiazepines are popular among those past their late twenties; in younger patients, marijuana, cocaine, and opioids may be preferred. For most alcoholics, however, these substances are merely ancillary; alcohol remains the "drug of choice."

Other disorders are often seen concurrent with alcoholism, including major depression, panic disorder (with or without agoraphobia), social phobia (of the generalized type), and, somewhat less commonly, bipolar disorder and schizophrenia. Of the personality disorders, antisocial personality disorder occurs in male alcoholics more often than one would expect by chance; the same is true for borderline personality disorder among female alcoholics.

Alcohol abusers are similar to alcoholics in that they continue to drink despite serious adverse consequences. But abusers are different from alcoholics in two ways. First, most alcohol abusers do not develop neuroadaptation as manifested by tolerance or withdrawal; the sustained drinking generally required to produce these phenomena is for the most part seen only in alcoholism. Exceptions, however, exist as some people seem particularly prone to developing withdrawal and may in fact have the shakes after only a few weeks of drinking, only then to become and remain abstinent. Such people probably do not have alcoholism. Second, one may inquire as to whether the drinker experiences a craving for alcohol rather than merely a desire for it. The alcohol abuser wants to drink and looks forward to it. The same may be true of the alcoholic at times; however, the alcoholic also has a craving for alcohol and because of that craving the ability to choose whether to drink or not is lost. At times the alcoholic simply "has to" drink. Consequences may deter the alcohol abuser, and the abuser may decide to stop because of them and then go ahead and stop. For the alcoholic, however, drinking persists despite the most disastrous consequences; some may continue to drink even while they lie on their death-bed in the hospital.

COURSE

Alcoholism may run an episodic or a chronic course. The alcoholic who experiences an episodic course is often referred to as a binge drinker. The binges themselves may last for days or weeks; in between them the alcoholic may go for months or a year or more without drinking at all. The alcoholic with a chronic course may drink on a regular daily basis or have brief periods of abstinence. The "weekend alcoholic" falls in this category. The pattern may change from episodic to chronic over many years. In most cases the complications of alcoholism tend to add up after 10 to 15 years: women tend to experience a more rapid progression than men.

Spontaneous remissions do occur in alcoholism, and they may be missed in epidemiologic surveys, as patients are generally reluctant to discuss their previous drinking. The general clinical impression, however, is that a full spontaneous remission is relatively rare.

The overall course of alcohol abuse is not as clearly understood: some may stop or successfully moderate their drinking; some may continue to drink abusively for an indefinite period of time without ever developing a craving and neuroadaptation, while some may develop these phenomena, thereby prompting a revision of the diagnosis to one of alcoholism.

COMPLICATIONS

The complications of alcoholism and alcohol abuse are exceedingly numerous. The population of our jails and hospitals would be dramatically reduced without alcoholism.

Both alcoholics and alcohol abusers are liable to arrests for public intoxication and driving while intoxicated, and both are more likely to have motor vehicle accidents, to lose jobs and to face separation from their loved ones. Other complications seen in both groups (albeit more commonly in the heavier-drinking alcoholics) include blackouts, alcohol withdrawal (the "shakes"), gastritis and fatty liver.

Alcoholics, in addition to the foregoing complications, are also at much higher risk for other complications, including the following.

Suicide is relatively common in active alcoholics, occurring in perhaps 15%. Risk factors include male sex, depression, unemployment, lack of social supports, and significant general medical illnesses, such as pancreatitis, cirrhosis, and others. An alcohol-induced depression may occur, and indeed such a "secondary" depression is seen in at least one-half of all alcoholics.

Drinking during pregnancy exposes unborn children to the risk of prematurity, low birth weight, and fetal alcohol syndrome.

Other complications of alcoholism include seizures ("rum fits"), delirium tremens, alcohol hallucinosis, alcoholic paranoia and alcoholic dementia. Head trauma, often with subdural hematoma, may be quite common.

Thiamine deficiency may be followed by Wernicke's encephalopathy, with a subsequent Korsakoff's syndrome.

Alcoholic cerebellar degeneration, polyneuropathy, and myopathy may completely disable the patient.

Alcoholic hepatitis is common, and cirrhosis may occur in something less than 10% of alcoholics with the subsequent development of bleeding esophageal varices. Recurrent bouts of pancreatitis are not uncommon.

Alcoholics are more prone to infections of all sorts; aspiration pneumonia is common, bacterial meningitis less so.

Laboratory abnormalities are common and may or may not be associated with symptoms. These include the following: hypomagnesemia, hypoprothrombinemia, megaloblastic anemia, thrombocytopenia, hypoglycemia, and ketoacidosis. The combination of an otherwise unexplained increase in mean corpuscular red blood cell volume and an elevation of the serum gamma-glutamyl transferase (SGGT) level is very suggestive of alcoholism. Another "marker" for alcoholism is an elevated carbohydrate-deficient transferrin (CDT) level in the absence of significant hepatic disease.

Alcoholic cardiomyopathy is a rare but often fatal complication.

Central pontine myelinolysis and Marchiafava-Bignami disease are extremely rare complications but carry a high morbidity and mortality. Tobacco-alcohol amblyopia may occur. Occasionally, desperate alcoholics may seek intoxication with isopropyl (rubbing) alcohol or with methanol (wood alcohol), with consequences as described in their respective chapters.

ETIOLOGY

Family history, twin and adoption studies leave little doubt as to the importance of inheritance in alcoholism, which may account for up to 60% of the risk. Genetic studies, however, have not as yet yielded conclusive results. Earlier studies suggesting an association with certain polymorphisms at the dopamine D2 receptor (DRD2) gene have not been consistently replicated; whether more recent studies suggesting associations with various polymorphisms at the genes for the serotonin transporter or for neuropeptide Y will stand the test of time is uncertain.

Clinical studies of the non-alcoholic sons of alcoholics have yielded some interesting findings, as might be expected given the evidence for inheritance. Electrophysiologic studies have demonstrated a reduced P300 wave and a reduction in alpha activity while not drinking coupled with an increase in alpha activity while drinking. Of more interest from a clinical point of view, however, is the response of sons of alcoholics to a drink as compared to controls. As a group, these non-alcoholic sons of alcoholics had a lower degree of intoxication than did controls. Furthermore, over long-term follow-up the sons with the lowest response had a 60% chance of developing alcoholism; by contrast, in the sons with the most normal response the chance of developing alcoholism was only 15%. Clearly, among sons of alcoholics, being able to "hold one's liquor" is an ominous prognostic sign.

The reduced prevalence of alcoholism among some Asian groups, noted earlier, is related to a differential inheritance pattern of certain normally occurring alleles for aldehyde dehydrogenase. Ethanol is normally metabolized by alcohol dehydrogenase to acetaldehyde, which in turn is rapidly metabolized by aldehyde dehydrogenase to acetic acid. A majority of Asians, however, have forms of aldehyde dehydrogenase which are slow acting, thus allowing for an accumulation of this toxic intermediary metabolite with the production of an extremely dysphoric "Antabuse" reaction as described in the chapter on disulfiram. Naturally such individuals would be unlikely to pursue further intoxication, and thus less likely to become alcoholics.

DIFFERENTIAL DIAGNOSIS

The main impediments to the diagnosis of alcoholism are the denial seen in alcoholics and the low index of suspicion held by most physicians. All patients should be directly asked how much they drink, and whenever there is a history of arrests, job loss or separation and divorce, this point should be pursued with vigor: when appropriate, this history should be pursued with significant others. Other "red flags" include any of the other complications mentioned earlier, including especially otherwise unaccounted for tremor, gastritis or hepatitis. Another "red flag" of some note is a combination of an elevated MCV and SGGT, which is strongly suggestive of alcoholism.

In cases where the course of alcoholism or alcohol abuse is clearly episodic, one must consider whether these might be occurring "secondary" to some other disorder which also has an episodic course, such as major depression or bipolar disorder. Patients with a depression of major depression or bipolar disorder may "drink to drown their sorrows" and patients with mania, as in bipolar disorder, in their overall exuberant excessiveness, often also drink to excess. In these cases a careful history may reveal the onset of a mood disturbance before the onset of excessive drinking, and a subsequent spontaneous moderation of alcohol intake when the mood disturbance resolves. In cases of concurrent alcoholism and depression where it is not clear whether the depression is primary or occurring secondary to the alcoholism, it may be necessary to observe the patient into abstinence to make the correct diagnosis: whereas a depression of major depression typically persists well into abstinence, an alcohol-induced secondary depression generally undergoes a spontaneous remission within four weeks.

A similar diagnostic strategy may be adopted in cases where there is significant antisocial or "borderline" behavior and it is not clear whether these represent an independent personality disorder of complications of alcoholism. This is especially true when the onset of alcoholism occurs in middle or early teenage years. Alcoholics often commit many antisocial acts to continue drinking: lying, stealing, using aliases (if under age), and consistently failing to meet family or work responsibilities are common. Repeated intoxication also seriously impairs the alcoholic's ability to form lasting relations or a stable sense of identity. Whether a personality disorder diagnosis is warranted depends on whether these symptoms persist despite a prolonged period of abstinence.

TREATMENT

The goal of treating alcoholism is abstinence. Attempts have been made to enable the alcoholic to continue drinking in a controlled fashion, but without sustained success. This goal must be stated to alcoholics clearly, simply, and unmistakably. With regard to alcohol abuse, there is debate as to whether the goal should be abstinence or controlled drinking. Although some alcohol abusers are able to moderate their drinking to a "social" level, it is not possible to predict which of them will be able to accomplish this. Given this unpredictability, and the potentially grievous complications of alcohol abuse, it may be prudent to approach alcohol abusers in the same way as alcoholics.

Some alcoholics, by an extraordinary act of will, are able to stop on their own, but this is rare, and the vast majority of alcoholics will continue to drink unless they receive help. In such cases various psychosocial measures are helpful and may be offered. Drugs, such as disulfiram, naltrexone and topiramate, are discussed later, but it must be borne in mind that their usefulness here is limited.

Various counseling methods, including notably cognitive-behavioral therapy, have been successful in a minority of cases. For patients who fail to achieve abstinence with counseling, the physician should consider referral to Alcoholics Anonymous (AA).

Alcoholics Anonymous is the oldest treatment approach to alcoholism, and, if participated in fully, has the best success. Patients should be instructed to attend "ninety meetings in ninety days" and to get an AA "sponsor." Given the wide variety of AA meetings, most patients, by sampling a large number, will find somewhere they feel "at home." Many patients, though initially accepting such a prescription for AA, will fail to follow through, and attend only a few meetings. Here, a failure to achieve sobriety, rather than serving as evidence for the ineffectiveness of AA, is simply a manifestation of non-compliance.

At some point most alcoholics are hospitalized, either to effect a period of enforced abstinence or to treat one of the complications of alcoholism. The goal of an admission, in addition to treatment of any complications, should be to engage the patient in a psychosocial treatment program, such as AA. Although 4-week inpatient rehabilitation programs were once popular throughout the United States, they have not been shown to increase the chances of long-term abstinence. Questions have been raised as to whether most alcoholics are even capable of understanding the sort of educational program offered during these 4-week stays. Most recently detoxified alcoholics experience a very mild delirium, the "fog," that may last for weeks. Until this "mental fog" lifts, truly the only new idea that befogged alcoholics may be able to grasp is that if they want to stay sober they should go to 90 meetings in the 90 consecutive days after discharge, starting with a meeting on the day of discharge.

Family and friends should be encouraged to stop "enabling" patients by rescuing them or otherwise shielding them from the consequences of their drinking. Most family and friends hate to see alcoholics suffer, but in alcoholism the experience of consequences is the best, and sometimes the only, effective teacher. Thus when family or friends "protect" alcoholics, they only enable them to stay in denial and continue drinking, thus hastening the alcoholic's demise. Those family and friends who find it difficult to stop "enabling" may benefit from attendance at Al-Anon, a group for family and friends that is allied with AA.

Three drugs, namely disulfiram, naltrexone, and, possibly, topiramate, may be of some benefit to some patients, but cannot be relied on in the absence of psychosocial methods.

Disulfiram, by inspiring patients with a fear of an "Antabuse" reaction should they drink, may make for enough sober time for patients to benefit from a psychosocial approach. Given the risks associated with disulfiram, cases must be highly selected, and disulfiram should generally not be prescribed to patients who are not committed to sobriety, as they generally end up drinking while taking it. This includes patients who want disulfiram so that they can "dry out" for a few weeks and recover their health preparatory to resuming drinking, and also patients who are requesting the drug at the behest of others, whether it be a spouse or an employer. The use of disulfiram is discussed in detail in that chapter.

Naltrexone, in a dose of 50 mg daily, may, by reducing craving and damping the reinforcing euphoria of a drink should the patient "slip", reduce the number of drinking days and increase the chances of abstinence. These effects, however, are modest at best, and may, indeed, in the case of severe alcoholism, be negligible.

Topiramate, in a dose of from 100 to 200 mg, was recently demonstrated, in one double-blind comparison with placebo, to reduce drinking days, and the amount consumed on drinking days, and to increase the number of abstinent days. If these results are replicated, then topiramate will assume a place in the treatment on alcoholism: its effectiveness relative to either disulfiram or naltrexone, however, remains to be seen.

Although the role of the physician in the treatment of alcoholism per se is limited, medical attention to concurrent psychiatric disorders may be critically important. Depression, mania, frequent panic attacks, or schizophrenia may all so incapacitate patients that they are unable to participate in rehabilitative efforts. By relieving patients of the symptoms of the concurrent disorder, the physician may enable them to fully involve themselves in their efforts at sobriety. If medications are used, their purpose must be clearly stated. Many patients fondly hope that taking a medicine will obviate the need for rehabilitative psychosocial work. Such hopes must be dashed; patients must understand clearly that no medicine for alcoholism itself exists. One must not prescribe sedative-hypnotics, including benzodiazepines, to outpatient alcoholics. Although these have a place in the treatment of alcohol withdrawal, as described in that chapter, they are contraindicated

for outpatients. Furthermore, when nonhabituating medicines, such as antidepressants or antipsychotics, are prescribed patients must be informed that they cannot get "hooked" on them. It is also prudent to tell patients that some members of AA, lumping nonhabituating and habituating medicines in the same group, frown on taking medication of any sort. Patients therefore should be advised to confine their discussions about medication to their prescribing physician.

During the first few months of abstinence, patients who went through alcohol withdrawal often complain of persisting symptoms, such as insomnia, easy startability, and other autonomic symptoms, and difficulty remembering or thinking clearly. In such cases, patient's may be reasssured that these symptoms generally clear in a matter of months, generally never lasting more than six months. In cases, however, where such symptoms are disruptive to the patient's rehabilitative efforts, treatment with divalproex, as discussed in the chapter on alcohol withdrawal, may be indicated. If symptoms persist beyond six months despite abstinence, then another disorder must be sought.

Relapses are common; most occur in the first 6 months. Only about 50% of alcoholics achieve a year of continuous abstinence. The physician therefore must guard against becoming frustrated and must likewise help the patient avoid demoralization. A "slip" should not be taken as an indication of failure but rather as an indication to redouble one's efforts at treatment.

BIBLIOGRAPHY

Anonymous. Matching alcoholism treatments to client heterogeneity: Project MATCH posttreatment drinking outcomes. *Journal of Studies on Alcohol* 1997;58:7-29.

Anton RF. Carbohydrate-deficient transferrin for detection and monitoring of sustained heavy drinking. What have we learned? Where do we go from here? *Alcohol* 2001;25:185-188.

Cadoret RJ, Cain CA, Grove WM. Development of alcoholism in adoptees raised apart from alcoholic biologic relatives. *Archives of General Psychiatry* 1980;37:561-563.

Charness ME, Simon RP, Greenberg DA. Ethanol and the nervous system. *The New England Journal of Medicine* 1989;321:442-454.

Hasin DS, Grant BF. Major depression in 6050 former drinkers: association with past alcohol dependence. *Archives of General Psychiatry* 2002;59:794-800.

Helzer JE, Robins LN, Taylor JR, et al. The extent of long-term moderate drinking among alcoholics discharged from medical and psychiatric treatment facilities. *The New England Journal of Medicine* 1985; 312:1678-1682.

Johnson BA, Ait-Daoud N, Bowden CL, et al. Oral topiramate for treatment of alcohol dependence: a randomized controlled trial. *Lancet* 2003;361:1677-1685.

Krystal JH, Cramer JA, Krol WF, et al. Naltrexone in the treatment of alcohol dependence. *The New England Journal of Medicine* 2001; 345:1734-1739.

Schuckitt MA, Smith TL. An 8-year follow-up of 450 sons of alcoholic and control subjects. *Archives of General Psychiatry* 1996;53:202-210.

Schuckitt MA, Smith TL, Anthenelli R, et al. Clinical course of alcoholism in 636 male inpatients. *The American Journal of Psychiatry* 1993;150:786-792.

Sigvardsson S, Bohman M, Cloninger CR. Replication of the Stockholm Adoption Study of alcoholism. Confirmatory cross-fostering analysis. *Archives of General Psychiatry* 1996;53:681-687.

Alcohol Intoxication (DSM-IV-TR #303.00)

The intoxicated patient is a familiar sight in any emergency room, and the determination of a blood alcohol level (BAL) is a commonplace procedure.

BAL by convention may be expressed as milligrams per deciliter, or, as it is often charted, milligrams percent (mg%). Roughly speaking, in a 70 kg person BAL rises anywhere from 15 to 25 mg/dl with every 15 ml of rapidly ingested pure ethyl alcohol. This amount of ethanol is found in 1 ounce of 100 proof liquor, one 12-ounce bottle of beer, or about one glass (6 ounces) of wine. Given that most "social drinkers," or alcohol-naive persons, become intoxicated at a BAL of 100 mg/dl, simple arithmetic shows that for such a person only about four drinks, or beers, or glasses of wine are required to produce intoxication. As will be noted later, however, heavy drinkers may develop tolerance, and a much higher BAL is needed to produce intoxication.

A small percentage of ingested alcohol is metabolized by alcohol dehydrogenase located in the gastric mucosa; of the remainder, about 25% is absorbed through the gastric mucosa and 75% in the small intestine. Over 90% of absorbed alcohol is metabolized in the liver, the rest being excreted unchanged via the skin, lungs and kidneys. Hepatic metabolism is primarily via alcohol dehydrogenase to acetaldehyde which in turn is metabolized by acetaldehyde dehydrogenase to acetate.

In a normal 70 kg person, alcohol is metabolized in the liver at a constant rate of anywhere from 5 to 10 ml of pure ethanol/hour. Thus in such a person who has ingested 4 ounces of 100 proof whiskey (equivalent to 60 ml of pure ethanol), BAL will reach negligible levels in anywhere from 6 to 12 hours.

Women tend to have higher BALs than men for any given amount of ethanol ingested, and this appears to result from a relative deficiency of gastric alcohol dehydrogenase.

ONSET

The time to onset of any signs or symptoms of intoxication is determined primarily by the rapidity with which alcohol is absorbed. The severity of the intoxication, in turn, is a product of not only the absolute BAL reached but also of how rapidly it is reached. Food delays absorption significantly: on an empty stomach, 4 ounces of 100 proof liquor might produce intoxication in anywhere from 20 to 30 minutes; on a full stomach, however, the maximum BAL may be delayed for 2 or more hours. Furthermore, even if the same BAL is reached, the symptoms of intoxication are significantly less than in a person who rapidly ingests the alcohol on an empty stomach.

CLINICAL FEATURES

In mild intoxication most individuals feel somewhat euphoric. They talk more and tend to shed their inhibitions. Reckless and boisterous behavior may be seen; sexual indiscretion may be evident; irritability may occur. Some individuals, however, may not fare so well. A suspicious person, if intoxicated, may develop ideas of persecution; a mildly depressed person may become tearful and morose.

In moderate intoxication behavior tends to become coarse; improprieties are commonplace. Thinking is slow; inattentiveness occurs, and the person is slow in responding to anything, even dangerous situations. The face is flushed, the conjunctivae reddened, and the pupils dilated. Slurred speech, nystagmus, ataxia, and generalized incoordination are present.

In severe intoxication stupor may occur. Ataxia is so severe that standing is impossible. Vertigo is common, and persistent vomiting may occur.

Eventually if the BAL continues to rise, coma will supervene. Respiratory depression may occur, and death may ensue from respiratory arrest.

In the alcohol-naive person, a BAL of 100 mg/dl generally produces a mild degree of intoxication; 200 mg/dl a moderate degree; and 300 mg/dl a severe degree. In the alcohol-naive person, 400 mg/dl usually causes coma, and 500 mg/dl may cause respiratory arrest. Those who drink frequently and chronically, however, usually develop tolerance. For them a much higher BAL is needed to produce the various degrees of intoxication: some are still up and walking with levels over 300 mg/dl, and some have survived levels over 700 mg/dl. For legal purposes, the BAL is often expressed as a percent weight to volume of plasma, and hence the corresponding values would be 0.1% for a mild degree of intoxication, 0.2% for a moderate degree, etc.

If sleep should come to the intoxicated person, it tends to be heavy and dreamless. As the BAL falls the person often wakes up and has trouble falling back asleep.

After the intoxication has passed most experience a "hangover." Headache is common, as is a pervasive dysphoria and malaise. Mild tremulousness and diaphoresis may occur; nausea is common, and the person may vomit. Depending on the degree of intoxication, a hangover may last anywhere from several hours up to almost the entire day.

COURSE

The signs and symptoms of intoxication wane as the BAL falls; many people simply "sleep it off." Interestingly, for any given BAL the degree of intoxication is less when the BAL is falling than when it is rising. Furthermore as the BAL falls the euphoria is generally replaced by dysphoria. Some people seek to remedy the situation by further drinking in the hopes of recapturing the euphoria; however, the attempt is generally in vain.

The duration of intoxication is proportionate to the degree to which the BAL is elevated above the person's "threshold" for intoxication, and it may vary from just a few hours up to a day or more.

COMPLICATIONS

Ataxia may lead to falls; patients may incur bruises, fractures, or a subdural hematoma. Delayed reaction time, poor coordination, and stupor lead to erratic driving and accidents. Alcohol impairs hepatic gluconeogenesis and significant hypoglycemia may develop during intoxication.

Intoxication may also be a factor in homicidal behavior; over half of incarcerated murderers committed their crimes while intoxicated. Similarly about a quarter of all suicides occur during intoxication. Alcohol may directly cause death from respiratory arrest or aspiration of vomitus.

ETIOLOGY

Alcohol, like many anesthetics, increases membrane fluidity, with consequent changes in ion channel function, and this may, in part, underlie its intoxicating effect. More recent work has focused, however, on alcohol's ability to both sensitize GABA receptors and inhibit NMDA glutamate receptors.

DIFFERENTIAL DIAGNOSIS

Huntington's disease, multiple sclerosis, cerebellar disease of any cause, or lithium intoxication may cause a syndrome of dysarthria, ataxia, and poor coordination very similar to that seen in alcohol intoxication. Here, however, the symptoms are either chronic or are unaccompanied by euphoria.

In pathologic intoxication, symptoms of intoxication occur after drinking only a small amount and with a low BAL. Furthermore the behavior of the pathologically intoxicated individual is generally quite out of character.

Intoxication with sedative-hypnotics, ethylene glycol, isopropyl alcohol and methanol all produce a condition similar to alcohol intoxication. Neither sedative-hypnotic intoxication nor ethylene glycol intoxication produce the distinctive odor of alcohol on the breath; furthermore in the case of sedative-hypnotic intoxication there is no conjunctival injection and in the case of ethylene glycol intoxication the anion gap is increased. Both isopropyl alcohol and methanol cause an odor of alcohol on the breath, but in both cases there is also prominent nausea and vomiting; furthermore, in methanol intoxication one finds the development of dimming of vision.

The overall clinical condition of alcohol-intoxicated patients may also be exacerbated by one of many alcohol-related complications, including head trauma, hypoglycemia, hepatic failure with hepatic encephalopathy, anemia due to bleeding esophageal varices, pneumonia and meningitis, and these must always be borne in mind, especially when the expected recovery from alcohol intoxication appears delayed.

TREATMENT

A BAL should be obtained, and an estimate made as to the time of the last drink. Given the rapidity with which alcohol is absorbed, lavage is rarely indicated and emesis is relatively contraindicated given the risk of aspiration. In stupor or coma, the patient is placed in the "postop" lateral decubitus position to reduce the risk of aspiration; respiratory depression may require intubation.

In the vast majority of cases supportive care is all that is required; most patients "sleep it off," recover, and may be discharged. Very rarely hemodialysis may be indicated. If the BAL is over 600 mg% and hepatic function is impaired, the risk of waiting for the patient to recover may outweigh the risk of dialysis.

There are anecdotal reports of alcohol-induced stupor or coma being reversed by high-dose flumazenil (e.g., 2 to 5 mg), and trying this would not be unreasonable in cases where it appears that intubation may be required. Importantly, however, in patients with a history of seizures, or those taking drugs which lower the seizure threshold, flumazenil may cause a seizure.

BIBLIOGRAPHY

Adachi J, Mizoi Y, Fukunaga T, et al. Degrees of alcohol intoxication in 117 hospitalized cases. *Journal of Studies on Alcohol* 1991;52:448-453.

Frezza M, de Padova C, Pozzato G, et al. High blood alcohol levels in women. The role of decreased gastric alcohol dehydrogenase activity and first-pass metabolism. *The New England Journal of Medicine* 1990;322:95-99.

Heatley MK, Crane J. The blood alcohol concentration at post-mortem in 175 fatal cases of alcohol intoxication. *Medicine, Science, and the Law* 1990;30:101-105.

Hoaken PN, Pihl RO. The effects of alcohol intoxication on aggressive responses in men and women. *Alcohol and Alcoholism* 2000;35:471-477.

Koch-Weser J, Sellers EM, Kalant H. Alcohol intoxication and withdrawal. *The New England Journal of Medicine* 1976;294:757-762.

Lheureux P, Askenasi R. Efficacy of flumazenil in acute alcohol intoxication: double blind placebo-controlled evaluation. *Human & Experimental Toxicology* 1991;10:235-239.

Minion GE, Slovis CM, Boutiette L. Severe alcohol intoxication: a study of 204 consecutive patients. *Journal of Toxicology, Clinical Toxicology* 1989;27:375-384.

47 Blackouts

Blackouts are characterized by a dense anterograde amnesia. During the blackout intoxicated individuals appear outwardly unchanged; however, for the duration of the blackout, events fail to enter their memory. After "coming to" these individuals have no recollection of what was said or done during the blackout. Although the vast majority of blackouts occur during alcohol intoxication, they may also occasionally be seen in intoxication with other sedative-hypnotics, in particular high-potency benzodiazepines. Importantly, although most patients with blackouts are alcoholics, this is not always the case, as blackouts may also occur in social drinkers who simply consume more than is typical for them.

ONSET

In general the blackout begins abruptly.

CLINICAL FEATURES

Upon recovery from a blackout, drinkers often recount that they remember everything up to a certain time and then "went blank." Some patients go to sleep during a blackout, and when they awaken wonder how they got home or got to bed. Often, however, drinkers remain awake throughout the blackout; their emergence from the blackout is often quite abrupt, and in the amnestic wake of the blackout they may be quite startled and unnerved. Some may "come to" in the midst of a conversation with someone else. The other person may not notice any change at all, yet the person emerging from a blackout has no idea of what he was talking about or how the conversation began.

Observers may never suspect that a blackout is occurring. Blacked-out individuals continue to act "in character," and though they do not store memories of events during the blackout, usually they can recall quite well what happened before the blackout. Formal memory testing during the blackout, however, reveals typical findings. Long-term recall is good; blacked-out individuals may tell you what they had for lunch or who they met with when they began drinking that day. Immediate memory is likewise good, and they may display a normal digit span. Short-term memory, however, is generally negligible; often they cannot recall any words they were asked to memorize after the passage of just a few minutes.

Upon recovery from a blackout, most patients are worried about what they did during the blackout. The car may be checked for evidence of an accident; indirect questions may be put to others in a discreet effort to find out if anything untoward happened.

Occasionally, patients may experience only a partial blackout, wherein, upon recovery, there is some, albeit spotty, memory for events that transpired during the event: these episodes are often referred to as "brownouts."

COURSE

Blackouts may last anywhere from minutes to several hours, or even up to a day or more. Those who experience lengthy blackouts may speak of the "lost weekend."

COMPLICATIONS

Complications are similar to those for alcohol intoxication. In addition, some individuals may get into trouble for not following up on any agreements or events occurring during the blackout.

ETIOLOGY

It is not clear why some individuals have blackouts and others do not, given the same degree of intoxication. One study suggested that low plasma tryptophan levels constituted a risk factor, but this has not as yet been replicated.

DIFFERENTIAL DIAGNOSIS

Blackouts must be distinguished from other causes of transient anterograde amnesia. Transient global amnesia is distinguished by the fact that these patients are disturbed by their amnesia, and during the episode will typically repeatedly ask what the matter is. Complex partial seizures are marked by "out of character" behavior, including automatisms, such as chewing, lip-smacking and the like. The rare instances of "pure epileptic amnesia" are suggested by a history of other seizure types, e.g., typical complex partial seizures or grand mal seizures. Above all, however, all these other causes may cause transient amnesia in sober people, in contrast to blackouts, which only occur during intoxication.

TREATMENT

Patients should be observed until the restoration of short-term memory indicates that the blackout has remitted. The concurrent alcohol intoxication is treated as described in that chapter.

Upon recovery from the intoxication, all patients should be evaluated for the presence of alcoholism and treated accordingly; in those uncommon instances of blackouts occurring in social drinkers, patients should be instructed to either remain abstinent, or, when they are unwilling to do so, to moderate their alcohol intake.

BIBLIOGRAPHY

Branchey L, Branchey M, Zucker D, et al. Association between low plasma tryptophan and blackouts in male alcoholic patients. *Alcoholism, Clinical and Experimental Research* 1985;9:393-395.

Goodwin DW. Two species of alcoholic "blackout". *The American Journal of Psychiatry* 1971;127:1665-1670.

Goodwin DW, Crane GB, Guze SB. Phenomenological aspects of the alcoholic "blackout." *The British Journal of Psychiatry* 1969;115:1033-1038.

Goodwin DW, Crane GB, Guze SB. Alcoholic "blackouts": a review and clinical study of 100 alcoholics. *The American Journal of Psychiatry* 1969;126:191-198.

Greenblatt DJ, Harmatz JS, Shapiro L, et al. Sensitivity to triazolam in the elderly. *The New England Journal of Medicine* 1991;324:1691-1698.

Meilman PW, Stone JE, Gaylor MS, et al. Alcohol consumption by college undergraduates: current use and 10-year trends. *Journal of Studies on Alcohol* 1990;51:389-395.

Tamerin JS, Weiner S, Poppen R, et al. Alcohol and memory: amnesia and short-term memory function during experimentally induced intoxication. *The American Journal of Psychiatry* 1971;128:1659-1664.

48 Pathological Intoxication

Classically, pathological intoxication is said to occur when, after consuming a relatively small amount of alcohol, drinkers undergo a marked change in behavior, often becoming agitated or violent, afterwards having at best a spotty memory for the event. This is a controversial diagnosis, not only because it lends itself to malingerers, but also because it has been difficult to replicate it in the laboratory setting. If it does exist in this classical form, it is probably rare.

ONSET

Episodes of pathologic intoxication may occur at any age; the onset of the episode itself is often quite abrupt.

CLINICAL FEATURES

Occurring after as little as one or two drinks, the change in behavior may be dramatic. A hitherto polite and unassuming person may start a fist fight; a well-mannered person may suddenly take offense if a date happens to look at someone else, flying into a jealous rage. This change may persist for only a few minutes, or up to hours. Upon recovery the drinker typically has difficulty in recalling everything that happened, and occasionally may report complete amnesia for the event.

COURSE

The clinical impression is that if someone has already experienced one episode of pathologic intoxication, that it is likely to recur with further alcohol consumption.

COMPLICATIONS

Various injuries, even homicide, may occur.

ETIOLOGY

Brain damage of any cause, particularly to the temporal lobes, may predispose to pathologic intoxication. In the majority of reported cases, however, there is no evidence for this, and the cause in these cases is not known.

DIFFERENTIAL DIAGNOSIS

In blackouts no significant change in the drinker's behavior is seen.

Complex partial seizures may be associated with violence, especially if attempts are made to restrain the patient during the ictus.

Malingerers may claim pathologic intoxication to escape responsibility for violent behavior.

Moderate degrees of alcohol intoxication may in some people be accompanied by violent behavior. Here, however, the behavior is usually "in character" for the person in question. Furthermore, one typically sees signs of moderate intoxication, such as ataxia and dysarthria, which are generally absent in pathologic intoxication.

TREATMENT

Patients should be secluded, or restrained if necessary, until the episode passes. Medication is generally not indicated.

BIBLIOGRAPHY

Anonymous. Pathological intoxication. *The American Journal of Psychiatry* 1971;128:660-661.

Bach-y-Rita G, Lion JR, Ervin FR. Pathological intoxication: clinical and electroencephalographic studies. *The American Journal of Psychiatry* 1970;127:698-703.

Banay RS. Pathologic reaction to alcohol. I. Review of the literature and original case reports. *Quarterly Journal of Studies on Alcohol* 1944;4:580-605.

Coid J. Mania à potu: a critical review of pathological intoxication. *Psychological Medicine* 1979;9:709-719.

Maletzky BM. The diagnosis of pathological intoxication. *Journal of Studies on Alcohol* 1976;37:1215-1228.

May PRA, Ebaugh FG. Pathological intoxication, alcoholic hallucinosis, and other reactions to alcohol: a clinical study. *Quarterly Journal of Studies on Alcohol* 1953;14:200-227.

Perr IN. Pathological intoxication and alcohol idiosyncratic intoxication—Part I: Diagnostic and clinical aspects. *Journal of Forensic Sciences* 1986;31:806-811.

Perr IN. Pathological intoxication and alcohol idiosyncratic intoxication—Part II: Legal aspects. *Journal of Forensic Sciences* 1986;31:812-817.

49 Alcohol Withdrawal (DSM-IV-TR #291.8)

Alcohol withdrawal, commonly known as "the shakes," may occur in anyone after excessive, prolonged use of alcohol. Although such drinking is far more common among alcoholics, alcohol withdrawal may also be seen in alcohol abusers.

ONSET

Withdrawal symptoms gradually appear as the blood alcohol level falls below the person's threshold for intoxication. Consequently in some patients withdrawal symptoms may appear after merely a reduction in alcohol intake, rather than actual cessation. In most cases withdrawal begins within 4 to 12 hours after the last drink. When drinkers fall asleep while intoxicated, they may awaken in the early morning hours, anxious and tremulous.

CLINICAL FEATURES

In full-blown alcohol withdrawal, drinkers are apprehensive, anxious, and easily startled; they may pace agitatedly up and down the hall. Depressed mood and irritability are common. The tremor is quite characteristic; it tends to be coarse and is evident not only in the hands but also in the lips, tongue, and eyelids. In severe cases drinkers may literally "shake like a leaf" and be unable to hold things or even at times to stand up. Diaphoresis, at times profuse, is often present.

Most have trouble concentrating and thinking clearly; memory tends to be poor. Although fatigue is prominent, most are also unable to sleep.

Headache, dry mouth, anorexia, nausea, and vomiting are common; diarrhea may occur.

On examination the temperature, pulse, respirations, and systolic blood pressure may all be elevated. The pupils are dilated, and the deep tendon reflexes are hyperactive. Rarely, one may see transient myoclonus, choreiform movements or parkinsonism.

Occasionally patients may have isolated, brief, vague, visual hallucinations or illusions, or rarely a few auditory hallucinations. If these do occur they tend to appear as the withdrawal symptoms reach their height.

Most people in withdrawal recognize that a drink would "solve" their problem. Such a recognition may or may not be accompanied by a strong craving for alcohol; when the craving does occur, taking the "morning drink" becomes much more likely.

COURSE

Symptoms tend to peak in a couple of days, and most people begin to experience some reduction in symptoms after another 2 or 3 days have passed. Most have substantial relief after a week. With abstinence those with relatively less intense drinking histories, such as alcohol abusers, may be completely recovered. However, among heavy drinkers, such as alcoholics, cognitive difficulties, such as poor concentration and memory, may persist for a month or more, and in some patients signs of autonomic hyperactivity, especially easy startability and insomnia, may persist for up to 6 months.

COMPLICATIONS

Most people experiencing alcohol withdrawal are unable to consistently do well socially or occupationally; their tremor alone is enough to preclude this.

Those with preexisting epilepsy are at higher risk for breakthrough seizures during withdrawal, and those with panic attacks are far more likely to have attacks while in withdrawal.

Preexisting cardiac disease, especially an arrhythmia, is likely to be exacerbated.

ETIOLOGY

Although the etiology of alcohol withdrawal is not known with certainty, it is suspected that with chronic intoxication there is either an up-regulation of post-synaptic glutamate receptors, or a down-regulation of post-synaptic GABA receptors, or both: in such a situation, an absence of alcohol would entail excessive neuronal activity and, presumably, the symptomatology seen during withdrawal.

DIFFERENTIAL DIAGNOSIS

Significant hypoglycemia may occasionally appear similar to alcohol withdrawal. The absence of a history of alcohol ingestion and the relief provided by food, however, suggest the correct diagnosis.

"Thyroid storm" as seen in hyperthyroidism may appear similar to alcohol withdrawal and may have an acute presentation. The presence of proptosis or thyromegaly, however, suggests the correct diagnosis.

Withdrawal from sedatives and hypnotics is for the most part indistinguishable from alcohol withdrawal.

Delirium tremens is accompanied by autonomic hyperactivity identical to that seen in alcohol withdrawal; however, here one also finds confusion and disorientation. Furthermore the hallucinations are prominent and well formed.

TREATMENT

Apart from routine supportive care, not all withdrawing patients require or even wish pharmacologic treatment for withdrawal symptomatology. For some alcoholics and alcohol abusers the "shakes" may be a valuable lesson, increasing the motivation toward sobriety; in such cases, only supportive care is indicated. Supportive care should include parenteral administration of 100 mg of thiamine; potassium, magnesium and calcium levels should be determined and replenishment provided if levels are significantly below normal; the glucose level should also be determined, but glucose should not be given until at least two hours have elapsed from when thiamine was given. Nausea, vomiting or diarrhea may be treated symptomatically, and intravenous fluids may be required in severe cases.

When autonomic symptoms are intolerable, serve no instructive point, or are a threat to the patient (for example, a patient with epilepsy or cardiac disease), treatment to reduce them is indicated. Benzodiazepines have long since replaced the barbiturates as the commonly accepted treatment. Occasionally a beta-blocker, such as propranolol, is used adjunctively. Either carbamazepine or divalproex may also be used, and indeed may be preferable to benzodiazepines.

If treatment with a benzodiazepine is indicated a typical protocol, using lorazepam as an example, is as follows. Oral administration is preferred; however, if the patient is NPO or unable to keep anything in his stomach, the same dose may be given intramuscularly. Initially 2 mg is given (or less in the elderly or debilitated), and an order is left to continue lorazepam 2 mg every 2 hours until the tremor is acceptably controlled. The next day the patient is prescribed a regular total daily dose equal to the amount required on the first day, with this dose administered in three or four divided doses. Provision is also made for supplementary doses of 1 to 2 mg every 2 hours should the regular dose not control the tremor. On succeeding days the total regular daily dose is increased by an amount approximately equal to that required in supplementary doses over the previous 24 hours. This procedure is followed until a full day has passed with no need for supplementary doses. The patient is subsequently placed on a tapering schedule whereby the dose is decreased on a daily basis by an amount approximately equal to 20% of the final regular total daily dose. Supplementary doses are generally not given during the tapering. In this way the patient is tapered in 4 or 5 days; coupled with the 2 or 3 days required to suppress tremor, the entire procedure takes about 1 week. Equivalent oral doses of other benzodiazepines are 5 to 10 mg of diazepam, 25 to 50 mg of chlordiazepoxide, and 30 to 60 mg of oxazepam: both diazepam and chlordiazepoxide are available for parenteral use, but their absorption after intramuscular administration is erratic. Such a withdrawal program usually requires admission. Most outpatients simply are unable to discipline themselves to it and end up aborting the tapering by taking supplementary doses or by resuming alcohol use. In general, patients should not be taking potentially addicting medicines before discharge.

Propranolol or other beta-blockers reduce certain autonomic symptoms, such as tremor, palpitations, and hypertension; however, in contrast to the benzodiazepines the beta-blockers do not reduce anxiety, easy startability, insomnia, and the like, nor is the risk of having a seizure reduced. Propranolol may be given in dosages of 20 mg every 90 minutes until tremor is controlled; the total daily dose and subsequent tapering may then be conducted in a manner analogous to that just described for the benzodiazepines.

Both carbamazepine and divalproex are each as effective as a benzodiazepine in suppressing the autonomic symptomatology of withdrawal. It has not, however, been demonstrated that they are effective in preventing alcohol withdrawal seizures or delirium tremens. In patients with normal hepatic function, carbamazepine may be started at 200 mg tid or qid, and divalproex at 20mg/kg/d in two or three divided doses, with subsequent dose adjustments of either agent made on the basis of clinical response and side-effects. As both these agents may take a day or two to quell the autonomic symptoms, it is generally appropriate to allow prn doses of lorazepam, as described above, until symptoms are controlled by the antiepileptic drug, after which no further lorazepam is given. Regardless of whether carbamazepine or divalproex is used, treatment should be continued for at least a week, that is to say for a sufficient period of time to allow the withdrawal syndrome to run its course, after which the drug may be tapered and discontinued over two or three days. In cases of persistent withdrawal symptomatology, as may be seen in severe alcoholics, there is evidence, in the case of divalproex, that long-term treatment may facilitate the achievement of long-term sobriety.

There is debate as to whether to rely on benzodiazepines or either carbamazepine or divalproex. One very clear advantage of the antiepileptics is that they are non-addicting and provide no euphoria and hence obviate the struggle that often occurs with drug-seeking patients being treated with a benzodiazepine. Hopefully future research will determine whether they are as effective as benzodiazepines in preventing alcohol withdrawal seizures or delirium tremens: if they are, then they should replace the benzodiazepines in the treatment of alcohol withdrawal.

BIBLIOGRAPHY

Bailly D, Servant D, Blandin N, et al. Effects of beta-blocking drugs in alcohol withdrawal: a double-blind comparative study with propranolol and diazepam. *Biomedicine & Pharmacotherapy* 1992;46:419-424.

Daeppen JB, Gache P, Landry U, et al. Symptom-triggered versus fixed-schedule doses of benzodiazepine for alcohol withdrawal: a randomized treatment trial. *Archives of Internal Medicine* 2002;162:1117-1121.

Drake ME. Recurrent spontaneous myoclonus in alcohol withdrawal. *Southern Medical Journal* 1983;76:1040-1042.

Fornazzari L, Carlen PL. Transient choreiform dyskinesias during alcohol withdrawal. *The Canadian Journal of Neurological Sciences* 1982;9:89-90.

Malcom R, Ballenger JC, Sturgis ET, et al. Double-blind controlled trial comparing carbamazepine to oxazepam treatment of alcohol withdrawal. *The American Journal of Psychiatry* 1989;146:617-621.

Miller WC, McCurdy L. A double-blind comparison of the efficacy and safety of lorazepam and diazepam in the treatment of the acute alcohol withdrawal syndrome. *Clinical Therapeutics* 1984;6:364-371.

Reoux JP, Saxton AJ, Malte CA, et al. Divalproex sodium in alcohol withdrawal: a randomized, double-blind placebo-controlled trial. Alcoholism, *Clinical and Experimental Research* 2001;25:1324-1329.

Shandling M, Carlen PL, Lang AE. Parkinsonism in alcohol withdrawal: a follow-up study. *Movement Disorders* 1990;5:36-39.

Stuppaeck CH, Pycha R, Miller C, et al. Carbamazepine versus oxazepam in the treatment of alcohol withdrawal: a double-blind study. *Alcohol and Alcoholism* 1992;27:153-158.

50 Alcohol Withdrawal Seizures

Alcohol withdrawal seizures, also known as "rum fits," are a rare accompaniment of the alcohol withdrawal syndrome. They generally occur only after many years of heavy drinking and repeated episodes of withdrawal and are seen in from 1% to 3% of patients withdrawing from alcohol.

ONSET

Seizures may occur anywhere from hours to 2 days after either cessation or a marked reduction in alcohol use.

CLINICAL FEATURES

For the most part, alcohol withdrawal seizures present as otherwise unremarkable generalized tonic-clonic seizures. In about a quarter of the cases, however, the seizures have a focal onset.

Most patients have just one seizure; occasionally, however, patients have a cluster of two or three and rarely as many as six. Rarely, status epilepticus occurs.

COURSE

As noted above, most alcohol withdrawal seizures occur fairly promptly; rarely would one see them after 2 or 3 days of total abstinence.

COMPLICATIONS

These are the same as for tonic-clonic seizures of any cause.

ETIOLOGY

Apart from the fact that these seizures are in some way causally related to alcohol withdrawal, little is known of their etiology. "Rum fits" with focal features probably represent a combination of a localized cortical lesion, perhaps secondary to previous head trauma, and the increased cortical irritability seen in alcohol withdrawal.

One recent epidemiologic study suggested that seizures may be associated with intoxication itself, in the absence of withdrawal symptoms, relative or otherwise. This seems doubtful, and replication is required.

DIFFERENTIAL DIAGNOSIS

Preexisting epilepsy is likely to become exacerbated during alcohol withdrawal; a history of seizures before the onset of alcoholism suggests the diagnosis.

Several other alcohol-related disorders may present with seizures. These include Wernicke's encephalopathy, head trauma with or without subdural hematoma, Marchiafava-Bignami disease, hypoglycemia, hypomagnesemia, and meningitis.

TREATMENT

Lorazepam, 2 mg IV, if given immediately after a first "rum fit," will significantly reduce the chances of a second one occurring over the ensuing six hours; however, as most patients will have no more than one or two fits, it is unclear if this should be a routine practice. What is clear is that the associated alcohol withdrawal syndrome should be aggressively treated, as described in the preceding chapter. Should status epilepticus occur, treatment should include intravenous lorazepam.

For a patient who has only alcohol withdrawal seizures, long-term preventive treatment is not indicated. Alcoholics who are actively drinking do not take medication, and if they are sober they do not need it.

BIBLIOGRAPHY

Brennan FN, Lyttle JA. Alcohol and seizures: a review. *Journal of the Royal Society of Medicine* 1987;80:571-573.

D'Onofrio G, Rathlev NK, Ulrich AS, et al. Lorazepam for the prevention of recurrent seizures related to alcohol. *The New England Journal of Medicine* 1999;340:915-919.

Earnest MP, Feldman H, Marx JA, et al. Intracranial lesions shown by CT scans in 259 cases of first alcohol-withdrawal seizures. *Neurology* 1988;38:1561-1565.

Hillbom ME, Hjelm-Jager M. Should alcohol withdrawal seizures be treated with anti-epileptic drugs? *Acta Neurologica Scandinavica* 1984;69:39-42.

Lambie DJ, Johnson RH, Vijayasenan ME, et al. Sodium valproate in the treatment of the alcohol withdrawal syndrome. *The Australian and New Zealand Journal of Psychiatry* 1980;14:213-215.

Rathlev NK, D'Onofrio G, Fish SS, et al. The lack of efficacy of phenytoin in the prevention of recurrent alcohol-related seizures. *Annals of Emergency Medicine* 1994;23:513-518.

51 Delirium Tremens (alcohol withdrawal delirium, DSM-IV-TR #291.0)

Delirium tremens, also known as alcohol withdrawal delirium and more commonly as "DTs," develops in the setting of the alcohol withdrawal syndrome, and is seen in about 5% of hospitalized alcoholics. It is characterized by gross accentuation of the tremor and autonomic signs and by the development of confusion, disorientation, and hallucinations.

ONSET

The interval between either a cessation of alcohol use, or merely a marked reduction in consumption, and the onset of delirium tremens ranges from several hours to up to a week and a half, with most cases occurring within 2 or 3 days. In about 10% of cases, the DTs are ushered in by an alcohol withdrawal seizure; furthermore, it appears that a history of DTs predicts a shorter interval to the onset of the current episode.

Delirium tremens is rarely seen outside of alcoholism; most patients with delirium tremens have been drinking excessively for years and have a history of repeated episodes of the alcohol withdrawal syndrome.

CLINICAL FEATURES

The patient is generally agitated, markedly tremulous, and very easily startled; mydriasis and generalized hyperreflexia are prominent, as are such autonomic signs as diaphoresis, tachycardia, elevated blood pressure, and increased respirations. Visual hallucinations are very common; they tend to be extremely vivid and complex. Often the patient sees insects or animals: dogs circle the bed; rats eat at the toes; bugs crawl on the arms and face. The patient may cringe in fear or try to swat them away. At times the patient may see simply a benign procession of animals, which he may watch from the bed as if it were an amusing procession. Curiously one also often sees a predilection for hallucinating strings or threads; the patient may pick them out of the air or warn the physician to avoid running into one stretched across the hospital room. Often the visual hallucinations may be provoked by suggestion. In the classic "string test" the examiner holds her hands about a foot and a half apart, the thumbs and index fingers apposed, several feet in front of the patient and asks if the patient sees anything. After the patient reports seeing nothing, the examiner asks "Don't you see the string?," whereupon the patient does indeed see a string stretched between the examiner's hands.

Tactile hallucinations may accompany the visual ones: the skin is ripped by teeth; spiders bite; bugs are felt crawling all over. The patient may complain of electric shocks or of pins being stuck into the toes.

Auditory hallucinations are common. Patients may hear bells, whistles, or alarms. If voices are heard, they tend to be critical, persecutory, or warning of dire events. Patients hear accusations of neglecting their children; the children are starving because the patients spent their paychecks on drink. The death sentence is pronounced; the physician is revealed as the executioner.

Delusions are common and tend to be persecutory. Murderers are outside the door; the nurse is bringing poison to the patient; other patients talk about and conspire against the patient.

Disorientation always occurs, often to both time and place. At times this disorientation is intensified by hallucinations. The patient refuses the bedtime medicine offered by the nurse and announces that it must be morning as the birds are chirping; if questioned as to orientation to place, the patient, seeing the clouds out the window, may report being in an airplane or perhaps an air ambulance.

Confusion waxes and wanes; often it is worse after dark. The patient appears befogged. Attention can be gained only with greatest difficulty.

Memory tends to be severely disturbed. Digit span is reduced. The patient is unable to recall the name of the physician or of the hospital. Recall of events before admission is also often quite spotty.

The behavior of these patients is commensurate with their symptoms. Some may sit tremulously on the bed, picking at the bed sheets or brushing away insects. They may grasp at strings in the air and mumble agitatedly about events occurring outside the window. Others may strike out at their "persecutors"; they may attempt to escape through the door or jump out the window.

In contrast one may occasionally encounter a "quiet" delirium tremens. Here the tremor and autonomic signs and symptoms are minimal, and the patient, all the while experiencing sometimes fantastic visual hallucinations, may lie relatively quietly in bed.

COURSE

In anywhere from 5% to 20% of patients delirium tremens is fatal, with death caused by various events, such as aspiration pneumonia, hepatic failure, cardiac arrhythmia (e.g., ventricular fibrillation) or hypovolemic shock. Those who survive generally have a gradual remission of symptoms over about 2 or 3 days; occasionally remission occurs in only a day. On the other extreme, in some cases symptoms may persist for 2 or even 3 weeks. Often remission comes when the patient begins to sleep. Upon recovery, there may be partial amnesia for the events; however, at times memory is quite vivid.

COMPLICATIONS

The complications of delirium tremens include those described in the chapter on delirium. Additionally, more so than the average delirious patient, patients with delirium tremens tend to be dangerous to themselves or others. Patients may jump out of windows to escape their imagined persecutors; at other times they may turn and attack.

ETIOLOGY

The likelihood of the DTs increases with the severity of alcoholism, severity of the preceding withdrawal syndrome, the presence of alcohol withdrawal seizures and, perhaps most importantly, the presence of a concurrent significant general medical illness, such as pneumonia, hepatic failure or severe anemia. It also appears likely that "kindling" plays a role in the genesis of delirium tremens, in that repeated episodes of severe withdrawal or delirium tremens may "sensitize" the cerebrum such that the development of delirium is more likely during subsequent episodes of alcohol withdrawal.

DIFFERENTIAL DIAGNOSIS

Both hypoglycemia and thyroid storm may cause delirium in the setting of heightened autonomic activity. Other disorders, not uncommonly seen in alcoholics, which may cause delirium include Wernicke's encephalopathy, hepatic encephalopathy, pneumonia, subdural hematoma and meningitis. It must also be kept in mind that an identical syndrome may occur during withdrawal from sedative-hypnotics such as benzodiazepines.

TREATMENT

Intravenous access, if possible, should be obtained. Lorazepam may be given in doses of 2 mg every 1 to 2 hours parenterally until the patient is lightly sedated, and it must be borne in mind that massive doses may be required. Diazepam or chlordiazepoxide may also be used, in doses of 10 or 50 mg, respectively; however, these should not be relied on for intramuscular use, given their erratic and often slow absorption. If the patient is already receiving carbamazepine or divalproex, these may be continued, but it must be emphasized that in the case of delirium tremens they may not constitute an adequate substitute for benzodiazepines. Thiamine is given in a dose of 100 mg parenterally, with parenteral doses continued for three days, after which oral administration may be used.

While benzodiazepine treatment is initiated, certain laboratory tests should be obtained on a routine basis, including CBC, electrolytes, glucose, BUN, liver enzymes, bilirubin, ammonia, calcium, magnesium, stool for occult blood, and an EKG. Further testing is based on clinical suspicion: if pneumonia is suspected, a chest x-ray; if pancreatitis, amylase and lipase levels; if a subdural hematoma, a CT scan.

Vomiting, diaphoresis and diarrhea may cause profound dehydration, and massive fluid replenishment may be required. Importantly, glucose should be withheld, if possible, until at least 2 hours have passed after the parenteral administration of thiamine.

The overall management of delirium is discussed in that chapter. If antipsychotics are required, haloperidol is probably most suitable.

Once symptoms have been brought under control, the total daily dose of the benzodiazepine may be cautiously reduced in daily increments of roughly 10% of the original dose.

BIBLIOGRAPHY

Ferguson JA, Suelzer CJ, Eckert GJ, et al. Risk factors for delirium tremens development. *Journal of General Internal Medicine* 1996;11:410-414.

Fisher J, Abrams J. Life-threatening ventricular tachyarrythmias in delirium tremens. *Archives of Internal Medicine* 1977;137:1238-1241.

Lundquist G. Delirium tremens: a comparative study of pathogenesis, course and prognosis. *Acta Psychiatrica Scandinavica* 1961;36:443-466.

Nielsen J. Delirium tremens in Copenhagen. *Acta Psychiatrica Scandinavica* 1965;41(Suppl 187):1-92.

Nolop KB, Natow A. Unprecedented sedative requirements during delirium tremens. *Critical Care Medicine* 1985;13:246-247.

Palmstierna T. A model for predicting alcohol withdrawal delirium. *Psychiatric Services* 2001;52:820-823.

Palsson A. The efficacy of early chlormethiazole medication in the prevention of delirium tremens. A retrospective study of the outcome of different drug treatment strategies at the Helsingborg clinics, 1975-1980. *Acta Psychiatrica Scandinavica* 1986;329:140-145.

Wernicke's encephalopathy, in its classic, fully developed state, is characterized by the classic triad of delirium, nystagmus, and ataxia and is secondary to chronic thiamine deficiency. Although seen primarily in alcoholics, it may occur in other disorders, such as hyperemesis gravidarum. An occasionally seen older synonym is polioencephalitis hemorrhagica superior.

ONSET

In general the onset is subacute, occurring over several days; nystagmus may be one of the early signs. Occasionally, however, one may see an acute onset over hours, and this may follow a glucose load, either orally or by infusion, in a thiamine-deficient patient.

CLINICAL FEATURES

Delirium is characterized by disorientation to time and place and confusion, which is often severe. Lethargy is common, and stupor or coma may occur.

Nystagmus is generally horizontal; however, vertical nystagmus may also be seen. With progression a bilateral, often asymmetric, sixth nerve palsy appears; and the patient may complain of diplopia. In extreme instances total ophthalmoplegia may occur.

Truncal and lower limb ataxia tend to follow nystagmus and may be so severe that the patient is unable to stand or sit up. Dysarthria and upper limb ataxia are less common.

It must be emphasized that the "classic" triad is the exception rather than the rule. In clinical practice, the most common presentation is with delirium alone, followed by combinations of delirium and nystagmus or delirium and ataxia: the classic triad is seen in less than 20% of autopsy-proven cases.

Convulsions may occur, as may sudden death.

The temperature is usually decreased, and the heart rate increased; postural hypotension is frequent. The pupils remain reactive but are often sluggish.

Occasionally the cerebrospinal fluid protein level is increased. On T2-weighted MRI scanning, the mammillary bodies generally display increased signal intensity on T-2 weighted scans (Figure 52-1).

COURSE

Untreated, up to one half of these patients die; those who survive are generally left with residual symptoms, as described below.

COMPLICATIONS

In addition to the complications described in the chapter on delirium, most patients upon recovery are left with some residual symptoms. About a third have nystagmus, a half some ataxia, and perhaps three quarters have some degree of memory defect. Of these three quarters, a significant percentage evidence Korsakoff's syndrome.

ETIOLOGY

Thiamine is converted into thiamine pyrophosphate, which in turn is an essential cofactor for the enzyme transketolase. With significant thiamine deficiency enzymatic activity is lost, and characteristic lesions, as described below, develop. In some patients, a genetically determined reduction in the affinity of transketolase for thiamine pyrophosphate exists, and such patients may develop symptoms with a relatively mild degree of thiamine deficiency.

Acutely, capillary dilatation and petechiae are seen in the hypothalamus (particularly the mammillary bodies), the thalamus (particularly the medial dorsal nucleus and the pulvinar), the peri-aqueductal gray and the adjacent oculomotor nucleus, the pons, especially the abducens nuclei, and in the anterior superior vermis of the cerebellum. In chronic cases these areas display neuronal loss, gliosis, and occasionally cystic changes.

Thiamine is found in many foods, and 1 or 2 mg is sufficient to meet most daily needs. Total body stores are only about 30 mg, however, and, in the absence of adequate intake, deficiency may appear in a matter of weeks or months. Such a deficiency is common in alcoholism, and for two reasons: first, most alcoholics are malnourished and obtain much of their calories from alcohol rather than from foods rich in thiamine; second, alcohol itself inhibits thiamine absorption from the gut. Other, less common, causes of thiamine deficiency include prolonged fasting, as may occur in anorexia nervosa, prolonged vomiting, as may be seen in hyperemesis gravidarum or after gastric surgery, or with prolonged parenteral nutrition in the absence of vitamin supplementation.

DIFFERENTIAL DIAGNOSIS

A viral encephalitis may initially mimic Wernicke's encephalopathy; however, here one generally finds an elevated temperature and often a stiff neck, findings not seen in Wernicke's encephalopathy.

Delirium tremens and Wernicke's encephalopathy may appear concurrently; from a practical point of view all delirious alcoholics should be treated as if they had Wernicke's encephalopathy and given parenteral thiamine.

The acute encephalopathic form of pellagra, as described in that chapter, may suggest Wernicke's encephalopathy.

TREATMENT

All alcoholic patients should receive 100 mg of thiamine intra-muscularly upon admission. In cases of suspected or definite Wernicke's encephalopathy this should be given slowly intra-venously. Barring a severe degree of hypoglycemia, food and glucose solutions should be withheld until at least several hours after thiamine administration because a glucose load can precipitate or worsen Wernicke's encephalopathy. Thiamine is subsequently given in a dosage of 100 mg twice daily parenterally until substantial improvement is seen, after which oral supplementation is used.

With adequate thiamine replacement, nystagmus and abducens palsy begin to clear the first day, sometimes within hours; the

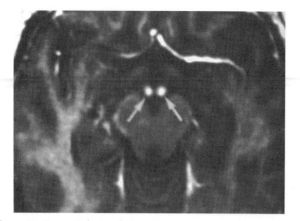

FIG. 52-1. Increased signal intensity in the mammillary bodies in Wernicke's encephalopathy. (From Osborn AG. *Diagnostic neuroradiology*, St. Louis, 1994, Mosby.)

ataxia and delirium clear within a few days. About 1 to 4 weeks may be required to obtain maximum improvement.

No improvement within the first day may indicate hypomagnesemia, and administration of magnesium sulfate, as described in the chapter on hypomagnesemia, may result in improvement.

Given the devastation of this disease and its sequelae, notably Korsakoff's syndrome, it is surprising that governments have not taken the simple step of requiring the supplementation of all alcoholic beverages with small amounts of thiamine. The results would be as dramatic as when flour was "enriched"

with niacin and the scourge of endemic pellagra was thereby eradicated.

BIBLIOGRAPHY

Blass JP, Gibson GE. Abnormality of a thiamine-requiring enzyme in patients with Wernicke-Korsakoff syndrome. *The New England Journal of Medicine* 1977;297:1367-1370.

Caine D, Halliday GM, Krill JJ, et al. Operational criteria for the classification of chronic alcoholics: identification of Wernicke's encephalopathy. *Journal of Neurology, Neurosurgery, and Psychiatry* 1997;62:51-60.

Chu K, Kang DW, Kim HJ, et al. Diffusion-weighted imaging abnormalities in Wernicke encephalopathy: reversible cytotoxic edema? *Archives of Neurology* 2002;59:123-127.

Cirignotta F, Manconi M, Mondini S, et al. Wernicke-Korsakoff encephalopathy and polyneuropathy after gastroplasty for morbid obesity: report of a case. *Archives of Neurology* 2000;57:1356-1359.

Doherty MJ, Watson NF, Uchino K, et al. Diffusion abnormalities in patients with Wernicke encephalopathy. *Neurology* 2002;58:655-657.

Harper C. Wernicke's encephalopathy: a more common disease than realized. A neuropathological study of 51 cases. *Journal of Neurology, Neurosurgery, and Psychiatry* 1979;42:226-231.

Harper C. The incidence of Wernicke's encephalopathy in Australia—a neuropathological study of 131 cases. *Journal of Neurology, Neurosurgery, and Psychiatry* 1983;46:593-598.

Harper CG, Giles M, Finlay-Jones R. Clinical signs in the Wernicke-Korsakoff complex: a retrospective analysis of 131 cases diagnosed at necropsy. *Journal of Neurology, Neurosurgery, and Psychiatry* 1986;49: 341-345.

Ogershok PR, Rahman A, Nestor S, et al. Wernicke encephalopathy in nonalcoholic patients. *The American Journal of the Medical Sciences* 2002;323:107-111.

53 Korsakoff's Syndrome (alcohol-induced persisting amnestic disorder, DSM-IV-TR #291.1)

Korsakoff's syndrome, also known as Korsakoff's psychosis, is characterized by a striking inability to form new memories, with the subsequent "blank spots" often filled in with confabulations. Although most frequently seen as a sequela of Wernicke's encephalopathy in alcoholism (wherein it is also referred to as alcohol-induced persisting amnestic disorder, or simply alcohol amnestic disorder), Korsakoff's syndrome may be secondary to other disorders, for example herpes simplex encephalitis. Korsakoff's syndrome is thought to be rare, but clinically the impression is that a large number of mild cases go undiagnosed.

ONSET

When secondary to thiamine deficiency Korsakoff's syndrome is left as a residual of Wernicke's encephalopathy: confusion clears, and alertness is restored, yet the patient, although attentive, is no longer able to memorize things.

CLINICAL FEATURES

The memory loss is of the short-term variety; although digit span is unimpaired, the patient's ability to recall anything after a few minutes (such as the physician's name) is grossly impaired. Long-term memory is relatively spared, and often exhibits a "temporal gradient" wherein events of the distant past are better recalled than those that occurred more recently. Remarkably patients are generally unconcerned with this inability to remember things; it is nothing to them, and if their attention is called to it the trouble may be laughed off. Confabulations are typically present and may at times be quite fabulous.

During casual questioning, these patients may not appear ill. They may talk appropriately about their surroundings, comment on the weather as they look out the window, or compliment the physician's taste in clothing. Some may be mildly euphoric, others bland and apathetic. A few direct questions, however, disclose the memory defect and the tendency to confabulate. For example, if the physician asks the patient if they have ever met before, the patient generally responds in the affirmative and may go on to describe an encounter with the physician earlier, perhaps a week ago, at a local bar, where they played pool, had a bite to eat, and a few drinks.

A degree of disorientation to time and place is invariably present; however, no confusion is seen.

When Korsakoff's syndrome is secondary to thiamine deficiency, one generally also finds other sequelae of Wernicke's encephalopathy, such as nystagmus or ataxia. Other alcohol-related disorders, such as alcoholic polyneuropathy and alcoholic myopathy, are also often present.

COURSE

Korsakoff's syndrome occurring as a sequela to Wernicke's encephalopathy is generally chronic: perhaps one-quarter of patients gradually show substantial improvement over the first year, whereas the remainder show little or no recovery. The course of Korsakoff's syndrome of other etiologies is dependent on the underlying cause.

COMPLICATIONS

Lifelong supervision is often required, often in an institution.

ETIOLOGY

Korsakoff's syndrome may occur secondary to lesions in any of the following structures: the hippocampus, fornix, mammillary bodies, mammillothalamic tract, and the dorsomedial nucleus of the thalamus. In almost all cases there are bilateral lesions; in those rare instances where the precipitating insult is unilateral, one can almost always demonstrate an older lesion in the opposite structure.

The most common cause of Korsakoff's syndrome, as noted earlier, is the thiamine deficiency seen in alcoholism. Here the dorsomedial nucleus of the thalamus and the mammillary bodies are damaged: the atrophy of the mammillary bodies may be visualized on coronal MRI scans.

Other causes include the following: infarction or tumor of any of the structures noted above, destruction of the hippocampi by herpes simplex encephalitis or during status epilepticus, and widespread insults, such as limbic encephalitis, cerebral anoxia or closed head injury.

DIFFERENTIAL DIAGNOSIS

In contrast to transient global amnesia and to dissociative amnesia, amnesia in Korsakoff's syndrome is continuously antegrade and is characterized by confabulation.

TREATMENT

In cases of Korsakoff's syndrome secondary to Wernicke's encephalopathy, oral thiamine is appropriate, not because this will reverse the amnesia, but because one wishes to forestall the development of thiamine deficiency in the future. Pharmacologic treatment of the syndrome itself is generally unavailing: although two small double-blinded studies of clonidine showed modest benefit, an attempt at replication in a larger sample yielded negative results. Neither fluvoxamine nor methylphenidate are of any value here.

BIBLIOGRAPHY

Albert MS, Butters N, Levin J. Temporal gradients in the retrograde amnesia of patients with alcoholic Korsakoff's disease. *Archives of Neurology* 1979;36:211-216.

Halliday G, Cullen K, Harding A. Neuropathological correlates of memory dysfunction in the Wernicke-Korsakoff syndrome. *Alcohol and Alcoholism* 1994;2:245-251.

Kopelman MD. The Korsakoff syndrome. *The British Journal of Psychiatry* 1995;166:154-173.

McEntee WJ, Mair RG. Memory enhancement in Korsakoff's psychosis by clonidine: further evidence for a noradrenergic deficit. *Annals of Neurology* 1980;7:466-470.

Mair RG, McEntee WJ. Cognitive enhancement in Korsakoff's syndrome by clonidine: a comparison with L-dopa and ephedrine. *Psychopharmacology* 1986;88:374-380.

Mair WG, Warrington EK, Weiskranz L. Memory disorder in Korsakoff's psychosis: a neuropathological and neuropsychological investigation of two cases. *Brain* 1979;102:749-783.

Malamud N, Skillicorn SA. Relationship between the Wernicke and the Korsakoff syndrome. *Archives of Neurology and Psychiatry* 1956;76: 585-591.

O'Carroll RE, Moffoot A, Ebmeier KP, et al. Korsakoff's syndrome, cognition and clonidine. *Psychological Medicine* 1993;23:341-347.

O'Carroll RE, Moffoot AP, Ebmeier KP, et al. Effects of fluvoxamine treatment on cognitive functioning in the alcoholic Korsakoff syndrome. *Psychopharmacology* 1994;116:85-88.

O'Donnell VM, Pitts WM, Fann WE. Noradrenergic and cholinergic agents in Korsakoff's syndrome. *Clinical Neuropharmacology* 1986;9:65-70.

Victor M, Adams RD, Collins GH. *The Wernicke-Korsakoff Syndrome and Related Neurologic Disorders Due to Alcoholism and Malnutrition*, ed 2, Philadelphia, 1989, FA Davis.

54 Alcoholic Dementia (alcohol-induced persisting dementia, DSM-IV-TR #291.2)

Alcoholism is one of the most common causes of dementia, accounting for perhaps one fifth of all cases; furthermore, at least 10% of all alcoholics have some degree of it. It may be more common among men than women. This disorder has also been referred to as alcohol-induced persisting dementia and dementia associated with alcoholism.

ONSET

Alcoholic dementia appears insidiously after many years, often decades, of heavy drinking.

CLINICAL FEATURES

Alcoholic dementia often presents with a personality change. Patients become coarse and heedless of social convention; they may become apathetic, and judgment is poor. Cognitive deficits eventually appear; short-term memory fails, and patients gradually have increasing difficulty in recalling events of the distant past. Thinking becomes concrete. With continued drinking the dementia may become profound. At times, minor "cortical" signs are seen such as apraxia, agnosia, and aphasia; however, these are not a prominent part of the clinical picture.

CT or MRI studies generally demonstrate both cortical atrophy and ventricular dilitation.

COURSE

Should alcohol consumption continue, the course is one of relentless progression. Such patients are much more prone to delirium tremens. With abstinence some improvement in cognitive functioning may occur; however, permanent deficits remain.

COMPLICATIONS

Complications include those outlined in the chapter on dementia. In addition, thus cognitively impaired, these patients are much less able to participate in any rehabilitation endeavor such as Alcoholics Anonymous.

ETIOLOGY

This dementia may occur regardless of the nutritional status of the patient. Thus, although thiamine deficiency may play a role, in all likelihood alcohol itself has a direct toxic effect on the cerebral cortex.

CT and MRI studies, as noted earlier, have demonstrated cortical atrophy and ventricular dilitation. Interestingly, with prolonged abstinence, one often sees some resolution of these changes, and this correlates with the accompanying clinical improvement. The basis for this resolution is not clear: although it may be due in part to fluid shifts, this alone does not account entirely for the changes

seen. Autopsy studies have demonstrated loss of cerebral white matter, and some, but not all, have also identified a loss of cortical neurons in the prefrontal cortex.

DIFFERENTIAL DIAGNOSIS

Given the sometimes persistent cognitive defects accompanying the alcohol withdrawal syndrome or delirium tremens, a diagnosis of dementia should generally be withheld until the patient has been abstinent for at least 1 month.

The differential diagnosis for dementia occurring in an alcoholic is the same as that for dementia occurring in a nonalcoholic and is summarized in the chapter on dementia. Certain disorders, not uncommonly seen in chronic alcoholics, should be especially considered, including subdural hematoma, acquired non-Wilsonian hepatocerebral degeneration and pellagra. Korsakoff's syndrome is distinguished by the absence of a generalized decrement in intellectual functioning.

TREATMENT

Adequate nutrition, vitamin supplementation, especially thiamine, and, above all, abstinence are required. If the patient is compliant, as noted earlier, some improvement will be seen, and this tends to occur in the first half year. Custodial care may be required until the patient has recovered sufficient cognitive ability to participate in rehabilitative efforts.

BIBLIOGRAPHY

Harper C. The neuropathology of alcohol-specific brain damage, or does alcohol damage the brain? *Journal of Neuropathology and Experimental Neurology* 1998;57:101-110.

Harper CG, Krill JJ, Holloway RL. Brain shrinkage in chronic alcoholics: a pathological study. *British Medical Journal* 1985;290:501-504.

Jensen GB, Pakkenberg B. Do alcoholics drink their neurons away? *Lancet* 1993;342:1201-1204.

Krill JJ, Halliday GM, Svodoba MD, et al. The cerebral cortex is damaged in chronic alcoholics. *Neuroscience* 1997;79:983-998.

Lishman WA. Cerebral disorder in alcoholism: syndromes of impairment. *Brain* 1981;104:1-20.

Mann K, Mundle G, Langle G, et al. The reversibility of alcoholic brain damage is not due to rehydration: a CT study. *Addiction* 1993;88:649-653.

Nicolas JM, Estruch R, Salamero M, et al. Brain impairment in well-nourished alcoholics is related to ethanol intake. *Annals of Neurology* 1997;41:590-598.

Pfefferbaum A, Sullivan EV, Mathalon DH, et al. Longitudinal changes in magnetic resonance imaging brain volumes in abstinent and relapsed alcoholics. *Alcoholism, Clinical and Experimental Research* 1995; 19:1177-1191.

Pfefferbaum A, Sullivan EV, Rosenbloom MJ, et al. A controlled study of cortical gray matter and ventricular change in alcoholic men over a 5-year interval. *Archives of General Psychiatry* 1998;55:905-912.

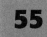

55 Alcohol Hallucinosis (alcohol-induced psychotic disorder with hallucinations, DSM-IV-TR #291.3)

Alcohol hallucinosis, also known as alcohol-induced psychotic disorder with hallucinations, is seen only in alcoholics, and then only after one or more decades of heavy alcohol consumption. Hallucinations, generally auditory, are often accompanied by delusions of reference and persecution and appear relatively suddenly, persisting for variable periods of time, well past the resolution of the withdrawal symptoms and regardless of whether the patient is abstinent.

This is an uncommon disorder; it is more common in men than in women; however, this may merely reflect the sex ratio seen in alcoholism.

ONSET

Most patients are in their late thirties or early forties when symptoms begin. Rarely in those who developed alcoholism in their early teens, one may see an onset in the twenties. The onset itself is generally abrupt, occurring over 2 or 3 days. In many cases, the symptoms appear to have had their inception within an episode of alcohol withdrawal or delirium tremens, and then persisted well after all the withdrawal symptoms per se had long remitted.

CLINICAL FEATURES

Auditory hallucinations constitute the principal symptom of alcohol hallucinosis. These are often extremely vivid and clear; the patient has no doubt as to their reality and does not believe that the physician does not hear them. For the most part they are critical, deprecatory, and often persecutory. Generally more than one voice is heard, and curiously the voices often talk among themselves about the patient. At times one may observe patients straining to overhear what the voices are saying.

What the patients hear, or overhear, is often quite distressing or frightening. They are accused of murder; the food will be poisoned; their relatives are selling all their goods and will leave them destitute and in the street.

Delusions of persecution and reference often accompany the auditory hallucinations and are generally congruent with them. Family members talk about the patient; they conspire against the patient to force her to sign documents, but she knows the documents are in fact cleverly worded confessions and refuses to sign them. Police follow the patient; they await any excuse to arrest her.

Such patients are often constrained and very watchful. They tend to be irritable and querulous. Should they feel too threatened, they may turn on their supposed persecutors.

Occasionally, visual hallucinations occur, but these are far less prominent than the auditory ones.

Should this disorder prove to be chronic, symptoms often undergo a gradual transformation over many months or a year or more. Although the voices persist, they seem not to bother the patients as much. Likewise the delusions lose their force; they become like mundane facts that excite little worry. The irritable constraint fades and may be replaced by complacency, even at times by a certain sense of humor. Such patients, if generally undisturbed, may be able to hold a job and, to casual observation, show no abnormalities.

COURSE

The course of alcohol hallucinosis is in large part a function of the subsequent use of alcohol. If after symptoms first appear the patient remains abstinent, in most cases a gradual remission occurs within anywhere from 3 weeks to 6 months or more. Should drinking resume after such a remission the probability that another episode will occur is higher; likewise such a subsequent episode generally lasts longer. With persistent drinking, episodes become progressively longer lasting until eventually the symptoms become chronic. In such cases, even with abstinence, symptoms may persist indefinitely.

COMPLICATIONS

Violence to supposed persecutors may occur; querulousness and uncooperativeness may preclude effective social or occupational functioning.

ETIOLOGY

Alcohol hallucinosis does not appear related to schizophrenia; indeed the prevalence of schizophrenia among first-degree relatives of patients with alcohol hallucinosis is no higher than that found in controls. Although the etiology of this disorder is not clear, it does appear that the risk of developing it rises in direct proportion to the severity of the patient's alcoholism and to the frequency with which alcohol withdrawal and delirium tremens have occurred. With this in mind, some investigators have proposed that alcohol hallucinosis is the product of an epileptogenic-like focus which has been kindled in the temporal lobes during the repeated autonomic storms of alcohol withdrawal.

DIFFERENTIAL DIAGNOSIS

Delirium tremens and the alcohol withdrawal syndrome are distinguished by the presence of autonomic signs and symptoms, which are absent in alcohol hallucinosis. Furthermore patients in delirium tremens are confused and forgetful, in contrast to the generally clear sensorium seen in alcohol hallucinosis.

Paranoid schizophrenia may present a clinical picture very similar to alcohol hallucinosis. The main differential point is whether the symptoms begin before heavy drinking. In those rare cases where alcoholism began in the early teens and hallucinations in the early twenties, one must look closely for symptoms such as loosening of associations, bizarre behavior, or mannerisms, all of which are not found in alcohol hallucinosis.

TREATMENT

Abstinence is essential if recovery is to be hoped for. Antipsychotics, used in the same fashion as for the treatment of schizophrenia, are helpful in reducing symptoms, and depot injections are often required because of noncompliance. If the patient remains symptom-free for a substantial period of time, the dose should be tapered and, if no symptoms appear, stopped to ascertain if a spontaneous remission has occurred.

BIBLIOGRAPHY

Schuckitt MA. The history of psychotic symptoms in alcoholism. *The Journal of Clinical Psychiatry* 1982;43:53-57.
Schuckit MA, Winokur G. Alcoholic hallucinosis and schizophrenia: a negative study. *The British Journal of Psychiatry* 1971;119:549-550.
Soyka M. Psychopathological characteristics in alcohol hallucinosis and paranoid schizophrenia. *Acta Psychiatrica Scandinavica* 1990;81: 255-259.
Surawicz FG. Alcoholic hallucinosis: a missed diagnosis. Differential diagnosis and management. *Canadian Journal of Psychiatry* 1980;25: 57-63.
Tsuang JW, Irwin MR, Smith TL, et al. Characteristics of men with alcoholic hallucinosis. *Addiction* 1994;89:73-78.
Victor M, Hope J. The phenomenon of auditory hallucinations in chronic alcoholism. *The Journal of Nervous and Mental Disease* 1958;126: 451-458.

56 Alcoholic Paranoia (alcohol-induced psychotic disorder with delusions, DSM-IV-TR #291.5)

■

The diagnosis of alcoholic paranoia, also known as alcohol-induced psychotic disorder with delusions, has remained controversial for over a century, and some have even doubted the existence of such an entity.

ONSET

The onset appears to be gradual, occurring after many years of alcoholism.

CLINICAL FEATURES

Classically, alcoholic paranoia is characterized by delusions of jealousy. The spouse is suspected of infidelity; absences from the house are seen as proof of it; the spouse's desire to keep apart from the patient during the patient's intoxicated rages is seen as a mere excuse. Rules are laid down; the spouse is neither allowed outside the house alone nor allowed to speak in private on the telephone. When drunk the patient may turn on the spouse, sometimes in a murderous fashion. In other cases the illness may be characterized by persecutory delusions: the police have begun to hound the patient. Yet another charge of driving under the influence of alcohol is trumped up; unmarked police cars cruise down the streets. The neighbors have been recruited to spy on the patient from behind their shades.

Occasionally hallucinations may occur, but they play only a minor role. Footsteps and sirens are heard at night; something moves in the attic. The food tastes spoiled, rotten, perhaps even poisoned. Strange people approach the house in the dead of night.

COURSE

In general, with continued drinking there is a gradual worsening of the psychosis; however, in some cases, a "plateau" of severity is reached and further deterioration does not occur despite ongoing drinking.

With abstinence, patients improve, with symptoms very gradually lessening over many months, in some cases disappearing entirely.

COMPLICATIONS

The irritable, and at times assaultive, behavior engendered by the delusions serves only to further isolate the alcoholic and at times may occasion incarceration or dismissal from work.

ETIOLOGY

The mechanism whereby these symptoms occur in alcoholism is not known; whether the etiology is similar to that proposed for alcohol hallucinosis is not known.

DIFFERENTIAL DIAGNOSIS

Active alcoholics do alienate people, and spouses often do turn to others for comfort, and hence the question often becomes whether the alcoholic's suspicions are well grounded or delusional. Getting alcoholics to elaborate on their suspicions often solves the problem, as those who have developed alcoholic paranoia will typically provide details that stretch past the bounds of credulity. For example, even though nosy neighbors may pry, they rarely hide out in the attic, waiting for the alcoholic to come home. Furthermore, even though spouses do have affairs, they rarely hide their lovers in the basement.

Delusional disorder, or paranoia, may present a similar picture to alcoholic paranoia. Here, however, the delusions appear to be more systematized, and a history of alcoholism is lacking.

Paranoid schizophrenia is betrayed by the bizarre nature of its symptoms and by the relative prominence of auditory hallucinations.

Alcohol hallucinosis is likewise distinguished by the prominence of auditory hallucinations.

Paranoid personality disorder is distinguished by the presence of symptoms before the onset of the alcoholism and by the absence of persistent delusions.

TREATMENT

The most effective treatment is abstinence, the achievement of which is discussed in the chapter on alcoholism. Antipsychotics may be of some use, and because many patients are not compliant with oral medication, the use of a decanoate preparation should be considered. Involuntary admission may be required to protect others from the patient.

BIBLIOGRAPHY

Albers A, Mirza S, Mirza KAH, et al. Morbid jealousy in alcoholics. *The British Journal of Psychiatry* 1995;167:668-672.
Kraepelin E. *Clinical Psychiatry*, ed 7, translated by Diefendorf AR, New York, 1981, Scholars Facsimiles and Reprints.
Langfeldt G. The erotic jealous syndrome: a clinical study. *Acta Psychiatrica Scandinavica* 1961;36(Suppl 151):7-36.
Soyka M, Naber G, Volcker A. Prevalence of delusional jealousy in different psychiatric disorders. *The British Journal of Psychiatry* 1991;158:549-553.

57 Alcoholic Polyneuropathy

A sensorimotor polyneuropathy, at times with an autonomic component, may occur secondary to chronic, heavy alcohol use and may be seen in about 10% of alcoholics.

ONSET

The onset is usually subacute. After years of heavy alcohol use, often painful paresthesias may gradually appear over several weeks, only to be followed later by a motor component.

CLINICAL FEATURES

Paresthesias begin distally, first in the feet and calves, later in the hands. Associated lancinating pains may occur. Hyperesthesia may also be present, and even the touch of a bed sheet on the soles of the feet may be more than the patient can tolerate. On examination vibratory sense is lost first, followed by other modalities; the ankle jerks are diminished or lost and the Romberg test is positive.

With continued drinking, patients develop motor weakness; this may be seen in as few as several weeks after sensory symptoms appear. Distal musculature is affected first, the lower extremities before the upper. Foot drop with a steppage gait is common; wrist drop may also occur. Atrophy of the calves and forearms may be seen. Although motor signs are bilateral, their severity is often asymmetric.

In advanced cases signs of peripheral autonomic neuropathy may occur, with impotence, postural dizziness, and rarely incontinence.

Alcoholic polyneuropathy is found not uncommonly in association with an alcohol-induced Korsakoff's syndrome.

Very rarely, alcoholic polyneuropathy may present acutely, over a week or two, with an ascending flaccid paralysis, reminiscent of the Guillain-Barre syndrome.

COURSE

With continued drinking, symptoms progress; with abstinence and proper nutrition, improvement may be seen in weeks, reaching a maximum in from 6 to 12 months.

COMPLICATIONS

Foot drop may lead to falls, especially when climbing stairs.

ETIOLOGY

Microscopically, axonal degeneration is seen, beginning distally; in severe cases this may progress to involve the anterior and posterior roots. This degeneration may occur secondary to a direct toxic effect of alcohol itself or to an associated deficiency of thiamine.

DIFFERENTIAL DIAGNOSIS

The differential diagnosis is the same as that for any polyneuropathy; disulfiram rarely may be implicated.

TREATMENT

Abstinence from alcohol is essential and all patients should be given thiamine, 100 mg/d. Benfotiamine, a fat-soluble analogue of thiamine, may also be given, in a dose of 50 mg/d. Mexiletine is effective for associated lancinating pain, but should generally not be used, given its ability to cause ventricular arrhythmias.

BIBLIOGRAPHY

Barter F, Tanner AR. Autonomic neuropathy in an alcoholic population. *Postgraduate Medical Journal* 1987;63:1033-1036.

Hawley RJ, Kurtzke JF, Armbrustmacher VW, et al. The course of alcoholic-nutritional peripheral neuropathy. *Acta Neurologica Scandinavica* 1982;66:582-589.

Koike H, Mori K, Misu K, et al. Painful alcoholic polyneuropathy with predominant small-fiber loss and normal thiamine status. *Neurology* 2001;56:1727-1732.

Nishiyama K, Sakuta M. Mexilitene for painful alcoholic neuropathy. *Internal Medicine* 1995;34:577-579.

Tredici G, Minazzi M. Alcoholic neuropathy. An electron-microscopic study. *Journal of the Neurological Sciences* 1975;25:333-346.

Woelk H, Lehri S, Bitsch R, et al. Benfotiamine in treatment of alcoholic polyneuropathy: an 8-week randomized controlled study (BAP I Study). *Alcohol and Alcoholism* 1998;33:631-638.

Wohrle JC, Spengos K, Steinke W, et al. Alcohol-related acute axonal polyneuropathy: a differential diagnosis of Guillain-Barre syndrome. *Archives of Neurology* 1998;55:1329-1334.

58   Alcoholic Cerebellar Degeneration

Alcoholic cerebellar degeneration, also known as "parenchymatous" or "secondary" cerebellar degeneration, presents with ataxia, most prominently in the lower extremities, after many years of heavy drinking. Although accurate figures as to clinical prevalence are not available, there is evidence from autopsy studies that close to one-half of severe alcoholics are affected. It is much more common in men than in women; however, this may merely reflect the sex ratio of alcoholism itself.

ONSET

The onset is subacute, with symptoms appearing over weeks, or at times months.

CLINICAL FEATURES

Ataxia of gait is the first symptom. Initially this may present with unsteadiness and a tendency to fall; eventually the patient develops a broad-based staggering gait. The heel to knee to shin test is positive, but, unless there is an associated polyneuropathy, the Romberg test is negative.

Truncal instability may accompany the gait ataxia. Ataxia of the upper extremities, dysarthria, and nystagmus all may occur but are relatively uncommon.

Cerebellar cortical atrophy may be seen on MRI or CT scanning (Figure 58-1).

There may or may not be an associated alcoholic polyneuropathy.

COURSE

With continued alcohol consumption, patients tend to worsen over the ensuing months, and then their condition tends to stabilize, even if drinking continues.

COMPLICATIONS

Falls, fractures, and eventually a fear of walking may ensue.

ETIOLOGY

Atrophy is seen in the anterior and superior segments of the vermis (Figure 58-2) and, less frequently, in the anterior lobe of the cerebellum. Microscopically, there is a loss of neuronal elements, in particular Purkinje cells. Cell death may be due to either a direct toxic effect of alcohol itself or to an associated thiamine deficiency.

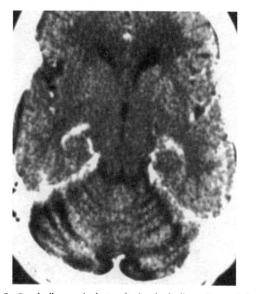

FIG. 58-1. Cerebellar cortical atrophy in alcoholism. (From Osborn AG. *Diagnostic neuroradiology*, St. Louis, 1994, Mosby.)

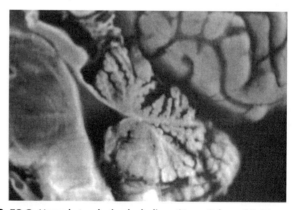

FIG. 58-2. Vermal atrophy in alcoholism. (From Osborn AG. *Diagnostic neuroradiology*, St. Louis, 1994, Mosby.)

DIFFERENTIAL DIAGNOSIS

Sensory ataxia, as may occur in alcoholic polyneuropathy, is suggested by the positive Romberg's test.

There are a host of other conditions that may cause ataxia of subacute or gradual onset, but these may generally be distinguished from alcoholic cerebellar degeneration by the presence of distinctive associated features or by the fact that they are generally relentlessly progressive. Subacute onsets may be seen with paraneoplastic cerebellar degeneration, Creutzfeldt-Jakob disease and Gerstmann-Straussler-Scheinker disease. Gradual onsets may occur with the autosomal dominant disorders spinocerebellar ataxia (SCA) and dentatorubropallidoluysian atrophy (DRPLA), and the olivo-ponto-cerebellar variant of multiple system atrophy. Consideration must also be given to lithium intoxication, chronic phenytoin use, chronic inhalant abuse, hypothyroidism, and a tumor of the posterior fossa. From a practical point of view, all patients, in addition to close clinical follow-up, should also undergo MRI imaging and thyroid function testing.

TREATMENT

With abstinence and thiamine replacement some improvement may be seen over months; however, significant residual symptoms are common.

BIBLIOGRAPHY

Allsop J, Turner B. Cerebellar degeneration associated with chronic alcoholism. *Journal of the Neurological Sciences* 1966;3:238-258.

Diener HC, Dichgans J, Bacher M, et al. Improvement of ataxia in alcoholic cerebellar atrophy through alcohol abstinence. *Journal of Neurology* 1984;231:258-262.

Hillbom M, Muuronen A, Holm L, et al. The clinical versus radiological diagnosis of alcoholic cerebellar degeneration. *Journal of the Neurological Sciences* 1986;73:45-53.

Karhunen PJ, Erkinjuntti T, Laippala P. Moderate alcohol consumption and loss of cerebellar Purkinje cells. *British Medical Journal* 1994;25:1663-1667.

Nicolas JM, Fernandez-Sola J, Robert J, et al. High ethanol intake and malnutrition in alcoholic cerebellar shrinkage. *Quarterly Journal of Medicine* 2000;93:449-456.

Phillips SC, Harper CG, Kril J. A quantitative histological study of the cerebellar vermis in alcoholic patients. *Brain* 1987;110:301-314.

Torvik A, Torp S. The prevalence of alcoholic cerebellar atrophy. A morphometric and histological study of an autopsy material. *Journal of the Neurological Sciences* 1986;75:43-51.

59 Alcoholic Myopathy

Excessive alcohol intake may be followed by an alcoholic myopathy that preferentially affects proximal limb musculature, producing variable degrees of weakness and atrophy; among alcoholics, some degree of this myopathy is present in over 50%.

ONSET

The onset may range from acute to insidious, with acute onsets typically associated with a binge.

CLINICAL FEATURES

The presentation of alcoholic myopathy varies dramatically with the mode of onset. Acute onsets are typically associated with myalgia, cramping, swelling and tenderness; insidious onsets, however, are generally characterized by a gradually progressive weakness without associated symptoms. Regardless of the mode of onset, the myopathy is generally bilaterally symmetric and tends to involve the lower more than the upper extremities, with the proximal musculature being more involved than the distal musculature. The CK and AST levels are generally elevated during acute onsets, but may be normal in insidious cases.

Rhabodmyolysis may occur during acute cases, with myoglobinuria, and, in a minority, acute renal failure.

Most patients will also have an alcoholic polyneuropathy and an alcoholic cardiomyopathy.

COURSE

With abstinence, roughly 50% will gradually recover almost full strength over the first year, with the remainder showing considerable improvement. With substantial moderation of alcohol intake, the deficit may remain chronic, without progression; with continued heavy drinking, however, progression is almost inevitable.

COMPLICATIONS

Ambulation, especially when climbing stairs, may become difficult or impossible.

ETIOLOGY

Alcohol appears to be directly toxic to skeletal muscle; microscopically, there is atrophy and, during acute cases, necrosis, primarily affecting Type II fibers.

DIFFERENTIAL DIAGNOSIS

Hypokalemia and hypomagnesemia, not uncommon in alcoholics, may also cause a myopathy; consideration may also be given to various drugs (e.g., steroids, emetine), AIDS and hyperthyroidism.

TREATMENT

Abstinence and adequate nutrition are essential.

BIBLIOGRAPHY

Estrcuh R, Sacanella E, Fernandez-Sola J, et al. Natural history of alcoholic myopathy: a 5-year study. *Alcoholism, Clinical and Experimental Research* 1998;22:2023-2028.

Fernandez-Sola J, Estruch R, Grau JM, et al. The relation of alcoholic myopathy to cardiomyopathy. *Annals of Internal Medicine* 1994; 120:529-536.

Martin F, Ward K, Slavin G, et al. Alcoholic skeletal myopathy, a clinical and pathological study. *Quarterly Journal of Medicine* 1985;55:233-251.

Pall HS, Williams AC, Heath DA, et al. Hypomagnesemia causing myopathy and hypocalcemia in an alcoholic. *Postgraduate Medical Journal* 1987;63:665-667.

Preedy VR, Adachi J, Ueno Y, et al. Alcoholic skeletal myopathy: definitions, features, contribution of neuropathy, impact and diagnosis. *European Journal of Neurology* 2001;8:677-687.

Rubenstein AE, Wainapel SF. Acute hypokalemic myopathy in alcoholism. A clinical entity. *Archives of Neurology* 1977;34:553-555.

Sacanella E, Fernandez-Sola J, Cofan M, et al. Chronic alcoholic myopathy: diagnostic clues and relationship with other ethanol-related diseases. *Quarterly Journal of Medicine* 1995;88:811-817.

60 Central Pontine Myelinolysis

Classically, central pontine myelinolysis is characterized by the development of a combination of flaccid quadriparesis and delirium, with demyelinization in the central portion of the basis pontis, two or three days after overly rapid correction of chronic hyponatremia, and classically it is seen most commonly in alcoholics. Exceptions to this classical picture, however, as described below, do occur, with prominent demyelinization occurring in extra-pontine sites, and this has prompted some authors to suggest alternative names for the syndrome, such as "central pontine and extrapontine myelinolysis" or, more generally, the "osmotic demyelination syndrome."

ONSET

The onset of the syndrome is subacute, anywhere from one to seven days (averaging two or three days) after rapid correction of chronic hyponatremia.

CLINICAL FEATURES

In classic cases, delirium and a flaccid symmetric quadriparesis develop, with symptoms gradually worsening over to a peak intensity over perhaps a week; cranial nerve palsies and pseudobulbar palsy may appear, and, in severe cases, the "locked-in" syndrome may occur wherein the patient is totally paralyzed except for vertical eye movements. Within two or three days of the onset, the flaccidity begins to resolve, to be replaced by increased deep tendon reflexes and extensor plantar responses. MRI scanning may be normal for one to three days, but eventually reveals changes in the central pons, with increased signal intensity on T2-weighted imaging and decreased signal intensity on T1-weighted scans (as illustrated in Figure 60-1). Importantly, CT scanning is very insensitive here, and may remain consistently normal despite florid symptomatology.

Exceptions to this classic picture occur when demyelinization is prominent in extra-pontine sites. Thus, one may see delirium alone, ataxia or, if the striatum is involved, parkinsonism or dystonia, and in these cases of striatal involvement, there may be a long delay between the rapid correction of hyponatremia and the appearance of a movement disorder, lasting weeks or even months. MRI scanning in cases characterized by parkinsonism or dystonia generally reveals signal changes in the putamina bilaterally.

COURSE

In fully-developed classic cases, death may occur in a matter of days; for those who survive, recovery begins within a week or two of the syndrome reaching its peak, with about one-third being left with severe complications, one-third with less severe complications, and one-third with significant or full recovery.

Parkinsonism may persist or, after months, resolve. Dystonia may resolve, persist, or, in some cases, progressively worsen.

COMPLICATIONS

In severe cases, patients may be left with dementia or permanent quadraparesis, and institutional care may be required.

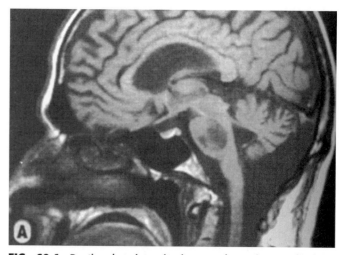

FIG. 60-1. Pontine hypointensity in central pontine myelinolysis. (From Kucharczyk W, ed. *MRI: central nervous system*, New York, 1990, Gower.)

ETIOLOGY

Classically, one finds a history of a rapid correction of chronic hyponatremia, and it is hypothesized that the resulting osmotically mediated intracellular to extracellular fluid shift is particularly damaging to oligodendroglia, resulting in the death of these cells and the subsequent loss of myelin sheathes. This scenario was first identified in alcoholics and chronically malnourished patients and even today alcoholism constitutes the most fertile ground for the development of central pontine myelinolysis. Other clinical settings that constitute a high risk for this syndrome include post-liver transplantation, prolonged vomiting or diarrhea, SIADH (as may be seen secondary to drugs such as carbamazepine, oxcarbazepine, SSRIs, etc.), and compulsive polydipsia.

On pathologic examination of classic cases, one finds an area of demyelinization in the basis pontis, which, in some cases, may extend dorsally into the tegmentum pontis or superiorly into the mensecephalon. This demyelinization is most intense centrally and spreads out symmetrically towards the periphery. In all cases, however, there is a rim of preserved white matter between the area of demyelinization and the periphery of the pons. Importantly, there is no inflammatory response, and despite the massive demyelinization, there is relative sparing of axons themselves.

In addition to this classic pathologic picture, extrapontine foci of demyelinization are also seen, involving the centrum semiovale, thalamus, striatum and cerebellum. In the striatum, demyelinization occurs primarily in the putamen, involving fibers which originated in the caudate.

Although it is clear that rapid correction of hyponatremia is at fault in most cases, recent cases have been reported, primarily in burn patients, where there had been no hyponatremia to begin with. In such cases, it appears that the preceding insult is the rapid development of a hyperosmolar state, and hence it may well be that central pontine myelinolysis is not tightly bound etiologically to hyponatremia or its rapid correction, but rather represents the end result of rapid increases in extracellular osmolality from any mechanism.

DIFFERENTIAL DIAGNOSIS

Infarction in the area of distribution of the basilar artery may produce a similar picture but is distinguished clinically by its sudden onset and, in most cases, by an asymmetry of the resulting paresis; furthermore, on MRI scanning the lesion in infarction is also often asymmetric and also extends to the periphery of the pons.

TREATMENT

Because no treatment exists, prevention is required. As discussed in the chapter on hyponatremia, slowly developing hyponatremia is generally well tolerated. Sodium concentrations of 120 or 115 mEq/L do not necessarily demand correction with normal saline and a diuretic, or with hypertonic saline. Fluid restriction is generally adequate. If saline is required in such cases, it should be administered slowly, as described in the chapter on hyponatremia, such that the serum sodium level is corrected at a rate no faster than 0.4 mEq/L/h.

BIBLIOGRAPHY

Adams RD, Victor M, Mancall TL. Central pontine myelinolysis: a hitherto undescribed disease occurring in alcoholics and malnourished patients. *Archives of Neurology and Psychiatry* 1959;81:154-172.

Estoll CJ, Faris AA, Martinez AJ, et al. Central pontine myelinolysis after liver transplantation. *Neurology* 1989;39:493-498.

Hadfiled MG, Kubal WS. Extrapontine myelinolysis of the basal ganglia without central pontine myelinolysis. *Clinical Neuropathology* 1996;15:96-100.

Karp BI, Laureno R. Pontine and extrapontine myelinolysis: a neurologic disorder following rapid correction of hyponatremia. *Medicine* 1993;72:359-373.

Lampl C, Yazdi K. Central pontine myelinolysis. *European Neurology* 2002;47:3-10.

McKee AC, Winkelman MD, Banker BQ. Central pontine myelinolysis in severely burned patients: relationship to serum hyperosmolality. *Neurology* 1988;38:1211-1217.

Maraganore DM, Folger WN, Swanson JW, et al. Movement disorders as sequelae of central pointine myelinolysis: report of three cases. *Movement Disorders* 1992;7:142-148.

Menger H, Jorg J. Outcome of central pontine and extrapontine myelinolysis (n=44). *Journal of Neurology* 1999;246:700-705.

Seiser A, Schwarz S, Aichinger-Steiner MM, et al. Parkinsonism and dystonia in central pontine myelinolysis and extrapontine myelinolysis. *Journal of Neurology, Neurosurgery, and Psychiatry* 1998;65:119-121.

Steller U, Koschorek F, Strenge H. Cerebellar ataxia with recovery related to central pontine myelinolysis. *Journal of Neurology* 1988;235:379-381.

Sterns RH, Riggs JE, Schochet SS. Osmotic demyelination syndrome following correction of hyponatremia. *The New England Journal of Medicine* 1986;314:1535-1542.

Sullivan AA, Chervin RD, Albin RL. Parkinsonism after correction of hyponatremia with radiological central pontine myelinolysis and changes in the basal ganglia. *Journal of Clinical Neuroscience* 2000;7:256-259.

Yoshida Y, Akanuma J, Tochikubo S, et al. Slowly progressive dystonia following central pontine and extrapontine myelinolysis. *Internal Medicine* 2000;39:956-960.

61 Marchiafava-Bignami Disease

Marchiafava-Bignami disease, also known as primary degeneration of the corpus callosum, is a very rare disorder seen generally only in alcoholic men, which may present in one of two fashions: acutely, with a delirium, or insidiously, with a dementia.

ONSET

The onset, as noted, may be either acute or insidious and tends to occur in middle-aged or older men after at least a decade of heavy drinking.

CLINICAL FEATURES

Acute-onset cases are characterized by delirium or stupor, often associated with seizures and various focal signs (e.g., hemiparesis, aphasia or ataxia).

Insidious-onset cases are typified by a slowly progressive dementia with prominent frontal lobe features such as apathy, disinhibition and primitive reflexes (e.g., snout and grasp reflexes); dysarthria may also be present, as may various focal signs such as apraxia or agnosia. Of interest, one often also sees classic callosal "disconnection" signs such as left-sided apraxia or agnosia.

In acute-onset cases, MRI scanning may reveal increased signal intensity on T2-weighted scans in the corpus callosum; among patients who survive the acute onset, and among patients with insidious onsets, MRI scanning reveals an area of decreased signal intensity on T1-weighted scans in the central portion of the corpus callosum, corresponding to the areas of demyelination described below.

COURSE

Patients with acute onsets generally progress to coma and death within days or weeks; those with insidious onsets, should they continue to drink, experience a steady decline, over six to eight years, into stupor, coma and death.

COMPLICATIONS

Those who survive acute onsets are generally left demented, and, like those with insidious onsets who progress, often require institutional care.

ETIOLOGY

Demyelinization, with relative axonal sparing, is found in the central portion of the corpus callosum, sparing the dorsal and ventral portions, and may extend laterally, in a symmetric fashion, to involve adjacent areas of the centrum semiovale. Demyelinization may also be seen in the anterior and posterior commisures and the middle cerebellar peduncles. In severe cases, cystic necrosis may occur.

The etiology of this demyelinization is not known. Originally, it was felt that there was an association with consumption of cheap red wine by Italian men, as most of the original cases fit this description; however, it is now clear that the syndrome may occur in alcoholics who consume whiskey, beer or wine of another variety, and may also occur in non-Italians. Indeed there are rare, but undoubtable, cases of the syndrome occurring in malnourished, but non-alcoholic patients. Presumably the demyelinization occurs

secondary to a vitamin deficiency of some sort or to one of the various metabolic derangements that can occur with severe malnutrition, and the occasional association of Marchiafava-Bignami disease with Wernicke's encephalopathy, pellagra or central pontine myelinolysis strengthens this presupposition.

DIFFERENTIAL DIAGNOSIS

Acute-onset cases may be mimicked by infarction in the area of the anterior cerebral artery, and insidious-onset cases by a tumor of the corpus callosum, and in each case the differential may rest on MRI findings. Overall, the diagnosis of Marchiafava-Bignami disease in life is difficult. Certainly, it should be on the differential for delirium or dementia occurring in an alcoholic.

TREATMENT

Abstinence, adequate nutrition, and adequate replenishment of thiamine and niacin are essential, and, if accomplished, may be followed by a stabilization of the clinical picture, and, over long periods of time, by a variable degree of recovery.

BIBLIOGRAPHY

Baron R, Heuser K, Marioth G. Marchiafava-Bignami disease with recovery diagnosed by CT and MRI: demyelination affects several CNS structures. *Journal of Neurology* 1989;236:364-366.

Caparros-Lefebvre D, Pruvo P, Josien B, et al. Marchiafava-Bignami disease: use of contrast media in CT and MRI. *Neuroradiology* 1994;36:509-511.

Chang KH, Cha SH, Han MH, et al. Marchiafava-Bignami disease: serial changes in corpus callosum on MRI. *Neuroradiology* 1992;34:480-482.

Helenius J, Tatlisumak T, Soinne L, et al. Marchiafava-Bignami disease: two cases with favorable outcome. *European Journal of Neurology* 2001;8:269-272.

Ironside R, Bosanquet FD, McMenemy WH. Central demyelination of the corpus callosum (Marchiafava-Bignami disease): with report of a second case in Great Britain. *Brain* 1961;64:212-230.

Kalckreuth W, Zimmerman P, Preilowski B, et al. Incomplete split-brain syndrome in a patient with chronic Marchiafava-Bignami disease. *Behavioural Brain Research* 1994;64:219-228.

Koeppen AH, Barron KD. Marchiafava-Bignami disease. *Neurology* 1978;28:290-294.

Leong AS. Marchiafava-Bignami disease in a non-alcoholic Indian male. *Pathology* 1979;11:241-249.

Lhermitte F, Marteau R, Serdaru M, et al. Signs of interhemispheric disconnection in Marchiafava-Bignami disease. *Archives of Neurology* 1977;34:254-257.

Rosa A, Demiati M, Cartz L, et al. Marchiafava-Bignami disease, syndrome of interhemispheric disconnection, and right-handed agraphia in a left-hander. *Archives of Neurology* 1991;48:986-988.

62 Tobacco-Alcohol Amblyopia

Tobacco-alcohol amblyopia is a rare disorder generally seen in patients with both nicotine dependence and alcoholism.

ONSET

The amblyopia generally occurs in middle years after long-term excessive use of alcohol and tobacco. The onset is generally subacute, occurring over weeks or a month or more.

CLINICAL FEATURES

Typically there is a painless, bilateral reduction in visual acuity, accompanied by central scotomas and temporal pallor of the optic discs.

COURSE

Within days or weeks, even without abstinence or any change in eating habits, the vision eventually stabilizes somewhere short of total blindness.

COMPLICATIONS

Complications are directly related to the degree of visual loss.

ETIOLOGY

Demyelinization is seen in the optic nerves, chiasm, and tract and chiefly affects the maculopapular bundle.

The cause of the demyelinization is not entirely clear: nutritional deficiencies (esp. of B vitamins) and a toxic effect of tobacco smoke have both been cited.

DIFFERENTIAL DIAGNOSIS

Of the various possible causes of painless loss of visual acuity, Leber's hereditary optic neuropathy is most likely to mimic tobacco-alcohol amblyopia, and may be diagnosed with genetic testing.

Visual loss in alcoholics always raises the question of methanol intoxication; however, in methanol intoxication the visual loss is generally abrupt in onset, and generally more severe than that seen in tobacco-alcohol amblyopia, often progressing to blindness.

TREATMENT

Replenishment of B vitamins, especially thiamine and vitamin B_{12}, may be followed by partial improvement in vision. Although improvement has been seen in patients who continue to drink and smoke, abstinence is also indicated, as this may be followed by further improvement.

BIBLIOGRAPHY

Cullom ME, Heher KL, Miller NR, et al. Leber's hereditary optic neuropathy masquerading as tobacco-alcohol amblyopia. *Archives of Ophthalmology* 1993;111:1482-1485.

Jestico JV, O'Brien MD, Teoh R, et al. Whole blood cyanide levels in patients with tobacco amblyopia. *Journal of Neurology, Neurosurgery, and Psychiatry* 1984;47:573-578.

Krumsiek J, Kruger C, Patzold U. Tobacco-alcohol amblyopia: neuro-ophthalmological findings and clinical course. *Acta Neurologica Scandinavica* 1985;72:180-187.

Rizzo JF, Lessell S. Tobacco amblyopia. *American Journal of Ophthalmology* 1994;117:817-819.

63 Methanol Intoxication

Methanol, also known as methyl alcohol or wood alcohol, is found in "canned heat" preparations, such as "Sterno," in certain solvents and paint thinners, and as a denaturant added to ethanol, which is then sold tax free as denatured alcohol for cleaning purposes.

Desperate alcoholics may occasionally resort to methanol when no other means of intoxication are possible. Methanol intoxication is also occasionally seen with inhalation of fumes, or absorption through the skin, or accidental ingestion.

A very small fraction of methanol is excreted unchanged in the urine; the vast majority is metabolized in the liver, first by alcohol dehydrogenase to formaldehyde then by aldehyde dehydrogenase to formic acid. As may be recalled, this is the same metabolic pathway utilized by ethanol, and it is of some clinical importance that ethanol, by virtue of its more avid binding to alcohol dehydrogenase, will delay the metabolism of methanol to formic acid. Methanol itself is relatively non-toxic; formic acid, however, is highly toxic and responsible for the life-threatening nature of methanol intoxication.

ONSET

The onset of intoxication by methanol generally occurs within several hours of ingestion; however, as noted below, if ethanol is ingested concurrently, the appearance of toxic formic acid may be delayed for up to a day, depending on how long it takes for the ethanol to be cleared.

CLINICAL FEATURES

The clinical features of methanol intoxication follow a more or less biphasic course. Initially, and before methanol can be metabolized to formic acid in appreciable amounts, one sees a mild ethanol-like euphoria, with an odor of alcohol on the breath and, in some patients, headache and nausea. As formic acid begins to accumulate, however, toxicity supervenes.

Toxicity is characterized by delirium, restlessness, dizziness, nausea and abdominal pain, which may be severe, and by the development of clouding and dimming of vision. With more severe intoxication seizures, coma, respiratory depression and shock may occur.

Methanol levels are generally above 30 mg/dL and a metabolic acidosis is present, with an increased anion gap created by the presence of formic acid.

COURSE

Untreated, about one-third of patients with methanol toxicity die; those who survive generally recover in from one to three days, but are typically left with one of the following complications.

COMPLICATIONS

Those who suffered visual dimming during the intoxication may have some improvement over a week or so, but are generally left with significant visual impairment. Severe intoxications may also be followed by a dementia or parkinsonism.

ETIOLOGY

In addition to causing the metabolic acidosis, it appears that formic acid is also directly neurotoxic, and widespread hemorrhages may be seen in the optic nerve and putamina, and, in more severe cases, the cerebral white and gray matter, particularly affecting the frontal and parietal lobes.

DIFFERENTIAL DIAGNOSIS

Ethanol intoxication may be distinguished by its more rapid onset, by the relative prominence of the euphoria, and by the absence of visual loss.

A confusing diagnostic picture may emerge when both ethanol and methanol are imbibed, as may occur if denatured alcohol is drunk. As noted earlier, ethanol inhibits the metabolism of methanol to formic acid, and hence the onset of the toxicity of methanol intoxication may be delayed significantly. Clinically, one initially sees a reassuring resolution of intoxication only to be followed by a deterioration in the patient's condition.

TREATMENT

If less than 2 hours have elapsed from ingestion, gastric lavage is performed.

Initially, and throughout treatment, one must monitor pH, bicarbonate levels, the anion gap, and the methanol level. Methanol levels above 20 mg/dL are generally considered toxic, and levels above 50 mg/dL potentially life-threatening.

The cornerstone of treatment rests on impeding the metabolism of methanol to formic acid. In the past this was accomplished by giving ethanol, which, as noted earlier, binds with greater affinity than methanol to alcohol dehydrogenase. A better approach, however, is to administer the newly approved intravenous fomepizole, a drug which inhibits alcohol dehydrogenase. Should fomepizole not be available, one may give an IV bolus of 0.6 to 1.0 mL/kg of 100% ethanol diluted in D5W to a 10% solution, followed by a maintenance dose of approximately 0.125 mL/kg of 100% ethanol (similarly diluted) with the dose adjusted to keep the BAL between 100 and 150 mg/dL. It is critical, in such a situation, to also give intravenous thiamine in a dose of 100 mg, in order to avoid precipitating a Wernicke's encephalopathy. In desperate situations where hospital care is not immediately available, one may begin treatment with oral alcohol by giving approximately 100 mL of a 50% ("100 proof") alcoholic beverage, such as whiskey, vodka or gin, combined with a suitable "mixer" to ensure palatability. Regardless of which method is used to retard the metabolism of methanol to formic acid, treatment should be continued until the methanol level has fallen below 10 mg/dL.

Folic acid hastens the metabolism of formic acid, and may be given in doses of 50 mg IV every six hours.

Bicarbonate is given to reduce acidosis, and large amounts may be required.

In cases where formic acid production and the resulting acidosis cannot be controlled by the foregoing methods, hemodialysis may be used.

BIBLIOGRAPHY

Anderson CA, Rubinstein D, Filley CM, et al. MR enhancing brain lesions in methanol intoxication. *Journal of Computer Assisted Tomography* 1997;21:834-836.

Anderson TJ, Shuaib A, Becker WJ. Methanol poisoning: factors associated with neurologic complications. *The Canadian Journal of Neurological Sciences* 1989;16:432-435.

Brent J, McMartin K, Phillips S, et al. Fomepizole for the treatment of methanol poisoning. *The New England Journal of Medicine* 2001;344:434-429.

McCormick MJ, Mogabgab E, Adams SL. Methanol poisoning as a result of inhalational solvent abuse. *Annals of Emergency Medicine* 1990;19:639-642.

McLean DR, Jacobs H, Mielke BW. Methanol poisoning: a clinical and pathological study. *Annals of Neurology* 1980;8:161-167.

Mittal BV, Desai AP, Khade KR. Methyl alcohol poisoning: an autopsy study of 28 cases. *Journal of Postgraduate Medicine* 1991;37:9-13.

Naraqui S, Dethlefs RF, Slobodniuk RA, et al. An outbreak of acute methyl alcohol intoxication. *The Australian and New Zealand Journal of Medicine* 1979;9:65-68.

64 Isopropyl Alcohol Intoxication

Isopropyl alcohol, also known as isopropanol, is found in after-shave lotion, hand lotion, hair tonics, and in "rubbing alcohol." Among desperate alcoholics it is known as "rubby-dubby" or "blue heaven," the latter referring to the coloring of hospital isopropyl alcohol. In part, isopropyl alcohol is metabolized in the liver via alcohol dehydrogenase to acetone; overall the half-life is about 3 to 6 hours.

ONSET

Intoxication begins shortly after ingestion.

CLINICAL FEATURES

The euphoria seen in isopropyl alcohol intoxication is not as pronounced as that seen with ethanol. Patients have headaches, dizziness, ataxia, and an odor of alcohol on the breath. Depending on the degree of acetonemia, there may also be a "fruity" aspect to the patient's breath. Typically, isopropyl alcohol also produces a severe gastritis, with nausea, vomiting, hematemesis, and melena. Aspiration pneumonia may occur.

A lethal dose in nontolerant patients is about 250 ml, but in alcoholics who have developed tolerance it may be much higher. Coma may occur, as may arrhythmias, hypotension, and respiratory depression, which may be fatal.

Acetonemia and acetonuria are found, and the anion gap is increased.

COURSE

For those who survive, coma typically clears within 12 hours, with full recovery within 2 to 3 days.

COMPLICATIONS

These are similar to those described in the chapter on alcohol intoxication.

ETIOLOGY

The mechanism whereby isopropyl alcohol produces intoxication is not known.

DIFFERENTIAL DIAGNOSIS

The prominent gastritis and the presence of acetonemia and acetonuria help distinguish isopropyl alcohol intoxication from ethanol or methanol intoxication.

Ethylene glycol ingestion is suggested by a picture of intoxication without the odor of alcohol on the breath.

TREATMENT

If instituted within 2 hours of ingestion, gastric lavage is useful. Hemodialysis may be used when supportive measures fail or when the isopropyl alcohol level is higher than 400 mg/dl.

BIBLIOGRAPHY

Abramson S, Singh AK. Treatment of the alcohol intoxications: ethylene glycol, methanol and isopropanol. *Current Opinion in Nephrology and Hypertension* 2000;9:695-701.

Freierich AW, Cinque TJ, Xanthaky G, et al. Hemodialysis for isopropanol poisoning. *The New England Journal of Medicine* 1967;277:699-700.

Lacouture PG, Wason S, Abrams A, et al. Acute isopropyl alcohol intoxication. Diagnosis and management. *The American Journal of Medicine* 1983;75:680-686.

Rich J, Scheife RT, Katz N, et al. Isolpropyl alcohol intoxication. *Archives of Neurology* 1990;47:322-324.

65 Other Alcohol Related Disorders

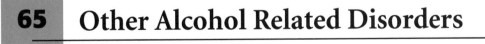

The neurologic and general medical complications seen in alcoholism are extensive; in addition to those described in the foregoing chapters, clinicians should be mindful of the following possibilities.

Head trauma is very common among alcoholics, and chronic subdural hematoma is a not uncommon cause of seizures or dementia in these patients.

Gastritis induced by alcohol is also common among alcoholics; hematemesis and persistent nausea and vomiting may occur.

Hepatic injury may take any one or a combination of three forms: fatty liver, hepatitis, and cirrhosis. Fatty liver is found in a majority of alcoholics. Although hepatomegaly and modest elevation of enzymes may be present, fatty liver is generally asymptomatic and with abstinence resolves without residuals in a few weeks. Hepatitis is less common and generally presents with nausea and vomiting, jaundice, abdominal pain, tender hepatomegaly, and marked elevation in liver enzymes and bilirubin. With abstinence the hepatic inflammation generally remits, but with some residual scarring possible. Alcoholic cirrhosis appears to be the result of chronic or repeated alcoholic hepatitis occurring in a patient genetically predisposed to develop this cirrhosis. Although cirrhosis may be asymptomatic, the majority of patients develop symptoms, the most severe of which are secondary to portal hypertension and portal-systemic shunting. Ascites and bleeding esophageal varices are common; the mortality rate is over 50% in those who continue to drink. One of the most feared consequences of cirrhosis or severe hepatitis is hepatic encephalopathy, which is described in detail in that chapter.

Pancreatitis may occur in an alcoholic after particularly heavy alcohol use and generally presents with the acute onset of nausea and vomiting with steady, severe upper abdominal pain that may radiate to the back. The amylase level is almost always elevated, the lipase level somewhat less frequently. With recurrent attacks pancreatic insufficiency may occur, with diabetes and malabsorption.

Hypoglycemia may result from a combination of an alcohol-induced impairment of hepatic gluconeogenesis and reduced oral intake as a result of nausea or vomiting. Hypoglycemia is discussed in detail in that chapter; generally the hypoglycemia seen in alcoholics is not severe enough to produce significant symptoms. However, if treatment is indicated, thiamine replenishment should be accomplished first to prevent precipitating Wernicke's encephalopathy.

Ketoacidosis may occur in an alcoholic after particularly heavy alcohol use. Kussmaul breathing, nausea and vomiting, and confusion may be seen. The arterial pH is reduced, and excess beta hydroxybutyric acid and lactic acid increase the anion gap. The glucose level may be normal, low, or elevated. Other causes of acidosis with an increased anion gap include the following: poisoning with methanol, ethylene glycol, salicylates, or paraldehyde; starvation; diabetes; and lactic acidosis secondary to shock, septicemia, and the like. Alcoholic ketoacidosis generally responds to supportive measures, such as administration of normal saline and, if hypoglycemia is present, glucose, provided that thiamine has been given first.

Hypomagnesemia may occur secondary to decreased intake, poor absorption, or vitamin D deficiency, and is described in detail in that chapter. The prothrombin time may be increased in alcoholics, and bleeding may occur. This may be due to either decreased intake of vitamin K or to a loss of hepatocytes to an extent that, even with a sufficient supply of vitamin K, vitamin K-dependent clotting factors are no longer synthesized in adequate number. If intramuscular administration of 10 to 25 mg of vitamin K does not significantly correct the prothrombin time, then hepatic insufficiency is the likely cause.

Rarely the acute encephalopathic form of pellagra, as described in that chapter, may be seen.

Thrombocytopenia may occur in alcoholics, with internal bleeding and easy bruisability. Administration of 1 to 2 mg of folic acid daily may help, but abstention is required for correction.

A megaloblastic anemia is quite common in alcoholics, and may be caused by a direct toxic effect of alcohol itself on the bone marrow or by folate or B_{12} deficiency.

Infections are particularly common in alcoholics and may be caused by deficient leukocyte functioning. Alcoholics are overrepresented among adults with bacterial meningitis. Aspiration pneumonia is particularly common and may involve gram-negative bacilli.

A dilated cardiomyopathy may occur secondary to the toxic effect of chronic alcohol use. Patients present with symptoms typical of congestive heart failure; sudden death may occur secondary to ventricular arrhythmia. Diuretics or vasodilators may help; digoxin is usually not helpful. With persistent alcohol use, over three quarters of these patients die within 3 years.

BIBLIOGRAPHY

Diamond I, Messing RO. Neurologic effects of alcoholism. *The Western Journal of Medicine* 1994;161:279-287.

Lieber CS. Hepatic and other medical disorders of alcoholism: from pathogenesis to treatment. *Journal of Studies on Alcohol* 1998;59:9-25.

Lieber CS. Medical disorders of alcoholism. *The New England Journal of Medicine* 1999;333:1058-1065.

Rubino FA. Neurologic complications of alcoholism. *The Psychiatric Clinics of North America* 1992;15:359-372.

Schenker S, Bay MK. Medical problems associated with alcoholism. *Advances in Internal Medicine* 1998;43:27-78.

Smith JW. Medical manifestations of alcoholism in the elderly. *International Journal of Addiction* 1995;30:1749-1798.

66 Anabolic Steroid Abuse

Anabolic steroids, if taken in large amounts over long periods of athletic training, do indeed increase muscle mass and improve athletic performance. Such use began in the 1950s among weightlifters, and since then use has spread among athletes in almost all sports. It is prominent in football, baseball, and basketball and is now also seen in track and field. The lifetime prevalence of any anabolic steroid use is about 0.5% in the United States. Although what percentage of these develop a pattern of abusive use is not known, it is clear that amongst competitive athletes a pattern of abusive use may be found in up to one-half.

Anabolic steroid abusers do not use these drugs for intoxication; rather they seek to improve their body build or performance. Unfortunately, however, a significant percentage of these users eventually develop serious untoward effects, most notably manic symptoms. Furthermore, after cessation of prolonged use a withdrawal syndrome may occur, consisting primarily of depressive symptoms.

A variety of different agents are abused for their anabolic effects. Although all are referred to as "anabolic" steroids, these agents are more properly referred to as androgens with varying mixtures of androgenic and anabolic activity. Testosterone is the prototype of such agents, but since it undergoes such a significant "first pass" effect, it is generally not used. Rather, athletes resort to either intramuscular long-acting esterified testosterone preparations or 17-alpha alkylated compounds, which, as they resist hepatic metabolism, may be taken orally.

These agents are typically taken in high doses, anywhere from 3 to 100 times the dosage used therapeutically; a list of commonly used preparations is supplied in the box on this page.

A large number of other agents are obtained in foreign countries and smuggled into the United States. They include norethandrolone and clostebol, both for parenteral use, testosterone undecanoate which may be used either intramuscularly or orally, and a large number of oral agents, such as mesterolone, oxymesterone, methenolone, formebolone, and an oral preparation of norethandrolone. Desperate patients may at times even resort to veterinary preparations, such as boldenone and mibolerone.

Although the vast majority of anabolic steroid users are male, a growing number of female athletes are also resorting to their use, despite the virilization that occurs secondary to the androgenic activity.

ONSET

Most patients begin to use steroids in their mid to late teenage years.

CLINICAL FEATURES

Steroids are obtained either by prescription or on the black market. Most users "cycle" their use, wherein they take higher dosages for months or more, then abstain for a matter of weeks or more, and then begin a new "cycle." During the cycle patients may "stack" drugs, using two or more at the same time; they may also "pyramid" the dosage or dosages, initially increasing then gradually tapering the dosage as the cycle is brought to a close. If training is intense during the cycle, a significant amount of muscle mass may be added, particularly in the chest and the shoulders.

Prolonged, high dose use of anabolic steroids may cause a mood disturbance, generally with manic features, in up to one-quarter of users. Euphoria and heightened sexuality may be seen; more problematic, however, is hostility and irritability, which at times may be quite pronounced and have a certain rigid quality to it. Grandiose ideation may be prominent: patients may feel themselves to be the meanest, the strongest, the "baddest." A sense of invulnerability may occur, and some patients may become reckless. In some cases steroid abusers may experience exaltation, racing thoughts, heightened energy, and decreased need for sleep. Delusions, either persecutory or grandiose, may occur, and voices may be heard. In some cases violent behavior, even homicide, may

Anabolic Steroids

INTRAMUSCULAR PREPARATIONS:	ORAL PREPARATIONS:
testosterone enanthate	methandienone
testosterone cypionate	(methandrostenolone)
testosterone phenpropionate	stanazol
nandrolone decanoate	methyltestosterone
	nandrolone
	fluoxymesterone
	oxymetholone
	oxandrolone
	mesterolone
	danazol

occur. Rarely, delusions of hallucinations may occur in the absence of manic symptomatology.

In some patients a withdrawal syndrome may occur following long-term use. This is characterized by depressed mood, fatigue, lack of interest, loss of appetite, insomnia, and a pronounced displeasure at the gradual loss of muscle mass that ensues. Suicidal ideation may occur. During this time the desire to resume use may be particularly strong. Interestingly, though, no "craving" per se for the drug or for the affective changes that may occur with its use occur. Rather the desire is to increase muscle mass again. These depressive symptoms are self-remitting after weeks or months.

During use, fluid retention may occur, and some patients take diuretics to relieve this. Males may develop acne and oligospermia. Rarely among males who use testosterone preparations, a degree of gynecomastia (which may be irreversible) may occur, and testicular atrophy may appear with any of these agents. Lutenizing hormone and follicle-stimulating hormone levels fall, and after cessation of use testosterone levels may be low for several weeks or more.

Virilization may occur among females. Initially acne, hirsutism, deepening of the voice, and irregular periods may develop. Over time, male-pattern baldness and clitoral enlargement may occur.

Prepubertal children who take anabolic steroids may initially show enhanced linear growth; however, epiphyseal closure occurs prematurely, and the eventual adult height is often less than it might have been.

COURSE

Anabolic steroid abuse appears to be long term, lasting years or a decade or more.

COMPLICATIONS

Long-term use of the 17-alpha alkylated compounds is often accompanied by some degree of cholestasis, and jaundice may occur. Rarely peliosis hepatitis may occur and even more rarely a hepatoma.

Some patients who use injectable preparations may share needles, thus incurring the risk of infection with hepatitis or AIDS.

With long-term use an increase in blood pressure and a fall in high-density lipoproteins may occur. Stroke and myocardial infarction have been reported, and they may be related to these changes.

Females who use anabolic steroids during pregnancy, especially during the first trimester, may give birth to masculinized female children.

The complications of the mania and depression are similar to those described in the chapter on bipolar disorder. Violent behavior may lead to incarceration.

DIFFERENTIAL DIAGNOSIS

Manic symptoms, or depressive symptoms, occurring in a "bulked-up" athlete or bodybuilder, though consistent, of course, with a primary mood disorder such as bipolar disorder or major depression, should always suggest anabolic steroid abuse.

ETIOLOGY

In a small minority of cases the recurrent use of anabolic steroids among body builders may be a kind of "reverse anorexia." Here the patient, although "bulked up," still fears being thin and weak and is compelled by this fear to continue steroid use. In most cases, however, apart from the obvious thirst for muscle mass, no specific etiology has been identified.

TREATMENT

Manic or psychotic symptoms may require antipsychotics; the effect of mood stabilizers such as divalproex or lithium on manic symptoms is not clear. Depressive symptoms may require treatment with an antidepressant, and anecdotally SSRIs, such as fluoxetine, have been used with success. In some cases, hospitalization may be required, but prolonged pharmacologic treatment, given the self-remitting nature of the mood symptoms, is not necessary.

The overall goal of treatment is abstinence; psychotherapy has been advocated to help the patient accept a less than "perfect" build; however, controlled studies are lacking.

BIBLIOGRAPHY

Copeland J, Peters R, Dillon P. Anabolic-androgenic steroid use disorders among a sample of Australian competitive and recreational users. *Drug and Alcohol Dependence* 2000;60:91-96.

Forbes GB, Porta CR, Herr BE, et al. Sequence of changes in body composition induced by testosterone and reversal of changes after drug is stopped. *The Journal of the American Medical Association* 1992;267:397-399.

Gruber AJ, Pope HG. Psychiatric and medical effects of anabolic-androgenic steroid use in women. *Psychotherapy and Psychosomatics* 2000;69:19-26.

Malone DA, Dimeff RJ. The use of fluoxetine in depression associated with anabolic steroid withdrawal: a case series. *The Journal of Clinical Psychiatry* 1992;53:130-132.

Pope HG, Katz DL. Homicide and near-homicide by anabolic steroid users. *The Journal of Clinical Psychiatry* 1990;51:28-31.

Pope HG, Katz DL. Psychiatric and medical effects of anabolic-androgenic steroid use. A controlled study of 160 athletes. *Archives of General Psychiatry* 1994;51:375-382.

Pope HG, Katz DL, Herman JI. Anorexia nervosa and "reverse anorexia" among 108 male bodybuilders. *Comprehensive Psychiatry* 1993;34:406-409.

Su TP, Pagliaro M, Schmidt PJ, et al. Neuropsychiatric effects of anabolic steroids in male normal volunteers. *The Journal of the American Medical Association* 1993;269:2760-2764.

SCHIZOPHRENIA AND OTHER PSYCHOTIC DISORDERS

67 Schizophrenia (DSM-IV-TR #295.1-295.3, 295.90)

Schizophrenia is a chronic, more or less debilitating illness characterized by perturbations in cognition, affect and behavior, all of which have a bizarre aspect. Delusions, also generally bizarre, and hallucinations, generally auditory in type, also typically occur. The original name for this illness, "dementia praecox," was coined by Emil Kraepelin, a German psychiatrist in the late nineteenth and early twentieth century, whose description of the illness remains a guiding force for modern investigators.

Schizophrenia is a relatively common disorder, with a lifetime prevalence of about 1%. Although the overall sex ratio is almost equal, males tend to have an earlier onset than females, a finding accounted for by the later age of onset in those females who lack a family history of the disease.

ONSET

Although most patients fall ill in late teenage or early adult years, the range of age of onset is wide: childhood onset may occur, and in some instances symptoms may not appear until the sixties.

There may or may not be a prodrome before the actual onset of symptoms. In some cases the "pre-morbid personality" appears completely normal. In others, however, peculiarities may have been apparent for years or even decades before the onset. In cases where the prodrome began in childhood, the history may reveal introversion and peculiar interests. In cases where the prodrome began later, after the patient's personality was formed, family members may recall a stretch of time wherein the patient "changed" and was no longer "the same." Prior interests and habits may have been abandoned and replaced by a certain irritable seclusiveness, or perhaps suspiciousness.

The onset of symptoms per se may be acute or insidious. Acute onsets tend to span a matter of weeks or months and may be characterized by confusion or at times by depressive symptoms. Patients may recognize that something is wrong, and they may make some desperate attempts to bring some order into the fragmenting experience of life. By contrast, in cases with an insidious onset the patient may not be particularly troubled at all. Over many months or a year or more, evanescent changes may occur: fleeting whispers, vague intimations, or strange occurrences.

CLINICAL FEATURES

Although the clinical presentation of schizophrenia varies widely among patients, certain signs and symptoms, though present to different degrees, are consistently present, and these include *hallucinations*, *delusions*, *disorganized speech* and *catatonic* or *bizarre behavior*. "Negative" symptoms (e.g., flattening of affect) are often also seen but in some cases are quite mild. Generally, based on the constellation of symptoms present, one may classify any given case of schizophrenia into one of several *subtypes*, namely the *paranoid*, *catatonic*, *hebephrenic* ("disorganized") and *simple* subtypes, with a large proportion of patients, however, failing to clearly fit any subtype and being characterized as having "*undifferentiated*" schizophrenia.

Hallucinations are very common in schizophrenia. Patients may hear things, often voices, or they may see things; hallucinations of taste, touch, and smell may also occur. But of all these, the hearing of voices is most characteristic of schizophrenia.

The voices may come from anywhere. They come from the air; God or angels send them. They may come from the television or radio; wiring may emanate the voices. Special devices may be planted in the walls or furniture. Sometimes they are in clothing; often they are localized to certain parts of the body. They come from the bowels, the liver, from "just behind the ear." They may be male or female; the patient may or may not be able to recognize the identity of the speaker. It is a sibling, or a dead parent. Most often, though, the voices are not recognized as belonging to anyone; they are from strangers. They may be clear and easily understood; sometimes they are deafening and compelling—"everything else is shut out." At other times they may be soft, "just a mumbling," indistinct and fading.

What the voices say is extremely varied: however, certain themes are relatively common. Voices may comment on what the patient is doing. Often two voices argue with one another about the patient. Often the voice echoes or repeats what the patient thought. Thoughts are "audible"; they are "heard out loud"; they are repeated on the television.

At times "command hallucinations," or voices that tell the patient what to do, may be heard. At times these are imperious and irresistible; at other times they are soft, "suggestive only." Sometimes they command innocuous things; the patient may be directed to shave again. At other times they may command the patient to commit suicide or to hurt others. Usually the commands can be resisted, but not always. Sometimes they are overwhelmingly compelling—"they must be obeyed."

The patients generally hear only short phrases, perhaps single words. Only very rarely do the voices speak at length in a coherent way. Often the patient is tortured by the voices. Patients may hear threats of death, accusations of unspeakable sins, or announcements that the gallows are being erected.

Rarely patients are encouraged or comforted by the voices. An angel's voice may proclaim their divinity; seductive voices may whisper enticement; their names may be praised. Unutterable joys are set aside for them. Patients who hear such voices may have a beatific countenance.

Most patients find the voices as real sounding as the voice of any other person. They may talk back to them out loud or may even argue with them. At times when the voices are unpleasant, the patient may try to drown them out by listening to music or to the television.

In addition to hearing voices patients may also hear sounds, such as a creaking or a rattling of chains. Footsteps or a tapping on the windows is heard. Hissing and whistling also may be heard. Sometimes a ringing of church bells or an explosion is heard. Hammering means the gallows are being constructed. Very rarely the patient may hear music.

Visual hallucinations, though common, play a relatively less prominent part in the clinical picture of schizophrenia than do auditory hallucinations. They may be poorly formed, indistinct, seen only "out of the corner of the eye." They may, however, be vivid and compellingly realistic. Strange people walk the halls; the devil in violent red appears in front of the patient; heads float through the air. Reptilian forms appear in the bath; things crawl in the food; a myriad of insects appear in the bedding. The electric chair is made ready; torturers approach; a chorus of sympathetic angels is seen.

Hallucinations of smell and taste, though not common, may be particularly compelling to the patient. Poison gas is smelled; it seems to be coming from the heating ducts. The patient smells putrefied flesh, so the corpses must be buried nearby. At times inexpressibly beautiful perfumes are appreciated, a seduction seems close at hand.

Tastes, often foul and bitter, may appear on the tongue "from nowhere." Often, however, something is detected in food or drink. Patients detect something brackish, a poisonous or medicinal taste. Patients may refuse all food and drink and declare that they have had enough poison already.

Hallucinations of touch, also known as haptic or tactile hallucinations, are relatively common. Something is crawling on them; a pricking is coming from behind. At night all manner of things are felt. Fluids are poured over the body; a caressing is felt, as are lips on all parts. Electrical sensations may be felt at any time. Sometimes patients may feel things inside their bodies. Their intestines shrivel up; the ovaries burst; the brain is pressed upon.

Delusions are almost universal in schizophrenia. The content of the delusions is extremely varied: patients may feel persecuted; they may have grandiose ideas; all manner of things may refer and pertain to them; thoughts may be broadcast, withdrawn, or inserted into them; they may feel influenced and controlled by outside forces; bizarre, loathsome events may occur. These beliefs may grow in the patient slowly. At first there may be only an inkling, a suspicion; only with time does conviction occur. Conversely, sudden enlightenment may occur; all may be immediately clear. Sometimes patients may have lingering doubts about the truth of these beliefs, but for most they are as self-evident

as any other belief. Occasionally patients may argue with those who disagree, but for the most part they do not press their case on the unbeliever. Most often the delusions are poorly coordinated with each other; typically they are contradictory and poorly elaborated. Occasionally, however, they may be systematized, and this is especially the case in the paranoid subtype.

Delusions of persecution are particularly common. There is a conspiracy against the patient; the FBI has coordinated its efforts with the local police. Plain-clothes officers follow the patient. At times the surveillance is covert. Satellites are used. Listening devices have been placed in the walls; the telephone is tapped. The patient is followed by cars; headlights blink on and off to indicate that capture is imminent. The food is poisoned. Electrical currents are passed through the body at night; internal organs are horribly manipulated during sleep. Tortures are prepared; escape is not possible. Sometimes patients may stoically endure their persecution, and at other times they may fight back. To the patient, this unprovoked assault may be a justifiable defense. Other patients attempt to flee their persecutors and may move to another state. For a time they may feel less insecure, but eventually they see signs that they have been found and again the persecution begins. Some patients attempt to protect themselves against noxious influences by armoring themselves or their apartments. One patient who believed that persecutors sent electrical charges down through the ceiling at night papered the entire ceiling with aluminum foil and for a time felt protected.

Grandiose delusions also occur frequently, often in conjugation with delusions of persecution. Patients are attacked by jealous enemies who seek to bar them from the throne. They are to be exalted; the angel of the Lord has visited them. Millions of dollars are kept secretly away from them. They embark for Washington; the President wishes their advice. Commonly most patients do not act on their delusions; rather they seem content to be comforted and sustained by them. Exceptions do occur, of course. One patient announced a plan for world happiness in a full-page newspaper ad; another sent a letter of advice to the Secretary of State.

Delusions of reference are intimately tied to delusions of persecution or of grandeur. Here patients believe that otherwise chance occurrences or random encounters have special meaning for them. What was done refers to them; it pertains to them. A busboy leaves a particle of food on the table; it is an intentional offense to the patient. The street lights blink on; it is a sign for the persecutors to close in for the final attack. The television newscaster speaks in code; the songs on the radio hold special meaning for the patient. There are no more coincidences in life, no accidental happenings. To the grandiose patient the events of creation are exalting; to the persecuted patient, walking the streets can provoke a terrifying self-consciousness. Everything is pregnant with meaning.

Some patients may develop some peculiarly bizarre beliefs about thinking itself, known as thought broadcasting, thought withdrawal, and thought insertion. In thought broadcasting patients experience thoughts as being broadcast from their heads, as if by electricity. "It is like radio broadcasting," explained one patient. These thoughts may then be picked up by others. Some patients compare it to telepathy; some feel they can receive others' thoughts. "There is mind reading going on," commented one patient. Sometimes the television may broadcast their thoughts back to them. In thought withdrawal the patients' thoughts are removed, taken from them. The mind is left blank. "There are no thoughts anymore," complained one patient. Magnetic devices may be used; the thoughts are never returned.

Patients who experience this symptom of thought withdrawal may concurrently, if they happen to be speaking their thoughts, display the sign known as "thought blocking." Here, patients in the middle of speaking abruptly cease talking, and this happens precisely because they abruptly find themselves with no thoughts to express. In thought insertion, a phenomenon opposite to that of thought withdrawal occurs. Here patients experienced the insertion of thoughts into their minds. The thoughts are alien, not their own; they were placed there by some other agency. The thoughts are transmitted toward them electrically; they can feel a tingling as they enter their brain. They cannot rid themselves of them.

Allied to the foregoing three delusions are what are known as delusions of influence, or control. Patients experience their thoughts, emotions, or actions to be directly controlled by some outside force or agency. They are made to experience or do these things; they are like robots or automatons, without any independence of will. The influence may emanate from the television broadcast tower; a spell may be cast on them; a massive computer has merged its workings into them. They are not themselves anymore.

Other delusions may occur. In fact any imaginable belief may be held, no matter how fantastic. Angels live in the patient's nose; sulphur is cast on the body during sleep; parents have risen from their graves; all fluids have evaporated from the body. Another delusion is the delusion of doubles, also known as the "Capgras phenomenon," or the delusion of impostors. Here the patient believes that someone, or something, has occupied the body of another. Although the body looks the same and the voice is the same, indeed, for all intents and purposes, it is the same person, yet the patient knows without doubt that it is an impostor. The patient may see subtle signs of it elsewhere; it is part of the conspiracy. The senses cannot be trusted anymore; appearances must be doubted. Doubles may be used for one's spouse or children; no one is immune. The patient must be on guard at all times.

Disorganized speech is the next symptom to consider. Here, we are concerned not so much with the content of the patient's speech, that is to say with delusions, but rather with the form of speech. This "formal thought disorder" is most often characterized as "loosening of associations"; less frequently it is referred to as incoherence or "derailment." The patient's speech becomes illogical; ideas are juxtaposed that have no conceivable connection. A family member may say that the patient "doesn't make sense." At its extreme, loosening of associations may present as a veritable "word salad." An example of loosening of associations follows. A patient was asked to report the previous day's activities; the patient replied, in part, "The sun bestrides the mouse doctor. In the morning, if you wish. Twenty-five dollars is a lot of money! Large faces and eyes. Terrible smells. Rat in the socket. Can there be darkness? Oh, if you only knew!" Here any inner connection among the various ideas and concepts is lost; it is as if they came at random. Or to put it another way the thoughts are no longer "goal-directed"; they no longer cohere in pursuit of a common purpose. If patients are pressed to explain what they mean, they are unable to offer a satisfactory reply. The question may be responded to, but only with another incoherent utterance. Interestingly, also, these patients seem little concerned about their incoherence. They seem oblivious to it and make little if any effort to clarify what they say.

Allied to loosening of associations are neologisms. These are words that occur in the normal course of the patient's speech and that the patient treats as an integral part of it, but that convey no more meaning to the listener than if they were from a long-dead foreign language. To the patient, however, they have as much meaning and status as any other word, but that meaning is private and inaccessible to the listener. When one patient was offered a cup of coffee, the reply was, "Yes, doctor, thank you. With bufkuf." When asked the meaning of "bufkuf," the patient replied "Oh, you know," and made no further effort to define or explain it.

Catatonic symptoms include negativism, certain peculiar disturbances of voluntary activity known as catalepsy, posturing, stereotypies and echolalia or echopraxia.

Negativism is characterized by a mulish, automatic, almost instinctual opposition to any course of action suggested, demanded, or merely expected. In some cases this negativism is passive: if food is placed in front of patients, they do not eat; if their clothes are set out for them, they do not dress; if a question is asked, they do not answer, and a bizarre scowl may mar the facial expression. In more extreme cases the negativism becomes active, and patients may do the exact opposite of what is expected: if shown to their room, they may enter another; if asked to open their mouths, they may clamp shut; if asked to walk from a burning room, they may walk back in. Such active negativism seems neither thought out nor done for a purpose; rather it appears instinctual, as if the patients themselves had no choice but to do the opposite. Remarkably, in some patients one may see the exact opposite of negativism in the symptom known as "automatic obedience." Here, patients do whatever they are told to do, regardless of what it is. In the nineteenth century, one way to test for this symptom was to tell a patient that you wished him to stick the tongue out so that it might be pierced with a needle. Patients would protrude their tongues and not flinch when pierced by the needle.

Catalepsy, or, as it is also known, waxy flexibility, is characterized by a state of continual and most unusual muscular tension. If one attempts to bend the patient's arm, it is as if one were bending a length of thick metal wire, like soldering wire. Definite resistance, though not great enough to hinder movement, is nevertheless present. The remarkable aspect here is that, as in bending the wire, the patient retains whatever position the limb, or for that matter, the body, is placed in. This happens regardless of whether the patient is instructed to maintain the position or not. In this way the most uncomfortable, grotesque, and strenuous positions may be maintained for hours. This symptom, rarely seen in modern times, was common before the advent of antipsychotic medicines in the middle of the twentieth century. The back wards of state hospitals housed many catatonic patients who held their bodies in positions throughout each nursing shift, day in and day out.

Posturing is said to occur when the patient, for no discernible reason, assumes and maintains a bizarre posture. One may keep the arms cocked; another stood bent at the waist to the side.

Stereotypies are constituted by bizarre, perseverated behaviors. A patient may march back and forth along the same line for hours; another may repeatedly dress and undress. Other persons may be approached again and again, each time being asked the same question. The same piece of paper may be folded and unfolded until it disintegrates. Most patients can offer no reason for their senseless activity. When asked, a patient replied, "it must be so."

Echolalia and echopraxia are said to occur when the patient's behavior mirrors that of the other person, and, importantly, when this happens automatically, and in the absence of any request. If asked a question the echolalic patient will simply repeat it, sometimes over and over again. The echopraxic patient may clumsily mirror the gestures and posture of the interviewer and, as in echolalia, may continue to do this long after the other person has left, as if uncontrollably compelled to maintain the same activity. Here it as if the ability to will something independent of the environment has been lost, and the patient is thus left enslaved in a mimicry of whatever is close at hand.

Bizarre behavior may manifest as mannerisms, bizarre affect or an overall disorganization and deterioration of behavior.

Mannerisms are bizarre or odd caricatures of gestures, speech, or behavior. In manneristic gesturing patients may offer their hands to shake with the fingers splayed out, or the fingers may writhe in a peculiar, contorted way. In manneristic speech, cadence, modulation, or volume are erratic and dysmodulated. One patient may speak in a sing-song voice, another in a telegraphic style, and yet another with pompous accenting of random syllables. Overall behavior may become manneristic. Rather than walking, some patients may march in bizarre, stiff-legged fashion.

Bizarre affect appears to represent a distortion of the normal connection between felt emotion and affective expression. Often, facial expression appears theatrical, wooden, or under a peculiar constraint. Patients may report feeling joy, yet the rapturous facial expression may appear brittle and tenuous. Conversely patients may report grief, and indeed tears may be present, yet the emotion lacks depth, as if patients were merely wearing a mask of grief that might disappear at any moment. Inappropriate affect may also be seen. Here the connection between the patient's ideas and affect seems completely severed. A young patient, grief stricken at a parent's funeral, was seen to snicker; another patient, relating the infernal tortures suffered just the night before, smiled beatifically.

Another, very important form of bizarre affect is unprovoked and mirthless laughter. For no apparent reason patients may break into bizarre and unrestrainable laughter. Though appearing neither happy nor amused, the laughter continues. Some patients report that they were unable to not laugh, that the laughter moved itself no matter how they felt.

The overall deterioration of behavior in schizophrenia is what often makes these patients "stand out" in public. Patients become untidy and may neglect to bathe or wash their clothes; the fingernails may become very long. Dress and grooming may become bizarre. Several layers of clothing are often worn, even during the summer. Bits of string or cloth may festoon the patient's hair or garments; makeup may be smeared on. Not uncommonly, paranoid patients shave their heads, and this often reliably predicts an oncoming exacerbation of illness, and also some form of self-mutilation. Patients may pluck out their eyelashes or cut deep gouges in their legs. Some seem to be almost completely analgesic: an eye may be plucked out; pieces of flesh may be bitten off; in extreme cases, self-evisceration may occur, "just to see" what the intestines look like. Although most often no purpose seems to drive this bizarre behavior, at times the patient may offer a reason. One patient wallpapered the walls, ceiling, and floors with aluminum foil "to keep the rays out"; another kept cotton in the ears "to keep the voices away."

Negative symptoms include flattening of affect, alogia (also commonly known as poverty of speech and thought), and avolition.

Flattening of affect, also known, when less severe, as "blunting" of affect, is characterized by a lifeless and wooden facial expression accompanied by an absence or diminution of all feelings. This is quite different from a depressed appearance. In depression patients appear drained or weighted down; there is a definite sense of something there. In flattening, however, patients seem to have nothing to express; they are simply devoid of emotion. They appear unmoved, wooden, and almost at times as if they were machines.

Poverty of speech is said to occur when patients, though perhaps talking a normal amount, seem to "say" very little. There is a dearth of meaningful content to what they say and speech is often composed of stock phrases and repetitions. Poverty of thought is characterized by a far-reaching impoverishment of the entire thinking of the patient. The patient may complain of having "no thoughts," that "the head is empty," that there are no "stirrings." Of its own accord nothing "comes to mind." If pressed by a question the patient may offer a sparse reply, then fail to say anything else.

Avolition, referred to by Kraepelin as "annihilation of the will," is said to be present when patients have lost the capacity to embark on almost any goal-directed activity. Bills are not paid; the house is not cleaned; infants are neither changed nor fed. This is not because patients feel inhibited, lack interest, or suffer from fatigue, but rather because the ability to will an action has become deficient.

Before leaving this discussion of the individual signs and symptoms of schizophrenia and proceeding to a discussion of subtypes, two other symptoms, neither of which fit neatly into the categories employed above, should be mentioned, namely ambivalence and "double bookkeeping."

Ambivalence may render patients incapable of almost any volitional activity. Here, patients experience two opposed courses of action at the same time, and for lack of ability to decide between them, do nothing. One patient stood at the washstand for hours unable to decide whether to shave or to use the toothbrush. This "paralysis of will," however, may at times be easily removed if another person gives directions. In this case an aide simply told the patient to brush his teeth and then put the toothbrush in the patient's hand. Immediately and with peculiar alacrity the patient then set to brushing his teeth. This kind of ambivalence found in schizophrenia is to be distinguished from the indecisiveness seen at times in depression and the "normal" ambivalence that anyone may experience. The depressed patient's inability to embark on decision-making stems more from a lack of energy and initiative; unlike the patient with schizophrenia, the depressed patient generally is not able to act when others make the decision. In normal circumstances competing desires may leave the patient unable to decide. With time, however, a normal person makes a decision because the capacity to do so is not lost. In schizophrenia, however, it is this very capacity that is no longer present.

"Double bookkeeping," a phenomenon first identified by Bleuler, refers to the patient's ability to, as it were, live in two worlds at the same time. On the one hand is the world of voices, visions, and delusions, and on the other hand, and quite coincident with this psychotic world, is the world as perceived by others. To the patient both worlds seem quite real. For example, a patient may hear a voice as clearly as the voice of the physician and believe it just as real, yet at the same time acknowledge that the physician does not hear it. Or the grandiose patient who fully believed that a coronation was imminent may yet continue to work at a janitor's job and go on doing so, living in two worlds, and feeling little if any conflict between them. A variant of double bookkeeping, known as "double orientation," or "delusional disorientation," may at times mislead the interviewer into thinking that the patient is disoriented. For example, a grandiose patient believed that he was John F. Kennedy, and when asked what year it was replied 1962. Later on, however, when filling out a form, he put down the correct year.

Subtypes of schizophrenia are characterized by particular constellations of symptoms and include the following: paranoid, catatonic, hebephrenic (or "disorganized"), and simple (which has also been referred to as "simple deteriorative disorder"). Patients whose illness does not fall into any of these subtypes are said to have an "undifferentiated" subtype. Subtype diagnosing is not an academic exercise, for, as discussed under Course, the different subtypes may have different prognoses. Furthermore, knowing the subtype allows one to predict with better confidence how any given patient might react in any specific situation.

Paranoid schizophrenia, which tends to have a later onset than the other subtypes, is characterized primarily by hallucinations and delusions. Other symptoms, such as loosening of associations, bizarre behavior, or flattened or inappropriate affect, are either absent or relatively minor. The hallucinations are generally auditory and typically hostile or threatening. The delusions are generally persecutory and referential. Voices warn patients that their supervisors plot against them. They begin to suspect that their co-workers talk about them behind their backs and laugh quietly as they pass by. Newspaper headlines pertain to them; the CIA is involved; meal portions at the factory cafeteria are secretly poisoned, and patients may refuse to eat at work. At times these patients may appeal to the police for help, or they may suffer their slights in rigid silence. Their attitude becomes one of intense, constrained anger and suspiciousness. Occasionally they may move away to escape their persecutors, yet eventually they are "followed." At times they may turn on their supposed attackers, and violent outbursts may be seen.

In paranoid schizophrenia, more so than in the other subtypes, the delusions may be somewhat systematized, even plausible. In most cases, however, inconsistencies appear, which, however, have no impact on the patients. Often, along with persecutory delusions, one may also see some grandiose delusions. Patients believe themselves persecuted not for a trivial reason; others now know that the patient recently acquired a controlling interest in the company. Rarely, grandiose delusions may be more prominent than persecutory ones and may dominate the entire clinical picture. A patient may believe herself anointed with holy oil; trumpets blared forth her appearance as a prophet. She has a message that will save the world, and sets about spreading it.

Catatonic schizophrenia manifests in one of two forms: stuporous catatonia or excited catatonia. In the stuporous form one sees varying combinations of immobility, negativism, mutism, posturing, and waxy flexibility. One patient curled into a rigid ball and lay on the bed, unspeaking, for days, moving neither for defecation nor urination, and catheterization was eventually required. Saliva drooled from the mouth, and as there was no chewing, food simply lay in the oral cavity and there was danger of aspiration. Another patient stood praying in a corner, mumbling very softly. A degree of waxy flexibility was present, and the patient's arm would, for a time, remain in any position it was placed, only eventually to slowly return to the position of prayer.

In the excited form of catatonia one may see purposeless, senseless, frenzied activity, multiple stereotypies, and at times extreme impulsivity. Patients may scream, howl, beat their sides repeatedly, jump up, hop about, or skitter back and forth. A patient leaped up and attacked a bystander for no reason, then immediately returned to a corner and restlessly marched in place, squeaking loudly. Often speech is extremely stereotyped and bizarre. Patients may shout, declaim, preach, and pontificate in an incoherent fashion. Words and phrases may be repeated hundreds of times. Typically, despite their extreme activity, these patients remain for the most part withdrawn. They often make little or no effort to interact with others; they keep their excitation to themselves, perhaps in a corner, perhaps under a bed. Rarely Stauder's lethal catatonia may occur. Here, as the excitation mounts over days or weeks, autonomic changes occur with hyperpyrexia, followed by coma and cardiovascular collapse.

Although some patients with catatonic schizophrenia may display only one of these two forms, in most cases they are seen to alternate in the same patient. In some cases a form may last days, weeks, or longer, before passing through to the other. In other cases, however, a rapid and unpredictable oscillation from one form to another may occur. A stuporous patient suddenly, without warning, jumped from his bed, screamed incoherently, and paced agitatedly from one wall of the room to another. Then, in less than an hour, the patient again rapidly fell into mute immobility.

Hebephrenic schizophrenia tends to have an earlier onset than the other subtypes and tends to develop very insidiously. Although delusions and hallucinations are present, they are relatively minor, and the clinical picture is dominated by bizarre behavior, loosened associations, and bizarre and inappropriate affect. Overall the behavior of these patients seems at times a caricature of childish silliness. Senselessly they may busy themselves first with this, then with that, generally to no purpose, and often with silly, shallow laughter. At other times they may be withdrawn and inaccessible. Delusions, when they occur, are unsystematized and often hypochondriacal in nature. Some may display very marked loosening of associations to the point of a fatuous, almost driveling incoherence.

Simple schizophrenia has perhaps the earliest age of onset, often first beginning in childhood, and shows very gradual and insidious progression over many years. Delusions, hallucinations, and loosening of associations are sparse, and indeed are for the most part absent. Rather the clinical picture is dominated by the annihilation of the will, impoverishment of thought, and flattening of affect. Gradually over the years these patients fall away from their former goals and often become cold and distant with their former acquaintances. They may appear shiftless, and some are accused of laziness. Few thoughts disturb their days, and they may seem quite content to lie in bed or sit in a darkened room all day. Occasionally some bizarre behavior or a fragmentary delusion may be observed. For the most part, however, these patients do little to attract any attention; some continue to live with aged parents; others pass from one homeless mission to another.

Undifferentiated schizophrenia is said to be present when the clinical picture of any individual case does not fit well into one of the foregoing subtypes. This is not uncommonly the case, and it also appears that in some instances the clinical picture, which initially did "fit" a subtype description, may gradually change such that it no longer squares with one of the specific subtypes: this appears to be more common with the catatonic and hebephrenic subtypes than with paranoid or simple schizophrenia.

Before leaving this discussion of subtypes, it is appropriate to briefly discuss another proposal for subdividing schizophrenia, which is said by some to have more predictive and heuristic value than the classical subtyping just discussed. Two subdivisions are proposed: "good prognosis," "reactive," or "type I" schizophrenia, and "poor prognosis," "process," or "type II" schizophrenia. The contrasting characteristics of these two subdivisions are outlined in Table 67-1. "Positive" symptoms are hallucinations, delusions and disorganization of speech, whereas "negative" symptoms consist of flattening of affect, poverty of thought and avolition.

Although this "good prognosis"/"poor prognosis" scheme is useful, many patients do not fit neatly into type I or type II but rather evidence a mixture of features of both types. Indeed, whether this typology represents an advance over the old "classical" subtypes is not yet clear. One might, for example, argue that the type I patient

■ **TABLE 67-1.** Type I and Type II Schizophrenia

	Type I	Type II
Premorbid personality	Normal	Poor adjustment
Age of onset	Late, often adult years	Early
Mode of onset	Acute	Gradual and insidious
Symptoms associated with onset	Confusion and depression	Few
Kind of symptoms	Positive	Negative
Ventriculomegaly on CT scan	Absent	Present
Course	More favorable	Unfavorable

has paranoid schizophrenia and the type II patient has simple schizophrenia. Further research is needed.

COURSE

Schizophrenia is a chronic disease, and, in most cases, exhibits one of two overall patterns. In one, the course of symptoms is waxing and waning, whereas in the other there is a more or less stable chronicity.

The waxing and waning course is marked by exacerbations and partial remissions. The pattern of these changes is often quite irregular, as are the durations of the exacerbations and partial remissions, ranging from weeks, to months, or even years. Some patients, during episodes of partial remission of the "positive" symptoms, may develop a sustained and pervasive depressed mood accompanied by typical vegetative symptoms. This condition, often referred to as a "postpsychotic depression," increases the risk of suicide. Importantly, such a postpsychotic depression should not be confused with the frequent, transient, and isolated depressive symptoms seen during an exacerbation of the other symptoms of the illness.

At times, exacerbations may be precipitated by life stresses; however, at other times they simply happen. Among the stresses that can precipitate exacerbations, living in a family with high "expressed emotion" is important. Such family members tend to be intrusive, critical, and over-involved, and patients exposed to such an onslaught, even when provided with optimum medical treatment, are likely to relapse. Some patients experience this fluctuating course for their entire lives; in many others, however, after 5 to 20 years, this pattern gives way to one of stable chronicity.

The stable chronicity seen in some patients may appear in some cases after the initial onslaught of symptoms seen at the onset of the disease has dampened, and in others, as for example those with simple schizophrenia, it may be apparent from the onset itself. Over long periods of time, patients with this course may show very slow progression until the disease eventually "burns out" leaving them in a deteriorated state.

The classical subtype diagnosis may allow for some prediction as to course. Those with paranoid or catatonic schizophrenia tend to pursue a fluctuating course, and of the two the eventual outcome appears to be worse for the catatonic subtype. The hebephrenic and simple subtypes tend to pursue either a stable or progressively deteriorating chronicity, and of the two the simple subtype seems to often undergo the greatest deterioration.

As noted earlier one may also make predictions as to course by subdividing cases into Type I and Type II, with the Type I cases showing a waxing and waning course and the Type II cases undergoing a more or less chronic deterioration.

Before leaving this discussion of the course of the disease, it is appropriate to consider whether or not schizophrenia, in the natural course of events, and in the absence of antipsychotic treatment, ever undergoes a full and complete remission. Certainly, far-reaching remissions have been documented; indeed, in many cases patients may appear at first glance to be recovered, and if one's definition of "recovery" or "remission" is broad enough, as is the case in many published studies, one might say that a remission did occur. However, on closer inspection one may generally find lingering residual symptoms in these "recovered" patients, such as fleeting hallucinations, odd thoughts, mannerisms or a certain poverty of thought. Thus, although "social" recoveries in the absence of treatment, although rare, do occur, it is very unlikely that, in the natural course of the disease, there is ever a *restitutio ad integrum*.

COMPLICATIONS

Academic and business failure are common; most patients are incapable of sustaining intimate relationships. About half attempt suicide, and about 10% succeed. Most suicides occur early in the course of the illness; depressive symptoms, as are seen in postpsychotic depression, male sex and unemployment increase the risk.

A not uncommon, but often overlooked, complication is hyponatremia. Some patients become "compulsive water drinkers"; however, the hyponatremia appears not to be caused solely by excessive intake of water. The renal tubule cells appear to be hypersensitive to ADH, leading to a urine osmolality that is less than maximally dilute relative to the degree of hyponatremia. Symptoms are as described in the chapter on hyponatremia.

ETIOLOGY

CT and MRI scans have conclusively demonstrated ventricular dilitation and cortical atrophy in schizophrenia; furthermore there is a good correlation between the degree of atrophy of the posterior portion of the left superior temporal gyrus and the severity of auditory hallucinations and speech disorganization. Some studies have also demonstrated atrophy of the thalamus; however, these findings are not as robust. Enlargement of the basal ganglia, demonstrated in earlier studies, now appears to be an artifact of antipsychotic treatment. Interestingly, the ventricular dilitation and cortical atrophy are present at the onset of the disease, and some studies have also suggested that they may progressively worsen over time.

Neuropathologic findings in schizophrenia have been notoriously difficult to replicate; however, certain findings appear to be standing the test of replication. First, it appears that there is neuronal loss in the mediodorsal nucleus of the thalamus. Second, there is, in the subcortical white matter in the frontal and temporal lobes, an increased number of residual neurons, neurons which, in the normal course of development, either undergo apoptotic death or migrate on through the white matter to settle in the overlying cortex.

Inheritance plays a very large part in schizophrenia. The lifetime prevalence of schizophrenia, as noted earlier, is about 1%; in first-degree relatives of patients, however, it is about 5%. Furthermore, whereas among dizygotic twins the concordance rate is from 10 to 15%, the concordance in monozygotic twins is roughly 50%. These findings, of course, could also be explained on the basis of environmental influence; however, adoption studies have clearly demonstrated that the influence here is genetic. Despite this evidence for inheritance; however, it has been extraordinarily difficult to conclusively identify any specific genes or establish linkage for schizophrenia. This being said, however, there is some evidence for linkage to loci on chromosomes 6, 8 and 22.

Taking these findings together, it is not unreasonable to consider that schizophrenia is a neurodevelopmental disorder characterized by defective neuronal migration, leading to thalamic and cortical atrophy, and that this defect is, at least in part, determined genetically. Environmental factors, however, are clearly at work, given that the monozygotic concordance rate is only 50%.

Of the multiple environmental factors investigated, there is reasonably good evidence for two. First, it appears clear that patients with schizophrenia are more likely to have had a difficult birth or to have suffered obstetrical trauma, and such events are capable of disrupting neuronal migration, which continues long after birth. Second, it also appears that there is an excess of winter births in patients with schizophrenia. Clearly, many factors could account for this, but one that has stood out has been the possibility of a seasonal viral infection that could have affected patients in utero. Fetal viral infections can clearly distort neuronal migration, and it has been speculated that what is inherited in schizophrenia is a vulnerability of neurons to viruses which, in normal circumstances, are not neurotropic.

This "neurodevelopmental" theory of the etiology of schizophrenia, though reasonable in light of the evidence, is not without controversy, and the reader is encouraged to watch the literature closely.

DIFFERENTIAL DIAGNOSIS

Given the broad range of symptoms that may occur in schizophrenia, it is not surprising that the differential diagnosis is quite large.

A manic episode of a bipolar disorder may "cross-sectionally" appear similar to hebephrenia, excited catatonia, or paranoid schizophrenia. If, however, one has an accurate history, the diagnosis is relatively straightforward. In schizophrenia, which is a chronic illness, psychotic symptoms almost always precede the excitation; in mania, which occurs as an episodic illness, however, affective symptoms appear first, and psychotic ones only appear as the patient progresses into the acute stage of mania and on up to the height of a manic episode, delirious mania. When a history is lacking, certain symptomatic differences may allow for a differential diagnosis. The mood and affect of a patient with mania are typically "infectious" and well developed. By contrast, the mood of an excited hebephrenic is one of silly, shallow hilarity, which, rather than provoking laughter, might leave the interviewer with a sense of puzzlement. Furthermore the activity of a manic patient is outgoing and extroverted; this is in striking contrast to an excited catatonic who, though hyperactive, remains withdrawn and may actually avoid contact with others. Finally, the irritable manic is "on the attack," whereas the agitated patient with paranoid schizophrenia is "on guard." Both are dangerous, the manic recklessly so, the schizophrenic only if approached in what appears to the patient to be a hostile manner.

During depressive episodes, occurring either as part of a major depression or bipolar disorder, one may see delusions and hallucinations. Here, however, the psychotic symptoms are preceded by the depressive ones and only occur when the depressive symptoms are severe. By contrast, whereas depressive symptoms may occur in schizophrenia, no invariable relationship exists between them and the psychotic symptoms. In schizophrenia one sees psychotic symptoms both when the patient is depressed and also when free of depressive symptoms. Should this history regarding the course of the depression be unavailable, certain "cross-sectional" features may assist in the differential diagnosis. Delusions, when they appear in a depressive episode, tend to be "mood congruent"; that is, they make sense given the way the patient is feeling. Conversely, in schizophrenia the delusions tend to be bizarre and generally unrelated to the mood.

The differential diagnosis between a catatonic stupor and a psychomotorically retarded depression may be facilitated if the patient is closely observed for movement over an extended period of time. In stupor one may occasionally see rapid movements as the negativism briefly remits; by contrast, in a psychomotorically retarded depression all movements are always slowed down.

The differential diagnosis between schizoaffective disorder and schizophrenia rests on a thorough and accurate history of the course of the illness. Both illnesses are characterized by chronic psychotic symptoms, such as hallucinations and delusions; however, in schizoaffective disorder one also sees the occurrence of full and sustained affective episodes (depressive, manic or mixed manic) during which, importantly, one also sees an exacerbation of the pre-existing psychotic symptoms. Although schizophrenia may also be marked by mood disturbances, these tend to be transient and not severe. One exception to this is the post-psychotic depression, described earlier under "Course," which is sustained and may be quite severe. Here, however, there is not an exacerbation of psychotic symptoms and it is this which distinguishes the depression of post-psychotic depression in schizophrenia from the depression seen in schizoaffective disorder.

As alcoholism and schizophrenia not uncommonly occur in the same patient, the differential diagnosis between alcohol hallucinosis or alcoholic paranoia and schizophrenia may be difficult. Certainly, if the psychotic symptoms began before the patient started to drink or relatively early on in the drinking career, then the diagnosis of schizophrenia would be favored. When, however, psychotic symptoms begin after many years of alcoholism and repeated episodes of delirium tremens, the differential between paranoid schizophrenia and alcohol hallucinosis or alcoholic paranoia may be difficult. The presence of mannerisms, stereotypies, or loosened associations favor schizophrenia; a remission of symptoms after 6 months or more of abstinence would favor alcohol hallucinosis or alcoholic paranoia.

Delusional disorder, or paranoia, is distinguished from paranoid schizophrenia by the systematization and "plausibility" of the delusions in paranoia and by the absence of symptoms typical of schizophrenia, such as loosening of associations, mannerisms, and stereotypies. Hallucinations, though they may appear in paranoia, play only a minor role in contrast with paranoid schizophrenia, where they are often abundant.

Paranoid personality disorder may be very difficult to distinguish from paranoid schizophrenia. Certainly the presence of delusions or hallucinations would favor a diagnosis of schizophrenia; however, in both disorders patients may be very guarded and secretive, and the interviewer may not be able to reliably determine if psychotic symptoms are present. In such instances the overall demeanor and behavior of the patient may help. The patient with paranoid personality disorder presents a fully integrated and internally consistent behavioral repertoire; indeed one may get the sense of a seamless fabric of anger and resentment. By contrast, the patient with paranoid schizophrenia often displays some fragmentation: affect may be somewhat dysmodulated or inappropriate; associations may be somewhat loosened; a mannerism may be seen.

Schizotypal personality disorder is distinguished from most of the subtypes of schizophrenia by the absence of psychotic symptoms. Differentiation from simple schizophrenia may not be possible on the basis of "cross-sectional" data. The course of the illness, however, enables a differential diagnosis: the patient with schizotypal personality disorder presents a stable clinical picture over time, whereas the patient with simple schizophrenia presents a clinical picture marked by progressive deterioration.

Patients with borderline personality disorder when under great stress may occasionally experience hallucinations and delusions. By contrast, in schizophrenia these symptoms, though exacerbated by stress, are present also in calm times.

Obsessions and compulsions may occasionally be seen in the prodrome to schizophrenia; the eventual appearance of unrelated psychotic symptoms, however, clarifies their differential import.

Autism may at times be difficult to distinguish from schizophrenia of childhood onset. Certainly, if symptoms appear before the age of 3 years, autism is the more likely diagnosis, as the earliest noted age of onset of schizophrenia is 5 years of age. The presence of hallucinations and delusions indicates schizophrenia; their absence, however, does not rule against schizophrenia, as young children may not be able to report such symptoms. Conversely the presence of typical autistic symptoms, such as gaze avoidance or a "flapping" tremor, argues strongly for a diagnosis of autism.

Mental retardation and schizophrenia are two not uncommon illnesses, and their coincidence in the same patient is not rare. Such "engrafted" schizophrenia may be heralded by a deterioration in a previously stable condition or by the appearance of delusions, hallucinations, or loosening of associations, features that are not seen in straightforward mental retardation. However, in patients with severe or profound mental retardation, such symptoms may not be ascertainable at all. In such instances close examination should be made for signs such as bizarre or flattened affect, echopraxia, and waxy flexibility.

Intoxication with phencyclidine, stimulants, or cocaine may produce psychotic symptoms; the prior history of substance use, a compatible urine or serum toxicology, and the remission of symptoms with enforced abstinence make the diagnosis.

Folie à deux, as described in that chapter, is distinguished by the presence of a "dominant" partner who does have schizophrenia, and by recovery with forced separation of the patient from this dominant partner. Malingering or factitious illness may at times cause diagnostic difficulty. Certainly the presence of mannerisms and similar symptoms would argue for schizophrenia because these symptoms are generally not known to the public at large and in any case are very difficult to fake.

Psychosis may also occur secondary to a large number of neurologic disorders, as discussed in the chapter on Secondary Psychosis. Of these, the most likely to be confused with schizophrenia are the chronic interictal psychosis, Huntington's disease, Wilson's disease and metachromatic leukodystrophy.

Before leaving this section on differential diagnosis, a word is in order regarding the putative entities known as "brief psychotic disorder" and "schizophreniform disorder," each of which are discussed in more detail in their own chapters. Both these illnesses are characterized by symptoms essentially identical to those which may be seen in schizophrenia: where they differ is in their supposed course. Patients who experience a full and complete remission of their psychosis in less than one month are said to have brief psychotic disorder and those whose psychosis persists past one month but fully remits before six months are said to have schizophreniform disorder. There is debate as to whether either disorder actually exists. Certainly there are patients with psychosis who remit fully with antipsychotic treatment, but whether there are patients who remit fully and completely, without a lingering trace of psychosis, without treatment, has not been demonstrated conclusively. Although by convention a diagnosis of schizophrenia is withheld until the patient has been ill for at least six months, one should always be prepared to revise the diagnosis of brief psychotic disorder and schizophreniform disorder as the months go by and the patient, as is almost always the case, remains ill.

TREATMENT

The treatment of schizophrenia almost always involves the use of an antipsychotic drug. Patients may also be seen in supportive psychotherapy, either on an individual basis or in a group, and in social skills training groups. A "token economy" approach may be required for severely debilitated patients. Families may also be seen, not only for educational purposes, but also to enable them to lessen the kinds of family interactions that tend to be followed by relapse. Assistance may be required to enable the patient to secure housing and employment.

The antipsychotics may be broadly divided into two groups, namely "first generation," or "typical" drugs, and "second generation," or "atypical" drugs. All of these agents are covered in detail in their respective chapters in the Section on Psychopharmacology, and discussion here will be limited to only a few. Commonly used first generation antipsychotics include haloperidol, fluphenazine and chlorproamzine. There is an ever growing number of second generation drugs, which now includes clozapine, olanzapine, risperidone, quetiapine, ziprasidone and aripiprazole. Clozapine, olanzapine and risperidone are probably all therapeutically superior to the first generation agents (especially with regard to negative symptoms), and, in the cases of olanzapine and risperidone, are generally better tolerated. Although quetiapine, ziprasidone and aripiprazole are also in general better tolerated than the first generation agents, it is not as yet clear that they are therapeutically superior.

All other things being equal, it is probably best to begin treatment with a second generation agent, such as olanzapine or risperidone; clozapine, although therapeutically superior to either of these, has such severe side-effects that it is generally held in reserve for treatment-resistant patients, as discussed below. The other second generation agents (quetiapine, ziprasidone and aripiprazole) cannot be as strongly recommended: although they are in general better-tolerated than the first generation drugs, there is not yet good evidence for their therapeutic superiority over the first generation agents. The choice between olanzapine and risperidone is not easy, as it is not as yet clear whether one is therapeutically superior to the other. In terms of side effects, olanzapine carries the risks of weight gain, diabetes and hyperlipidemia, whereas risperidone is more likely than olanzapine to cause extrapyramidal side effects such as akathisia or parkinsonism. Olanzapine may be used in doses ranging from 10 to 30 mg daily, and in the case of risperidone a dose of 4 mg daily appears optimal.

In some cases, it may be appropriate to use a first generation agent. Cost is an issue for many patients: the oral preparations of the first generation agents, unlike the second generation ones, are all available in generic form, and the cost differences can be very large. Another issue is a history of a good response: for patients who have done perfectly well on a first generation agent, there may be little reason to change. Finally, there is the availability of two of the first generation agents, haloperidol and fluphenazine, in long-acting injectable decanoate preparations: noncompliance with oral medications is very common in schizophrenia, and in some cases the use of a long-acting injectable is the only way to maintain the patient in the community. Although a long-acting injectable form of risperidone has been developed, it has not, as of this writing, been released in the United States; if it is released, then this reason for using a first generation agent may well disappear. Choosing among the first generation agents is simplified, as discussed in that chapter, by dividing them into "low potency" drugs, such as chlorpromazine, and "high potency" drugs, such as haloperidol or fluphenazine. Low potency agents tend to cause sedation, hypotension and anticholinergic effects (e.g., dry mouth, blurry vision, constipation, urinary hesitancy), but have a lower tendency to cause extrapyramidal side effects (e.g., parkinsonism, dystonia, akathisia); high potency drugs, by contrast, exhibit a high potential for extrapyramidal side effects, but are relatively benign otherwise. Sometimes the choice between low and high potency drugs may be made on the basis of side effects: for example, a patient with postural dizziness probably should not be given a low potency agent that might exacerbate postural hypotension; on the other hand a patient in traction might not tolerate a dystonia very well at all and might be better served by a low potency agent. In cases where side effects are not a compelling issue, then using either haloperidol or fluphenazine is probably best, as this would facilitate transition to a decanoate form should that become necessary.

Once an antipsychotic has been chosen, it should be given at an adequate trial, not only in terms of duration but also dose. In general, presuming the dose is adequate, two weeks is long enough to see an initial response. Adequate doses for risperidone and olanzapine were discussed earlier; doses for the other atypicals are discussed in the respective chapters. Adequate oral doses for haloperidol and fluphenazine are 5 to 15 mg/d, and for chlorpromazine 100-300 mg. Obviously, lower doses are indicated for the elderly and frail and for patients with significant hepatic dysfunction or for those with significant general medical illnesses. In some cases, in particular with agitated or assaultive patients, one may have to use adjunctive treatments at the start, and continue them until the antipsychotic has had a chance to take effect. Divalproex, given in a loading dose of 15 to 20 mg/kg/d for otherwise healthy patients, is effective, as is use of as needed doses of a benzodiazepine, such as lorazepam at 2 mg orally roughly every four hours. In some cases one may also simply use much higher doses of the antipsychotic; however, this always incurs the risk of worse side effects. Although experience with high dose risperidone and olanzapine is limited, haloperidol has been given in doses of 60 mg daily and chlorpromazine in doses of up to 3000 mg daily. These issues are more thoroughly discussed in the chapter on Rapid Pharmacologic Treatment of Agitation.

If the patient gets an initial good response, then the agent may be continued as maintenance treatment, as discussed below. If the response is only partial, but otherwise promising, one may continue treatment for an additional four weeks. At that point, if the response is good one may move to maintenance treatment. If the response is less than adequate, then one should first review the case, and make sure the diagnosis is correct. Assuming the diagnosis is correct, then one should consider significantly increasing the dose, and observing the patient for another couple of weeks. If the response is still inadequate or if side effects are unacceptable, then one may consider switching to another agent. Certainly, if the patient had not been given a trial of risperidone or olanzapine, one of these should be considered, and if one of these two had been used and found wanting, then the other should be given a trial.

A good response is followed by maintenance treatment; an inadequate response should prompt consideration of clozapine.

Clozapine is superior to every other antipsychotic, and may succeed where all the others have failed. Enthusiasm for its use, however, is tempered by its many side effects, most notably the risk of agranulocytosis and the necessity for routine CBCs. Details regarding clozapine are covered in the respective chapter.

Maintenance treatment is appropriate for almost all patients. Initially, patients should be maintained on a dose similar, if not identical, to that which initially provided relief. Once patients are stable in the community, cautious dose adjustments may be considered once every three or four months. As noted earlier, in many cases the course of schizophrenia is characterized by a waxing and waning of symptoms, and in these cases, it is appropriate to attempt to "titrate" the dose to the underlying severity of the disease. Furthermore, some patients may become so distressed at side effects that they find a mild increase in the symptoms of the disease a reasonable price to pay for a reduction in the intensity of side effects. Should patients become almost symptom free, some psychiatrists may elect to decrease the dose in a step-wise fashion every 3 months until either symptoms reappear or drug discontinuation is achieved, with the patient being left with only mild, residual symptoms. Unfortunately, however, even when patients and family members are instructed regarding the "early warning signs" of relapse, troublesome symptom recurrence is common; therefore, chronic maintenance treatment, albeit with low doses, may be better than intermittently attempting trials at drug discontinuation. In general, over long term follow-up it is appropriate to keep the dose overall as low as possible to reduce the risk of tardive dyskinesia. This side effect, discussed in its own chapter, occurs in a significant minority of patients who take antipsychotics over the long haul, and hence the physician must always be alert to the emergence of any abnormal involuntary movements.

Should a post-psychotic depression occur, it is appropriate to give an antidepressant, such as an SSRI, and to treat the patient in the same fashion as one would acutely treat a depressive episode that occurred in a major depression, as described in the chapter. One must always be careful, however, to distinguish between a depression and a antipsychotic-induced bradykinesia (or akinesia), as may be seen especially when high potency first generation agents are used. Bradykinesia, as discussed in the chapter on first generation neuroleptics, when occurring in isolation, may appear similar to a psychomotorically-retarded depression. ECT may also be helpful in post-psychotic depression. Interestingly, ECT is also at times effective in catatonic schizophrenia, whether excited or stuporous, regardless of whether depressive symptoms are present.

Before leaving the subject of antipsychotic treatment, a word is in order regarding akathisia. This extrapyramidal side-effect, also discussed in more detail in the chapter on first generation antipsychotics, may "masquerade" as an exacerbation of psychosis, and if this diagnosis is missed then the clinician, mistakenly believing that the exacerbation of psychotic symptoms is resulting from an exacerbation of the underlying illness, might go ahead and increase the dose of the antipsychotic, thus increasing the akathisia and initiating a downwardly spirally therapeutic misadventure.

After antipsychotics have brought more florid symptoms under control, patients may profit from cognitive-behavioral therapy and, if still in contact with family, family therapy. Insight or psychoanalytically oriented psychotherapy is contraindicated. Not only does it not help, but also indeed some patients may worsen while being thus treated.

When families are involved, psychoeducationally oriented multiple-family groups are very helpful. Parents should be clearly told that they did not "cause" the illness and that no connection exists between child-rearing or early childhood events and the appearance of schizophrenia. When family members are critical, intrusive, and over-involved, behavioral family therapy aimed at reducing these behaviors is very helpful and reduces the number of hospital stays required.

Hospitalization is required for most patients at some point in their illness, and in some cases, repeated admissions occur. Involuntary admission may be required and may be lifesaving. Partial hospitalization services are available in many areas and have enabled many former "back ward" patients to survive and maintain themselves in the community.

BIBLIOGRAPHY

Andreasen NC. Negative symptoms in schizophrenia: definition and reliability. *Archives of General Psychiatry* 1982;39:784-788.

Barta PE, Pearlson GD, Powers RE, et al. Auditory hallucinations and smaller superior temporal gyral volume in schizophrenia. *The American Journal of Psychiatry* 1990;147:1457-1462.

Black DW, Boffeli TJ. Simple schizophrenia: past, present and future. *The American Journal of Psychiatry* 1989;146:1267-1273.

Byne W, Buchsbaum MS, Mattiace LA, et al. Postmortem assessment of thalamic nuclear volume in subjects with schizophrenia. *The American Journal of Psychiatry* 2002;159:59-65.

Cahn W, Pol HE, Lems EB, et al. Brain volume changes in first-episode schizophrenia: a 1-year follow-up study. *Archives of General Psychiatry* 2002;59:1002-1010.

Csernansky JG, Mahmoud R, Brenner R, et al. A comparison of risperidone and haloperidol for the prevention of relapse in patients with schizophrenia. *The New England Journal of Medicine* 2002;346:16-22.

Fenton WS, McGlashan TH. Natural history of schizophrenia subtypes. I. Longitudinal study of paranoid, hebephrenic, and undifferentiated schizophrenia. *Archives of General Psychiatry* 1991;48:969-977.

Kane JM, Davis JM, Schooler N, et al. A multidose study of haloperidol decanoate in the maintenance treatment of schizophrenia. *The American Journal of Psychiatry* 2002;159:554-560.

Kasai K, Shenton ME, Salisbury DF, et al. Progressive decrease of left superior temporal gyrus gray matter volume in patients with first-episode schizophrenia. *The American Journal of Psychiatry* 2003;160:156-164.

Kelleher JP, Centorrino F, Albert MJ, et al. Advances in atypical antipsychotics for the treatment of schizophrenia: new formulations and new agents. *CNS Drugs* 2002;16:249-261.

Marder SR. Integrating pharmacological and psychosocial treatments for schizophrenia. *Acta Psychiatrica Scandinavica* 2000;102(Suppl):87-90.

Pilling S, Bebbington P, Kuipers E, et al. Psychological treatments in schizophrenia: I. Meta-analysis of family intervention and cognitive behavior therapy. *Psychological Medicine* 2002;32:763-782.

Pilling S, Bebbington P, Kuipers E, et al. Psychological treatments in schizophrenia: II. Meta-analyses of randomized controlled trials of social skills training and cognitive remediation. *Psychological Medicine* 2002;32:783-791.

Rioux L, Nissanov J, Lauber K, et al. Distribution of microtubule-associated protein MAP2-immunoreactive interstitial neurons in the parahippocampal white matter in subjects with schizophrenia. *The American Journal of Psychiatry* 2003;160:149-155.

Sawa A, Snyder SH. Schizophrenia: diverse approaches to a complex disease. *Science* 2002;296:692-695.

Shenton ME, Kikinis R, Jolesz FA, et al. Abnormalities of the left temporal lobe and thought disorder in schizophrenia: a quantitative magnetic resonance imaging study. *The New England Journal of Medicine* 1992; 327:604-612.

Thakar GK, Carpenter WT. Advances in schizophrenia. *Nature Medicine* 2001;7:667-671.

Volavka J, Czobor P, Sheitman B, et al. Clozapine, olanzapine, risperidone, and haloperidol in the treatment of patients with chronic schizophrenia and schizoaffective disorder. *The American Journal of Psychiatry* 2002;159:255-262.

68 Schizophreniform Disorder (DSM-IV 295.40)

Schizophreniform disorder is described as an illness which resembles schizophrenia in every respect except course: whereas schizophrenia is a chronic, lifelong illness, schizophreniform disorder is said to undergo a full, complete and spontaneous remission within six months. Estimates as to the lifetime prevalence of such a disorder vary widely, from as high as 0.2% to exceedingly rare; indeed, some skeptics doubt whether it exists at all.

ONSET

Prior to the onset, the patient's premorbid functioning may or may not have been normal. The onset is said to occur in late teenage or early adult years, and to be characterized by a more or less lengthy prodrome, marked by peculiar behavior or a change in personality, after which psychotic symptoms appear.

CLINICAL FEATURES

Psychotic symptoms are essentially identical to those seen in schizophrenia, and include hallucinations, delusions, loosening of associations, bizarre behavior or catatonia. In some cases, these psychotic symptoms may be accompanied by considerable confusion or perplexity, or by flattening or blunting of affect.

COURSE

In the natural course of events, the illness is said to last at least one month, but no longer than six months: importantly, this six month period encompasses not only the time during which the patient had psychotic symptoms, but also any prodrome before that, and any residuals afterward. At the end of this six months, patients are said to be fully restored to health, without psychotic symptoms, residual peculiarities or any impairment at all.

COMPLICATIONS

The complications are similar to those described for schizophrenia.

ETIOLOGY

Presumably, such an illness would have an etiology similar to that of schizophrenia; importantly, though, there has been relatively little research in this regard, and no conclusions can be drawn.

DIFFERENTIAL DIAGNOSIS

A secondary psychosis, as described in that chapter, must be ruled out, with particular attention to those cases wherein, in the natural course of events, the secondary psychosis may resolve spontaneously in a relatively short time, as for example with substance intoxications.

A manic episode of bipolar disorder, at its height, may be characterized by profound confusion and psychotic symptoms, with very little in the way of such classic manic symptoms as heightened mood, pressured speech or hyperactivity. Provided one can get a good history, however, there should be little diffi-culty in correctly diagnosing such patients. In most cases, there will be a history of classic manic symptoms for at least several days, and generally much longer, before the confusion and psychotic symptoms appear, and it is the existence of these earlier manic symptoms which suggests the correct diagnosis. Some difficulty may arise in those uncommon cases of mania wherein the onset is explosive and the height of mania is attained within hours. However, it is this very lack of any symptoms preceding the psychosis, of any prodrome at all, which distinguishes such explosive onset manias from schizophreniform disorder, wherein there is a prodrome preceding the psychotic symptoms.

A depressive episode of either bipolar disorder or major depression may also be complicated by psychotic symptoms; however, here one may always find prominent and typical depressive symptoms, not only accompanying the psychotic ones, but preceding them for weeks or months.

Brief psychotic disorder, another controversial diagnostic category, is distinguished, by definition, from schizophreniform disorder by its brevity, in that it lasts for less than one month.

Schizophrenia and schizoaffective disorder are both chronic illnesses, which do not, in the natural course of events, remit within six months.

Above all, when considering the diagnosis of schizophreniform disorder, it must be borne in mind that the diagnosis cannot be made with confidence until after one has observed a full, complete and spontaneous remission within six months. Prior to that the diagnosis must be considered provisional. In this regard, one must not mistake a superb response to antipsychotic treatment for a spontaneous remission. In cases of psychosis where treatment was instituted within six months of the onset and patients recovered completely with treatment, one would have to, in order to confidently make the diagnosis of schizophreniform disorder, discontinue treatment at some point after six months from the onset: if the patient remained well, then indeed one may have a case of schizophreniform disorder; if symptoms recurred, however, then the diagnosis is ruled out. Certain features, known as "good prognostic features," may predict a favorable outcome, namely normal premorbid functioning, an acute onset of psychotic symptoms with a prodrome of less than four weeks, the presence of perplexity or confusion while psychotic symptoms are present, and an absence of flattening of affect.

TREATMENT

The same treatments recommended for schizophrenia may also be utilized here.

BIBLIOGRAPHY

Benazzi F. DSM-III-R schizophreniform disorder with good prognostic features: a six-year follow-up. *Canadian Journal of Psychiatry* 1998;43: 180-182.

Bergem AL, Dahl AA, Guldberg C, et al. Langfeldt's schizophreniform psychoses fifty years later. *The British Journal of Psychiatry* 1990;157: 351-354.

Strakowski SM. Diagnostic validity of schizophreniform disorder. *The American Journal of Psychiatry* 1994;151:815-824.

Zarate CA, Tohen M, Land ML. First-episode schizophreniform disorder: comparisons with first-episode schizophrenia. *Schizophrenia Research* 2000;46:31-34.

Zhang-Wong J, Beiser M, Bean G, et al. Five-year course of schizophreniform disorder. *Psychiatry Research* 1995;59:109-117.

69 Brief Psychotic Disorder (DSM-IV 298.8)

Brief psychotic disorder is a controversial diagnostic category reserved for patients who experience a psychosis which, while lasting at least a day, undergoes a full, complete and spontaneous remission within one month. This diagnosis is rarely given in developed countries, and some skeptics question whether such a disorder actually exists. In the past, this was known as "brief reactive psychosis" in deference to the belief that marked psychosocial stressors played a prominent role in its onset: the word "reactive" was dropped from

the name in order to widen the diagnostic concept to include cases that occur in the absence of significant stressors.

ONSET

The onset is said to occur in either adolescents or adults, most notably in those in the third and fourth decades, and to be rapid: although most cases are said to be immediately preceded by marked psychosocial stressors, occurrences in the absence of such stressors is also allowed.

CLINICAL FEATURES

Delusions, hallucinations, loosening of associations and bizarre or catatonic behavior are described, generally in the setting of profound confusion, emotional turmoil and intense and labile affect.

COURSE

By definition, brief psychotic disorder, while enduring for at least a day, undergoes a spontaneous remission within a month with a full and complete return to the premorbid level of functioning.

COMPLICATIONS

Patients are said to experience marked impairment in their ability to function and to have an increased risk of suicide.

ETIOLOGY

There is a dearth of research here, and nothing can be said with confidence.

DIFFERENTIAL DIAGNOSIS

Patients with borderline, paranoid or schizotypal personality disorders not uncommonly experience brief psychotic episodes while under stress; however, as this is an integral part of these disorders it does not warrant the additional diagnosis of brief psychotic disorder.

Secondary psychoses, especially those due to substance intoxication, may cause diagnostic confusion, and in all suspected cases of brief psychotic disorder toxicology screens and a careful attention to recent drug use are essential.

In cases where confusion dominates the clinical picture the diagnosis of delirium must be considered, followed by an evaluation as described in that chapter.

Mania, at its height, may be characterized by psychotic symptoms occurring in the midst of profound confusion, with little in the way of such classic manic symptoms as heightened mood, pressured speech or hyperactivity. A careful history taking, with special attention to both the possibility of classic manic symptoms preceding the psychosis and to a history of more typical manic episodes in the past, is required to make this differential.

Malingering or factitious illness must be considered whenever there is a suspicion that the patient has something to gain from the illness, even if it is merely to satisfy a desire to be a patient in the hospital: these conditions are discussed fully in the respective chapters.

Since by definition brief psychotic disorder remits spontaneously within one month, the diagnosis must be provisional until such a remission has been observed. Importantly, one must not mistake an excellent response to an antipsychotic as a spontaneous remission: in such cases it would be necessary to discontinue the antipsychotic and demonstrate prolonged normal functioning before making the diagnosis with confidence. Should symptoms persist beyond one month, then consideration would have to be given to schizophreniform disorder, schizophrenia or schizoaffective disorder.

TREATMENT

Most patients who carry this diagnosis are treated in a fashion similar to that described for schizophrenia.

BIBLIOGRAPHY

Beighley PS, Brown GR, Thompson JW, et al. DSM-III-R brief reactive psychosis among Air Force recruits. *The Journal of Clinical Psychiatry* 1992;53:283-288.

Hansen H, Dahl AA, Bertelsen A, et al. The Nordic concept of reactive psychosis—a multicenter reliability study. *Acta Psychiatrica Scandinavica* 1992;86:55-59.

Modestin J, Sonderegger P, Erni T. Follow-up study of hysterical psychosis, reactive/psychogenic psychosis and schizophrenia. *Comprehensive Psychiatry* 2001;42:51-56.

Munoz RA, Amado H, Hyatt S. Brief reactive psychosis. *The Journal of Clinical Psychiatry* 1987;48:324-327.

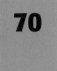

70 Schizoaffective Disorder (DSM-IV-TR #295.70)

The term "schizoaffective disorder" has had many definitions since it was first introduced by Kasanin in 1933. As conceived here, schizoaffective disorder is characterized by the presence of chronic, unremitting psychotic symptoms, upon the course of which are superimposed either episodes of depression alone (schizoaffective disorder, depressed type), or episodes of mania and episodes of depression (schizoaffective disorder, bipolar type). The prevalence of schizoaffective disorder is not known with certainty; it is probably far less common than schizophrenia.

ONSET

Onset typically occurs in the late teens or early twenties.

CLINICAL FEATURES

Viewed over time schizoaffective disorder appears to represent a superimposition of a mood disorder, such as major depression or bipolar disorder, upon schizophrenia. Thus these patients are chronically psychotic and never without some of the typical symptoms of schizophrenia, such as delusions, hallucinations, or some loosening of associations. Periodically, however, these chronic symptoms are joined either by a depressive episode (as described in the chapter on major depression) or by a manic episode (as described in the chapter on bipolar disorder). Typically, whenever an episode of depression or of mania does appear, the chronically persistent psychotic symptoms become more severe, only to return approximately to their previous level of intensity once the episode of depression or mania has run its course.

COURSE

The course of schizoaffective disorder, as conceived here, presents an amalgamation of the courses of schizophrenia and either bipolar disorder or major depression. The critical point is that in the intervals between affective episodes the patient remains ill with non-mood-congruent psychotic symptoms. In most cases the long-term outcome of patients with schizoaffective disorder is not as good as that for patients with a mood disorder, yet not as grave as that for patients with schizophrenia.

COMPLICATIONS

Complications are as described in the chapters on schizophrenia, bipolar disorder, and major depression.

ETIOLOGY

Family studies suggest that schizoaffective disorder results from a "double" genetic loading for both schizophrenia and a mood disorder.

DIFFERENTIAL DIAGNOSIS

Given that patients with schizoaffective disorder are chronically psychotic, a diagnosis of schizophrenia is often entertained. The critical differential point is the presence of a full affective episode (depressive, manic, or mixed-manic) with an accompanying increase in "positive" or "productive" psychotic symptoms in schizoaffective disorder; such episodes are not seen in schizophrenia. Naturally, one must be careful not to mistake flattened affect, negativism, or catatonic stupor for depression, nor must one be misled by the "postpsychotic depression" seen in some patients with schizophrenia, which occurs in the absence of an exacerbation of the "productive" symptoms. One must also be careful not to mistake paranoid agitation, hebephrenic silly euphoria, or catatonic excitement for mania.

At times when the interval psychotic symptoms are mild or perhaps easily concealed by the patient, the illness of a patient with schizoaffective disorder may at first glance appear to consist only of affective episodes, thus leading to an incorrect diagnosis

of a mood disorder. Prolonged close observation reveals the chronic psychotic symptoms, thus enabling the correct diagnosis to be made.

TREATMENT

As this illness appears to be an amalgamation of schizophrenia and an affective disorder, the treatment borrows heavily from the treatments for these two disorders. In general, then, most patients take an antipsychotic chronically: in many cases an antipsychotic alone will not only control the psychotic symptoms but will also substantially reduce the mood symptoms; in this regard olanzapine appears superior to the other antipsychotics. When affective symptoms persist despite antipsychotic treatment, one may add a mood stabilizer (e.g., lithium, divalproex or carbamazepine) in the case of mania, or an antidepressant (e.g., an SSRI) in the case of a depression. Importantly, in the case of schizoaffective disorder, bipolar type, when the patient is in the midst of a depressive episode, it is necessary to "cover" the patient first with a mood stabilizer before adding an antidepressant in order to reduce the risk of precipitating a manic episode. After the affective episode has run its course, the decision as to whether to offer maintenance treatment with a mood stabilizer or an antidepressant may be made according to the principles for maintenance treatment as outlined in the chapters on bipolar disorder and major depression. Other modalities of treatment specified in the chapters on schizophrenia, major depression, and bipolar disorder are utilized as needed.

BIBLIOGRAPHY

Andreasen NC, Rice J, Endicott J, et al. Familial rates of affective disorder: a report from the National Institute of Mental Health Collaborative Study. *Archives of General Psychiatry* 1987;44:461-469.

Benabarre A, Vieta E, Colom F, et al. Bipolar disorder, schizoaffective disorder and schizophrenia: epidemiologic, clinical and prognostic differences. *European Psychiatry* 2001;16:167-172.

Greil W, Ludwig-Mayerhofer W, Erazo N, et al. Lithium vs carbamazepine in the maintenance treatment of schizoaffective disorder: a randomized study. *European Archives of Psychiatry and Clinical Neuroscience* 1997;247:42-50.

Janicak PG, Keck PE, Davis JM, et al. A double-blind, randomized, prospective evaluation of the efficacy and safety of risperidone versus haloperidol in the treatment of schizoaffective disorder. *Journal of Clinical Psychopharmacology* 2001;21:360-368.

Kendler KS, McGuire M, Gruenberg AM, et al. Examining the validity of DSM-III-R schizoaffective disorder and its putative subtypes in the Roscommon Family Study. *The American Journal of Psychiatry* 1995;152:755-764.

Tohen M, Zhang F, Keck PE, et al. Olanzapine versus haloperidol in schizoaffective disorder, bipolar type. *Journal of Affective Disorders* 2001;67:133-140.

Tran PF, Tollefson GD, Sanger TM, et al. Olanzapine versus haloperidol in the treatment of schizoaffective disorder. Acute and long-term therapy. *The British Journal of Psychiatry* 1999;174:15-22.

Delusional Disorder (DSM-IV-TR #297.1)

Delusional disorder is a chronic disorder characterized by the gradual appearance of one or more delusions that gradually elaborate into a coherent system. In contrast to the delusions found in other disorders, these have a certain plausibility, and the eventual system is within itself often quite logical. Considered apart from their delusions, these patients are otherwise often remarkably normal.

The traditional name for this disorder and the name originally bestowed on it by Kraepelin is "paranoia." The modern synonym, "delusional disorder," has two advantages: first, it emphasizes the cardinal aspect of the disorder, namely the presence and prominence of delusions; second, it avoids the unfortunate association between "paranoid" and "persecutory" and reminds one that the delusions seen here may be of any type. Despite these advantages, however, the traditional name has a certain felicity, and it is often used in this text.

Delusional disorder is an uncommon disorder, with a lifetime prevalence falling between 0.01 and 0.05%.

ONSET

The illness usually begins between the ages of 20 and 50, and although certain conditions might precipitate it, such as immigration or deafness, one is often unable to find any precipitating event. Generally, these patients experience a lengthy and insidiously progressive prodrome, often lasting years before the illness is apparent to others. At first they may experience only heightened sensitivity; events that heretofore passed unnoticed now assume a certain meaning. Things begin to change; intentions and motives are seen underlying everyday events; chance remarks take on significance. Coincidences no longer exist, but things eventually begin to display an inner purpose to these patients, and they begin to search for further evidence of their growing suspicions. Eventually the suspicions become convictions, delusions appear, and the illness assumes its definitive form. This transition from prodrome to active illness may at times be sudden. Some patients may experience a sudden "epiphany," as all their lurking suspicions crystallize into definite beliefs. Often, however, the transition from prodrome to active illness is gradual, almost furtive.

CLINICAL FEATURES

Although the most common type of delusion seen in paranoia is that of persecution, other themes may be prominent: jealousy, grandiosity, erotic longing, litigiousness, and bodily concerns may all occur. Regardless of which delusional theme is most prominent, however, each case has one thing in common, namely the systematization of the patient's delusions into a corpus of beliefs that is internally coherent and, within its own boundaries, logical. Furthermore, although the premise from which this corpus of belief grows may be recognized by the observer as a delusion, it yet may have a certain plausibility about it, which the patient will defend mightily if questioned.

Evolving from one or a few delusional premises, this systematic corpus of belief is elaborated and strengthened by a constant misinterpretation of events in the patients' lives. This process, whereby the systematic corpus of delusions is elaborated, is not confined to the present. Often, memories of past events are misinterpreted or reinterpreted, and the patient may come to "see" that in fact the current troubles began in the distant past. Years ago as a teenager the patient may have been let go from a job. At the time it meant nothing to the patient who went ahead and found another without any difficulty. Yet now, in retrospect, the patient sees it as the first evidence of the persistent malevolent plan to take away all means of support. "Pseudomemories" may also occur. Here, as far as the examiner is concerned, the memory is unquestionably false, yet for the patient it has the same quality as any other memory. The patient may report that the President came secretly to the house to offer support.

The behavior of these patients is generally quite predictable. When events in the world about them touch upon an aspect of their delusional system, their reaction is entirely consistent with their beliefs. A firm handshake and a sincere thank you to the grandiose patient is yet another indication of your deep adoration; an abrupt goodbye to a patient with delusions of persecution is taken as an indication of underlying hatred. Yet outside of the system, in areas of life that do not touch upon the delusions, the patient generally behaves normally and does not appear ill. Though fearful of the persecutions at the factory, the patient may otherwise lead an unremarkable life, sing in the choir, coach a Little League team, and be regarded as a good, if perhaps somewhat distant, neighbor.

Hallucinations may or may not occur in paranoia. If hallucinations do occur, they are at most a minor part of the clinical picture and in general are consistent with the patient's delusions. Voices may be heard; the persecuted patient may hear the execution date announced. Visions, though less common than voices, may also occur. The erotomanic patient may see erotic dancers. Tactile and olfactory hallucinations may also occur, especially in patients with bodily concerns: the patient convinced of an infestation may feel bugs on the skin and the patient convinced of severe halitosis may smell foul odors.

Mood and affect are consistent with the delusions and are normal if the patient is not influenced by the delusions. The patient experiencing grandiose delusions may be euphoric; the persecuted patient may be irritable, even hostile.

Traditionally, paranoia has been divided into several subtypes, namely persecutory, litigious, grandiose, erotomanic, jealous, and somatic, and these are described below. These divisions, however, are somewhat artificial because, whereas in each patient one delusional theme may dominate, other themes are almost always present.

In the persecutory subtype the dominant delusion is that one is persecuted or conspired against. Patients feel singled out; they are watched and followed; people on the street talk about them. The FBI and the CIA are involved; the local police cannot be trusted. Family members, friends, or the physician may all be trusted for a time, but eventually they too may be enrolled in the conspiracy. These patients may move to a different part of the country to escape their persecutors, but inevitably, their persecutors find them. Their new neighbors begin to look the other way; the mail seems tampered; listening devices are suspected. Eventually, the patient may move again, only to be tracked down once again. Patients with persecutory paranoia may be quite dangerous. Surrounded and hounded, the patient may turn and attack the imagined persecutors in self-defense.

The litigious subtype is considered by some to be a variant of the persecutory subtype and may be the most difficult to diagnose, as the initiating delusion seems at times almost entirely plausible, and the systematically elaborated delusions that follow upon it have an almost unassailable logic to them. During the outbreak of the illness these patients are generally involved in legal proceedings that go badly for them. The suit may be lost or, if won, the award may seem too low. Patients become convinced that someone is at fault. Their attorneys are incompetent; the judges are biased; the juries are prejudiced. The patients may pore over the trial transcripts until finally some irregularity, no matter how trivial, is found. New attorneys are hired, appeals are filed, and a series of legal proceedings is embarked on. With each failure the patients' convictions grow that the legal system as a whole is conspiring in the denial of justice. Eventually the disparity between the magnitude of these patients' sense of being unjustly wronged and the trivial, insignificant nature of the inciting insult to their sense of justice brings to light the pathologic nature of their behavior.

In the grandiose subtype the dominant theme, grandiosity, may be evident in any of several ways. Patients may believe themselves to be secret captains of industry whose advice is sought by the financial community. Bankers seek them out; the Secretary of the Treasury asks for a special meeting. Delusions of high descent are common. The patient's mother, a fabulously wealthy heiress, gives birth to the patient out-of-wedlock and, out of shame, gives the patient up for adoption to a poor family. Now as an adult the patient feels no need to work as it is only a matter of time before the inheritance is received. Another patient spends great amounts of time working on inventions, believing that those in the scientific community are consumed by envy and too ashamed to acknowledge the patient's genius. Consequently, the patient toils on, recognizing the immense value of such a work to humanity. Fantastic diagrams and sketches may litter the walls where such patients work.

In the erotomanic subtype (also known as de Clerambault's syndrome), patients come to believe that they are loved by someone else, someone usually of very high social station. The clinical picture is dominated by the patient's belief that she is loved by another who, for any number of reasons, cannot openly express that love. This imagined lover is generally of high station; mayors, governors, singers, or movie stars are frequent candidates. The patient has a certain feeling about this person; the patient begins to suspect that the mayor, for example, is attracted. She sees the mayor at a political rally; the mayor turns away, and this is a sign that in fact the mayor is fighting against the urge to gaze at her. The newspaper hints at a strain in the mayor's marriage, and the patient recognizes that except for the mayor's high moral character, the marriage would be dissolved immediately. This attitude of hopeful expectation can continue for years; occasionally she may send a letter or wait across the street from the mayor's house, but often the mere assurance of the mayor's love is enough. At times, however, patients may become violent. One patient, convinced that a movie star was being forcibly detained by a jealous spouse, accosted the star's spouse one day in a parking lot, threatening death unless the star was released immediately.

In the jealous subtype of paranoia the patient becomes convinced that his spouse or lover is unfaithful. The patient not only sees "evidence" for the supposed infidelity but also may at times actually seek it. Sheets and underclothing are inspected for stains; telephone conversations are listened in on; a private detective is hired and surveillance is set up. Evidence begins to abound: the spouse is a few minutes late in getting home because the lovemaking was too passionate to stop; a car parked across the street means that the lover is waiting; the phone rings twice to indicate that all is ready. The patient may insist upon the spouse staying home; in some instances the spouse becomes a virtual prisoner.

In the somatic subtype patients believe, despite reassurances to the contrary from physicians, that they have a serious disease. They are not merely worried that they might be sick or overly concerned with minor aches and pains. Rather these patients are convinced that they have a severe disease, a tumor, a disfigurement, or a lethal infection. Two variations of this somatic subtype deserve mention: the olfactory reference syndrome and parisittosis. In the olfactory reference syndrome patients are convinced that they are emanating a foul odor from the mouth or some other orifice: they may hallucinate a stench and anxiously ask others if they smell it also. In parasittosis patients believe that their skin is infested: they may complain of feeling the bugs crawling, and may dig under the skin to find them.

COURSE

For the most part, delusional disorder appears to pursue a chronic, waxing and waning course. Whether spontaneous remissions ever truly occur is unclear; however, in some instances partial remissions lasting months or years do occur, and symptoms may be quite minimal indeed during these times. In the persecutory subtype these partial remissions may occur when the patient moves to another locale to escape the persecutors; however, as described earlier, symptoms eventually recur.

COMPLICATIONS

The severity of complications bears a direct relationship to the type of delusions and to the areas wherein the patient's system overlaps with daily life. In some cases the patient's life may seem almost totally undisturbed. A patient with grandiose paranoia might spend hours a day in the basement, concocting elaborate schemes, yet engage in quite normal conduct with the family and at work. In other cases severe disruption may occur. The patient with jealous paranoia sends threatening letters to a superior whom he is convinced is having an affair with his spouse, and gets fired.

The most severe complication, homicide, may be seen in the erotomanic and the persecutory subtypes. A patient convinced that a movie star is held captive by a movie director kills the director, or, in the persecutory subtype, the "persecuted" may become the "persecutor" and turn on the tormentors in the final act of self-defense.

ETIOLOGY

Paranoia appears to run in families; importantly there does not appear to be a familial relationship with either schizophrenia or one of the mood disorders.

DIFFERENTIAL DIAGNOSIS

Schizophrenia may present with delusions; however, on close inspection these are qualitatively different from those seen in paranoia. Often they are implausible or frankly bizarre. A patient with schizophrenia may indeed have a delusion of jealousy, but with further questioning one may find that the patient believes the spouse to be copulating with aliens. Furthermore, the delusions in schizophrenia are often illogical, contradictory, and fragmentary. The systematization seen in paranoia is lacking. In addition to presenting with qualitatively different delusions, schizophrenia almost always causes other symptoms not seen in paranoia. The presence of flattened or inappropriate affect, loosening of associations, mannerisms, and so forth should immediately rule out the diagnosis of paranoia. The presence of hallucinations, however, does not necessarily rule out paranoia, for these at times may be seen in this illness. However, as noted earlier, when hallucinations do occur in paranoia, they are at best a minor part of the overall clinical picture. In schizophrenia, on the other hand, they may dominate the picture.

One subtype of schizophrenia, namely paranoid schizophrenia, may present special diagnostic difficulties. Here the patient's guardedness and suspiciousness may be such that only the fact of the "conspiracy" is leaked to the physician, with all else held in secret. In time some patients may reveal some of their bizarre experiences, thus facilitating the diagnosis; however, some may stonewall. However, this refusal to talk with the physician and the immediate inclusion of the physician among the persecutors suggest the correct diagnosis. The delusions seen in paranoia are rarely so mercurial; patients with paranoia size the physician up for hours, if not days, before making a decision and may in fact eventually come to trust the examiner. In paranoid schizophrenia, however, the decision about the examiner is often immediate and abrupt, resulting in almost instant distrust.

In a depressive episode, either as part of major depression or bipolar disorder, one may also see delusions. Persecutory and somatic delusions are not uncommon. Patients report that they are condemned, that the execution date is set; they may complain of being lightheaded, that they have a brain tumor. The distinguishing feature here is that these delusions occur within the context of the vegetative symptoms of depression, which always precede the delusion. The delusions themselves also often have a distinctive quality to them, as if soaked in guilt. It is as if the depressed patient feels that the execution is deserved, or that the tumor is divine punishment. Patients with paranoia, however, feel quite differently. To them, the execution is unfair and unjustified; the disease is something someone else should have gotten.

In a manic episode, both grandiose and persecutory delusions are common. However, here, as in depression, the delusions occur within the context of an affective disturbance, with the typical manic symptoms preceding the appearance of the delusion.

In both hypochondriasis and Briquet's syndrome, patients have unfounded concerns about their health, and thus may appear similar to the patient with the somatic subtype of paranoia. However, patients with these disorders, unlike those with paranoia, are not deluded. They can be reasoned with, albeit with difficulty.

The very important differential diagnosis between the somatic subtype of delusional disorder and dysmorphophobia, or body dysmorphic disorder, is discussed in that chapter.

Paranoid personality disorder may pose special difficulties. These patients are logical and coherent, and their sense of being wronged, pressed upon, or injured, though not in fact delusional, may be so strongly felt and experienced as to mislead the examiner into thinking that a delusion is actually present. A major difference between paranoid personality disorder and paranoia is the lack of "encapsulation" in the personality disorder. In paranoia the abnormal behavior is seen only within the "capsule" of the delusional system; in other areas of their lives these patients may get along adequately with others. To the contrary, patients with paranoid personality disorder are constantly on edge, tense, and watchful in all situations. They take offense at the behavior of almost everyone; their guard must be up no matter who they are with or where they are. No "geographic cure" exists for a patient with a paranoid personality disorder.

Dementia may often be complicated by persecutory delusions; however, here the presence of concurrent cognitive deficits allows for the correct diagnosis.

Alcoholic paranoia may present with delusions of persecution or, more commonly, delusions of jealousy. A long history of heavy alcohol use, however, suggests the correct diagnosis.

A stimulant-induced psychosis, as may occur with amphetamines or cocaine, may resemble the persecutory subtype of paranoia: here, however, one may find evidence of prior use; furthermore, these substance-induced psychoses, unlike paranoia, do not pursue a chronic course but typically remit within days to weeks of abstinence.

TREATMENT

Patients with paranoia rarely seek treatment with a psychiatrist on their own initiative. Lawyers, internists, family practitioners, and private detectives all may be consulted, but as these patients see nothing wrong with their own beliefs, they see no reason to see a psychiatrist.

The first step in treatment is the creation of a physician-patient relationship that neither directly threatens the patient's beliefs nor cripples the psychiatrist's efforts at altering those beliefs. Establishing such a relationship requires great tact and diplomacy. Arguing with these patients about their beliefs or attempting to offer any insight is to no avail and must be avoided; conversely, one must also avoid speaking so that patients feel one is in full accord with the delusions. A tendency toward reservation of judgment, a benign "wait and see attitude," often works best.

Within such a nonthreatening, yet nonacquiescing relationship, it may be possible to get the patient to take an antipsychotic. Generally, the indications for medication must be put in terms that do not clash with the patient's delusions. Whereas the patient may accept a prescription for "nerves" or for "sleep," a prescription for "paranoia" will never be accepted. Except in emergencies one should start with a low dose, as these patients are quick to find that any side effects are unacceptable. The dose is then very gradually titrated against the patient's symptoms. In general, one should avoid sedating antipsychotics, as sedation is rarely acceptable to these patients. Second generation agents such as risperidone and olanzapine are reasonable choices, given their overall effectiveness and generally favorable side effect profile.

There are scattered reports of successful treatment with antidepressants, especially with clomipramine in the somatic subtype. This course might be considered in the somatic subtype or when some concurrent vegetative symptoms are evident.

Efforts at guidance and direction must likewise be made with circumspection; when tactfully approached, however, these patients are often willing to follow the physician's advice. The goal is to build some restraint into the patient's life so that delusions are not acted upon.

Occasionally, hospitalization may be required. This is most often true in the persecutory and jealous subtypes, wherein the patient may become dangerous to others. Despite the fact that these admissions are often court-ordered and involuntary, patients often accept treatment and at discharge may be less dangerous.

BIBLIOGRAPHY

Hsiao MC, Liu CY, Yang YY, et al. Delusional disorder: retrospective analysis of 86 Chinese outpatients. *Psychiatry and Clinical Neurosciences* 1999;53:673-676.

Kendler KS, Gruenberg AM, Strauss JS. An independent analysis of the Copenhagen sample of the Danish Adoption Study of Schizophrenia. III. The relationship between paranoid psychosis (delusional disorder) and the schizophrenia spectrum disorders. *Archives of General Psychiatry* 1982;38:987-997.

Kendler KS, Masterson CC, Davis KL. Psychiatric illness in first-degree relatives of patients with paranoid psychosis, schizophrenia and medical illness. *The British Journal of Psychiatry* 1985;147:524-531.

Kennedy HG, Kemp LI, Dyer DE. Fear and anger in delusional (paranoid) disorder: the association with violence. *The British Journal of Psychiatry* 1992;160:488-492.

Tandon R. Delusional disorder: paranoia and related illnesses. *The American Journal of Psychiatry* 2000;157:1898-1899.

Wada T, Kawakatsu S, Nadaoka T, et al. Clomipramine treatment of delusional disorder, somatic type. *International Clinical Psychopharmacology* 1999;14:181-183.

Watt JAG. The relationship of paranoid states to schizophrenia. *The American Journal of Psychiatry* 1985;142:1456-1458.

Winokur G. Familial psychopathology in delusional disorder. *Comprehensive Psychiatry* 1985;26:241-248.

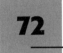

72 Postpartum Psychosis

Postpartum psychosis, also known as puerperal psychosis, is a rare disorder, occurring in perhaps less than 1 or 2 per 1000 deliveries. It is more common in primiparous than multiparous women.

Debate exists regarding the diagnostic validity of this entity. Many believe that it merely represents an entrainment of manic episodes to the postpartum period and that these patients in fact have nothing other than bipolar disorder. Undoubtedly, as noted in the section on differential diagnosis, such an entrainment may occur. However, many of these patients never experience another psychotic illness unless they again become pregnant, suggesting that perhaps a certain percentage of postpartum women who become psychotic do indeed suffer from a distinct illness, namely postpartum psychosis.

The classification of this disorder in DSM-IV is problematic. The category "Brief Psychotic Disorder" allows for a specifier of "with postpartum onset"; however, as noted below, cases of postpartum psychosis may endure longer than one month, thus passing beyond the time limit for a diagnosis of brief psychotic disorder. In such cases this disorder would, for coding purposes, have to be subsumed under "psychotic disorder not otherwise specified."

ONSET

Symptoms generally appear abruptly within about 3 days to several weeks after delivery.

CLINICAL FEATURES

Mood may be heightened or depressed and is often labile; agitation, increased activity, and insomnia may also occur. Delusions may appear; the baby may be seen as an embodiment of evil or as the Messiah; auditory hallucinations may also occur and may be command, at times commanding the patient to kill the baby. Infanticide may occur. Often patients experience confusion and disorientation.

COURSE

In the natural course of events, symptoms gradually undergo a spontaneous remission over weeks or months. A substantial minority of these patients, perhaps close to half, will have another episode after the next delivery.

COMPLICATIONS

A tremendous strain is placed on the family and on the development of a normal mother-infant bond. Suicide may occur and, in as many as 4%, infanticide.

ETIOLOGY

The etiology is not known. Attempts at correlating symptoms with changing hormonal levels have not been successful.

DIFFERENTIAL DIAGNOSIS

As noted in the chapter on bipolar disorder, bipolar patients are at higher risk for relapse during the postpartum period. A history of manic episodes before delivery, or at a subsequent time outside the postpartum period, would indicate this diagnosis.

Patients with schizophrenia may undergo an exacerbation in the postpartum period. Here, however, one would see signs of the illness before delivery.

The rare postpartum eclampsia may present with delirium. Here, however, one finds hypertension and proteinuria, and seizures are common. Rarely, a psychosis may occur secondary to bromocriptine, as may be used to suppress lactation.

The presence of chorea suggests the occurrence of chorea gravidarum, which, rarely, may be accompanied by psychotic symptoms.

TREATMENT

Hospitalization is generally indicated. Patients with a definitely manic-like presentation may be treated as outlined in the chapter on bipolar disorder for the acute treatment of mania, and in this regard, loading with divalproex is a reasonable strategy. In other cases, patients may be treated as outlined in the chapter on schizophrenia. Regardless of which pharmacologic treatment is used, it is always possible, given the natural course of the illness, to eventually taper and discontinue the medication.

As the patient begins to improve, an experienced nurse may gradually guide the patient into appropriate interaction with the infant. In some settings the infant is admitted to the same hospital, but not in the same room. Breast-feeding is generally contraindicated.

Subsequent to recovery the patient should be counseled regarding the risk of recurrence. If she does elect a second pregnancy, she should be very closely observed postpartum. If antimanic agents had been used previously with success, a case could be made for their preventive use immediately after delivery.

BIBLIOGRAPHY

Austin MP. Puerperal affective psychosis: is there a case for lithium prophylaxis? *The British Journal of Psychiatry* 1992;161:692-694.

Bagedahl-Strindlund M. Postpartum mental illness: timing of illness onset and its relation to symptoms and sociodemographic characteristics. *The American Journal of Psychiatry* 1986;74:490-496.

Brockington IF, Cernik KF, Schofield EM, et al. Puerperal psychosis. Phenomena and diagnosis. *Archives of General Psychiatry* 1981;38:829-833.

Canterbur RJ, Haskins B, Kahn N, et al. Postpartum psychosis induced by bromocriptine. *Southern Medical Journal* 1987;80:1463-1464.

Kumar R, Issacs S, Meltzer E. Recurrent postpartum psychosis: a model for prospective clinical investigation. *The British Journal of Psychiatry* 1983;142:618-620.

Rohde LA, Marneros A. Postpartum psychoses: onset and long-term course. *Psychopathology* 1993;26:203-209.

73 Folie à Deux (shared psychotic disorder, DSM-IV-TR #297.3)

■

In folie à deux, a patient, usually dependent and impressionable, having fallen under the influence of a dominant person who has a psychosis, comes to adopt and believe in the delusions expressed by the dominant person. These "imposed" false beliefs of the patient with folie à deux, however, are not to be considered delusions, because the patient gradually loses belief in them if separated from the dominant partner. Also known as "induced paranoid disorder," "shared paranoid disorder," "double insanity," or, more recently, "shared psychotic disorder," folie à deux is in all likelihood a rare disorder; it may be slightly more common in females than males. Typically, only one person has come under the sway of the dominant person; hence the disorder has been referred to as "à deux." Rarely, two or more may come under the influence, and then one may speak of folie à trois, à quatre, and so on, or even folie à famille.

ONSET

Folie à deux is typically of gradual onset, and although it may occur at any time from late childhood to old age, the average age of onset is in the late forties.

CLINICAL FEATURES

Typically, the patient has lived in intimate association with the dominant person for a prolonged period of time. The most common relationships are among parents and children, spouses, and siblings. The dominant person almost always has a chronic psychotic illness, often delusional disorder or paranoid schizophrenia, and typically the patient has lived with this dominant person in isolation, cut off from the rest of society.

The dominant person is possessed by a persecutory delusion that often evolves from, and in some fashion makes "sense" of, some past experience that the dominant person and the patient went through together; occasionally a grandiose delusion may be shared. Having heard the delusion expressed over and over, the patient, often impressionable and dependent and perhaps suffering from some other disorder such as depression, dementia, or mental retardation, gradually comes to believe in it. Although initially the patient may have resisted it, eventually, however, the dominant person's delusion is accepted as true, and the patient may even come to defend it against criticism or questioning from outsiders.

The patient with an established folie à deux typically lives on in a passive relationship with the dominant person, and may in fact resist any outside efforts to separate them. However, should a prolonged separation occur, the patient, especially if kept in relation with normal people, gradually falls away from the delusion of the dominant person, begins to question it, and loses belief in it entirely.

COURSE

This is determined by the longevity of the relationship between the patient and the dominant person, and, as this tends to be long lasting, folie à deux likewise tends to be chronic.

COMPLICATIONS

In general, few direct complications occur, as the patient tends to live in the shadow of the dominant person.

ETIOLOGY

The dependence, submissiveness, and passivity of the patient are fertile soil for the imposition of the dominant person's strongly held and strongly voiced delusion; however, as noted earlier, the patient's false belief is not considered a delusion, for rather than being autonomous it flourishes only for as long as the patient is under the sway of the dominant person.

DIFFERENTIAL DIAGNOSIS

Folie à deux is distinguished from delusional disorder and paranoid schizophrenia by its self-remitting course subsequent to separation from the dominant person. It may be suspected when interviews with the patient's close relatives disclose a dominant psychotic person who holds the same beliefs as the patient does but much more strongly and contentiously.

TREATMENT

Separation from the dominant person and immersion into normal social interaction is generally sufficient to effect a disappearance of the patient's false belief. Should separation not be possible, successful treatment of the dominant person's psychotic illness with antipsychotics may also be helpful.

BIBLIOGRAPHY

Dippel B, Kemper J, Berger M. Folie a six: a case report on induced psychotic disorder. *Acta Psychiatrica Scandinavica* 1991;83:137-141.

Kashiwase H, Kato M. Folie a deux in Japan—analysis of 97 cases in the Japanese literature. *Acta Psychiatrica Scandinavica* 1997;96:231-234.

Partridge M. One operation cures three people: effect of prefrontal leucotomy on a case of folie à deux et demie. *Archives of Neurology and Psychiatry* 1950;54:792-796.

Silveira JM, Seeman MV. Shared psychotic disorder: a critical review of the literature. *Canadian Journal of Psychiatry* 1995;40:389-395.

Waltzer H. A psychotic family—folie à douze. *The Journal of Nervous and Mental Disease* 1963;137:67-75.

MOOD DISORDERS

74 Major Depressive Disorder (DSM-IV-TR #296.2-296.3)

Major depressive disorder, or as it is often called, "major depression," is characterized by the presence of one or more depressive episodes during the patient's lifetime. Typically, a depressive episode lasts anywhere from months to years, after which most patients are generally left again in their normal state of health. Although some patients may have only one episode during their lifetime, the majority have two or more. Thus major depression is a periodic, or cyclic, illness with the patient "cycling" down into, and then up out of periods of depression. Exceptions, however, do occur. For example, in a minority of cases the depressive episode may be chronic, and an episode once begun may persist throughout the patient's life.

Synonyms for this disorder include unipolar affective disorder; melancholia; and manic-depressive illness, depressed type. "Unipolar" highlights the critical difference between major depression and bipolar disorder, namely the fact that the patient with major depression cycles in only one direction, toward the depressive "pole," in contrast to the patient with bipolar disorder, who cycles at times not only to the depressive pole but also at other times to the manic pole. "Melancholia" is the most ancient term for this disorder, coming to us from the Greek, meaning black bile. However, over the centuries its meaning has changed, and hence it remains open to misinterpretation. "Manic-depressive illness, depressed type," is perhaps the least satisfactory of these synonyms. Kraepelin, as best as can be made out, felt that patients with only recurrent depression and those with both episodes of depression and episodes of mania had in fact the same illness, which he called "manic-depressive insanity." Later clinicians, recognizing that this was probably not the case, separated the "depressed" type of "manic-depressive illness" from the "circular" type; however, this continued to cloud the fundamental distinction between these two groups of patients. Currently, at least in the United States, when one speaks of manic-depressive illness, most often one is referring to bipolar disorder, and, at least for now, this developing convention should probably be honored, and the term "manic-depressive illness, depressed type," should probably be left in the history books.

Major depression is a common disorder. Prevalence figures vary according to methodology, but at least 5% of the general adult population has this disorder. Given, however, the relapsing and remitting nature of the depressive episodes, a lower percentage of the population is actually in the midst of a depressive episode at any given time. Again, estimates vary, with point prevalence figures ranging anywhere from 2 to 5%.

Amongst adults, major depression is seen twice as frequently among women as men; however, among children the sex ratio is equal.

ONSET

Although the first depressive episode generally occurs in the mid-twenties, not uncommonly the first episode is seen in adolescence or, on the other extreme, in old age. Indeed in rare instances the onset may be seen in early childhood or as late as the ninth decade.

Most depressive episodes appear gradually and insidiously. Typically, a long prodrome occurs, sometimes lasting months or in rare instances years, characterized by indefinite and at times fleeting symptoms such as moodiness, anxiety, or fatigue. Furthermore, when depressive symptoms finally do settle in, their several severities accrue and worsen often haltingly or imperceptibly, and it is the rare patient who can date the onset with any precision. This is not to say that acute onsets are never seen. To the contrary, they do occur, and some patients describe a rapid fall from emotional well-being into a depressive episode in as little as a few weeks. Such acute onsets of depressive episodes, however, are the exception rather than the rule for major depression.

In major depression a stressful life event, typically a serious loss, not uncommonly precedes and apparently triggers a depressive episode. Examples include the death of a loved one, divorce, the loss of a job, and the like. At times, however, close inquiry may reveal that the stressful life event, rather than actually precipitating the depressive episode, was to the contrary itself caused by the depressive episode. For example, a married patient in the midst of a prodrome may be sufficiently irritable to cause the spouse to leave. Here the patient may blame the depression on the separation; however, it appears that the depression itself led to the separation. In that group of patients where an independent precipitating stress occurs, subsequent episodes tend to become independent and autonomous and occur whether there is a stressor or not.

CLINICAL FEATURES

From a clinical point of view the core symptoms of a depressive episode include the following: depressed mood; loss of energy; difficulty with concentration and short-term memory and decision making; loss of interest in heretofore pleasurable activities; insomnia or, less commonly, hypersomnia; anorexia and weight loss or, less commonly, hyperphagia and weight gain; psychomotor agitation or, less commonly, retardation; and, finally, a pessimistic outlook that is often accompanied by suicidal ideation. Not uncommonly, patients also describe a diurnal variation in their symptoms: they feel markedly worse in the morning and experience some degree of relief as the afternoon or evening comes on. In the following paragraphs each of these symptoms is discussed in some detail.

Mood is depressed or sometimes irritable. Some patients may complain of anxiety, and irascibility may occur. Some, however, despite a dejected facial expression, may deny feeling depressed at all. Rather they may speak of a sense of discouragement, or complain of a sense of lassitude or heaviness, of being weighted down. The patients' affect generally reflects their mood. The facial musculature may sag lifelessly; they may have copious tears. At other times, particularly in anxious patients, a "pained" facial expression is evident, and occasionally one may see the classic "omega sign" of depression wherein the brow is so peculiarly furrowed and pinched as to create the Greek letter omega on the forehead, arising up from between the eyes. Some patients may attempt to hide their mood by feigning a cheerful affect, thus presenting the so-called smiling depression.

Energy is lacking. Patients complain of feeling tired, fatigued, lifeless, or drained. The exhaustion may at times be so extreme that patients are unable to complete their chores or even dress themselves. Occasionally a patient may complain of too much energy; however, on close questioning, a "nervous energy," akin to agitation, is apparent. This energy is useless to the patient and is always shadowed by a sense of imminent and impending exhaustion.

Thinking becomes difficult; patients complain of difficulty concentrating, remembering, or in making decisions. A dull, heavy-headedness, "like a fog," impairs the patient's ability to concentrate. Memory fails, and patients are unable to recall where they put things or what was said earlier in the day. Attempts to read or watch television may end in miserable failure. The same paragraph may be read again and again, without the patient being able to grasp its meaning or recall what had just preceded. Making decisions, even simple ones, may become an insuperable task. Everything appears too complicated to the patient, with too many options and possibilities. In severe cases patients may be unable to decide what shirt to wear and may remain in front of their closet until someone else makes the decision for them.

Patients lose interest in former things and have no curiosity for what is new in life. They take no pleasure in their activities; nothing arouses them. Libido is diminished. They must force themselves to do what they formerly enjoyed doing, and they go about their day lifeless and desolate.

Insomnia is common, and may be a particular torment to the patient. Although many complain of what is technically known as initial insomnia, or trouble falling asleep, the most characteristic kind of insomnia comes later in the night as either middle insomnia or early-morning awakening. In middle insomnia the patient awakens for no apparent reason and then has difficulty falling back asleep, lying awake for an hour or more until sleep finally returns. Early-morning awakening comes later in the night; here the patient awakens well before the customary hour and then cannot fall back asleep at all. Many, as they lie awake, experience ruminations or racing, restless thoughts. Finally, when morning comes, patients arise unrefreshed, exhausted, as if they had not slept at all. Rarely, patients with major depression complain of hypersomnia; however, as is noted in the section on differential diagnosis, this symptom should always raise the possibility of bipolar disorder.

Appetite is routinely lost, and many patients lose weight, sometimes in substantial amounts. Food may lose its taste or become unpalatable. Patients may complain it tastes like cardboard or that it leaves them nauseated. Some force themselves to eat; however, others do not and may lose 10 to 30 or more pounds. Uncommonly, some patients complain of increased appetite and weight gain, at times of substantial degree. As with hypersomnia, however, this is somewhat more common in bipolar disorder.

Constipation is common. Patients may also complain of headaches and myalgia. In severe cases the body temperature may fall, and menstruation may cease. The patient may appear to have aged precipitously: the skin appears dry, roughened, and wrinkled; the hair loses its luster, and the eyes appear dull. The overall effect may be shocking to an acquaintance who has not seen the patient since before the onset of the depressive episode.

Psychomotor agitation or, less commonly, retardation may be seen. Agitation, when slight, may be confined to a certain inner restlessness. When more severe, hand-wringing and nervous pacing about may occur. Patients complain of being unable to keep still; they may lament their fate out loud, and some may give way to wailing and repetitive pleas for help. The tension of these patients may be extreme, almost palpable, and yet, despite their pitiful pleas for help, they cannot be comforted, no matter what is done for them. Some may loudly berate themselves over and over again, confessing and accusing themselves of the worst sins and derelictions. Some may beg to be put out of their misery.

If psychomotor retardation occurs, the patient, drained of all vigor, may slip into a torpor. Speech, when it occurs, is slow and halting, and in some cases may cease altogether as if the effort to go on were simply too great. Some patients may sit immobile for hours; efforts to take them to the bathroom or to meals may be met with reluctance, even irritation. Left undisturbed, they may neither bathe nor change clothes, even though they may have defecated or urinated on themselves.

The attitude and outlook of these patients may become profoundly negative and pessimistic. They have no hope for themselves or for the future. They see no way out. Self-esteem sinks, and the workings of conscience become prominent. Patients see themselves as worthless, as having never done anything of value. Rather they see their sins multiply before them. Indeed, in reviewing their past they seem blind to their accomplishments and fix only on their misdeeds or shortcomings, which, as they recall them, become magnified at times to heinous proportions. Some may begin to ruminate: failings, defects, and gloomy predictions of the future may repeat themselves again and again in an implacable litany.

Thoughts of suicide are almost always present. At times these may be passive, and patients may wish aloud that they might die of some disease or accident. Conversely, they may be active, and patients consider hanging or shooting themselves, jumping from tall buildings, or overdosing on dangerous medicines. Often the risk of a suicide attempt is greatest as patients begin to recover. Still seeing themselves as worthless and hopeless sinners, these patients, now rising from their fatigue, may have enough energy to carry out the plan. Tragically, some also take their families with them. In their profound pessimism, they may see family members as equally hopeless, and take their lives to spare them their misery.

In addition to these core symptoms of depression some patients have panic attacks. Others may experience obsessions or compulsions. A particularly common compulsion is the "horrific temptation" to use a knife or gun to kill a loved one, and a consequent overwhelming necessity to rid the house of such objects and to avoid coming into contact with them outside the house.

A minority, perhaps 15%, of depressive episodes are characterized by delusions or hallucinations. Typically, these episodes are severe, with prominent psychomotor change. Those inclined to agitation may wail ceaselessly, pacing agitatedly about their room, begging for deliverance. Those who develop psychomotor retardation may fall into a profound stupor. They may lie immobile for hours or days, mute, at times incontinent, seemingly lifeless. Consciousness is clouded, and upon recovery some patients may not be able to recall their experiences during this time.

The delusions are mood congruent in that they are in some fantastic, extreme way appropriate to the patients' mood and to their view of themselves. Guilt becomes extreme, and patients may confess to unspeakable, impossible sins. They have poisoned their children; family and friends are imprisoned for some crime the patient committed. They believe they are condemned to hell; they have only hours to live; death is deserved and is near. Persecutory delusions are also common and have a peculiar twist to them. Here patients fully believe that they deserve such persecution for their miserable sins and shortcomings. Neighbors whisper about them as they leave the house; the police have been alerted; a warrant is drawn up; the electric chair is readied; a trial is not necessary, for their guilt is self-evident.

Delusions of poverty and nihilistic delusions may occur and are consonant with patients' view of themselves as worthless and hopeless. They are without funds; bills cannot be paid, and the family will be destitute. Having them look at a favorable bank statement is to no avail; they know more bills are due, that it is a fraud. Allied with these delusions of poverty are nihilistic delusions. Patients believe themselves either dead or near death; their insides have turned to dust or concrete; their brains have shriveled; the heart has dried up for lack of blood. In extreme cases patients may assert that they are in fact dead. In other cases they may insist that everyone about them is dead. Death has covered the world leaving only robots or automatons.

Auditory hallucinations may occur and generally reflect the patients' delusions. Voices may accuse them or announce their execution. They may hear the hum of the electric chair as it is readied for their execution. Visual hallucinations, though less common, also occur. Beheaded corpses may appear. Olfactory, gustatory, and tactile hallucinations are rare. Some may smell rotting flesh.

All the foregoing descriptions apply most particularly to adults. The presentation of a depressive episode in childhood years or later years or in those with mental retardation may be somewhat different. In prepubertal children one of the first indicators of depression may be a lack of weight gain. One may also see irritability. Some children may also develop severe anxiety over the prospect of being separated from their parents, and they may have numerous complaints of headaches, stomachaches, and general malaise. Among adolescents serious misconduct may appear. Rebelliousness and irritability may be seen. Grades fall as concentration is impaired, and patients may fall in with others who have a conduct disorder and adopt their attitudes and behavior. Among the elderly, agitation and hypochondriacal concerns are common, and indeed the patient may deny feeling depressed at all. Memory and concentration may be so impaired in the elderly that a dementia occurs. In the past this has been called a "pseudodementia," presumably to distinguish it from other kinds of dementia. However, a better, more recent term is "dementia syndrome of depression." Mentally retarded patients may be unable to describe their mood or how they view themselves. Hence the presentation may be with unexplained weight loss, insomnia, agitation, and other signs.

Recently, much attention has been focused on patients whose affective episodes seem entrained to the changing seasons. Patients with major depression who exhibit this seasonal pattern tend to have their depressive episodes in fall or winter and seem more likely to have hyperphagia and hypersomnia. It must be kept in mind that, although a major depression may exhibit a seasonal pattern, such a seasonal pattern is more commonly found in bipolar disorder.

COURSE

Major depression is a relapsing and remitting illness, characterized in most patients by the recurrence of depressive episodes throughout life, in between which the patient remains more or less in a normal state of health.

In perhaps one-half of cases, the depressive episode gradually undergoes a full remission within 6 to 12 months; in the remainder one sees either a partial remission or a persistence of the full syndrome. Overall, however, the long-term outlook for a given episode of depression is good, with less than one-tenth of episodes persisting in full form past two years.

After the first episode of depression has remitted, it is difficult to predict when the next is destined to occur: in some patients, it may appear in less than a year whereas, on the other extreme, in some patients the next episode may not be destined to occur until after the patient dies of some unrelated cause, thus perhaps accounting for those cases wherein only one depressive episode is seen in the patient's entire life. Despite this wide variability, it does appear that, on average, the interval between episodes is about five years. Over time, however, and with repeated occurrences of episodes, this interval becomes shorter, and the duration of the episode longer, until, in some cases, after many years, the episodes "merge" to create a chronic depression.

COMPLICATIONS

Work performance typically declines. Fatigue and lack of interest leave patients falling behind, and difficulty with memory, concentration, and decision making impair their ability to complete any task they may attempt. Patients may miss promotions, be put on notice, or even be fired. Children and adolescents do poorly in school for similar reasons and, as noted earlier, become at risk for drifting down toward those whose misconduct may then become a compelling pattern for the patient.

Relations with family and friends typically suffer. Parents may be unable to care for children. Marital discord is common, and separation or divorce may occur.

"Self-medication," typically with alcohol or benzodiazepines, is relatively common, and in those so predisposed may occasion a pattern of abusive use or may result in substance dependence.

Faulty, regrettable decisions are not uncommon. Convinced of their pessimistic outlook patients may decide against taking offered opportunities, or may withdraw from a current enterprise that to them now seems doomed.

Those with other illnesses may lose hope in recovery from those illnesses and stop their medicines or withdraw from treatment, thus occasioning further suffering.

The overall suicide rate in major depression is about 4%; among hospitalized patients, however, the risk rises to 9%.

ETIOLOGY

Major depression appears in part to be inherited. Among the first-degree relatives of patients with major depression, the prevalence of major depression is some two to three times higher than among the first-degree relatives of normal controls. Furthermore, whereas the concordance rate for dizygotic twins is about 20%, the rate for monozygotic twins rises to about 50%. Adoption studies further support a role for heredity in major depression. Despite these findings, however, genetic studies have not as yet identified any loci or genes which can be confidently associated with this illness, indicating that in all likelihood major depression is genetically complex, involving not only multiple genes, but also possibly multiple modes of inheritance.

Abnormalities in the hypothalamic-pituitary axis are clearly present in major depression, and the great majority of patients will demonstrate non-suppression on the dexamethasone suppression test, blunting of the TSH response to TRH or blunting of the growth hormone response to clonidine. DST non-suppression has been most extensively studied, and it is clear that this is related to hypothalamic changes: the concentration of corticotrophin releasing factor (CRF) in the hypothalamic paraventricular and supraoptic nuclei is elevated, and the response of ACTH to exogenous CRF is blunted, as would be expected with chronic over-stimulation of the pituitary by endogenous CRF. In a similar vein, it appears that the blunted TSH response to TRH is also likely related to hypothalamic changes, as the CSF concentration of TRH is elevated in depressed patients.

Abnormalities of sleep architecture, as might be expected, are also present, and of these the most interesting is a shortened REM latency. REM sleep, in normals, may be induced by the infusion of cholinergic agents, and patients with major depression exhibit an enhanced sensitivity to two cholinergic agents, arecoline and donepezil, with a prompter onset of REM sleep after infusion.

Neuroanatomic abnormalities may or may not be present in major depression: as yet MRI studies have not yielded conclusive results. PET studies have generally indicated bilateral hypofrontality, which, in some studies, has been more pronounced on the left side.

The undoubtable success of various antidepressants has focused attention on the biogenic amines: given that all antidepressants have effects on either noradrenergic or serotoninergic functioning, it appears reasonable to assume that there is a complementary disturbance in these amines in patients with major depression. Despite enormous research effort, consistent findings implicating these amines have been difficult to obtain. One exception is the finding that, in patients with major depression currently in an SSRI-induced remission, a depletion of tryptophan, the dietary precursor of serotonin, is generally followed by a rapid relapse of depressive symptoms.

Inheritance, though of great importance in major depression, cannot account for all cases, and environmental factors are clearly important. Among the various factors postulated, it appears that early childhood loss may be the most important. Significant loss, as for example through death or divorce, also appears important as a precipitant for episodes in adult life. The importance of precipitants, however, tends to wane with successive episodes, such that after repeated episodes, little or nothing by way of a precipitant may be required for the next episode to make its appearance.

Integrating the foregoing etiologic factors into a coherent theory is problematic, and typically involves some speculation. With this caveat in mind, however, it appears reasonable to say that major depression is characterized by an inherited abnormality of noradrenergic, serotoninergic or cholinergic functioning, of variable degree, in the hypothalamus (or related limbic structures) and certain brainstem structures (such as the noradrenergic locus ceruleus, the serotoninergic dorsal raphe nucleus and the cholinergic pedunculopontine nucleus), which, though spontaneously reversible early on, eventually becomes permanent with repeated episodes. It also appears plausible to say that the experience of loss in childhood or adult years may exacerbate this inherited abnormality, or even possibly, in some cases, cause it, but that once these abnormalities appear, that they persist.

DIFFERENTIAL DIAGNOSIS

In the normal course of life, adverse events, especially losses, are followed by depressive symptoms. A common example is bereavement following upon the death of a loved one. At times, however, especially when these symptoms are severe or long lasting, the clinician is asked to decide whether the patient is still in the midst of a "reactive" depression, that is to say a "normal" reaction to the event, or whether the event has precipitated a depressive episode that would perpetuate symptoms long after the patient would "normally" have recovered and "gotten over it." Four differential points aid in this distinction. First, consider whether the severity of the symptoms is out of proportion to the event. Severe symptoms are to be expected after the death of a child, but not after failing to win a promotion. Second, consider the duration of symptoms. Assuming that the adverse event is not ongoing, a duration beyond 6 months and certainly beyond a year is highly suggestive that another process has supervened. Third, be alert to symptoms that, though not uncommon in a depressive episode, are unusual for a "normal" or "reactive" depression, such as severe and unremitting guilt and self-deprecation; profound and prolonged psychomotor change; middle insomnia or early-morning awakening; and, most assuredly, delusions or hallucinations of any sort. Fourth, and finally, consider whether a personal or family history of major depression exists, as this increases the likelihood that a depressive episode may have supervened. In general, one is looking to see whether the patient's symptoms in some way or other have become "autonomous" and have achieved a life of their own, independent of whatever event may have triggered them.

Dysthymia is characterized by chronic, yet generally mild, depressive symptoms. At times when mild depressive symptoms arise de novo from euthymic functioning, the diagnostician may wonder whether this is a dysthymia or perhaps only a long prodrome to a depressive episode. Certainly, if the patient has had previous depressive episodes, one would lean toward the diagnosis of a prodrome; if the patient lacks this history, however, one may have to diagnose a dysthymia, but remain alert to the occurrence of an episode that would prompt a diagnostic revision.

The distinction between a depressive episode occurring as part of a major depression and a depressive episode occurring as part of a bipolar disorder is critical and at times very difficult. Certainly, with a history of mania, a diagnosis of major depression is definitely ruled out. Obtaining this history, however, may be very difficult. Depressed patients suffused with pessimism and hopelessness may simply be unable to recall having been manic. The experience of euphoria or increased energy may simply be so far from their current existence that it does not come to mind. Here careful questioning of relatives and friends is very important. Furthermore, even if one can say with certainty that no history of mania exists, then the question still arises as to whether or not a manic episode might occur in the years to come. The majority of patients with bipolar disorder begin their illness with a depressive episode, and they may have more than one before the first manic episode occurs. Four ways are used to assess the risk of a future manic episode. First, determine both the number of previous depressive episodes, if any, and the length of time from the first one to the current one. A history of five or more prior depressive episodes, or a duration of 10 or more years from the first to the current depressive episode, makes the likelihood of a future manic episode very low. Second, determine whether an episode of major depression occurred in childhood or early adolescence: patients with depressive episodes of such early onset are far more likely to have a manic one in their lifetimes than are patients whose first depressive episode did not occur until adult years. Third, inquire as to a family history of mania. Although this may be found among the relatives of patients with a major depression, it is far more common among relatives of those with a bipolar disorder. Fourth, examine closely the onset and symptomatology of the current episode itself for features that, though certainly possible in a depressive episode of a major depression, are nonetheless more commonly seen in a bipolar depression. Bipolar depressions tend to be of acute onset, in contrast to those in major depression, which are generally gradual. In terms of symptoms, bipolar depression tends to be characterized by psychomotor retardation, hyperphagia, and hypersomnia, whereas in major depression one tends to see agitation, insomnia, and anorexia with weight loss; furthermore, although psychotic symptoms may occur in major depression, they are far more common in bipolar depression. Another important point to keep in mind when evaluating depressive symptomatology is that "a hint of mania" means that, rather than a depressive episode, one is actually seeing a "mixed-manic" episode with a heavy preponderance of depressive symptoms. Examples include the following: "racing thoughts" or "flight of thought" that may be confused with incessant ruminations occurring in major depression, prominent mood lability, and a certain tense inner excitement that may be confused with agitation of major depression. Certainly, if the depressed patient appears wearing a garland in her hair, or a gay boutonniere in his jacket, even if only for a few moments, one would begin to doubt this is a "pure" depressive episode.

Atypical depression is a controversial entity: earlier authorities believed it to be a disorder separate from major depression, whereas current thinking holds it to be a variant. In this book, it is treated separately in Chapter 76. Whether one considers it to be a separate disorder or a variant, there is general agreement on what constitute atypical features, namely mood reactivity, rejection sensitivity, leaden fatigue, hypersomnia and hyperphagia.

Postpartum depression, as discussed in that chapter, is generally diagnosed only when the depressive episodes are "entrained" exclusively to the immediate postpartum period and do not occur at other times.

Premenstrual dysphoric disorder, as discussed in that chapter, is distinguished by the prompt remission of symptoms with the onset of menstrual flow.

Obsessive-compulsive disorder is often accompanied by depressive symptoms, yet here the obsessions and compulsions long precede the depressive symptoms. By contrast the occasional isolated obsessions or compulsions that sometimes complicate a depressive episode are preceded by prominent depressive symptoms. Posttraumatic stress disorder, Briquet's syndrome, and hypochondriasis may all be complicated by depressive symptoms.

Yet here, as in obsessive-compulsive disorder, the depressive symptoms occur within the context of the other symptoms of these illnesses.

Schizoaffective disorder, depressed type, is distinguished from major depression by the persistence of psychotic symptoms throughout the intervals between depressive episodes.

Severe generalized anxiety disorder is distinguished from an agitated depressive episode by the relative absence of such symptoms as fatigue, loss of interest, guilt, and middle insomnia or early-morning awakening.

Secondary depression, such as may occur in Cushing's syndrome, hypothyroidism, and so forth, is discussed in that chapter.

Active alcoholism, alcohol withdrawal, and withdrawal from cocaine or stimulants are all typically complicated by depressive symptoms, which may be severe. Here, however, within 3 or 4 weeks of abstinence, symptoms begin to clear spontaneously.

In anorexia nervosa significant weight loss is generally accompanied by depressive symptoms. However, the depressive symptoms clear fairly promptly with weight restoration.

In the elderly a depression often manifests with prominent loss of memory and concentration, with other symptoms being at times relatively insignificant. This "dementia syndrome of depression" may be suspected when there is a history of prior episodes of depression or when the incorrect answers on the mental status examination seem to stem from an inability to put forth the effort to answer them. The possibility of a concurrence of both a dementia syndrome of depression and another dementing disease, such as Alzheimer's disease, must also be kept in mind.

TREATMENT

The overall treatment of major depression is conveniently divided into three phases: "acute" treatment directed at the current depressive episode, "continuation" treatment directed at preventing a relapse into the current episode, and, "prophylactic," or "maintenance," treatment directed at the prevention of future episodes.

Regarding acute treatment for a depressive episode, one may, in addition to routine supportive psychotherapy, use either antidepressant medications or a specific psychotherapeutic method, such as cognitive therapy, or at times a combination of these two approaches. Since cognitive therapy (and an allied approach, interpersonal psychotherapy) has been demonstrated to be effective only in patients with mild to moderately severe depressive episodes, it is not the first choice for patients who are severely depressed or in those with psychotic symptoms, such as hallucinations or delusions. Antidepressants, however, are effective regardless of severity, and the following scheme for their use is now presented.

The initial step in this scheme is to select an antidepressant from the various available groups of antidepressants, each of which is discussed in detail in its respective chapter in the section on Psychopharmacology. These groups include the SSRIs (e.g., citalopram), the tricyclics (e.g., nortriptyline), the MAOIs (e.g., phenelzine) and a miscellaneous group including venlafaxine, mirtazapine, bupropion, nefazodone and trazodone. Several considerations come into play when making this selection, including: first, overall effectiveness; second, a personal or family history of antidepressant treatment with special attention to effectiveness and tolerability; third, anticipated side effects; fourth, potential drug-drug interactions; and, fifth, lethality in overdose.

First, overall, it appears that the various antidepressants are, by and large, of equal effectiveness in relieving depression. There may, however, be certain exceptions to this rule. There is some evidence for superior effectiveness of venlafaxine and tricyclics over other agents. In addition, it appears that trazodone may be somewhat less effective than the others. These possible differences in effectiveness, however, are of no more than modest degree.

Second, inquire closely as to a personal or family history of treatment with an antidepressant, with particular reference not only to effectiveness but also the occurrence of side effects. History tends to repeat itself and if a patient responded well to a certain agent in the past, with no or modest side effects, then it makes sense to strongly consider using this agent again. Family history is less strong as a predictor, but still has some effect.

Third, consider the burden of anticipated side effects. Weight gain can be a significant factor over the long haul, and in this regard an SSRI is probably preferable to a tricyclic or mirtazapine. Sexual side effects (e.g., erectile dysfunction, decreased lubrication, delayed orgasm) are common with most antidepressants, with the notable exceptions of mirtazapine, bupropion and nefazodone. Orthostatic hypotension, with possible falls or "watershed" cerebral infarctions in the elderly, is unlikely with SSRIs, venlafaxine, bupropion and mirtazapine, but not uncommon with tricyclics. Cardiac arrhythmias may be induced or exacerbated by tricyclics, but SSRIs carry little risk in this regard. The seizure threshold is reduced by tricyclics (especially maprotilene and clomipramine), bupropion and venlafaxine, and this consideration is especially important in those with a history of seizures or, in the case of bupropion, in patients with a history of bulimia, as such patients, for unclear reasons, may be especially prone to seize if treated with bupropion. Another side effect to consider is sedation, which tends to be more prominent with tricyclics (with the exception of nortriptyline, protriptyline and desipramine), mirtazapine, nefazodone and trazodone than with other agents, such as SSRIs. In the past, it was felt that this side effect could be put to good use in agitated patients, as it was believed that agitation responded better to a sedating drug, such as a tricyclic, than to other agents, such as an SSRI: as it turns out, however, tricyclics are no better in treated "agitated" depressions than are SSRIs.

Fourth, consider possible drug-drug interactions with other medications the patient is taking, or is likely to. In this regard, the "cleanest" agents are the SSRIs citalopram and escitalopram, and by far the most problematic are the MAOIs. Indeed the list of medications (and foods) that must be avoided when taking one of the currently available MAOIs is of such length that these agents are generally a last choice in the treatment of major depression.

Fifth, and finally, consider the potential lethality of these agents in the case of overdose. In this regard, the SSRIs are unquestionably the safest agents, followed by venlafaxine, mirtazapine, and nefazodone: the tricyclics and MAOIs are by far the most dangerous.

Clearly, given the large number of antidepressants available, and the multiple considerations involved in choosing among them, arriving at the best first choice for any given patient is a complex task that must be individualized. All other things being equal, however, several good choices stand out, including the SSRI escitalopram, the tricyclic nortriptyline, and, from the miscellaneous group, bupropion, mirtazapine or venlafaxine.

Once an agent is chosen, it must be given an "adequate trial," assuming of course that no unacceptable side effects are seen. An "adequate trial" means treatment with an "adequate" dose for an "adequate" period of time. In general, one increases the dose as tolerated up to the "average" dose for that agent, as described in their respective chapters, always keeping in mind that reduced doses are indicated for the elderly, the debilitated, and those with

significant hepatic disease. At this point blood levels are not required, with the exception of nortriptyline, which probably has a "therapeutic window." In general one should not expect to see much improvement for the first 1 or 2 weeks after reaching an "average" dose; if none is seen by the end of the third week, then one may assume that, at least at the current dose, the medicine probably will not be that helpful. In cases, however, where improvement is seen by 3 weeks, one must tell a patient that it may take up to 3 months to see the full effect.

If, after approximately 3 weeks, there is minimal or no improvement, one should, if not already done, check thyroxine and TSH levels. Hypothyroidism, even if only "chemical," perhaps being manifest only by an elevated TSH level, will blunt the response to antidepressants and must be corrected. Presuming that both thyroxine and TSH levels are normal, one may, if side effects are tolerable, consider increasing the dose of the antidepressant. With the exception of nortriptyline, which, as noted earlier, has a "therapeutic window," it appears that for most other antidepressants the dose-response curve is generally linear, and thus one may gradually increase the dose up to the maximum described for each agent in its respective chapter.

If the patient does not respond to high dose treatment and the thyroid status is normal, or if side-effects preclude a significant dose increase, then one may consider either switching to another antidepressant or trying a combination. Switching antidepressants is a viable option, but in so doing one should probably switch to an antidepressant from a different group. In some cases, one must be careful of potential drug-drug interactions in making a transition: for example, given the long half-life of some SSRIs and their ability to inhibit the metabolism of tricyclics, one should generally, if switching from an SSRI to a tricyclic, phase in the tricyclic relatively slowly after stopping the SSRI. Combination treatment is also viable, but only a small number of combinations have been shown to be effective in double-blinded studies, including the following: lithium plus either a tricyclic or an SSRI; olanzapine (in a dose of 10 mg) plus fluoxetine; triiodothyronine (in a dose of 50 mcg) plus a tricyclic; and, finally, a tricyclic plus an MAOI. This last combination is potentially quite dangerous, and should probably be considered the last option. Regardless of whether one substitutes another single agent, or tries a combination, one must then again provide an "adequate trial," ensuring that doses are adequate and that at least three weeks are allowed to see if a response will occur.

At this point, should the response be minimal or less, one might consider different single agents or different combinations. How far one goes at this point depends largely on the severity of the depression. If it is tolerable, one could consider further medication trials. If, however, there is substantial morbidity or significant risk of death, one should consider ECT.

Although the foregoing schema is in general applicable to most cases, exceptions do occur. First, in severe cases requiring hospitalization, one might consider immediately checking thyroid status and beginning with a rapid titration of a single agent or a combination. Second, for the highly suicidal patient or in those cases where the depression is otherwise life threatening (for example, because of extreme weight loss), moving immediately to ECT may be appropriate, as it remains the most effective and rapid treatment for depression. Third, some debate exists over whether antipsychotics are required for depressive episodes accompanied by psychotic symptoms. In some cases aggressive treatment using the schemas outlined above effects a remission, not only of the typical depressive symptoms but also of delusions and hallucinations. Certainly, this is the case when ECT is used. Most clinicians however will treat such patients with a combination of a second generation antipsychotic and an SSRI.

Before leaving this discussion of acute treatment of a depressive episode with antidepressants, some words are required regarding alprazolam, buspirone, "alternative" treatments such as St. John's wort (hypericum), and certain experimental treatments. Alprazolam in doses of 3 to 6 mg may be as effective as a single-agent antidepressant for mildly to moderately severe depressions. The risk of neuroadaptation and the often extreme difficulty in withdrawing from alprazolam, however, makes this a less than attractive alternative. Buspirone, in high doses (for example, 60 mg or more), likewise appears to be effective in mildly to moderately severe depressions. Its effectiveness relative to other agents, however, is not as yet clear. Of the "alternative" agents, St. John's wort may be helpful with mild depressions; however, its effectiveness in moderate or severe depressions is doubtful. Experimental treatments include transcranial mangnetic stimulation and vagus nerve stimulation. Both have shown promise in treatment-resistant cases, but experience with them is still too limited to justify their routine use. Certainly, if one were contemplated, transcranial magnetic stimulation, a relatively benign procedure, is probably a first choice, given the invasiveness of vagal nerve stimulation.

Once "acute" treatment has effected a symptomatic remission of depressive symptoms, "continuation" treatment is in order. It must be kept in mind that these treatments do not alter the natural course of the depressive episode itself. Rather they merely suppress symptoms. Consequently, if treatment is discontinued shortly after symptoms remit, those symptoms almost invariably return, generally within a few weeks or perhaps a month or longer. Consequently, "continuation" treatment is required until such time as the depressive episode itself has gone into a spontaneous remission. In general this involves a continuation of the "acute" treatment; however, in a minority of cases scaling down the intensity of treatment without a return of symptoms may be possible. For example, if a combination of two or more antidepressants is required, one of the agents may be dropped off and the patient maintained on a single agent or, if a single agent was effective from the start, the dose reduced. One must be cautious here, however, for in most cases patients require for "continuation" treatment a regimen very close or identical to that which worked acutely. If ECT was used, one has the option of either continuing "maintenance" ECT, perhaps on a once-monthly basis, or of using an antidepressant: both paroxetine and a combination of nortriptyline and lithium have been found effective in this regard. Most patients opt for the antidepressant. However, though this is generally effective some patients do relapse, and in these cases a trial of maintenance ECT is probably indicated.

As noted, continuation treatment should persist for as long as the depressive episode would last in the natural course of events. In cases where the patient has a prior history of depressive episodes of fairly uniform and discrete length, this may be taken as a reliable guide for the duration of the current episode. In most cases, however, such guidance is not available. Either no prior episodes occurred, or, if they did, they were of such indistinct onset and remission that their length could not be reliably estimated. In these cases prolonged continuation of treatment until the patient has been symptom free for at least four consecutive months is prudent. This guideline, empirically determined, rests on several assumptions: first, that no acute treatment is perfect; second, that given the waxing and waning nature of depressive symptoms, in the natural course of events, at times symptom severity is expected to rise to a "peak" that could "break through" the treatment and cause some symptoms in the patient; and third, the longer a patient goes

without a "breakthrough," the more likely the depressive episode is finally undergoing a natural remission. When the time does come to cease continuation treatment, given the fact that a small risk of relapse still exists, one may want to time the cessation of treatment with respect to events in the patient's life. For example, a patient may not wish to be exposed to any risk of relapse when starting a new job, assuming any major new responsibility, or facing any major stress. In most cases it is prudent to hold off cessation of continuation treatment until the patient feels that life has become manageable and is likely to remain so. In any case one may want to see the patient at least one more time, perhaps 2 or 3 months after cessation of continuation treatment to make sure that the depressive episode has indeed remitted.

Given that the majority of patients have a subsequent episode, asking the patient to consider preventive treatment is appropriate. Such preventive treatment is generally recommended when either the euthymic interval between episodes is less than 2 years or, based on past experience, one can predict that a future episode would be sufficiently severe as to cause significant suffering or complications. Another impetus for the recommendation of preventive treatment are recent studies suggesting that episodes "beget" future episodes in a "kindling" process, suggesting that control of present episodes may reduce the risk of an increased frequency of episodes in the future. If the patient does opt for preventive treatment, an extension of the continuation regimen of an antidepressant is usually effective; whether cognitive-behavior therapy or ECT is effective is not clear. Should patients decline preventive treatment, one should review the prodromal symptoms experienced in the past. Thus explicitly forewarned, patients may be better able to recognize early symptoms in the future and secure treatment before the symptoms become severe and disabling.

Upon first examining the patient, one should consider all three phases of treatment: acute, continuation, and preventive. For many physicians the choice of treatment for the acute phase is influenced by what has been shown effective in both the continuation and preventive phases. Clearly then, antidepressant treatment currently appears best suited; if an antidepressant regimen works for acute treatment, then in all likelihood the treatment will be effective for both the continuation and preventive phases.

An additional treatment option involves phototherapy. Mounting evidence supports the use of phototherapy for patients whose depressive episodes display a seasonal pattern with onset in the winter and remission in the spring. Patients are exposed to full-spectrum light at 2500 lux for about 2 hours every morning. If a response is not seen within about a week, consideration might be given to increasing the duration to 4 or even 6 hours. Although some patients appear to respond to exposure at other times, for example at midday or in the evening, or to shorter durations with higher intensity of exposure (to as little as a half hour at 10,000 lux), starting with the 2-hour morning "dose" and proceeding from there is prudent. Some patients with a seasonal pattern may respond to phototherapy, both as acute treatment and as continuation treatment. Some, however, require the addition of an antidepressant to achieve full relief. Because phototherapy is time consuming and for many patients simply impractical, one should bear in mind that major depression whose course is marked by a seasonal pattern also responds to antidepressants without the use of phototherapy.

Indications for hospitalization include the following: a significant risk of suicide; significant disability caused by symptoms of depression, making patients unable to maintain themselves at home or at work; significant concurrent illness (for example, certain cardiac conditions) that requires intensive monitoring; or acute treatment with ECT (continuation treatment with ECT generally may be done on an outpatient basis). At times the decision to hospitalize is easy, for example when the patient has recently made a suicide attempt, is in danger of being fired because fatigue and poor concentration make work impossible, or has recently had a myocardial infarction. Most patients, however, fall into a "gray zone," and in these cases carefully considered clinical judgment is required.

Deciding when to discharge a patient also requires considerable judgment. Though one may wish to wait until the depressive symptoms are fully remitted, such a strategy is usually grossly impractical given the burden, financial and otherwise, attendant on a long hospital stay. In practice, one waits until an uninterrupted "trend" toward improvement has been established. Given that setbacks often occur early in treatment, one should not discharge the patient at the first blush of improvement. Rather one may want to wait until the patient has been definitely "on the mend" for at least 3 or 4 days in a row before considering discharge. The patient's support system must also be considered. Those with little outpatient support may require longer inpatient care to allow for a fuller degree of recovery before discharge. When the patient is discharged with a potentially lethal prescribed medicine, one may want to limit the number of tablets dispensed to a sublethal amount.

BIBLIOGRAPHY

Aberg-Wistedt A, Husselmark L, Stain-Malmgren R, et al. Serotoninergic "vulnerability" in affective disorder: a study of the tryptophan depletion test and relationships between peripheral and central serotonin indexes in citalpopram responders. *Acta Psychiatrica Scandinavica* 1998;97:374-380.

Banki CM, Bissette F, Arato M, et al. Elevation of immunoreactive CSF TRH in depressed patients. *The American Journal of Psychiatry* 1988;145:1526-1531.

Beigel A, Murphy DL. Unipolar and bipolar affective illness: differences in clinical characteristics accompanying depression. *Archives of General Psychiatry* 1971;24:215-220.

Brown GW, Harris TO, Hepworth C. Life events and endogenous depression: a puzzle reexamined. *Archives of General Psychiatry* 1994;51:525-534.

Cascalenda N, Perry JC, Looper K. Remission in major depressive disorder: a comparison of pharmacotherapy, psychotherapy, and control conditions. *The American Journal of Psychiatry* 2002;159:1354-1360.

Dunner DL, Fleiss JL, Fieve RR. The course of development of mania in patients with recurrent depression. *The American Journal of Psychiatry* 1976;133:905-908.

Janicak PG, Dowd SM, Martin B. Repetitive transcranial magnetic stimulation versus electroconvulsive therapy for major depression: preliminary results of a randomized trial. *Biological Psychiatry* 2002;51:659-667.

Joffe RT, Singer W, Levitt AJ, et al. A placebo-controlled comparison of lithium and triiodothyronine augmentation of tricyclic antidepressants in unipolar refractory depression. *Archives of General Psychiatry* 1993;50:387-393.

Katona CL, Abou-Saleh MT, Harrison DA, et al. Placebo-controlled trial of lithium augmentation of fluoxetine and lofepramine. *British Journal of Psychiatry* 1995;166:80-86.

Lauritzen L, Odgaard K, Clemmesen L, et al. Relapse prevention by means of paroxetine in ECT-treated patients with major depression: a comparison with imipramine and placebo in medium-term continuation therapy. *Acta Psychiatrica Scandinavica* 1996;94:241-251.

Marangell LB. Switching antidepressants for treatment-resistant major depression. *The Journal of Clinical Psychiatry* 2001;62(Suppl 18): 12-17.

Marangell LB, Rush AJ, George MS, et al. Vagus nerve stimulation (VNS) for major depressive episodes: one year outcome. *Biological Psychiatry* 2002;51:280-287.

Mitchell PB, Wilhelm K, Parker G, et al. The clinical features of bipolar depression: a comparison with matched major depressive disorder patients. *The Journal of Clinical Psychiatry* 2001;62:212-216.

Perlis ML, Smith MT, Orff JH, et al. The effects of an orally administered cholinergic agonist on REM sleep in major depression. *Biological Psychiatry* 2002;51:457-462.

Prien RF, Kupfer DJ. Continuation drug therapy for major depressive episodes: how long should it be maintained? *The American Journal of Psychiatry* 1986;143:18-23.

Raadsheer FC, van Heerikhuize JJ, Lucassen PJ, et al. Corticotropin-releasing mRMA levels in the paraventricular nucleus of patients with Alzheimer's disease and depression. *The American Journal of Psychiatry* 1995;152:1372-1376.

Sackheim HA, Haskett RF, Mulsant BH, et al. Continuation pharmacotherapy in the prevention of relapse following electroconvulsive therapy: a randomized controlled trial. *The Journal of the American Medical Association* 2001;285:1299-1307.

Shelton RC, Keller MB, Gelenberg A, et al. Effectiveness of St John's wort in major depression: a randomized controlled trial. *The Journal of the American Medical Association* 2001;285:1978-1986.

Shelton RC, Tollefson GD, Tohen M, et al. A novel augmentation strategy for treating resistant major depression. *The American Journal of Psychiatry* 2001;158:131-134.

Tollefson GD, Greist JH, Jefferson JW, et al. Is baseline agitation a relative contraindication for a selective serotonin reuptake inhibitor? A comparative trial of fluoxetine versus imipramine. *Journal of Clinical Psychopharmacology* 1994;14:385-391.

Videbech P. PET measurements of brain glucose metabolism and blood flow in major depressive disorder: a critical review. *Acta Psychiatrica Scandinavica* 2000;101:11-20.

Zisook S, Schucter SR. Uncomplicated bereavement. *The Journal of Clinical Psychiatry* 1993;54:365-372.

75 Dysthymia (dysthymic disorder, DSM-IV-TR #300.4)

In dysthymia, patients present with extremely chronic yet low-level depressive symptoms that seem to pervade their entire existence—past, present, and probably future.

Dysthymia is 1½ to 3 times more frequent among females than males, and appears to be a common condition, with a lifetime prevalence of about 6%.

Considerable debate exists as to whether dysthymia represents a disorder sui generis or is rather merely a mild form of major depression. The fact that the vast majority of patients with dysthymia also at some point experience a full depressive episode argues for an identity between the two disorders; however, a small percentage of patients with dysthymia never experience a full depressive episode throughout their lives.

ONSET

Dysthymia typically has an insidious onset in childhood or teenage years, less commonly in adulthood. Customarily, those with an onset at or before the age of 21 are said to have an "early onset," whereas those with an onset past the age of 21 are said to have a "late onset."

CLINICAL FEATURES

Mood is typically depressed and sorrowful; at times some querulousness or irritability may occur. The outlook is pessimistic, even somber. Everything is taken too seriously, and life is seen as an opportunity only for toil. Though joyous occasions, such as a promotion, graduation, or the birth of a child, may temporarily lift these patients to some warmth and appreciation, they typically sink again quickly back into misery.

Self-confidence is lacking. New tasks or stresses seem hopelessly difficult, and although patients may shoulder their burdens with grim determination, in their hearts they expect only failure.

Thinking is difficult. Patients may complain of feeling heavy-headed and slow and of not being able to concentrate. Irresolution is common, and decisions may be postponed, again and again.

Fatigue is common, and patients may complain of feeling exhausted much of the time.

Hypochondriacal concerns may appear. Patients may worry over minor headaches or gastrointestinal upset, and this may occasion numerous trips to the physician. Appetite may suffer, and some patients may lose weight. Difficulty falling asleep is common, and some patients complain of restless, broken sleep.

Concurrent personality disorders are common, including histrionic and borderline types. Concurrent panic disorder may also be seen.

COURSE

Dysthymia typically pursues a chronic course, with symptoms typically waxing and waning over many years: although most patients will, at times, experience periods of euthymia, these euthymic intervals are generally brief, lasting no longer than days or weeks, and rarely more than a month. As noted earlier the vast majority of patients will also develop a full depressive episode at some point, and this is seen in about three-quarters of patients within five years of onset and an even larger proportion within a decade.

COMPLICATIONS

Through lack of self-confidence and difficulty thinking, many patients fall short of accomplishments otherwise within their reach. Marriages and friendships are rarely as rewarding as they might be.

Similar complications occurring in childhood or adolescence can have devastating and far-reaching effects on the course of the patient's life.

ETIOLOGY

Dysthymia and major depression run in the same families, and it is currently felt that they have similar, if not identical, etiologies. Indeed, one may conceive of dysthymia as an extremely long-lasting depressive episode that also happens to be of quite low severity.

DIFFERENTIAL DIAGNOSIS

The appearance of a manic or hypomanic episode rules out dysthymia in favor of a diagnosis of bipolar disorder or cyclothymia, respectively.

In hypochondriasis, depressive symptoms may also occur. However, here the patient's suspicion of a serious illness is paramount, and the depressive symptoms are fleeting. By contrast the dysthymic patient accepts the physician's reassurances and continues then with the chronic depressive symptoms.

Normal human unhappiness may at times be very difficult to distinguish from dysthymia. Some patients truly do suffer recurrent reversals in life, illnesses, and misfortunes to a degree that their chronic depression seems understandable. Generally, though, for most, life is not consistently filled with misfortune, and by careful questioning of the patient and long-term acquaintances one may usually find a period of time that was unburdened with such misfortune. Here if one finds that the patient gradually felt better, and stayed that way until the next unavoidable misfortune, one may rule for unhappiness and against dysthymia. The converse ruling would apply, of course, if the patient failed to "perk up." If one does not find a history of such a period of tranquility, one may want to attempt a "diagnosis by treatment response" and place the patient on an antidepressant.

The differential between dysthymia and major depression is, to say the least, problematic, as in positing that there are two disorders here we may be guilty of the logical sin of making a distinction where there is no difference. Current custom dictates that when patients with chronic, low-level depressive symptoms go on to develop a full depressive episode that we make two diagnoses, namely dysthymia plus major depression, thus characterizing these patients as having "double depressions." It would appear, however, just as reasonable, in such cases, to simply revise the diagnosis from dysthymia to major depression, with an explanatory note that the current depressive episode had an extraordinarily long prodrome.

TREATMENT

Both tricyclics and SSRIs are effective, and treatment may proceed as outlined in the chapter on major depression for the acute and continuation phases of treatment of a depressive episode. Given the mild nature of symptoms seen in dysthymia, one may also consider a psychotherapy such as cognitive behavior therapy.

BIBLIOGRAPHY

Akiskal HS. Dysthymia: clinical and external validity. *Acta Psychiatrica Scandinavica* 1994;89(suppl 383):19-23.

Dunner DL. Duration of periods of euthymia in patients with dysthymia. *The American Journal of Psychiatry* 1999;156:1992-1993.

Keller MB. Dysthymia in clinical practice: course, outcome, and impact on the community. *Acta Psychiatrica Scandinavica* 1994;89(suppl 383): 24-34.

Klein DN, Riso LP, Donaldson SK, et al. Family study of early-onset dysthymia. Mood and personality disorders in relatives of outpatients with dysthymia and episodic major depression and normal controls. *Archives of General Psychiatry* 1995;52:487-496.

McCullough JP, Braith JA, Chapman RC, et al. Comparison of early and late onset dysthymia. *The Journal of Nervous and Mental Disease* 1990;178:577-581.

Ravindram AV, Guelfi JD, Lane RM, et al. Treatment of dysthymia with sertraline: a double-blind, placebo-controlled trial in dysthymic patients without major depression. *The Journal of Clinical Psychiatry* 2000;61:821-827.

Vanelle JM, Attar-Levy D, Poirier MF, et al. Controlled efficacy study of fluoxetine in dysthymia. *The British Journal of Psychiatry* 1997;170: 345-350.

76 Atypical Depression

Atypical depression has a controversial nosologic status: originally conceived of as a unique disorder separate from major depression, it is currently considered by most authorities to represent merely a variant of major depression, or, as it is called, major depressive disorder with atypical features. Given that definitive studies, however, have not as yet been done, it is treated as a separate disorder in this book.

The cardinal feature of atypical depression is the presence of mood reactivity and rejection sensitivity: patients typically brighten up when they feel loved and cared for, but are extraordinarily sensitive to any hint of rejection, and always vulnerable to depressive symptoms should rejection occur, or even merely threaten.

Although the prevalence of atypical depression is not known, the clinical impression is that it is not rare; it is probably three times more common in females than males.

ONSET

The onset is probably in the late teenage or early adult years.

CLINICAL FEATURES

The mood reactivity, as noted above, plays itself out in the extraordinary rejection sensitivity seen in these patients. These patients seek to be the center of attention and the object of admiration, and when this position feels threatened, or if others actually do abandon them, they rapidly plunge into a depression. When depressed these patients also complain of one or more of the following "atypical" features. Anergia is very common, and patients may complain of a profound fatigue, often likened to a "leaden" paralysis. Need for sleep is increased, and patients also have an increased appetite, often for sweets, particularly chocolates. Despite the often severe nature of these depressive symptoms, mood reactivity, again, is not lost, and if patients once again find themselves loved and admired, these symptoms may rapidly clear.

Frequently, these patients' lives are characterized by multiple, often rapidly changing, romantic entanglements, and many of these patients also meet the criteria for borderline personality disorder.

COURSE

The rejection sensitivity appears to be chronic; whether or not it lessens with age is not known.

COMPLICATIONS

Long-term relationships, if they develop at all, are particularly difficult to sustain. During the depressions themselves, these patients may be unable to complete their work. Some may gain a substantial amount of weight.

ETIOLOGY

Although the etiology is not known, preliminary data suggest a disturbance in noradrenergic functioning.

DIFFERENTIAL DIAGNOSIS

As noted above, it is not clearly established whether such patients should receive a diagnosis of atypical depression or major depression with atypical features; the DSM-IV-TR calls for the latter, and this is how it should be coded for official purposes; however, an open mind on this nosologic question is still appropriate.

Patients with a borderline personality disorder are often extremely sensitive to rejection; however, their reaction is usually one of anger in contrast to the triad of leaden fatigue, hypersomnia, and hyperphagia seen in atypical depression.

Patients with a histrionic personality disorder likewise are often extremely sensitive to rejection and may feel depressed in its wake.

In this personality disorder, however, one rarely sees the triad mentioned above; indeed the depression of the patient with a histrionic personality disorder seems rather a tool that the personality disordered patient uses to manipulate others, rather than something that controls the patient.

TREATMENT

Phenelzine, in doses of 60 mg or more per day, is clearly superior to imipramine, and, by extension, probably also to other tricyclics. Fluoxetine, though not superior therapeutically to imipramine, is better tolerated. Cognitive therapy appears to offer a viable alternative to phenelzine for many patients.

BIBLIOGRAPHY

Annis GM, McGinn LK, Sanderson WC. Atypical depression: clinical aspects and noradrenergic function. *The American Journal of Psychiatry* 1995;152:31-36.

Jarrett RB, Schaffer M, McIntire D, et al. Treatment of atypical depression with cognitive therapy or phenelzine: a double-blind, placebo-controlled trial. *Archives of General Psychiatry* 1999;56:431-437.

McGrath PJ, Stewart JW, Janal MN, et al. A placebo-controlled study of fluoxetine versus imipramine in the acute treatment of atypical depression. *The American Journal of Psychiatry* 2000;157:344-350.

Nierenberg AA, Alpert JE, Pava J, et al. Course and treatment of atypical depression. *The Journal of Clinical Psychiatry* 1998;59(Suppl 18): 5-9.

Pande AC, Birkett M, Fechner-Bates S, et al. Fluoxetine versus imipramine in atypical depression. *Biological Psychiatry* 1996;40:1017-1020.

Quitkin FM, McGrath PJ, Stewart JW, et al. Atypical depression, panic attacks, and response to imipramine and phenelzine. A replication. *Archives of General Psychiatry* 1990;47:935-941.

Stewart JW, Tricamo E, McGrath PJ, et al. Prophylactic efficacy of phenelzine and imipramine in chronic atypical depression: likelihood of recurrence on discontinuation after 6 months' treatment. *The American Journal of Psychiatry* 1997;154:31-36.

77 Premenstrual Dysphoric Disorder

Premenstrual dysphoric disorder is a classic example of an episodic, or cyclic, disorder. Women suffering from it experience recurrent, discrete symptomatic episodes that are tightly entrained to events of the menstrual cycle. Though the time of onset of the episode is variable, ranging from hours to two weeks before menstruation begins, the time of closure of the episode is almost invariable, with symptoms remitting within the first few days of menstrual flow. During the episode itself, patients experience depressive symptoms and complain of bloating, mastalgia, and related phenomena.

Although the prevalence of premenstrual dysphoric disorder is not known with certainty, it probably occurs in from 3 to 8% of menstruating females.

ONSET

The onset of this disorder typically occurs somewhere between menarche and the late twenties, although later onsets have been noted. Some patients date the onset to the few months following childbirth.

CLINICAL FEATURES

Many patients (or sometimes those around them) are able to predict accurately when menses will begin by counting forward from when their premenstrual symptoms appear. Mood is variously described as depressed, sad, or anxious. Often some lability occurs, such as inexplicable, uncontrollable crying spells or irritability and unwanted anger; many patients complain that they feel "out of control." Patients complain of fatigue, even lethargy; interest in work or sexual activities is lost, and they often have great difficulty in concentrating and paying attention. Appetite may change and is often increased; many report intense cravings for sweets or chocolates. Sleep disturbance is also common with either insomnia or

hypersomnia. Other typical complaints include any or all of the following: headaches, breast swelling and tenderness, bloating, swelling of the hands or feet, clumsiness, nausea, or constipation.

The duration of these symptoms, as noted earlier, is quite variable. In most cases they occupy the few days before menstrual flow begins; however, as noted, some may suffer for 10 days, and, in rare instances, the episode may begin up to 3 weeks before menses, leaving the patient with only a week or so of relief during each menstrual cycle.

COURSE

In the vast majority of cases episodes continue to occur, and indeed may worsen in severity or duration, until menopause, when they cease.

COMPLICATIONS

Complications are similar to those outlined in the chapter on major depression. Patients may voluntarily isolate themselves in order to spare others their irritability, and, in a similar vein, some family members may learn to "leave well enough alone" during that part of the menstrual cycle.

ETIOLOGY

Premenstrual dysphoric disorder is familial, and among patients with this disorder one also finds an increased incidence of major depression relative to control females. Serotonin appears to play a role in this disorder, as evidenced by the fact that dietary tryptophan depletion and administration of a serotonin receptor blocker worsen symptoms and that the SSRIs constitute effective treatments.

DIFFERENTIAL DIAGNOSIS

Many other disorders may undergo an exacerbation premenstrually, and this is particularly true of dysthymia or a depressive episode of either major depression or bipolar disorder. However, in contrast to the symptoms of premenstrual dysphoric disorder, the symptoms of these disorders do not undergo a complete remission with the onset of menses; rather they simply return back to their baseline. In doubtful cases, the utilization of a daily symptom diary for two or three consecutive menstrual cycles may be helpful.

Patients with dysmenorrhea complain of cramping, bloating, headaches, and the like. However, these symptoms occur not before, but after the onset of menses, and are not accompanied by depressive symptoms.

TREATMENT

SSRIs constitute the mainstay of treatment, and of these fluoxetine at 20 mg/d and sertraline, at 100 mg/d, have the most support: in both cases it is often possible to restrict medication to the luteal phase of the cycle without any loss of effectiveness. Venlafaxine, in doses of 150 mg/d, may also be effective, but there is little support for bupropion, desipramine or other antidepressants. Alprazolam was also effective in doses of from 0.75 to 4.0 mg daily given during the luteal phase.

Various hormonal treatments have been attempted, with variable success. Although estrogen preparations may be effective, progesterone probably isn't. Gonadotropin releasing hormone analogues may be effective, but induce anovulation in the majority of cases. Other treatments, including bromocriptine, pyridoxine and beta blockers, have not found strong support.

BIBLIOGRAPHY

Bloch M, Schmidt PJ, Rubinow DR. Premenstrual syndrome: evidence for symptom stability across cycles. *The American Journal of Psychiatry* 1997;154:1741-1746.

Cohen LS, Miner C, Brown EW, et al. Premenstrual daily fluoxetine for premenstrual dysphoric disorder: a placebo-controlled, clinical trial using computerized diaries. *Obstetrics and Gynecology* 2002;100:435-444.

Freeman EW, Rickels K, Sondheimer SJ, et al. A double-blind trial of oral progesterone, alprazolam, and placebo in treatment of severe premenstrual syndrome. *The Journal of the American Medical Association* 1995;274:51-57.

Freeman EW, Rickels K, Sondheimer SJ, et al. Differential response to antidepressants in women with premenstrual syndrome/premenstrual dysphoric disorder: a randomized controlled trial. *Archives of General Psychiatry* 1999;56:932-939.

Freeman EW, Rickels K, Yonkers KA, et al. Venlafaxine in the treatment of premenstrual dysphoric disorder. *Obstetrics and Gynecology* 2001;98:737-744.

Grady-Weliky TA. Premenstrual dysphoric disorder. *The New England Journal of Medicine* 2003;348:433-438.

Halbreich U, Bergeron Y, Yonkers KA, et al. Efficacy of intermittent, luteal phase sertraline treatment of premenstrual dysphoric disorder. *Obstetrics and Gynecology* 2002;100:1219-1229.

Menkes DB, Coates DC, Fawcett JP. Acute tryptophan depletion aggravates premenstrual syndrome. *Journal of Affective Disorders* 1994;32:37-44.

Roca CA, Schmidt PJ, Rubinow DR. A follow-up study of premenstrual syndrome. *The Journal of Clinical Psychiatry* 1999;60:763-766.

Roca CA, Schmidt PJ, Smith MJ, et al. Effects of metergoline on symptoms in women with premenstrual dysphoric disorder. *The American Journal of Psychiatry* 2002;159:1876-1881.

Wittchen HU, Becker E, Lieb R, et al. Prevalence, incidence and stability of premenstrual dysphoric disorder in the community. *Psychological Medicine* 2002;32:119-132.

78 Postpartum Blues (Maternity Blues)

Perhaps half of all postpartum women experience the "baby blues." Although such a high incidence may suggest that this is a "normal" reaction, the fact that the clinical symptomatology is often strikingly out of character for the patient argues rather that the "blues" may represent a specific disorder.

ONSET

The onset is usually fairly acute, occurring within the first few days postpartum.

CLINICAL FEATURES

The patient may be depressed, irritable, or fearfully anxious. Crying spells are frequent, and at times a striking lability of mood and affect may occur: crying spells may come and go with rapidity; at times the patient may actually be laughing and claim to be happy with her delivery, yet be absolutely unable to stop the tears cascading down past her smile.

The patient may also experience some minor fatigue, difficulty with concentration, and insomnia.

COURSE

Symptoms peak within a few days and then gradually go into remission by two weeks postpartum.

Although the postpartum blues may recur after subsequent pregnancies, they are generally less severe.

COMPLICATIONS

Symptoms may place a strain on the marriage, and the mother may have difficulty in caring for the infant.

ETIOLOGY

Though the postpartum blues are undoubtedly related to the endocrinologic and neurophysiologic changes that occur in the postpartum period (such as falls in progesterone and estrogen levels and a rise in prolactin levels), endocrinologic studies have not, as yet, yielded solid findings: the most promising finding, however, is an association between the occurrence of the blues and a deeper fall of progesterone levels immediately postpartum. Two studies have found elevated alpha-2 receptors on platelets in patients as compared to unaffected postpartum women, suggesting disturbances on biogenic amine function.

DIFFERENTIAL DIAGNOSIS

Postpartum depression has a later onset, less lability, and more typical "vegetative" symptoms. Importantly, given the high prevalence of postpartum blues, a not insignificant proportion of women with postpartum blues will go on to develop a postpartum depression, and hence any persistence of depressive symptoms beyond two weeks postpartum should prompt a clinical re-evaluation.

TREATMENT

Support from family and friends is indicated; a short half-life benzodiazepine may be used for a few days if insomnia is severe. Antidepressants are not indicated, given the fact that the postpartum blues generally remit before an antidepressant could become effective.

BIBLIOGRAPHY

Best NR, Wiley M, Stump K, et al. Binding of tritiated yohimbine to platelets in women with maternity blues. *Psychological Medicine* 1988;18:837-842.

Harris B, Lovett L, Newcombe RG, et al. Maternity blues and major endocrine changes: Cardiff puerperal mood and hormone study II. *British Medical Journal* 1994;308:949-953.

Iles S, Gath D, Kennedy H. Maternity blues. II. A comparison between post-operative women and post-natal women. *The British Journal of Psychiatry* 1989;155:363-366.

Kennerly H, Gath D. Maternity blues. I. Detection and measurement by questionnaire. *British Journal of Psychiatry* 1989;155:356.

Metz A, Stump K, Cowen PJ, et al. Changes in platelet alpha 2-adrenocreceptor binding post partum: possible relation to maternity blues. *Lancet* 1983;1:495-498.

O'Hara MW, Schlechte JA, Lewis DA, et al. Prospective study of the postpartum blues, biological and psychosocial factors. *Archives of General Psychiatry* 1991;48:801.

Pitt B. Maternity blues. *British Journal of Psychiatry* 1973;122:431.

Rohde LA, Busnello E, Wolf A, et al. Maternity blues in Brazilian women. *Acta Psychiatrica Scandinavica* 1997;95:231-235.

Yalom ID, Lunde DT, Moos RH, et al. "Post partum blues" syndrome: a description and related variables. *Archives of General Psychiatry* 1968; 18:16.

79   Postpartum Depression

Depressive episodes may occur in from 10-15% of women in the immediate postpartum months, and it appears that two disorders may be occurring here. On the one hand, a proportion of these women have a history of depressive episodes occurring outside the puerperium, and such cases are probably best characterized as having what the DSM-IV terms a major depression "with postpartum onset." On the other hand, there are also women who only have depressive episodes in the puerperium and it may well be that these women have a distinct disorder, namely postpartum, or postnatal depression.

ONSET

The onset of symptoms occurs gradually anywhere from several weeks to several months after delivery. An episode of the postpartum blues may or may not precede it.

CLINICAL FEATURES

The symptoms are similar to those of a depressive episode as described in the chapter on major depression: patients complain of a depressed mood, anxiety, fatigue, anhedonia, difficulty concentrating, crying spells, anorexia, and initial insomnia. There may however, be some differences: anxiety tends to be worse during a postpartum depression and, when obsessions occur during a postpartum depression, they tend to be more violent: classically, patients experience "horrific temptations" to kill their baby.

Typically, the patient feels inadequate in her ability to care for the infant.

COURSE

The course is variable; most recover within months to a year; however, in some cases symptoms become chronic. Patients have a significant chance of recurrence during subsequent postpartum periods.

COMPLICATIONS

Typically, patients may experience difficulty in establishing a mutually satisfying bond with the infant. In some cases suicide may occur, and, rarely, infanticide.

ETIOLOGY

Postpartum depression may represent an unusual sensitivity of mood-regulating structures within the central nervous system to the profound hormonal changes seen postpartum. One study looked at two groups of women: both groups had a history of depressive episodes, but in one they were confined to the puerperium whereas in the other they occurred outside the puerperium. All patients were euthymic at the time of the study, and all received chronic treatment with supraphysiologic doses of estradiol and progesterone for 8 weeks, after which the medications were abruptly discontinued. In the group of women with a history of postpartum depression, the withdrawal of gonadal steroids was followed by a depression in the majority, whereas in the group with a history of depression outside the puerperium, no depression occurred.

There are also reports demonstrating an association between the presence of anti-thyroid peroxidase antibodies antenatally with the occurrence of depression postnatally, regardless of whether TSH or thyroxine levels were normal or not. Treatment of women with thyroxine in the puerperium is ineffective in preventing postpartum depression, and the import of these findings of anti-thyroid antibodies is unclear.

DIFFERENTIAL DIAGNOSIS

The postpartum blues begin earlier and for the most part remit before the typical time of onset of postpartum depression. Furthermore, vegetative symptoms are less common in the postpartum blues.

Sheehan's syndrome is distinguished by deficient lactation, an absence of menstruation, and often by loss of pubic and axillary hair.

Patients with a preexisting major depression may, as noted above, experience an episode of depression in the postpartum period. These patients are distinguished from those with postpartum depression by the course; patients with major depressive disorder have episodes outside of the postpartum period, whereas the episodes of patients with postpartum depression occur only within the postpartum period. Patients with bipolar disorder may also have a depression in the postpartum period, and the same reasoning applies here as for the differential diagnosis of major depression.

TREATMENT

Fluoxetine, 20 mg, cognitive-behavioral therapy and interpersonal therapy have all been shown to be effective. In the case of fluoxetine, treatment should be continued until the patient has been asymptomatic for a matter of months, after which it may be discontinued and the patient observed closely for any signs of relapse. Of interest, a double-blinded study also demonstrated the effectiveness of estradiol patches, 0.2 mg daily. There are no comparison studies of fluoxetine and estradiol, and hence the decision between them might best be made in light of the patient's overall obstetric and gynecologic care.

Attempts have been made to prevent depression in women with a history of the postpartum depression by giving an antidepressant (e.g., nortriptyline) immediately postpartum, but the results were no better than with placebo. Whether fluoxetine would work better is an open question.

Provision must be made for care for the infant, with a gradual transition back to full parenthood as the patient recovers. If antidepressants are used, breast-feeding is generally contraindicated.

BIBLIOGRAPHY

Appleby L, Warner R, Whitton A, et al. A controlled trial of fluoxetine and cognitive-behavioral counseling in the treatment of postnatal depression. *British Medical Journal* 1997;314:932-936.

Bloch M, Schmidt PJ, Danaceau M, et al. Effects of gonadal steroids in women with a history of postpartum depression. *The American Journal of Psychiatry* 2000;157:924-930.

Chaudron LH, Klein MH, Remington P, et al. Predictors, prodromes and incidence of postpartum depression. *Journal of Psychosomatic Obstetrics and Gynaecology* 2001;21:103-112.

Cooper PJ, Murray L. Course and recurrence of postnatal depression. Evidence for the specificity of the diagnostic concept. *The British Journal of Psychiatry* 1995;166:191-195.

Gregoire AJ, Kumar R, Everitt B, et al. Transdermal oestrogen for treatment of severe postnatal depression. *Lancet* 1996;347:930-933.

Harris B, Oretti R, Lazarus J, et al. Randomized trial of thyroixine to prevent postnatal depression in thyroid-antibody-positive women. *The British Journal of Psychiatry* 2002;180:327-330.

Hendrick V, Altshuler L, Strouse T, et al. Postpartum and nonpostpartum depression: differences in presentation and response to pharmacologic treatment. *Depression and Anxiety* 2000;11:66-72.

Kuijpens JL, Vader HL, Drexhage HA, et al. Thyroid peroxidase antibodies during gestation are a marker for subsequent depression postpartum. *European Journal of Endocrinology* 2001;145:579-584.

O'Hara MW, Stuart S, Gorman LL, et al. Efficacy of interpersonal psychotherapy for postpartum depression. *Archives of General Psychiatry* 2000;57:1039-1045.

Wisner KL, Peindl KS, Gigliotti T, et al. Obsessions and compulsions in women with postpartum depression. *The Journal of Clinical Psychiatry* 1999;60:176-180.

Wisner KL, Perel JM, Peindl KS, et al. Prevention of recurrent postpartum depression: a randomized clinical trial. *The Journal of Clinical Psychiatry* 2001;62:82-86.

Wisner KL, Parry BL, Piontek CM. Postpartum depression. *The New England Journal of Medicine* 2002;347:194-199.

80 Bipolar Disorder (DSM-IV-TR #296.0-296.89)

Bipolar disorder is characterized by the occurrence of at least one manic or mixed-manic episode during the patient's lifetime. Most patients also, at other times, have one or more depressive episodes. In the intervals between these episodes, most patients return to their normal state of well-being. Thus bipolar disorder is a "cyclic" or "periodic" illness, with patients cycling "up" into a manic or mixed-manic episode, then returning to normal, and cycling "down" into a depressive episode from which they likewise eventually more or less recover.

Bipolar disorder is probably equally common among men and women and has a lifetime prevalence of from 1.3 to 1.6%.

Bipolar disorder in the past has been referred to as "manic depressive illness, circular type." As noted in the introduction to the chapter on major depression, the term "manic depressive illness," at least in the United States, has more and more come to be used as equivalent to bipolar disorder. As this convention, however, is not worldwide, the term "bipolar" may be better, as it clearly indicates that the patient has an illness characterized by "swings" to the manic "pole" and generally also to the depressive "pole."

ONSET

Bipolar disorder may present with either a depressive or a manic episode, and the peak age of onset for the first episode, whether depressive or manic, lies in the teens and early twenties. Earlier onsets may occur; indeed some patients may have their first episode at 10 years of age or younger. After the twenties the incidence of first episodes gradually decreases, with well over 90% of patients having had their first episode before the age of 50. Onsets as late as the seventies or eighties have, though very rare, been seen.

Premorbidly, these patients may either be normal or display mild symptoms for a variable period of time before the first episode of illness.

CLINICAL FEATURES

The discussion of signs and symptoms proceeds in three parts: first, a discussion of a manic episode; second, a discussion of a depressive episode; and, third, a discussion of a mixed-manic episode.

Manic Episode

The nosology of the various stages of a manic episode has changed over the decades. In current DSM-IV nomenclature, hypomanic episodes are separated from the more severe full manic episodes, which in turn are characterized as either mild, moderate, severe, or severe with psychotic features. Kraepelin, however, divided the "manic states" into four forms—hypomania, acute mania, delusional mania, and delirious mania—and noted that his observation revealed "the occurrence of gradual transitions between all the various states." In a similar vein, Carlson and Goodwin, in their elegant paper of 1973, divided a manic episode into "three stages": hypomania, or stage I; acute mania, or stage II; and delirious mania, or stage III. As this "staging" of a manic episode is very useful from a descriptive and differential diagnostic point of view, it is used in this chapter. Thus, when the term "manic episode" is used it may refer to any one of the three stages of mania: hypomania, acute mania, or delirious mania.

Manic episodes are often preceded by a prodrome, lasting from a few days to a few months, of mild and often transitory and indistinct manic symptoms. At times, however, no prodromal warning signs may occur, and the episode starts quite abruptly. When this occurs, patients often unaccountably wake up during the night full of energy and vigor—the so-called "manic alert."

The cardinal symptoms of mania are the following: heightened mood (either euphoric or irritable); flight of ideas and pressure of speech; and increased energy, decreased need for sleep, and hyperactivity. These cardinal symptoms are most plainly evident in hypomania. In acute mania they exacerbate and may be joined by delusions and some fragmentation of behavior, and in delirious mania only tattered scraps of the cardinal symptoms may be present, otherwise being obscured by florid and often bizarre psychotic symptoms. Although all patients experience a hypomanic stage, and almost all progress to at least a touch of acute mania, only a minority finally are propelled into delirious mania. The rapidity with which patients pass from hypomania through acute mania and on to delirious mania varies from a week to a few days to as little as a few hours. Indeed, in such hyperacute onsets, the patient may have already passed through the hypomanic stage and the acute manic stage before he is brought to medical attention. The duration of an entire manic episode varies from the extremes of as little as a few days or less to many years, and rarely even to a decade or more. On the average, however, most first episodes of mania last from several weeks up to 3 months. In the natural course of events, symptoms tend to gradually subside; after they fade many patients feel guilty over what they did and perhaps are full of self-reproach. Most patients are able to recall what happened during hypomania and acute mania; however, memory is often spotty for the events of delirious mania. With this brief general description of a manic episode in mind, what follows now is a more thorough discussion of each of the three stages of mania.

Hypomania. In hypomania the mood is heightened and elevated. Most often these patients are euphoric, full of jollity and cheerfulness. Though at times selfish and pompous, their mood nevertheless is often quite "infectious." They joke, make wisecracks and delightful insinuations, and those around them often get quite caught up in the spirit, always laughing with the patient, and not at him. Indeed, when physicians find themselves unable to suppress their own laughter when interviewing a patient, the diagnosis of hypomania is very likely. Self-esteem and self-confidence are greatly increased. Inflated with their own grandiosity, patients may boast of fabulous achievements and lay out plans for even grander conquests in the future. In a minority of patients, however, irritability may be the dominant mood. Patients become demanding, inconsiderate, and intemperate. They are constantly dissatisfied and intolerant of others, and brook no opposition. Trifling slights may enrage the patient, and violent outbursts are not uncommon. At times, pronounced lability of mood may be evident; otherwise supremely contented patients may suddenly turn dark, churlish, and irritable.

In flight of ideas the patient's train of thought is characterized by rapid leaps from one topic to another. When flight of ideas is mild, the connections between the patient's successive ideas, though perhaps tenuous, may nonetheless be "understandable" to the listener. In somewhat higher grades of flight of ideas, however, the connections may seem to be illogical and come to depend more on puns and word plays. This flight of ideas is often accompanied by pressure of thought. Patients may report that their thoughts race, that they have too many thoughts, that they run on pell-mell. Typically, patients also display pressure of speech. Here the listener is deluged with a torrent of words. Speech may become imperious, incredibly rapid, and almost unstoppable. Occasionally, after great urging and with great effort, patients may be able to keep silent and withhold their speech, but not for long, and soon the dam bursts once again.

Energy is greatly, even immensely, increased, and patients feel less and less the need for sleep. They are on the go, busy and involved throughout the day. They wish to be a part of life and to be involved more and more in the lives of those around them. They are strangers to fatigue and are still hyperactive and ready to go when others must go to bed. Eventually, the patients themselves may finally go to sleep, but within a very brief period of time they then awaken, wide-eyed, and, finding no one else up, they may seek someone to wake up, or perhaps take a whistling stroll of the darkened neighborhood, or, if alone, they may spend the hours before daybreak cleaning out closets or drawers, catching up on old correspondence, or even paying bills.

In addition to these cardinal symptoms, hypomanic patients are often extremely distractible. Other conversations and events, though peripheral to the patients' present purposes, are as if glittering jewels that they must attend to, to take as their own, or simply to admire. In listening to patients, one may find that a fragment of another conversation has suddenly been interpolated into their flight of ideas, or they may stop suddenly and declare their unbounded admiration for the physician's clothing, only then again to become one with the preceding rush of speech.

Hypomanic patients rarely recognize that anything is wrong with them, and though their judgment is obviously impaired they have no insight into that condition. Indeed, as far as hypomanic patients are concerned, the rest of the world is sick and impaired; if only the rest of the world could feel as they do and see as clearly as they do, then the rest of the world would be sure to join them. These patients often enter into business arrangements with unbounded and completely uncritical enthusiasm. Ventures are begun, stocks are bought on a hunch, money is loaned out without collateral, and when the family fortune is spent, the patient, undaunted, after perhaps a brief pause, may seek to borrow more money for yet another prospect. Spending sprees are also typical. Clothes, furniture, and cars may be bought; the credit card is pushed to the limit and checks, without any foundation in the bank, may be written with the utmost alacrity. Excessive jewelry and flamboyant clothing are especially popular. The overinvolvement of patients with other people typically leads to the most injudicious and at times unwelcome entanglements. Passionate encounters are the rule, and hypersexuality is not uncommon. Many a female hypomanic has become pregnant during such escapades. If confronted with the consequences of their behavior, hypomanic patients typically take offense, turn perhaps indignantly self-righteous, or are quick with numerous, more or less plausible excuses. When hypomanic patients are primarily irritable rather then euphoric, their demanding, intrusive, and injudicious behavior often brings them into conflict with others and with the law.

Acute Mania. The transition from hypomania to acute mania is marked by a severe exacerbation of the symptoms seen in hypomania, and the appearance of delusions. Typically, the delusions are grandiose: millions of dollars are held in trust for them; passersby stop and wait in deferential awe as they pass by; the President will announce their elevation to cabinet rank. Religious delusions are very common. The patients are prophets, elected by God for a magnificent, yet hidden, purpose. They are enthroned; indeed God has made way for them. Sometimes these grandiose delusions are held constantly; however, in other cases patients may suddenly boldly announce their belief, then toss it aside with laughter, only to announce yet another one. Persecutory delusions may also appear and are quite common in those who are of a predominantly irritable mood. The patients' failures are not their own but the results of the treachery of colleagues or family. They are persecuted by those jealous of their grandeur; they are pilloried, crucified by the enemy. Terrorists have set a watch on their houses and seek to destroy them before they can ascend to their thrones. Occasionally, along with delusions, patients may have isolated hallucinations. Grandiose patients hear a chorus of angels singing their praises; the persecuted patients hear the resentful muttering of the envious crowd.

The mood in acute mania is further heightened and often quite labile. Domineeringly good-natured one moment, the patient, if thwarted at all, may erupt into a furious rage of screaming, swearing, and assaultiveness. Furniture may be smashed and clothes torn apart. The already irritable patient may become consistently, and very dangerously, hostile.

Flight of ideas and pressured speech become very intense. Patients seem unable to cease talking; they may scream, shout, bellow, sing in a loud voice or preach in a declamatory fashion to anyone whose ear they can catch.

Hyperactivity becomes more pronounced, and the patient's behavior may begin to fragment. Impulses come at cross purposes, and patients, though increasingly active, may be unable to complete anything. Fragments of activity abound: patients may run, hop in place, roll about the floor, leap from bed to bed, race this way and then that, or repeatedly change their clothes at a furious pace.

Occasionally, patients in acute mania may evidence a passing fragment of insight: they may suddenly leap to the tops of tables and proclaim that they are "mad," then laugh, lose the thought, and jump back into their pursuits of a moment ago. Some may devote themselves to writing, flooding reams of paper with an extravagant handwriting, leaving behind an almost unintelligible, tangential flight of written ideas. Patients may dress themselves in the most fantastic ways. Women may decorate themselves with garlands of flowers and wear the most seductive of dresses. Men may be festooned with ribbons and jewelry. Unrestrainable sexuality may come to the fore. Patients may openly and shamelessly proposition complete strangers; some may openly and exultantly masturbate. Strength may be greatly increased, and sensitivity to pain may be lost.

Delirious Mania. The transition to delirious mania is marked by the appearance of confusion, more hallucinations, and a marked intensification of the symptoms seen in acute mania. A dreamlike clouding of consciousness may occur. Patients may mistake where they are and with whom. They cry out that they are in heaven or in hell, in a palace or in a prison; those around them have all changed—the physician is an executioner; fellow patients are secret slaves. Hallucinations, more commonly auditory than visual, appear momentarily and then are gone, perhaps only to be replaced by another. The thunderous voice of God sounds; angels whisper secret encouragements; the devil boasts at having the patient now; the patient's children cry out in despair. Creatures and faces may appear; lights flash and lightning cracks through the room. Grandiose and persecutory delusions intensify, especially the persecutory ones. Bizarre delusions may occur, including Schneiderian delusions. Electrical currents from the nurses' station control the patient; the patient remains in a telepathic communication with the physician or with the other patients.

Mood is extremely dysphoric and labile. Though some patients still are occasionally enthusiastic and jolly, irritability is generally quite pronounced. There may be cursing, and swearing; violent threats are made, and if patients are restrained they may spit on those around them. Sudden despair and wretched crying may grip the patient, only to give way in moments to unrestrained laughter.

Flight of ideas becomes extremely intense and fragmented. Sentences are rarely completed, and speech often consists of words or short phrases having only the most tenuous connection with the other. Pressure of speech likewise increases, and in extreme cases the patient's speech may become an incoherent and rapidly changing jumble. Yet even in the highest grades of incoherence, where associations become markedly loosened, these patients remain in lively contact with the world about them. Fragments of nearby conversations are interpolated into their speech, or they may make a sudden reference to the physician's clothing or to a disturbance somewhere else on the ward.

Hyperactivity is extreme, and behavior disintegrates into numerous and disparate fragments of purposeful activity. Patients may agitatedly pace from one wall to the other, jump to a table top, beat their chest and scream, assault anyone nearby, pound on the windows, tear the bed sheets, prance, twitter, or throw off their clothes. Impulsivity may be extreme, and the patient may unexpectedly commit suicide by leaping from a window.

Self-control is absolutely lost, and the patient has no insight and no capacity for it. Attempting to reason with the patient in delirious mania is fruitless, even assuming that the patient stays still enough for one to try. The frenzy of these patients is remarkable to behold and rarely forgotten. Yet in the height of delirious mania, one may be surprised by the appearance of a sudden calm. Instantly, the patient may become mute and immobile, and such a catatonic stupor may persist from minutes to hours only to give way again to a storm of activity. Other catatonic signs, such as echolalia and echopraxia and even waxy flexibility, may also be seen.

As noted earlier not all manic patients pass through all three stages; indeed some may not progress past a hypomanic state. Regardless, however, of whether the peak of severity of the individual patient's episode is found in hypomania, in acute mania, or in delirious mania, once that peak has been reached, a more or less gradual and orderly subsidence of symptoms occurs, which to a greater or lesser degree retraces the same symptoms seen in the earlier escalation. Finally, once the last vestiges of hypomanic symptoms have faded, the patient is often found full of self-reproach and shame over what he has done. Some may be reluctant to leave the hospital for fear of reproach by those they harmed and offended while they were in the manic episode.

In current nomenclature, those patients whose manic episodes never pass beyond the stage of hypomania are said to have "Bipolar II" disorder, in contrast with "Bipolar I" disorder wherein the mania does escalate beyond the hypomanic stage. Recent data indicate that bipolar II disorder may be more common than bipolar I disorder; however, should a patient with bipolar II disorder ever have a manic episode wherein stage II or III symptoms occurred, then the diagnosis would have to be revised to bipolar I.

Occasionally the age of the patient may influence the presentation of mania. Adolescents and children, for example, seem particularly prone to the very rapid development of delirious mania. On the other extreme, in the elderly, one may see little or no hyperactivity. Some elderly manic patients may sit in the same chair all day long, chattering away in an explosive flight of ideas. Mental retardation may also influence the presentation of mania. Here in the absence of speech one may see only increased, seemingly purposeless, activity.

Depressive Episodes

The depressive episodes seen in bipolar disorder, in contrast to those typically seen in a major depression, tend to come on fairly acutely, over perhaps a few weeks, and often occur without any significant precipitating factors. They tend to be characterized by psychomotor retardation, hyperphagia, and hypersomnolence and are not uncommonly accompanied by delusions or hallucinations. On the average, untreated, these bipolar depressions tend to last about a half year.

Mood is depressed and often irritable. The patients are discontented and fault-finding and may even come to loathe not only themselves but also everyone around them.

Energy is lacking; patients may feel apathetic or at times weighted down.

Thought becomes sluggish and slow. Patients cannot concentrate to read and cannot remember what they do read. Comprehending alternatives and bringing themselves to decisions may be impossible.

Patients may lose interest in life; things appear dull and heavy and have no attraction.

Many patients feel a greatly increased need for sleep. Some may succumb and sleep 10, 14, or 18 hours a day. Yet no matter how much sleep they get, they awake exhausted, as if they had not slept at all. Appetite may also be increased and weight gain may occur, occasionally to an amazing degree. Conversely, some patients may experience insomnia or loss of appetite.

Psychomotor retardation is the rule, although some patients may show agitation. In psychomotor retardation the patient may lie in bed or sit in the chair for hours, perhaps all day, profoundly apathetic and scarcely moving at all. Speech is rare; if a sentence is begun, it may die in the speaking of it, as if the patient had not the energy to bring it to conclusion. At times the facial expression may become tense and pained, as if the patient were under some great inner constraint.

Pessimism and bleak despair permeate these patients' outlooks. Guilt abounds, and on surveying their lives patients find themselves the worst of failures, the greatest of sinners. Effort appears futile, and enterprises begun in the past may be abandoned. They may have recurrent thoughts of suicide, and impulsive suicide attempts may occur.

Delusions of guilt and of well-deserved punishment and persecution are common. Patients may believe that they have let children starve, murdered their spouses, poisoned the wells. Unspeakable punishments are carried out: their eyes are gouged out; they are slowly hung from the gallows; they have contracted syphilis or AIDS, and these are a just punishment for their sins.

Hallucinations may also appear and may be quite fantastic. Heads float through the air; the soup boils black with blood. Auditory hallucinations are more common, and patients may hear the heavenly court pronounce judgment. Foul odors may be smelled, and poison may be tasted in the food.

In general a depressive episode in bipolar disorder subsides gradually. Occasionally, however, it may come to an abrupt termination. A patient may arise one morning, after months of suffering, and announce a complete return to fitness and vitality. In such cases, a manic episode is likely to soon follow.

Mixed-Manic Episode

Mixed-manic episodes are not as common as manic episodes or depressive episodes, but tend to last longer. Here one sees various admixtures of manic and depressive symptoms, sometimes in sequence, sometimes simultaneously. Euphoric patients, hyperactive and pressured in speech, may suddenly plunge into despair and collapse weeping into chairs, only to rise again within hours to their former elated state. Even more extraordinary, patients may be weeping uncontrollably, with a look of unutterable despair on their faces, yet say that they are elated, that they never felt so well in their lives, and then go on to execute a lively dance, all the while with tears still streaming down their faces. Or a depressed and psychomotorically retarded patient may consistently dress in the brightest of clothes, showing a fixed smile on an otherwise expressionless face. These mixed-manic episodes must be distinguished from the transitional periods that may appear in patients who "cycle" directly from a manic into a depressive episode, or vice versa, without any intervening euthymic interval. These transitional periods are often marked by an admixture of both manic and depressive symptoms; however, they do not "stand alone" as episodes of illness unto themselves, but are always both immediately preceded and followed by a more typical episode of homogenous manic or homogenous depressive symptoms. In contrast the mixed-manic episode "stands alone." It starts with mixed symptoms, endures with them, and finishes with them, and is neither immediately preceded nor immediately followed by an episode of mania or by an episode of depression.

At this point, before proceeding to a consideration of course, two other disorders that are strongly associated with bipolar disorder should be mentioned, namely alcoholism and cocaine addiction. During manic episodes, patients with these addictions are especially likely to take cocaine or drink even more heavily, and the effects of these substances may cloud the clinical picture.

COURSE

Bipolar disorder is an episodic or, as noted earlier, "cyclical" illness, being characterized in most patients by the intermittent lifelong appearance of episodes of illness, in between which most patients experience a "euthymic" interval during which they more or less return to their normal state of health.

The pattern and sequencing of successive episodes is quite variable among patients. The duration of the euthymic interval varies from as little as a few weeks or days to as long as years, or even decades. In contrast, however, to the extreme variability of the euthymic intervals among patients, finding a certain regular pattern in the history of any given patient is not unusual. Indeed in some patients the euthymic interval is so regular that patients can predict sometimes to the month when the next episode will occur. The postpartum period is a time of increased risk. Occasionally, one may also see a "seasonal" pattern, with manic episodes more likely in the spring or early summer and depressive ones in the fall or winter.

Early on in the overall course of the illness the cycle length, or time from the onset of one episode to the onset of the next, tends to shorten. Specifically, whereas the duration of the episodes themselves tends to be stable, the euthymic interval shortens, so episodes come progressively closer together. With time, however, the duration of the euthymic interval stabilizes.

Patients who have four or more episodes of illness in any one year are customarily referred to as "rapid cyclers." Although only about 10% of all patients with bipolar disorder display such a pattern of rapid cycling, these patients are nevertheless clinically quite important as they tend to be relatively "resistant" to many currently available treatments. On the other extreme, the euthymic interval may be so long, lasting many decades, that the patient dies before the second episode is "due," thereby having only one episode of illness during an entire lifespan.

The sequence of episodes is also quite variable among patients. Rarely would one find a patient whose course is characterized by regularly alternating manic and depressive episodes; most patients show a preponderance of either depressive episodes or of manic ones. For example, in an extreme case a patient may have throughout life perhaps six depressive episodes and only one manic one. On the other extreme, another patient might have up to a dozen episodes of mania and only one depressive one. Indeed one may encounter a patient who has only manic episodes and never any depressive ones. Such "unipolar manic" patients are very rare. In general, a depressive preponderance is more common in females, and a manic one in males.

As noted earlier, for most patients the interval between episodes is euthymic and free of symptoms. In at least a quarter of all cases, however, the interval may be "colored" by very mild symptoms, and the direction of this "coloring," or its "polarity," correlates with the preponderance of episodes. For example, a patient with very mild subhypomanic symptoms during the interval is likely to have more manic episodes than depressive ones, and the converse holds true for the patients whose interval is clouded with mild depression or fatigue. In general, among women the preponderance of episodes are depressive; among men, manic.

In perhaps a quarter of all cases, the course exhibits "coupling." Here a manic episode may invariably and immediately be followed by a depressive one, or vice versa. In such cases the transition from one episode to the next may be marked by a mixture of symptoms, as if the various symptoms of the preceding episode trailed off at different rates, while the various symptoms of the following episode appeared also at varying rates, such that the two coupled episodes in a sense overlapped and interdigitated with each other, with this interdigitation presenting as the mixture of symptoms. Such "overlap" or transitional experiences must, as noted earlier, be distinguished from mixed-manic episodes proper, which stand on their own.

Occasionally, one may find bipolar patients in whom certain conditions, pharmacologic and otherwise, can more or less reliably precipitate a manic episode. These include serotoninergic agents such as tryptophan or 5-hydroxytryptophan; noradrenergic agents, such as cocaine, stimulants, or sympathomimetics, or situations in which noradrenergic tone is increased as in alcohol or sedative-hypnotic withdrawal or in the abrupt discontinuation of long-term treatment with clonidine; dopaminergic agents such as L-dopa or bromocriptine; and treatment with exogenous steroids, such as prednisone. Older antidepressants, such as the MAOIs and tricyclics, are particularly notorious for precipitating manic episodes in bipolar patients, and some evidence suggests that these antidepressants, in addition to being capable of precipitating a manic episode, may also alter the fundamental course of bipolar disorder and increase the frequency with which future episodes occur: newer antidepressants, such as SSRIs, bupropion and venlafaxine, do not appear as likely to precipitate mania. Phototherapy may also induce manic episodes in those patients whose course exhibits a "seasonal pattern."

COMPLICATIONS

In mania, spending sprees and ill-advised business ventures may land patients in serious debt, or even bankruptcy. Hypersexuality may lead to unplanned and unwanted pregnancies or ill-considered marriages. A reckless exuberance may carry the patient past all speed limits and into conflict with the law; accidents are common. Irritable manics are likewise often in conflict with the law and may pick fights and create disputes with whomever they come in contact. Friendships may be broken, and divorce may occur.

Suicide occurs in from 10 to 20% of patients with bipolar disorder and appears to be more common in those who have only hypomanic episodes (i.e., those with bipolar II disorder) than in those whose manic episodes progress beyond the first stage (i.e., those with bipolar I disorder). Although most suicides appear to occur during episodes of depression, patients in a mixed-manic episode may be at an even higher risk.

The complications of a depressive episode are as outlined in the chapter on major depression.

ETIOLOGY

Genetic factors almost certainly play a role in bipolar disorder. A higher prevalence of bipolar disorder exists among the first-degree relatives of patients with bipolar disorder than among the relatives of controls or the relatives of patients with major depression, and the concordance rate among monozygotic twins is significantly higher than that among dizygotic twins. Similarly and most tellingly, adoption studies have demonstrated that the prevalence of bipolar disorder is several-fold higher among the biologic parents of bipolar patients than among the biologic parents of control adoptees.

Genetic studies in bipolar disorder have been plagued by failures of replication. In all likelihood, multiple genes on multiple different chromosomes are involved, each conferring a susceptibility to the disease.

Autopsy studies, likewise, have often yielded inconsistent results. Perhaps the most promising finding is of a reduced neuronal number in the locus ceruleus and median raphe nucleus.

Endocrinologic studies have yielded robust findings, similar to those found in major depression, including non-suppression on the dexamethasone suppression test and a blunted TSH response to TRH infusion.

Other robust findings include a shortened latency to REM sleep upon infusion of arecoline and the remarkable ability of intravenous physostigmine to not only bring patients out of mania but also to cast them down past their baseline and into a depression.

Taken together, these findings are consistent with the notion that bipolar disorder is, in large part, an inherited disorder characterized by episodic perturbations in endocrinologic, noradrenergic, serotoninergic and cholinergic function, with these in turn possibly being related to subtle microanatomic changes in relevant brainstem structures.

DIFFERENTIAL DIAGNOSIS

In distinguishing bipolar disorder from other disorders, the single most useful differential feature is the course of the illness. Essentially no other disorder left untreated presents with recurrent episodes of mood disturbance at least one of which is a manic episode, with more or less full restitution to normal functioning between episodes. Thus if the patient in question has had previous episodes and if the available history is complete, then one can generally state with certainty whether the patient has bipolar disorder. However, these are two big "ifs," and in clinical practice history may either be absent or unobtainable, and herein arises diagnostic difficulty.

Occasionally a patient in a manic episode is brought to the emergency room by police with no other history except that he was arrested for disturbing the peace. If the patient is in the stage of acute mania with perhaps irritability and delusions of persecution, one might wonder if the patient is currently in the midst of the onset of paranoid schizophrenia or of its exacerbation. Here the behavior of the patient when left undisturbed is helpful: left to themselves, patients with paranoid schizophrenia often sit quietly, patiently waiting for the next assault, whereas patients with acute mania continue to display their hyperactivity and pressured speech. If the patient is in the stage of delirious mania, the differential would include an acute exacerbation of catatonic schizophrenia and also a delirium from some other cause. The quality of the hyperactivity seen in the excited subtype of catatonic schizophrenia is different from that seen in mania. The catatonic schizophrenic, no matter how frenzied, remains self-involved and has little contact with those around him. By contrast, manic patients, no matter how fragmented their behavior, show a desire and a compelling interest to be involved with others. In the highest grade of delirious mania, the patient, as noted earlier, may lapse

into a confusional stupor. At this point, the differential becomes very wide, as discussed in the chapter on delirium. At times, a "cross-sectional" view of the patient, say in the emergency room, may allow an accurate diagnosis; however, a "longitudinal" view is always more helpful. As noted earlier, all patients in delirious mania or acute mania have already passed from relatively normal functioning through the distinctive stage of mania. Obtaining a history of this progression from normal through and past stage I hypomania allows for a more certain diagnosis.

The distinction between secondary mania and a manic episode of bipolar disorder is discussed in that chapter.

At times patients with schizoaffective disorder, bipolar type, may be very difficult to distinguish from those with bipolar disorder. Here a precise interval history is absolutely necessary. In schizoaffective disorder psychotic symptoms, such as delusions, hallucinations, or incoherence, persist between the episodes, in contrast to the "free" intervals seen in bipolar disorder. The interval psychotic symptoms seen in schizoaffective disorder may be very mild indeed, and thus close and repeated observation over extended periods of time may be required to ascertain their presence.

Cyclothymia may at times present diagnostic difficulty, for it also presents a history of discrete individual episodes. The difference is that in cyclothymia the manic symptoms are very mild. The possibility also exists, however, that the apparently cyclothymic patient is presenting, in fact, with a very long prodrome to bipolar disorder. Thus continued observation over many years may necessitate a diagnostic revision if a manic episode should ever occur.

The differential between a postpartum psychosis and a bipolar disorder that has become "entrained" to the postpartum period is discussed in that chapter.

The persistence of very mild affective symptoms between episodes might suggest, depending on the polarity of the symptoms, a diagnosis of dysthymia or of hyperthymia. Here, however, temporal continuity of these symptoms with a full episode of illness betrays their true nature, that of either a prodrome or of a condition of only partial remission of a prior episode.

The distinction between a depressive episode occurring as part of a major depression and one occurring as part of bipolar disorder is considered in the chapter on major depression.

TREATMENT

The overall treatment of bipolar disorder is conveniently approached by considering, in turn, the treatment of the manic or mixed-manic episode first, then the treatment of the depressive episode, in each instance considering three phases of treatment: acute, continuation, and preventive. As will be seen, of all the medications useful in bipolar disorder, lithium is probably the best choice as it is the only one which has been shown to be effective for all three phases of treatment for both manic and depressive episodes.

Manic or Mixed-Manic Episodes

Acute Treatment. The acute treatment of a manic or mixed-manic episode almost always involves the administration of either a mood stabilizer (i.e., lithium, valproate or carbamazepine) or an antipsychotic (i.e., olanzapine, risperidone, aripiprazole, quetiapine or ziprasidone), or most commonly, a combination of a mood stabilizer and an antipsychotic. Although there are no hard and fast rules for choosing among these agents, some general guidelines may be offered. Certainly, if the patient has a history of an excellent response to a particular agent, then it should be seriously considered. Lacking such a history, and assuming there are no significant contraindications, the first choice among the mood stabilizers is probably lithium, as it has the longest track record. Divalproex is a close second, and, in the case of episodes with a significant depressive component, and certainly in the case of a mixed-manic episode, is actually superior to lithium. Another advantage of divalproex is the rapidity with which it becomes effective when a "loading" strategy is used, with patients often responding in a matter of days, in contrast with the week or two required with lithium. Carbamazepine is probably a little less effective than lithium, and, in general, is not as well-tolerated. Among the antipsychotics, the first choice is probably olanzapine in that it has the longest track record among these second generation agents in this regard and has also, in contrast with the other second generation agents, been shown to be effective in preventive treatment.

When symptoms are relatively mild, that is to say of hypomanic intensity, utilization of a mood stabilizer alone may be sufficient. However, when the mania has escalated into stage II or III, a mood stabilizer alone is generally not capable of controlling the clinical storm quickly enough, and in such cases it is common practice to initiate treatment with a combination of a mood stabilizer and one of the second-generation antipsychotics. In emergent situations, one may also employ one of the protocols outlined in the chapter on rapid pharmacologic treatment of agitation. Consideration should also be given to ECT: bilateral ECT is effective for mania and is indicated when the foregoing treatments are not successful or in life-threatening situations where urgent improvement is absolutely required. Should ECT be utilized, lithium should not be administered concurrently, as it may enhance ECT-induced confusion.

Many manic patients require admission to a locked unit. Stimulation, including visitors, mail, and phone calls, should be kept to an absolute minimum, as it routinely exacerbates manic symptoms. Indeed, occasional patients in acute mania, still possessed of a few tattered shreds of insight, may demand to be put in seclusion. Isolated from all stimuli, they gradually improve, although their symptoms only partially abate. A calm, patient, and nonconfrontive manner is generally best; sometimes sharing the patient's jokes may be calming and helpful in enlisting cooperation. At times, however, a "show of force" may be necessary; indeed violent, irritable, and very agitated patients, though completely unfazed by routine measures, may calm down immediately upon the appearance of several formidable male orderlies, who, though calm, clearly "mean business." Restraints, however, may be required.

Continuation Treatment. Once acute treatment has been successful in bringing the manic symptoms under control, continuation treatment is begun. As noted earlier the average duration of the first manic episode is about 3 months, and that of a mixed-manic episode a little longer. The purpose of continuation treatment is to prevent a breakthrough of symptoms until such time as the episode itself has run its course. Generally this is accomplished by continuing the regimen that was effective during the acute phase. If lithium is used it may be necessary during the continuation phase to reduce the dose. In many patients even though the dose of lithium is held constant, the blood level rises when the manic symptoms eventually come under complete control. The unexpected appearance of side effects to lithium may indicate this and should prompt a blood level determination. If ECT were used, a mood stabilizer should be started after treatment is terminated.

If the patient decides not to enter into a preventive phase of treatment, one must estimate when the patient's current episode, in all likelihood, will go into a spontaneous remission. A prior history of manic episodes may provide some guidance here; if that is lacking, one is guided by the duration of an average episode, mentioned earlier. Clearly, if the patient is having breakthrough manic symptoms, no matter how mild, treatment should continue. Furthermore, even when the estimated date of remission has passed, one should continue treatment if the patient's life is unstable, and wait until a period of relative stability has occurred before exposing the patient to the risk, however small, of relapse. If lithium was utilized, it is important to taper the dose over a few weeks time, as it appears that abrupt discontinuation of lithium predisposes to a recurrence of mania. Although the need for tapering has not been demonstrated for the other agents, prudence dictates the use of a gradual taper here also.

Preventive Treatment. The decision to embark on preventive treatment is based on several factors including the following: frequency of episodes, severity of episodes, rapidity with which episodes develop, and side effects of the agent used. Frequent episodes, perhaps occurring more than once every 2 years, usually constitute an indication for preventive treatment; a frequency of one every 5 or 10 years, however, may be such that the risk to the patient of another episode is outweighed by the trouble of taking medicine and any attendant side effects. Severe episodes, however, no matter how infrequent, may warrant prevention. Whereas the patient's employer and family may be able to tolerate a manic episode limited to a hypomanic stage, a mania that enters a delirious stage is usually so destructive that it should be guarded against. Patients whose episodes tend to develop very slowly, over perhaps weeks or a month, may be able to "catch" themselves before their insight and judgment are lost. By making timely application for treatment, they may be able to bring the episode under control on an outpatient basis. Those whose episodes come on acutely over a few days or even hours, however, are defenseless and thus more appropriate for preventive treatment.

If preventive treatment is elected, then the patient should be treated with a mood stabilizer (lithium, divalproex or carbamazepine) or olanzapine. Among the mood stabilizers, lithium has the longest track record and is therefore a reasonable first choice. Divalproex and carbamazepine may also be considered; however, the data supporting the use of divalproex as a preventive agent are not that good and carbamazepine is generally not very well tolerated. If lithium is used, it is important to keep the serum level between 0.6 and 1.0 mEq/L. The optimum dose for valproate and for carbamazepine for prophylaxis has not as yet been determined; prudence suggests using a dose similar to that which was effective for continuation treatment. When "breakthrough" symptoms of mania occur it is imperative to determine the patient's thyroid status: hypothyroidism, even if manifest by only a slight rise in TSH, will blunt the response to any mood stabilizer, and must be corrected. When breakthrough mania occurs despite normal thyroid status and good compliance, consideration may be given to switching to monotherapy with another mood stabilizer or to using a combination of mood stabilizers such as lithium plus divalproex or lithium plus carbamazepine. Given the possibility of such "breakthrough" manias, it is generally prudent, in the case of reliable patients being maintained on a mood stabilizer, to prescribe a supply of adjunctive medication (e.g., olanzapine) to take at home in order to abort an episode and obviate the need for admission. In this regard, outpatients should be clearly instructed to call the physician should they even experience a "hint" of manic symptoms.

Olanzapine has recently been shown to be effective in preventive treatment, and thus may be considered as an alternative to a mood stabilizer. It must be borne in mind, however, that, as compared with the mood stabilizers, especially lithium, the experience with olanzapine is limited; furthermore, emerging data regarding the risks of diabetes and hyperlipidemia with olanzapine may also temper enthusiasm for the long-term use of this agent.

As noted in the section on course, various pharmacologic conditions, such as the use of sympathomimetics, the abrupt discontinuation of long-term treatment with clonidine, and the like, may precipitate manic episodes, and these conditions should be avoided whenever possible. Furthermore, as noted earlier, insomnia, or simply voluntarily going without sleep, may also precipitate a manic episode, and consequently, good sleep hygiene should be promoted.

Recently it has been shown that cognitive behavioral therapy may, when used in conjunction with preventive pharmacologic treatment, reduce the frequency of breakthrough episodes. The mechanism here is not clear, and it also must be kept in mind that no form of psychotherapy is effective for either acute or continuation treatment of mania.

Depressive Episodes

Acute Treatment. When a depressive episode occurs in a patient with bipolar disorder the first step in the acute phase of treatment is to ensure that the patient is taking an antimanic drug, such as lithium, valproate, or carbamazepine, in a dose that would be effective in the acute treatment phase of mania. If the depression is not severe, one may want to wait 2 or 3 weeks to see if the depressive symptoms begin to clear, as this may often happen when one of these three agents is used. When depressive symptoms persist or when they are so severe to begin with that one cannot wait, one may add an antidepressant or consider adding lamotrigine or perhaps topiramate. Traditionally an antidepressant has been used; however, though effective, all the antidepressants entail the risk of precipitating a manic episode; a strategy for choosing and utilizing an antidepressant is discussed in the chapter on major depression. Neither lamotrigine nor topiramate carry a risk of inducing a manic episode, and between the two, the evidence for the effectiveness of lamotrigine is much stronger. In mild cases of depression, one may also consider the use of cognitive-behavioral therapy.

Continuation Treatment. Once the depressive symptoms are relieved, treatment should be continued until the patient has been asymptomatic for a significant period of time. If an antidepressant were added to a mood stabilizer, one should probably consider discontinuing the antidepressant after the patient has been asymptomatic for a matter of months. Given the ongoing risk of a "precipitated" mania, it is preferable to discontinue the drug as soon as possible: if depressive symptoms recur, one may always restart it. In the case of topiramate or lamotrigine, the optimum duration of continuation treatment is not clear. Prudence suggests that if one knows, from history, how long the patient's depressive episodes tend to last, that treatment be continued somewhat past the expected date of spontaneous remission of the depression.

Preventive Treatment. Lithium, carbamazepine and lamotrigine are all effective in preventing future depressive episodes. Preventive treatment with antidepressants in bipolar disorder is generally not justified, given the ongoing risk of precipitating a manic episode.

Other Treatment Considerations

Pregnancy. Pregnancy constitutes a special challenge in the treatment of bipolar disorder. None of the mood stabilizers are safe during pregnancy (especially the first trimester). First generation antipsychotics, such as haloperidol, are probably less teratogenic; the teratogenic potential of olanzapine is not as yet clear. If mania does occur during pregnancy, then the risks to the fetus must be carefully weighed against the risks inherent in a manic episode. ECT should be carefully considered given that, with proper anesthetic technique, it is of low risk to the fetus.

Bipolar women currently in the preventive phase of treatment may often be safely managed into and through a planned pregnancy. Preventive treatment may be continued up to a few days before conception is attempted. If conception does not occur, preventive treatment is restarted and continued until the couple again wishes to conceive. Once conception does occur, preventive treatment is withheld, to be restarted immediately upon delivery; indeed, barring obstetric complications, it should be restarted within hours. In collaboration with the obstetrician, adjunctive treatment is then made available should manic symptoms appear. In cases where the risk of a relapse of mania is high and outweighs the risk to the fetus, one may consider restarting a mood stabilizer after the first trimester. With regard to breast feeding, no firm advice can be given: although maternal use of lithium, valproate and carbamazepine have all been rarely associated with adverse effects in breast-fed infants, large, controlled studies are lacking. Consequently the decision to breast feed or not should be made in light of the entire clinical picture, including the mother's illness and response to treatment.

Substance Use. As noted earlier, alcohol abuse or alcoholism and cocaine addiction are not infrequently associated with bipolar disorder, and these must also be treated.

BIBLIOGRAPHY

Baumann B, Bogerts B. Neuroanatomical studies on bipolar disorder. *The British Journal of Psychiatry* 2001;(Suppl 41):142-147.

Blackwood DH, Visscher PM, Muir WJ. Genetic studies of bipolar affective disorder in large families. *The British Journal of Psychiatry* 2001;(Suppl 41):134-136.

Bowden CL, Brugger AM, Swann AC, et al. Efficacy of divalproex vs lithium and placebo in the treatment of mania. The Depakote Mania Study Group. *The Journal of the American Medical Association* 1994;271:918-924.

Bowden CL, Calabrese JR, McElroy SL, et al. A randomized, placebo-controlled 12-month trial of divalproex and lithium in treatment of outpatients with Bipolar I disorder. Divalproex Maintenance Study Group. *Archives of General Psychiatry* 2000;57:481-489.

Bunney WE, Murphy D, Goodwin FK, et al. The "switch process" in manic depressive illness. I. A systematic study of sequential behavior change. *Archives of General Psychiatry* 1972;27:295-302.

Calabrese JR, Bowden CL, Sachs GS, et al. A double-blind placebo-controlled study of lamotrigine in outpatients with bipolar I depression. Lamictal 602 Study Group. *The Journal of Clinical Psychiatry* 1999;60:79-88.

Carlson GA, Goodwin FK. The stages of mania: a longitudinal analysis of the manic episode. *Archives of General Psychiatry* 1973;28:221-228.

Chaudron LH, Jefferson JW. Mood stabilizers during breastfeeding: a review. *The Journal of Clinical Psychiatry* 2000;61:79-90.

Craddock N, Jones I. Molecular genetics of bipolar disorder. *The British Journal of Psychiatry* 2001;(Suppl 41):128-133.

Gelenberg AJ, Kane JM, Keller MB, et al. Comparison of standard and low serum levels of lithium for maintenance treatment of bipolar disorder. *The New England Journal of Medicine* 1989;321:1489-1493.

Goodwin FK. Rationale for long-term treatment of bipolar disorder and evidence for long-term lithium treatment. *The Journal of Clinical Psychiatry* 2002;63(Suppl 10):5-12.

Greil W, Ludwig-Mayerhofer W, Erazo N, et al. Lithium versus carbamazepine in the maintenance treatment of bipolar disorders—a randomized study. *Journal of Affective Disorders* 1997;43:151-161.

Himmelhoch JM, Mulla D, Neil JF, et al. Incidence and significance of mixed affective states in a bipolar population. *Archives of General Psychiatry* 1976;33:1062-1066.

Janowsky DS, El-Yousef K, David JM, et al. Parasympathetic suppression of manic symptoms by physostigmine. *Archives of General Psychiatry* 1973;28:542-547.

Joffe RT, MacQueen GM, Marriott M, et al. Induction of mania and cycle acceleration in bipolar disorder: effect of different classes of antidepressant. *Acta Psychiatrica Scandinavica* 2002;105:427-430.

Keck PE, Versiani M, Potkin S, et al. Ziprasidone in the treatment of acute mania: a three-week, placebo-controlled, double-blind, randomized trial. *The American Journal of Psychiatry* 2003;160:741-748.

Kramlinger KG, Post RM. Adding lithium carbonate to carbamazepine: antimanic efficacy in treatment-resistant mania. *Acta Psychiatrica Scandinavica* 1989;79:378-385.

Lam DH, Watkins ER, Hayward P, et al. A randomized controlled study of cognitive therapy for relapse prevention for bipolar affective disorder: outcome of the first year. *Archives of General Psychiatry* 2003;60:145-152.

Lipkin KM, Dyrud J, Meyer GG. The many faces of mania: therapeutic trial of lithium carbonate. *Archives of General Psychiatry* 1970;22:262-267.

Lusznat RM, Murphy DP, Nunn CM. Carbamazepine vs lithium in the treatment and prophylaxis of mania. *The British Journal of Psychiatry* 1988;153:198-204.

McElroy SL, Keck PE, Stanton SP, et al. A randomized comparison of divalproex oral loading versus haloperidol in the initial treatment of acute psychotic mania. *The Journal of Clinical Psychiatry* 1996;57:142-146.

McIntyre RS, Mancini DA, McCann S, et al. Topiramate versus bupropion SR when added to mood stabilizer therapy for the depressive phase of bipolar disorder: a preliminary single-blind study. *Bipolar Disorders* 2002;4:207-213.

Meehan K, Zhang F, David S, et al. A double-blind, randomized comparison of the efficacy and safety of intramuscular injections of olanzapine, lorazepam, or placebo in treating acutely agitated patients diagnosed with bipolar mania. *Journal of Clinical Psychopharmacology* 2001; 21:389-397.

Mukherjee S, Sackheim HA, Schnur DB. Electroconvulsive therapy of acute manic episodes: a review of 50 years' experience. *The American Journal of Psychiatry* 1994;151:169-176.

Muller-Oerlinghausen B, Berghofer A, Bauer M. Bipolar disorder. *Lancet* 2002;359:241-247.

Swann AC, Bowden CL, Morris D, et al. Depression during mania. Treatment response to lithium or divalproex. *Archives of General Psychiatry* 1997;54:37-42.

Tohen M, Baker RW, Altshuler LL, et al. Olanzapine versus divalproex in the treatment of acute mania. *The American Journal of Psychiatry* 2002;159:1011-1017.

Tohen M, Ketter TA, Zarate CA, et al. Olanzapine versus divalproex sodium for the treatment of acute mania and maintenance of remission: a 47-week study. *The American Journal of Psychiatry* 2003;160:1263-1271.

Zajecka JM, Weisler R, Sachs G, et al. A comparison of the efficacy, safety, and tolerability of divalproex sodium and olanzapine in the treatment of bipolar disorder. *The Journal of Clinical Psychiatry* 2002;63:1148-1155.

81 Cyclothymia (cyclothymic disorder, DSM-IV-TR #301.13)

Cyclothymia, or "cycloid temperament," is a chronic disorder characterized by the sequential appearance of periods of very mild manic symptoms and periods of mild depressive ones. Although in all likelihood it represents a forme fruste of bipolar disorder, it is considered, in deference to current DSM-IV usage, in its own chapter.

Prevalence figures for cyclothymia range from 0.4% to 1%; it is probably equally common among males and females.

ONSET

The onset is usually quite insidious, occurring in adolescence or early adult years.

CLINICAL FEATURES

These mild manic and depressive periods typically alternate in an irregular fashion, lasting for days or weeks; the euthymic intervals between the periods range in duration from a month or more to hours or less. Indeed in some cases, no euthymic interval exists at all, and the patient demonstrates continuous cycling.

During manic periods patients may be enthusiastic and overhappy, or at times irritable. Energetic and overactive, these patients tend to become overinvolved with projects or with other people. In gifted individuals this may result in heightened productivity; however, in those with average talents or in those with a predominantly irritable mood, conflicts with others or with authority abound.

During depressive periods patients are moody, irritable, and unduly sensitive to slights and to criticism. Fatigue and apathy hamper their efforts, and modest changes in appetite and sleep may be seen, with a tendency toward hypersomnia.

Borderline personality disorder, histrionic personality disorder, and substance use disorder, particularly involving alcohol, cocaine, or stimulants, are often seen in association with cyclothymia.

COURSE

Cyclothymia is a chronic disorder; in some patients it may be lifelong.

COMPLICATIONS

Some patients, particularly if their symptoms are mild, may escape complications entirely. Indeed, as noted earlier, some, thrust along by their mild manic symptoms, may succeed brilliantly.

In other patients the mood fluctuations are so extreme that friendships, marriages, and business relationships are repeatedly fractured by them. Irritable patients may come into so much conflict with the law that incarceration occurs.

ETIOLOGY

As noted in the introduction, cyclothymia is probably a forme fruste of bipolar disorder. The prevalence of bipolar disorder is increased among the biologic relatives of patients with cyclothymia as compared to the relatives of controls.

DIFFERENTIAL DIAGNOSIS

Certain patients with borderline or histrionic personality disorder may at times present such a tumultuous clinical picture as to suggest cyclothymia. In personality disorders, however, mood changes are always intimately and inextricably tied to events in the patient's life. By contrast, in cyclothymia, the mood changes are autonomous and independent from changes in the patient's life. However, some patients may have both a personality disorder and cyclothymia, with their mood changes at times bound up with, and at times autonomous from, events around them.

In adolescence, cyclothymia may lead to extreme misconduct, suggesting a diagnosis of conduct disorder.

Similar mood changes may occur as either a lengthy prodrome to bipolar disorder or as residual symptoms in the interval between full-blown manic episodes, and indeed about one third of patients with a history compatible with cyclothymia eventually have a manic episode of stage I or greater intensity, or a full depressive one, in which case the diagnosis is revised to bipolar disorder.

TREATMENT

Both lithium and divalproex are reportedly useful; however, there are no double-blinded trials of either agent. Antidepressants often precipitate mania in these patients and thus should be used with caution, and never without the patient first being "covered" with a mood stabilizer.

BIBLIOGRAPHY

Akiskal HS. Dysthymia and cyclothymia in psychiatric practice a century after Kraepelin. *Journal of Affective Disorders* 2001;62:17-31.

Akiskal HS, Djenderedjian AH, Rosenthal RH, et al. Cyclothymic disorder: validating criteria for inclusion in the bipolar affective group. *The American Journal of Psychiatry* 1977;134:1227-1233.

Howland RH, Thase ME. A comprehensive review of cyclothymic disorder. *The Journal of Nervous and Mental Disease* 1993;181:485-493.

Jacobsen FM. Low-dose valproate: a new treatment for cyclothymia, mild rapid cycling disorders, and premenstrual syndrome. *The Journal of Clinical Psychiatry* 1993;54:229-234.

Kraepelin E. *Manic depressive insanity and paranoia,* translated by Barclay RM, New York, 1976, Arno Press.

Levitt AJ, Joffe RT, Ennis J, et al. The prevalence of cyclothymia in borderline personality disorder. *The Journal of Clinical Psychiatry* 1990;51: 335-339.

Peselow ED, Dunner DL, Fieve RR, et al. Lithium prophylaxis of depression in unipolar, bipolar II, and cyclothymic patients. *The American Journal of Psychiatry* 1982;139:747-752.

82   Hyperthymia

Hyperthymia, also known as hyperthymic temperament or hypomanic personality, is a relatively rare, chronic disorder and probably represents a forme fruste of bipolar disorder.

ONSET

Onset is usually in early adolescence.

CLINICAL FEATURES

These patients seem always more or less energetically on the go. Talkative and often ebullient, they are full of plans, schemes, and new ideas and are often able to "infect" others with their overconfidence and thus establish a certain following. Their careless disregard of the inevitable pitfalls in any venture, however, and their blind enthusiasm often lead them into disastrous financial and personal entanglements. Sexuality is often greatly increased, and promiscuity may occur.

When challenged or thwarted, some hyperthymic patients may "laugh it off"; however, more often than not they become irritable, rude, and dogmatically insistent on their way of doing things.

Abuse of or addiction to either alcohol or cocaine is not uncommonly associated with hyperthymia.

COURSE

Hyperthymia is apparently chronic and may be lifelong.

COMPLICATIONS

Business failure and sometimes disastrous romantic affairs may occur.

ETIOLOGY

Hyperthymia probably represents a very chronic "subhypomanic" episode with an etiology presumably the same as that of bipolar disorder.

DIFFERENTIAL DIAGNOSIS

Some individuals with a "sunny" disposition may seem unfazed by life's misfortunes; however, here one fails to see the push and pressure of thoughts and activity seen in hyperthymia. The sunny person takes life as it comes; the patient with hyperthymia reaches out and grasps it.

Patients with bipolar disorder may exhibit a lengthy prodrome of very mild manic symptoms, and these may also occur after a manic episode has only gone into partial remission. Thus any patient who appears to have hyperthymia must be watched closely for the development of a manic episode and the consequent need to revise the original diagnosis.

TREATMENT

No controlled studies of the treatment of hyperthymia exist. By analogy with bipolar disorder, one may try lithium or divalproex, and, should one of these agents work, consider chronic treatment, given the chronicity of the disorder.

BIBLIOGRAPHY

Brieger P, Marneros A. Dysthymia and cyclothymia: historical origins and contemporary development. *Journal of Affective Disorders* 1997;45:117-126.

Cassano GB, Akiskal HS, Savino M, et al. Proposed subtypes of bipolar II and related disorders: with hypomanic episodes (or cyclothymia) and with hyperthymic temperament. *Journal of Affective Disorders* 1992;26:127-140.

Deltito JA. The effect of valproate on bipolar spectrum temperamental disorders. *The Journal of Clinical Psychiatry* 1993;54:300-304.

Kraepelin E. *Manic depressive insanity and paranoia*, translated by Barclay RM, New York, 1976, Arno Press.

Kwapil TR, Miller MB, Zinser MC, et al. A longitudinal study of high scorers on the hypomanic personality scale. *Journal of Abnormal Psychology* 2000;109:222-226.

Lemere F, Smith JW. Hypomanic personality trait in cocaine addiction. *The British Journal of Addictions* 1990;85:575-576.

83 Panic Disorder (panic disorder with or without agoraphobia, DSM-IV-TR #300.01, 300.21)

Panic disorder is characterized by the repeated occurrence of discrete panic attacks. Between attacks these patients are often well, although most, after repeated attacks, develop some persistent apprehension, or anticipatory anxiety, regarding the possibility of another attack; in turn, about one half of these patients eventually develop agoraphobia.

This is a relatively common disorder and has a lifetime prevalence of from 1 to 2%. It is several times more common in women than in men. In the past these patients might have received many different diagnoses including the following: DaCosta's syndrome, "effort heart," neurocirculatory asthenia, neurasthenia, and acute anxiety neurosis. However, in reading old reports keep in mind that these are not actual synonyms for panic disorder but rather loosely defined terms that include not only patients who today would be diagnosed as having panic disorder but also many other patients suffering sometimes from quite disparate disorders.

ONSET

Although some patients, in retrospect, report feeling vaguely unwell in the weeks or months before their first panic attack, most experience no prodrome, and the onset of the illness is heralded by the occurrence of the first attack. This experience is often recalled in vivid detail, and patients may be able to describe precisely the circumstances in which the attack occurred. This first attack generally occurs in late adolescence or the early twenties; however, later onsets, up to the thirties, are not uncommon. Rarely, onset may occur in childhood or over the age of 40.

CLINICAL FEATURES

The panic attack itself usually comes on acutely, often within a minute, and crescendos rapidly. Symptoms generally last only 5 to 15 minutes, or sometimes less, and very rarely up to an hour, and then recede over minutes. After the attack most patients feel "shaken," and may feel drained and apprehensive for a long time, sometimes hours. During the attack itself, patients may experience any of the symptoms listed in the box on p. 159. These symptoms may appear in any combination, and a patient rarely experiences all of these symptoms during any one attack.

The anxiety may take any of several forms. Some patients experience the classic "sense of impending doom," as if something terrible were about to happen. Some fear they are having a heart attack or a stroke, and this may occasion multiple visits to the emergency room. Some fear they will "go crazy." For others the anxiety may be only a minor part of the symptomatology of the attack; rarely, patients do not have any anxiety at all during the attack, only a sense of discomfort. The existence of these cases, dubbed "panic attacks without panic," was initially controversial. However, in every other respect they are typical attacks, and as no other etiology than panic disorder can be established for them, one must assume that in rare instances a patient may experience a panic attack without undue anxiety at all.

Tremor may or may not be a complaint; some patients complain more of a sense of internal shakiness.

The palpitations and chest discomfort often prove most alarming to patients. The discomfort itself may be quite severe and sometimes radiates to the left shoulder or the left side of the neck. Such complaints, of course, also cause discomfort in the emergency room physician. The palpitations are often described as "racing," and less often as "skipped beats."

The other symptoms require little discussion. Patients describe them in the most varied terms, and one may inquire specifically after each term to become familiar with the range of descriptions possible.

In most patients the attacks are without precipitating factors, and this is perhaps one of the most striking features of panic attacks. They seem to "come out of the blue" and strike without warning. Although patients may recall with vivid clarity the exact circumstances surrounding the first attack, they are generally unable to identify anything that could conceivably have caused the attack. Many patients, after repeated attacks, may come to fear being in situations where help might not be readily available should another attack occur. Thus they may have anxiety about driving on limited access freeways, or bridges, or in tunnels. Flying or boating may likewise be avoided. In describing their fear of these situations, patients may give the impression that they are afraid that the situation itself might cause a panic attack. However, on closer questioning one can see that what they are afraid of is not so much that the situation will cause the attack but that they might have an attack in that situation and be unable to get to help

Panic Attack Symptoms

Anxiety	Hot and cold flushes
Tremor	Dyspnea
Palpitations	Dizziness or faintness
Chest discomfort	Nausea or abdominal distress
Diaphoresis	Acral paresthesias

immediately. In some patients, as noted below, agoraphobia may develop.

Nocturnal panic attacks are not uncommon; however, as patients may not report them, one should inquire after them specifically. Polysomnography has revealed that these nocturnal attacks tend to arise from non-REM sleep.

COURSE

The frequency with which panic attacks occur varies widely, and it appears that the long-term course falls more or less into one of two patterns. In one pattern, the frequency gradually waxes and wanes (anywhere from once daily to once every few months), over many years or decades, without the patient ever experiencing any prolonged attack-free intervals. In the other pattern one does see prolonged attack-free intervals, and in this pattern it may be appropriate to speak of an "episodic" course, wherein episodes, characterized by panic attacks occurring with varying frequency, are separated by intervals free of attacks.

COMPLICATIONS

The most common complication of panic disorder is agoraphobia, and this is seen in anywhere from one-third to one-half of all patients, generally within the first year. Here the anticipatory anxiety becomes so severe and attached to so many different situations that patients begin to more or less severely restrict their travels. Truck drivers may give up their long-distance routes and restrict themselves to local deliveries; traveling salespersons may quit their routes altogether. At its worst these patients may become housebound.

Abuse of alcohol, benzodiazepines, or other tranquilizers or sedatives is a serious risk. Patients may use these to quell anticipatory anxiety; others may take them during the panic attack itself in the mistaken belief that blood levels sufficient to have an effect will occur before the attack remits spontaneously. This complication may compound itself if tolerance and withdrawal occur. During withdrawal, panic attacks are more likely to occur, which in turn could spur further use of a tranquilizer, thus setting up a vicious cycle.

Patients who suffer from both panic disorder and major depression may be at higher risk for suicide than those with major depression alone. However, contrary to earlier reports, those with panic disorder alone do not appear to be at higher risk for a suicide attempt.

ETIOLOGY

Panic disorder appears to run in families. As the degree of consanguinity increases from general population to first-degree relatives, or from dizygotic to monozygotic twins, so too does the risk of having panic disorder. Although this is consistent with a hereditary basis, the effects of a shared environment cannot be ruled out, and until adoption studies are done, the basis for the familial occurrence of panic disorder remains uncertain. Genetic and linkage studies, to date, have not yielded robust findings.

The discovery of panicogens has been one of the major fruits of research in panic disorder. These are substances that, though innocuous to normal controls, reliably produce panic attacks in patients with panic disorder. These induced panic attacks are essentially identical to the naturally occurring ones. Furthermore, these induced attacks may be prevented by the same medications that are effective in preventing the naturally occurring attacks.

Several substances have been shown to be panicogenic. They include sodium lactate, inhalation of 5% or 35% carbon dioxide, cholecystokinin tetrapeptide, caffeine, yohimbine, isoproterenol, and the benzodiazepine antagonist, flumazenil. Of these the best studied is sodium lactate infusion. In light of the family studies noted above, it is of interest that the inhalation of 35% carbon dioxide by the asymptomatic and not-ill relatives of probands induces panic attacks, an effect not seen in normal controls.

Various neurotransmitters have also been investigated. The noradrenergic system is strongly implicated by the panicogenic efficacy of adrenergic agents such as yohimbine and isoproterenol, and this is further supported by studies demonstrating a blunted GH response to clonidine administration. The serotoninergic system is implicated not only by the undoubted efficacy of serotoninergic antidepressants in the treatment of panic disorder, but also by studies involving manipulation of brain serotonin levels. For example, depletion of tryptophan, the dietary precursor of serotonin, increases the effectiveness of a panicogen such as flumazenil, whereas the administration of 5-hydroxytryptophan, which increases serotonin levels, will blunt the effectiveness of CO_2 inhalation as a panicogen. The GABA-ergic system is strongly implicated by the effectiveness of flumazenil as a panicogen and by the effectiveness of benzodiazepines in the treatment of panic disorder, and is supported by a recent finding of reduced GABA levels in the occipital cortex of panic disorder patients.

Functional MRI studies, although not entirely in agreement, suggest strongly that the hippocampus and parahippocampal gyrus are abnormally activated in panic disorder.

Integrating these findings into a coherent etiologic theory is problematic and requires some speculation. However, it appears plausible to say that panic disorder represents an inherited disturbance in the overall function of noradrenergic, serotoninergic or GABAergic systems in one or more of those central nervous system structures responsible for anxiety. Candidate structures include the locus ceruleus, dorsal raphe nucleus, parahippocampus, hippocampus and amygdala. The locus ceruleus is noradrenergic, the dorsal raphe nucleus serotoninergic, and both send fibers to a large number of structures, including the parahippocampus, hippocampus and amygdala, structures rich in GABA receptors. Stimulation of these limbic structures, in turn, is well known to produce fear and anxiety. If one assumes that overactivity of the amygdala is the "final common pathway," then disturbance in any one of the other structures, or the amygdala itself, could cause a panic attack.

It has been proposed that one possible "trigger" for the activation of this neuronal circuit is an abnormal sensitivity to disturbances of acid-base balance in the brainstem. Such a sensitivity, if it did exist, could explain the efficacy of panicogens such as lactate infusion and CO_2 inhalation, maneuvers which both induce changes in acid-base balance. This "false suffocation alarm" could then lead to overactivation of either the locus ceruleus or dorsal raphe nucleus.

Before leaving this discussion of the etiology of panic disorder a word is in order regarding the association of panic disorder with mitral valve prolapse. Although this association has not been consistently replicated, most studies do support it. It appears unlikely, however, that mitral valve prolapse causes panic or that, vice versa, panic causes prolapse; rather the association is probably secondary to some commonly shared abnormality, the nature of which is unclear.

DIFFERENTIAL DIAGNOSIS

Panic attacks may be seen in simple phobia, social phobia, posttraumatic stress disorder, and obsessive-compulsive disorder. In these disorders, however, the panic attacks are precipitated. For example, if the simple phobic has to approach a snake, the social phobic public speaking, the posttraumatic patient a situation reminiscent of the original trauma, or the obsessive-compulsive patient a contaminated object, a severe panic attack may indeed occur. If, however, these patients can avoid the stimuli, there are no panic attacks. In such cases a separate diagnosis of panic disorder is not made.

Occasionally an otherwise normal individual experiences a spontaneous panic attack; to qualify, however, for a diagnosis of panic disorder, the attacks must be either severe enough to cause marked distress or be frequent, occurring generally once a month or more.

Panic attacks are also seen with some frequency in patients suffering from a depressive episode either as part of major depression or bipolar disorder. In some cases the panic attacks may actually predate the onset of the depressive symptoms, and when they are concurrent with depressive symptoms, no relationship between them and the severity of the depressive symptoms is evident. In such cases a separate panic disorder is occurring in addition to the depressive disorder, and consequently, two diagnoses are given.

A number of conditions may produce symptomatic episodes that may very closely resemble panic attacks, thus engendering some diagnostic confusion (see the box on this page). Usually, however, certain differential points allow a correct diagnosis.

Parkinson's disease is associated with panic attacks when patients are treated with levodopa and have a prominent "on-off" effect. Here, as the preceding dose of levodopa wears off and the parkinsonism worsens, patients may have a panic attack very similar to those seen in panic disorder.

Patients suffering a myocardial infarction or an attack of angina pectoris may complain of chest pain, dyspnea, nausea, diaphoresis, and often a sense of impending doom. Radiation of pain to the neck or arm is not an infallibly reliable diagnostic point, since this may also occur during a panic attack. The general medical setting of the illness is often diagnostically helpful. Clearly, if the patient is elderly, with known cardiac disease or multiple coronary risk factors, one might lean toward a diagnosis of myocardial insufficiency. Conversely, if the patient is young, with no risk factors, one might be inclined toward a diagnosis of panic disorder, especially with a history of numerous prior identical attacks.

At the moment of lodgment of a relatively large pulmonary embolus, patients may have a sudden onset of chest discomfort, dyspnea, nausea, diaphoresis, and significant anxiety, thus presenting a clinical picture quite similar to a panic attack. The disproportionate emphasis on dyspnea relative to other symptoms is a helpful diagnostic point for pulmonary embolus. Likewise, hemoptysis or wheezing point immediately to the correct diagnosis; however, these latter two symptoms are often not present. As is the case with myocardial ischemia, the setting of the illness may be a helpful point. Prolonged immobilization, thrombophlebitis or cardiac failure would make one's index of suspicion higher for pulmonary embolus, especially if this were a first episode.

Paroxysmal supraventricular tachycardia (SVT), also known as paroxysmal atrial tachycardia, occasionally may cause diagnostic problems because the patient may become quite anxious during an attack of tachycardia. Two diagnostic points strongly suggest SVT: first, a hyperacute onset (often less than a second) and, second, the ability of the patient to terminate the attack by a Valsalva maneuver. Holter monitoring will help establish the diagnosis; however, it is important to utilize "event monitoring" so that the episode is not missed.

Simple partial seizures may occasionally be characterized by a panic attack. Clues to this diagnosis include not only the occurrence, at other times, of other seizure types (e.g., grand mal or complex partial) but also the exquisitely paroxysmal nature of the ictal panic attack: whereas panic attacks in panic disorder take minutes to crescendo, the ictal anxiety peaks within seconds. An EEG may or may not be helpful in such cases, as it may be normal even while the patient is having the seizure.

Episodic hypoglycemia may be very difficult to distinguish from a panic attack. Symptomatic episodes of hypoglycemia, however, tend to have a slower onset than a panic attack and tend to last longer. Relief of symptoms with orange juice or some other sugar is a helpful diagnostic point. The setting is also helpful; the suspicion for hypoglycemia is higher in a patient taking insulin or an oral hypoglycemic and in those in whom the attacks tend to occur postprandially.

A minority of patients with pheochromocytoma have paroxysmal attacks that very closely resemble panic attacks. Typically, though, in contrast to patients with panic attacks, these patients have a prominent headache. Furthermore, hypertension is always present during the attack and is often also present between the attacks. Furthermore, although paroxysms in pheochromocytoma may occur spontaneously, at times they are precipitated by abdominal compression or micturition, factors that clearly distinguish them from panic attacks.

Mastocytosis may present with episodes of light-headedness, palpitations, headaches, dyspnea, chest pain, and nausea. Though these episodes, in these respects, are similar to panic attacks, certain points suggest the correct diagnosis. Patients with mastocytosis almost always experience intense flushing during the episode. Interestingly, though this can be profound, they rarely complain of it and must be questioned directly about the presence or absence of flushing. Furthermore, after the attack most patients experience profound lethargy to the point of prostration, which may last for days or longer. Such post-attack prostration is not seen after a panic attack. Finally, physical examination generally reveals

---

Conditions that may Produce Symptomatic Episodes that Resemble Panic Attacks

Parkinson's disease	Simple partial seizures
Myocardial infarction	Hypoglycemia
Angina pectoris	Pheochromocytoma
Supraventricular tachycardia	Mastocytosis
Pulmonary embolus	Carcinoid syndrome

urticaria pigmentosa, although not all patients with mastocytosis have this.

Carcinoid syndrome is often included in the differential diagnosis of panic attacks, but it would appear difficult to confuse the two. The flushing and diarrhea that are hallmarks of the carcinoid syndrome are relatively minor in a panic attack.

Certain other disorders are often included on the differential diagnosis for panic disorder, including hyperthyroidism, certain drug intoxications, and certain drug withdrawals; however, the anxiety seen in these disorders is generally not paroxysmal. The anxiety of hyperthyroidism may wax and wane, but is not episodic. Drugs such as caffeine, cocaine, amphetamines and various over-the-counter sympathomimetics may produce an episode of anxiety, but, unless the durg is injected intravenously or taken by inhalation, the onset is usually gradual. Withdrawal from alcohol, benzodiazepines or other sedative-hypnotics is often accompanied by anxiety which may at times undergo an episodic surge similar to a panic attack. In such cases, these "attacks" subside with abstinence.

As may be gathered from the foregoing discussion, the differential diagnosis in patients suspected of panic disorder is rather extensive. The task of differential diagnosis here, however, is not as formidable as it may seem. A careful history generally points in the right direction. If one is lucky enough to have the patient under observation during an attack, one should, in addition to a careful description of symptoms and cutaneous signs, note blood pressure, pulse, and if possible obtain an ECG, blood for a glucose level, and, if suspicious of mastocytosis, a histamine level. Determination of CBC and cardiac enzymes depends on the level of suspicion of cardiac or pulmonary disease. Other tests (such as a pulmonary scan, arteriography, Holter monitor, electroencephalogram, glucose tolerance test, plasma norepinephrine and epinephrine, and 24-hour urine for 5-hydroxyindoleacetic acid or histamine and its metabolites) should be used only as indicated by one's diagnostic suspicions.

TREATMENT

The goal of treatment in panic disorder is twofold: to prevent future attacks and to relieve anticipatory anxiety and enable patients to overcome any avoidance behavior they may have developed. Both cognitive-behavioral treatment and medication have a role; medications are discussed first.

When initiating pharmacologic treatment one must impress on the patient the fact that, short of intravenous medication, probably nothing is available that reliably aborts an attack once it has begun, and that therefore the thrust of drug treatment is to prevent future attacks.

Once the patient has decided on prophylactic treatment, the next step is to select the prophylactic agent best suited for the patient. Two groups of medicines provide effective prophylaxis: certain benzodiazepines and most of the currently available antidepressants. Which group to choose has been the subject of intense debate. Buspirone is not effective.

Four benzodiazepines are clearly effective: alprazolam, clonazepam, lorazepam and diazepam. The benzodiazepines offer certain advantages. They have a rapid onset of action, generally few side effects, and often serve to reduce the anticipatory anxiety that most patients with panic disorder experience. The total daily dose is gradually titrated up until symptoms are controlled: alprazolam may be started at from 0.75 to 1.5 mg, with most patients responding to doses of from 1.5 to 6 mg; comparable figures for clonazepam are 0.5 to 1.5 mg to start, titrating to from 1.0 to 4.0 mg, for lorazepam 1 to 2 mg to start, titrating to from 2 to 6 mg, and for diazepam 4 to 10 mg to start, titrating to from 10 to 60 mg. Alprazolam, if given in the extended-release formulation, may be given once daily; otherwise the total daily dose must be divided into three or more administrations; clonazepam and diazepam are generally given in two divided doses.

Given the risk of neuroadaptation with benzodiazepines, many clinicians prefer to start with an antidepressant, choosing an SSRI, tricyclic or MAOI. The SSRIs are generally better tolerated than the tricyclics, and the MAOIs, though undoubtedly effective, are generally held in reserve given their side-effect profile and dietary requirements. Regardless of which antidepressant is chosen it is generally prudent to start with a low dose: although in most cases a full "antidepressant" dose is required, starting at or near such a dose often precipitates either agitation or a "flurry" of panic attacks, and consequently one should begin with a dose from one-tenth to one-third of the "full" dose, followed by an upward titration, in similar increments, every week or so. Importantly, although most patients do indeed both tolerate and require a titration to a "full dose" there is a small minority of patients who do not tolerate more than a small amount but yet do get a good anti-panic effect from it. Unfortunately, one cannot as yet tell prospectively which patients will have this sort of response. Once an optimum dose has been reached, a response may not be seen for weeks, and a full response may be delayed for up to 3 months. Given this potentially long delayed response, many clinicians will begin treatment with a combination of a benzodiazepine and an SSRI (e.g., clonazepam and sertraline) and then taper off the benzodiazepine once the SSRI has had a chance to become effective.

Among the SSRIs, the following (with their average doses) have been shown to be effective in double-blinded studies: paroxetine (40 mg), fluoxetine (20 mg), fluvoxamine (150 mg), citalopram (20 mg), escitalopram (10 mg) and sertraline. In the case of sertraline, it appears that any dose between 50 and 200 mg is effective.

Of the tricyclics, imipramine, in doses of 150 to 200 mg, although effective, and indeed the "gold standard," is generally poorly tolerated over the long haul. Nortriptyline, in doses of from 50 to 150 mg, desipramine, in doses of from 150 to 200 mg, and clomipramine, in doses of from 50 to 150 mg, are alternatives.

Of the MAOIs, phenelzine, in doses of 30 to 90 mg, is effective. Two other reversible MAOIs, not yet available in the United States, are also effective, namely brofaromine and moclobemide.

Other medications that may be considered include propranolol and inositol. Propranolol, in total daily doses of roughly 180 mg, may be effective, but the clinical impression is that it is less reliably so than a benzodiazepine or an antidepressant. Inositol is an isomer of glucose which serves as a precursor for inositol, an intracellular "second messenger": remarkably, in a double-blinded comparison, with doses of roughly 6000 mg bid, it was more effective than fluvoxamine. Clearly, this is very promising, and bears watching for replication.

Response to medical treatment is usually quite good. Many patients become completely free of panic attacks. However, a large percentage continue to have attacks, albeit much less frequently and of much less severity.

Cognitive-behavior therapy, used either independently or in conjunction with medical treatment, should also be considered, especially in light of the fact that in addition to reducing the frequency of panic attacks, it is also an effective treatment for agoraphobia.

BIBLIOGRAPHY

Bakker A, van Dyck R, Spinhoven P, et al. Paroxetine, clomipramine, and cognitive therapy in the treatment of panic disorder. *The Journal of Clinical Psychiatry* 1999;60:831-838.

Bakker A, van Balkom AJ, Spinhoven P. SSRIs vs. TCAs in the treatment of panic disorder: a meta-analysis. *Acta Psychiatrica Scandinavica* 2002;106:163-167.

Bell C, Forshall S, Andover M, et al. Does 5-HT restrain panic? A tryptophan depletion study in panic disorder patients recovered on paroxetine. *Journal of Psychopharmacology* 2002;16:5-14.

Bisaga A, Katz JL, Antonini A, et al. Cerebral glucose metabolism in women with panic disorder. *The American Journal of Psychiatry* 1998;155:1178-1183.

Finn CT, Smoller JW. The genetics of panic disorder. *Current Psychiatry Reports* 2001;3:131-137.

Fleet RP, Martel JP, Lavoie KL, et al. Non-fearful panic disorder: a variant of panic in medical patients? *Psychosomatics* 2000;41:311-320.

Goddard AW, Mason GF, Almai A, et al. Reductions in occipital cortex GABA levels in panic disorder detected with 1h-magnetic resonance spectroscopy. *Archives of General Psychiatry* 2001;58:556-561.

Gorman JM, Kent JM, Sullivan GM, et al. Neuroanatomical hypothesis of panic disorder, revised. *The American Journal of Psychiatry* 2000;157:493-505.

Kampman M, Keijsers GP, Hoogduin CA, et al. A randomized, double-blind, placebo-controlled study of the effects of adjunctive paroxetine in panic disorder patients unsuccessfully treated with cognitive-behavioral therapy alone. *The Journal of Clinical Psychiatry* 2002;63:772-777.

Katerndahl DA. Panic and prolapse: meta-analysis. *The Journal of Nervous and Mental Disease* 1993;181:539-544.

Lessmeier TJ, Gamperling D, Johnson-Liddon V, et al. Unrecognized paroxysmal supraventricular tachycardia. Potential for misdiagnosis as panic disorder. *Archives of Internal Medicine* 1997;157:537-543.

Mellman TA, Uhde TW. Patients with frequent sleep panic: clinical findings and response to medication treatment. *The Journal of Clinical Psychiatry* 1990;51:513-516.

Palatnik A, Frolov K, Fux M, et al. Double-blind, controlled, crossover trial of inositol versus fluvoxamine for the treatment of panic disorder. *Journal of Clinical Psychopharmacology* 2001;21:335-339.

Russell JL, Kushner MG, Beitman BD, et al. Non-fearful panic disorder in neurology patients validated by lactate challenge. *The American Journal of Psychiatry* 1991;148:361-364.

Schruers K, van Diest R, Overbeek T, et al. Acute L-5-hydroxytryptophan administration inhibits carbon dioxide-induced panic in panic disorder patients. *Psychiatry Research* 2002;113:237-243.

Sheehan DV. The management of panic disorder. *The Journal of Clinical Psychiatry* 2002;63(Suppl 14):17-21.

84 Agoraphobia (panic disorder with agoraphobia, DSM-IV-TR #300.21, and agoraphobia without history of panic disorder, DSM-IV-TR #300.22)

Agoraphobia is taken from the Greek and literally means a "fear of the marketplace" or, more generally, of open spaces. However, on questioning, what becomes apparent is that patients do not fear a particular place or situation but rather the possibility of suddenly becoming ill or incapacitated in some fashion and either not being able to escape or not being able to receive immediate help.

Probably more than one kind of agoraphobia exists. In one kind, patients fear having a panic attack, and in such cases the agoraphobia represents a complication of panic disorder. In another, patients seem unable to describe how they might fall ill; they deny ever having a panic attack, and indeed may never have had any illness other than the agoraphobia itself.

The lifetime prevalence of agoraphobia is somewhat controversial, ranging from a conservative estimate of a little less than 1% to as much as 5%. It is probably two to four times more common in females than males.

ONSET

The onset is usually in the twenties or thirties. In cases where the agoraphobia appears subsequent to panic disorder, anywhere from a few days up to a year may elapse between the first panic attack and the onset of the agoraphobia. In general, agoraphobic symptoms gradually worsen over time.

CLINICAL FEATURES

Any number of situations or places may be feared and avoided. Examples include the following: riding across bridges or through tunnels, riding in airplanes or trains, going on a trip anywhere, being in elevators or on escalators, riding in a two-door car in the back seat, or simply waiting in line. In extreme cases patients may fear being anywhere except in the safety of home; the prospect of merely walking around the block, or even of stepping out on the stoop to get the paper, may fill the patient with incapacitating fear. Some patients become completely housebound and may never set foot outside the house for years.

In many cases patients may be able to temporarily overcome their agoraphobia if they take their "safety" with them when they leave home. The companionship of a friend or family member is often sufficient reassurance to quell their fear.

COURSE

Agoraphobia appears to be a chronic disorder. In those cases associated with panic disorder, remission of the agoraphobia does not occur so long as the panic attacks continue.

COMPLICATIONS

Jobs, friendships, and anything that requires leaving the home may be lost. Substance abuse and depression may also occur.

ETIOLOGY

In cases occurring secondary to panic disorder, the "anticipatory anxiety" suffered by the patient with panic attacks becomes so severe that it cannot be borne by the patient outside the relative safety of home.

In those cases where agoraphobia occurs in the absence of a panic attack the etiology is not known.

DIFFERENTIAL DIAGNOSIS

In social phobia of the generalized subtype, patients may fear and avoid many different situations; the difference here is that social phobics fear that they will do something embarrassing or humiliating, whereas agoraphobics fear rather that something will happen to them, such as a panic attack.

In illnesses characterized by ideas or delusions of reference or persecution, widespread avoidance of situations may occur. This may be seen in schizophrenia, schizoaffective disorder, the persecutory subtype of paranoia, certain depressive disorders, and so forth. Here, however, the patient fears that others will do something harmful to him, in contrast to the agoraphobic who fears that some symptoms will occur in him.

TREATMENT

Agoraphobia may be treated with cognitive behavioral therapy or a behavioral program of "graded exposure" wherein the patient gradually and sequentially takes progressively greater steps toward and into the feared situation. The housebound patient may as a first step simply stand outside on the porch and then do that for a set amount of time every day until the anxiety is minimal or absent. The next step would be to go to the end of the front walk, and then farther until the patient is walking around the block, then going to a local store, and so on. Such plans must be tailored to the patient's specific symptoms and the locale in which the plan is to be implemented. In some cases the presence of a therapist is required, in others that of a friend or acquaintance, but the goal remains independent travel anywhere away from home.

The occurrence of a panic attack during such a behavioral program generally sets the patient back, often right back to a housebound state. Thus, it is prudent to treat patients who have panic attacks as outlined in the chapter on panic disorder. However, antipanic agents, of themselves, usually have little or no effect on the agoraphobia itself and cannot substitute for a behavior program.

BIBLIOGRAPHY

Breier A, Charney DS, Heninger GR. Agoraphobia with panic attacks. Development, diagnostic stability, and course of illness. *Archives of General Psychiatry* 1986;43:1029-1036.

Fava GA, Zielezny M, Savron G, et al. Long-term effects of behavioral treatment for panic disorder with agoraphobia. *The British Journal of Psychiatry* 1995;166:87-92.

Fava GA, Rafanelli C, Grandi S, et al. Long-term outcome of panic disorder with agoraphobia treated by exposure. *Psychological Medicine* 2001; 31:891-898.

Goisman RM, Warshaw MG, Steketee GS, et al. DSM-IV and the disappearance of agoraphobia without a history of panic disorder: new data on a controversial diagnosis. *The American Journal of Psychiatry* 1995; 152:1438-1443.

Horwarth E, Lish JD, Johnson J, et al. Agoraphobia without panic: clinical reappraisal of an epidemiologic finding. *The American Journal of Psychiatry* 1993;150:1496-1501.

Ito LM, de Araujo LA, Tess VL, et al. Self-exposure therapy for panic disorder with agoraphobia: randomized controlled study of external v. interoceptive self-exposure. *The British Journal of Psychiatry* 2001;178:331-336.

85 Specific Phobia (DSM-IV-TR #300.29)

The patient with a specific or, as it is also called, a simple phobia experiences extreme anxiety when approaching something that for others arouses little or no apprehension. Although adult patients acknowledge the irrationality of the fear, they nevertheless go out of their way to avoid contact with the feared object. First described by Hippocrates, this condition is apparently quite common. Accurate prevalence figures are difficult to establish because many patients simply do not admit their phobias; however, the lifetime prevalence appears to be about 10%. Simple phobias are about twice as common in females as in males.

In the past it was fashionable to name the various specific phobias according to the feared object. Thus one reads about claustrophobia, acrophobia, arachnophobia, and the like. Such names, however, add little to our understanding of specific phobia and are thus probably best reserved for displays of erudition. One exception to this, however, as is seen later, is the "blood-injury" phobia that indeed may be different from the other specific phobias.

ONSET

No premorbid abnormalities are evident, nor is a prodrome generally found. The onset of the illness is heralded by the first time the patient experiences the characteristic irrational anxiety. Occasionally, a precipitant may be apparent. For example, a stressful life event may precipitate it; however, for many patients no precipitating factor whatsoever exists, and they are at a loss as to how to explain becoming so frightened. Both animal phobias and blood-injury phobia tend to have an onset in childhood; the others may first appear either in childhood or early adult years.

CLINICAL FEATURES

Although the number of objects and situations that patients have come to be phobic about is extraordinarily large, each individual patient usually fears only one or, at the most, several things. Common among the phobias are fears of snakes, spiders, air travel, train travel, being in closed spaces, heights, darkness, and storms.

On approaching the phobic object (or at times even on merely imagining such an approach), the patient experiences extreme anxiety, often accompanied by autonomic symptoms such as tachycardia, tremor, diaphoresis, and piloerection. Depersonalization may occur. Some patients may be able to steel themselves to this and stay nearby, but for the most part the fear is so great that they must escape no matter how humiliating or embarrassing such behavior might be to them. Most adolescent and adult patients make no attempt to justify their behavior; they realize that it is irrational yet they feel powerless over it. Children, however, may not appreciate the irrationality of their reaction and may have temper tantrums or be excessively clinging.

Blood-injury phobia, as mentioned earlier, appears different from the other phobias. A common example is found in patients who are phobic about having a venipuncture. If these patients can force themselves to hold still for a phlebotomist, the symptomatic response is biphasic. First they have anxiety, tachycardia, and hypertension, and these are symptoms similar to what is seen in the other specific phobias. Second, however, one sees a parasympathetic response with a drop in blood pressure and a "vaso-vagal" syncope. It is this second phase of response which clinically differentiates the blood-injury phobia from the other specific phobias.

COURSE

The later the age of onset, the more chronic the phobia tends to be; in many cases they are lifelong. Phobias with an onset in childhood, however (for example, the common animal phobias), tend to remit spontaneously over a few months or a year. When the childhood onset phobia persists into teenage years, however, the course tends to be chronic.

COMPLICATIONS

Depending on how the phobic object figures in the patients' life, complications may range from trivial to disabling. The life of the sailor may not be disturbed at all by a fear of snakes; a coal miner, however, who developed a fear of closed spaces would be disabled.

ETIOLOGY

The specific phobias, most especially the blood-injury type, are familial, and although environmental factors are clearly important, it appears that genetic factors also play a role: some authors assert that children "learn" phobias by modeling their parents' behavior, whereas others believe that certain specific phobias may be "innate" and a vestigial remnant from our earlier evolutionary history, when the possession of certain automatic fearful responses, such as a fear of snakes, might indeed have conferred a selective advantage. In support of the evolutionary hypothesis is the fact that certain monkeys who have never had any contact with a snake react with fear upon seeing one.

In the case of blood-injury phobia, it appears that there is an underlying, chronic, autonomic dysfunction that predisposes these patients to a vaso-vagal response.

DIFFERENTIAL DIAGNOSIS

Social phobia may be distinguished from specific phobia by the fact that in social phobia what is feared is humiliation or embarrassment, rather than the thing itself. For example, the patient with a fear of eating in public is not afraid of the act of eating itself; indeed, if alone, the patient demonstrates faultless conduct at the table. What the patient does fear is the possible public scrutiny should the meal be eaten in public. In a similar vein one may distinguish a "school phobia" from a specific phobia. In "school phobia," or separation anxiety disorder, what is feared is separation from home and parents, not going to school itself.

Occasionally one may see otherwise typical phobias in the course of a depressive episode, or at times early in the course of schizophrenia. As these phobias subside with adequate treatment of the underlying disorder, their presence does not necessitate a second diagnosis of specific phobia.

TREATMENT

An element common to all successful treatments for specific phobia is persuading the patient to confront the phobic object or situation. The patient who fears flying must fly; the patient who fears closed spaces must spend time in one. It is the only way they eventually become convinced, in a meaningful way, of the baselessness of their fear.

Often this goal may be accomplished by supportive psychotherapy alone. For many patients, gentle, encouraging prodding by a confident physician may be all that is needed to bring them in contact with what they fear. Often, however, more specific techniques may be required.

Traditionally, systematic desensitization has been employed, and there is now evidence that computer-generated "virtual reality" exposure may also be effective. Recently, cognitive therapy has been successfully employed for specific phobias, and this may be comparable in effectiveness to desensitization.

Drug treatment of specific phobia has not been extensively studied. In practice many patients are prescribed a benzodiazepine; however, this has not been formally studied, and one must be wary of the dangers of neuroadaptation: one exception to this caution would be in "one time" situations, e.g., when a patient with claustrophobia must undergo an MRI study in a "closed" system, when a mildly sedating dose of a rapid-acting benzodiazepine would be appropriate. A recent small, but double-blinded, study found that paroxetine, in a dose of 20 mg, was more effective than placebo, but replication is required: if successfully replicated then a comparison study of paroxetine and cognitive or behavioral treatments would be very interesting.

BIBLIOGRAPHY

Accurso V, Winnicki M, Shamsuzzaman AS, et al. Predisposition to vasovagal syncope in subjects with blood/injury phobia. *Circulation* 2001;104:903-907.

Benjamin J, Ben-Zion IZ, Karbofsky E, et al. Double-blind placebo-controlled pilot study of paroxetine for specific phobia. *Psychopharmacology* 2000;149:194-196.

Fyer AJ, Mannuzza S, Gallops MS, et al. Familial transmission of simple phobias and fears. A preliminary report. *Archives of General Psychiatry* 1990;47:252-256.

Hollenhorst J, Munte S, Friedrich L, et al. Using intranasal midazolam spray to prevent claustrophobia induced by MR imaging. *American Journal of Roentgenology* 2001;176:865-868.

Marks I. Blood-injury phobia: a review. *The American Journal of Psychiatry* 1988;145:1207-1213.

Ost LG, Alm T, Brandberg M, et al. One vs five sessions of exposure and five sessions of cognitive therapy in the treatment of claustrophobia. *Behaviour Research and Therapy* 2001;39:167-183.

Rothbaum BO, Hodges LF, Kooper R, et al. Effectiveness of computer-generated (virtual reality) graded exposure in the treatment of acrophobia. *The American Journal of Psychiatry* 1995;152:626-628.

86 Social Phobia (DSM-IV-TR #300.23)

In social phobia patients fear that if they attempt to do things in public they will appear inept, foolish, or inadequate and thus suffer shame, embarrassment, or humiliation. Feeling this way, patients, although admitting that the fears are irrational and groundless, nevertheless become intensely anxious upon approaching these situations and may go to great lengths to avoid them.

Estimates of the lifetime prevalence of social phobia in the United States range from 2.6 to 13.3%; it is more common in females than in males.

ONSET

Onset ranges from late childhood to early adult years, with most patients falling ill in their midteens. Premorbidly, some of these patients tend to be shy and to blush easily. The actual onset itself is heralded by the first wave of irrational anxiety over doing something in public.

CLINICAL FEATURES

There are two subtypes of social phobia, namely generalized and circumscribed. The generalized subtype, also known as social anxiety disorder, is characterized by fears that span multiple situations: such patients may be fearful of answering questions in class, asking others out for dates, attending meetings or, in severe cases, of interacting socially at all. The circumscribed subtype, also known as the discrete or non-generalized subtype, by contrast, is characterized by a fear of acting ineptly or foolishly in only very circumscribed situations. Among the circumscribed social phobias a fear of public speaking is by far the most common, followed by fears of trembling when writing in public, choking when eating in public, and being unable to urinate when others are around.

Regardless of the subtype, however, it is not so much the act itself that is feared, but rather, it is the doing of the act in public which arouses the fear. The patient paralyzed into muteness by a fear of public speaking may be able, provided that the hall is empty, to mount the podium and deliver the speech flawlessly.

If patients do approach the phobic situation (or even sometimes merely imagine approaching it), they experience intense anxiety, often accompanied by tremor, diaphoresis, palpitations, and dyspnea. In some cases patients may be able to endure these symptoms and go through with the situation. In other cases, however, the symptoms are overwhelming and patients may refuse to go on. In extreme cases a full-blown panic attack may occur.

One specific social phobia, erythrophobia, deserves special mention, as it appears to be much more common in females than in males. Here the patient's fear is of blushing in public. At times, in fact, the patient may blush scarlet; however, often the blush is not noted by others and is experienced privately by the patient as a flush or an uncomfortable sense of rising warmth.

Major depression, dysthymia, and alcohol abuse and alcoholism may also be present.

COURSE

Social phobia appears to be chronic; whether or not spontaneous remissions occur with any frequency is not known.

COMPLICATIONS

Complications vary depending on the juxtaposition of the phobia and the patient's occupation, or the social demands placed upon them. For a patient with a phobia of public speaking, a promotion may be refused if the new position involves giving speeches. Some patients with the fear of urinating in public rest rooms may refuse family trips.

Finally, anxiety and autonomic symptoms may in fact impair performance to the point where it is inept. A patient phobic about writing in public may tremble so much that handwriting does indeed become illegible.

ETIOLOGY

Most research has focused on the generalized subtype of social phobia. The risk of social phobia is clearly higher in first-degree relatives of patients, and there may be an increased concordance in twins. Various studies have implicated different neurotransmitters in social phobia. Fenfluramine, an indirect serotonin agonist, causes an enhanced release of cortisol, suggesting a hypersensitivity of serotonin receptors. The endogenous benzodiazepine system has also been implicated by the finding of a reduced density of benzodiazepine receptors on platelets from patients with social phobia. Finally, abnormalities of dopaminergic function have been strongly suggested by two studies, one of which found a reduced density of dopamine reuptake transporters and another which found a reduced binding capacity of post-synaptic dopamine receptors. Although no structural changes have been found on MRI scanning, functional MRI studies have demonstrated a greater activation of the amygdala and related areas to social stress in patients than in controls. Given these findings, it is plausible that the generalized subtype of social phobia results from an inherited disturbance of neurotransmitter functioning leading to an enhanced responsiveness of those central nervous structures, such as the amygdala, which mediate anxiety in social situations.

Regarding the circumscribed subtype of social phobia, it appears that there might be an enhanced sensitivity of norepinephrine receptors.

DIFFERENTIAL DIAGNOSIS

Simple, or specific, phobias may be readily distinguished from social phobias by asking patients if they are able to engage in the fearful behavior in private: the patient with a simple phobia, say a fear of snakes, is no more able to approach the snake in private than in public; however, the patient with a social phobia, say a fear of public speaking, may be able to perform perfectly a speech in private which would be terrifying if done in public.

"School phobia," more properly known as "separation anxiety disorder," may be distinguished from a social phobia by examining what the child is afraid of. In school phobia, the fear is not so much of entering the social situation of school but rather is of being separated from the mother or father.

Agoraphobia is distinguished from the generalized subtype of social phobia by the nature of the patient's fear. In agoraphobia the fear is not of doing something humiliating or embarrassing in public spaces, but is rather that something awful might happen while being out in a public space.

Dysmorphophobia, also known as body dysmorphic disorder, is, like the generalized subtype of social phobia, characterized by a fear of humiliation or embarrassment on being in public, but in dysmorphophobia the fear arises from the patient's belief that they are in some way misshapen, rather than from a concern that they might act in an embarrassing way.

Certain psychotic disorders, such as schizophrenia, may be accompanied by a fear of going out into public, but here the fear arises from delusions, such as delusions of reference or persecution. Of interest, clozapine may also, as a side-effect, induce behavioral changes similar to those seen in social phobia.

Certain disorders, by their very symptoms, may occasion some embarrassment, and in such cases a separate diagnosis of social phobia is not made. Examples include essential tremor, developmental stuttering and anorexia nervosa.

One must distinguish between social phobia and a "normal" fear of doing something in public. Most people experience some apprehension or stage fright when first approaching certain situations. However, the anxiety is not potentially disabling. Furthermore, the anxiety tends to abate with a reasonable amount of exposure or a few "dress rehearsals."

Before leaving this discussion of differential diagnosis, a word is in order regarding avoidant personality disorder. It is not clear whether social phobia and avoidant personality disorder are, in fact, distinct disorders, and may authors consider avoidant personality disorder to be an extreme example of a generalized social phobia.

TREATMENT

With regard to the generalized subtype, multiple treatment options are available, including SSRIs, venlafaxine, clonazepam, MAOIs, gabapentin and various psychotherapies. Among the SSRIs, sertraline (50-150 mg/d), paroxetine (20-40 mg/d) and fluvoxamine (150-200 mg/d) are all effective, fluoxetine; however, was not found effective in a double-blinded study. Venlafaxine may be given in doses of from 150 to 225 mg daily. Clonazepam, in a dose of 2-3 mg/d, is effective, but must be tapered slowly to avoid withdrawal anxiety. Of the MAOIs, phenelzine, in doses of 60-90 mg/d, is effective; brofaromine, a reversible MAOI not available in the United States, is also effective. Gabapentin, in doses of 2800 mg/d or less, is more effective than placebo, and generally very well tolerated. Choosing among these various options is difficult, in large part because there are no comparison studies. The SSRIs, venlafaxine, clonazepam and gabapentin are all easy to use and generally well tolerated, and it is reasonable to start with one of these and switch to another in case of non-response: given that the SSRIs have the most experimental backing, it is reasonable to begin with one of these. The MAOI phenelzine is difficult to use, and thus generally held in reserve. Of the psychotherapies, cognitive-behavioral group therapy is comparable to clonazepam and phenelzine, but both medications outperformed the psychotherapy on several measures.

With regard to the circumscribed subtype, patients troubled by prominent autonomic symptoms (e.g., tremor or tachycardia) may be treated with propranolol in doses of from 20-60 mg on a "prn" basis about an hour before the social situation. In cases where the social situation will outlast the half-life of immediate-release propranolol, a long-acting preparation may be used. Psychotherapy is also useful in the circumscribed subtype, typically involving some form of in vivo or imaginal desensitization.

BIBLIOGRAPHY

Brantigan CO, Brantigan TA, Joseph N. Effect of beta blockade and beta stimulation on stage fright. *The American Journal of Medicine* 1982; 72:88-94.

Davidson JR, Potts N, Richichi E, et al. Treatment of social phobia with clonazepam and placebo. *Journal of Clinical Psychopharmacology* 1993;13:423-428.

Fyer AJ, Mannuzza S, Chapman TF, et al. A direct interview family study of social phobia. *Archives of General Psychiatry* 1993;50:286-293.

Greist JH. The diagnosis of social phobia. *The Journal of Clinical Psychiatry* 1995;56(Suppl 5):5-12.

Hartley LR, Ungapen S, Davie I, et al. The effect of beta adrenergic blocking drugs on speakers' performance and memory. *The British Journal of Psychiatry* 1983;142:512-517.

Heimberg RG, Liebowitz MR, Hope DA, et al. Cognitive behavioral group therapy vs phenelzine therapy for social phobia: 12-week outcome. *Archives of General Psychiatry* 1998;55:1133-1141.

Jefferson JW. Social phobia: everyone's disorder? *The Journal of Clinical Psychiatry* 1996;57(Suppl 6):28-32.

Jefferson JW. Benzodiazepines and anticonvulsants for social phobia (social anxiety disorder). *The Journal of Clinical Psychiatry* 2001; 62(Suppl 1):50-53.

Johnson MR, Marazziti D, Brawman-Mintzer O, et al. Abnormal peripheral benzodiazepine receptor density associated with generalized social phobia. *Biological Psychiatry* 1998;43:306-309.

Katzelnick DJ, Kobak KA, Greist JH, et al. Sertraline for social phobia: a double-blind, placebo-controlled crossover study. *The American Journal of Psychiatry* 1995;152:1368-1371.

Kobak KA, Greist JH, Jefferson JW, et al. Fluoxetine in social phobia: a double-blind, placebo-controlled pilot study. *Journal of Clinical Psychopharmacology* 2002;22:257-262.

Lieb R, Wittchen HU, Hofler M, et al. Parental psychopathology, parenting styles, and the risk of social phobia in offspring: a prospective-longitudinal community study. *Archives of General Psychiatry* 2000;57:859-866.

Liebowitz MR, Schneier F, Campeas R, et al. Phenelzine vs atenolol in social phobia. A placebo-controlled comparison. *Archives of General Psychiatry* 1992;49:290-300.

Lott M, Greist JH, Jefferson JW, et al. Brofaromine for social phobia: a multicenter, placebo-controlled, double-blind study. *Journal of Clinical Psychopharmacology* 1997;17:255-260.

Otto MW, Pollack MH, Gould RA, et al. A comparison of the efficacy of clonazepam and cognitive-behavioral group therapy for the treatment of social phobia. *Journal of Anxiety Disorders* 2000;14:345-358.

Pallanti S, Quercioli L, Rossi A, et al. The emergence of social phobia during clozapine treatment and its response to fluoxetine augmentation. *The Journal of Clinical Psychiatry* 1999;60:819-823.

Pande AC, Davidson JR, Jefferson JW, et al. Treatment of social phobia with gabapentin: a placebo-controlled study. *Journal of Clinical Psychopharmacology* 1999;19:341-348.

Schneier FR, Liebowitz MR, Abi-Dargham A, et al. Low dopamine D(2) receptor binding potential in social phobia. *The American Journal of Psychiatry* 2000;157:457-459.

Stein DJ, Stein MB, Goodwin W, et al. The selective serotonin reuptake inhibitor paroxetine is effective in more generalized and in less generalized social anxiety disorder. *Psychopharmacology* 2001;158:267-272.

Stein DJ, Versiani M, Hair T, et al. Efficacy of paroxetine for relapse prevention in social anxiety disorder: a 24-week study. *Archives of General Psychiatry* 2002;59:1111-1118.

Stein MB, Fyer AJ, Davidson JR, et al. Fluvoxamine treatment of social phobia (social anxiety disorder): a double-blind, placebo-controlled study. *The American Journal of Psychiatry* 1999;156:756-760.

Stein MB, Goldin PR, Sareen J, et al. Increased amygdala activation to angry and contemptuous faces in generalized social phobia. *Archives of General Psychiatry* 2002;59:1027-1034.

Tancer ME, Mailman RB, Stein MB, et al. Neuroendocrine responsivity to monaminergic system probes in generalized social phobia. *Anxiety* 1994;1:216-223.

Tiihonen J, Kuikka J, Bergstrom K, et al. Dopamine reuptake site densities in patients with social phobia. *The American Journal of Psychiatry* 1997;154:239-242.

Walker JR, Van Ameringen MA, Swinson R, et al. Prevention of relapse in generalized social phobia: results of a 24-week study in responders to 20 weeks of sertraline treatment. *Journal of Clinical Psychopharmacology* 2000;20:636-644.

87 Obsessive-Compulsive Disorder (DSM-IV-TR #300.3)

Obsessive-compulsive disorder, once known as "obsessive-compulsive neurosis," and occasionally referred to by subtype designations, such as "délire de doute" or "délire de toucher," is a relatively common disorder, with a lifetime prevalence of from 2 to 3%. It is probably equally common among males and females.

Patients with this disorder are plagued with recurrent obsessions or compulsions, often with both. Obsessions may manifest as recurrent thoughts, ideas, images, impulses, fears, or doubts. The obsessions are autonomous; although patients who find themselves obsessing may resist them, they are unable to stop them; they come and go on their own. Compulsions, likewise, may manifest in a variety of ways. Patients may feel compelled to touch, to count, to check, to have everything symmetrically arranged, or to repeatedly wash their hands. Attempts to resist the compulsion are met with crescendoing anxiety, which is relieved as soon as the patient gives in to the compulsion.

With the exception of children, most patients at some point recognize the senselessness of their obsessions and compulsions; yet, though their lives may be consumed by them, patients find themselves unable to stop or resist them.

Most patients with this disorder are ashamed of their experience. This shame may be especially profound in the case of certain compulsions, as, for example, the compulsive washer who spends 6 or 8 hours a day in the bathroom, or in certain obsessions, especially those with violent or sexual themes. Such shame makes patients reluctant to report their symptoms, and this may account for the fact that earlier epidemiologic studies reported this to be a rare disorder, with a traditional prevalence figure being about 0.05%.

Before the 1980s these patients had little hope. The extremity of their suffering is perhaps hinted at by the fact that many patients seriously entertained the option of lobotomy, and some underwent it. Modern behavioral treatment and pharmacologic treatment, however, may now provide relief for a majority of sufferers, and as this news has spread in the general population, more and more patients are overcoming their shame and revealing their symptoms to their physicians.

ONSET

In some cases the onset seems to follow an "understandable" precipitating factor. A compulsion to wash, for example, may follow contact with a particularly foul substance. Even with precipitants, however, the symptoms that follow are clearly out of all reasonable proportion. A normal person may feel "compelled" to wash his hands twice, or perhaps even three times, after touching something putrid; this, however, is a far cry from the patient who for years washes his hands dozens of times each day.

Most patients fall ill in adolescent or early adult years; onset in childhood is not rare, but onset past the age of 40 is quite rare.

CLINICAL FEATURES

The majority of patients with obsessive-compulsive disorder experience both obsessions and compulsions; somewhat less than 25% have only obsessions, and about 5% have only compulsions. Very rarely one finds a patient with a subtype known as primary obsessive slowness.

Although the subject matter of an obsession may be neutral, for example recurrent meaningless phrases or songs, one often finds violent or sexual themes. Patients may be horrified to find themselves obsessing over such things; they do their utmost to will the obsession away, and when that fails, as it usually does, they may avoid situations that might bear a relationship to the subject of their obsessions. A young mother could not stop imagining her toddler being crushed to death by a truck; she would not let him from her sight, and when crossing the street she insisted on carrying him. A seminary student experienced a horrible impulse to utter obscenities upon approaching others; the apprehension that this urge might not be controllable was so great that the student left the seminary. Some patients experience what are known as obsessive-ruminative states, wherein they continuously, ploddingly ponder over abstruse religious or philosophic speculations.

Compulsions spring from recurrent doubts or fears that something awful has happened or will happen. Patients are often subtyped according to what they feel compelled to do. Common subtypes include checkers, washers, touchers, counters, and arrangers. Although patients recognize the senselessness of their compulsive behavior, they are unable to resist acting on the compulsion. If they try to resist, the anxiety associated with their fear or doubt may become so intolerable that they have to give into the compulsion and go back to check, touch, count, or wash. In one case, a patient, upon driving over a bump in the road, was filled with the fear that someone might have been run over and thus was compelled to go back and check to see if there was a body in the road. The relief at not finding one was only momentary, however, because almost immediately the fear arose that the victim had not been killed but simply badly injured and had crawled off the road, and this fear gave birth to the compulsion to check behind the bushes at the roadside, then in nearby backyards, and so on. Other common checkings include going back to see if the door is locked or if the gas is turned off; one patient could not mail a letter because of the need to open it repeatedly to check if everything had been spelled correctly in the letter itself.

Washers generally fear that they have been contaminated by germs, dirt, or excrement; they feel compelled to wash repetitively no matter what the circumstance. To one office worker, doorknobs were a source of contagion, and if one were ever touched a trip to the bathroom was absolutely necessary to repeatedly wash the hands, even if it meant keeping the boss waiting.

Compulsions may or may not have a certain logic to them. In some cases one may "understand" the patient's feelings. For example, one can empathize with the patient who fears contamination and experiences a compulsion to wash. What passes empathy, of course, is the fact that the patient feels compelled to wash repeatedly, whereas the normal individual would be satisfied with one or perhaps two washings. Other compulsions, however, seem to defy logic. At times some magical thinking may be associated with them. In fact in some instances, patients themselves have difficulty describing the motive for their compulsive behavior. Arrangers, touchers and counters often fall in this group. One "arranger" felt compelled to have things organized "just so" in the closet before going to bed. Shoes had to be arranged in a certain way, the ties all hanging perfectly straight, none of the suit jackets touching each other as they hung from the rod. Repeatedly the patient would get back out of bed to adjust an article of clothing, moving it this way or that, sometimes only a fraction of an inch. Retiring again, the patient would be seized with the fear that things were not perfectly symmetric, and again would have to get up and go to the closet. When pressed by the exasperated spouse for an explanation of this behavior, the patient could say no more than that he felt a premonition that something awful would happen if the compulsion were not given in to. Another patient, a toucher, felt compelled to touch every hardbound book that came into view; though feeling foolish in doing so and acknowledging that the fear was even more foolish,

the patient could not shake the idea that someone would die if the books failed to be touched.

Although most compulsive behaviors are observable, at times "silent" mental rituals may occur. Examples include the patient who had to think "The Lord's Prayer" a precise number of times, or another who was compelled to imagine a certain sequence of scenes.

Initially, at least, almost all patients view their compulsions as senseless, and out of embarrassment, shame, or simply annoyance at having so much time consumed by them, they resist carrying them out. The growing tension that accompanies this resistance, however, is generally unbearable, and indeed many patients eventually give up trying; they eventually either put up no resistance or only a token one and eventually simply give in. In obtaining a history, therefore, one should ask not only about the patient's current response to the compulsion but also the initial one. Rarely, patients with obsessive-compulsive disorder become psychotic. For example, a compulsive washer may develop the delusion that indeed a contamination is present and that the repetitive washings therefore make perfect sense.

In primary obsessive slowness, routine daily activities become transformed into lengthy, meticulous rituals. Dressing or perhaps preparing and eating breakfast may take hours. The sequence and form of each step in the process is carefully and scrupulously observed; they experience intense anxiety should any deviation occur or even threaten to occur. Only when perfectly satisfied that the job has been rightly done can the patient move on to the next task of the day. Patients with primary obsessive slowness also tend to have, or to have had earlier in life, other compulsions, such as checking or washing.

Three disorders associated with obsessive-compulsive disorder are major depression, Tourette's syndrome, and any of a number of different personality disorders. Perhaps one half of all patients with obsessive-compulsive disorder also have one or more depressive episodes in their lifetimes. About 5% of patients with obsessive-compulsive disorder also have Tourette's syndrome, and almost 25% have some form of tic. The relationship between obsessive-compulsive disorder and obsessive-compulsive personality disorder deserves special comment. Early writings held that the obsessive-compulsive personality style provided fertile soil for the development of true obsessions and compulsions and suggested an etiologic relation between the two disorders. Recent research, however, fails to support this notion. Although the majority of patients with obsessive-compulsive disorder indeed have one of the personality disorders, only a minority have an obsessive-compulsive personality disorder; other personality disorders, such as histrionic, passive-aggressive, and schizotypal, are more common.

COURSE

Although obsessive-compulsive disorder generally pursues a gradually waxing and waning course, exceptions do occur. In a small minority, perhaps 5%, symptoms will undergo a complete, or near-complete, spontaneous remission; in such cases, however, relapses generally occur in the following years. In another minority of cases, perhaps 10 to 15%, the course is progressively downhill until patients' lives are consumed by obsessions and compulsions and their responses to them.

COMPLICATIONS

The complications of obsessive-compulsive disorder are for the most part directly related to the time and energy consumed by the obsessions and/or the compulsions. In mild cases, especially if characterized primarily by obsessions, there may be little encroachment on the patient's work and family life. In severe cases, however, little time is left for other activities, and job and marriage may be lost. The hands of hand washers may become so raw, even bleeding, that dermatologic consultation may be sought. Unfortunately, often in such cases the dermatologist is kept in the dark about the cause of the lesion, and a fruitless search for a primary dermatologic disorder may be undertaken.

ETIOLOGY

Family studies have demonstrated an increased prevalence of obsessive-compulsive disorder in the first degree relatives of patients as compared to controls, and twin studies, though not conclusive, suggest a higher concordance rate in monozygotic as compared to dizygotic twins. There is also, in a subset of patients, a familial relation with Tourette's syndrome.

Serotoninergic transmission is disturbed in obsessive-compulsive disorder. The only currently available medicines that are consistently effective in obsessive-compulsive disorder, clomipramine and the SSRIs, all preferentially affect serotoninergic transmission, with noradrenergic and dopaminergic transmission being relatively unaffected directly. Medications such as desipramine, which have a preferential affect on noradrenergic transmission, are ineffective. Furthermore, m-chlorophenylpiperazine (mCPP), a mixed serotonin agonist/antagonist, has been shown in some studies to increase the severity of obsessions and compulsions.

PET scanning has strongly implicated involvement of the orbito-frontal cortex, the caudate nucleus and the thalamus: remarkably, the increased metabolic activity found in these structures reverts toward normal in successfully treated patients.

Overall, it appears plausible to say that in most cases, obsessive-compulsive disorder represents an inherited abnormality of serotoninergic functioning in the fronto-striato-thalamo-cortical circuit; the molecular nature of this abnormality, however, is not as yet clear.

In a minority of cases, it appears that obsessive-compulsive disorder occurs as a sequela to Sydenham's chorea. As noted in the section on differential diagnosis, below, prominent obsessions and compulsions are seen in the majority of patients with Sydenham's chorea, and it appears that, in an as yet unknown proportion of these cases, obsessions and compulsions may reappear in the future, unaccompanied by chorea. One clue to the diagnosis of this etiologic variant of obsessive-compulsive disorder is a "triggering" of obsessions or compulsions by a preceding group A beta-hemolytic streptococcal pharyngitis.

DIFFERENTIAL DIAGNOSIS

The first diagnostic task is to determine whether or not patients have true obsessions or compulsions. Once it has been established that they do, then a differential diagnosis of these "true" symptoms must be pursued.

Various disorders may produce symptoms quite similar to true obsessions and compulsions; however, with close inquiry, these "look-alikes" may be correctly identified.

Paraphilias, alcoholism, bulimia nervosa, pathologic gambling, or pyromania are all accompanied by a sense, on the patient's part, of being "compelled" to do something, whether it be aberrant sexual acts, drinking, eating, gambling or fire-setting. Importantly, however, in these conditions, in contrast with obsessive-compulsive disorder,

gratification or pleasure is involved in giving in to the "compulsion." Paraphiliacs enjoy giving in to the compulsion to, say, engage in sadomasochistic behavior, and alcoholics enjoy the drink they feel compelled to take. By contrast, although the patient with obsessive-compulsive disorder may experience some relief at giving in to the compulsion, say, to wash, there is no actual pleasure in the act of washing itself.

Obsessive-compulsive personality disorder is characterized by an "obsession" with detail and a "compulsion" to do things perfectly; these drives, however, are not "true" obsessions and compulsions: unlike "true" obsessions and compulsions, which patients view as senseless and try and resist, the drives for order and perfection seen in the personality disorder are experienced as quite purposeful, and, rather than being resisted, are often pursued with righteous vigor.

Social phobia may resemble obsessive-compulsive disorder in those cases where patients are obsessed with doing something potentially embarrassing. For example, a patient obsessed with a fear of cursing may avoid giving lectures, and thus appear similar to the patient with a social phobia of public speaking. The difference here is that whereas patients with obsessive-compulsive disorder worry about what they might do to the audience, e.g., curse, patients with social phobia worry about what the audience might do to them, e.g., laugh at their trembling hands and quavering voice.

Depression may be characterized by brooding or rumination, which may appear similar to obsessions. Here, however, in contrast to the attitude of patients with obsessive-compulsive disorder regarding obsessions, the depressed patient considers the ruminations quite sensible; the endless repetitive thoughts of guilt, sin, and punishment strike such a patient as quite fitting.

Various psychoses, such as schizophrenia, may be characterized by the Schneiderian First Rank delusion of "thought insertion," which may appear very similar to an obsession. Here, however, the patient experiences the thought as alien, as being "inserted" by "outside forces." Furthermore, patients with this psychotic symptom may have further unusual beliefs related to the source of the thought, believing it to be induced by computers, rays, or UFOs.

Once it has been established that the patient, indeed, does have obsessions or compulsions, the following should be considered in the differential diagnosis.

Lesions of the basal ganglia are especially prone to cause obsessions or compulsions, as may be seen with infarction, closed head injury, Fahr's syndrome, or subsequent to cerebral anoxia or viral encephalitis. Lesions of the right parietal lobe may, albeit less commonly, also be at fault. Second generation antipsychotics, including clozapine, risperidone and olanzapine, may also be responsible. Simple partial seizures may manifest with recurrent, intrusive thoughts; here the correct etiology is suggested by a history of other, more obvious, epileptic phenomena, such as complex partial or grand mal seizures.

Sydenham's chorea is especially important in the differential of obsessions and compulsions: up to 70% of patients with Sydenham's will have these, and in most cases they appear before chorea does. Here, a history of other rheumatic manifestations (e.g., arthritis), and, of course, the eventual appearance of the chorea, make the diagnosis.

Tourette's syndrome, schizophrenia and depression are often complicated by obsessions or compulsions, but in such cases the accompanying symptomatology serves to indicate the correct diagnosis.

Finally, it must be kept in mind that the occasional obsession or compulsion is part of normal life. Most people, at some point, complain of a "song I can't stop thinking about" or of wondering whether or not they locked the door or turned off the gas. Here, however, the obsessions or compulsions are of brief duration and do not cause any disability.

TREATMENT

Effective treatment involves using behavior therapy, cognitive therapy, or a serotoninergic medication such as clomipramine, or one of the SSRIs of fluoxetine, fluvoxamine, paroxetine, sertraline, citalopram or escitalopram; in most cases patients are best served by a combination of behavior or cognitive therapy plus a medication.

Behavioral techniques, such as exposure and response prevention, are quite effective, and although clinician-guided therapy is most successful, many patients also benefit from a computer-guided self-help therapy accessed through an interactive telephone system. Cognitive therapy is likewise successful, and indeed, if added in cases of treatment failure with medication, may turn a non-responder into a responder.

SSRIs are by and large equally as effective as clomipramine, and, because they are generally better tolerated, are usually a first choice. The effective dose for fluoxetine is from 20 to 60 mg, for fluvoxamine 100 to 300 mg, for paroxetine 40 to 60 mg, for sertraline 50 to 200 mg, for citalopram 10 to 40 mg, and for escitalopram 5 to 20 mg. Clomipramine is given in a dose from 150 to 300 mg. Importantly, up to six weeks may be required for an initial response, and three months for a full response to any given dose.

In cases where patients do not respond, consideration may be given to using a higher dose, provided it is tolerated. Should that be unfeasible or ineffective, one option is to switch to a different medication, e.g., from an SSRI to clomipramine, or vice versa. Importantly, if one is switching from an SSRI to clomipramine, it is generally prudent to wait until the SSRI has "washed out" before starting clomipramine in order to avoid an SSRI-induced elevation in clomipramine blood level. Another option is to add either risperidone or haloperidol. Risperidone may be effective in low doses of from 2 to 3 mg daily; haloperidol, in doses of perhaps 5 mg, may also be effective, but only in those cases where there is a history of tics. Importantly, these antipsychotics are effective only as augmenting agents; used by themselves they do not relieve obsessions or compulsions. Some clinicians will also combine an SSRI and clomipramine; however, this approach has not been demonstrated effective in double-blinded trials. In disabling cases, where treatment with combinations of medications and either behavior or cognitive therapy are ineffective, consideration may be given to a neurosurgical procedure, such as cingulotomy, anterior capsulotomy or chronic electrical stimulation of the anterior capsules.

BIBLIOGRAPHY

Asbahr FR, Negrao AB, Gentil V, et al. Obsessive-compulsive and related symptoms in children and adolescents with rheumatic fever with and without chorea: a prospective 6-month study. *The American Journal of Psychiatry* 1998;155:1122-1124.

Bergeron R, Ravindran AV, Chaput Y, et al. Sertraline and fluoxetine treatment of obsessive-compulsive disorder: results of a double-blind, 6-month treatment study. *Journal of Clinical Psychopharmacology* 2002;22:148-154.

Berthier ML, Kulisevsky J, Gironell A, et al. Obsessive-compulsive disorder associated with brain lesions: clinical phenomenology, cognitive function, and anatomic correlates. *Neurology* 1996;47:353-361.

Broocks A, Pigott TA, Hill JA, et al. Acute intravenous administration of ondansetron and m-CPP, alone and in combination, in patients with obsessive-compulsive disorder (OCD): behavioral and biological results. *Psychiatry Research* 1998;79:11-20.

Chacko RC, Corbin MA, Harper RG. Acquired obsessive-compulsive disorder associated with basal ganglia lesions. *The Journal of Neuropsychiatry and Clinical Neurosciences* 2000;12:269-272.

de Haan L, Beuk L, Hoogenboom B, et al. Obsessive-compulsive symptoms during treatment with olanzapine and risperidone: a prospective study of 113 patients with recent-onset schizophrenia or related disorders. *The Journal of Clinical Psychiatry* 2002;63:104-107.

Dougherty DD, Baer L, Cosgrove GR, et al. Prospective long-term follow-up of 44 patients who received cingulotomy for treatment-refractory obsessive-compulsive disorder. *The American Journal of Psychiatry* 2002;159:269-275.

Greist JH, Jefferson JW, Rosenfeld R, et al. Clomipramine and obsessive compulsive disorder: a placebo-controlled double-blind study of 32 patients. *The Journal of Clinical Psychiatry* 1990;51:292-297.

Greist JH, Jefferson JW, Kobak KA, et al. A 1 year double-blind placebo-controlled fixed dose study of sertraline in the treatment of obsessive-compulsive disorder. *International Clinical Psychopharmacology* 1995;10:57-65.

Greist JH, Marks IM, Baer L, et al. Behavior therapy for obsessive-compulsive disorder guided by a computer or by a clinician compared with relaxation as a control. *The Journal of Clinical Psychiatry* 2002;63:138-145.

Kampman M, Keijsers GP, Hoogduin CA, et al. Addition of cognitive-behavior therapy for obsessive-compulsive disorder patients non-responding to fluoxetine. *Acta Psychiatrica Scandinavica* 2002;106:314-319.

Kobak KA, Greist JH, Jefferson JW, et al. Behavioral versus pharmacological treatments of obsessive compulsive disorder: a meta-analysis. *Psychopharmacology* 1998;136:205-216.

Lopez-Ibor JJ, Saiz J, Cottraux J, et al. Double-blind comparison of fluoxetine versus clomipramine in the treatment of obsessive-compulsive disorder. *European Neuropsychopharmacology* 1996;6:111-118.

McDougle CJ, Epperson CN, Pelton GH, et al. A double-blind, placebo-controlled study of risperidone addition in serotonin reuptake inhibitor-refractory obsessive-compulsive disorder. *Archives of General Psychiatry* 2000;57:794-801.

Mundo E, Rouillon F, Figuera ML, et al. Fluvoxamine in obsessive-compulsive disorder: similar efficacy but superior tolerability in comparison with clomipramine. *Human Psychopharmacology* 2001;16:461-468.

Nesdadt G, Lan T, Samuels J, et al. Complex segregation analysis provides compelling evidence for a major gene underlying obsessive-compulsive disorder and for heterogeneity by sex. *American Journal of Human Genetics* 2000;67:1611-1616.

Perlmutter SJ, Leitman SF, Garvey MA, et al. Therapeutic plasma exchange and intravenous immunoglobulin for obsessive-compulsive and tic disorders in childhood. *Lancet* 1999;354:1153-1158.

Perse TL, Greist JH, Jefferson JW, et al. Fluvoxamine treatment of obsessive-compulsive disorder. *The American Journal of Psychiatry* 1987;144:1543-1548.

Saxena S, Brody AL, Ho ML, et al. Differential cerebral metabolic changes with paroxetine treatment of obsessive-compulsive disorder vs major depression. *Archives of General Psychiatry* 2002;59:250-261.

Stein DJ. Obsessive-compulsive disorder. *Lancet* 2002;360:397-405.

Zohar J, Judge R. Paroxetine versus clomipramine in the treatment of obsessive-compulsive disorder. OCD Paroxetine Study Investigators. *The British Journal of Psychiatry* 1996;169:468-474.

88 Posttraumatic Stress Disorder (DSM-IV-TR #309.81)

Posttraumatic stress disorder (PTSD), formerly known as "traumatic neurosis," may occur in practically anyone who has been exposed to an overwhelmingly traumatic event. Subsequent to the trauma, whether it be a life-threatening accident, torture, a natural disaster, or some other extraordinary calamity, patients re-experience the event over and over again as if unable to lay it to rest. A general withdrawal from present life occurs, and patients tend to be anxious and easily startled. They may have recurrent dreams of the event or experience intrusive recollection of it during the day. In extreme instances patients seem in fact to be actually reliving the event, and they may act accordingly. For example, a combat veteran may dive for cover if a child sets off a firecracker in the park.

Figures for the lifetime prevalence of this disorder vary widely according to the diagnostic criteria used, with estimates ranging from 1 to 9%. It is probably more common in females than males.

ONSET

As trauma may occur at any age, from childhood to senescence, so too can posttraumatic stress disorder. However, given that the most common precipitating traumas, such as combat, occur in early adult years, most cases have an onset in the twenties.

Symptoms may appear either acutely, within days or weeks after the trauma, or in a delayed fashion, after a latency of months or years, and appear to be more likely in situations wherein the patient, during the actual trauma, experienced dissociation, in particular a distorted perception of time. In cases of delayed onset the latency period is generally, but not always, characterized by dysphoria and occasionally by a tendency to avoid situations reminiscent of the trauma. Occasionally the latent period abruptly ends if the patient experiences a new trauma similar to the first one.

CLINICAL FEATURES

In one fashion or another, these patients become numb to the world around them. Events that used to arouse their interest now leave them unaffected and unmoved. They may complain of feeling dead inside or of having no feelings at all; some may appear listless and detached.

The experience of the trauma lives on in these patients. They have intense, vivid memories of it. Nightmares are common, and, unlike most nightmares, they have little of the fantastic in them; rather they tend to stick to the persistently disturbing facts. At times the waking recollection of the trauma may be more vivid and compelling than the patients' actual surroundings, and they may experience a "flashback" wherein they act as if the trauma were actually recurring. In extreme cases illusions or actual visual and auditory hallucinations recreate the trauma.

Situations that remind the patient of the trauma tend to be avoided. Veterans may refuse to see war films, World War II concentration camp survivors may avoid anything German. If unavoidably trapped in the situation, patients become intensely anxious, even to the point of having a panic attack.

These patients tend to be anxious, tense, and easily startled. Though often fatigued, they struggle to remain alert, as if on guard against some fresh onslaught. Most complain of difficulty with concentration. Insomnia is common. The mood is often labile. Irritability is common, and patients may become enraged with little or no provocation.

Major depression is not uncommon.

Many patients use alcohol to excess, and alcohol abuse or alcoholism may occur, with a concurrent florid exacerbation of the symptoms of posttraumatic stress disorder.

The presentation of posttraumatic stress disorder in childhood is somewhat different from that just described for adults. Many children recreate the trauma while playing. A tortured child may again and again torture dolls or stuffed animals. Nightmares may be less connected with the trauma; they may simply be "scary dreams." Some children come to believe that they will die young; they may seem resigned to it and be disinclined to plan or talk about careers, marriage, or family.

COURSE

In about one half of all cases, symptoms remit spontaneously within months, and this appears to be more often the case when the onset is acute.

A chronic course, however, is not uncommon. A delayed onset tends to predict this, as does a persistence of symptoms for more than a half year. When the course is chronic, symptoms may persist in a waxing and waning fashion for years or decades.

COMPLICATIONS

Preoccupied and more involved with the trauma than with their present life, these patients may let marriage and career slip away from them. Their anxiety and irritability often strain whatever relationships remain; violence may incur legal consequences.

ETIOLOGY

By far the best predictor of posttraumatic stress disorder is the type and severity of the trauma itself. Products of human cruelty, such as torture, or incarceration in a death camp, commonly produce this disorder. Events that catch persons by surprise and then leave them with no social support afterward, such as a typhoon that devastates a community, likewise provide fertile ground for the development of posttraumatic stress disorder. Conversely, certain traumatic events, such as car accidents, are less likely to produce this disorder.

The fact that, regardless of the severity of the trauma, not all survivors develop posttraumatic stress disorder indicates that other factors are involved. Twin studies have suggested a genetic susceptibility; however, it is not clear whether the inherited factor is a susceptibility to the development of posttraumatic stress disorder *per se* or rather a tendency to become involved in high-risk activities.

Biochemical and endocrinologic studies of patients have yielded interesting findings. Noradrenergic activity is clearly abnormal. CSF levels of norepinephrine are increased, and there is a generalized increased reactivity of the sympathetic nervous system; furthermore, administration of yohimbine, a noradrenergic agonist, will often provoke symptoms, such as "flashbacks." Serotoninergic activity is also abnormal, as suggested by a decreased number of paroxetine binding sites on platelets and the ability of mCPP, a serotonin mixed agonist/antagonist, to induce flashbacks. The hypothalamo-pituitary-adrenal cortex axis has been extensively studied, and shows unique abnormalities. CSF levels of CRF are increased, and this is similar to what is found in depression. However, in stark contrast to what is seen in depression, basal cortisol levels are decreased in posttraumatic stress disorder and the low-dose dexamethasone suppression test shows an enhanced suppression of cortisol.

MRI studies, though not entirely in agreement, strongly suggest that the hippocampi of patients with posttraumatic stress disorder are slightly smaller than those of controls. Initially, it was felt that this might be related to the stress of the disorder itself, perhaps being mediated by the high cortisol levels normally seen in times of great stress. The finding, however, of reduced cortisol levels, as noted above, makes this explanation unlikely, and raises the possibility that this subtle hippocampal atrophy might have preceded the stress.

Overall, it appears reasonable to invoke a "stress-diathesis" model for the etiology of posttraumatic stress disorder. However, although the "stress" is clear, the nature of the "diathesis" is not. Conceivably, however, there may be subtle alterations in noradrenergic or serotoninergic activity in those central nervous system structures, such as the amygdala, hippocampus and hypothalamus that mediate anxiety, remembrance and hormonal tone.

DIFFERENTIAL DIAGNOSIS

Diagnostic difficulty may arise if a depressive episode happens to occur after a significant trauma. In such cases patients may be withdrawn, agitated, and tend to ruminate over their misfortune, and thus appear similar to patients with a posttraumatic stress disorder. However, certain qualitative differences exist. The depressed mood contrasts with the detached "numb" experience seen in posttraumatic stress disorder and depressive ruminations are heavy, leaden, and plodding, in sharp contrast to the starkly vivid nature of the intrusive recollections of posttraumatic stress disorder.

Should head injury occur during the trauma, one may see a contribution of a postconcussion syndrome to any difficulty with memory and concentration.

Malingerers or those with factitious illnesses may present a history compatible with posttraumatic stress disorder. Examination of records, particularly military service records, often exposes the lie. In cases where in fact a trauma occurred, a diagnosis of malingering may remain in doubt until symptoms resolve after adjudication of the lawsuit.

Before leaving this discussion of differential diagnosis, some words are in order regarding the putative entity "acute stress disorder." As described in DSM-IV, this diagnosis is given to patients whose illness is essentially clinically identical to posttraumatic stress disorder with the exception of course: when the illness undergoes a spontaneous remission within one month of the trauma, one is asked to make a diagnosis of "acute stress disorder";

however, if the illness persists beyond that time one is supposed to revise the diagnosis to posttraumatic stress disorder. Given that most patients diagnosed with "acute stress disorder" remain ill beyond a month and thus have to have their diagnosis revised, this distinction between "acute stress disorder" and posttraumatic stress disorder may in fact be artificial and unwarranted. It would perhaps be more appropriate to simply say that some cases of posttraumatic stress disorder run a rapid course, resolving within weeks, and let it go at that.

TREATMENT

Both cognitive therapy and behavioral therapy are beneficial. Certain medications are also effective; however, there have not, as yet, been controlled comparisons of medications with either cognitive or behavior therapy. Fluoxetine in doses of 60 mg, paroxetine in doses of 20 to 50 mg, and sertraline in doses of 50 to 200 mg have all been found effective. Both imipramine and phenelzine are also effective; however, their side-effect profiles argue against using them as first line agents. Recent work has also focused on pharmacologic treatment of the troubling nightmares seen in this disorder, and two medications are useful here: cyproheptadine may be given in doses of from 4 to 12 mg hs; prazosin may be started at 1 mg hs and increased in similar increments every few days until patients obtain relief or limiting side-effects occur; most patients respond to a dose of approximately 10 mg. Interestingly, prazosin, in addition to reducing the frequency of nightmares, also led to a diminution of other symptoms.

As noted earlier, alcoholism or alcohol abuse not uncommonly accompanies posttraumatic stress disorder, and when this is the case, it is critical to treat the substance use disorder either first or concurrently with the posttraumatic stress disorder.

BIBLIOGRAPHY

Adler A. Neuropsychiatric complications in victims of Boston's Coconut Grove disaster. *Journal of the American Medical Association* 1943; 123:1098-1101.

Baker DG, West SA, Nicholson WE, et al. Serial CSF corticotropin-releasing hormone levels and adrenocortical activity in combat veterans with posttraumatic stress disorder. *The American Journal of Psychiatry* 1999;156:585-588.

Bryant RA, Harvey AG. Delayed-onset posttraumatic stress disorder: a prospective evaluation. *The Australian and New Zealand Journal of Psychiatry* 2002;36:205-209.

Frank JB, Kosten TR, Giller EL, et al. A randomized clinical trial of phenelzine and imipramine for posttraumatic stress disorder. *The American Journal of Psychiatry* 1988;145:1289-1291.

Geracioti TD, Baker DG, Ekhator NN, et al. CSF norepinephrine concentrations in posttraumatic stress disorder. *The American Journal of Psychiatry* 2001;158:1227-1230.

Harvey AG, Bryant RA. Two-year prospective evaluation of the relationship between acute stress disorder and posttraumatic stress disorder following mild traumatic brain injury. *The Australian and New Zealand Journal of Psychiatry* 2000;157:626-628.

Horowitz M, Willner N, Kaltreider N, et al. Signs and symptoms of posttraumatic stress disorder. *Archives of General Psychiatry* 1980; 37:85-92.

Jacobs-Rebhun S, Schnurr PP, Friedman MJ, et al. Posttraumatic stress disorder and sleep difficulty. *The American Journal of Psychiatry* 2000;157:1525-1526.

Kanter ED, Wilkinson CW, Radant AD, et al. Glucocorticoid feedback sensitivity and adrenocortical responsiveness in posttraumatic stress disorder. *Biological Psychiatry* 2001;50:238-245.

Kinzie JD, Fredrickson RH, Ben R, et al. Posttraumatic stress disorder among survivors of Cambodian concentration camps. *The American Journal of Psychiatry* 1984;141:645-650.

Lee KA, Vaillant GE, Torrey WC, et al. A 50-year prospective study of the psychological sequelae of World War II combat. *The American Journal of Psychiatry* 1995;152:516-522.

Marks I, Lovell K, Noshirvani H, et al. Treatment of posttraumatic stress disorder by exposure and/or cognitive restructuring: a controlled study. *Archives of General Psychiatry* 1998;55:317-325.

Martenyi F, Brown EB, Zhang H, et al. Fluoxetine versus placebo in posttraumatic stress disorder. *The American Journal of Psychiatry* 2002;63:199-206.

Raskind MA, Peskind ER, Kanter ED, et al. Reduction of nightmares and other PTSD symptoms in combat veterans by prazosin: a placebo-controlled study. *The American Journal of Psychiatry* 2003;160:371-373.

Southwick SM, Krystal JH, Bremner JD, et al. Noradrenergic and serotoninergic function in posttraumatic stress disorder. *Archives of General Psychiatry* 1997;54:749-758.

Stein MB, Jang KL, Taylor S, et al. Genetic and environmental influences on trauma exposure and posttraumatic stress disorder symptoms: a twin study. *The American Journal of Psychiatry* 2002;259:1675-1681.

Tucker P, Zaninelli R, Yehuda R, et al. Paroxetine in the treatment of chronic posttraumatic stress disorder: results of a placebo-controlled, flexible-dosage trial. *The Journal of Clinical Psychiatry* 2001;62:860-868.

Villarreal G, Hamilton DA, Petropoulos H, et al. Reduced hippocampal volume and total white matter volume in posttraumatic stress disorder. *Biological Psychiatry* 2002;52:119-125.

Zohar J, Amital D, Miodownik C, et al. Double-blind placebo-controlled pilot study of sertraline in military veterans with posttraumatic stress disorder. *Journal of Clinical Psychopharmacology* 2002;22:190-195.

89 Generalized Anxiety Disorder (DSM-IV-TR #300.02)

Generalized anxiety disorder (GAD), also known as "chronic anxiety neurosis," is characterized by chronic "free-floating anxiety," accompanied by such autonomic symptoms as tremor, tachycardia, and diaphoresis.

The lifetime prevalence of generalized anxiety disorder has been estimated at about 5%, and the female to male ratio at about 2:1. Some doubt, however, has been expressed about these figures, as it appears that in the epidemiologic surveys patients with depression may have been misdiagnosed as having generalized anxiety disorder.

ONSET

Onset is usually in adolescence or childhood years; however, it may also first appear in early adult years. Symptoms tend to evolve gradually and insidiously.

CLINICAL FEATURES

Commonly the patient complains of anxiety, sometimes with bitterness, and often has already consulted several other physicians in the search for relief. The patient is easily startled and jumpy, and loud noises or sudden movements may be particularly alarming. Unable to relax, the patient may spend restless hours at night waiting for sleep.

The patient often complains of a sense of shakiness and may have a fine tremor of the hands. Some patients may "shake like a leaf." The heart may race uncomfortably, "like a bird fluttering in the chest." They may have a lump in the throat, and cold clammy skin is evident upon a handshake.

Patients often complain of indigestion and cramping. They may have constipation or diarrhea. Frequent urination is common. Some may complain of lightheadedness and a fear that they might faint. The completion of minor tasks requires an inordinate degree of effort, and patients often complain of feeling exhausted and of being unable to concentrate.

Patients may volunteer "reasons" why they are anxious; however, on close inspection, either their concerns are unjustified or, if in fact they have an actual occasion for worry, their anxiety and other symptoms are all out of proportion to the facts. Indeed often the free-floating anxiety has "attached" itself to part of the patient's life, or the patient, in a desperate attempt to "make sense" of this experience, has decided that this or that thing is the "cause" of the anxiety.

COURSE

This appears to be a chronic disorder, with symptoms waxing and waning over the years or decades. Whether or not this could be an episodic illness, with long symptom-free intervals, is not clear.

COMPLICATIONS

When symptoms are mild, they may constitute but little interference in the patient's life. In severe cases, however, patients may be completely "paralyzed" by their anxiety and may be unable to function in almost any capacity.

ETIOLOGY

Both family and twin studies support a genetic role in generalized anxiety disorder, and although it is not entirely clear what is inherited, several findings support the presence of abnormalities in GABAergic and noradrenergic activity. GABAergic dysfunction is suggested by the effectiveness of benzodiazepines in this disorder and by the finding of reduced benzodiazepine binding sites, not only on peripheral blood lymphocytes but also within the left temporal pole. Noradrenergic dysfunction is suggested by the similarity of the symptoms of the disorder with those seen upon infusion of noradrenergic drugs and by the presence of a reduced number of alpha-2 adrenergic receptor sites on platelets.

DIFFERENTIAL DIAGNOSIS

An agitated depressive episode, especially during its prodrome, or an agitated dysthymia may present with a clinical picture very similar to that of generalized anxiety disorder, and these two disorders probably occasion most of the many incorrect diagnoses of generalized anxiety disorder. However, certain qualitative differences are noted between the symptomatology of depression and that of generalized anxiety disorder that may allow for the correct diagnosis. Although depressed patients may be anxious, they also experience pervasive despair, hopelessness, or melancholy—affects that are at the most only transiently present in generalized anxiety disorder. The sense of fatigue is likewise different in these disorders. Depressed patients complain of feeling drained or chronically leaden and weighted down; in contrast the patient with generalized anxiety disorder may not experience fatigue until an actual attempt is made to do something. Crying spells, which are common in depression, are not often seen in generalized anxiety disorder.

Patients with panic disorder may develop considerable anticipatory anxiety; however, here the anxiety is over the prospect of having another attack, and panic attacks are not part of the symptomatology of generalized anxiety disorder. Thus in any chronically anxious patient one must take a painstaking history in search of a panic attack.

Patients with specific phobia, social phobia, or obsessive-compulsive disorder may likewise experience considerable anxiety; however, here the symptoms are clearly in direct proportion to the patient's proximity to the dreaded event. Such a clear and predictable correlation between symptoms and events is not seen in generalized anxiety disorder.

In hypochondriasis, anxiety may be pervasive; however, in contrast to generalized anxiety disorder, the symptoms are always intimately connected with one thing, namely the patient's apprehension that she may have an underlying serious disease.

Patients dependent on alcohol, sedative-hypnotics, or anxiolytics may repeatedly find themselves in the midst of withdrawal symptoms characterized by anxiety and autonomic symptoms. Should their substance use be secret, a diagnosis of generalized anxiety disorder might be considered. One clue would be a marked fluctuation in symptoms occurring over hours. Such a course is not seen in generalized anxiety disorder but is quite typical of an intoxication fading rapidly into withdrawal.

A variety of drugs if taken chronically may produce a constant set of side effects that may mimic generalized anxiety disorder. These include caffeine, sympathomimetics, yohimbine, and certain of the "alerting" antidepressants, such as desipramine, bupropion, and the SSRIs. Antipsychotic-induced akathisia may also at times cause some diagnostic uncertainty.

A number of general medical conditions may also cause chronic anxiety, and in most cases the diagnosis is suggested by their associated signs and symptoms. Examples include chronic obstructive pulmonary disease, congestive heart failure, Cushing's syndrome and as a sequela to cerebral infarction in the right hemisphere. Hyperthyroidism is suggested by proptosis, and in many cases by a simple handshake: in contrast to the generalized anxiety patient whose handshake is cold and clammy, the hyperthyroid patient's hand is warm and sweaty. Given, however, the subtlety of many cases of hyperthyroidism, it is appropriate in all cases to get a thyroid profile. Hypocalcemia may also present with chronic anxiety, and may or may not be accompanied by other signs and symptoms such as tetany, Chvostek's or Trousseau's sign, cataracts, calcification of the basal ganglia or a movement disorder.

TREATMENT

Either cognitive behavior therapy or medications may be utilized, and it is not clear which is more effective. Medications include antidepressants, buspirone, benzodiazepines, hydroxyzine and propranolol.

Effective antidepressants, with their average effective doses, include venlafaxine (as the extended release preparation in a dose of ~225 mg), paroxetine (20-40 mg) and imipramine (150 mg); trazodone (250 mg) is also more effective than placebo, but probably not as effective as the other antidepressants. Given the lack of head-to-head comparisons of venlafaxine, paroxetine and imipramine, the choice among them is often made on the basis of their side-effect profile, and with this in mind, most clinicians will choose either venlafaxine or paroxetine.

Buspirone may be used in low doses of 5 mg tid; however, higher doses, in the range of 15 to 20 mg tid, are probably more effective.

Among the benzodiazepines, effective agents include diazepam (15-25 mg daily), alprazolam (1 to 4 mg) and lorazepam (1 to 4 mg). Among these, diazepam is probably preferable, as, given its long half-life, there is a lower probability of withdrawal symptoms.

Hydroxyzine, an antihistamine similar to diphenhydramine, is more effective than placebo when given in a total daily dose of approximately 50 mg.

Propranolol, although generally ineffective against the experience of anxiety *per se*, may relieve the "peripheral" manifestations of anxiety, such as tremor and tachycardia; the effective dose ranges between 60 and 240 mg.

Choosing among these various medications is not straightforward. The antidepressants and buspirone all require weeks to become effective, and on this score the benzodiazepines are definitely preferable, as they work almost immediately. This enthusiasm for benzodiazepines, however, is tempered by the fact that after a month or so of treatment they are less effective than antidepressants for anxiety *per se*; furthermore, and most importantly, the benzodiazepines carry with them the risk of neuroadaptation and withdrawal symptomatology. Hydroxyzine, like the benzodiazepines, is immediately effective, and has the advantage of not causing neuroadaptation. Propranolol, given its relative ineffectiveness against anxiety *per se*, is generally a last choice for monotherapy.

All other things being equal, it seems preferable to start with either an antidepressant, such as venlafaxine or paroxetine, or with buspirone. Should these be ineffective, it is appropriate to consider a benzodiazepine, such as diazepam, or hydroxyzine: in patients with substance abuse, hydroxyzine should be used. Propranolol might be considered as monotherapy in cases where the "peripheral" symptoms were the most troubling to patients; in most cases, however, if it is used at all, it is employed as an adjunct to one of the other medications. In some cases, serial trials of one agent after another are justified in an attempt to find an optimum regimen. Importantly, when either switching from a benzodiazepine to another agent, or simply stopping a benzodiazepine, it is critical to gradually taper the dose to mitigate withdrawal; furthermore, one may consider "covering" the patient during this tapering with either imipramine or buspirone, as either agent will blunt the exacerbation of anxiety symptoms typically seen during a benzodiazepine taper.

BIBLIOGRAPHY

Borkovec TD, Ruscio AM. Psychotherapy for generalized anxiety disorder. *The Journal of Clinical Psychiatry* 2001;62(Suppl 11):37-42.

Cameron OG, Smith CB, Lee MA, et al. Adrenergic status in anxiety disorders: platelet alpha 2-adrenergic receptor binding, blood pressure, pulse, and plasma catecholamines in panic and generalized anxiety disorder patients and in normal subjects. *Biological Psychiatry* 1990;28:3-20.

Delle Chiaie R, Pancheri P, Casacchia M, et al. Assessment of the efficacy of buspirone in patients affected by generalized anxiety disorder, shifting to buspirone from prior treatment with lorazepam: a placebo-controlled, double-blind study. *Journal of Clinical Psychopharmacology* 1995;15:12-19.

Elie R, Lamontagne Y. Alprazolam and diazepam in the treatment of generalized anxiety. *Journal of Clinical Psychopharmacology* 1984;4:125-129.

Enkelmann R. Alprazolam versus buspirone in the treatment of outpatients with generalized anxiety disorder. *Psychopharmacology* 1991;105:428-432.

Hettema JM, Prescott CA, Kendler KS. A population-based twin study of generalized anxiety disorder in men and women. *The Journal of Nervous and Mental Disease* 2001;189:413-420.

Hoehn-Saric R, McLeod DR, Zimmerli WD. Differential effects of alprazolam and imipramine in generalized anxiety disorder: somatic versus psychic symptoms. *The Journal of Clinical Psychiatry* 1988;49:293-301.

Keller MB. The long-term clinical course of generalized anxiety disorder. *The Journal of Clinical Psychiatry* 2002;63(Suppl 8):11-16.

Laakmann G, Schule C, Lorkowski G, et al. Buspirone and lorazepam in the treatment of generalized anxiety disorder in outpatients. *Psychopharmacology* 1998;136:357-366.

Lader M, Scotto JC. A multicentre double-blind comparison of hydroxyzine, buspirone and placebo in patients with generalized anxiety disorder. *Psychopharmacology* 1998;139:402-406.

Montgomery SA, Mahe V, Haudiquet V, et al. Effectiveness of venlafaxine, extended release formulation, in the short-term and long-term treatment of generalized anxiety disorder: results of a survival analysis. *Journal of Clinical Psychopharmacology* 2002;22:561-567.

Noyes R, Clarkson C, Crowe RR, et al. A family study of generalized anxiety disorder. *The American Journal of Psychiatry* 1987;144:1019-1024.

Pollack MH, Zaninelli R, Goddard A, et al. Paroxetine in the treatment of generalized anxiety disorder: results of a placebo-controlled, flexible-dosage trial. *The Journal of Clinical Psychiatry* 2001;62:350-357.

Rickels K, Downing R, Schweizer E, et al. Antidepressants for the treatment of generalized anxiety disorder. A placebo-controlled comparison of imipramine, trazodone, and diazepam. *Archives of General Psychiatry* 1993;50:884-895.

Rickels K, DeMartinis N, Garcia-Espana F, et al. Imipramine and buspirone in treatment of patients with generalized anxiety disorder who are discontinuing long-term benzodiazepine therapy. *The American Journal of Psychiatry* 2000;157:1973-1979.

Rocca P, Beoni AM, Eva C, et al. Peripheral benzodiazepine receptor messenger RNA is decreased in lymphocytes of generalized anxiety disorder patients. *Biological Psychiatry* 1998;43:767-773.

Tiihonen J, Kuikka J, Rasanen P, et al. Cerebral benzodiazepine receptor binding and distribution in generalized anxiety disorder: a fractal analysis. *Molecular Psychiatry* 1997;2:463-471.

90 Briquet's Syndrome (somatization disorder, DSM-IV-TR #300.81)

In Briquet's syndrome, first described by Paul Briquet in 1859, patients feel that they have been sickly most of their lives and complain of a multitude of symptoms referable to numerous different organ systems. This conviction of illness persists despite repeatedly negative and unrevealing consultations, hospitalizations, and diagnostic procedures, and patients continue to seek medical care, to take prescription medicines, and to submit to needless diagnostic procedures.

Briquet's syndrome, also known as somatization disorder, is rare in males; indeed some conservative diagnosticians doubt that it ever occurs in males. Among females, estimates of the lifetime prevalence range from 0.2% to 3%.

ONSET

Most patients gradually fall ill in their teenage years. Common initial complaints are of headache, dysmenorrhea, and abdominal pain. Onset past the age of 30 is extremely rare.

CLINICAL FEATURES

These patients tend to be excessively vague or dramatic as they relate their medical history. They move restlessly from one symptom to another, never lingering long enough on any one symptom to give an adequately detailed account. Often one finds that the patient has seen many other physicians and has been hospitalized multiple times. A history of frequent surgeries is not uncommon, and on abdominal examination one may find a "battlefield abdomen" with an incredible number of surgical scars. The physician often becomes exasperated, as repeated attempts to isolate the problem are frustrated. Occasionally the only reliable conclusion that may be drawn from the interview is that the review of systems is "diffusely positive."

Patients are often fatigued, weak all over, and plagued with headaches. They may have dizzy spells and pain in the chest. The heart may beat "wildly," and attacks of dyspnea may occur. Patients experience pains in the arms and legs, the back, and in many joints. Vague and poorly localized abdominal pain is common; nausea may be intense, and bloating may be complained of bitterly. Constipation is common, diarrhea somewhat less so, and the patient often has a list of foods that cannot be eaten except at peril to the stomach and intestines. Irregular, painful, or heavy menstruation is almost always a complaint, and patients with children may complain that they vomited every day throughout the entire pregnancy. Most patients have little interest in sex, and females may complain of dyspareunia or frigidity. Occasionally, burning pain in the rectum or vagina occurs.

Conversion symptoms, as described in the chapter on conversion disorder, are frequently present. Common complaints include syncope, blurry vision, blindness, aphonia, globus hystericus, deafness, paralysis, anesthesia, seizures, and varying degrees of urinary retention.

Ongoing controversy exists as to how many symptoms are required for a definitive diagnosis of Briquet's syndrome. The fourth edition of the DSM divides the various symptoms into four groups, namely pain, gastrointestinal symptoms, sexual dysfunction, and conversion symptoms, and requires, as noted in the box on p. 177, anywhere from one to four symptoms from each group.

The physician may approach the physical examination with a mixture of relief and weariness: relief because, finally, reliable data may be obtained, and weariness because lengthy and excruciatingly detailed examinations are required to follow up the patient's numerous complaints. Perhaps a few abnormalities may be found, but none that could reasonably account for the patient's complaints.

Rather than being relieved to hear that "nothing is wrong," the patient may become angry, even resentful, and demand further tests. Goaded, the physician may then begin an ever-escalating series of diagnostic tests. Quickly passing through phlebotomies, cardiograms, stress tests, and x-rays, one progresses to CT or MRI scanning. Endoscopies and exploratory surgeries may follow, and some patients may even come to neurosurgery. Eventually "fired" by the exasperated physician, the patient then moves on to the next.

The demandingness of these patients is typically seen not only in medical settings but also in their personal lives. Family members must be solicitous and attentive; if patients feel that the illness is no longer the center of attention, they may become self-pitying and aggrieved. Further sacrifices are demanded, and a pall of guilt and resentment often hangs over the entire family. Bitter divorces are not uncommon as the patient carries the tyranny of illness from one marriage to another. Along the way, depressive symptoms almost always occur, and suicide gestures or attempts are not uncommon. Panic attacks may occur. Alcohol abuse and at times alcoholism may also be seen. A concurrent personality disorder may also be found, especially of the borderline, antisocial, or histrionic types.

Symptoms Seen in Briquet's Syndrome

PAIN (≥4)
Headache
Abdominal pain (often vague
   and poorly localized)
Backache
Arthralgia
Chest pain
Rectal pain
Painful menstruation
Dyspareunia
Dysuria
	SEXUAL SYMPTOMS (≥1)
	Decreased libido
	Impotence
	Ejaculatory disturbance
	Irregular menses
	Heavy menstrual bleeding
	Prolonged and frequent vomiting
	   during pregnancy

GASTROINTESTINAL SYMPTOMS (≥2) Nausea Bloating Vomiting Diarrhea Constipation Multiple food intolerances	**CONVERSION SYMPTOMS (≥1)** Ataxia Weakness or paralysis Dysphagia or globus Aphonia Urinary retention Anesthesia Blurry vision Diplopia Blindness Deafness Pseudoseizures Amnesia Dizzy spells Syncope Non-syncopal loss of consciousness

COURSE

Briquet's syndrome is chronic, and although symptoms are most numerous and severe in early adult years, they persist indefinitely in a gradually waxing and waning fashion.

COMPLICATIONS

These patients rarely consider themselves well enough to work, and should they have a job, their repeated sick days eventually get them fired. Medical expenses often become a crippling burden, and unnecessary procedures, such as laparotomies, may bring their own complications.

ETIOLOGY

Briquet's syndrome is clearly familial: the prevalence in first degree female relatives may be as high as 20%, and adoption studies indicate both genetic and environmental factors. There may also be a relationship with antisocial personality disorder, which is more common in the male relatives of females with Briquet's syndrome, and some authors have suggested that both Briquet's syndrome and antisocial personality disorder have the same genetic background with a sex-mediated expression, producing Briquet's syndrome in females and antisocial personality disorder in males.

DIFFERENTIAL DIAGNOSIS

During a depressive episode, certain patients, especially the elderly, are likely to complain of multiple aches and pains. The existence of vegetative symptoms before the onset of these complaints suggests the correct diagnosis. Furthermore, should the complaints assume a nihilistic, delusional character, the diagnosis of Briquet's syndrome is almost ruled out.

Patients with schizophrenia may similarly complain of multiple aches and pains; however, here one finds not only symptoms typical of schizophrenia but also bizarre and implausible complaints.

In hypochondriasis, the patient is not so much concerned with the illness and its symptoms, as is the patient with Briquet's syndrome, but rather with what the symptoms imply, namely a terrible and as yet undiagnosed disease. The patient with Briquet's syndrome would rest content with a physician who eschewed diagnostic measures and concentrated on numerous symptomatic treatments. By contrast the patient with hypochondriasis "doctor shops" until an aggressive diagnostician is found.

In conversion disorder the number of symptoms is small, often only one, and is generally referable to only one organ system, typically the central nervous system. By contrast the patient with Briquet's syndrome has a multitude of symptoms that range widely over many different organ systems.

Malingerers and those with factitious illness typically also lack the number and range of symptoms presented by the patient with Briquet's syndrome.

A variety of diseases, for example systemic lupus erythematosus, multiple sclerosis, sarcoidosis, and so forth, may all produce a large number of symptoms and thus mimic Briquet's syndrome. Indeed some patients with one of these disorders may become quite embittered and demanding after a succession of physicians have all failed to uncover the underlying disease. Thus a thorough and patient examination and laboratory follow-up is always indicated in pursuing the diagnosis of Briquet's syndrome.

Finally, in those patients with Briquet's syndrome who have come to surgery, one must keep in mind that new symptoms subsequent to the surgery may, rather than being part of Briquet's syndrome, represent a complication of the surgery itself.

TREATMENT

Every effort is made to establish these patients in a long-term relationship with one primary care physician. Regularly scheduled "checkups" are indicated, and a conservative diagnostic and therapeutic stance is taken. Without such a relationship, overuse of narcotics and the creation of iatrogenic illnesses are almost certain to occur.

Both ongoing psychiatric consultation to the primary care physician and group therapy have each been found effective in reducing the severity of symptoms, and preliminary work also suggests that cognitive behavioral therapy may also be effective.

Should depressive symptoms be prominent, antidepressants may be helpful. Care must be taken to choose an antidepressant that has few, if any, side effects.

Any potentially addicting substances are to be avoided, as they may be abused by these patients.

BIBLIOGRAPHY

Allen LA, Woolfolk RL, Lehrer PM, et al. Cognitive behavior therapy for somatization disorder: a preliminary investigation. *Journal of Behavior Therapy and Experimental Psychiatry* 2001;32:53-62.

Golding JM, Smith GR, Kashner TM. Does somatization disorder occur in men? Clinical characteristics of women and men with multiple unexplained somatic symptoms. *Archives of General Psychiatry* 1991;48:231-235.

Guze SB, Cloninger CR, Martin RL, et al. A follow-up and family study of Briquet's syndrome. *The British Journal of Psychiatry* 1986;149:17-23.

Kashner TM, Rost K, Cohen B, et al. Enhancing the health of somatization disorder patients. Effectiveness of short-term group therapy. *Psychsomatics* 1995;36:462-470.

Kroll P, Chamberlain KR, Halpern J. The diagnosis of Briquet's syndrome in a male population: the Veteran's Administration revisited. *The Journal of Nervous and Mental Disease* 1979;167:171-174.

Mai FM, Merskey H. Briquet's Treatise on Hysteria. A synopsis and commentary. *Archives of General Psychiatry* 1980;37:1401-1405.

Quill TE. Somatization disorder. One of medicine's blind spots. *The Journal of the American Medical Association* 1985;254:3075-3079.

Smith GR, Monson RA, Ray DC. Psychiatric consultation in somatization disorder. A randomized controlled study. *The New England Journal of Medicine* 1986;314:1407-1413.

91 Conversion Disorder (DSM-IV-TR #300.11)

Conversion disorder is characterized by the occurrence of certain signs or symptoms that are clearly inconsistent with what is known about anatomy and pathophysiology. For example, the patient may complain of blindness, yet cortical visual evoked potentials are normal. Or a patient may complain of complete anesthesia of the left upper extremity and go on to describe the boundary of the anesthesia as being a clear-cut line encircling the elbow. Other common complaints include hemiplegia, deafness, and seizures.

On close inspection the specific symptomatology in each case corresponds with the patient's particular conception of how an illness might manifest itself. Take for example a patient who complains of such unsteadiness that walking is impossible; the patient's conception of the malady, however, simply does not encompass the symptomatology evident at bedside examination that the physician's knowledge of pathophysiology would predict. Thus, although the patient stumbles and lurches in the attempt to cross from chair to the bed, in bed there is no truncal ataxia and no deficiency on finger-to-nose or heel-to-knee-to-shin testing.

Patients who find themselves with such symptoms, however, are not to be confused with malingerers or those with factitious illness. Patients who suffer conversion symptoms do not intentionally feign such symptoms, as malingerers do; they experience them as genuine, and their distress over them may be as genuine as that of the patient whose unsteadiness is produced by a midline cerebellar tumor.

A synonym for conversion disorder is "hysterical neurosis, conversion type." Both terms are to a degree unfortunate. The term "conversion" has its roots in psychoanalysis and connotes a specific etiologic theory that has not been substantiated. "Hysterical," though an ancient term, has so many different meanings and is such a pejorative term that it might best be allowed to rest in peace.

The lifetime prevalence of conversion disorder is not known with certainty, and estimates range from 0.01% to 0.5% of the general population; it is more common in females, with female to male ratios ranging from 2:1 up to 10:1.

ONSET

Although conversion disorder may appear at any time from early childhood up to old age, most patients experience their first symptoms during adolescence or early adult years. In most cases the actual onset of symptoms is abrupt and typically follows a major stress in the patient's life.

CLINICAL FEATURES

In general, at any given time most patients with conversion disorder have only one symptom. Some of the more common ones are listed in the box on p. 179, and most of these are described in detail below.

Conversion anesthesia may occur anywhere, but it is most common on the extremities. One may see a typical "glove and stocking" distribution; however, unlike the "glove and stocking" distribution that may occur in a polyneuropathy, the areas of conversion anesthesia have a very precise and sharp boundary, often located at a joint. The same nonphysiologic sharp boundary may be seen in conversion hemianesthesia, wherein the boundary precisely bisects the body on a sagittal plane. Other anomalies may appear on examination. Patients who complain of total lack of all sensory modalities (including vibratory sense) in the hand or foot may nevertheless have intact position sense at the index finger or the great toe. Furthermore, patients who complain of a similar complete lack of feeling in their legs are nonetheless able to walk normally and have a negative Romberg test. Some patients, when asked to close their eyes and say "yes" if they feel something and "no" if they don't, will reliably say "no" every time the "anesthetic" area is touched. Deep tendon reflex testing fails to show the expected hyporeflexia. In doubtful cases somatosensory evoked potentials may be helpful. Anesthesia may also occur on the cornea and on the palate. Indeed in the nineteenth and early twentieth centuries these symptoms were accorded a special place among the "stigmata" of "hysteria."

In conversion paralysis one may see the same sort of anomalous boundary as seen in conversion anesthesia. For example, the weakness may extend up to the elbow and end precisely there. In conversion hemiplegia, other abnormalities may be seen; for example, though weak for many months the affected arm may hang limply at the side, rather than displaying the typical physiologic flexion posture. Patients with conversion hemiplegia may also display the "wrong-way tongue" sign wherein the protruded tongue, instead of deviating toward the hemiplegic side, as in "true" hemiplegia, deviates instead toward the normal side. Furthermore, on observation of gait one finds that the weakened leg is dragged, rather than circumducted. On formal testing of muscle strength in the lower extremities, an attempt to elicit Hoover's sign may be helpful. Here, with the patient recumbent, the examiner's hands, palms up, are placed under the heel of the weakened leg and likewise under the heel of the unaffected leg,

Common Conversion Symptoms

Anesthesia	Parkinsonism
Paralysis	Syncope
Ataxia	Coma
Tremor	Anosmia
Tonic-clonic pseudoseizures	Nystagmus
Deafness	Convergence spasm
Blindness	Facial weakness
Aphonia	Ageusia
Globus hystericus	

and the patient is then asked to exert as much effort as possible in raising the affected leg from the bed. In the case, say, of weakness secondary to a stroke, although the affected leg does not move, the examiner feels considerable pressure upon the hand underneath the unaffected leg as the patient puts maximum effort into the task. In cases of conversion paralysis, however, Hoover's sign is present, and the examiner does not feel any pressure on the hand underneath the unaffected leg. Finally, in conversion paralysis the Babinski sign is absent, and the deep tendon reflexes are not increased.

In conversion paraplegia, one finds normal, rather than increased, deep tendon reflexes, and the Babinski sign is absent; in doubtful cases the issue may be resolved by demonstrating normal motor evoked potentials.

In conversion ataxia (or, as it has been classically called, astasia-abasia), a patient, upon attempting to stand or walk, lurches and staggers forward, arms flinging and trunk swaying, always barely making it to the safety of bed or chair. Yet when examined in bed, one finds no limb or truncal ataxia.

Conversion tremor tends to be coarse and irregular and generally disappears when the patient is distracted.

Conversion seizures, also known as "hysterical fits" or "non-epileptic seizures," may mimic either grand mal or complex partial seizures.

Conversion grand mal seizures display multiple anomalies. Their onset is gradual rather than sudden; if the patient cries out at the onset it usually consists of intelligible screaming rather than an inarticulate cry. The movements during a conversion seizure are extremely varied but generally purposeful. The patient may thrash about, strike at the walls, or break one piece of furniture over another, all in contrast to the rhythmic, simple tonic-clonic activity seen in most grand mal seizures. Most patients do not bite their tongue during a conversion seizure, and only those with considerable medical sophistication pass urine. Most conversion seizures end gradually rather than abruptly, and afterwards patients display neither confusion nor somnolence.

Conversion seizures of the complex partial type may be more difficult to diagnose. One differential point is that true complex partial seizures typically start with a motionless stare or with automatisms (such as chewing) before the onset of complex behavior, whereas conversion seizures of the complex partial type typically begin with complex behavior.

Other findings helpful in distinguishing conversion seizures from "true" seizures include a post-ictal Babinski sign, an elevated prolactin or neuron-specific enolase level, and a positive ictal or post-ictal EEG. Babinski signs are almost universal after "true" grand mal seizures, and are seen also in about one-fifth of patients after complex partial seizures. Prolactin and neuron-specific enolase

levels are generally elevated after either type of seizure, and both are useful to obtain 15 to 30 minutes post-ictally. Surface EEGs are always appropriate: the ictal EEG is always abnormal during a grand mal seizure and almost always so during a complex partial seizure; post-ictal EEGs generally also show slowing after either type of seizure. As negative findings accrue (i.e., the absence of a Babinski sign, normal prolactin and neuron-specific enolase levels, and normal ictal and post-ictal EEGs) the likelihood that the event in question was a pseudoseizure increases. In doubtful cases, one may consider placebo induction, for example with an infusion of normal saline.

In conversion deafness the blink reflex to a loud and unexpected sound is present, thus demonstrating the intactness of the brain stem. Should one suspect the vanishingly rare bilateral cortical deafness, a brain stem auditory evoked potential will resolve the issue.

Bilateral conversion blindness may be suspected when the patient, though complaining of recent onset of blindness, neither sustains injury while maneuvering around the office nor displays any of the expected bruises or scrapes. The pupillary reflex is present, thus demonstrating the intactness of the optic nerve, chiasm, tract, lateral geniculate body, and mesencephalon. Should one suspect cortical blindness, a visual evoked potential will resolve the question.

In cases of monocular conversion blindness, one need only demonstrate two things to make the correct diagnosis: first, that the peripheral fields are full in the unaffected eye; and second, that the pupillary response is normal in both eyes.

Conversion aphonia may be suspected when the patient is asked to cough, for example, during auscultation of the lungs. In contrast with other aphonias, the cough is normally full and loud.

A synonym for "globus hystericus" might be conversion dysphagia; however, this term fails to convey the essence of the patient's chief complaint, which is a most distressing sense of having a lump in one's throat. Finding that the patient can swallow solid food with little difficulty or even that swallowing liquid may ease the discomfort argues strongly for a diagnosis of globus. In doubtful cases a chest x-ray, video esophogram, and esophageal manometry may be required to rule out other conditions.

Conversion parkinsonism differs from most "true" parkinsonian conditions in several respects: onset is usually abrupt and the course nonprogressive, in contrast with the gradual onset and progressive downhill course seen in conditions such as Parkinson's disease or diffuse Lewy body disease; cogwheeling is absent, and although there may be a loss of associated arm movements when walking, the arm is typically held at the side, rather than in flexion; and finally, tremor, rather than diminishing with action, may actually increase in severity. In doubtful cases, and provided that appropriate help is available, one may vigorously check for retropulsion with a sudden, unexpected and forceful push backward to the patient's chest: if the patient with conversion parkinsonism does begin to fall back, one often sees an extreme loss of balance accompanied by a telltale rapid and fluid upswing of the arms.

In conversion syncope one fails to see autonomic changes, such as pallor. Furthermore, the conversion faint itself often has a "swooning" character to it, which typically heightens the drama of the moment and never results in injury.

In conversion coma a number of distinctive findings may be present, including the following: fluttering of the eyelid when the eyelashes are lightly stroked, resistance to eyelid opening and an abrupt closure of the lids when they are released, and normal pupillary responses. In doubtful cases one may resort to a surprise touch to the face with an ice cube. If the issue is still in doubt, a normal EEG will help resolve the issue.

Other conversion symptoms, of course, are possible. Like the foregoing, most suggest central or peripheral nervous system disease, such as strokes, tumors, and the like. Conversion anosmia, nystagmus, ocular bobbing, convergence spasm, facial weakness, and ageusia may occur. Conversion symptoms suggesting disease outside the nervous system, such as conversion vomiting, pseudo-cyesis, or cough, are decidedly uncommon. Regardless of the symptoms, however, the physician with enough ingenuity is generally able to demonstrate how each particular conversion symptom "violates" the laws of anatomy or pathophysiology.

Patients with conversion disorder may or may not display the classic "la belle indifference," the attitude of casual disregard for normally alarming symptoms such as blindness or hemianesthesia. Even when present, this sign is not reliable because it may be confused with the studied stoicism seen in patients with other illnesses or with the symptom of anosognosia.

Conversion disorder may occur in isolation; however, in many instances a personality disorder is also seen, most commonly histrionic, passive-aggressive, borderline, or, in males, antisocial. Dysthymia or major depression may also occur concurrently.

COURSE

Conversion disorder may pursue either an episodic or chronic course, with the initial conversion symptom remitting spontaneously, often within weeks or months. In such cases a subsequent episode may be expected in the years to come; should such a subsequent episode occur, the conversion symptom itself may be different from the initial one.

A minority of patients experience their conversion symptoms chronically; this tends to be the case with an associated personality disorder.

COMPLICATIONS

Should patients take to bed or restrict their activities because of conversion symptoms, jobs may be lost and relationships strained. Potentially dangerous diagnostic procedures, such as arteriography, may be undergone. In chronic cases of conversion paralysis, disuse atrophy or contractures may occur.

ETIOLOGY

Conversion symptoms are more common among the uneducated and unsophisticated; the actual conversion symptom itself is generally a reflection or extension of symptoms that the patient has seen in another or has personally experienced.

In most instances, consequent upon the appearance of the conversion symptom there is a reduction in the patient's level of anxiety. Close inspection reveals that conversion symptoms are not, however, premeditated—they simply happen—and although observers may feel a "purpose" is behind them, the patient himself is unaware of any such thing. Many clinicians feel that the symptom itself may be a kind of "sign language," or a sort of hieroglyphic that conveys what the patient is unable to put into words.

Recent PET scanning has demonstrated that in patients with conversion hemiplegia or hemianesthesia, there is a decreased activation of the contralateral basal ganglia and thalamus. The pathophysiologic relevance of this, however, is unclear. It may represent a premorbid susceptibility to the development of conversion symptoms or might, in turn, merely be epiphenomenal and unrelated to the underlying cause or causes.

DIFFERENTIAL DIAGNOSIS

The diagnosis of conversion disorder cannot be made unless one can demonstrate with certainty that the patient's symptomatology clearly violates the laws of anatomy and pathophysiology. To demonstrate merely that no explanation for the symptom can be found is not sufficient, as many diseases may present in a most subtle and deceptive way. Examples include multiple sclerosis, systemic lupus erythematosus, polyarteritis nodosa, and sarcoidosis. Certain disorders, such as early torsion dystonia, akinetic seizures, or supplementary motor seizures, may tax the skills of even the most experienced diagnostician. Furthermore, it is not uncommon for patients with conversion seizures to also have "true" seizures. Where doubt persists after an exhaustive workup, one should defer on diagnosis and observe the patient over time until the clinical picture crystallizes. This is especially the case when the patient's complaint is of pain. Although conversion pain does exist, such a diagnosis should be entertained only after a scrupulously exhaustive examination.

When the symptoms fall clearly outside the realm of anatomic possibility, one must then rule out both malingering and factitious illness. In both these cases, in contrast to conversion disorder, the patient premeditates the symptoms and intentionally feigns them with a clearly conceived purpose in mind. In malingering the purpose is to avoid some unpleasantness, such as jail. In factitious illness the purpose is to be a patient and under medical care. Demonstrating such purposefulness and premeditation is difficult and often requires prolonged observation and repeated interviews.

At this point, assuming that one has demonstrated both that the symptom lies outside the bounds of anatomic possibility and that it is neither premeditated nor does it serve any purpose that the patient is aware of, then one may with reasonable confidence say that the patient has a conversion symptom. Before making a diagnosis of conversion disorder, however, one must rule out two other disorders that may produce conversion symptoms, namely schizophrenia and Briquet's syndrome. Schizophrenia is distinguished by the bizarreness, hallucinations, and delusions characteristic of that illness. In Briquet's syndrome one generally finds not merely one conversion symptom at a time, as is the case in conversion disorder, but multiple conversion symptoms. Furthermore, in Briquet's syndrome the conversion symptoms are only a part, and often a minor part at that, of a much larger fabric of multiple complaints referable to multiple organ systems other than the nervous system.

TREATMENT

After the diagnosis is made, one should inform the patient in a gentle and nonjudgmental, yet quietly authoritative, way that neither the examination nor the diagnostic tests have revealed any damage to the brain or nerves. One may then confess honestly that, although medicine does not know the cause of the symptoms, it is nevertheless known that patients tend to recover in a few weeks. With such support and reassurance, a majority of patients will experience a remission during a hospital stay, and this is especially likely when the conversion symptoms have been of acute onset and short duration, and were preceded by an obvious psychosocial precipitant. In certain instances a few sessions with a physical therapist who is knowledgeable about these patients may expedite the remission, often providing a sort of "face saving" device. At all costs one must avoid pejorative statements such as "there is nothing really wrong with you," as these only serve to undermine the physician-patient relationship.

When these measures fail, alternative techniques may be used. Hypnosis may effect a remission; however, early relapses tend to occur. Another approach involves viewing the symptoms as a kind of "sign language," deciphering what the sign means, and then assisting the patient in putting that meaning into words and taking appropriate action. Such an approach is often labor intensive, yet the clinical impression is that it may produce solid results.

BIBLIOGRAPHY

Baker AH, Silver JR. Hysterical paraplegia. *Journal of Neurology, Neurosurgery, and Psychiatry* 1987;50:375-382.

Couprie W, Wijdicks EF, Rooijmans HG, et al. Outcome on conversion disorder: a follow up study. *Journal of Neurology, Neurosurgery, and Psychiatry* 1995;58:750-752.

Keane JR. Wrong-way deviation of the tongue with hysterical hemiparesis. *Neurology* 1986;36:1406-1407.

Keane JR. Hysterical gait disorders: 60 cases. *Neurology* 1989;39:586-589.

Lang AE, Koller WC, Fahn S. Psychogenic parkinsonism. *Archives of Neurology* 1995;52:802-810.

Moene FC, Spinhoven P, Hoogduin KA, et al. A randomised controlled clinical trial on the additional effect of hypnosis in a comprehensive treatment programme for in-patients with conversion disorder of the motor type. *Psychotherapy and Psychosomatics* 2002;71:66-76.

Roelofs K, Hoogduin KA, Keijsers GP, et al. Hypnotic susceptibility in patients with conversion disorder. *Journal of Abnormal Psychology* 2002;111:390-395.

Speed J. Behavioral management of conversion disorder: retrospective study. *Archives of Physical Medicine and Rehabilitation* 1996;77:147-154.

Vuilleumier P, Chicherio C, Assal F, et al. Functional neuroanatomical correlates of hysterical sensorimotor loss. *Brain* 2001;124:1077-1090.

92 Hypochondriasis (DSM-IV-TR #300.7)

In hypochondriasis patients come to believe, or at least to very strongly suspect, that they are sick with a serious, perhaps life-threatening disease. Minor symptoms or anomalies support and augment their concern. A muscle ache or perhaps an accidental bruise indicates the dreaded diagnosis. Their concerns persist despite the reassurances of their physicians. The preoccupation with illness may become all-consuming; some patients become invalids, bed-bound not by their symptoms, but by their fear of having a disabling illness.

Hypochondriasis has a lifetime prevalence somewhere between 1 and 5%, and appears to be equally common in males and females.

ONSET

Hypochondriasis may begin anywhere from teenage to older years. The peak age of onset is in the twenties and thirties.

As yet, no apparent premorbid or prodromal changes have been identified. In some cases, however, precipitating factors appear to play a role. Witnessing someone else suffer or die of a disease seems at times to trigger hypochondriasis. In some cases a serious illness in the patient's own life may precede the onset of the hypochondriasis. The postmyocardial infarction patient who becomes a "cardiac cripple" is a familiar example.

CLINICAL FEATURES

Patients with hypochondriasis come to the physician already certain that they have a serious disease. A cough has appeared; it is a sure sign of pneumonia. The pulse quickens, and the patient is sure that the heart will fail; a discomfort in the chest, and the patient is convinced that a heart attack is occurring; some nausea, and the patient becomes convinced that an ulcer has eaten through the stomach; the bowels are sluggish, and the patient fears cancer of the colon. Diffuse aches and pains are to the patient a sure sign of AIDS.

Often patients present their complaints in minute detail. They may bring lists or calendars with them. If they have been to other physicians, as is often the case, they may complain about the other physicians' refusals to take them seriously and their failure to order more tests. Often the examining physician feels uncomfortable, as if under attack. An appropriate interview and examination are generally unrevealing, or if findings diagnostic of a certain disease are evident, the patients' complaints are all out of proportion to what one generally sees with that disease. Indeed the patients themselves are often dissatisfied with the diagnosis. For example, patients convinced that they have serious heart disease may receive the diagnosis of costochondritis with skepticism, if not thinly veiled hostility. They may demand some tests, convinced that something has been missed. They have read about cardiac catheterization and are willing to undergo it.

"Doctor shopping" is predictably common in patients with hypochondriasis. They may bring photostatic copies of all their records with them. Their symptoms change with time, and this may be presented as grounds for a new round of tests. Occasionally the careful, meticulous physician may be able to get the patient to admit that perhaps in fact little is wrong and that further testing is not appropriate. However, such a fragile alliance between physician and patient rarely lasts. Indeed within minutes after leaving the physician's office, doubts may enter the patient's mind. The physician-patient relationship generally deteriorates; the patient becomes resentful, and the physician becomes at the least irritated with the demanding patient who will not accept reassurance.

The symptoms of hypochondriasis, though perhaps most clearly highlighted in the physician's office, are often present in all facets of the patient's life. The preoccupation with minor symptoms, the persistent conviction that one suffers a serious (though perhaps undiagnosed) disease, and the ineffectiveness of medical reassurance may be evident at the dinner table, the office, or the club. Similar to "doctor shopping," patients with hypochondriasis tend to "people shop" until they find someone who is willing to listen to their tale of woe with a sympathetic ear. Some degree of anxiety and depression are common in these sufferers; at times they may appear irritable, beaten down, a picture of suffering.

COURSE

Once established, hypochondriasis tends to be a chronic lifelong illness, with symptoms waxing and waning over the months or years. Patients may have interludes of partial remission during which, though still worried, they may make few demands on the physician. Rarely, true remissions may occur.

COMPLICATIONS

Hypochondriasis may indeed be disabling. Convinced of their illness, patients may quit work or refuse to travel. Their unreasonable demands may drive away friends and family. Unwary physicians may consent to provide various diagnostic procedures with the subsequent risk of iatrogenic illness. Some patients eventually opt for admission to a nursing home.

ETIOLOGY

Although personal or vicarious experience of illness is suspected to be related to hypochondriasis, as yet nothing certain is known about the etiology of this disorder, except that it is not familial. In retrospect, one may find that as children these patients were quite ill, perhaps with severe recurrent bronchitis or asthma. Alternatively one may find that these children were subject to maternal overprotectiveness and oversolicitousness regarding minor complaints such as stomachaches and the like.

The same experiences may be found in adulthood. Perhaps the best known is the case of the "cardiac cripple," wherein, after recovering from a myocardial infarction and being given clearance by the cardiologist to resume activities, the patient, un-reassured and consumed with the fear of having another heart attack, remains an invalid.

DIFFERENTIAL DIAGNOSIS

In Briquet's syndrome, patients present their symptoms in a colorful, dramatic, and often maddeningly vague fashion, in contrast to the often carefully detailed description given by patients with hypochondriasis. Furthermore, in Briquet's syndrome the emphasis is not so much on what the symptoms imply, namely having a serious disease, as it is on the seriousness of the symptoms themselves.

In conversion disorder the presenting complaint generally relates to a loss of ability or function, such as blindness, anesthesia, or focal weakness, rather than to misinterpreting a minor symptom, such as a bruise, as indicating a serious illness. Furthermore, some patients with conversion disorder display "la belle indifference" to their symptoms, in striking contrast to the anxious concern displayed by the patient with hypochondriasis.

Body dysmorphic disorder and hypochondriasis may be distinguished with reference to the underlying motivation of the patient's concerns. In hypochondriasis a blemish is of no concern per se; rather what is of concern is what the blemish means, namely that it is a sign of some serious underlying disease. In contrast, in body dysmorphic disorder the disfiguring effect of the blemish itself is the source of the concern.

In both malingering and factitious illness a purpose may be discerned behind the patient's complaints. In malingering, the purpose, such as financial gain or avoidance of responsibility, may be obvious. In factitious illness, the patient's intent, which is none other than to be under medical care or hospitalized, may be harder to discern. One clue may be the patient's attitude toward repeated, and ever more dangerous, tests: though both hypochondriacal and factitious patients accept these, and may even request them, the hypochondriacal patient approaches them with anxiety and trepidation, whereas the factitious patient typically shows little concern or apprehension.

In depression, patients may sink into a conviction that they are ill, and minor changes in function may solidify that belief. Simple constipation may convince the patient that the bowels are locked with cancer; elderly depressed patients are particularly likely to express such "hypochondriacal" concerns, and in fact may deny feeling depressed at all. Indeed such hypochondriacal concerns are what often bring the patient first to medical attention, as they seek consultation with their primary care physician. In such cases a vigilant attention on the part of the primary care physician to other symptoms of depression may enable the correct diagnosis to be made and spare the patient a fruitless workup for other causes.

Other differential points between hypochondriasis and depression are the presence of delusions and an episodic course. In some cases of depression the hypochondriacal concerns may become delusional and resistant to all reassurance, in contrast to hypochondriasis, where reassurance is always effective, at least for a time. The course of the patient's concerns is also important; as noted earlier, true and full remissions are rare in hypochondriasis: thus, if there are long intervals wherein the patient is free of hypochondriacal concerns, the diagnosis of depression, which is more commonly episodic, is much more likely.

In histrionic personality disorder, the patient's presentation may be laced with hypochondriacal complaints; however, these constitute only a minor theme in the overall drama.

In schizophrenia and at times in schizotypal personality disorder, patients may be convinced that they have some other disease. These convictions, however, in contrast with hypochondriasis, are often either delusional or bizarre. The patient with hypochondriasis may complain of abdominal pain; the patient with schizophrenia may complain of "movements, like snakes" in the belly.

Transient hypochondriacal concerns are relatively common, are seen as normal variants, and should not prompt a diagnosis of hypochondriasis. The various "doctor's diseases" suffered by medical students are a good example.

Finally, one must be alert to the possibility that the minor symptoms do in fact indicate a serious disease. The patient who complains of chest pain may not be having a myocardial infarction; however, he may be experiencing pleurisy secondary to systemic lupus erythematosus: each complaint must be evaluated on its own merits.

TREATMENT

If patients can be convinced to attend, group psychotherapy appears to reduce "doctor shopping" and invalidism, and recent data also suggest an effectiveness for individual cognitive behavioral therapy. In all cases, one must inform the patient's other physicians of the diagnosis.

Most patients with hypochondriasis, unfortunately, do not accept a referral for psychotherapy. In these cases, the primary care physician should see the patient for an appropriate examination on a regularly scheduled basis. If patients are not seen on a regularly scheduled basis, but told to come back only if they "need to," the hypochondriasis often worsens. Overall, medical management should be very conservative.

Benzodiazepines are often prescribed, but their usefulness here is doubtful. A preliminary, open investigation suggested that fluoxetine, in doses of 60 to 80 mg, may reduce hypochondriacal concerns.

BIBLIOGRAPHY

Barsky AJ. Clinical practice. The patient with hypochondriasis. *The New England Journal of Medicine* 2001;345:1395-1399.

Barsky AJ, Cleary PD, Sarnie MK, et al. The course of transient hypochondriasis. *The American Journal of Psychiatry* 1993;150:484-488.

Barsky AJ, Fama JM, Bailey ED, et al. A prospective 4- to 5-year study of DSM-III-R hypochondriasis. *Archives of General Psychiatry* 1998;55:737-744.

Bouman TK, Visser S. Cognitive and behavioral treatment of hypochondriasis. *Psychotherapy and Psychosomatics* 1998;67:214-221.

Clark DM, Salkovskis PM, Hackmann A, et al. Two psychological treatments for hypochondriasis. A randomized controlled trial. *The British Journal of Psychiatry* 1998;173:218-225.

Fallon BA, Liebowitz MR, Salman E, et al. Fluoxetine for hypochondriacal patients without major depression. *Journal of Clinical Psychopharmacology* 1993;13:438-441.

Noyes R, Kathol RG, Fisher MM, et al. The validity of DSM-III-R hypochondriasis. *Archives of General Psychiatry* 1993;50:961-970.

Noyes R, Holt CS, Happel RL, et al. A family study of hypochondriasis. *The Journal of Nervous and Mental Disease* 1997;185:223-232.

93 Body Dysmorphic Disorder (DSM-IV-TR #300.7)

In body dysmorphic disorder (BDD) patients become overly concerned, or at times convinced, that in some fashion or other they are misshapen or deformed, despite all evidence to the contrary. Given these concerns, patients rarely seek treatment from psychiatrists, preferring to visit dermatologists or cosmetic surgeons. Although the lifetime prevalence of this disorder is not known, anywhere from 2 to 6% of patients seen in dermatology or cosmetic surgery clinics are affected.

Historically, and still in the United Kingdom and Europe, this disorder has been known as dysmorphophobia; whether or not the cumbersome phrase "body dysmorphic disorder," as used in the DSM-IV, is preferable to the mellifluous "dysmorphophobia" is a matter of debate.

ONSET

The morbid concern that one has a defect typically has an insidious onset in midteenage to late teenage years.

CLINICAL FEATURES

Patients are generally concerned about some aspect of their appearance or with the possibility that they have some deformity. Different patients express different concerns, and most have more than one; in most cases the concerns focus on the face or the head. Facial and scalp hair are not right; the nose is misshapen or too large; the skin is scarred or pimpled or deformed by wrinkles; the eyes may be too far apart. The breasts are too large or too small; they are unequal in size or asymmetric. Blemishes are seen on the hands or the face; the hips are too large.

On examination the physician finds either no abnormality at all or, if one is present, it is trivial and would pass unnoticed by almost anyone else.

Reassurance from the physician, however, that "there is nothing wrong" or "nothing to be concerned about" has little lasting effect on these patients. Only a small minority recognize the groundlessness of their concerns; the vast majority are more or less convinced, and in a significant proportion the conviction becomes a delusion. Patients are often in torment over their "defect," and the majority repeatedly check themselves in mirrors: in some cases such "mirror-checkers" may be so distressed by what they see that they may avoid mirrors, or cover them up. Most patients avoid contact with others, and a minority become housebound; ideas or delusions of reference may appear. A majority of patients eventually seek treatment from plastic surgeons or dermatologists, with uniformly disappointing results and a tendency to seek legal redress.

Most patients have concurrent disorders, such as major depression or obsessive-compulsive disorder.

COURSE

Dysmorphophobia pursues a chronic, waxing and waning course in most patients; although over long periods of time, the "focus" of concern may change, nevertheless the concern with appearance, *per se*, remains constant.

COMPLICATIONS

As noted, social withdrawal is common, and patients may be unable to work or to sustain relationships with others. Suicidal ideation is common, and completed suicide may occur.

ETIOLOGY

Although the etiology is not known, the response to SSRIs and the similarity of an "obsession" with a defective appearance with the obsessions seen in obsessive-compulsive disorder suggest that dysmorphophobia may be one of the "obsessive-compulsive spectrum" disorders.

DIFFERENTIAL DIAGNOSIS

A heightened concern about appearance is normal during adolescence; the fact that it passes with time or a change in circumstances differentiates it from dysmorphophobia.

In narcissistic personality disorder, one may see an excessive concern with maintaining a perfect facial appearance; however, this interest in appearance is only part of a more pervasive drive to perfection that affects almost every aspect of the patient's life. By contrast, patients with dysmorphophobia are content with being "merely normal" in other aspects of their lives.

In those cases where the concern is delusional, a diagnosis of delusional disorder, somatic subtype, may be considered. Here, however, the typical nonpsychotic symptomatology preceding the development of the delusion enables the correct diagnosis. The fact that these patients with psychotic dysmorphophobia are in every way similar to nondelusional patients, including response to treatment, further argues against making a diagnosis of delusional disorder.

Patients with transsexualism are convinced of the defective nature of their sexual characteristics; however, here the concern is secondary to the patient's conviction either that he is actually a female and that his penis is a mistake or, conversely, that she is actually a male and that her breasts are a mistake.

Anorexia nervosa is characterized by a pervasive concern with shape and size, that at times may be quite focal: the hips are too big; the cheeks are too chubby. However, the anorexic's goal is not to become normal in appearance, but rather to succeed in the pursuit of thinness.

In hypochondriasis patients may be overly concerned about blemishes and the like. Their concern is not so much with being unattractive as it is with the possibility that the blemish indicates the presence of a severe underlying disease.

In the midst of a depressive episode, patients may become concerned or convinced that they are deformed. This conviction, however, is intimately connected with the patient's notion of sin and guilt, notions that are not part of dysmorphophobia.

Patients with schizophrenia may have all manner of concerns about their appearance; however, these tend to be bizarre and unusual and are accompanied by the other symptoms typical of the disease not found in dysmorphophobia.

TREATMENT

As patients with dysmorphophobia are loath to consider their pathologic concerns per se, they rarely stay in treatment.

Both fluoxetine and clomipramine are effective in reducing the intensity of the patients' concerns, and there is some preliminary evidence for the effectiveness of behavior therapy. Importantly, both clomipramine and fluoxetine are as effective in the psychotic subtype of dysmorphophobia as they are in the non-psychotic subtype.

BIBLIOGRAPHY

Hollander E, Allen A, Kwon J, et al. Clomipramine vs. desipramine crossover trial in body dysmorphic disorder: selective efficacy of a serotonin reuptake inhibitor in imagined ugliness. *Archives of General Psychiatry* 1999;56:1033-1039.

McElroy SL, Phillips KA, Keck PE, et al. Body dysmorphic disorder: does it have a psychotic subtype? *The Journal of Clinical Psychiatry* 1993;54:389-395.

McKay D. Two-year follow-up of behavioral treatment and maintenance for body dysmorphic disorder. *Behavior Modification* 1999;23:620-629.

Phillips KA, McElroy SL, Keck PE, et al. Body dysmorphic disorder: 30 cases of imagined ugliness. *The American Journal of Psychiatry* 1993;150:302-308.

Phillips KA, McElroy SL, Keck PE, et al. A comparison of delusional and nondelusional body dysmorphic disorder in 100 cases. *Psychopharmacology Bulletin* 1994;30:179-186.

Phillips KA, Brant J, Siniscalchi J, et al. Surgical and nonpsychiatric medical treatment of patients with body dysmorphic disorder. *Psychosomatics* 2001;42:504-510.

Phillips KA, Albertini RS, Rasmussen SA. A randomized placebo-controlled trial of fluoxetine in body dysmorphic disorder. *Archives of General Psychiatry* 2002;59:381-388.

Thomas CS, Goldberg DP. Appearance, body image and distress in facial dysmorphophobia. *Acta Psychiatrica Scandinavica* 1995;92:231-236.

94 Dissociative Amnesia (DSM-IV-TR #300.12)

Dissociative amnesia, also known as "psychogenic amnesia," is characterized by a fully reversible retrograde amnesia, usually associated with some form of psychological or emotional stress. The prevalence of this disorder is currently a matter of great controversy. Traditionally it has been considered rare; more recently some authors have claimed that it is quite common.

ONSET

Patients typically present in adolescence or early adult years.

CLINICAL FEATURES

The retrograde memory defect of dissociative amnesia may occur in one of four different types: localized, continuous, generalized, and systematized.

In the localized type, which is by far the most common, patients are unable to recall events that transpired during a specific period of time in the past, ranging anywhere from hours to days, or even longer. In a variant of this, known as "selective" amnesia, the patient's inability to recall events that transpired during this specific period of time is "patchy" such that some of the events may be brought to mind whereas others, perhaps the most emotionally charged, are inaccessible to memory.

In the continuous type, patients are unable to recall events for a period of time stretching from the present back to a specific time in the past. This type is in many respects similar to the "localized" type, the main difference being that the "continuous" amnesia stretches up to the moment of the interview.

In the generalized type, patients are unable to recall anything at all from their entire past.

In the systematized type, when patients look back it appears that events of a certain class have been, as it were, systematically removed from memory. For example, patients may report being unable to recall any of numerous instances of abuse stretching back for years or decades: they can recall events that transpired up until the episode of abuse began, and events that occurred after the episode of abuse stopped, but not the abuse itself.

Some patients may also suffer from depersonalization, depression, conversion disorder, or a personality disorder, often of the borderline type.

COURSE

In most cases, without treatment the amnesia is permanent.

COMPLICATIONS

Patients' failure to address adequately the traumatic events surrounding the amnestic period may lead to an inability to address similar situations adequately in the future.

ETIOLOGY

These patients tend to be easily hypnotized, and PET scanning has demonstrated different patterns of activation during memory tasks in patients as compared to controls. Most authors invoke concepts of dissociation or repression; however, these terms are in essence descriptive only and do not help to elucidate any underlying pathologic process.

DIFFERENTIAL DIAGNOSIS

Delirium and dementia are distinguished by the presence of other cognitive deficits, such as confusion, disorientation, and difficulties with calculations and abstracting.

Depression may be characterized by great difficulty with memory; however, here one sees accompanying vegetative signs, such as fatigue, anhedonia, and changes in appetite and sleep, all of which are not characteristic of dissociative amnesia.

Multiple personality disorder may be associated with amnesia, but in multiple personality disorder, in contrast to dissociative amnesia, there is an assumption of a new identity during the amnestic period. Dissociative fugue may also, in some cases, be associated with the assumption of a new identity, but even when this is absent, there is some confusion about personal identity, a finding absent in dissociative amnesia.

The localized type of amnesia must be distinguished from several other neuropsychiatric disorders. Alcoholic blackouts are suggested by the accompanying intoxication, and the amnesia seen with concussion by the history of head trauma. Transient global amnesia is suggested by the older age of onset and by the fact that during the episode itself, patients typically are quite concerned and ask repeatedly what the matter is. Pure epileptic amnesia is suggested by a history of other, more obvious, seizure types, such as grand mal or complex partial seizures.

The continuous type of amnesia must be distinguished from a Korsakoff's syndrome as may be seen in alcoholism or any other condition associated with thiamine deficiency.

The generalized and systematized types are unique, and are not mimicked by any other disorders.

TREATMENT

The optimum approach to patients with dissociative amnesia is not clear. Some clinicians advocate the dramatic intervention of hypnosis or an amobarbital interview, whereas others prefer to engage the patient in psychotherapy, suggesting frequently that the patient will indeed remember what happened: often, with support, and while in an emotionally "safe" environment, patients will begin to recall the forgotten events.

BIBLIOGRAPHY

Izumi SI, Yasueda M, Hihara N, et al. An individual patient comparison of response to a memory training program—psychogenic v organic amnesia: brief report. *American Journal of Physical Medicine & Rehabilitation* 1998;77:458-462.

Kapur N. Amnesia in relation to fugue states—distinguishing a neurological from a psychogenic basis. *The British Journal of Psychiatry* 1991;159: 872-877.

Kopelman MD, Panayiotopoulos CP, Lewis P. Transient epileptic amnesia differentiated from psychogenic "fugue": neuropsychological, EEG, and PET findings. *Journal of Neurology, Neurosurgery, and Psychiatry* 1994;57:1002-1004.

Merckelbach H, Dekkers T, Wessel I, et al. Dissociative symptoms and amnesia in Dutch concentration camp survivors. *Comprehensive Psychiatry* 2003;44:65-69.

Pope HG, Hudson JI, Bodkin JA, et al. Questionable validity of "dissociative amnesia" in trauma victims. Evidence from prospective studies. *The British Journal of Psychiatry* 1998;172:210-215.

Sengupta SN, Jena S, Saxena S. Generalized dissociative amnesia. *The Australian and New Zealand Journal of Psychiatry* 1993;27: 699-700.

Yasuno F, Nishikawa T, Nakagawa Y, et al. Functional anatomical study of psychogenic amnesia. *Psychiatry Research* 2000;99:43-57.

95 Dissociative Fugue (DSM-IV-TR #300.13)

In "dissociative fugue" (also known as "psychogenic fugue") patients suddenly travel away from their accustomed surroundings and experience either confusion or uncertainty regarding their personal identity or actually develop a new identity of varying degrees of complexity. This is probably a rare disorder and appears to be equally common among males and females.

ONSET

Fugue generally appears in adolescence or early adulthood.

CLINICAL FEATURES

An episode of fugue typically appears quite suddenly and is often precipitated by some major personal stress. Whether at home or at work, patients leave off what they are doing and begin to travel. Though still alert and intelligent and possessed of all their former skills, if questioned, patients are not able to tell the interviewer their names, nor anything regarding their personal past. Curiously, if this deficit is brought to light and pointed out, patients may evidence little concern about it.

Some patients may travel only across town. On the other extreme, some may go cross-country or travel to other countries. When travel ceases, the patient may set up residence, take on a new name, get a job, and essentially set up a more or less completely new life, carrying on as if nothing had happened. Generally, the new life is simple and unassuming, and little about the patient might attract attention.

An episode of fugue generally ends as abruptly as it began. Patients suddenly "come to" and undergo an abrupt change. Now, they have no recollection of what happened during the fugue, and their most recent memory is of what happened just before the fugue began. Possessed of their original identity and having no knowledge of their behavior during the fugue, patients are surprised and baffled at finding themselves in a "strange" place and may be baffled by finding a paycheck for work that they have no recollection of doing.

COURSE

What portion of patients will experience recurrent episodes of fugue is not clear.

COMPLICATIONS

Apart from missed work and the distress of family members, there are generally few complications.

ETIOLOGY

Although it is assumed that the phenomenon of dissociation underlies psychogenic fugue, nothing is known with certainty regarding the underlying pathophysiology.

DIFFERENTIAL DIAGNOSIS

In dissociative amnesia, patients may forget their personal identity and undertake travel. However, here patients are often distressed about their inability to recall personal information, and a new identity is not developed.

Multiple personality disorder, or dissociative identity disorder, is characterized by the appearance of a new identity; however, in contrast to fugue, often more than one new identity appears, and generally the patient, while in the new identity, is aware of the original one. Additional differential points include an often rapid shifting from one identity to another and a life that is often chaotic and grossly disturbed.

Complex partial seizures, though generally manifest with confusion and simple purposeless behavior, such as lip-smacking and picking at clothing, may occasionally manifest in more or less purposeful travel, even to the point of driving fairly long distances, thus resembling fugue. In contrast with fugue, however, in a complex partial seizure one always finds some degree of confusion and one never finds the assumption of a new identity. Furthermore, in the history of "wandering" epileptic patients, one generally also finds evidence of more obvious seizure types, such as grand mal seizures.

Demented or delirious patients may wander away from home or the hospital and have little recollection of prior events; however, here, in contrast to fugue, one finds either a generalized intellectual deficit or confusion.

Malingerers may assert symptoms compatible with fugue and indeed may be quite convincing. In contrast to fugue, however, the patient often stands to gain should others believe his story.

TREATMENT

The approach to patients is quite different depending on whether or not they are still in the fugue.

If the episode of fugue has already remitted, the precipitating stress is identified and measures are taken to prevent its recurrence.

If, however, the episode of fugue is ongoing, efforts are directed to helping patients recollect what happened before they entered the fugue. Supportive and gently inquisitive psychotherapy and hypnosis have both been successful; amobarbital interviews, once popular, are probably no more effective than hypnosis.

BIBLIOGRAPHY

Akhtar S, Brenner I. Differential diagnosis of fugue-like states. *The Journal of Clinical Psychiatry* 1979;40:381-385.

Coons PM. Psychogenic or dissociative fugue: a clinical investigation of five cases. *Psychological Reports* 1999;84:881-886.

Macleod AD. Posttraumatic stress disorder, dissociative fugue and a locater beacon. *The Australian and New Zealand Journal of Psychiatry* 1999; 33:102-104.

Mayeux R, Alexander MP, Benson DF, et al. Poriomania. *Neurology* 1979;29:1616-1619.

Riether AM, Stoudemire A. Psychogenic fugue states: a review. *Southern Medical Journal* 1988;81:568-571.

96　Multiple Personality Disorder (dissociative identity disorder, DSM-IV-TR #300.14)

In multiple personality disorder patients undergo sudden, profound, and far-reaching changes in personality, and for all intents and purposes they appear to become different people, with different memories, attitudes, and habits. Generally, often more than one such alternate personality appears, and "switching" from one to another is common. The original personality often has no direct knowledge of the alternate personalities; the times wherein the alternate personalities are present appear to the original personality as amnestic blank spots frequently referred to as "lost time."

This disorder, also known as dissociative identity disorder, is anywhere from three to nine times more common in females than males. Its prevalence is a matter of great controversy. Some believe that it has been greatly underdiagnosed; others, however, are skeptical that it ever occurs on other than an iatrogenic basis.

ONSET

Multiple personality disorder generally has an onset in adolescence or early adult years. In most cases years pass before medical attention is sought. In some cases the onset appears to follow a specific traumatic event, such as abuse, which often appears to have been sexual.

CLINICAL FEATURES

Most patients manifest more than one personality; indeed 10 or more is not uncommon. The transitions or "switches" from one personality to another are generally sudden, occurring in minutes or even seconds. Rarely the transition may be protracted over hours or even a day. These transitions are often precipitated by events that are stressful to the patient; they may also be precipitated by hypnosis.

Each personality represents a cohesive character structure, which is unique to it and clearly different from the other personalities. Memories, attitudes, habits, facial expressions, postures, gestures, and even tone of voice all cohere into a meaningful whole. Indeed were one prevented from recognizing the patient by sight, the observer would have little reason to doubt that, at separate times, one was talking to separate people.

Often, while in one personality the patient engages in behavior that is totally "out of character" and unacceptable to another personality. For example, a patient who, in the original personality, leads a reserved, almost cloistered life may be found to engage in all manner of promiscuous behavior while in an alternate personality.

The various personalities may differ from each other along other dimensions. One may see differences in age, intelligence, race, and even gender. One personality may be able to function effectively at work, whereas another cannot. Often each personality has a different name.

Generally one can identify an "original," or "primary," personality; that is to say, the one that developed in infancy and earliest childhood, well before the onset of the disorder. As noted earlier, this original personality generally has no knowledge of the alternate personalities. The patient may complain about "lost time" or periods of amnesia corresponding to those times when other personalities were evident. Generally, however, one or more of the alternate personalities is knowledgeable of the original personality and perhaps of some of the alternates. In these cases one may find actual conflict between personalities, with a secondary personality actively thwarting what an original one is doing. For example, a libertine secondary personality may cancel a reservation for a weekend religious retreat. Upon reappearance, the original personality, prim, reserved, and anxious to go on the retreat, is at a loss to explain what happened to the reservation. Incidents such as these, wherein the original personality finds evidence of another personality at work, are often what first indicate to the patient that something is desperately wrong.

Often the life of the patient is chaotic and unstable, reflecting the maladaptive character structures of some of the alternate personalities. In one case, a parent in the original personality was tender and attentive toward the baby; however, while in an alternate personality they would spill shards of glass into the crib. In another case, a patient who in the original personality was content with marriage would in an alternate personality become irritable and verbally abusive toward the spouse. When transformations such as these take place frequently, personal and family relationships are unlikely to remain stable for any period of time.

COURSE

Multiple personality disorder is a chronic lifelong disorder. Over the decades, however, the frequency of "switching" tends to decrease, and one of the personality structures tends to become more dominant.

COMPLICATIONS

Complications are in direct proportion to the frequency of switching and the degree of maladaptiveness of the various personalities. Marriage and work often suffer or fail.

ETIOLOGY

Multiple personality disorder appears to be more common among first-degree relatives of patients than in the general population. Whether this represents environmental or genetic factors is not known. Evidence suggests that most patients, as children, were subjected to abuse, often sexual in nature.

Patients with multiple personality disorder are as a rule readily hypnotized, and some have suggested that many, if not most, cases are "induced" by the treating physician.

DIFFERENTIAL DIAGNOSIS

Borderline personality disorder is often mistaken for multiple personality disorder. The lives of borderline patients are as chaotic and unstable as those of patients with multiple personality disorder, and borderline patients typically not only lack a stable sense of identity but also act "as if" they were someone else, and in some cases may refer to themselves by another's name. Indeed, some clinicians believe that most patients diagnosed with multiple personality disorder in fact have a primary borderline personality disorder.

In dissociative amnesia one does not see the appearance of a new identity. In fugue the patient may assume a new personality and be amnestic for events before the fugue; however, important differences are evident with multiple personality disorder. In fugue the new personality usually develops very slowly, over days or weeks, in contrast to the sudden appearance of a full personality in multiple personality disorder. Furthermore, in fugue the patient wanders away and establishes residence elsewhere, whereas this is not common in multiple personality disorder. Most multiple personality disorder patients remain in the same locale. Finally, one does not see the switching back and forth in fugue that is so common in multiple personality disorder.

Patients with prolonged complex partial seizures may complain of "lost time," and others may report uncharacteristic behavior during the seizure. In complex partial seizures, however, patients do not assume a new identity.

Malingering is difficult to rule out. Adept individuals have been able to mislead even experienced observers into incorrectly diagnosing multiple personality disorder. Given the current media attention devoted to this disorder, one should look for any gain, financial or otherwise, that the patient may obtain by virtue of receiving the diagnosis.

TREATMENT

Most patients are treated with individual psychotherapy, and, anecdotally, this has been successful. Treatment with group psychotherapy generally does not work, as the multiple personality transformations are too disruptive to the group process. If hospitalized, these patients tend to get worse; thus hospitalization should be brief. Most clinicians find these patients extraordinarily difficult to treat; such an endeavor is not recommended for novices.

Medications are indicated for any concurrent disorders, such as depression or cyclothymia. They have no direct effect on the disorder itself.

BIBLIOGRAPHY

Fahy TA. The diagnosis of multiple personality disorder. A critical review. *The British Journal of Psychiatry* 1988;153:597-606.

Lauer J, Black DW, Keen P. Multiple personality disorder and borderline personality disorder. Distinct entities or variations on a common theme? *Annals of Clinical Psychiatry* 1993;5:129-134.

Merskey H. The manufacture of personalities. The production of multiple personality disorder. The British Journal of Psychiatry 1992;160:327-340.

Piper A. Multiple personality disorder. *The British Journal of Psychiatry* 1994;164:600-612.

Powell RA, Gee TL. The effects of hypnosis on dissociative identity disorder: a reexamination of the evidence. *Canadian Journal of Psychiatry* 1999;44:914-916.

Rifkin A, Ghisalbert D, Dimatou S, et al. Dissociative identity disorder in psychiatric inpatients. *The American Journal of Psychiatry* 1998; 155:844-845.

97 Depersonalization Disorder (DSM-IV-TR #300.6)

Depersonalization may occur either on an idiopathic basis, in which case one speaks of "depersonalization disorder," or secondary to some other disorder, such as depression, schizophrenia, or epilepsy. Infrequent episodes of depersonalization may also be seen in normal individuals; indeed such appears to be the case in a third to a half of all college students.

Depersonalization disorder is probably rare, and may be more common among females than males.

ONSET

Depersonalization disorder usually has an onset in mid to late teenage years; it may also first appear in early adult years, but onset in middle or older age is decidedly rare.

CLINICAL FEATURES

In most cases depersonalization begins suddenly. Patients almost abruptly find themselves detached from themselves. Though they continue to do what they were doing—to talk, work, eat, or whatever—they seem to be observing these things happening, without actually participating in them, as if they were observing an automaton that just moments earlier had been themselves. At times the body or the arms or legs may appear distorted, enlarged, or shrunken. Time may appear to slow down. Some report the experience of observing themselves from above, as if suspended or floating several feet up in the air.

Frequently, depersonalization is accompanied by the closely allied experience of derealization. Here, though the person clearly perceives the surrounding world, suddenly it appears as if all life and reality were drained or withdrawn from it. Objects and people appear strange, dead, lifeless, and without substance.

The experience of depersonalization may be profoundly unnerving and anxiety provoking, and many fear they are "going insane." Some patients bear it stoically but others may desperately engage in behavior designed to engender a sense of reality. They may raise their voice, as if the volume can stamp their words with a sense of reality. Some, experiencing derealization, may repetitively touch or grasp persons or things in the hopes of imbuing their lifeless perceptions with a sense of solidity and substance.

COURSE

In the majority of cases, depersonalization, though waxing and waning in intensity, is chronic. In a minority, an episodic course is seen, with the episodes themselves enduring anywhere from seconds to days before gradually resolving.

COMPLICATIONS

Depersonalization may impair a patient's ability to remain at task in the work place, and some may become reluctant to leave home or the company of close acquaintances for fear of being alone during an episode.

ETIOLOGY

Patients with depersonalization disorder are readily hypnotized and display a decreased galvanic skin response to unpleasant scenes; furthermore, preliminary PET scanning suggests a preferential activation of the right parietal lobe. Synthesizing these findings into a coherent theory is problematic, and further research is needed.

DIFFERENTIAL DIAGNOSIS

Depersonalization, as noted earlier, is commonly seen in normal life, and this is especially the case during dangerous events, such as motor vehicle accidents. It is also common in panic disorder (wherein it occurs as part of a panic attack), depression, schizophrenia, posttraumatic stress disorder and multiple personality disorder. Various drugs may induce this symptom, such as quetiapine, indomethacin, cannabis and LSD, and in the case of cannabis and LSD, depersonalization may also occur as a "flashback." Hypoglycemia may provoke depersonalization, and a significant minority of head trauma patients may also be affected. Depersonalization may also constitute the aura to a migraine headache or to a complex partial or grand mal seizure, and in such cases the subsequent headache or seizure immediately discloses the diagnosis. More problematic from a differential point of view is the fact that depersonalization may also constitute the sole symptomatology of a simple partial seizure. In this situation, finding a history of other, more obvious, seizure types, such as grand mal or complex partial, is especially helpful. In doubtful cases, an ictal surface EEG (with anterior temporal leads) may be obtained, but it must be borne in mind that this is often normal: in such cases an MRI may be considered in order to see whether there is a lesion present that could reasonably be expected to cause such seizures. In some cases, where the suspicion of a seizure is high, but the EEG and MRI are both normal, an attempt to make a "diagnosis by treatment response" to an antiepileptic drug may be justified.

TREATMENT

Clonazepam, fluoxetine and clomipramine have all, anecdotally, been found effective; clomipramine was also compared to desipramine in a double-blinded study with inconclusive results. Many patients are also taken into psychotherapy.

BIBLIOGRAPHY

Grigsby J, Kaye K. Incidence and correlates of depersonalization following head trauma. *Brain Injury* 1993;7:507-513.

Hollander E, Liebowitz MR, DeCaria C, et al. Treatment of depersonalization with serotonin reuptake blockers. *Journal of Clinical Psychopharmacology* 1990;10:200-203.

Lambert MV, Sierra M, Phillips ML, et al. The spectrum of organic depersonalization. *The Journal of Neuropsychiatry and Clinical Neurosciences* 2002;14:141-154.

Mathew RJ, Wilson MH, Humphreys D, et al. Depersonalization after marijuana smoking. *Biological Psychiatry* 1993;33:431-434.

Sarkar J, Jones N, Sullivan G. A case of depersonalization-derealization syndrome during treatment with quetiapine. *Journal of Psychopharmacology* 2001;15:209-211.

Segui J, Marquez M, Garcia L, et al. Depersonalization in panic disorder: a clinical study. *Comprehensive Psychiatry* 2000;41:172-178.

Simeon D, Gross S, Guralnik O, et al. Feeling unreal: 30 cases of DSM-III-R depersonalization disorder. *The American Journal of Psychiatry* 1997;154:1107-1113.

Simeon D, Stein DJ, Hollander E. Treatment of depersonalization disorder with clomipramine. *Biological Psychiatry* 1998;44:302-303.

Simeon D, Guralnik O, Hazlett EA, et al. Feeling unreal: a PET study of depersonalization disorder. *The American Journal of Psychiatry* 2000; 157:1782-1788.

SEXUAL AND GENDER IDENTITY DISORDERS

98 Decreased Libido (including: hypoactive sexual desire disorder, DSM-IV-TR #302.71, and female and male hypoactive sexual desire disorder due to a general medical condition, DSM-IV-TR #625.8, 608.89)

Decreased libido may be "primary" and due to psychologic causes, in which case it is referred to as "hypoactive sexual desire disorder," or secondary to any of a large number of other causes, in which case one speaks of "hypoactive sexual desire disorder due to a general medical condition."

The lifetime prevalence of hypoactive sexual desire disorder is roughly 15% in males and 30% in females.

ONSET

Decreased libido may occur at any age from adolescence to senescence.

CLINICAL FEATURES

Although exceptions occur, libido tends to gradually decrease with age, and this must be taken into account in evaluating any patient. For example, what might be a normal degree of libido for an elderly person would perhaps be considered decreased for an adolescent.

The patient's lack of interest may be complained of either by the patient or by the patient's partner. In general, the frequency of coitus falls; however, this is not always seen. In some couples the patient may "go along" just to please the partner.

COURSE

The course is extremely variable and in large part determined by the etiology.

COMPLICATIONS

The patient's partner may become aggrieved, and if marital conflict is not already present, it generally follows.

ETIOLOGY

The primary form of decreased libido, that is to say hypoactive sexual desire disorder, may follow sexual trauma, conflict in a sexual relationship, or ensue upon a reduced frequency of sexual activity, as may occur when another sexual dysfunction, such as erectile dysfunction or premature ejaculation, is present. It also appears that a reduced testosterone level is associated with decreased libido in both males and females.

"Secondary" causes of decreased libido include depression, schizophrenia and the inter-ictal personality syndrome, orbito-frontal or hypothalamic lesions, hepatic failure, alcoholism, most antipsychotics and antidepressants (with the notable exceptions of nefazodone, mirtazapine and bupropion), various antihypertensives, carbonic anhydrase inhibitors and anabolic steroids, and a number of endocrinologic conditions, notably hypothyroidism, testosterone deficiency, hyperprolactinemia and menopause.

DIFFERENTIAL DIAGNOSIS

Decreased sexual activity per se need not indicate a decreased libido. Some patients may have very active sexual fantasies and for one reason or another not act on them.

TREATMENT

Hypoactive sexual desire disorder, that is to say primary reduced libido, may be treated with individual or couples psychotherapy, often using specific sex techniques. One preliminary study in females suggested that some patients may improve with bupropion, regardless of whether depression is present or not.

Secondary reduced libido is approached by treating, if possible, the underlying cause. Specifically, with testosterone deficiency, testosterone replacement is indicated, and in the case of hyperprolactinemia, treatment with bromocriptine may restore libido. Menopausal patients may benefit from hormone replacement therapy, and in this respect tibolone appears very effective in restoring libido.

BIBLIOGRAPHY

Davis SR. The effects of tibolone on mood and libido. *Menopause* 2002;9: 162-170.

Guay AT, Jacobson J. Decreased free testosterone and dehydroepiandrosterone-sulfate (DHEA-S) levels in women with decreased libido. *Journal of Sex & Marital Therapy* 2002;28(Suppl 1):129-142.

Schiavi RC, Schreiner-Engel P, White D, et al. Pituitary-gonadal function during sleep in men with hypoactive sexual desire and in normal controls. *Psychosomatic Medicine* 1988;50:304-318.

Segraves RT, Croft H, Kavoussi R, et al. Bupropion sustained release (SR) for the treatment of hypoactive sexual desire disorder (HSDD) in nondepressed women. *Journal of Sex & Marital Therapy* 2001;27: 303-316.

Wallace TR, Fraunfelder FT, Petursson GJ, et al. Decreased libido—a side effect of carbonic anhydrase inhibitor. *Annals of Ophthalmology* 1979;11:1563-1566.

Warnock JJ. Female hypoactive sexual desire disorder: epidemiology, diagnosis and treatment. *CNS Drugs* 2002;16:745-753.

Weizman A, Weizman R, Hart J, et al. The correlation of increased serum prolactin levels with decreased sexual desire and activity in elderly men. *Journal of the American Geriatrics Society* 1983;312: 485-488.

99 Female Sexual Arousal Disorder (DSM-IV-TR #302.72)

Female sexual arousal disorder is characterized by insufficient sexual arousal and lubrication occurring secondary to emotional distress, and may occur in up to one-third of all adult women. Reduced sexual arousal in women may also occur secondary to several general medical conditions, as noted below under "differential diagnosis." In the past the condition of reduced sexual arousal was referred to as "frigidity"; however, this term is rarely seen in current medical literature.

ONSET

This disorder may occur at any time from adolescence to old age.

CLINICAL FEATURES

Most women at some point in their lives experience a transient lack of lubrication. In female sexual arousal disorder, however, the patient, despite having a more or less normal libido, complains that she has been unable for a long time to get "turned on" or aroused. Both she and her partner may complain of the dryness, which in turn may lead to dyspareunia and a disinclination to attempt further intercourse.

COURSE

Onset in adolescence is associated with a chronic course; when the onset occurs after a significant period of normal sexual functioning, the prognosis is much better.

COMPLICATIONS

Shame for the patient and discord for the couple are not uncommon.

ETIOLOGY

Sexual ignorance, guilt, anxiety or anger, inadequate foreplay and marital discord may all play a role. Women with decreased libido will also generally experience a failure of arousal and lubrication.

DIFFERENTIAL DIAGNOSIS

"Secondary" cases of reduced sexual arousal in women may be seen in postmenopausal atrophic vaginitis, diabetes mellitus, pelvic arteriosclerosis, pelvic radiotherapy, sacral cord lesions and partial or complete cord transections, partial epilepsy, depression, and with various medications including anticholinergics, clonidine, some antihistamines, some antihypertensives, low-potency first-generation neuroleptics, and certain antidepressants.

TREATMENT

Sex therapy, often utilizing the "sensate focus" technique, is generally successful and typically combined with some form of individual or couples psychotherapy. Lubricants are often employed, at least initially, and may facilitate progress. Recent work also supports the use of sildenafil in doses of 25 or 50 mg.

BIBLIOGRAPHY

Caruso S, Intelisano G, Lupo L, et al. Premenopausal women affected by sexual arousal disorder treated with sildenafil: a double-blind, cross-over, placebo-controlled study. *International Journal of Obstetrics and Gynaecology* 2001;108:623-628.

Meston CM, Gorzalka BB, Wright JM. Inhibition of subjective and physiological sexual arousal in women by clonidine. *Psychosomatic Medicine* 1997;59:399-407.

Morrell MJ, Sperling MR, Stecker M, et al. Sexual dysfunction in partial epilepsy: a deficit in physiologic sexual arousal. *Neurology* 1994;44: 243-247.

Sipski ML, Alexander CJ, Rosen R. Sexual arousal and orgasm in women: effects of spinal cord injury. *Annals of Neurology* 2001;49:35-44.

Traish AM, Kim NN, Munarriz R, et al. Biochemical and physiological mechanisms of female genital sexual arousal. *Archives of Sexual Behavior* 2002;31:393-400.

100 Erectile Dysfunction (male erectile disorder, DSM-IV-TR #302.72; male erectile disorder due to a general medical condition, DSM-IV-TR #607.84)

Men with erectile dysfunction fail to have erections of sufficient rigidity and duration to allow for completion of sexual intercourse. Erectile dysfunction may be due to emotional distress, in which case it is considered "primary" and referred to as "male erectile disorder" or may occur secondary to any of a large number of general medical conditions, as for example diabetes mellitus. The prevalence of erectile dysfunction increases with age, ranging from 7% to 9% for young men and up to 25% to 50% for those over 55.

In the not-distant past, an inability to have or sustain an erection was referred to as impotence; however, this term is rapidly being supplanted by "erectile dysfunction," in large part because the latter term has never garnered the stigma that the term impotence has, and thus is more acceptable to patients and physicians alike.

Neural elements relevant to erection include the limbic system, descending parasympathetic pathways down the cord to the sacral segments, and sacral parasympathetic efferents, traveling eventually through the nervi erigentes to the penis. This complex system in turn is dependent on adequate levels of circulating testosterone. Erection itself is dependent on an anatomically normal penis, an adequate vascular supply, and parasympathetically mediated engorgement of the corpora cavernosa and the corpus spongiosum.

The relative percentages of primary and secondary erectile dysfunction change with age; among younger men, perhaps 80% of cases are primary, whereas among older men, perhaps only 50% are primary, the other 50% being clearly secondary to some other disorder.

ONSET

Erectile dysfunction may occur at any age, from adolescence through senescence. In general, primary erectile dysfunction tends to be of relatively acute onset, whereas secondary erectile dysfunction tends to occur insidiously.

CLINICAL FEATURES

Erectile dysfunction, whether partial or complete, is at the least an anxiety-provoking event, and for some men may be emotionally devastating. Certain historical features may help to differentiate primary from secondary erectile dysfunction. Primary erectile dysfunction tends to be selective, perhaps occurring only with a certain partner, or transient, with the capacity to have erections waxing and waning over time. Secondary erectile dysfunction tends to be persistent and pervasive, and these men report not having erections regardless of who they are with or what they are doing. Thus one must ask the patient complaining of erectile dysfunction whether he has ever had an adequate erection since the onset of the erectile dysfunction, with special attention to masturbation, "wet dreams," or morning erections.

When it is difficult to differentiate primary from secondary erectile dysfunction, measurement of nocturnal penile tumescence and rigidity in a sleep laboratory may be helpful. In general, most men with primary erectile dysfunction have normal erections during REM sleep, and most men with secondary erectile dysfunction do not. Exceptions, however, do occur. For example, men suffering from a major depression may not exhibit nocturnal penile tumescence; conversely, men impotent secondary to hyperprolactinemia may show nocturnal penile tumescence.

COURSE

The natural course of primary erectile dysfunction tends to vary according to the mode of onset. Those with acute onset following specific precipitating factors tend to recover spontaneously. In contrast, those with an insidious onset and without an identifiable precipitant tend to run a chronic course, and this is particularly the case in those uncommon cases where the patient has apparently been impotent since puberty.

The course of secondary erectile dysfunction is determined by the underlying cause.

COMPLICATIONS

When single men have erectile dysfunction, they may avoid relationships that could become sexual. Those who are married or in stable sexual relationships may face the dissolution of their relationship.

ETIOLOGY

Primary erectile dysfunction often occurs when a man is anxious, perhaps out of a fear of not being able to perform, or when he feels guilty. If angry at a partner, most men are unable to have or sustain an erection. Regardless of which circumstance occasions the erectile dysfunction, the man faces a risk that a vicious cycle will be established, wherein, out of fear of repeat instances of erectile dysfunction, the man becomes so anxious that he is again unable to perform.

The causes of secondary erectile dysfunction are conveniently organized in several categories: cerebral, spinal, peripheral nervous, vascular, endocrinologic, those caused by local disease of the penis, drug induced, and finally a miscellaneous group.

Cerebral lesions, especially those affecting the temporal lobes or limbic system, may cause erectile dysfunction and are often also associated with decreased libido. These include multiple sclerosis, tumors, infarctions, and neurosyphilis. Parkinsonian conditions, as for example Parkinson's disease or multiple system atrophy, may also may be associated with erectile dysfunction.

Spinal cord lesions also may cause erectile dysfunction, but generally do not decrease libido. These include amyotrophic lateral sclerosis, tabes dorsalis, spina bifida, and subacute combined degeneration as seen in hypovitaminosis B_{12}. Plaques of multiple sclerosis or tumors of the conus medullaris also may cause erectile dysfunction, as may lesions of the cauda equina. Lesions causing paraplegia, such as tumors, infarctions, or transverse myelitis, may or may not cause erectile dysfunction, depending on the level. For example, in thoracic lesions, the patient may have "reflex" erections unassociated with any pleasurable feelings.

Peripheral autonomic polyneuropathy, as may be seen in alcoholism or amyloidosis, may cause erectile dysfunction but generally spares libido. Diabetic polyneuropathy is a very common cause; however, as noted below, the erectile dysfunction in diabetes may also be caused by vascular lesions. Genital herpes may be associated with erectile dysfunction, possibly due to a herpetic infection of the nervi erigentes. Various surgical procedures may lead to erectile dysfunction due to nerve damage. These include radical cystectomy, abdominal perineal colon resection, and radical prostatectomy. Transurethral prostatectomy, on the other hand, is generally not associated with erectile dysfunction.

Arteriosclerosis of large or small vessels may cause erectile dysfunction but generally does not diminish libido. The Leriche syndrome is an example of large vessel arteriosclerosis affecting selectively the aortoilial vessels and is characterized by erectile dysfunction and claudication of the buttocks, thighs, and occasionally the calves. Diabetes may lead to arteriolar disease and erectile dysfunction, and this is often in conjunction with a diabetic autonomic polyneuropathy. Radiation therapy may cause erectile dysfunction secondary to vascular damage. In patients with early vascular disease, a "steal" phenomenon may be seen. When the patient is at rest, a normal erection may occur, but with increased blood flow to the lower extremities during pelvic thrusting, penile perfusion pressure may fall below a critical level, with loss of erection. Finally, both sickle cell anemia and severe hypertriglyceridemia may, by reducing blood flow in small vessels, also cause erectile dysfunction.

Testosterone deficiency is generally associated with both erectile dysfunction and decreased libido and may be secondary to disturbances at the level of the hypothalamus, pituitary, or testes. Hypothalamic lesions may include various tumors or granulomatous infiltrations. Gonadotropin secretions from the pituitary may be reduced secondary to tumors of the pituitary gland, including prolactinomas. When tumors do compromise pituitary endocrine function, gonadotrophic secretion generally falls first, followed by growth hormone, thyrotropin, and ACTH. Hemochromatosis may cause selective deposition of iron in gonadotropin-secreting cells. Excessive steroids, whether from Cushing's syndrome or high-dose exogenous steroids, may inhibit gonadotropin release. Testicular failure per se may occur secondary to orchiectomy (as may be performed for prostatic cancer), mumps orchitis, Klinefelter's syndrome, malnutrition, myotonic dystrophy, lead poisoning, and a variety of chronic debilitating diseases, such as cirrhosis of the liver, renal failure, respiratory failure, or widespread malignancy. Erectile dysfunction may also be seen in hypothyroidism and rarely in hyperthyroidism.

Local diseases of the penis, such as Peyronie's disease or chordee, may cause erectile dysfunction. It may also occur as a sequel to priapism.

A large number of drugs may produce erectile dysfunction in a minority of patients. These include the following: certain antihypertensives, including propranolol, clonidine, reserpine, methyldopa, guanethidine, hydralazine, and phentolamine; certain diuretics, such as hydrochlorothiazide; antipsychotics; tricyclic antidepressants (especially clomipramine); monoamine oxidase inhibitors; selective serotonin reuptake inhibitors; lithium; various drugs of abuse including opioids, stimulants, cannabis, and alcohol; digoxin; cimetidine; statins and fibrates; and various antimetabolites.

Miscellaneous causes include schizophrenia, depression and obstructive sleep apnea.

Primary and secondary causes of erectile dysfunction may coexist in the same patient. For example, a patient with erectile dysfunction secondary to an antihypertensive medication may be so anxious about his next attempt that he remains unable to sustain an erection even after the offending drug is stopped. Another example is a diabetic patient who heretofore could have an erection despite a certain amount of anxiety, but now, with a modest compromise of penile blood flow because of diabetic vasculopathy, is able to perform only when free of anxiety, being unable to at other times.

DIFFERENTIAL DIAGNOSIS

Given a reliable history, one should have no difficulty in diagnosing the presence of erectile dysfunction per se. Difficulty occurs, however, when some patients confuse erectile dysfunction with loss of libido or with ejaculation that is premature, retrograde, or delayed. Careful, specific questioning is required.

TREATMENT

In primary erectile dysfunction, consideration may be given to psychotherapy. Sometimes simple reassurance is curative, and this is especially likely in instances where the erectile dysfunction was preceded by normal sexual functioning, was clearly related to a psychosocial precipitating factor, and was of acute onset. When reassurance is ineffective, sex therapy, utilizing a "sensate focus" approach, may be successful, and, in cases where there is considerable friction in the relationship, couples therapy may be indicated. In cases where psychotherapy is ineffective or impractical, sildenafil, discussed below, is indicated as it is effective in erectile dysfunction of either primary or secondary type. There is some evidence to support the use of yohimbine for primary erectile dysfunction, and its use is discussed in that chapter.

In secondary erectile dysfunction the underlying condition, if treatable, is addressed. Some points deserve emphasis. In vascular erectile dysfunction, revascularization is of benefit only in primarily large vessel disease. In testosterone deficiency, oral testosterone preparations are generally not used due to the risk of hepatotoxicity. Transdermal testosterone or injections of testosterone enanthate or proprionate are preferred. Testosterone treatment is relatively contraindicated in those with prostatic hypertrophy and is absolutely contraindicated in those with prostatic cancer. In hyperprolactinemia, testosterone treatment may fail, whereas treatment with bromocriptine may be successful. When erectile dysfunction is caused by an antidepressant, consideration should be given to switching to one of the agents not likely to be associated with erectile dysfunction, namely bupropion, nefazodone, trazodone or mirtazapine. If antihypertensive medication is at fault, then an ACE inhibitor or a calcium channel blocker may be considered, as they are less likely to cause erectile dysfunction than other agents.

Various pharmacologic options are available, and of all these the first choice is the phosphodiesterase-5 inibitor, sildenafil. Provided that the vascular supply to the penis is not severely compromised, sildenafil is effective in both primary and almost all secondary forms of erectile dysfunction: contraindications include the coadministration of nitrates, the presence of significant autonomic failure (as may be seen in multiple system atrophy) and any condition, such as sickle cell anemia, which may predispose to priapism. Two other phosphodiesterase inhibitors, tadalafil and vardenafil, will probably be available soon; however, it is not as yet clear how they compare with sildenafil. In the case of patients who tolerate sildenafil but achieve little benefit, consideration may be given to combination treatment with prn sildenafil and a daily dose of doxazosin: if doxazosin is used, one must start at a low dose or perhaps 1 mg and increase only gradually, in order to avoid symptomatic hypotension, to the average effective dose of 4 mg daily. For patients who cannot tolerate sildenafil, or who simply do not benefit from it even after eight or more trials, consideration may be given to either apomorphine or alprostadil. Sublingual apomorphine (not yet available in the United States) in a prn dose of 2 to 4 mg, is often beneficial, but may cause troubling nausea. Alprostadil may be given by intracavernous injection, via a miniature urethral suppository, or as a cream applied to the glans penis: most patients find the injection overall most satisfactory.

Non-pharmacologic options include a vacuum constrictor device and either rigid or semi-rigid prostheses.

BIBLIOGRAPHY

De Rose AF, Giglio M, Traverso P, et al. Combined oral therapy with sildenafil and doxazosin for the treatment of non-organic erectile dysfunction refractory to sildenafil monotherapy. *International Journal of Impotence Research* 2002;14:50-53.

Dula E, Bukofzer S, Perdok R, et al. Double-blind, crossover comparison of 3 mg apomorphine SL with placebo and with 4 mg apomorphine SL in male erectile dysfunction. *European Urology* 2001;39:558-563.

Eardley I, Morgan R, Dinsmore W, et al. Efficacy and safety of sildenafil citrate in the treatment of men with mild to moderate erectile dysfunction. *The British Journal of Psychiatry* 2001;78:325-330.

Fink HA, MacDonald R, Rutks IR, et al. Sildenafil for male erectile dysfunction: a systematic review and meta-analysis. *Archives of Internal Medicine* 2002;162:1349-1360.

Gresser U, Gleiter CH. Erectile dysfunction: comparison of efficacy and side effects of the PDE-5 inhibitors sildenafil, vardenafil and tadalafil—review of the literature. *European Journal of Medical Research* 2002;7:435-446.

Hussain IF, Brady CM, Swinn MJ, et al. Treatment of erectile dysfunction with sildenafil citrate (Viagra) in parkinsonism due to Parkinson's disease or multiple system atrophy with observations on orthostatic hypotension. *Journal of Neurology, Neurosurgery, and Psychiatry* 2001;71:371-374.

Levine LA, Dimitriou RJ. Vacuum constriction and external erection devices in erectile dysfunction. *The Urologic Clinics of North America* 2001;28:335-341.

Nurnberg HG, Gelenberg A, Hargreave TB, et al. Efficacy of sildenafil citrate for the treatment of erectile dysfunction in men taking serotonin reuptake inhibitors. *The American Journal of Psychiatry* 2001;158:1926-1928.

Shabsigh R, Anastasiadis AG. Erectile dysfunction. *Annual Review of Medicine* 2003;54:153-168.

101 Female Anorgasmia (female orgasmic disorder, DSM-IV-TR #302.73)

Anorgasmia, or the inability to achieve orgasm despite adequate arousal, may be primary and related to emotional distress, in which case one speaks of "female orgasmic disorder," or secondary to some general medical condition, as for example certain spinal cord injuries. Primary anorgasmia is very common, and may be seen in up to 30% of all women.

ONSET

Primary anorgasmia may have an onset at puberty and be lifelong, or it may be acquired, and in such cases this usually follows significant stress in the patient's sexual relationship. The age of onset of secondary anorgasmia is determined by the underlying cause.

CLINICAL FEATURES

Despite normal libido, adequate lubrication, and otherwise adequate stimulation, the patient reports an inability to achieve orgasm. This anorgasmia may be situational, as for example when a woman is able to experience orgasm with masturbation but not intercourse, or may be generalized, in which case orgasm is not possible in any situation.

COURSE

In cases of primary anorgasmia where orgasm has never been achieved, the course tends to be relatively chronic. With age, however, progressively more women become orgasmic.

COMPLICATIONS

Frustration and dissatisfaction may lead to marital discord.

ETIOLOGY

Most cases of anorgasmia are primary and related to psychologic factors; for example, the patient may feel guilty over having pleasure, or may be afraid to "let go," for fear of losing control.

Secondary anorgasmia may be due to various drugs, including antihypertensives, antipsychotics, and most antidepressants. In the case of antidepressants, it appears that those with a more pronounced serotoninergic effect, such as the SSRIs or clomipramine, are more likely to cause this problem. Other causes of secondary anorgasmia include injury to the vagina or clitoris and some cases of spinal cord damage; there are also case reports of women with cataplexy who would not allow themselves to reach orgasm for fear of provoking a cataplectic attack.

DIFFERENTIAL DIAGNOSIS

A failure to achieve orgasm during intercourse is not considered anorgasmia if the foreplay is inadequate or the man suffers from erectile dysfunction or premature ejaculation.

TREATMENT

In cases of primary anorgasmia individual and couples therapy is often indicated; furthermore, in lifelong cases, directed masturbation is often used adjunctively. In a preliminary single-blind study, bupropion, in doses of 150 to 300 mg, was also helpful; furthermore there are anecdotal reports of increased orgasmic potential secondary to treatment with trazodone.

In secondary cases the underlying cause is attended to. In cases of antidepressant-induced anorgasmia, consideration may be given to bupropion, mirtazapine or nefazodone, all of which are generally free of sexual side-effects.

BIBLIOGRAPHY

Modell JG, May RS, Katholi CR. Effect of bupropion-SR on orgasmic dysfunction in nondepressed subjects: a pilot study. *Journal of Sex & Marital Therapy* 2000;26:231-240.

Monteiro WO, Noshirvani HF, Marks IM, et al. Anorgasmia from clomipramine in obsessive-compulsive disorder. A controlled trial. *The British Journal of Psychiatry* 1987;151:107-112.

Riley AJ, Riley EJ. A controlled study to evaluate directed masturbation in the management of primary orgasmic failure in women. *The British Journal of Psychiatry* 1978;133:404-409.

Roy A. Anorgasmia and cataplexy. *Archives of Sexual Behavior* 1977;6: 437-439.

Segraves RT. Antidepressant-induced orgasm disorder. *Journal of Sex & Marital Therapy* 1995;21:192-201.

Sipski ML, Alexander CJ, Rosen RC. Orgasm in women with spinal cord injuries: a laboratory-based assessment. *Archives of Physical Medicine and Rehabilitation* 1995;76:1097-1112.

Sovner R. Anorgasmia associated with imipramine but not desipramine. *The Journal of Clinical Psychiatry* 1983;44:345-346.

102   Inhibited Male Orgasm (male orgasmic disorder, DSM-IV 302.74)

In inhibited male orgasm, also known as retarded ejaculation, a man, despite otherwise adequate stimulation, finds himself unable to ejaculate. Inhibited male orgasm may be primary and the result of emotional distress, in which case it is referred to as "male orgasmic disorder," or it may occur secondary to a number of medications or general medical conditions. Primary inhibited male orgasm is a relatively uncommon condition.

ONSET

Primary inhibited male orgasm may have an onset at puberty and be lifelong, or may be "acquired" in that it occurs after a period of normal sexual functioning, usually in the context of considerable emotional distress. The age of onset of secondary inhibited male orgasm is determined by the underlying cause.

CLINICAL FEATURES

Primary inhibited male orgasm may be either situational, as for example when a man is able to ejaculate with masturbation but not intravaginally, or generalized, wherein ejaculation is delayed or absent in all situations. In some cases, patients, rather than orgasm and ejaculation, may experience rather a slow and pleasureless seepage.

COURSE

Primary inhibited male orgasm of pubertal onset tends to remain chronic; the course of the situational type is quite variable. With regard to secondary inhibited male orgasm, the course is determined by the underlying cause.

COMPLICATIONS

Both the man and woman may feel frustrated. In addition the woman may feel rejected or inadequate.

ETIOLOGY

Severe guilt, a fear of impregnation, or hostility toward a woman have all been associated with primary inhibited male orgasm.

Secondary inhibited male orgasm may be caused by certain antidepressants (particularly clomipramine and SSRIs), antipsychotics (including risperidone and, particularly, thioridazine), and antihypertensives. It may also occur as a sequel to prostatectomy or secondary to lesions in the conus medullaris or low sacral cord, which may leave erection intact but make ejaculation impossible.

DIFFERENTIAL DIAGNOSIS

In retrograde ejaculation, although no ejaculate is seen, orgasm and detumescence do occur.

TREATMENT

In primary inhibited male orgasm, sex therapy is generally helpful. In secondary cases, the underlying cause is addressed: in the case of antidepressant-induced inhibited male orgasm, consideration may be given to switching to bupropion, mirtazapine or nefazodone, all of which are generally free of sexual side effects.

BIBLIOGRAPHY

Raja M. Risperidone-induced absence of ejaculation. *International Clinical Psychopharmacology* 1999;14:317-319.

Segraves RT. Effects of psychotropic drugs on human erection and ejaculation. *Archives of General Psychiatry* 1989;46:275-284.

Waldinger MD, Hengeveld MW, Zwiderman AH, et al. Effect of SSRI antidepressants on ejaculation: a double-blind, randomized, placebo-controlled study with fluoxetine, fluvoxamine, paroxetine, and sertraline. *Journal of Clinical Psychopharmacology* 1998;18:274-281.

Waldinger MD, Zwinderman AH, Olivier B. Antidepressants and ejaculation: a double-blind, randomized, placebo-controlled, fixed-dose study with paroxetine, sertraline, and nefazodone. *Journal of Clinical Psychopharmacology* 2001;21:293-297.

Waldinger MD, Zwinderman AH, Olivier B. SSRIs and ejaculation: a double-blind, randomized, fixed-dose study with paroxetine and citalopram. *Journal of Clinical Psychopharmacology* 2001;21:556-560.

103 Premature Ejaculation (DSM-IV-TR #302.75)

In premature ejaculation, a man consistently ejaculates earlier than he wishes to, with relatively little sexual stimulation, and either before, or shortly after, penetration, and before his partner reaches orgasm. This is a common problem, occurring in 30% or more of men.

ONSET

Although premature ejaculation may occur at any age, it is most common among adolescents.

CLINICAL FEATURES

Although preferring that the woman climax before he ejaculates, the premature ejaculator finds himself persistently ejaculating before that, and sometimes well before that, either during foreplay, penetration, or after a few thrusts.

COURSE

Untreated, premature ejaculation tends to become chronic.

COMPLICATIONS

Shame and humiliation may prompt the man to avoid intercourse; the woman, dissatisfied, may become resentful.

ETIOLOGY

In most cases, premature ejaculation is psychologically determined. The man may have apprehension that he will not be able to satisfy the woman, or have a fear of being overwhelmed by her. Guilt or fear of discovery may make a man want to get it over with; the presence of any hostility also makes for a brief union.

Although antidepressants and neuroleptics, if they have any effect on the rapidity of ejaculation, tend to delay ejaculation, in some cases they have caused it.

Prostatitis is common in men with premature ejaculation; however, it is unclear if treatment of prostatitis by itself will relieve the condition.

Rarely, premature ejaculation may be associated with Parkinson's disease or with lesions of the sacral cord.

DIFFERENTIAL DIAGNOSIS

Should a woman have anorgasmia, ejaculation is always, in a sense, "premature." The boundary between premature ejaculation and anorgasmia is sometimes hard to draw; as a general rule, most women on the average experience orgasm within 10 minutes of intercourse.

TREATMENT

In most cases of psychologically determined premature ejaculation, sex therapy, using the "squeeze" or "stop-and-start" techniques, is quite successful. Should this fail, or should marital conflict be evident, then individual or couples therapy is indicated.

Various pharmacologic agents are also effective. Of the SSRIs, paroxetine (20 mg), sertraline (50 mg), fluoxetine (20 mg) and citalopram (20 mg) are all effective, and of these, paroxetine is the most effective. Clomipramine, 50 mg, may be more effective than paroxetine; however, side-effects often make it a second choice. Although the foregoing medications are generally taken on a daily basis, it has recently become clear that, at least in the case of paroxetine, sertraline and clomipramine, they may also be taken on a prn basis, 3 to 5 hours before anticipated intercourse. It has also recently been shown that sildenafil on a prn basis is effective for premature ejaculation, and indeed in one study was more effective than the SSRIs.

BIBLIOGRAPHY

Abul-Hamid IA, Naggar EA, El Gilany AH. Assessment of as needed use of pharmacotherapy and the pause-squeeze technique in premature ejaculation. *International Journal of Impotence Research* 2001;13:41-45.

Berkovitch M, Keresteci AG, Koren G. Efficacy of prilocaine-lidocaine cream in the treatment of premature ejaculation. *The Journal of Urology* 1995;154:1360-1361.

Kim SC, Seo KK. Efficacy and safety of fluoxetine, sertraline and clomipramine in patients with premature ejaculation: a double-blind, placebo controlled study. *The Journal of Urology* 1998;159:425-427.

Screponi E, Carosa E, Di Stasi SM, et al. Prevalence of chronic prostatitis in men with premature ejaculation. *Urology* 2001;58:198-202.

Waldinger MD, Hengeveld MW, Zwinderman AH, et al. Effect of SSRI antidepressants on ejaculation: a double-blind, randomized, placebo-controlled study with fluoxetine, fluvoxamine, paroxetine and sertaline. *Journal of Clinical Psychopharmacology* 1998;18:274-281.

Waldinger MD, Zwinderman AH, Olivier B. Antidepressants and ejaculation: a double-blind, randomized, placebo-controlled, fixed-dose study with paroxetine, sertaline and nefazodone. *Journal of Clinical Psychopharmacology* 2001;21:293-297.

Waldinger MD, Zwinderman AH, Olivier B. SSRIs and ejaculation: a double-blind, randomized, fixed-dose study with paroxetine and citalopram. *Journal of Clinical Psychopharmacology* 2001;21:556-560.

104 Female Dyspareunia (DSM-IV-TR #302.76)

Dyspareunia, or persistent pain in the genitalia during or shortly after intercourse, may be either primary and psychologically determined or secondary to a number of general medical conditions, such as vaginitis. Dyspareunia is very common, occurring in up to 30% of all women.

ONSET

Dyspareunia may occur at first intercourse or at any time subsequent.

CLINICAL FEATURES

The location of the pain, its relationship to the depth of thrusting, and its association, if any, with a lack of lubrication are all important diagnostic clues. Some women, perhaps out of embarrassment or a sense that intercourse no matter how painful is their duty, may not be forthcoming with this complaint or may be reluctant to provide a detailed account.

COURSE

The course is variable and dependent in large part on the cause.

COMPLICATIONS

Dissatisfaction and marital strain may occur; many women avoid intercourse, and in some, vaginismus may develop.

ETIOLOGY

Primary dyspareunia is often related to sexual guilt.

Secondary dyspareunia may occur in the following conditions: vaginismus, vulvar vestibulitis, hymenal remnants, post-operative scarring, vaginal dryness (as may be seen in atrophic vaginitis or in Sjorgen's syndrome), vaginitis, endometriosis, adnexal masses or infections, other intra-abdominal processes (e.g., celiac disease), urethritis or cystitis, and allergic reactions to semen, condoms or lubricants.

Since most cases of dyspareunia are either in part or wholly secondary to some general medical condition, a thorough gynecologic examination, which may include laparoscopy, is required in all cases.

DIFFERENTIAL DIAGNOSIS

Dyspareunia may occur as an integral part of Briquet's syndrome.

TREATMENT

In cases of secondary dyspareunia, treatment is directed at the underlying cause; in primary, psychologically determined, dyspareunia, sex or couples therapy is generally required.

BIBLIOGRAPHY

Graziottin A. Clinical approach to dyspareunia. *Journal of Sex & Marital Therapy* 2001;27:489-501.

Heim LJ. Evaluation and differential diagnosis of dyspareunia. *American Family Physician* 2001;63:1535-1544.

Meana M, Binik YM. Painful coitus: a review of female dyspareunia. *The Journal of Nervous and Mental Disease* 1994;182:264-272.

Peckham BM, Maki DG, Patterson JJ, et al. Focal vulvitis: a characteristic syndrome and cause of dyspareunia. Features, natural history and management. *American Journal of Obstetrics and Gynecology* 1986;154:855-864.

Tayal SC, Watson PG. Dyspareunia in undiagnosed Sjorgen's syndrome. *British Journal of Clinical Practice* 1996;50:57-58.

105 Vaginismus (DSM-IV-TR #306.51)

In vaginismus a woman persistently experiences an uncontrollable spasm of the outer third of the vagina that makes intromission either difficult or impossible. Severe cases of vaginismus are not common, occurring in less than 10% of women; milder degrees, however, may be much more common.

ONSET

Vaginismus may occur at any time from adolescence to old age.

CLINICAL FEATURES

Despite the fact that the patient desires intercourse, and may indeed even experience a normal degree of arousal and lubrication, the vagina becomes so tight that intromission is uncomfortable, difficult, or impossible.

Vaginismus may also be apparent on gynecologic examination; spasm may be so intense that neither the speculum nor the physician's finger can be inserted.

COURSE

A chronic course appears common, with the severity of vaginal spasm waxing and waning over time.

COMPLICATIONS

Marital discord may become extreme; in severe cases, impregnation may be impossible, and the couple may remain childless.

ETIOLOGY

Vaginismus is said to be primary when it occurs on the basis of guilt or anxiety, which in turn is typically related to a history of witnessing or being the victim of a sexual assault. Vaginismus may also occur secondary to a general medical condition, as for example dyspareunia, wherein repeated episodes of painful intercourse leave the patient anxious about further attempts.

DIFFERENTIAL DIAGNOSIS

Scarring or vaginal atresia are evident on pelvic examination.

TREATMENT

If a preceding dyspareunia is present, it must be treated first. Couples therapy, combined with the use of either in-office or at home insertion of progressively larger dilators, is generally successful.

BIBLIOGRAPHY

de Kruiff ME, ter Kuile MM, Weijenborg PT, et al. Vaginismus and dyspareunia: is there a difference in clinical presentation? *Psychosomatic Obstetrics and Gynecology* 2000;21:149-155.

O'Sullivan K. Observations on vaginismus in Irish women. *Archives of General Psychiatry* 1979;36:824-826.

Schnyder U, Schneider-Luthi C, Ballinari P, et al. Therapy for vaginismus: in vivo versus in vitro desensitization. *Canadian Journal of Psychiatry* 1998;43:941-944.

Silverstein JL. Origins of psychogenic vaginismus. *Psychotherapy and Psychosomatics* 1989;52:197-204.

van der Velde J, Evereard W. The relationship between involuntary pelvic floor muscle activity, muscle awareness and experienced threat in women with and without vaginismus. *Behaviour Research and Therapy* 2001;39:395-408.

106 Male Dyspareunia (DSM-IV-TR #302.76)

Dyspareunia in the male is quite uncommon and is usually secondary to a general medical condition, such as prostatitis, rather than being primary and related to psychologic factors.

ONSET

The onset is determined by the etiology.

CLINICAL FEATURES

Pain in the penis, testicle, or perineum may be experienced either during intercourse or during or just after ejaculation.

COURSE

The course is determined by the etiology.

COMPLICATIONS

Depending on the severity of the pain, some men may avoid intercourse, leading to marital discord.

ETIOLOGY

Secondary male dyspareunia may be due to herpes or other rashes, urethritis, prostatitis, chordee, or Peyronie's disease. Painful ejaculation may also occur as a result of treatment with MAOIs, tricyclic antidepressants, SSRIs, venlafaxine and certain antipsychotics.

In the rare cases of primary dyspareunia, the pain is usually post-ejaculatory and associated with involuntary spasm of the perineal musculature; these patients often harbor guilt or shame regarding sexual pleasure.

DIFFERENTIAL DIAGNOSIS

Assuming an accurate history, there can be little diagnostic confusion.

TREATMENT

Treatment is directed to the underlying cause. In the case of primary male dyspareunia, individual psychotherapy is generally offered; however, there have been no controlled outcome studies. In cases secondary to antidepressants, case reports note relief upon treatment with the alpha-1 antagonist, tamsulosin.

BIBLIOGRAPHY

Aizenberg D, Zenishlany Z, Hermesh H, et al. Painful ejaculation associated with antidepressants in four patients. *The Journal of Clinical Psychiatry* 1991;52:461-463.

Berger SH. Trifluoperazine and haloperidol—sources of ejaculatory pain? *The American Journal of Psychiatry* 1979;136:350.

De Leo D, Magni G. Sexual side effects of antidepressant drugs. *Psychosomatics* 1983;24:1076-1082.

Demyttenaere K, Huygens R. Painful ejaculation and urinary hesitancy in association with antidepressant therapy: relief with tamsulosin. *European Neuropsychopharmacology* 2002;12:337-341.

Kaplan HS. Post-ejaculatory pain syndrome. *Journal of Sex & Marital Therapy* 1993;19:91-103.

107   Paraphilias (DSM-IV-TR #302.1-302.4, 302.81-302.84, 302.9)

All the paraphilias, also known as sexual deviations or sexual perversions, share certain common characteristics. In each one the patient finds repeatedly that the preferred object of sexual desire is something other than mutually enjoyable sexual activity with a postpubertal consenting partner. Examples of such paraphilias include the following: the voyeur who prefers peeping; the exhibitionist who prefers exposing his genitals; the frotteur who prefers rubbing or touching an unsuspecting female; the fetishist who may prefer shoes or lingerie; the transvestic fetishist who prefers to dress like a woman; the sadist or masochist who prefers pain, humiliation, or suffering; and the pedophile who prefers children. These patients are often capable of normal sexual activity; indeed about half of them are married. Yet normal sexual behavior pales in attraction when compared with the insistent urge prompted by the paraphilic object.

Because the paraphilic behaviors are generally illegal and at times embarrassing or shameful to the patient, obtaining accurate data regarding these disorders is very difficult; it is clear, however, that the vast majority of patients are male. Much of the available data comes from specialized clinics whose patients are there, by and large, under legal duress. Thus what follows may or may not be representative of the entire group of paraphilias.

Most patients seen in clinics have more than one paraphilia. Voyeurism, exhibitionism, frotteurism, and fetishism are found almost exclusively in males; indeed, transvestic fetishism is found only in heterosexual males and never in females. Sexual sadism is almost never seen in females; and male masochists greatly outnumber female masochists. Occasionally, one finds a female

pedophiliac. The only paraphilia wherein females are found almost as often as males is zoophilia.

No reliable figures are available regarding the prevalence of the various paraphilias. Although these patients are rarely treated in a general practice, the clinical impression is that some of them, such as voyeurs and exhibitionists, are common. Some of the others, such as sexual sadists or pedophiles, may be just as common, but the fear of consequences serves to deter many patients from following their paraphilic inclinations.

The patient with a paraphilia may or may not feel ashamed or embarrassed about what he wants to do. Those who do may confine themselves to only imagining the indulgence of the paraphilic desires. Such fantasies, indeed, may be required for the patient to engage in normal sexual behavior. For example, the pedophile may be unable to sustain an erection and engage in intercourse unless he imagines his partner to be a child; likewise the sexual masochist may be unable to achieve orgasm unless enthralled by the fantasy of being bound and whipped. Some patients seek out prostitutes who act out their paraphilic fantasies with them.

Many patients see nothing wrong with their paraphilic behavior. The degree of denial and rationalization may be extreme. The exhibitionist may assert that he was only attempting to educate women about sexual anatomy; the voyeur insists that the women wanted to be seen or else they would have closed all the blinds; the pedophile may describe his victim as at least willing, if not indeed provocative.

Other disorders found in patients with paraphilias include antisocial personality disorder and borderline personality disorder. Alcoholism and other substance use disorders are also seen.

ONSET

In a majority of cases the paraphilic behavior begins in adolescence or earlier, and this is routinely the case with voyeurism, exhibitionism, frotteurism, fetishism, and transvestic fetishism. Indeed, in fetishism and transvestic fetishism the onset may often be traced into childhood years. Patients with sexual sadism or sexual masochism generally experience their characteristic fantasies in childhood, yet often not until early adult years does the sadistic or masochistic behavior become firmly established.

Pedophilia may be an exception to this rule of early onset for paraphilias. Although some cases begin in adolescence, the majority appear to begin in the thirties and some report onsets in the fifties. Although patients with an apparent later age of onset may deny ever having been sexually attracted to children before the age of 30, their self-reports may not be reliable given society's attitude toward such inclinations.

CLINICAL FEATURES

In voyeurism the patient takes his pleasure at a distance, watching women while they dress or undress or as they engage in foreplay or intercourse. The voyeur may masturbate while watching, or he may wait until he gets home, only to masturbate there as he recalls the scene. Voyeurs, though often capable of normal sexual relations, often find such activity far less stimulating than their voyeuristic exercises, and indeed their partners may feel neglected.

The exhibitionist generally shows care as he prepares to expose himself; the victim should be attractive, unsuspecting, and a stranger to the patient. The place of the deed must allow for rapid escape. Unfrequented parks or deserted public places are favorite spots. Often, before exposing his genitals, the patient is thrilled as he imagines how his victim will react. The patient often masturbates during the exposure, or he may wait until he gets home before stimulating himself. These patients, though fearful of legal consequences, often take few pains to conceal their identity. Rarely do they attempt to disguise themselves with masks, and, if a car is involved, they often make no attempt to hide it or the license plates. Like voyeurs, exhibitionists often are capable of normal sexual relations, yet like voyeurs they may neglect their regular partners as they are repetitively drawn to seek out unsuspecting victims.

The frotteur often scrutinizes the crowd at a bus or subway station until he finds an attractive female, generally one wearing tight clothing. Insinuating himself through the crowd he may then maneuver himself until he is pressed up against her in the crowded subway or bus. Then he may rub his hands or his erect penis against her buttocks or legs until he ejaculates, all the while imagining that he and his victim are sexually involved. Moments may pass before the victim realizes what is happening and makes an attempt to stop him.

The fetishist may take any of a number of objects as his fetish. Shoes, lingerie, a lock of hair, even amputated hands or feet may excite him. He may get a particular pleasure in stealing the fetish. Simply viewing the fetish may be sufficient for masturbation, or the patient may wish to touch it with his penis during masturbation. Some fetishists may insist that their sexual partner wear the fetish during intercourse. The strength of the fetish becomes clear when one observes that the patient may not be able to sustain an erection unless his partner wears the shoes, lingerie, or whatever the fetish might be.

The transvestic fetishist, though seeing himself as a heterosexual male, is unable to reliably sustain an erection unless he cross-dresses, either partially or completely, in women's clothes. Most of these patients keep a supply of lingerie or dresses; they may insist on wearing at least some article of women's clothing during intercourse, and at times their wives or girlfriends may agree to this. At other times the transvestic fetishist cross-dresses while alone in order to masturbate. Despite such fantasies, however, transvestic fetishists do not consider themselves homosexual and remain attracted to women. These patients often also evidence sexual masochism.

The sexual sadist and the sexual masochist are similar to one another in that normal sexual play or intercourse generally leaves the patient cold. Rather, to become aroused, these patients require the fantasy of or the actual infliction of pain, suffering, or humiliation. Indeed most sexual sadists will at one time or another engage in masochistic behavior, and a substantial minority of sexual masochists at times venture into sadistic behavior.

The sexual sadist may take his pleasure from any number of sadistic acts: partners may be beaten, bound, made to wear diapers, urinated or defecated on, caged, or even tortured. Prostitutes may be used. At times willing partners, masochists themselves, may be found. A substantial minority of sexual sadists rape. In extreme cases, where nothing less than the death of the partner suffices to excite the patient, lust murder may occur.

The sexual masochist may incite, provoke, or, failing these, demand sadistic behavior from his partner. Tenderness and normal foreplay simply fail to arouse these patients. Lacking a cooperative partner, some sexual masochists may imagine or even practice sadism on themselves in order to masturbate. In extreme cases, patients may practice autoerotic asphyxiation wherein they hang themselves to the point of orgasm, hoping to remove the noose before losing consciousness. In milder cases simply imagining being sadistically attacked may allow the masochistic patient to become aroused by normal touching, caressing, or intercourse.

In pedophilia, the patient finds himself preferentially aroused by children. Most pedophiles prefer children of the opposite sex; a minority prefer those of the same sex; a sizable number find themselves attracted to either sex. Often the patient is known by the victim; indeed some patients seek out children by working at daycare centers or schools, or even by adopting them. Sexual contact, for the most part, is limited to looking, touching, fondling, exposing, or masturbating in the presence of the child. Less commonly, the child may be forced into fellatio or cunnilingus. Oral or vaginal penetration is rare, except in those situations where the victim is a member of the patient's immediate family. In most instances the patient threatens the child to make sure that the child never tells.

A number of other paraphilias exist, about which relatively less is known. These include zoophilia, or intercourse with animals; coprophilia, or sexual play with feces; and necrophilia, or intercourse with corpses.

COURSE

Though for the most part the tendency to be preferentially aroused by paraphilic objects or actions persists for the life of the patient, the frequency with which the patient engages in the actual paraphilic behavior tends to decline with age, with paraphilic behaviors peaking between the ages of 15 and 25, and generally undergoing a gradual decline thereafter. An exception to this rule may occur in sexual sadism or masochism, where, at the least, the severity of the sadomasochistic behavior tends to actually increase with age.

The probability of legal consequences also directly affects the frequency of paraphilic behaviors. The fear of consequences may induce considerable restraint in exhibitionists, frotteurs, or pedophiliacs. The same may hold true for transvestic fetishists and sadists or masochists, unless of course they can find willing partners. By contrast, fetishists who practice alone and voyeurs are little affected by legal or social consequences.

Several factors may be helpful in determining a prognosis for an individual case. For any one patient, the earlier the age of onset, the greater the number of separate paraphilias, and the greater the number of paraphilic behaviors, the worse the prognosis. Furthermore, those with little shame or guilt or with extreme rationalization or denial tend to have poorer prognoses than those who have some compunction about their behavior. A history of excessive alcohol use, perhaps by virtue of a disinhibiting effect, worsens the prognosis. Finally, interest in and availability of partners interested in normal sexual activity appear to influence the outcome. Patients who have lost all ability to be aroused by normal sexual behavior or those for whom no willing normal partner is available, seem to have difficulty in sustaining a distance between themselves and their paraphilic inclinations.

COMPLICATIONS

As the patient pursues his paraphilic interest, gradually he loses interest in normal relations; girlfriends leave, divorces occur. In extreme cases the paraphilia itself may be lethal, as in autoerotic asphyxiation.

As most paraphilias are illegal, the paraphiliac faces arrest, trial, and punishment. The pedophile may face decades in prison; the sadistic lust murderer, execution.

ETIOLOGY

Theories abound as to how people could come to be preferentially aroused by things outside the range of normal sexual behavior; however, little is known with certainty. In the case of pedophilia, however, it does appear that the patients themselves were sexually assaulted in their boyhoods. Furthermore, in transvestic fetishism one often finds in taking the history that the patient, as a child, was forced to cross-dress as a punishment.

DIFFERENTIAL DIAGNOSIS

In mental retardation the patient may neither have the ability to restrain himself nor the capacity to distinguish between normal and paraphilic objects.

Likewise, in schizophrenia and in mania, a lack of impulse control may be evident. Furthermore, the patient may be driven by voices or delusions.

In dementia, disinhibition is common; pedophiliac behavior in patients with Alzheimer's disease may be frequent. There are also case reports of patients with Parkinson's disease who developed zoophilia and transvestitism with increased doses of dopaminomimetics, with resolution of the symptoms with a dose decrease.

Some patients with obsessive-compulsive disorder may experience an obsessive urge to engage in paraphilic behavior, for example to touch someone sexually. Yet here, in contrast to paraphilia, they have no pleasure in imagining this, and, further, the patient does not in fact act on the urge.

A certain amount of paraphilic behavior is normal among adolescent boys. Voyeurism, a fetishistic interest in lingerie, and even cross-dressing are not uncommon. For most boys, however, this is only playacting and recedes as they mature into adults. If the paraphilic interest seems unusually strong, however, only long-term observation enables the diagnostician to see whether the boy's sexual desires eventually fix on normal or paraphilic objects.

Transvestic fetishism must be distinguished from other conditions characterized by cross-dressing. A sexual masochist may willingly cross-dress, yet here the wearing of women's clothing itself is not what is exciting; rather, the patient is excited by the humiliation of dressing like a woman. Effeminate homosexuals may cross-dress, yet here the patient does so to attract another male, unlike the transvestic fetishist who is always heterosexual. Transsexuals cross-dress, yet in transsexualism the patient conceives of himself as a female, whereas the transvestic fetishist definitely considers himself a male.

Simple rape must be distinguished from sexual sadism. The simple rapist uses force and may beat or bind his victim. Yet here, in contrast to sexual sadism, the simple rapist uses force in the service of rendering his victim submissive, in contrast to the sadistic rapist who inflicts pain even when the victim is already submissive, because the infliction of pain itself is sexually arousing. Indeed sadistic rape is not common, accounting for less than 10% of all rapes.

Finally, one must distinguish between a paraphilia and normal sexual play. Most men are excited by viewing, touching, the use of lingerie, and even at times partial or complete cross-dressing. Yet these activities are all in the nature of foreplay and do not distract, but rather enhance, normal sexual behavior. Many couples likewise engage in sadomasochistic behavior, yet here such behavior remains within the realm of play and stops short of the actual infliction of pain, suffering, or humiliation.

TREATMENT

Most paraphiliacs come to treatment under duress. In many cases, arrest or shameful discovery is followed by a diminution of paraphilic urges, and the paraphiliac may pronounce himself cured. Yet such diminution is only temporary; within weeks or months the urges return.

Current treatment approaches focus on reducing the paraphilic urges and on increasing interest in normal sexual behavior. Depot medroxyprogesterone is useful in reducing the frequency of paraphilic behavior. Depot medroxyprogesterone is given in doses of 200 to 500 mg intramuscularly every week, with a subsequent fall in both testosterone levels and libido. The dose is titrated to the point where paraphilic urges can be resisted, but not to the point where libido is lost entirely, as most patients simply do not comply with such a regimen. Side effects, such as testicular atrophy, liver damage, diabetes, weight gain, and feminization, may occur, yet patients may accept them to avoid engaging in illegal behavior. Intramuscular gonadotropin-releasing hormones offer an alternative to medroxyprogesterone, and include leuprolide in a dose of approximately 7.5 mg or triptolerin in a dose of 3.75 mg, both given on a monthly basis. As there is typically an initial surge in testosterone levels with gonadotropin-releasing hormone therapy before the decline, it is generally advisable to give an anti-androgen, such as flutamide 250 mg tid, for the first two weeks.

Recent work has also suggested that SSRIs, such as fluoxetine, may reduce paraphilic urges; however, these were open studies. In one small, preliminary, double-blinded study, clomipramine was more effective than placebo in suppressing these urges.

In general, it is necessary to provide ongoing psychotherapy in addition to medication. Both group therapy and cognitive behavioral therapy have been advocated. Behavior therapy has also been utilized: patients may be taught to imagine adverse consequences whenever they get a paraphilic urge; others are instructed to sniff ammonia or to self-administer electric shocks whenever an urge appears; exhibitionists may be instructed to repeatedly expose themselves to a group of women trained to evidence boredom, thus depriving the exhibitionist of his reward, which is the shock displayed by his victim; finally, some patients are instructed to summon up a paraphilic fantasy and then to masturbate and to keep on masturbating long after orgasm and ejaculation, until the paraphilic fantasy itself begins to leave them cold.

Sex education and social skills training may help some paraphiliacs develop their interest in normal sexual behavior, leaving less time for the indulgence in, and strengthening of, their paraphilic urges.

Penile plethysmography is very useful in monitoring the success of treatment. Although some paraphiliacs are able to suppress erections, thus causing a "false negative test," the occurrence of an erection upon viewing a film of paraphilic behavior is generally reliable as positive evidence for the need for further treatment. Penile plethysmography also may be used to detect paraphilic interests that the patient has denied.

The use of alcohol or other substances or drugs that disinhibit the patient must be avoided. Likewise, stress and idle time, both of which are associated with an increase in paraphilic behavior, should be reduced whenever possible.

The treatment of the paraphiliac is extremely difficult and fraught with ethical conflict. When the general psychiatrist finds the patient unresponsive, referral to a specialist is indicated.

BIBLIOGRAPHY

Briken P, Nika E, Berner W. Treatment of paraphilia with lutenizing hormone-releasing hormone agonists. *Journal of Sex & Marital Therapy* 2001;27:45-55.

Chalkely AJ, Powell GE. The clinical description of forty-eight cases of sexual fetishism. *The British Journal of Psychiatry* 1983;142:292-295.

Cooper AJ, Sandhu S, Losztyn S, et al. A double-blind placebo controlled trial of medroxyprogesterone acetate and cyproterone acetate with seven pedophiles. *Canadian Journal of Psychiatry* 1992;37:687-693.

Fagan PJ, Wise TN, Schmidt CW, et al. Pedophilia. *The Journal of the American Medical Association* 2002;288:2458-2465.

Jimenez-Jimenez FJ, Sayed Y, Garcia-Soldevilla MA, et al. Possible zoophilia associated with dopaminergic therapy in Parkinson disease. *The Annals of Pharmacotherapy* 2002;36:1178-1179.

Kafka MP, Prentky R. Fluoxetine treatment of nonparaphilic sexual addictions and paraphilias in men. *The Journal of Clinical Psychiatry* 1992;53:351-358.

Kruesi MJ, Fine S, Valladares L, et al. Paraphilias: a double-blind crossover comparison of clomipramine versus desipramine. *Archives of Sexual Behavior* 1992;21:587-593.

Regestein QR, Reich P. Pedophilia occurring after onset of cognitive impairment. *The Journal of Nervous and Mental Disease* 1978;166:794-798.

Riley DE. Reversible transvestic fetishism in a man with Parkinson's disease treated with selegiline. *Clinical Neuropharmacology* 2002;25:234-237.

Rosler A, Witztum E. Treatment of men with paraphilia with a long-acting analogue of gonadotropin-releasing hormone. *The New England Journal of Medicine* 1998;338:416-422.

Spengler A. Manifest sadomasochism of males: results of an empirical study. *Archives of Sexual Behavior* 1977;6:441-456.

108 Transsexualism (gender identity disorder, DSM-IV-TR #302.6, 302.85)

In transsexualism, or "gender identity disorder," patients, despite having normal primary and secondary sexual characteristics, believe that in fact they are truly members of the opposite sex. A male transsexual, for example, may feel himself to be a female, dress and act like one, and view his genitalia with disgust. He may seek hormonal treatment to change his voice and habitus and may demand surgical removal of his penis and testes and creation of a vagina. The goal, eventually, is to become a woman and then to date and even marry a man. Such patients often say that they feel as if they have been "born into the wrong body," and in a sense all their efforts are directed at changing their body to match their inner sense of sexual identity.

Transsexualism is a rare disorder and is perhaps three times more common among males than females.

ONSET

In most cases the onset is in early childhood. Much less commonly, patients may initially experience a congruence between their sense of sexual identity and their anatomy for many years, even into adult years, before the notion dawns and takes root that in fact they are members of the opposite sex. In recognition of this initial period of normal development, such patients are often characterized as having "secondary" transsexualism, in contrast to those "primary" transsexuals with very early onset.

In the history of males with primary transsexualism, one finds that the boy preferred playing with girls rather than boys and preferred playing with dolls and the like rather than engaging in any roughhousing. Wishful fantasies of being a girl are common, and the boy may adopt the gestures and names of girls and may dress in girls' clothing. Some insist on sitting to urinate, and some say outright that they do not like their penis, and want to have a vagina and breasts.

By contrast, in the history of females with primary transsexualism, one finds that the girl often preferred roughhousing to playing with other girls or with dolls. Such girls often dress in boys' clothing and insist on acting like boys, even to the point of refusing to sit down to urinate. Some admit that they want a penis and that they never want to grow breasts or begin to menstruate.

Secondary transsexualism may appear in teenage or early adult years and often appears to follow upon a significant stress, such as being fired or going through a divorce. In secondary transsexualism the intensity of the patient's conviction of being "born into the wrong body" may either wax and wane over time or, as in the case of primary transsexualism, remain steady and unshakable.

CLINICAL FEATURES

Transsexual males believe that they are in fact females. They may wear makeup, dress in women's clothing, and imitate feminine gestures, voice, and manner. Some adopt a female name and attempt to live as a woman, perhaps taking stereotypically female jobs. Some openly seduce men, perhaps in bars or nightclubs, and some engage in prostitution, but only if the men they are prostituting themselves to are interested in anal intercourse. Many take estrogen and may undergo electrolysis to remove facial hair. They regard their penis and testes with disgust or revulsion and may seek sex reassignment surgery, undergoing penectomy and orchiectomy with the subsequent creation of a vagina. Some also seek breast implants.

Transsexual females believe that in fact they are males. They wear men's clothing and bind their breasts. They walk, talk, act like men, and some, after taking a masculine name, may engage in stereotypically masculine jobs. Many take testosterone, and some may seek a mastectomy. Some strap rubber phalluses onto the groin, and others may seek out sex reassignment surgery to create an artificial penis.

Character pathology is very common in male transsexuals, somewhat less so among female transsexuals, and a concurrent diagnosis of borderline personality disorder is often made.

Forme frustes of transsexualism are not uncommon. For example, some male transsexuals may be content with cross-dressing and electrolysis and be ambivalent about hormonal treatment or sex reassignment surgery.

COURSE

Transsexualism appears to be a chronic disorder. Symptoms, however, especially in those with secondary transsexualism, may wax and wane over time.

COMPLICATIONS

Those who are "discovered" may face ostracism and ridicule. The common borderline personality disturbances, however, cause most of the complications, and these are as described in that chapter.

ETIOLOGY

The etiology of transsexualism remains unknown. Efforts to find endocrinologic or chromosomal abnormalities have not yielded reproducible results, and imaging studies have been unrevealing. A recent autopsy study reported alterations in the number of neurons in the bed nucleus of the stria terminalis; however, this requires replication. Some speculate that male transsexuals overidentify with their mothers during infancy and early childhood, and that female transsexuals overidentify with their father. However, even if this were true, suggesting that it is causative may be incorrect. Rather, one might just as well say that the transsexual boy would naturally feel close to his mother, and that the unusually close bond was at the instigation of the boy and not his mother.

The character pathology seen in these patients as teenagers and adults may not be an integral part of transsexualism. Rather it may result from the inevitable conflicts that the transsexual child has with parents and peers.

DIFFERENTIAL DIAGNOSIS

Otherwise normal males with strong feelings of sexual inadequacy may at times make statements to the effect that they are "not much of a man." Here, however, the person still believes that in fact he is a man, and his statement reflects only his despair with his performance.

Transsexualism probably should not be diagnosed until the patient has passed puberty. Most children who express some confusion about their sexual identity do not emerge as transsexuals, but rather develop a sexual identity that is congruent with their anatomy.

Transvestic fetishism, on the surface, appears very similar to transsexualism. The fundamental difference here, however, is that the transvestic fetishist, even while cross-dressing, retains his sense of himself as being a male. Indeed the male transvestic fetishist dresses like a woman to get an erection, either to masturbate or to engage in intercourse with a woman. By contrast the transsexual male who cross-dresses does not seek an erection and may be dismayed if one occurs. The male transvestic fetishist values his penis; the transsexual, on the other hand, wishes to be rid of it. Likewise, homosexuals may cross-dress, not to change their identity, but rather to be more attractive. For example, an effeminate male homosexual may dress in women's clothing to attract the man he wants, but he never loses sight or appreciation of the fact that he too is a male. Like the transvestic fetishist, the effeminate male homosexual values his penis and would never seek out the sort of surgery that the male transsexual desires.

Patients with schizophrenia may develop the delusion that they are actually of the opposite sex; in such cases, however, other symptoms typical of schizophrenia, for example loose associations, indicate the correct diagnosis.

Patients with intersex states, such as pseudohermaphroditism, typically do not in fact present with transsexualism as adults. Most are reared as boys or girls, depending on the overall appearance of their primary and secondary sexual characteristics, and develop an identity consonant with them.

TREATMENT

Psychotherapy is indicated for those with secondary transsexualism. Some find that their conviction of belonging to the opposite sex wanes with time, and they may eventually become satisfied with their anatomy. When this is not the case, treatment may proceed as for primary transsexuals.

Primary transsexuals, in general, do not respond to any psychotherapeutic attempts to make them comfortable with their anatomy. Indeed they often resent such attempts and refuse to cooperate. In such cases patients may be referred to medical centers that specialize in sex reassignment surgery. Before surgery is offered, most patients are required to live as a member of the opposite sex for a prolonged period to demonstrate that in fact they are emotionally capable of doing so. Hormone therapy is then offered to both males and females, and males are offered electrolysis. Should the patient continue to function well and still desire surgery, it may then be offered, but only after detailed written informed consent is obtained.

Penectomy, orchiectomy, and creation of an artificial vagina are offered to male transsexuals. Surgical revision may be required, as the artificial vagina may be too short or may become stenotic, thus prohibiting intercourse.

Female transsexuals often undergo mastectomy, and some request a hysterectomy. As the results of surgery to create a penis are often disappointing, many women forgo this procedure.

Although most patients are satisfied with the results of sex reassignment surgery this is not inevitable, and some may live to regret what they did, and some may attempt, or even commit, suicide.

BIBLIOGRAPHY

Cohen-Kettenis PT, Gooren LJ. Transsexualism: a review of etiology, diagnosis and treatment. *Journal of Psychosomatic Research* 1999;46: 315-333.

Commander M, Dean C. Symptomatic transsexualism. *The British Journal of Psychiatry* 1990;156:894-896.

Kruijver FP, Zhou JN, Pool CW, et al. Male-to-female transsexuals have female neuron numbers in a limbic nucleus. *Journal of Clinical Endocrinology and Metabolism* 2000;85:2034-2041.

Marks I, Green R, Mataix-Cols D. Adult gender identity disorder can remit. *Comprehensive Psychiatry* 2000;41:273-275.

Rehman J, Lazer S, Benet AE, et al. The reported sex and surgery satisfactions of 28 postoperative male-to-female transsexual patients. *Archives of Sexual Behavior* 1999;28:71-89.

Smith YL, van Goozen SH, Cohen-Kettenis PT. Adolescents with gender identity disorder who were accepted or rejected for sex reassignment surgery: a prospective follow-up study. *Journal of the American Academy of Child and Adolescent Psychiatry* 2001;40:472-481.

EATING DISORDERS

109 Anorexia Nervosa (DSM-IV-TR #307.1)

In anorexia nervosa the patient, usually an adolescent female, embarks upon a relentless pursuit of thinness. By dieting and exercise, sometimes aided by vomiting and purging of the bowels, these patients sustain an alarming degree of weight loss, at times coming to resemble concentration camp survivors.

The name, "anorexia nervosa," is itself something of a misnomer, for these patients rarely lose their appetite. In fact, they often remain intensely interested in, even preoccupied with, food and food preparation. True anorexia only occurs when the self-induced starvation brings these patients to the point of inanition.

Anorexia nervosa occurs almost exclusively in females; males represent only about 5% of the cases. Estimates as to the lifetime prevalence of this disorder vary widely, depending on the strictness of the diagnostic criteria used: conservative criteria yield figures of from 0.3 to 0.5% of young females. Evidence suggests that the incidence of anorexia nervosa has increased during the latter part of the twentieth century. The reasons for this are not clear. Although often stated that this rising incidence is secondary to the value that modern society places on thinness, this has not been proven.

ONSET

Premorbidly, most patients are conscientious and perfectionistic. They often excel in academics or athletics, and parents may describe them as having been "model" children; furthermore, these perfectionistic traits typically persist after recovery. In general, there is no prodrome, per se. Most patients are "all right" up until the actual onset of the disorder. Precipitating factors may or may not be present. Occasionally a major event immediately precedes the onset, such as parents' divorce, a death in the family, or the birth of a new sibling. At times, however, the precipitating factor, though obviously integrally related to the decision to diet, may seem trivial. One teenage girl was trying on a new bathing suit at a department store. As she looked at herself in the mirror, she seemed to herself to be fat and decided that she must become thinner. Over the ensuing months, though she starved herself into emaciation, she insisted that she was still too fat to wear a bathing suit.

For most patients, actually being overweight is not a precipitating factor. In fact, only about one third of patients are overweight at onset, and most of them only to a mild degree. Indeed many patients were regarded as thin even before they began to diet. Onset usually occurs in teenage years, for females generally 4 or 5 years after menarche. Some cases with prepubertal or childhood onset

have been reported; and at the other extreme are reports of onset as late as the early thirties.

CLINICAL FEATURES

Patients with anorexia nervosa universally have a distorted body image, and although this is not unique to anorexia nervosa, it is most striking here. These patients persist in their belief that they are fat, no matter how much weight they lose. If asked to draw a self-portrait, an emaciated patient with anorexia nervosa may render a likeness that, if not obese, is at least plump. One cannot reason with patients on this point; although the physician may be able to circle the patient's waist with both hands, the patient refuses to give up the belief that she is fat.

In all cases, diet and exercise are utilized in pursuit of thinness. Some patients also attempt to rid themselves of calories by self-induced vomiting or by laxative-induced purging, but these actions generally play only a relatively minor role.

Patients pursue their diets with a heartbreaking relentlessness. Progressively smaller portions are requested, and a progressively smaller percentage of what they are served is eaten. The food is pushed here and there on the plate. Mealtimes become strained and tense; at times the dinner table may become a veritable battleground as parents insist that the patient eat more. Starches and sweets are anxiously avoided; most patients prefer vegetables and clear liquids. Seemingly paradoxically, however, these patients, rather than avoiding food altogether, seem to take a lively interest in it. They may spend hours in the kitchen baking cookies and cakes. They may collect recipes, and they may prepare sometimes elaborate meals. Their preoccupation with food may sometimes assume a peculiar stamp. They may hoard food; sometimes it may be hidden in the back of a closet or under a mattress. Occasionally, eating becomes ritualized: utensils must be placed just so and used only in a certain order.

Exercise is generally pursued with the same relentlessness evident in dieting. Running, jogging, and bicycling are preferred. Exercises that may increase muscle bulk, such as weightlifting or swimming, are generally avoided. At times, the need to keep exercising may be absolutely imperious; one patient, emaciated and absolutely exhausted to the point where standing without assistance was impossible, continued doing calisthenics while lying in a hospital bed.

Some patients self-induce vomiting to rid themselves of a meal. This is done in secret after mealtime. They may take themselves to their room, a closet, or the basement, where they stick their fingers down their throats to get relief. One may see peculiarities here also. Sometimes the vomitus is saved or hidden away. One patient vomited into plastic baggies and hid them under the bed. Many vomiters find that with time they no longer need to use their fingers. The vomiting just "sort of happens" without them actually having to do anything. Most patients are intensely embarrassed about their vomiting; some even deny it despite incontrovertible evidence to the contrary.

Purging of the bowels is another activity done in secret, with embarrassment. Generally, laxatives are used; patients only rarely resort to enemas. The amount of laxatives eventually required may be astounding. One patient took over 50 laxative tablets a day, and still felt uncomfortably full.

A minority of patients with otherwise typical anorexia nervosa occasionally are also subject to binge eating. The binges themselves are similar to those seen in bulimia nervosa, and, as is discussed in the section on differential diagnosis, some controversy exists as to how these patients should be diagnosed. A minority of patients also experience obsessions and compulsions.

The eventual amount of weight lost varies widely. Some patients with childhood onset may not actually lose weight but may simply not experience the normal weight gain of puberty. Other patients lose only a modest amount, dropping perhaps to only 15% to 20% below their "ideal body weight," and then stabilize there. Although clearly underweight even to a casual observer, they may yet be able to carry on with their daily life. For many patients, however, the pursuit of thinness carries them toward a profound degree of emaciation. When this occurs, most come to feel depressed and listless; they may have trouble concentrating and may experience insomnia. Some come to resemble living skeletons and sink into a profound lethargy and apathy.

The review of systems generally uncovers amenorrhea, which may be either primary or secondary. When secondary, the amenorrhea may commence before any weight loss, whereas in others it seems to be tied to the loss of body fat. In males, erectile dysfunction is commonly found, and infertility occurs. Constipation is the rule unless, of course, laxatives are used. Even then, laxative dependence may occur, and patients may still complain of constipation.

Physical examination is generally rewarded with a number of findings in addition to low weight and varying degrees of cachexia. Temperature, pulse, and blood pressure are all low. The skin may be dry and scaly. Widespread lanugo, or fine downy hair, may be seen. In vomiters, the teeth may be carious secondary to acid erosion, and the knuckles may be scarred where they have rubbed against the upper teeth during the induction of vomiting. Edema may be seen, and this may occur independent of hypoalbuminemia. In some patients the salivary glands may be enlarged. Indeed, enlargement of the parotid gland may mask the extent of facial emaciation.

Routine laboratory studies generally show abnormalities. The red blood cell, platelet, and white blood cell counts are generally depressed, and these patients are at increased risk for serious infections, such as pneumonia or septicemia. Hypokalemia is almost always present, and in vomiters or purgers may be profound and life threatening. Usually a degree of prerenal azotemia occurs, and AST, LDH, and alkaline phosphatase are generally elevated. Magnesium levels may be low, and up to one-fifth of patients may be thiamine deficient. In vomiters, amylase may also be increased. Serum beta-carotene levels may also be increased, and in these cases the skin may take on a yellowish tinge.

The electrocardiogram may show bradycardia, a prolonged QT interval, nonspecific ST changes, and occasionally U-waves. A variety of arrhythmias may be present, including ventricular fibrillation and asystole; syncopal episodes may occur, as may sudden cardiac death.

COURSE

In the natural course of events, roughly 40% of patients experience significant recovery, 25% improve somewhat, 20% remain severely ill, and the remainder die from suicide or medical complications. Even among those patients who do "recover" spontaneously, however, certain symptoms still persist, such as an unreasonable concern about weight, peculiar food preferences, and a preference for baggy clothing, no matter how unattractive or unfashionable. Factors indicating a poor prognosis include the following: older age at onset, chronic emaciation, and the presence of other psychiatric disorders.

COMPLICATIONS

In addition to the risks of suicide and the multiple medical complications described above, anorexia nervosa may produce devastating social complications. With weight loss, these patients generally stop dating. Likewise, as weight loss proceeds, grades tend to fall. They seem to once again become prepubertal and stay that way. They fail to develop into mature young adults, and although some may actually marry, they rarely have a satisfactory sexual relationship, as if their psychosexual development is stunted.

ETIOLOGY

Although the etiology of anorexia nervosa is not clear, several fairly robust findings provide suggestive clues.

As noted earlier, the prevalence of anorexia nervosa, strictly defined, among young females in general is no more than 0.5%. Among dizygotic twins, however, the concordance is about 10%, and for monozygotic twins it rises to almost 50%. Although this suggests a genetic factor, the effects of a shared environment cannot be ruled out until adoption studies are done.

Until recently, social class was thought to affect the prevalence of anorexia nervosa, as it appeared to be more common among the upper classes. More rigorous epidemiologic studies, however, have shown anorexia nervosa to be evenly distributed among the social classes.

Also, family structure has been thought to have an etiologic bearing on anorexia nervosa. Indeed the families of these patients appear to be "enmeshed" and rigid. Their parents do indeed appear controlling and intrusive. What is not clear, however, is whether this family pattern significantly predates the onset of the illness, or perhaps whether it is caused by the illness itself. Baffling and potentially life-threatening conditions in children have profound effects on parents and siblings, and the observed family structure may be a reaction to the illness, rather than a cause. The answer to this question awaits prospective studies of family structure, an admittedly formidable task.

Neuroendocrine studies have revealed a number of significant changes; however, most of them are seen also in starvation, regardless of cause. Luteinizing hormone levels are reduced, and the normal adult pulsatile pattern is lost or blunted. The TSH response to TRF is blunted, as is the growth hormone response to hypoglycemia. These findings normalize with weight restoration and do not appear to be unique to anorexia nervosa but can occur in starvation of any cause.

Investigation of the hypothalamic-pituitary-adrenal axis, however, has produced more significant findings. In both anorexia nervosa and starvation of other causes, the cortisol level is increased, and the low-dose dexamethasone suppression test is often positive. However, in anorexia nervosa one also finds that the ACTH response to CRF is blunted, and this is not seen in starvation from other causes. Furthermore, in anorexia nervosa the cerebrospinal fluid level of CRF is increased as compared to controls.

Multiple lines of evidence suggest a disturbance in serotoninergic functioning in anorexia nervosa. For example, among weight-restored patients PET scanning reveals a reduction in post-synaptic serotonin 2A receptor sites, and CSF levels of 5-HIAA, a metabolite of serotonin, are increased. Furthermore in recovered patients one also sees a unique response to the serotonin mixed agonist/antagonist mCPP with, as compared to placebo, an elevation of mood and an improvement in the distorted body image.

A relationship between anorexia nervosa and the mood disorders also appears to exist. The incidence of major depression and of bipolar disorder is higher in the relatives of patients with anorexia nervosa than in relatives of controls.

In summary, it appears plausible to say that anorexia nervosa represents an inherited disturbance in serotoninergic function, especially within the hypothalamus, which predisposes those so affected to develop the syndrome in the setting of certain, as yet undetermined, environmental changes.

DIFFERENTIAL DIAGNOSIS

Although many illnesses, in addition to anorexia nervosa, may be associated with substantial weight loss, only one might reasonably be confused with anorexia nervosa, namely schizophrenia. All others may be easily differentiated from anorexia nervosa by keeping in mind the cardinal feature of this disease, namely that the weight loss is caused by a fear of being fat and a relentless pursuit of thinness.

Of the many disorders that may cause weight loss in a teenage girl, the following are often listed as being potentially confused with anorexia nervosa, but in none of these is the weight loss caused by dieting: depression, neoplasms, tuberculosis, Crohn's disease, celiac sprue, Addison's disease, hyperthyroidism, diabetes mellitus, panhypopituitarism, and hypothalamic lesions, such as tumors or inflammatory infiltrates.

Very rarely, schizophrenia may present with a clinical picture very similar to anorexia nervosa. This may occur, for example, in cases where the patient has a delusion that weight loss is a holy or imperative goal. Occasionally, in these cases the avoidance of food and the weight loss may be so profound as to distract the physician from the other symptoms. Close questioning, however, elicits the symptoms characteristic of schizophrenia, such as delusions and hallucinations.

Assuming that the diagnosis of anorexia nervosa is firmly established, one must keep in mind that the patient may have more than one disorder and must be prepared to make more than one diagnosis. Two disorders occur with some frequency in patients with anorexia nervosa: major depression and bulimia nervosa.

As noted earlier, most patients with anorexia nervosa who experience substantial weight loss develop some of the vegetative signs of depression. In most cases, however, their listless apathetic state clears with weight restoration and thus should be considered secondary to starvation and not to depression. Instances occur,

however, where the depressive symptoms are independent of weight loss. In some cases they predate any weight loss; in others they persist long after weight restoration. In these cases an additional diagnosis of a depressive disorder is warranted, and proper treatment for it should be instituted.

Binge eating may also occur, as noted earlier, in anorexia nervosa, and a long-standing debate continues as to how these patients should be diagnosed. The problem appears to be in defining what the "threshold" should be for triggering an additional diagnosis of bulimia nervosa. Clearly, a patient with anorexia nervosa who experiences only several binges scattered over a year-long illness otherwise typical for anorexia nervosa should probably not receive the additional diagnosis of bulimia nervosa. On the other hand, a patient with anorexia nervosa who is binging several or more times a week would appear to have both disorders and thus merit both diagnoses. For most patients with anorexia nervosa, who also binge, however, the frequency of binging falls somewhere between these two extremes. As a precise diagnostic cutoff in terms of frequency has not as yet been established, clinical judgment is required. Two points may help suggest a correct diagnosis. First, patients with both disorders tend to bear a closer resemblance to a patient who has only bulimia nervosa than to a patient who has only a classical, "restricter," type of anorexia nervosa. The "restricter" type tends to be orderly, compulsive, rigid, and perfectionistic. This is in contrast to the patient with bulimia nervosa, who tends to be more unstable and impulsive. Second, if the binging either predates the pursuit of thinness or persists long after weight restoration, then the additional diagnosis would appear warranted.

TREATMENT

The goal of treatment is weight restoration and the reintegration of the patient into a normal family and social life. Without weight restoration, psychotherapy is not effective. Hence, initial efforts must be directed toward weight restoration. Both behavior therapy and medication have been used to facilitate this goal; however, of the two, behavior therapy is clearly superior.

Before beginning behavior treatment, however, one must decide whether or not to hospitalize the patient. Some patients may be managed with an outpatient behavior program; however, by the time most patients are brought to medical attention, either weight loss has become life threatening or such inanition has occurred that the patient is so listless that anything short of a structured inpatient program fails to have effect. In these instances, admission is indicated.

Before the institution of specific treatment, life-threatening conditions must be sought and corrected. Cardiac monitoring may be required; hypokalemia and hypomagnesemia must be corrected, and all patients should receive 200 mg of thiamine intramuscularly before refeeding, with continued oral supplementation of 100 mg daily thereafter. If the patient is so listless from weight loss that she cannot respond to a behavior program, temporary forced feeding may be required. Parenteral nutrition, given its risks, should be avoided if at all possible. Nasogastric feeding is preferred, using an appropriate low-osmolality supplement. Excessively rapid refeeding may lead to a "refeeding pancreatitis"; hence, moderation is in order. With refeeding, the patient may have a temporary rise in liver enzymes; however, this is generally not cause for alarm.

Once the patient is out of immediate danger and has regained sufficient energy to be able to respond to a behavior program, admission should be arranged to an inpatient adolescent psychiatric ward where staff are familiar with the behavioral treatment of anorexia nervosa. Although these patients can occasionally be managed in other settings, their chances are much better in a specialized setting. A number of behavior programs have proved successful; what follows is a sample program.

For the first few days, the patient is observed and integrated into the daily life of the ward. Careful note is made of those activities that appear most rewarding to the patient. Subsequently a "goal weight" is set for the patient. This figure is arrived at with reference to the following: "ideal body weight" tables, the patient's premorbid weight, the weight at which the patient might be able to feel comfortable, bone structure and general muscular development of the patient, and, finally, good clinical judgment. No neat formula can be used for arriving at the optimum goal weight; in general, it ends up being just somewhat below the premorbid weight, provided that the patient is not obese or, if obesity is present, just below an "ideal body weight." Most patients as they gain weight experience a disproportionate gain in the abdomen, hips, buttocks, or face, so the goal weight must not be so high as to leave them looking "fat" to their peers on the ward. One taunt from a teenager has been known to set a patient's progress back for weeks.

On the first and each succeeding day of the program, the patient is weighed after going to the toilet and before breakfast, on the same scale wearing nothing but a fresh hospital gown. The scale must be accurate to the nearest quarter pound or better, and the same scale always must be used. The patient is not allowed to wear her own clothing, as patients have been known to sew objects into hems to fake weight gain.

On the first day of the program the patient is allowed and expected to follow the normal ward routine, regardless of the weight that morning. On the second and succeeding days, the patient is deprived of significantly rewarding activities for exactly 24 hours unless at least one half pound has been gained over the previous day's weight. This is not to say that the patient must gain one half pound over the previous highest weight, but only that the weight must be at least one half pound greater than the weight exactly 24 hours earlier. Choosing which activities to withhold requires considerable judgment, and in many cases nothing short of isolation to her room is sufficient. If isolation is used, the only allowed activities are reading, writing, and listening to music; the patient is seen briefly by a physician every day and by a nurse once every shift, for no more than 15 minutes per visit. If at the end of the 24-hour period of isolation the patient has not gained at least one half pound over the previous day's weight, then the isolation continues for another 24 hours. This process continues until the patient gains at least one half pound over the previous day's weight, at which point the next 24 hours are spent following the regular ward routine, with full access to all rewarding activities.

Whether or not the patient should be excused from isolation to attend group or family psychotherapy is a matter of clinical judgment. Some patients may purposefully fail to gain weight to avoid psychotherapy; others may use a family therapy session while in isolation as an opportunity to play on the oftentimes raw sympathies of parents.

The patient is never encouraged to eat. If isolated, the patient receives a tray in her room; if not isolated, she can eat with other patients. Snacks are available ad lib.

Upon reaching and maintaining the goal weight, the patient is no longer isolated and may exercise routine ward privileges. Daily weigh-ins continue, however, and though the patient need not continue to gain weight, she must maintain the goal weight or else the program goes back into effect, beginning with isolation that day.

As soon as the patient has maintained the goal weight for 14 consecutive days, she may be discharged. During those 14 consecutive days the patient should take at least two overnight home passes.

Regardless of whether this or some other behavior program is used, certain other steps must be taken, or else the program may fail. Perhaps most important, one must review a written copy of the program with the patient, and then separately with the parents. One must be consistent and scrupulously honest. These patients are often extremely sensitive to anything perceived as unfair. Parents must be prepared for the sometimes heartbreaking complaints that their child may have about the program, or they may "side" with the patient and sabotage the treatment. The patient must be frequently reassured that she will not "overshoot" the goal weight and become obese; calm authoritative reassurance can go a long way toward gaining the patient's cooperation. Finally, parents must bring in successively larger-sized clothing for the patient to wear as weight gain occurs. Most patients will have altered the old clothing or simply thrown it away and bought new, smaller clothes, so this often means the parents must make several purchases of new wardrobes.

In general, most patients end up spending several days in isolation soon after the program is started. Once they realize, however, that they are not going to "win," progressive weight gain begins and continues up until the goal weight has been about halfway met. At that point most patients "dig their heels in" again and refuse further weight gain. A few more days of isolation often turns the tide, however, and then it is smooth sailing after that.

Many centers advocate the use of liquid nutritional supplements during a behavior program; however, this has drawbacks. When "regular" food is used, the patient learns how to moderate food intake to achieve the desired effect on weight. A patient's control may be very precise; some patients, toward the end of a 7-day period, may realize that they need to gain, say, $1\frac{1}{2}$ pounds, to obtain privileges, and gain precisely that much. Furthermore, once the goal weight is met, most patients have little difficulty in keeping their daily weight anywhere from $\frac{1}{2}$ to $1\frac{1}{2}$ pounds above the goal for the remaining 14 days. Since liquid nutritional supplements cannot reasonably be used at home or school, they do not afford the sort of learning experience these patients need, and hence are probably best avoided.

Occasionally, one may encounter a particularly stubborn patient who actually loses more weight after the program is begun. In such instances, one may have to establish a minimum weight below which the patient must not fall. The threat of tube feedings, should that minimum be passed, is often sufficient to motivate compliance with the program.

One instance where a behavior program using isolation is contraindicated is when the patient is suicidal. In such instances, other behavior contingencies must be established, using one's knowledge of those things that have proved reinforcing to the patient in the past. Such individualized programs are very difficult to devise and implement.

In addition to behavioral treatment, various medications have been used to facilitate weight gain. The only one with robust double-blinded support is cyproheptadine, eventually in high doses of up to 24 mg/d. Importantly, however, cyproheptadine is effective only in patients with a more or less classical "restrictor" pattern: patients with prominent binging may actually worsen with cyproheptadine.

If the patient does not require admission, an outpatient behavior program may be instituted. Though generally less elaborate than an inpatient program, an outpatient program may in fact be more difficult to enforce. A goal weight is established, using the principles outlined earlier. The program begins on a Friday afternoon, and on that first Friday afternoon and on each succeeding Friday the patient is weighed at the physician's office using the same scale (accurate to at least one quarter pound) and wearing the same clothing. For the first 7 days of the program the patient is free to pursue a normal routine. On the second and each succeeding Friday, however, if the patient has not gained at least 3 pounds over the weight obtained 7 days earlier, she is confined to the house until the following Monday morning. During the confinement the patient may not make telephone calls, have visitors or mail, watch TV, or listen to music. Once the patient reaches the goal weight and maintains it for at least two consecutive Fridays, then the program ends. Before the outpatient behavior program is started, a minimum weight, below which the patient must not fall, is established. The patient understands that if she is found below the weight at any of the Friday weigh-ins at the physician's office, hospitalization will occur immediately that day for institution of an inpatient weight restoration program.

After successful inpatient or outpatient weight restoration, the patient must be monitored for weight loss or gain. Although the weigh-ins must be scheduled, frequency may vary anywhere from weekly to monthly, depending on the clinical situation. As before, the weigh-in must be standardized, with the same scale and clothing, and should be done at the physician's office. Two minimum weights should be prospectively established, with provision for institution of an outpatient or inpatient behavior program, depending on which minimum is surpassed. Outpatient monitoring should be continued until the patient has maintained weight above the higher of the two minima for at least 6 months of consecutive weigh-ins.

Psychotherapy plays a critical part in recovery from anorexia nervosa. Although weight restoration is a necessary prerequisite for resumption of a normal life, it alone does not suffice. Concurrent with the pursuit of thinness, these patients often come to function at a prepubertal level, and after weight restoration they are faced again with the developmental tasks of adolescence. Their burden, however, is often made heavier by an enmeshment with often intrusive parents and by their own fear that they might fail again.

Of all the psychotherapies utilized in anorexia nervosa after weight restoration, family therapy has the most empirical support, and then only for patients under 18 who have been ill for a relatively brief period of time: older patients, or those of any age who have been chronically ill, are unlikely to benefit from family therapy.

Individual therapies, such as cognitive-behavioral therapy or psychodynamic psychotherapy, are often provided, especially to those over 18, but the evidence supporting their effectiveness is less robust.

Recently, it has also been shown that fluoxetine, 20 mg/d, if begun and continued after weight restoration, decreases the likelihood of relapse.

BIBLIOGRAPHY

Chipkevitch E. Brain tumors and anorexia nervosa syndrome. *Brain & Development* 1994;16:175-179.

Dare C, Eisler I, Russell G, et al. Psychological therapies for adults with anorexia nervosa: randomized controlled trial of out-patient treatments. *The British Journal of Psychiatry* 2001;178:216-221.

Duclos M, Corcuff JB, Roger P, et al. The dexamethasone-suppressed corticotrophin-releasing hormone stimulation test in anorexia nervosa. *Clinical Endocrinology* 1999;51:725-731.

Eisler I, Dare C, Russell GF, et al. Family and individual therapy in anorexia nervosa. A 5-year follow-up. *Archives of General Psychiatry* 1997;54: 1025-1030.

Frank GK, Kaye WH, Weltzin TE, et al. Altered response to meta-chlorophenylpiperazine in anorexia nervosa: support for a persistent alteration of serotonin activity after short-term weight restoration. *The International Journal of Eating Disorders* 2001;30:57-68.

Frank GK, Kaye WH, Meltzer CC, et al. Reduced 5-HT2A receptor binding after recovery from anorexia nervosa. *Biological Psychiatry* 2002;52: 896-906.

Goldberg SC, Halmi KA, Eckert ED, et al. Cyproheptadine in anorexia nervosa. *The British Journal of Psychiatry* 1979;134:67-70.

Halmi KA, Eckert E, LaDu TJ, et al. Anorexia nervosa. Treatment efficacy of cyproheptadine and amitriptyline. *Archives of General Psychiatry* 1986;43:177-181.

Kaplan AS. Psychological treatments for anorexia nervosa: a review of published studies and promising new directions. *Canadian Journal of Psychiatry* 2002;47:235-242.

Kaye WH, Nagata T, Weltzin TE, et al. Double-blind placebo-controlled administration of fluoxetine in restricting- and restricting-purging-type anorexia nervosa. *Biological Psychiatry* 2001;49:644-652.

Lowe B, Zipfel S, Buchholz C, et al. Long-term outcome of anorexia nervosa in a prospective 21-year follow-up study. *Psychological Medicine* 2001;31:881-890.

Srinivasagam NM, Kaye WH, Plotnicov KH, et al. Persistent perfectionism, symmetry, and exactness after long-term recovery from anorexia nervosa. *The American Journal of Psychiatry* 1995;152:1630-1634.

Steinhausen HC. The outcome of anorexia nervosa in the 20th century. *The American Journal of Psychiatry* 2002;159:1284-1293.

Winston AP, Jamieson CP, Madira W, et al. Prevalence of thiamin deficiency in anorexia nervosa. *The International Journal of Eating Disorders* 2000;28:451-454.

110 Bulimia Nervosa (DSM-IV-TR #307.51)

Bulimia nervosa is characterized by recurrent episodes of uncontrollable binge eating, followed by often desperate, compensatory measures to prevent weight gain. Those with the "purging type" of bulimia may self-induce vomiting or purge the bowels with laxatives; however, some patients, that is those with the "non-purging type," rather concentrate on fasting or exercise to control weight.

The lifetime prevalence of bulimia nervosa lies anywhere from 1 to 3%; over 90% of these patients are female.

ONSET

In females, binge eating usually begins in mid to late adolescence or perhaps early adult years; in males the onset is usually a few years later. Premorbidly, most patients are either of normal weight or only slightly overweight. Not uncommonly, these patients have fallen ill previously with anorexia nervosa. In such cases the anorexia nervosa often undergoes partial remission with some weight being regained before the onset of the bulimia nervosa.

CLINICAL FEATURES

The episode of binge eating itself may be of either gradual or acute onset. When the onset is gradual the patient may plan the binge, even to the point of going to the grocery store and buying the forbidden foods. However, when the onset is acute and the urge to binge is urgent and overwhelming, almost any food at hand may be pressed into service.

Ice cream, cakes, and cookies are often preferred; candies, breads, and rolls may also be sought. At times the patient may attempt to resist the urge to binge, yet only rarely is such an effort successful. In any case, once the first bite is taken, all semblance of control is generally lost. Shame and humiliation often accompany the thought of binging, and most binges are done in secret. The food is generally consumed voraciously; the patient's appetite seems impossible to satisfy. Some eat until literally no room is left in the stomach and no more food can be swallowed. On the average, a binge lasts for about an hour and most end before the patient is literally stuffed. Nausea or bloating may stop the patient; some may be overcome by guilt or self-disgust, and some may simply fall asleep.

At the conclusion of the binge, most patients feel guilty or anxious over what they have done and most do something to undo it. Self-induced vomiting is the most common means employed; some patients become so accustomed to this that eventually they no longer need to stick their fingers down their throats. The food simply regurgitates automatically. Bowel purging is the next most commonly employed means: enemas are rarely used; laxatives, however, are used with regularity and sometimes in enormous doses. Some patients take over 50 times the recommended dose of a stimulant laxative. A substantial minority of patients also use diuretics, often furosemide, to control their weight. A small percentage of patients use ipecac to induce vomiting.

Most patients binge several times a day. Some, however, may binge only twice a week, while at the other extreme some patients binge up to 50 times a week. Most experience an increased frequency of binging when under stress.

Some patients, rather than engage in vomiting or bowel purging, exercise vigorously or fast to offset the binge. These non-purging type patients often experience substantial weight fluctuation as their episodes of binges alternate with their strenuous efforts at weight loss.

There is also a large group of patients who, though engaging in binge eating, do not regularly engage in "compensatory" behaviors such as purging or strenuous exercise. Such patients are currently said to have "binge eating disorder"; however, the diagnostic and nosologic status of these patients is uncertain: they may simply have a mild form of bulimia nervosa or might perhaps be suffering from a different disorder.

Like patients with anorexia nervosa, most patients with bulimia nervosa have a distorted body image. All appearance to the contrary and all facts notwithstanding, most see themselves as fat.

Despite the fact that most of them experience only weight fluctuations rather than progressive weight gain, most fear that they will become fat.

Patients with bulimia nervosa often suffer from other disorders, such as major depression and panic disorder, with or without agoraphobia. Many patients with bulimia nervosa also have a borderline personality disorder or borderline traits. Some bulimics engage in rumination. Impulsivity is common; specifically, many patients engage in kleptomania. Self-mutilation may be seen. Abuse or dependence on alcohol or stimulants is not uncommon. Suicide attempts are seen in about 5% of patients.

Physical examination may reveal scarring of the knuckles from where they have been rubbed against the teeth during the induction of vomiting. Severe dental caries may be present secondary to erosion of the enamel by acidic gastric juices. Bilaterally symmetric hypertrophy of the parotid glands also may be found.

The amylase level may be elevated, and a rough correlation is seen between the extent of elevation and frequency of binging. Occasionally, serum potassium and magnesium are decreased.

COURSE

The course of bulimia nervosa may be either chronic, wherein binges recur at a regular frequency over many years, or episodic, wherein there are periods of regular binging separated by lengthy binge-free intervals. Overall, however, over the decades, binges tend to become less severe and less frequent, and by middle years most patients have substantially recovered.

COMPLICATIONS

Occasionally, during a particularly copious binge, patients may experience acute gastric dilatation. This presents with acute, severe abdominal pain and should be treated emergently with nasogastric suction to prevent gastric rupture.

Frequent vomiting may lead to severe caries, as noted above. Gastroesophageal reflux and esophagitis may occur; occasionally, esophageal tears may appear. Alcohol-intoxicated patients may aspirate during self-induced vomiting and develop pneumonia.

Hypokalemia may result from vomiting or diuretic use. Patients with concurrent anorexia nervosa are especially prone to this complication, which may produce life-threatening arrhythmias.

Extensive use of ipecac may lead to a cardiomyopathy.

Those who engage in extreme laxative use may become laxative dependent.

ETIOLOGY

Bulimia nervosa is clearly familial, and among the first degree relatives of patients one finds, in addition to bulimia nervosa, an increased rate of anorexia nervosa and mood disorders.

Multiple converging lines of evidence indicate a disturbance in serotoninergic functioning in bulimia nervosa: CSF levels of 5-HIAA (the metabolite of serotonin) are increased, PET scanning indicates a reduction in serotonin 2A binding receptor binding sites in the medial orbital frontal cortex, the response of patients to infusions of the mixed serotonin agonist/antagonist mCPP is different from that of controls, and, finally, acute tryptophan depletion will provoke an urge to binge.

Humoral factors involved in appetite and satiety may also play a role in the illness. Cholecystokinin (CCK) is a "satiety" hormone normally released from the gut after a meal. In patients, the CSF level of CCK is low and the rise of CCK after a meal is reduced as compared to controls.

Finally, although imaging studies have been normal, EEG studies have demonstrated an increased rate of epileptiform discharges.

Integrating these findings into a coherent theory is problematic; however, it seems plausible to say that bulimia nervosa is probably an inherited disorder characterized by a disturbance in serotoninergic functioning. The CCK findings may be epiphenomenal; however, the EEG findings, in light of the possible efficacy of phenytoin and topiramate, are of interest and suggest that perhaps in some cases the binges represent simple partial seizures.

DIFFERENTIAL DIAGNOSIS

Currently the diagnostic classification of patients who apparently have both bulimia nervosa and anorexia nervosa is being debated. This question is discussed at length in the chapter on anorexia nervosa.

Patients with borderline personality disorder may occasionally engage in binge eating. However, here the binges are an inherent part of the overall instability and impulsivity of this disorder and are generally not frequent.

Patients with schizophrenia may occasionally binge eat; the other symptoms of schizophrenia serve to make the diagnosis, and the binges generally cease upon adequate treatment of schizophrenia with antipsychotics.

Depressed patients, especially those with bipolar depression, occasionally experience hyperphagia, rather than anorexia. Although enormous quantities may be eaten, true binging does not occur. Unlike patients who binge, patients with hyperphagia do not experience discrete episodes of overeating; rather they tend to eat continuously, and rarely, if ever, engage in vomiting or bowel purging.

Hypothalamic lesions, for example tumors, or infiltrative processes such as sarcoidosis, may present with hyperphagia; however, as with the hyperphagia seen in depression, here the hyperphagia does not present as discrete binges.

Kleine-Levin syndrome is often included in the differential diagnosis of bulimia; however, it has several distinguishing features. First, it is rare in females; second, the hyperphagia seen here is prolonged and does not occur in discrete binges; and, finally, associated features such as hypersomnolence and hypersexuality are not typical of bulimia nervosa.

TREATMENT

A variety of treatments have been shown to be effective for bulimia nervosa, and these may generally be accomplished on an outpatient basis. Admission is generally not required and should be reserved for the following situations: failure of outpatient treatment, presence of a disabling depression or serious risk for suicide, and presence of a serious complication, such as esophageal tears, gastric dilatation, or significant hypokalemia.

Both psychotherapy and medications are effective in bulimia nervosa, and it may well be that the combination of the two is most effective.

The two most commonly used psychotherapeutic techniques are cognitive behavioral therapy and interpersonal therapy, and as between the two, cognitive behavioral therapy appears to be more effective.

Multiple medications have been shown effective in double-blinded studies; unfortunately, however, there are no comparative studies. Of the antidepressants, fluoxetine, desipramine, trazodone, imipramine, and phenelzine are all effective. Other effective medications include phenytoin, naltrexone, ondansetron, and inositol. Of all these medications, fluoxetine, in a dose of 60 mg, is the best studied, and should probably be the first choice. In cases where fluoxetine is not well tolerated or is ineffective consideration may be given to desipramine in a dose of 150 mg. Trazodone and imipramine are not as well tolerated, and the use of phenelzine in a patient who might binge on a tyramine-containing food is fraught with danger. Phenytoin might be considered in cases where the binge has a truly paroxysmal onset; the relative indications for naltrexone, 50 mg, ondansetron, 24 mg, or inositol, 18 gm, are as yet unclear.

Before leaving the subject of medication treatment, a word is in order regarding topiramate. Topiramate, in an average dose of 200 mg, is clearly effective in patients with "binge eating disorder," and a case series report suggested similar effectiveness in typical bulimia nervosa. Topiramate may be especially attractive in those cases where patients are obese, as it is also effective for weight loss in obese patients who do not binge.

Given the chronic nature of bulimia nervosa, long-term maintenance therapy is generally indicated.

BIBLIOGRAPHY

Agras WS, Rossiter EM, Arnow B, et al. Pharmacologic and cognitive-behavioral treatment for bulimia nervosa: a controlled comparison. *The American Journal of Psychiatry* 1992;149:82-87.

Agras WS, Walsh T, Fairburn CG, et al. A multicenter comparison of cognitive-behavioral therapy and interpersonal psychotherapy for bulimia nervosa. *Archives of General Psychiatry* 2000;57:459-466.

Barbee JG. Topiramate in the treatment of severe bulimia nervosa with comorbid mood disorders: a case series. *The International Journal of Eating Disorders* 2003;33:468-472.

Faris PL, Kim SW, Meller WH, et al. Effect of decreasing afferent vagal activity with ondansetron on symptoms of bulimia nervosa: a randomized, double-blind trial. *Lancet* 2000;355:792-797.

Gelber D, Levine J, Belmaker RH. Effect of inositol on bulimia nervosa and binge eating. *The International Journal of Eating Disorders* 2001;29:345-348.

Jacobs MB, Schneider JA. Medical complications of bulimia: a prospective evaluation. *Quarterly Journal of Medicine* 1985;54:177-182.

Kaye WH, Greeno CG, Moss H, et al. Alterations in serotonin activity and psychiatric symptoms after recovery from bulimia nervosa. *Archives of General Psychiatry* 1998;55:927-935.

Kaye WH, Frank GK, Meltzer CC, et al. Altered serotonin 2A receptor activity in women who have recovered from bulimia nervosa. *The American Journal of Psychiatry* 2001;158:1152-1155.

Lydiard RB, Brewerton TD, Fossey MD, et al. CSF cholecystokinin octapeptide in patients with bulimia nervosa and in normal comparison subjects. *The American Journal of Psychiatry* 1993;150:1099-1101.

McCann UD, Agras WS. Successful treatment of nonpurging bulimia nervosa with desipramine: a double-blind, placebo-controlled study. *The American Journal of Psychiatry* 1990;147:1509-1513.

McElroy SL, Arnold LM, Shapira NA, et al. Topiramate in the treatment of binge eating disorder associated with obesity: a randomized, placebo-controlled trial. *The American Journal of Psychiatry* 2003;160:255-261.

Marrazzi MA, Bacon JP, Kinzie J, et al. Naltrexone use in the treatment of anorexia nervosa and bulimia nervosa. *International Clinical Psychopharmacology* 1995;10:163-172.

Pope HG, Hudson JI, Jonas JM, et al. Bulimia treated with imipramine: a placebo-controlled, double-blind study. *The American Journal of Psychiatry* 1983;140:554-558.

Pope HG, Keck PE, McElroy SL, et al. A placebo-controlled study of trazodone in bulimia nervosa. *Journal of Clinical Psychopharmacology* 1989;9:254-259.

Romano SJ, Halmi KA, Sarkar NP, et al. A placebo-controlled study of fluoxetine in continued treatment of bulimia nervosa after successful fluoxetine treatment. *The American Journal of Psychiatry* 2002;159: 96-102.

Smith KA, Fairburn CG, Cowen PJ. Symptomatic relapse in bulimia nervosa following acute tryptophan depletion. *Archives of General Psychiatry* 1999;56:171-176.

Strober M, Freeman R, Lampert C, et al. Controlled family study of anorexia nervosa and bulimia nervosa: evidence of shared liability and transmission of partial forms. *The American Journal of Psychiatry* 2000;157:393-401.

Walsh BT, Gladis M, Roose SP, et al. Phenelzine vs placebo in 50 patients with bulimia. *Archives of General Psychiatry* 1988;45: 471-475.

Wermuth BM, Davis KL, Hollister LE, et al. Phenytoin treatment of the binge-eating syndrome. *The American Journal of Psychiatry* 1977;134: 1249-1253.

111 | Obesity

Obesity may be usefully conceived of as either primary and idiopathic or as secondary to some other disorder. Other disorders responsible for obesity are discussed in the section on etiology; examples include hypothalamic tumors or rare congenital disorders, such as Prader-Willi syndrome. The vast majority of cases, however, are of the idiopathic variety, and this type may be further subdivided according to the age of onset. The early-onset type begins in childhood or adolescence and tends to be severe; the late-onset type occurs often in middle age and is often of relatively modest degree.

The boundary between obesity and normal weight is not sharp. Since weight, like hypertension, varies along a continuum, any precise cut-off point, of necessity, is bound to be somewhat arbitrary. One common definition holds as obese anyone whose weight is 20% above the norm listed on the Metropolitan Life Table. Another common definition utilizes a formula, the body mass index, or BMI. The BMI is equal to the patient's weight in kilograms divided by the square of his height, measured in meters. Those with a BMI over 30 are often classified as obese.

The prevalence of obesity has increased in the United States, with anywhere from one-third to one-half of the adult population affected.

Among the mildly and moderately obese, men appear to outnumber women; however, among the severely obese the sex ratio is apparently equal.

ONSET

The ages of onset of the secondary forms of obesity are dictated by the underlying disorder.

Those with early-onset primary obesity often are overweight in infancy or childhood. The patient with late-onset primary obesity, however, often appears to represent an exaggeration of a normal weight gain seen as individuals age into the middle years.

CLINICAL FEATURES

Obesity is readily apparent to casual inspection. The distribution of the excess adipose tissue tends to vary according to sex and, in cases of primary obesity, with age of onset. Women tend to gain weight in the hips and thighs, whereas in men the abdomen is more often the repository. In late-onset primary obesity, the excess adipose tissue tends to be centrally located with relative sparing of the extremities. By contrast, in early-onset primary obesity there is a more even distribution between the trunks and the extremities.

For clinical purposes, obesity may be categorized as mild, moderate, or severe, corresponding, respectively, to 20% to 40% overweight or a BMI of from 30 to 34.9, 41% to 99% overweight or a BMI of 35 to 39.9, and 100% or more overweight or a BMI of 40 or more.

As a rule, obese patients tend to think poorly of themselves and often complain of feeling depressed and anxious. Those who are severely obese may come to hate themselves. Most moderate or severely obese patients meet with ridicule and rejection, and many come to lead isolated lives rather than face others.

COURSE

In most cases, weight gain progresses up to a certain point, which varies widely among patients, and then tends to plateau off, or perhaps continues, but at a much slower rate.

COMPLICATIONS

The complications of obesity are numerous and in some instances potentially catastrophic (see the box on p. 214).

ETIOLOGY

Although, as noted earlier, the vast majority of cases of obesity are of the idiopathic type, consideration must be given to the secondary causes, most of which are treatable.

Perhaps the most common secondary cause of obesity is a medication-related effect. Most of the tricyclic antidepressants can cause weight gain; of the tricyclics, however, desipramine, nortriptyline and protriptyline are less likely to have this side effect. Antipsychotics may also be at fault, and this is particularly true of the low-potency first generation agents (e.g., chlorpromazine) and the second generation agents olanzapine and clozapine: an exception to this rule is the first-generation agent molindone, which may actually be associated with slight weight loss. Lithium, valproate, and, to a lesser degree, carbamazepine and gabapentin may also cause weight gain. The weight gain associated with oral contraceptives may induce women to stop taking birth control pills.

Congenital and inherited conditions associated with weight gain include the following: Kleine-Levin syndrome, Prader-Willi syndrome, Bardet-Biedl syndrome, Alstrom's syndrome, Carpenter's syndrome, Blount's disease, Cohen's syndrome, and Frolich's syndrome.

Complications of Obesity

Osteoarthritis	Accelerated arteriosclerosis
Venous statis with varicosities and possible thrombophlebitis with pulmonary emboli	Pseudotumor cerebri
	Small increased risk of certain cancers
Insulin resistance and possible diabetes mellitus	
Snoring	*Women*
Obstructive sleep apnea*	Endometrial cancer
Pickwickian syndrome*	Breast cancer
Intertrigo	
Hyperlipidemia	*Men*
Cholesterol gallstones	Prostate cancer
Hypertension	Colorectal cancer

*Covered in the respective chapter.

Patients with Cushing's syndrome are often distinguished by the classic findings of central obesity and purple striae. However, up to one half of patients with Cushing's syndrome may also display weight gain in the extremities, and patients obese from other causes may have abdominal striae, which, however, tend to be pale rather than purple.

Weight gain in hypothyroidism is generally secondary to water retention and is relieved by thyroid replacement. Occasionally, however, excess adipose tissue may indeed form during hypothyroidism.

Lesions affecting the ventromedial nucleus of the hypothalamus may at times cause massive obesity. The most common cause is a craniopharyngioma; other causes include the basal meningitides of syphilis or sarcoidosis, infiltration in histiocytosis or leukemia, postencephalitic scarring, trauma, obstructive hydrocephalus, and lacunar infarctions. Obesity may also follow any surgical intervention in that area. Hypothalamic lesions affecting both the ventromedial nucleus and the tuber cinerum in infants or very young children may cause a syndrome of obesity and genital hypoplasia, known as Frolich's syndrome, or adiposogenital dystrophy.

Depression, especially when seen in bipolar disorder, may be associated with significant hyperphagia and weight gain.

Bulimia nervosa, in a minority of cases, may be associated with modest weight gain. "Binge eating disorder," which may be a variant of bulimia nervosa characterized by binge eating without "compensatory" measures such as purging or exercise, is commonly associated with obesity. Indeed, a significant minority of obese females, perhaps up to one-quarter, have this disorder.

Presuming that all these secondary causes have been ruled out, then in all likelihood the patient may be assumed to have primary obesity. The etiology of this disorder, although clearly not understood, appears to have both genetic and environmental aspects.

Both twin and adoption studies have clearly demonstrated a genetic factor; indeed in one combined twin-adoption study, most of the variance in weight was accounted for by genetic background rather than by the environment the patient was raised in. There are several theories as to what might be inherited. One suggests that in the metabolic pathways of obese patients excess calories are more likely to be stored in fat than to be burned off in thermogenesis. Another theory suggests that within the limbic system, perhaps within the ventromedial nucleus of the hypothalamus, a "set point" for satiety exists, and that some patients have inherited a higher "set point," so their hunger is not satisfied by meals that would sate others. A final theory suggests that what is inherited is the actual

number of adipocytes: those with a greater number of fat cells would be more likely to store excess calories as fat than those with a normal complement of these cells. Indeed, those with early-onset primary obesity tend to have "hyperplastic" obesity, characterized by an excessive number of adipocytes, whereas those with late-onset primary obesity experience a "hypertrophic" obesity, with an enlargement of individual fat cells but only a minimal increase in their actual number.

Environmental factors that may contribute to the development of obesity include one's lifestyle and certain child-rearing practices. A sedentary lifestyle is clearly a factor, and this is especially the case in children who spend time watching television rather than playing active sports. Contributory child-rearing practices include overfeeding on the part of the parent: some mothers appear to simply prefer "chubby babies" and overfeed an infant until the "ideal" is reached, whereas others appear to be particularly "pushy" about feeding. Pregnancy may also be a factor. Many women complain that they were never able to lose the excess weight they gained while pregnant.

DIFFERENTIAL DIAGNOSIS

Obesity is a condition of excess adipose tissue; thus not all patients who are overweight by comparison with standard tables or formulas are obese. Edema may lead to substantial weight gain. Well-muscled individuals may be quite "overweight" but have little or no adipose tissue.

TREATMENT

Losing weight is a difficult task for most patients and requires a high degree of motivation. For the mildly obese, diet and exercise may be sufficient; for those with moderate obesity, these measures must be supplemented by behavior therapy. For both the mildly and the moderately obese, programs such as Weight Watchers and the self-help organization known as TOPS (Take Off Pounds Sensibly) may be very helpful. Overeaters Anonymous, patterned after Alcoholics Anonymous, also appears to hold promise. When patients fail to make acceptable progress despite good compliance with the above measures, medication may be indicated. Some severely obese patients may respond to the foregoing measures; however, failures are more common in this group, and surgery, such as gastric binding, may be in order.

A 1- or perhaps 2-pound weight loss per week is a reasonable goal. Given that a pound of fat equates to about 3500 calories, a 500 calorie deficit/day is required for weight loss of about 1 pound a week. Setting a goal weight prospectively is important and should be done with due regard for such factors as "ideal" weight from tables, the patient's own preference, and, if the obesity is of late onset, the patient's premorbid weight. Exercise alone rarely is adequate, and a reducing diet is almost always required.

For most patients, a well-balanced 1200 to 1500 calorie diet is both effective and reasonably well tolerated. Low calorie diets in the range of 700 to 800 calories and very low calorie diets of about 300 calories are very difficult to maintain. Vitamins and mineral supplements are mandatory, and the protein must be of high quality, such as egg albumin, soya, or fish, to avoid complications. Such diets should probably be reserved for the very highly motivated patient and must be carried out under close medical supervision.

Although exercise, as compared to diet, is a relatively inefficient way to induce a caloric deficit, it should be a part of a weight loss program. In addition to the modest caloric deficit, it also promotes self-esteem and is at least one activity that is relatively incompatible with eating. Walking, bicycling, aerobics, swimming, and jogging are all excellent choices, and patients should be encouraged to participate in one of these activities for at least 45 minutes a day for at least 5 days a week.

A behavior modification program is indicated when patients, despite good motivation, find themselves unable to stick to the regimen of diet and exercise. Most behavior programs begin by having the patient keep a "food diary" for a couple of weeks, noting exactly what and how much they eat and the precise circumstances that surround their eating. Inspection of the food diary generally indicates areas where behavioral change is indicated. Common recommendations include the following: eating in only one place, not engaging in any other activity except conversation while eating, and putting down the fork or spoon between bites. Rewards, such as watching a favorite program later in the day, are provided for successful implementation of these recommendations, and the patients are encouraged by paying attention not so much to the rate of weight loss as to their daily adherence to the program of diet and exercise.

Group support is often helpful, and this may be done in a psychotherapy group or in one of the commercial or self-help programs mentioned above.

Medication should be reserved for those who, despite compliance with their program, are unable to maintain an acceptable rate of weight loss. It must be kept in mind, however, that drugs generally cannot substitute for diet and exercise, and that the weight loss caused by them, with the possible exception of topiramate, is modest at best, and often minimal. Sibutramine, in a dose of 10 to 20 mg daily, is the most popular agent in use today; however, it must be used with due regard to the risk of a serotonin syndrome if it is combined with other serotoninergic agents. Orlistat, a gastrointestinal lipase inhibitor, in a dose of 120 mg tid, is perhaps slightly less effective than sibutramine, and may be associated with diarrhea and a deficiency of such fat-soluble vitamins as A, D and E. Metformin, in a dose of 850 mg bid, may also cause weight loss and should clearly be considered in treating obese patients who have diabetes mellitus; although metformin also appears to cause weight loss in non-diabetics, its usefulness in these patients has not been extensively studied. Of the stimulant drugs, both phentermine and diethylpropion are effective; however, these should probably be considered second-line agents given their abuse potential. Topiramate, in an average dose of 200 mg, was recently shown effective in obesity associated with binge eating: this is an exciting development, as the weight loss seen with topiramate may be quite impressive. Recent work also supports a role for bupropion, in doses of 400 mg, and for zonisamide.

The optimum duration of drug treatment is not clear. It may be appropriate to continue an agent until either a goal weight is reached or the patient reaches a "plateau" which cannot be surpassed. The drug could then be discontinued and the patient observed on a diet and exercise program alone; should weight gain recur, then drug treatment may be reconsidered.

Obese patients who require treatment for a concurrent depression should be considered candidates for agents unlikely to cause weight gain, such as an SSRI (especially fluoxetine), bupropion, venlafaxine or nefazodone.

Most patients find it extremely difficult to remain compliant with a program of dieting and exercise. In general, those with early-onset "hyperplastic" obesity have more difficulty losing weight than those with "hypertrophic" late-onset obesity. Once the goal weight is reached, a maintenance program for weight stabilization should be continued. This should include ongoing regular exercise and a diet ranging anywhere from 1500 to 3000 calories/day. However, obese patients, especially those with early-onset primary obesity, tend to gain weight on a daily calorie regimen that would not induce weight gain in a nonobese patient. Without a weight stabilization program, almost all patients eventually regain their weight.

For the severely obese who repeatedly fail to lose weight with a program such as the one outlined above, surgery may be considered. Of the many procedures which have been used, gastric binding and bypass surgery are currently in favor. Although the weight loss seen with these procedures can be truly impressive, side effects are common; in particular deficiencies of folic acid and vitamin B12 must be watched for.

BIBLIOGRAPHY

Anderson JW, Greenway FL, Fujioka K, et al. Bupropion SR enhances weight loss: a 48-week double blind, placebo-controlled trial. *Obesity Research* 2002;10:633-641.

Bray GA, Gallagher TF. Manifestations of hypothalamic obesity in man: a comprehensive investigation of eight patients and a review of the literature. *Medicine* 1975;54:301-330.

Carney DE, Tweddell ED. Double blind evaluation of long acting diethylpropion hydrochloride in obese patients from a general practice. *The Medical Journal of Australia* 1975;1:13-15.

Eckersley RM. Losing the battle of the bulge: causes and consequences of increasing obesity. *The Medical Journal of Australia* 2001;174:590-592.

Finer N, James WP, Kopelman PG, et al. One-year treatment of obesity: a randomized, double-blind, placebo-controlled, multicentre study of orlistat, a gastrointestinal lipase inhibitor. *International Journal of Obesity and Related Metabolic Disorders* 2000;24:306-313.

Gadda KH, Francisyc DM, Wagner HR, et al. Zonisamide for weight loss in obese adults. A randomized controlled trial. *The Journal of the American Medical Association* 2003;289:1820-1825.

Glazer G. Long-term pharmacotherapy of obesity 2000: a review of efficacy and safety. *Archives of Internal Medicine* 2001;161:1814-1824.

Gokcel A, Gumurdulu Y, Karakose H, et al. Evaluation of the safety and efficacy of sibutramine, orlistat and metformin in the treatment of obesity. *Diabetes, Obesity & Metabolism* 2002;4:49-55.

James WP, Astrup A, Finer N, et al. Effect of sibutramine on weight maintenance after weight loss: a randomized trial. STORM study group. Sibutramine Trial of Obesity Reduction and Maintenance. *Lancet* 2000;356:2119-2125.

Lee A, Morely JE. Metformin decreases food consumption and induces weight loss in subjects with obesity with type II non-insulin-dependent diabetes. *Obesity Research* 1998;6:47-53.

McElroy SL, Arnold LM, Shapira NA, et al. Topiramate in the treatment of binge eating disorder associated with obesity: a randomized, placebo-controlled trial. *The American Journal of Psychiatry* 2003;160:255-261.

Malhotra S, McElroy SL. Medical management of obesity associated with mental disorders. *The Journal of Clinical Psychiatry* 2002; 63(Suppl 4):24-32.

Steinbeck K. Obesity: the science behind the management. *Internal Medicine Journal* 2002;32:237-241.

Stunkard AJ, Harris JR, Pedersen NL, et al. The body-mass index of twins who have been reared apart. *The New England Journal of Medicine* 1990;322:1483-1487.

Valle-Jones JC, Brodie NH, O'Hara H, et al. A comparative study of phentermine and diethylpropion in the treatment of obese patients in general practice. *Pharmatherapeutica* 1983;3:300-304.

Yanovski SZ, Yanovski JA. Obesity. *The New England Journal of Medicine* 2002;346:591-602.

112 Pica (DSM-IV-TR #307.52)

In pica, patients eat any of a variety of nonfood items, including dirt, clay, starch, ice, cloth, and so forth. Transient pica is very common in normal children, and may also be seen in about one-quarter of severely retarded patients. Pica may be seen in up to a third or more of pregnant women; it may also be endemic in certain culturally isolated groups, but is for the most part rare in otherwise normal adults.

ONSET

Pica may begin anywhere from infancy through adult years.

CLINICAL FEATURES

Children may eat paint, masonry, hair, clothing, dirt, sand, plastic cups, or tobacco. Retarded children may additionally eat feces or trash, and the severer the level of retardation, the worse the pica is likely to be. Pregnant women may eat ice, clay, or starch; clay and starch eating is also common in certain parts of the South.

Patients with pica usually also eat normal food and generally do not lose weight.

COURSE

Most non-retarded children eventually stop engaging in pica by the age of 6; pica rarely persists into adult years in this group. In contrast, those with mental retardation may continue this practice for many years.

Pica associated with pregnancy usually stops postpartum.

COMPLICATIONS

Sand or dirt may become impacted in the bowel and cause obstruction. Hair and cloth may give rise to bezoars. Sharp plastic may cause perforation. Ingestion of feces or dirt may be followed by infection with toxoplasma or toxocara. Clay itself may complex with iron in the gut and cause iron deficiency anemia. The most common and the most severe complication is lead poisoning from eating paint chips.

ETIOLOGY

In the case of non-retarded children, one often finds a history of neglect, inadequate supervision, or encouragement from adults to engage in this behavior.

Among the mentally retarded with pica, and perhaps also in some non-retarded individuals, a zinc deficiency may be found.

In the case of pica during pregnancy, one typically finds either a personal or family history of pica.

Among adults, pica (in particular pagophagia, or ice-eating) is a reliable sign of iron deficiency, being seen in almost one-half of all iron-deficient patients.

DIFFERENTIAL DIAGNOSIS

Infants typically eat anything they happen to find, and this is not considered pica. However, after the age of 3 or 4, the exclusive preference for food is normally established, and any persistent ingestion of nonfood items is considered to be pica.

Patients with schizophrenia, dementia, delirium, autism, Kleine-Levin syndrome and the Kluver-Bucy syndrome may eat any number of nonfood items; however, this behavior is seen as part of the overall illness and does not merit a separate diagnosis of pica.

TREATMENT

In non-retarded children, provision of adequate adult supervision is generally sufficient. Among the mentally retarded with pica, several behavior techniques appear successful. When immediately initiated, verbal reprimands, very brief physical restraint, blindfolding, or "over correction" (immediate vigorous oral hygiene) appear to diminish pica. Time-outs may also be used, as may rewards for abstention from pica. Among all adults with pica, especially those with pagophagia, iron status should be checked and any deficiency corrected. It may also be appropriate to consider determining a 24-hour zinc level, and providing zinc supplementation should it be low.

BIBLIOGRAPHY

Lofts RH, Schroeder SR, Maier RH. Effects of zinc supplementation on pica behavior of persons with mental retardation. *American Journal of Mental Retardation* 1990;95:103-109.

McLoughlin IJ. Pica as a cause of death in three mentally handicapped men. *The British Journal of Psychiatry* 1988;152:842-845.

Rector WG. Pica: its frequency and significance in patients with iron-deficiency anemia due to chronic gastrointestinal blood loss. *Journal of General Internal Medicine* 1989;4:512-513.

Rose EA, Porcerelli JH, Neale AV. Pica: common but commonly missed. *The Journal of the American Board of Family Practice* 2000;13:353-358.

Smulian JC, Motiwala S, Sigman RK. Pica in a rural obstetric population. *Southern Medical Journal* 1995;88:1236-1240.

Solyom C, Solyom L, Freeman R. An unusual case of pica. *Canadian Journal of Psychiatry* 1991;36:50-53.

113 Rumination (including rumination disorder, DSM-IV-TR #307.53)

Rumination, also known as merycism, is characterized by the regurgitation of food that is then rechewed and subsequently either swallowed or spat out. Most cases of rumination are seen in infants, and in such cases one speaks of "rumination disorder." It must be kept in mind, however, that rumination is not uncommon in mental retardation, being seen in up to 10% of those with severe or profound cases, and may also, albeit rarely, occur in otherwise normal children, adolescents or adults.

ONSET

In infants up to several months of age, occasional rumination is normal. In rumination disorder it either persists past the first year or recurs after at least a month's worth of normal feeding.

In other cases, including the mentally retarded and otherwise normal individuals, the onset may be in childhood, adolescence or early adult years.

CLINICAL FEATURES

Infantile ruminators tend to lie quietly for a brief time after eating. Forceful abdominal contractions may then be seen, and the young patients may then hold their heads back with their mouths open, almost straining the back, until the feeding is regurgitated and rechewing can begin. Most infants seem quite content as they savor their feeding the second time, and then either reswallow it or spit the rest out. In those who tend to spit, actual weight loss may occur despite more than adequate feeding, with some undue fussiness between feedings.

In those with childhood or later onset rumination, the regurgitation and rechewing are less dramatic, and in some adults of normal intelligence may be quite subtle.

COURSE

Although most infants with rumination experience a spontaneous remission, a substantial minority, perhaps a quarter or more, die from malnutrition if untreated.

Those with mental retardation may experience a chronic course, and in a small minority the disorder is fatal.

In those of normal intelligence, it appears that the disorder may either resolve spontaneously in a matter of months or endure chronically, for years or longer.

COMPLICATIONS

Among infants, as noted above, malnutrition may occur, and in those cases where it is not fatal, the child's development may be delayed. Regardless of whether malnutrition occurs, most parents are put off by the behavior, if not by the smell, and a certain tension may occur between the parent and child.

Among adult ruminators complications include esophagitis, aspiration pneumonia, caries and periodontal disease, halitosis, and, in those of normal intelligence, a sense of shame sufficient to lead a patient into isolation.

ETIOLOGY

Although regurgitation occurs consequent to relaxation of the lower esophageal sphincter and concurrent contractions of the diaphragm and abdominal musculature, the etiology of the entire ruminating act, including the rechewing, is not known. Some patients may find the rumination pleasurable.

In a minority of adolescent or adult onset cases, rumination is seen in association with bulimia nervosa or anorexia nervosa.

DIFFERENTIAL DIAGNOSIS

Pyloric stenosis, hiatal hernia, esophageal spasm or obstruction, or a Zenker's diverticulum may all be associated with regurgitation or vomiting, but in these cases one does not see the distinctive rechewing that characterizes rumination.

As noted in the chapter on mental retardation, occasional rumination may be seen in otherwise uncomplicated mental retardation; the additional diagnosis of rumination is made only if the behavior is persistent or severe.

TREATMENT

Among infants, the provision of a "substitute mother," who is able to both distract the infant before rumination can begin and lavish praise for nonruminating behavior, may effectively stop the rumination. In more severe cases the application of bitter lemon juice into ruminated food may be effective.

Among the mentally retarded, behavioral approaches are indicated, which may include the reinforcement of incompatible behaviors or vigorous tooth brushing.

In patients of normal intelligence various methods have been advocated, including reassurance, cognitive behavioral therapy and biofeedback.

BIBLIOGRAPHY

Chial HJ, Camilleri M, Williams DE, et al. Rumination syndrome in children and adolescents: diagnosis, treatment and prognosis. *Pediatrics* 2003; 111:158-162.

Malcolm A, Thumshirn MB, Camilleri M, et al. Rumination syndrome. *Mayo Clinic Proceedings* 1997;72:646-652.

Parry-Jones B. Merycism or rumination disorder. A historical investigation and current assessment. *The British Journal of Psychiatry* 1994; 165:303-314.

Starin SP, Fuqua RW. Rumination and vomiting in the developmentally disabled: a critical review of the behavioral, medical, and psychiatric treatment research. *Research in Developmental Disabilities* 1987; 8:575-605.

Tamburrino MB, Campbell NB, Franco KN, et al. Rumination in adults: two case histories. *The International Journal of Eating Disorders* 1995; 17:101-104.

114 Narcolepsy (DSM-IV-TR #347)

Narcolepsy is characterized by narcoleptic attacks and in most cases cataplectic attacks. Hypnogogic or hypnopompic hallucinations and sleep paralysis may also be seen. In addition to this traditional "tetrad" of symptoms, a certain percentage of patients also experience episodes of "automatic behavior."

Although narcolepsy is not a common disorder, occurring in from 0.02 to 0.16% of the adult population, it is one of the more common disorders seen in sleep disorders clinics; it is equally common in males and females.

ONSET

Although the age of onset of narcolepsy ranges from late childhood to over the age of 40, most cases appear during the teenage and early adult years, and the vast majority are apparent by the mid-thirties.

In most cases, narcoleptic attacks are the first symptom to appear; over the years, cataplectic attacks and other symptoms gradually accrue.

CLINICAL FEATURES

Patients with narcoleptic attacks may or may not experience other symptoms of narcolepsy. Although perhaps three quarters eventually also experience cataplectic attacks, only about a third experience sleep paralysis with a similar proportion experiencing hypnogogic or hypnopompic hallucinations. Only about a tenth of patients experience the full tetrad of narcolepsy, cataplexy, sleep paralysis, and hypnogogic hallucinations.

During a narcoleptic attack, the patient experiences an overwhelming, irresistible urge to go to sleep. The urge itself tends to occur in circumstances where most people might feel somewhat drowsy, such as lectures, driving on the highway, or in the midst of a long conversation. The attacks may be as brief as a few seconds, but tend to last a few minutes. Patients may be easily awakened by touch or by simply calling their name. When left undisturbed, patients may sleep for a half hour or more. Upon awakening, patients generally feel refreshed and may recall vivid dreams. Most patients have at least several narcoleptic attacks during the day, and these tend to cluster in the afternoon. A distinctive feature of these attacks is the fact that for the most part they consist of REM sleep. Paradoxically, many narcoleptic patients complain of insomnia. They may have multiple awakenings during the night, and the actual total 24-hour sleep time is generally no more than that of a nonnarcoleptic patient.

Cataplectic attacks are generally precipitated by sudden, strong emotion. Hearty laughter, a storm of anger, orgasm, a sudden surprise, or merely being tickled may all trigger an attack. During the attack, the patient suddenly becomes weak; the weakness itself may be generalized, leading to collapse, or at time localized, leading, if the neck musculature were involved, to a sudden drooping of the head, or if the hand and forearm musculature were involved, to dropping things. In all cases, however, diaphragmatic and extraocular muscle strength remains intact. Most attacks remit in less than a minute, and during the attack the patient remains completely awake and alert. Occasionally, however, an attack may be prolonged, sometimes for many minutes, and in these cases visual hallucinations may appear.

Hypnogogic hallucinations are those that occur at the onset of sleep; hallucinations that occur as the patient arouses from sleep are termed hypnopompic. These are almost always visual; however, at times auditory hallucinations may occur. Hallucinations tend to be complex and vivid, as if the patient were dreaming while yet still awake. They may be accompanied by sleep paralysis.

Episodes of sleep paralysis may occur either as the patient is falling asleep or immediately upon awakening. During the episode the patient, though awake, is paralyzed and unable to move arms, legs, or head, or to open the eyes. Occasionally the patient may be able to produce an inarticulate sound; however, to the observer the patient generally appears peacefully asleep. Initially, many patients are frightened during these episodes, particularly if they also have visual hallucinations during them. In time, however, most patients come to accept them and simply wait them out without significant distress. In general, they only last a minute or two, and they may be interrupted at any time, with full restoration of strength, by a touch or sometimes by merely calling the patient's name.

In recent years it has become apparent that a substantial minority of patients also experience what, for want of a better name, are called episodes of "automatic behavior." Clinically, these appear to represent a kind of prolonged transition between normal wakefulness and a narcoleptic attack, and they tend to occur in the same sorts of situations that are conducive to narcoleptic attacks. For example, a patient, while taking notes during an afternoon lecture, may suddenly come to and find the notebook filled with senseless or illegible writing. Or, while driving down a monotonous highway, a patient, becoming suddenly fully alert, is unable to recall the last miles, or even exits.

In addition to these symptoms, anywhere from one quarter to one half of all patients with narcolepsy also experience periodic limb movements of sleep, and perhaps a tenth of patients also display episodes of sleep apnea. A small minority also have REM sleep behavior disorder.

COURSE

For most patients, narcolepsy is a chronic disorder, and narcoleptic attacks and other symptoms, if they occur, tend to recur for the remainder of the life span. Occasionally, patients may have temporary remissions with several months passing without any attacks. Rarely, one may see a complete and permanent spontaneous remission.

COMPLICATIONS

Narcolepsy can be a disabling illness. Depending on the circumstances during which the narcoleptic attack occurs, one may see a variety of consequences: there may be automobile accidents; untimely "naps" on the job may lead to dismissal; and "falling asleep" during a family conversation, as for example at the dinner table, may be taken as a grave insult and lead to strained relations.

Cataplectic attacks, while driving or in other dangerous situations, may be followed by serious injury. Some patients may isolate themselves from others to avoid the strong emotion that may trigger an attack.

ETIOLOGY

Narcolepsy is an inherited disorder with low penetrance. There is a striking association with the HLA-DQB1*0602 antigen located on the short arm of chromosome 6: virtually all patients with narcolepsy are positive for this antigen, which is found in only about 20% of the general population.

Recently, it has become apparent that CSF levels of hypocretin (formerly known as orexin) are grossly reduced in narcolepsy with cataplexy, and two autopsy studies have demonstrated changes in the posterior hypothalamus: in one, a reduced amount of hypocretin mRNA was found, and in the other there was a reduced number of hypocretin-positive neurons. Mutations in the gene for hypocretin, however, have not been identified in human cases, and the mechanism underlying these changes is not known.

Most researchers believe that narcolepsy results from an as yet unidentified disturbance in the functioning of the pontine and mesenchephalic structures responsible for REM sleep.

DIFFERENTIAL DIAGNOSIS

In most instances the clinical history is sufficient to make a reliable diagnosis; indeed, the combination of sleep attacks and cataplexy is almost pathognomonic: in the English language literature there are only a few case reports of a similar picture, as for example with lesions of the hypothalamus, midbrain or pons.

Two methods are used to confirm the diagnosis; testing for the HLA-DQB1*0602 antigen and the multiple sleep latency test (MSLT). Finding the HLA-DQB1*0602 antigen supports the diagnosis; however, as it is present in about 20% of the general population, this finding does not make the diagnosis certain. An absence of the HLA-DQB1*0602 antigen, however, argues very strongly against the diagnosis of narcolepsy.

The MSLT is performed in conditions conducive to narcoleptic attacks. Most narcoleptic patients fall asleep within minutes, and in most instances the observed sleep is REM sleep. The test, however, is not completely reliable because not all narcoleptic attacks are accompanied by REM sleep. Furthermore, other disorders, such as a hypersomnic depression, may evidence rapid onset of sleep during an MSLT.

Excessive daytime sleepiness, which may mimic narcoleptic attacks, may be seen in a variety of disorders, including depression, alcoholism or sedative-hypnotic dependence, the Pickwickian syndrome, sleep apnea, nocturnal myoclonus, restless legs syndrome, certain hypothalamic lesions (for example, tumors or infiltrates), and the Kleine-Levin syndrome. In all these conditions, however, the excessive sleepiness neither occurs in discrete attacks, nor is it refreshing.

Atonic seizures may appear similar to cataplectic attacks; however, here consciousness is lost. "Drop attacks" as may be seen in vertebral basilar ischemia may be very similar to cataplectic attacks, with preservation of consciousness and complete paralysis. However, here one fails to find the precipitating surprise, which is an integral part of cataplexy.

TREATMENT

Activities such as driving or operating hazardous machinery are potentially dangerous and are to be avoided until the attacks are controlled. Educational counseling with the patient and those affected by the symptoms may be very helpful. Two or three "scheduled" naps during the day and a regular bedtime may reduce the frequency of narcoleptic attacks.

In most cases, pharmacologic treatment is required, and this generally involves one of the stimulant or stimulant-like drugs, including modafinil, methylphenidate and pemoline. Modafinil is currently preferred, as it has a very low liability of abuse, and does not appear to cause tolerance: most patients respond to 200 mg daily; in some cases 400 mg may be required, but this is associated with more side-effects, in particular nausea. Methylphenidate is given in divided doses, once in the morning and once in the early afternoon, with the total daily dose ranging from 20 to 60 mg. Pemoline is currently a third choice, in large part due to its potential hepatotoxicity; it may be given in a once daily dose of from 37.5 to 150 mg. Should tolerance occur to methylphenidate or pemoline, with an increase in narcoleptic attacks, the drug should be gradually withdrawn over a few days, followed by a subsequent "drug holiday" for a day or two, after which the drug may be gradually reintroduced. After a drug holiday, lower doses are relatively more effective.

Selegeline, in a dose of 20 mg daily, appears effective not only in the prevention of narcoleptic attacks but also cataplectic attacks. At this dose, however, it is a non-selective MAOI, and consequently all the dietary restrictions noted in the chapter on MAOIs are necessary.

Certain tricyclic antidepressants appear useful for cataplectic attacks, and may also reduce the frequency of narcolepsy. Clomipramine, in doses of 25 to 75 mg hs, is most commonly used. Other options include protriptyline, 10-40 mg hs and desipramine 25-75 mg hs.

A recent addition to the pharmacologic treatment of narcolepsy is sodium oxybate, formerly known as gamma-hydroxybutyrate. Given in divided doses of 3 to 4.5 gm at hs and 3 to 4.5 gm 2½ to 4 hours later, this agent reduces cataplexy and may also reduce narcolepsy. Unfortunately, however, sodium oxybate has a very high abuse potential.

On balance, in cases characterized by narcolepsy alone, it is appropriate to start with modafinil. In cases where cataplexy is also present, and clinically significant, one may begin with modafinil and add a tricyclic in low dose. An argument could be made in such cases, however, for starting with a tricyclic or selegeline, in hopes of killing two birds with one stone. Sodium oxybate, given its problematic dosing schedule and high abuse potential, is generally held in reserve.

BIBLIOGRAPHY

Malik S, Boeve BF, Krahn LE, et al. Narocolepsy associated with other central nervous sytem disorders. *Neurology* 2001;57:539-541.

Mayer G, Ewert Meier K, Hephata K. Selegeline hydrochloride treatment in narcolepsy. A double-blind, placebo-controlled study. *Clinical Neuropharmacology* 1995;18:306-319.

Mignot E, Lammers GJ, Ripley B, et al. The role of cerebrospinal fluid hypocretin measurement in the diagnosis of narcolepsy and other hypersomnias. *Archives of Neurology* 2002;59:1553-1562.

Mitler NM, Shafor R, Hajdukovich R, et al. Treatment of narcolepsy: objective studies on methylphenidate, pemoline, and protriptyline. *Sleep* 1986;9:260-264.

Peyron C, Faraco J, Rogers W, et al. A mutation in a case of early onset narcolepsy and a generalized absence of hypocretin peptides in human narcoleptic brain. *Natural Medicine* 2000;6:991-997.

Rogers AE, Aldrich MS, Lin X. A comparison of three different sleep schedules for reducing daytime sleepiness in narcolepsy. *Sleep* 2001;24:385-391.

Scammell TE. The neurobiology, diagnosis, and treatment of narcolepsy. *Annals of Neurology* 2003;53:154-166.

Shapiro WR. Treatment of cataplexy with clomipramine. *Archives of Neurology* 1975;32:653-656.

USD Modafinil in Narcolepsy Study Group. Randomized trial of modafinil as a treatment for the excessive daytime somnolence on narcolepsy. *Neurology* 2000;54:1166-1175.

115 Sleep Apnea (breathing-related sleep disorder, DSM-IV-TR #780.59)

Sleep apnea, also known as "breathing-related sleep disorder," may be of three types: obstructive, central and mixed. The common denominator among all three types is the appearance of frequent apneic episodes during sleep and complaints of either daytime sleepiness or, less commonly, insomnia.

In obstructive sleep apnea, the oropharyngeal airway closes, and, despite the ongoing inspiratory effort of the diaphragm and intercostal musculature, air flow at the mouth and nostrils ceases. By contrast, in central sleep apnea, cessation of air flow occurs not because of any obstruction, but because of cessation of inspiratory effort with inappropriately relaxed diaphragmatic and intercostal musculature. In mixed sleep apnea, one sees a combination of central and obstructive components. Typically, during the episode of absent nasal and oral air flow, one sees initially an inappropriate lack of respiratory effort, soon followed by activation of the diaphragmatic and intercostal musculature, which, due to airway obstruction, is not followed by inspiration.

Sleep apnea is one of the most common disorders seen in the sleep laboratory and has a prevalence ranging from 1% to 10% of the population. Of the three types, obstructive sleep apnea is by far the most common, followed by the mixed type, with the pure central type being relatively rare. Among adults, all three types are at least twice as common in males than females.

ONSET

Although obstructive sleep apnea can occur at almost any age, it generally first appears in middle years; among females the incidence tends to rise after menopause. The central type of sleep apnea typically has a later onset.

CLINICAL FEATURES

Apneic episodes may last anywhere from 10 seconds up to 2 minutes and may occur from 30 to several hundred times a night. Interestingly, although patients generally experience multiple, albeit brief, awakenings at the end of the apneic episode, often they have no clear recollection of these awakenings.

In obstructive sleep apnea, the patient, often an obese middle-aged man, presents with a chief complaint of daytime sleepiness, with or without complaints of broken sleep. Almost universal is a history of frequent loud snoring, which may have prompted correspondingly loud complaints from the patient's spouse. Upon observing these patients while they sleep, one sees a characteristic obstructive sleep apneic episode. Oral and nasal air flow ceases despite increasingly vigorous inspiratory effort, until finally the obstruction resolves with a loud, gasping snort, at which point the patient often partially awakens, perhaps for only a few seconds, then immediately falls back into sleep. The electroencephalogram reveals diminished or absent slow wave sleep.

In central sleep apnea the patient tends to complain of insomnia and restless sleep, with or without daytime drowsiness. As snoring and gasping are generally absent, the patient's spouse may have no complaints about the patient's sleep. The typical central sleep apneic episode is far less dramatic than an obstructive one. Patients with central sleep apnea simply stop breathing. Their chest and diaphragm are relaxed, and no nasal or oral air flow occurs. Eventually, however, the episode is terminated by a resumption of inspiratory effort, which is generally accompanied by transient awakening.

Mixed sleep apneic episodes, as noted in the introduction, pursue a biphasic course. After an initial period of central apnea, inspiratory effort begins but is met by airway obstruction, after which a period of obstructive apnea is seen. Clinically, these patients resemble more the obstructive, than the central, type, and often one hears complaints of excessive snoring and daytime drowsiness in cases of mixed sleep apnea.

In addition to complaints of insomnia or daytime drowsiness, patients with sleep apnea often experience a dry mouth and a dull headache on arising, and many also have "sleep drunkenness" wherein they experience a period of confusion as they struggle to become fully alert. Males may also experience erectile dysfunction. Rarely, enuresis may occur and there are isolated case reports of pseudotumor cerebri.

Difficulty with concentration during the day is common, and patients may complain of feeling "fuzzy" much of the day; short term memory may be impaired and patients may have difficulty making decisions. Rarely, these intellectual deficits may become severe and evolve into a dementia. Furthermore, and again rarely, some patients may present with delirium.

Depressive symptoms are also common in patients with sleep apnea.

Patients with sleep apnea may have a variety of arrhythmias, including the following: sinus bradycardia, sinus tachycardia, sinus arrest, atrial flutter, premature ventricular contractions, and ventricular tachycardia. Second-degree AV block may also be seen.

During an apneic episode, hypercapnia and hypoxia occur, and cyanosis may be seen. With frequent episodes of hypercapnia, pulmonary hypertension occurs, leading to cor pulmonale and an elevated hematocrit. Systemic hypertension also commonly occurs and tends to be diastolic.

Polysomnography is indicated not only to confirm the diagnosis but also to ascertain the presence and possible danger of arrhythmias.

COURSE

Sleep apnea appears to be a chronic condition.

COMPLICATIONS

Snoring may occasion marital conflict; daytime sleepiness may result in motor vehicle accidents or being fired for "sleeping on the job."

Sleep apnea may aggravate epilepsy, with a pronounced increase in the frequency of nocturnal seizures.

ETIOLOGY

Airway obstruction in obstructive sleep apnea may occur secondary to any number of conditions alone or in combination. These include the following: hypertrophy of the tonsils or adenoids; micrognathia, in which the tongue falls back to occlude the airway; lingual hypertrophy, as may be seen in myxedema or acromegaly; and, most commonly, obesity. Occasionally, no apparent cause is found for the obstruction, and in these cases defective brain stem mechanisms might allow inappropriate relaxation and collapse of the airway during inspiration.

Central sleep apnea is more common in obese patients, and in some cases may be secondary to lesions in the brainstem medulla, as may be seen with infarction, multiple sclerosis, tumors, syringobulbia and in the Shy-Drager variant of multiple system atrophy.

DIFFERENTIAL DIAGNOSIS

During normal sleep, up to 10 apneic episodes a night may occur; these apparently do not cause symptoms.

Narcolepsy may simulate the excessive daytime sleepiness seen typically in sleep apnea; however, narcolepsy is not typified by snoring, and sleep apnea is not accompanied by cataplexy, sleep paralysis, or hypnogogic hallucinations. Furthermore, narcoleptic sleep attacks tend to be briefer and more refreshing than those seen in sleep apneic patients.

Nocturnal myoclonus and restless legs syndrome may prompt complaints of restless sleep, as is typical in central sleep apnea. The history of jerkings, as provided by the spouse, or of a sense of akathitic restlessness, as provided by the patient, however, serve to make the diagnosis.

The Pickwickian syndrome is distinguished by the presence of hypercarbia during wakefulness: it must be borne in mind, however, that obstructive sleep apnea and the Pickwickian syndrome often co-exist.

Depression, especially if accompanied by hypersomnia and hyperphagia with weight gain, may simulate obstructive sleep apnea. Indeed, if the weight gain is substantial, it may actually cause obstructive sleep apnea.

TREATMENT

In obstructive sleep apnea, correction of any underlying condition, such as obesity, may be followed by significant relief. In mild cases, having patients sleep on their sides, a position that favors patency of the airway, may be helpful. Mild cases may also respond to protriptyline, 20 mg hs, paroxetine, 20 mg hs or oral medroxyprogesterone acetate, in doses of 20 to 60 mg daily. The benefit from medications is slight, however, and in moderate to severe cases they are of little use. In such cases, a first step in treatment is the use of a continuous positive airway pressure (CPAP) device. In patients who tolerate CPAP but still have some residual drowsiness, modafinil, in a dose of 200 mg, may offer further relief during the day. For those who either cannot tolerate CPAP or in whom it is ineffective, the use of orthodontic devices or surgery may be considered. Orthodontic devices serve to keep the jaw advanced, thus preventing the tongue from occluding the airway. Surgical options include uvulopalatopharyngoplasty and uvuloplasty, and, in limiting cases, trachesotomy.

In certain cases of central sleep apnea, acetazolamide in doses of 250 mg four times daily may provide some relief; however, its effectiveness may wane within a year. In selected cases, diaphragmatic pacing may be considered.

The treatment of mixed sleep apnea borrows from all the foregoing and is tailored to the particular sequence of events seen during the patient's mixed episode.

Regardless of the type of sleep apnea, agents that depress respiratory drive are generally contraindicated. Thus hypnotics, sedatives, anxiolytics, alcohol, opioids, and the like are generally not to be prescribed.

BIBLIOGRAPHY

Brownell LG, West P, Sweatman P, et al. Protriptyline in obstructive sleep apnea: a double-blind trial. *The New England Journal of Medicine* 1982;307:1037-1042.

Cutler MJ, Hamdan AL, Hamdan MH, et al. Sleep apnea: from the nose to the heart. *The Journal of the American Board of Family Practice* 2002;15:433-434.

Feuerstein C, Naegele B, Pepin JL, et al. Frontal lobe-related cognitive functions in patients with sleep apnea syndrome before and after treatment. *Acta Neurologica Belgica* 1997;97:96-107.

Flemons WW. Obstructive sleep apena. *The New England Journal of Medicine* 2002;347:498-504.

Karacan I, Karatas M. Erectile dysfunction in sleep apnea and response to CPAP. *Journal of Sex & Marital Therapy* 1995;21:239-247.

Kingshott RN, Vennelle M, Coleman EL, et al. Randomized, double-blind, placebo-controlled crossover trial of modafinil in the treatment of residual daytime sleepiness in the sleep apnea/hypopnea syndrome. *American Journal of Respiratory and Critical Care Medicine* 2001; 163:918-923.

Kraiczi H, Hedner J, Dahlof P, et al. Effect of serotonin uptake inhibition on breathing during sleep and daytime symptoms in obstructive sleep apnea. *Sleep* 1999;22:61-67.

Kramer NR, Bonitati AE, Millman RP. Enuresis and obstructive sleep apnea in adults. *Chest* 1998;114:634-637.

Lee AG, Golnik K, Kardon R, et al. Sleep apnea and intracranial hypertension in men. *Ophthalmology* 2002;109:482-485.

Lee JW. Recurrent delirium associated with obstructive sleep apnea. *General Hospital Psychiatry* 1998;20:120-122.

Malhotra A, White DP. Obstructive sleep apnea. *Lancet* 2002;360:237-245.

Malow BA, Levy K, Maturen K, et al. Obstructive sleep apnea is common in medically refractory epilepsy patients. *Neurology* 2000;55: 1002-1007.

White DP, Zwillich CW, Pickett CK, et al. Central sleep apnea. Improvement with acetazolamide therapy. *Archives of Internal Medicine* 1982;142:1816-1819.

116 Pickwickian Syndrome

The Pickwickian syndrome (also known as the "obesity hypoventilation syndrome"), named after the fat boy in Dickens' *The Pickwick Papers,* is characterized by severe obesity, alveolar hypoventilation, somnolence, and, often, sleep apnea. Although the prevalence of this syndrome is not known, such patients are not uncommon in pulmonary clinics.

ONSET

Although the onset may be at almost any age from adolescence to old age, most patients appear to be in their middle years. The onset itself is generally gradual and insidious.

CLINICAL FEATURES

These severely obese patients often complain of excessive sleepiness occurring throughout the day. They often appear lethargic and inattentive, and in severe cases confusion or seizures may occur.

Chronic alveolar hypoventilation leads to progressively worsening hypoxemia and hypercapnia. With exercise, hypoxemia worsens, and cyanosis may appear. Erythrocytosis occurs, and when this is severe, patients may develop a ruddy, plethoric complexion. Hypercapnia may cause pulmonary hypertension, and cor pulmonale may appear. With severe hypercapnia, intracranial pressure may rise, and, rarely, papilledema may be seen.

Although not invariably present, obstructive sleep apnea typically is present. Central sleep apnea, presumably secondary to the chronic hypercapnia, may also occur.

COURSE

As with obesity, the course of the Pickwickian syndrome is likewise generally chronic.

COMPLICATIONS

Complications are similar to those described in the chapter on sleep apnea. In addition, the pulmonary status of these patients is often so compromised that an otherwise trivial bronchitis may cause acute respiratory failure.

ETIOLOGY

The burden of excess adipose tissue encircling the chest and also pushing up the diaphragm from the obese abdomen below leads to the chronic alveolar hypoventilation. The resultant hypoxemia itself causes somnolence; should sleep apnea also occur, this would further worsen the somnolence.

DIFFERENTIAL DIAGNOSIS

The combination of somnolence, obesity, and erythrocytosis is quite distinctive.

Sleep apnea from causes other than severe obesity may cause a somnolence similar to that seen in Pickwickian syndrome, but here the arterial blood gases drawn while the patient is awake are normal in contrast to the often severe derangements seen in Pickwickian syndrome.

Acutely appearing or worsening preexisting somnolence in an obese patient may occur secondary to pulmonary emboli, a not infrequent event in the severely obese patient with venous stasis, varicosities, and thrombophlebitis.

TREATMENT

Treatment is directed at the underlying cause, which is obesity, and this is described in the chapter on obesity. If obstructive sleep apnea is also present, CPAP should be offered. Some patients will benefit from oral medroxyprogesterone acetate.

Although oxygen will relieve the daytime hypoxemia, it may also, in these chronically hypercapnic individuals, precipitate acute respiratory failure.

BIBLIOGRAPHY

Chiagn ST, Lee PY, Liu SY. Pulmonary function in a typical case of Pickwickian syndrome. *Respiration* 1980;39:105-113.

Harman E, Wynne JW, Block AJ, et al. Sleep-disordered breathing and oxygen desaturation in obese patients. *Chest* 1981;79:256-260.

Rapoport DM, Garay SM, Epstein H, et al. Hypercapnia in the obstructive sleep apnea syndrome. A reevaluation of the "Pickwickian syndrome." *Chest* 1986;89:627-635.

Sullivan CE, Berthon-Jones M, Issa FG. Remission of severe obesity-hypoventilation syndrome after short-term treatment during sleep with nasal continuous positive airway pressure. *American Review of Respiratory Diseases* 1983;128:177-181.

Sutton FD, Zwillich CW, Creagh CE, et al. Progesterone for outpatient treatment of Pickwickian syndrome. *Annals of Internal Medicine* 1975; 83:476-479.

117 Restless Legs Syndrome

The restless legs syndrome, also known as Ekbom's syndrome, is a common disorder, with a lifetime prevalence of approximately 5%. As the name implies, it is characterized by the experience of restlessness in the legs, an experience so uncomfortable that it keeps patients awake at night.

The restless legs syndrome occurs in two forms: a primary form which in all likelihood is inherited, and a secondary form occurring on the basis of numerous other disorders, most notably iron deficiency and uremia.

ONSET

The primary form generally has an onset in early adult years. The age of onset of the secondary form is of course determined by the underlying cause; however, in most cases these patients are older, generally having reached middle age.

CLINICAL FEATURES

Typically, when patients either sit down or, more especially, lie down, they feel a restlessness deep within the legs, generally in the calves. For some, this may be accompanied by an aching discomfort; formication may occur in others. Often the restlessness is so uncomfortable that the patient feels impelled to get up and walk around, a maneuver that brings at least some relief. Over time the restlessness may ascend to the arms.

At night, falling asleep may be almost impossible, and patients may either try to lie still and bear the discomfort or spend hours out of bed, often pacing about. Typically, symptoms are less severe toward early morning hours, and patients may finally get some restful sleep then.

Most of these patients also have periodic limb movements of sleep.

COURSE

Restless legs syndrome is generally chronic, and symptoms may either progressively worsen over time or pursue a waxing and waning course. Interestingly, certain medications, such as the SSRI paroxetine, may cause an exacerbation of the syndrome.

COMPLICATIONS

The resultant insomnia may leave the patient fatigued and irritable the next day.

ETIOLOGY

The primary form of the restless legs syndrome appears to be inherited in an autosomal dominant fashion in a large proportion of patients. Although it is not as yet clear what is inherited, there may be a disturbance in iron metabolism: CSF levels of ferritin are decreased while CSF transferrin levels are increased, and MRI studies have demonstrated a reduced iron content in the basal ganglia and substantia nigra. Importantly, these changes are seen in patients who are not anemic and who have normal peripheral iron stores. Despite these indications of CNS iron deficiency, however, the administration of iron to patients with the primary form of the syndrome is not helpful.

Secondary restless legs syndrome may be seen in peripheral sensory polyneuropathies of any cause, radiculopathies, spinal cord lesions, uremia, as a side-effect of chronic hemodialysis, in iron deficiency anemia, pregnancy and Parkinson's disease. Given that in many cases the responsible polyneuropathy may be subclinical, it may be appropriate, in cases where the diagnosis is in doubt, to screen patients with nerve conduction velocity (NCV) studies.

DIFFERENTIAL DIAGNOSIS

Akathisia, as may occur with antipsychotic treatment, may be difficult to distinguish from the restless legs syndrome. Two clues may be helpful: patients with antipsychotic-induced akathisia may "march in place," a phenomenon not seen in the restless legs syndrome; conversely, patients with the restless legs syndrome may get some relief by massaging their feet or calves, a maneuver that is useless in akathisia.

The syndrome of painful legs and moving toes is distinguished by the presence of pain and abnormal toe movements.

TREATMENT

In secondary cases of the restless legs syndrome, the underlying cause should, if possible, be treated. Importantly, in cases secondary to iron deficiency anemia, the administration of iron is often curative.

In the primary form, and in secondary forms where the underlying cause is untreatable or not responsive to treatment, a large number of pharmacologic agents have been shown to be superior to placebo, including certain dopaminergic agents, certain antiepileptic drugs, certain benzodiazepines, certain opioids, and clonidine.

Dopaminergic drugs have been most extensively studied in restless legs syndrome, and effectiveness has been found for levodopa (50 to 250 mg, typically with carbidopa), pergolide (0.05 to 1.0 mg), pramipexole (0.125-0.75 mg) and bromocriptine (1.25-7.5 mg). Although levodopa has traditionally been recommended, it has recently become apparent that with chronic levodopa treatment a phenomenon known as "augmentation" often occurs, wherein restlessness becomes more intense and begins to appear earlier in the evening, or even in the afternoon. Although this may also be seen with the direct-acting dopamine agonists, it is less pronounced.

Antiepileptic drugs effective in this syndrome include gabapentin and carbamazepine. Carbamazepine is rarely used, given its side effect burden; gabapentin, in contrast, is very well tolerated and is recommended in a total daily dose of approximately 1800 mg, with one-third the dose being given in the early afternoon and the remainder a couple of hours before bedtime.

Various benzodiazepines have been recommended; of them the best studied is clonazepam, in a does of from 0.5 to 2.0 mg hs.

Opioids effective for restless legs include propoxyphene, 65 mg hs, and oxycodone in a dose of 15 mg hs.

Clonidine, in a dose of 0.025 to 0.05 mg, is effective, but carries substantial side effects.

Choosing among these various agents is problematic, given that there has been only one double-blinded head to head comparison study done: this compared pergolide with levodopa and found pergolide to be superior. Traditionally, one begins with a dopaminergic agent, but given the phenomenon of augmentation, this may no longer be advisable: certainly if a dopaminergic agent were chosen, it is reasonable to consider pergolide. Of the remaining choices, gabapentin stands out, given its extraordinary ease of use and lack of drug-drug interactions. Clonazepam is also a reasonable alternative, but carries with it the risk of neuroadaptation: the same liability applies to opioids, which also carry a greater side effect burden. Clonidine is rarely used.

BIBLIOGRAPHY

Allen RP, Earley CJ. Augmentation of the restless legs syndrome with carbidopa/levodopa. *Sleep* 1996;19:205-213.
Allen RP, Barker PB, Wehrl F, et al. MRI measurement of brain iron in patients with restless legs syndrome. *Neurology* 2001;56:263-265.
Collado-Seidel V, Kazenwadel J, Wetter TC, et al. A controlled study of additional sr-L-dopa in L-dopa responsive restless legs syndrome with late-night symptoms. *Neurology* 1999;52:286-290.
Earley CJ. Restless legs syndrome. *The New England Journal of Medicine* 2003;348:2103-2109.
Ekbom KA. Restless legs syndrome. *Neurology* 1960;10:868-873.
Garcia-Borreguero D, Larrosa O, de la Llave Y, et al. Treatment of restless legs syndrome with gabapentin: a double-blind, cross-over study. *Neurology* 2002;59:1573-1579.
Krishnan PR, Bhatia M, Behari M. Restless legs syndrome in Parkinson's disease: a case-controlled study. *Movement Disorders* 2003;18:181-185.
Montplaisir J, Nicolas A, Denesle R, et al. Restless legs syndrome improved by pramipexole: a double-blind randomized trial. *Neurology* 1999;52:938-943.
Odin P, Mrowka M, Shing M. Restless legs syndrome. *European Journal of Neurology* 2002;9(Suppl 3):59-67.
Polydefkis M, Allen RP, Hauer P, et al. Subclinical sensory polyneuropathy in late-onset restless legs syndrome. *Neurology* 2000;55:1115-1121.
Saletu M, Anderer P, Saletu-Zyhlarz G, et al. Restless legs syndrome (RLS) and periodic limb movement disorder (PLMD): acute placebo-controlled sleep laboratory studies with clonazepam. *European Neuropsychopharmacology* 2001;11:153-161.
Sanz-Fuentenebro FJ, Huidobro A, Tehadas-Rivas A. Restless legs syndrome and paroxetine. *Acta Psychiatrica Scandinavica* 1996;94:482-484.
Staedt J, Wassmuth F, Siemann U, et al. Pergolide: treatment of choice in restless legs syndrome (RLS) and nocturnal myoclonus syndrome (NMS). A double-blind randomized crossover trial of pergolide versus L-Dopa. *Journal of Neural Transmission* 1997;104:461-468.
Telstad W, Sorenson O, Larsen S, et al. Treatment of restless legs syndrome with carbamazepine: a double blind study. *British Medical Journal, Clinical Research Edition* 1984;288:444-446.
Wagner ML, Walters AS, Coleman RG, et al. Randomized, double-blind, placebo-controlled study of clonidine in restless legs syndrome. *Sleep* 1996;19:52-58.
Walters AS, Hening WA, Kavey N, et al. A double-blind randomized crossover trial of bromocriptine and placebo in restless legs syndrome. *Annals of Neurology* 1988;24:455-458.
Walters AS, Hening W, Rubinstein M, et al. A clinical and polysomnographic comparison of neuroleptic-induced akathisia and the idiopathic restless legs syndrome. *Sleep* 1991;14:339-345.
Walters AS, Wagner ML, Hening WA, et al. Successful treatment of idiopathic restless legs syndrome in a randomized double-blind trial of oxycodone versus placebo. *Sleep* 1993;16:327-332.
Winkelmann J, Wetter TC, Collado-Seidel V, et al. Clinical characteristics and frequency of the hereditary restless legs syndrome in a population of 300 patients. *Sleep* 2000;23:597-602.
Winkelmann J, Muller-Myshok B, Wittchen HU, et al. Complex segregation analysis of restless legs syndrome provides evidence for an autosomal dominant mode of inheritance in early age at onset families. *Annals of Neurology* 2002;52:297-302.

118 Painful Legs and Moving Toes

■

As the name implies, this syndrome is characterized by pain in the legs, which may be excruciating, and by peculiar rhythmic abnormal involuntary movements of the toes; associated insomnia may be severe. This is a rare, but potentially devastating, disorder.

ONSET

In most cases the onset is in the sixth or seventh decades.

CLINICAL FEATURES

Symptoms appear when patients go to bed. Typically, the first symptom to appear is pain in the legs, which may be aching, burning, throbbing or crushing, and is often extraordinarily severe. The abnormal movements of the toes are generally rhythmic, and may consist of alternating clawing and fanning, circular movements or complex "piano-playing" motions. Although symptoms may begin unilaterally, bilateral spread is the rule.

Sleep is almost impossible, and walking about does not help relieve symptoms. When sleep finally does come, the abnormal movements cease.

COURSE

This is a chronic condition.

COMPLICATIONS

Both the pain and the insomnia may be debilitating.

ETIOLOGY

This syndrome has been noted with lesions of the spinal cord, posterior lumbar roots, cauda equina, peripheral nerves and soft tissues or bones of the feet; there is also one case report of an association with treatment with the antipsychotic molindone.

Although the mechanism underlying this disorder is not known, it is speculated to be similar to that underlying causalgia.

DIFFERENTIAL DIAGNOSIS

The restless legs syndrome is distinguished by the absence of pain and abnormal movements, and by the relief obtained with walking.

Causalgia is distinguished by the absence of abnormal movements.

TREATMENT

There are anecdotal reports of relief with transcutaneous electrical nerve stimulation (TENS) with or without vibratory stimulation, lumbar sympathetic block, epidural block, epidural spinal cord stimulation, baclofen and clonazepam.

BIBLIOGRAPHY

Dressler D, Thompson PD, Gledhill RF, et al. The syndrome of painful legs and moving toes. *Movement Disorders* 1994;9:13-21.

Guieu R, Tardy-Gervet MF, Blin O, et al. Pain relief achieved by transcutaneous electrical nerve stimulation and/or vibratory stimulation in a case of painful legs and moving toes. *Pain* 1990;42:43-48.

Okuda Y, Suzuki K, Kitajima T, et al. Lumbar epidural block for "painful legs and moving toes" syndrome: a report of three cases. *Pain* 1998;78:145-147.

Sandyk R. Neuroleptic-induced "painful legs and moving toes" syndrome: successful treatment with clonazepam and baclofen. *Italian Journal of Neurological Sciences* 1990;11:573-576.

Takahashi H, Saitoh C, Iwata O, et al. Epidural spinal cord stimulation for the treatment of painful legs and moving toes syndrome. *Pain* 2002;96:343-345.

119 Periodic Limb Movements of Sleep

■

Periodic limb movements of sleep is characterized by multiple jerkings of one or both legs during sleep, leading to sleep disruption. This disorder was traditionally known as nocturnal myoclonus; however, this is a misnomer, for, as pointed out under "differential diagnosis" below, the abnormal movements seen in periodic limb movements of sleep are not truly myoclonic in nature. Although the lifetime prevalence of this disorder is not known with certainty, it appears that up to one-third of patients over the age of 65 may have at least some periodic movements during sleep.

ONSET

Onset may occur at any age, from early adult years to senescence.

CLINICAL FEATURES

The jerking itself occurs in one or both lower extremities and is characterized by a "triple-flexion" movement lasting anywhere from 0.5 to 5 seconds. The foot undergoes dorsiflexion, and flexion occurs also at the knee and often at the thigh. Jerks tend to occur in episodes, wherein they may recur at intervals of anywhere from 20-40 seconds, with the episodes themselves lasting from minutes to hours.

Typically, the patient is unaware of the jerks, and complains only of poor sleep with multiple awakenings. Reliable history, therefore, must be obtained from the person sharing the patient's bed. If the patient sleeps alone, a history of finding the sheets in disarray in the morning may offer a clue.

A minority of these patients also have the restless legs syndrome.

COURSE

Periodic limb movements of sleep tends to be chronic.

COMPLICATIONS

Fatigue and irritability may compromise the patient's ability to function the next day.

ETIOLOGY

Periodic limb movements of sleep occurs in two forms, primary and secondary. The primary form may be inherited, and has been associated with a reduction of post-synaptic dopamine receptors within the basal ganglia. The strong resemblance of the jerk with a Babinski sign has prompted speculation that the jerks occur due to a pronounced deficiency of supraspinal inhibition during sleep.

The secondary form may be seen with spinal cord lesions, renal failure, folate deficiency, congestive heart failure and during pregnancy.

DIFFERENTIAL DIAGNOSIS

Hypnic jerks are a normal accompaniment of sleep onset. They differ from the jerks of periodic limb movements of sleep in that they are very brief, typically involve all four extremities, and occur only as the patient is falling asleep.

Myoclonus may be confused with the jerks of periodic limb movements of sleep; indeed, as noted earlier, this disorder used to be called "nocturnal myoclonus." Myoclonic jerks, however, are brief and lightning-like, in marked contrast to the relatively leisurely development of the jerks.

TREATMENT

In secondary cases, the underlying cause, if possible, is treated. In secondary cases where there is not possible, or not effective, and in primary cases, various medications may be considered. Levodopa (150-250 mg, usually in combination with carbidopa), pergolide (0.05 to 1.0 mg), pramipexole (0.125 to 0.75 mg), clonazepam (0.5 to 2 mg) and oxycodone (15 mg) are all effective, and gabapentin (1200-1800 mg) probably is also. Choosing among these medications is determined in large part by whether or not the patient also has the restless legs syndrome; if so, then either pergolide, clonazepam or gabapentin are reasonable choices. In cases of isolated periodic limb movements of sleep one might also consider levodopa.

BIBLIOGRAPHY

Garcia Borreguero D, Larrosa O, de la Llave Y, et al. Treatment of restless legs syndrome with gabapentin: a double-blind, cross-over study. *Neurology* 2002;59:1573-1579.

Lee MS, Choic YC, Lee SH, et al. Sleep-related periodic limb movements associated with spinal cord lesions. *Movement Disorders* 1996;11: 719-722.

Montplaisir J, Nicolas A, Denesle R, et al. Restless legs syndrome improved by pramipexole: a double-blind randomized trial. *Neurology* 1999; 52:938-943.

Peled R, Lavie P. Double-blind evaluation of clonazepam on periodic leg movements in sleep. *Journal of Neurology, Neurosurgery, and Psychiatry* 1987;50:1679-1681.

Smith RC. Relationship of periodic movement in sleep (nocturnal myoclonus) and the Babinski sign. *Sleep* 1985;8:239-243.

Staedt J, Stoppe G, Kogler A, et al. Nocturnal myoclonus syndrome (periodic movements in sleep) related to central dopamine D2-receptor alteration. *European Archives of Psychiatry and Clinical Neuroscience* 1995;245:8-10.

Staedt J, Wassmuth F, Ziemann U, et al. Pergolide: treatment of choice in restless legs syndrome (RLS) and nocturnal myoclonus syndrome (NMS). A double-blind randomized crossover trial of pergolide versus L-Dopa. *Journal of Neural Transmission* 1997;104:461-468.

Walters AS, Wagner ML, Hening WA, et al. Successful treatment of the idiopathic restless legs syndrome in a randomized double-blind trial of oxycodone versus placebo. *Sleep* 1993;16:327-332.

120 Circadian Rhythm Sleep Disorder (DSM-IV 307.45)

The onset and duration of sleep, like many other biologic rhythms, is regulated by the suprachiasmatic nucleus of the hypothalamus, which functions as the body's "internal clock." With respect to sleep, this internal clock is set by the environmental light-dark cycle, such that most normal individuals begin to feel sleepy after dark, are able to fall asleep sometime between 2000 and 2400 hours and then awaken, generally refreshed, some 7 or 8 hours later, when it gets light.

Whenever there is a mismatch between social demands for sleep or wakefulness and the internal clock, one speaks of a circadian rhythm sleep disorder. Such mismatches occur primarily via one of two mechanisms: first, there may be an abrupt and substantial change in social demands or the environmental light-dark cycle; or, second, the patient's "internal clock" may be incapable of matching up with the ongoing environmental light-dark cycle. Circadian rhythm sleep disorders occurring secondary to the first mechanism include the "shift work type" and the "jet lag type," and those occurring secondary to the second mechanism include the "delayed sleep phase type" ("night owls"), the "advanced sleep phase type" ("morning larks"), and others, including the "non-24 hour sleep-wake pattern type" and the "irregular sleep-wake pattern type."

Circadian rhythm sleep disorders, as a whole, are quite common, especially the shift work and jet lag types. The delayed sleep phase type may occur in up to 7% of adolescents; however, the remaining types are relatively uncommon.

ONSET

The shift work and jet lag types occur promptly upon beginning night shift work or eastward jet travel across five or more meridians.

The delayed sleep phase type generally appears in adolescence. The advanced sleep phase type, as noted below, may occur on either a familial or sporadic basis: familial cases generally appear in childhood or adolescence, whereas sporadic cases are generally confined to the elderly.

CLINICAL FEATURES

The shift work type occurs when individuals who normally work during daylight hours are rotated to a night shift. Although a minority may, after a few days, be able to adjust to this change, the majority cannot, and, under the ongoing influence of their internal clock, feel sleepy when at work during the night, and yet unable to sleep when at home during the day.

The jet lag type occurs when individuals, as noted above, fly eastward across five or more time meridians: at their destination, and under the influence of the internal clock, individuals begin to feel sleepy hours before the local bedtime. Although westward travel can also cause a mismatch (with individuals not feeling at all ready for bed at the local bedtime), this kind of jet lag is generally not as problematic.

The delayed sleep phase type is characterized by an inability to fall asleep at socially approved times, such that these individuals are unable to awaken early enough to comply with social demands. Thus, adolescent "night owls" may stay awake long past midnight and into the early morning and then be unable to awaken in time to get to school without significant drowsiness. Importantly, if such individuals are allowed to sleep in, as for example while on vacation, their sleep is in all respects normal, except for its timing.

The advanced sleep phase type is characterized by an urge to go to sleep early in the evening, long before others are ready to go to bed. These individuals, however, if allowed to go to bed early, sleep a normal duration, and then awaken with the morning larks, long before daylight.

In the non-24 hour sleep-wake pattern type, the patient's internal clock does not entrain to the environmental light-dark cycle but "runs free." In such cases, if the cycle of the internal clock is not 24 hours, but, as is usually the case, a little longer, the patient's sleep cycle will progressively appear later and later relative to the 24 hour day until it finally traverses the full 24 hour cycle, after which the progression once again occurs. In most cases, this failure of entrainment of the internal clock to the day-night cycle is because patients are totally blind.

In the irregular sleep-wake pattern type the relationship between the internal clock of the suprachiasmatic nucleus and sleep-producing structures of the brainstem is abnormal, and the urge to sleep seems to occur almost at random, without any reference to the environmental light-dark cycle or to any conceivable internally-generated cycle.

COURSE

In the jet lag type, provided that individuals adhere rigidly to the local bedtime, the internal clock gradually "resets" after a number of days roughly equal to the number of meridians crossed, after which individuals find themselves sleeping on the local schedule without difficulty.

In the shift work type, although there may be some improvement during the work week, sleep disruption generally does not resolve fully until individuals get off and stay off night work.

The delayed sleep phase type is fairly chronic, persisting for years or even decades.

The other types appear, in the natural course of events, to be chronic for the remainder of the individual's lifespan.

COMPLICATIONS

With the exception of the advanced sleep phase type, which generally has few complications, all the circadian sleep rhythm disorders produce drowsiness and inattentiveness at times when the social demands require wakefulness and alertness, thus setting the stage for motor vehicle accidents, injuries while using machinery, or simply falling asleep while at work or school. Furthermore, those with the shift work type have an increased risk of peptic ulcer and cardiovascular disease.

ETIOLOGY

The shift work and jet lag types are the normal results of suddenly having the environment shift by five or more hours. In the delayed sleep phase and advanced sleep phase types, genetics may play a role. In the delayed sleep phase type, there is an association with a polymorphism of the "circadian clock gene," hPer3 on chromosome 2, and in those cases of the advanced sleep phase type which are familial, mutations of the same gene have been found in some, but not all, families. The non-24 hour sleep-wake pattern type, as noted, is generally found in those who are totally blind, and here, given that entrainment to the light-dark schedule is simply not possible, the internal clock runs free at its own cycle length, which, as noted, is generally a little bit longer than 24 hours. The etiology of the irregular sleep-wake pattern type is not known.

DIFFERENTIAL DIAGNOSIS

The diagnosis in most cases is generally self-evident by history, and when there is doubt a "sleep diary" will generally clarify the picture; polysomnography is generally not required. In all cases, however, one must be alert to the possibility, especially in the case of adolescent night owls, of a voluntary departure from socially approved bedtimes. Further, in the case of the delayed sleep phase type, one must consider depression and excessive caffeine use.

Clinical pictures resembling the delayed sleep phase type and the non-24 hour sleep-wake pattern type have also occurred after traumatic brain injury.

TREATMENT

The shift work type may be partially alleviated by the use of moderately bright light (roughly 1200 Lux) for three hours during the night, and avoidance of daylight during the day by keeping the blinds drawn and by wearing dark goggles while outside. Hypnotics, such as zolpidem, may be helpful, and are preferable to drinking oneself to sleep; melatonin, although helpful in some cases, does not appear to be robustly effective.

The jet lag type is treated by rigidly adhering to the bedtime at the destination, and by the short term use, for five or so days, of a bedtime dose of either melatonin (in a dose of 5 mg) or a hypnotic (e.g., zolpidem in a dose of 5 or 10 mg). Although melatonin may not be quite as effective as zolpidem, it is better tolerated.

The delayed sleep phase type may be treated by imposing a rigid wake-up schedule at 0800 or earlier, administering two or more hours of bright light in the morning, keeping lights dim in the evening, and administering 5 mg of melatonin a couple of hours before the desired bedtime. Another option is what is known as "chronotherapy." Here, patients progressively set their sleep time three hours later each day, until, by going round the clock, they reach a socially acceptable bedtime. Although effective, chronotherapy is difficult to adhere to, and during the week it takes to get to the desired bedtime patients' sleep schedule is most definitely out of tune with social demands.

Treatment of the advanced sleep phase type is not clear, in large part because this type rarely requires treatment.

The treatment of the non-24 hour sleep-wake and irregular sleep-wake types is not clear; anecdotal reports suggest an effectiveness for melatonin.

Importantly, when melatonin is used for any of these types, the immediate-release formulation is more effective than the delayed-release preparation.

BIBLIOGRAPHY

Archer SN, Robilliard DL, Skene DJ, et al. A length polymorphism in the circadian clock gene Per3 is linked to delayed sleep phase syndrome and extreme diurnal preference. *Sleep* 2003;26:413-415.

Boivin DB, James FO, Santo JB, et al. Non-24-hour sleep-wake syndrome following a car accident. *Neurology* 2003;60:1841-1843.

Dahlitz M, Alverez B, Vignau J, et al. Delayed sleep phase syndrome responsive to melatonin. *Lancet* 1991;337:1121-1124.

Eastman CI, Stewart KT, Mahoney MP, et al. Dark goggles and bright light improve circadian rhythm adaptation to night-shift work. *Sleep* 1993; 17:535-543.

Kayumov L, Brown G, Jindal R, et al. A randomized, double-blind, placebo-controlled crossover study of the effect of exogenous melatonin on delayed sleep phase syndrome. *Psychosomatic Medicine* 2001;63:40-48.

Martin SK, Eastman CI. Medium-intensity light produces circadian rhythm adaptation to simulated night-shift work. *Sleep* 1998;21: 154-165.

Palm L, Blennow G, Wetterberg L. Correction of non-24-hour sleep/wake cycle by melatonin in a blind retarded boy. *Annals of Neurology* 1991;29:336-339.

Quinto C, Gellido C, Chokroverty S, et al. Posttraumatic delayed sleep phase syndrome. *Neurology* 2000;54:250-252.

Reid KJ, Chang AM, Dubocovich ML, et al. Familial advanced sleep phase syndrome. *Archives of Neurology* 2001;58:1089-1094.

Satoh K, Mishima K, Inoue Y, et al. Two pedigrees of familial advanced sleep phase syndrome in Japan. *Sleep* 2003;26:416-417.

Suhner A, Schlagenhauf P, Hofer I, et al. Effectiveness and tolerability of melatonin and zolpidem for the alleviation of jet lag. *Aviation, Space, and Environmental Medicine* 2001;72:638-646.

Watanabe T, Kajimura N, Kato M, et al. Effects of phototherapy in patients with delayed sleep phase syndrome. *Psychiatry and Clinical Neurosciences* 1999;53:231-233.

Wright SW, Lawrence LM, Wrenn KD, et al. Randomized clinical trial of melatonin after night-shift work: efficacy and neuropsychologic effects. *Annals of Emergency Medicine* 1998;32:334-340.

121 Primary Insomnia (DSM-IV 307.42)

Primary insomnia represents a diagnosis of exclusion and should be made only when other causes of insomnia, as discussed under Differential Diagnosis, below, have been ruled out.

Primary insomnia, as currently defined by DSM-IV, actually includes two different disorders, namely psychophysiologic insomnia and idiopathic insomnia. Psychophysiologic insomnia is very common, being found in anywhere from 1 to 10% of the general population and up to 25% of the elderly; idiopathic insomnia, by contrast, is rare.

ONSET

Psychophysiologic insomnia generally appears in adult or middle years, usually after some stressful life event. Idiopathic insomnia

has an onset in childhood, and in some cases may have been present in infancy.

CLINICAL FEATURES

Primary insomnia is characterized by difficulty falling asleep, multiple awakenings and an overall reduced total sleep time; patients are often fretful over their lack of sleep, and, while lying in bed, may be unable to stop worrying that they won't be able to fall asleep.

COURSE

Psychophysiologic insomnia lasts at least a month, and in well over half of all patients for longer than a year: in some cases it may pursue a chronic course, waxing and waning in intensity over the years.

Idiopathic insomnia is chronic.

COMPLICATIONS

Drowsiness and poor concentration during the day are common and patients may make errors at work or while driving.

ETIOLOGY

Psychophysiologic insomnia, as noted earlier, typically begins after a major life stress during which the individual had some trouble sleeping; although most individuals eventually start falling asleep again, some become anxious that they won't be able to sleep, and at this point a vicious cycle may appear, wherein the anxiety over sleep prevents sleep, thus causing more anxiety and perpetuating the insomnia. In this sense, psychophysiologic insomnia represents the end result of "negative conditioning," wherein the bed, rather than seeming an invitation to sleep, seems rather to arouse anxiety and concern. Interestingly, such patients often find that they are able to sleep better if they are not in their own bed, and may report better sleep while in a hotel or on their own living room couch.

Idiopathic insomnia is thought to occur secondary to dysfunction of brainstem structures responsible for the initiation and maintenance of sleep.

DIFFERENTIAL DIAGNOSIS

Before a diagnosis of primary insomnia is made, other causes of insomnia must be ruled out, including circadian rhythm sleep disorder, sleep apnea, restless legs syndrome, the syndrome of painful legs and moving toes, and nocturnal myoclonus: each of these is discussed in its own chapter.

Psychiatric disorders associated with insomnia must also be ruled out, including major depression, dysthymia, a depressive episode of bipolar disorder, generalized anxiety disorder, posttraumatic stress disorder and schizophrenia. In some cases, insomnia may constitute the presentation of a depressive or anxiety disorder, and here careful follow-up is required with special attention to the occurrence of other characteristic symptoms.

The use of caffeine, stimulants and some decongestants may all cause insomnia, as may alcohol or opioid withdrawal.

Painful conditions, such as gastroesophageal reflux or arthritis, may also prevent sleep.

"Short sleepers" are individuals who sleep relatively little at night, but have no complaints: they have no difficulty in falling asleep, and sleep through the night, and, for unclear reasons, "get by" with an amount of sleep that would be inadequate for most.

Finally, there is a condition known as "sleep state misperception" wherein, despite polysomnographically normal sleep, patients complain, and sometimes bitterly so, of insomnia. Before making this diagnosis, however, it must be borne in mind that, as noted earlier, some patients with psychophysiologic insomnia are better able to sleep while away from their bed than in it, and in such cases the sleep lab results will constitute a false negative. When this is suspected, home polysomnography may be required.

TREATMENT

Good sleep hygiene is essential. Patients should be discouraged from napping and encouraged to take daily exercise. Caffeine is forbidden except in the morning, and patients should engage in relaxing activity in the evening. The bedroom itself should be quiet and dark, and the bed should be used only for sleep or sexual activities. If sleep does not come, patients should do something else, perhaps read a boring book, until drowsiness sets in. Wake-up times should be strictly adhered to.

When improved sleep hygiene by itself is ineffective, cognitive behavioral therapy may be employed. Although this approach may take weeks to become effective, the results are generally good and persist after therapy is discontinued. Various medications may also be considered, including zolpidem (10 mg), zaleplon (10 mg), doxepin (25-50 mg), trazodone (25-100 mg) or an antihistamine, such as diphenhydramine (25 to 50 mg). Each of these can, and probably should, be used only on a prn basis. Zolpidem is very commonly used, and seems to lack a rebound insomnia effect; doxepin, on the other hand, may be followed, in a minority, by a severe rebound insomnia if stopped abruptly. Trazodone is very commonly used, and, unlike doxepin, does not disturb sleep architecture. Diphenhydramine is a common ingredient in over the counter hypnotics, and, while effective, may produce drowsiness the next morning.

BIBLIOGRAPHY

Edinger JD, Wohlgemuth WK, Radtke RA, et al. Cognitive behavioral therapy for treatment of chronic primary insomnia: a randomized controlled trial. *The Journal of the American Medical Association* 2001;285:1856-1864.

Hajak G, Rodenbeck A, Voderholzer U, et al. Doxepin in the treatment of primary insomnia: a placebo-controlled, double-blind, polysomnographic study. *The Journal of Clinical Psychiatry* 2001;62:453-463.

Riemann D, Voderholzer U. Primary insomnia: a risk factor to develop depression? *Journal of Affective Disorders* 2003;76:255-259.

Tsutsui S. A double-blind comparative study of zolpidem versus zopilcone in the treatment of chronic primary insomnia. *The Journal of International Medical Research* 2001;29:163-177.

Walsh JK, Roth T, Randazzo A, et al. Eight weeks of non-nightly use of zolpidem for primary insomnia. *Sleep* 2000;23:1087-1096.

122 Primary Hypersomnia (DSM-IV 307.44)

Primary, or idiopathic, hypersomnia is a diagnosis of exclusion which is made only after other causes of hypersomnia, noted under Differential Diagnosis, below, are ruled out.

Some authorities include not only chronic hypersomnia under the rubric of primary hypersomnia but also recurrent, or episodic, forms, such as the Kleine-Levin syndrome or menstruation-related hypersomnia. Given the fundamental difference in course here, this nosological "lumping" does not appear appropriate and these periodic forms are not discussed further in this chapter.

Although the prevalence of primary hypersomnia in the general population is not known, such cases do constitute 5 to 10% of patients seen in sleep clinics.

ONSET

The onset is gradual, and may occur anywhere from the age of 15 to 30 years.

CLINICAL FEATURES

In addition to sleeping long hours at night, patients also find themselves drowsy and napping during the day.

Total nocturnal sleep time may last from 8 to 14 hours, or even longer, and despite sleeping such long hours, patients awaken unrefreshed and often very groggy; sleep drunkenness may occur as patients attempt to wake up, with confusion, ataxia, and, at times, combativeness.

Drowsiness and grogginess persist through the day, and patients often slip into naps which, though lasting from 1 to 2 hours, leave them no more refreshed than before. Importantly, these naps do not occur as acute onset "attacks," but rather are preceded by gradually increasing drowsiness, which many patients are able, at times, to resist.

Nocturnal polysomnography, apart from revealing a reduced sleep latency and an increased total sleep time, is normal. The multiple sleep latency test fails to reveal any sleep-onset REM.

COURSE

Primary hypersomnia is chronic and persistent.

COMPLICATIONS

Grogginess and napping not only interfere with work and social activities but may also endanger patients when they drive or use dangerous machinery.

ETIOLOGY

Apart from the fact that primary hypersomnia is familial in over one third of cases, little is known of its etiology.

DIFFERENTIAL DIAGNOSIS

Narcoleptic attacks are distinguished from the naps of hypersomnia by their abrupt onset, relatively brief duration, refreshing nature and, on the Multiple Sleep Latency Test (MSLT), by the appearance of sleep-onset REM.

Other sleep disorders, each discussed in its own chapter, which may be associated with excessive daytime sleepiness include sleep apnea, the Pickwickian syndrome and circadian rhythm sleep disorder.

General medical conditions associated with excessive daytime sleepiness include respiratory failure, myotonic muscular dystrophy and hypothyroidism. Daytime sleepiness may also be seen after traumatic brain injury and with bilateral hypothalamic or paramedian thalamic lesions.

Various medications and substances may cause somnolence, including benzodiazepines, tricyclic antidepressants, some antipsychotics, some antihistamines, opioids and, of course, alcohol. Withdrawal from caffeine or stimulants may also be associated with daytime grogginess.

Some viral illnesses, especially mononucleosis, may leave a hypersomnolence in their wake that lasts for months.

Any condition which causes ongoing insomnia may leave patients chronically groggy during the day, including the restless legs syndrome and nocturnal myoclonus.

After going without sufficient sleep for a matter of days, daytime grogginess is normal; however, in these situations, a night or two of "catch-up" sleep is generally all that is required to restore normal daytime alertness.

"Long sleepers" are individuals who typically require more than 8 hours of sleep a night. These normal individuals, however, in contrast to patients with hypersomnia, awaken refreshed and do not feel groggy or take naps during the day.

TREATMENT

Modafinil or methylphenidate may be used as described in the chapter on narcolepsy, and although helpful, the response is not robust.

BIBLIOGRAPHY

Bassetti C, Aldrich MS. Idiopathic hypersomnia. A series of 42 patients. *Brain* 1997;120:1423-1435.

Bassetti C, Mathis J, Gugger M, et al. Hypersomnia following paramedian thalamic stroke: a report of 12 patients. *Annals of Neurology* 1996; 39:471-480.

Billiard M, Merle C, Carlander B, et al. Idiopathic hypersomnia. *Psychiatry and Clinical Neurosciences* 1998;52:125-129.

Eisensehr I, Noachter S, von Schlippenbach C, et al. Hypersomnia associated with bilateral posterior hypothalamic lesion. A polysomnographic case study. *European Neurology* 2003;49:169-172.

Sachs C, Persson HE, Hagenfeldt K. Menstruation-related periodic hypersomnia: a case study with successful treatment. *Neurology* 1982;32:1376-1379.

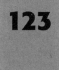

123 Nightmare Disorder (DSM-IV-TR #307.47)

The occasional nightmare, occurring perhaps once every few weeks, is not abnormal. When nightmares recur frequently, on an at least weekly basis, however, one speaks of "nightmare disorder."

ONSET

Nightmare disorder typically begins in childhood or adolescence, generally after an emotionally traumatic event.

CLINICAL FEATURES

Nightmares almost always arise from REM sleep, and they are more frequent during the middle and latter third of the night, when REM sleep is more frequent.

During a nightmare, patients for the most part lie still. Seldom is there any movement, and one never sees any thrashing about during the nightmare itself. During the nightmare, patients may be chased, attacked, tortured, or preyed on by any number of unspeakable apparitions. Typically, as the fear crescendos, patients awaken with a cry of fear and are shaky, mildly diaphoretic, and tachycardic. Within moments, full alertness and orientation occur, and patients may be able to give a vivid and emotional account of the nightmare. Some are able to go directly back to sleep, but others may be so frightened of having another nightmare that they stay awake for a half hour or more. The nightmares of nightmare disorder, as noted, tend to occur at least weekly, and in some cases they may occur multiple times a night. Some patients are plagued with the same nightmare, again and again. Fever, fatigue, emotional stress, and frightening shows or stories may all aggravate this condition.

COURSE

In most cases nightmares undergo a spontaneous remission; children seem to "grow out of it." For some patients, however, the disorder is chronic and may be lifelong.

COMPLICATIONS

Loss of sleep may impair daytime functioning, and for some patients the day is passed in a pervasive anticipatory dread of the nightmare that is sure to come that night.

ETIOLOGY

Frequent nightmares appear to be familial; although there is an association with schizotypal personality traits, in many patients there is no associated psychopathology.

DIFFERENTIAL DIAGNOSIS

An increased frequency of nightmares may occur as an integral part of a number of conditions including posttraumatic stress disorder, depressive episodes, schizophrenia, and delirium. Very rarely, simple partial seizures may present as nightmares.

Nightmares may occur as a side effect of a variety of drugs, including antidepressants (MAOIs, tricyclics and SSRIs), stimulants, antipsychotics, propranolol and other beta blockers, reserpine, clonidine, alpha-methyldopa, levodopa, bromocriptine, benzodiazepines, terfenadine and naproxen.

Nightmares may also occur as part of a REM rebound following discontinuation of REM-suppressant drugs such as monoamine oxidase inhibitors, tricyclic antidepressants, and benzodiazepines, and are also commonly found in alcohol withdrawal.

Night terror is occasionally confused with nightmare disorder; however, several features distinguish the night terror: its occurrence in non-REM sleep (often during the first third of the night); dramatic motor activity during the dream; and, upon arousal, intense sympathetic activity and at best only a very hazy recall of the dream. Furthermore, whereas the patient experiencing a nightmare may be easily awakened, often by a light touch, awakening the patient in the grip of a night terror is generally not possible.

Nocturnal panic attacks are distinguished by the general lack of any dream recall and by the greater intensity of the autonomic symptoms. Furthermore, most patients with nocturnal panic attacks also have attacks during waking hours.

TREATMENT

Avoidance of fatigue, frightening stories or shows, and, whenever possible, emotional stress, along with prompt treatment of any febrile illness, is generally indicated.

Behavioral treatments, including desensitization or dream rehearsal, are generally effective. In resistant cases, one may consider using a REM suppressing drug, such as a tricyclic anti-depressant or a benzodiazepine, keeping in mind that in some patients these agents may paradoxically cause nightmares. Cyproheptadine, in a dose of 16 to 24 mg hs, is also reported to be effective.

BIBLIOGRAPHY

Bakht FR, Miller LG. Naproxen-associated nightmares. *Southern Medical Journal* 1991;84:1271-1273.

Boller F, Wright DG, Cavalieri R, et al. Paroxysmal "nightmares." Sequel of a stroke responsive to diphenylhydantoin. *Neurology* 1975;25:1026-1028.

Brophy MH. Cyproheptadine for combat nightmares in post-traumatic stress disorder and dream anxiety disorder. *Military Medicine* 1991;156:100-101.

Burgess M, Gill M, Marks I. Postal self-exposure treatment of recurrent nightmares. Randomized controlled trial. *The British Journal of Psychiatry* 1998;172:257-262.

Hublin C, Kaprio J, Partinen M, et al. Nightmares: familial aggregation and association with psychiatric disorders in a nationwide twin cohort. *American Journal of Medical Genetics* 1999;20:329-336.

Kales A, Soldatos CR, Caldwell AB, et al. Nightmares: clinical characteristics and personality patterns. *The American Journal of Psychiatry* 1980; 137:1197-1201.

Kellner R, Neidhardt J, Krakow B, et al. Changes in chronic nightmares after one session of desensitization or rehearsal instructions. *The American Journal of Psychiatry* 1992;149:659-663.

Lepkifker E, Dannon PN, Iancu I, et al. Nightmares related to fluoxetine treatment. *Clinical Neuropharmacology* 1995;18:90-94.

Neidhardt EJ, Krakow B, Kellner R, et al. The beneficial effects of one treatment session and recording of nightmares on chronic nightmare sufferers. *Sleep* 1992;15:470-473.

Solomon K. Thiothixene and bizarre nightmares: an association? *Journal of Clinical Psychiatry* 1983;44:77-78.

Thompson DF, Pierce DR. Drug-induced nightmares. *The Annals of Pharmacotherapy* 1999;33:93-98.

124 Sleep Terror Disorder (DSM-IV-TR #307.46)

Sleep terror, also known as night terror or pavor nocturnus, occurs in from 1 to 4% of all children, and is probably more common in boys than girls.

ONSET

Sleep terrors usually appear between the ages of 4 and 12, with most occurring before the child reaches 9 years of age; occasionally a first attack may appear in early adult years.

CLINICAL FEATURES

The attack generally appears in the first third of the night, arising out of stage III or stage IV sleep, before the onset of the first REM episode. Patients suddenly cry out in terror and sit bolt upright in bed and typically appear agitated. Often one sees mydriasis, diaphoresis, and tachycardia. Patients never fully awaken during the attack and appear confused and dazed. The sheets may be grasped and patients may gasp for breath and cry for help. The whole attack generally lasts minutes, rarely more than 10 minutes, and throughout it the frightened parents are unable to comfort patients. Then, generally fairly abruptly, patients gain full consciousness, or may fall back into normal sleep without fully awakening.

After fully awakening, patients generally have no or at best a fragmentary recall of the events of the dream. Some may describe a sense of having struggled vainly to try and wake up. Most have a vivid recollection of their sense of terror yet nevertheless go right back to sleep. In the morning, they may have no recollection of the attack. Generally, parents are more shaken by the attack than are patients.

The frequency of attacks is quite variable, usually only one attack per night. Rarely they may occur over a few successive nights; more commonly they are scattered, seemingly at random, throughout the weeks and months. Occasionally, "pavor diurnus" occurs with sleep terrors during daytime naps. Anxiety, stress, fatigue, fever, and irregular sleep habits may increase the frequency of the attacks.

Occasionally, these patients may also display somnambulism, and this may occur either during or after the attack of pavor nocturnus. An association is evident with enuresis, migraine, and possibly Tourette's syndrome.

COURSE

If the disorder begins in childhood, as is usually the case, it generally remits spontaneously in early adolescence; occasionally, however, attacks may persist into adult years. By contrast, if the onset of sleep terror disorder is in adult years, it tends to be chronic.

COMPLICATIONS

Children in a dormitory situation, for example at camp, may be ridiculed for their unusual behavior. Parents, unlike the patients who are able to fall back asleep, may fret and lose sleep, leading to family tension.

ETIOLOGY

The etiology of sleep terror disorder is unclear. It is familial, and in an as yet undetermined number of cases, it appears that its expression is dependent on the presence of a coexisting obstructive sleep apnea.

DIFFERENTIAL DIAGNOSIS

Nightmares are quite different from sleep terrors. Unlike sleep terrors, nightmares arise from REM sleep in the middle or last third of the night. Nightmare patients are also easily awakened, and they do not exhibit a prolonged period of dazed confusion as seen with sleep terror. Furthermore, nightmare patients often have a vivid recollection of what happens in the dream, and because of that are often afraid to go back to sleep.

Patients with nocturnal panic attacks may awaken in an agitated panic, much like the patient with sleep terror. However, in a panic attack the patient is immediately fully alert and aware and can usually relate the attack to similar ones occurring during the day.

Nocturnal complex partial seizures may be extremely difficult to differentiate from pavor nocturnus. The occurrence of complex partial seizures during wakefulness, or of other seizure phenomena, whether nocturnal or not, should alert the clinician to the need for polysomnography. Other anomalies, such as automatic picking at the sheets while not agitated, may also provide a clue.

Isolated case reports indicate that, albeit rarely, sleep terror may occur as a side-effect of antidepressants, antipsychotics, and amantadine.

TREATMENT

Patients should be evaluated for obstructive sleep apnea, and if this is present it should be treated, as successful treatment of the sleep apnea is typically followed by a resolution of the sleep terrors. In other childhood onset cases, parents may be reassured that patients generally "grow out of it" and generally suffer no harmful consequences. In cases where treatment is required, although there are no blinded studies, several medications have, anecdotally, been effective, including diazepam, imipramine, paroxetine, or trazodone.

BIBLIOGRAPHY

Allen RM. Attenuation of drug-induced anxiety dreams and pavor nocturnus by benzodiazepines. *The Journal of Clinical Psychiatry* 1983;44:106-108.

Balon R. Sleep terror disorder and insomnia treated with trazodone: a case report. *Annals of Clinical Psychiatry* 1994;6:161-163.

Cooper AJ. Treatment of coexistent night-terrors and somnambulism in adults with imipramine and diazepam. *The Journal of Clinical Psychiatry* 1987;48:209-210.

Flaherty JA, Bellur SN. Mental side effects of amantadine therapy: its spectrum and characteristics in a normal population. *The Journal of Clinical Psychiatry* 1981;42:344-345.

Kales A, Soldatos CR, Bixler ED, et al. Hereditary factors in sleepwalking and night terrors. *The British Journal of Psychiatry* 1980;137:111-118.

Lillywhite AR, Wilson SJ, Nutt DJ. Successful treatment of night terrors and somnambulism with paroxetine. *The British Journal of Psychiatry* 1994;164:551-554.

Llorente MD, Currier MB, Norman SE, et al. Night terrors in adults: phenomenology and relationship to psychopathology. *The Journal of Clinical Psychiatry* 1992;53:392-394.

Lombroso CT. Pavor nocturnus of proven epileptic origin. *Epilepsia* 2000;41:1221-1226.

Montplaisir J, Laverdiere M, Saint-Hilaire JM, et al. Sleep and temporal lobe epilepsy: a case study with depth electrodes. *Neurology* 1981; 31:1352-1356.

Ohayon MM, Guilkleminault C, Priest RG. Night terrors, sleepwalking, and confusional arousals in the general population: their frequency and relationship to other sleep and mental disorders. *The Journal of Clinical Psychiatry* 1999;60:268-276.

Scheffer IE, Bhatia KP, Lopes-Cendes I, et al. Autosomal dominant frontal epilepsy misdiagnosed as sleep disorder. *Lancet* 1994;343:515-517.

125 Somnambulism (sleepwalking disorder, DSM-IV-TR #307.46)

Isolated episodes of sleepwalking are not uncommon, occurring in up to 30% of normal children. Frequent episodes, however, are not normal, and here one speaks of somnambulism or, as it is also called, "sleepwalking disorder." Somnambulism is not common, being present in perhaps only 2 to 3% of children, and far fewer adolescents or adults.

ONSET

The first somnambulistic episode typically occurs between the ages of 4 and 12; an onset in adult years is rare.

CLINICAL FEATURES

Somnambulism generally occurs during the first third or half of the night. Most episodes occur spontaneously; however, in some instances a disturbance, such as a loud noise, may precipitate one. The patient suddenly sits up in bed; the eyes may be either open or closed; and the patient often presents a blank stare and seems not to recognize the surroundings. Most patients repetitively and clumsily pick at the sheets or their pajamas. In some cases the episode terminates at this point; however, in most instances the patient goes on to get out of bed and begins to walk. Most patients seem to more or less avoid obstacles in their path; however, the patient may stumble over a chair or bump into something. Some patients may speak; however, for the most part their speech is mumbled or inarticulate. Occasionally, patients may engage in behavior far more complex than simply walking about the bedroom. Doors may be opened and closed; some patients may walk outside or climb out a window. Some get dressed or perhaps prepare a meal. Rarely, patients may drive a car or attempt to write a letter.

Attempts to talk with the patient or to awaken him are generally futile; indeed some patients may actively resist any interference. If the patient is awakened, however, one rarely hears a report of dreaming. Violent or dangerous behavior is uncommon during sleepwalking.

Somnambulistic episodes rarely last more than 15 or 30 minutes, and in many cases may terminate after only a few minutes. Toward the end of the episode, most patients return to bed; however, some fall back asleep somewhere else in the house, perhaps on the couch. Upon awakening in the morning, patients generally have either no, or only a very fragmentary, recollection of the episode and are often surprised to find evidence of their somnambulism, such as furniture knocked over or clothing pulled from drawers. Should patients actually awaken from an episode, they may experience a brief period of confusion, lasting perhaps a minute or two, after which consciousness fully returns, yet with little or no memory of what transpired.

Electroencephalographic monitoring reveals that somnambulistic episodes arise from non-REM, stage IV, or sometimes stage III sleep. No epileptiform activity is evident.

Some patients may also experience sleep terrors or nocturnal enuresis, and there is an association with Tourette's syndrome.

Adults with somnambulism are more likely to have some other form of psychopathology, such as a personality disorder.

COURSE

If the onset is in early childhood, spontaneous remission is likely in early adolescence. If, however, the onset is in late childhood, sleepwalking may persist into adult years. In some instances, after an apparent remission, sleepwalking may recur in the twenties, thirties, or even later. The frequency of episodes waxes and wanes over time, and is exacerbated by stress, sleep deprivation, or fever.

COMPLICATIONS

A child may refuse to sleep over at a friend's house for fear of ridicule. Injuries may occur if the patient falls or bumps into things; in some cases, death occurred after the patient crawled out a window.

ETIOLOGY

Somnambulism is clearly familial, and in some cases it appears that the underlying inherited tendency to sleepwalk is facilitated by the presence of obstructive sleep apnea.

DIFFERENTIAL DIAGNOSIS

Sleep drunkenness may resemble somnambulism; however, the episodes of sleep drunkenness are seen in the morning, as the patient struggles to awaken, in contrast to somnambulism, which is generally seen in the first half of the night.

Nocturnal complex partial seizures may be difficult to distinguish clinically; however, in most cases one also may obtain either a history of such events during wakefulness or a history of other, more obvious, epileptic phenomena, such as grand mal seizures. In doubtful cases, polysomnography is appropriate.

Fugue states are distinguished by the fact that they occur during wakefulness.

Various medications may precipitate sleepwalking, including chloral hydrate, methaqualone, methyprylon, doxepin, and thioridazine. It has also been associated with various combinations including amitriptyline and perphenazine, desipramine and chlorpromazine, and lithium and chlorpromazine, thiothixene, perphenazine, fluphenazine, or haloperidol.

TREATMENT

Parents and patients should be reassured regarding the generally benign nature of this disorder, and steps should be taken to ensure the safety of the patient. Windows should be locked, and the bedroom, if possible, should be on the ground floor. For young children, a portable gate may be placed in the bedroom doorway. For adolescents or adults, the bedroom door may be locked; if this is impractical, then the door to the house and all other windows should be securely locked and keys carefully hidden. Potentially dangerous items should be removed. Should these measures fail to protect the patient or should violent behavior occur, other measures may be implemented. In children, simply awakening the child shortly before the anticipated onset will often prevent the episode. When this is either ineffective or simply impractical, medications may be considered. Diazepam, in a dose of approximately 10 mg hs, has been shown effective in a blinded study. Anecdotally, clonazepam 0.5-1.0 mg, imipramine 10-50 mg, and paroxetine 20 mg are also effective.

BIBLIOGRAPHY

Barabas G, Mathews WS, Ferrari M. Somnambulism in children with Tourette syndrome. *Developmental Medicine and Child Neurology* 1984;26:457-460.

Cooper AJ. Treatment of coexistent night-terrors and somnambulism in adults with imipramine and diazepam. *The Journal of Clinical Psychiatry* 1987;48:209-210.

Frank NC, Spirito A, Stark L, et al. The use of scheduled awakenings to eliminate childhood sleepwalking. *Journal of Pediatric Psychology* 1997;22:345-353.

Kales A, Soldatos CR, Bisler EO, et al. Hereditary factors in sleepwalking and night terrors. *The British Journal of Psychiatry* 1980;137:111-118.

Kales A, Soldatos CR, Caldwell AB, et al. Somnambulism. Clinical characteristics and personality patterns. *Archives of General Psychiatry* 1980;37:1406-1410.

Kavey NB, Whyte J, Resor SR, et al. Somnambulism in adults. *Neurology* 1990;40:749-752.

Klackenberg G. Somnambulism in childhood—prevalence, course and behavioral correlations. A prospective longitudinal study (6-16 years). *Acta Paediatrica Scandinavica* 1982;71:495-499.

Lillywhite AR, Wilson SJ, Nutt DJ. Successful treatment of night terrors and somnambulism with paroxetine. *The British Journal of Psychiatry* 1994;164:551-554.

Reid WH, Haffke EA, Chu CC. Diazepam in intractable sleepwalking: a pilot study. *Hillside Journal of Clinical Psychiatry* 1984;6:49-55.

Schenck CH, Mahowald MW. A polysomnographically documented case of adult somnambulism with long-distance automobile driving and frequent nocturnal violence: parasomnia with continuing danger as a noninsane automatism? *Sleep* 1995;18:765-772.

126 REM Sleep Behavior Disorder (DSM-IV 307.47)

REM sleep behavior disorder (RBD) is a remarkable condition wherein patients, while asleep and dreaming, literally act out their role in the dream with the bedroom serving, as it were, as a stage. Although a rare condition in the general population, it is found in a significant minority of patients with such parkinsonian conditions as multiple system atrophy, Parkinson's disease and diffuse Lewy body disease.

ONSET

Most patients are middle-aged or older males.

CLINICAL FEATURES

Most episodes occur in the middle or last thirds of the night. Patients, while still asleep, rise up or get out of bed and, only dimly aware of their surroundings, act out their part in the dream, with variable consequences for furniture and other occupants. One patient, dreaming he was playing football, tackled a bedroom dresser, and another, dreaming he was choking a deer, was awakened by his wife's cries to find that he was choking her. Typically, patients can be awakened, and upon awakening are able to give a vivid account of the dream.

Polysomnography reveals REM sleep without atonia during the episode.

COURSE

Although the condition is chronic, the frequency of episodes varies widely, from several per night to once every few months.

COMPLICATIONS

Bed partners may be injured, furniture may be broken and patients themselves may incur fractures or head injuries. Some patients, to avoid these complications, will tie themselves to the bed before going to sleep.

ETIOLOGY

As noted earlier, RBD is not uncommon in such parkinsonian conditions as multiple system atrophy, Parkinson's disease and diffuse Lewy body disease, and in some cases may constitute the presentation of the disease, preceding parkinsonian symptoms by years or decades. In all likelihood cell loss in the locus ceruleus or substantia nigra represents the causative lesion.

There are reports of both mirtazapine and selegiline precipitating RBD in patients with parkinsonian conditions.

DIFFERENTIAL DIAGNOSIS

Somnambulism is distinguished by its occurrence during NREM sleep and by the absence of dreaming.

Nocturnal complex seizures are distinguished by an absence of dreaming and by difficulty in waking the patient. Furthermore, the history generally reveals complex partial seizures occurring during waking hours, or grand mal seizures occurring at any time. In doubtful cases, polysomnography will reveal ictal activity during the episode.

TREATMENT

Clonazepam, in doses from 0.5 to 2 mg at bedtime, is generally effective; both melatonin, in doses of 5 to 10 mg, and donepezil 10 mg have also been reported as effective.

Pending effective treatment, it is prudent to make the bedroom as safe as possible.

BIBLIOGRAPHY

Gagnon JF, Bedard MA, Fantini FL, et al. REM sleep behavior disorder and REM sleep without atonia in Parkinson's disease. *Neurology* 2002;59:585-589.

Loudon MB, Morehead MA, Schmidt HS. Activation by selegiline (Eldepryl) of REM sleep behavior disorder in parkinsonism. *The West Virginia Medical Journal* 1995;91:101.

Onofrj M, Luciano AL, Thomas A, et al. Mirtazapine induces REM sleep behavior disorder (RBD) in parkinsonism. *Neurology* 2003;60: 113-115.

Plazzi G, Corsini R, Provini F, et al. REM sleep behavior disorder in multiple system atrophy. *Neurology* 1997;48:1094-1097.

Ringman JM, Simmons JH. Treatment of REM sleep behavior disorder with donepezil: a report of three cases. *Neurology* 2000;55:870-871.

Takeuchi N, Uchimura N, Hashizume Y, et al. Melatonin therapy for REM sleep behavior disorder. *Psychiatry and Clinical Neurosciences* 2001;55:267-269.

Uchiyama M, Isse K, Tanaka K, et al. Incidental Lewy body disease in a patient with REM sleep behavior disorder. *Neurology* 1995;45: 709-712.

127 Nocturnal Head Banging

Nocturnal head banging, also known as jactatio nocturna capitis, is one of the rhythmic movement disorders and is characterized by head banging or bumping during the transition to sleep. Nocturnal head banging occurs in up to 15% of healthy infants and generally resolves by late childhood, with only rare cases of persistence into adolescence or adult years.

ONSET

Head banging generally begins in the first year of life, with an average age of onset of nine months.

CLINICAL FEATURES

Head banging is seen during the transition into sleep and may persist into Stage I or even Stage II sleep. The head movements themselves are rhythmic, with the head repeatedly making contact with the bed, bedrails or headboard.

COURSE

The vast majority of cases resolve before the age of 10 years.

COMPLICATIONS

Head banging in an adult may disturb a bed partner; actual head injury is exceedingly rare.

ETIOLOGY

The etiology is unknown.

DIFFERENTIAL DIAGNOSIS

Head banging during the day may be seen in autism, mental retardation and schizophrenia.

There is a case report of nocturnal head banging occurring after a closed head injury.

TREATMENT

Anecdotally, behavior therapy, imipramine (10 mg) and clonazepam (0.5-2 mg) have all been reported as effective; it must be borne in mind, however, that for the vast majority of cases simple reassurance is all that is required.

BIBLIOGRAPHY

Chisholm T, Morehouse RL. Adult head banging: sleep studies and treatment. *Sleep* 1996;19:343-346.
Drake ME. Jactatio nocturna after head injury. *Neurology* 1986;36:867-868.
Hashizume Y, Yoshijima H, Uchimura N, et al. Case of head banging that continued to adolescence. *Psychiatry and Clinical Neurosciences* 2002;56:255-256.
Kravitz H, Rosenthall V, Teplitz Z, et al. A study of head banging in infants and children. *Diseases of the Nervous System* 1960;21:203-208.

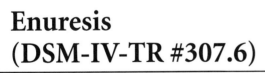 **128** Enuresis (DSM-IV-TR #307.6)

In the normal course of events 90% or more of children become dry during the night by the age of 5 or 6 years. Persistent, recurrent bedwetting past this age is considered abnormal and is termed enuresis. The prevalence of enuresis declines with age, from perhaps 5% at age 5 or 6 to about 1% at age 18. Enuresis is at least twice as common among males than females at all ages.

Enuresis occurs on both an idiopathic basis, which is over-whelmingly the most common, and secondary to any of a large number of general medical conditions, as for example a urinary tract infection.

ONSET

Idiopathic cases almost always have an onset in childhood years. In most of these cases, nighttime dryness was simply never established; these are referred to as "primary" cases, in contrast with the small minority of "secondary" cases wherein continence was established, and maintained for a year or more, after which bedwetting recurred.

Enuresis due to a general medical condition may have an onset in childhood or adult years.

CLINICAL FEATURES

Although bedwetting may occur at any time of the night and during any stage of sleep, it is more common during the first half of the night and during non-REM sleep. The child may or may not fully awaken during bedwetting; if the child does awaken, it is always after urination has begun. If the wetting occurs during REM sleep, the child may or may not recall the dream, which in turn may or may not have involved urination.

If the onset of enuresis follows a considerable period of dryness, one may find a precipitating stress, such as another illness, hospitalization for some reason, divorce of parents, or the birth of a sibling.

In idiopathic cases, the enuresis is often the only symptom; by contrast in enuresis due to a general medical condition, one often finds other symptoms such as dysuria, dribbling, or true polyuria.

COURSE

In the natural course of events, idiopathic enuresis undergoes a spontaneous remission. By the age of 12, only 3% of children and only about 1% of adults are enuretic.

The course of enuresis due to a general medical condition is determined by the underlying cause.

COMPLICATIONS

Most enuretic children are embarrassed and ashamed. Sleepovers and trips to summer camp may be avoided. Parents may feel humiliated and angered and resort to punitive measures, which may be severe. In rare instances the terrified child may so decidedly and consistently constrict the external urinary sphincter that bladder dilatation and hydronephrosis occur.

ETIOLOGY

Idiopathic enuresis, in about two-thirds of cases, is inherited as an autosomal dominant trait of high penetrance. Although it is not as yet clear what is inherited, several mechanisms have been proposed, including a delay in the normally developing capacity for continence, a smaller than normal "functional" bladder capacity, and either a reduced secretion of vasopressin or a decreased sensitivity of renal tubule cells to vasopressin. Idiopathic enuresis is not associated with any particular variety of toilet training or any definable personality traits.

Idiopathic enuresis may also be accompanied by other sleep disorders, such as somnambulism and sleep terrors.

The various general medical conditions capable of causing enuresis are listed in the box on this page. Many of these causes may be determined by history, general physical examination, neurologic examination, urinalysis with specific gravity, glucose, BUN, creatinine level, and CBC. The decision to perform invasive procedures, such as cystoscopy, is made in consultation with a urologist.

DIFFERENTIAL DIAGNOSIS

In mental retardation, toilet training is delayed, and in those who are severely or profoundly retarded it may never be achieved.

Some authors include daytime awake wetting under the rubric of enuresis; however, this is controversial. In such cases the wetting is often either intentional or secondary to a resistance to going to the bathroom, as may be seen in a young child who is reluctant to leave his friends on the playground.

TREATMENT

In enuresis due to a general medical condition, treatment is directed at the underlying cause.

In idiopathic enuresis the first step is to reassure the child and his parents regarding the benign nature and good prognosis of enuresis. A simple behavioral program should also be instituted. Caffeinated beverages are eliminated; fluids, except for ice chips and small sips of water for medicine or tooth brushing, are restricted for 3 hours before bedtime; and the child urinates just before retiring. If the child remains dry throughout the night, he or she is given a small treat the next morning, and a star is placed on a calendar. If bedwetting occurs, the child is neither punished nor shamed but is expected to strip the bed before breakfast. Many children respond favorably within a month. When this approach fails, it may be supplemented with an enuresis alarm. Use of these alarms, which are relatively inexpensive and are triggered by minute quantities of urine, is generally followed by gradual improvement over a few weeks to a few months. Once dryness has been maintained for a month, the behavioral program and the alarm may be discontinued. Somewhat more than a quarter of patients subsequently relapse; however, a second and sometimes even a third course of treatment generally provides lasting results.

If the foregoing measures fail, various medications may be considered. Double-blinded trials have established efficacy for the tricyclics imipramine and amitriptyline, desmopressin, the prostaglandin inhibitors indomethacin and diclofenac, and carbamazepine. Choosing among these medications is not straightforward. Of the tricyclics, imipramine has the most empirical support, and although there is some indication that a tricyclic may be superior to desmopressin, the difference is not great. The prostaglandin inhibitors are less effective than desmopressin, and experience with carbamazepine is very limited. Another agent often mentioned is oxybutynin, but the results of double-blinded studies here are mixed, and its use cannot be routinely recommended. Most clinicians recommend either imipramine or desmopressin. Overall, imipramine takes longer to work and is harder to tolerate, given its anticholinergic side effects; desmopressin, although rapidly effective and generally very well tolerated, has its own drawbacks, and there are cases of hyponatremic delirium and seizures secondary to its use. If imipramine is selected start at a dose of approximately 1 mg/kg 1 hour before bedtime and increase in approximately $\frac{1}{2}$ mg/kg increments every 2 weeks until acceptable control is achieved, limiting side effects occur, or a maximum dose of about 2.5 mg/kg is reached. Tricyclic levels provide a rough guide and responses have been associated with total imipramine and desipramine levels of between 60 and 80 nanograms/mL. Once continence has been achieved,

General Medical Causes of Enuresis

POLYURIA	SPASTIC BLADDER
Diabetes mellitus	Cerebral palsy
Diabetes insipidus	Spina bifida or other myelodysplastic
Cystic medullary disease	conditions
Sickle cell disease	
	PRESSURE ON BLADDER
ANATOMIC LESIONS	Pelvic masses
Bladder outlet obstruction	Impacted stool
Urethral valves	
Meatal stenosis	**MISCELLANEOUS CAUSES**
	Nocturnal seizures
	Sedating drugs given at bedtime
	Clozapine
	Obstructive sleep apnea

imipramine should be continued for from one to three months of continence, after which it may be tapered over three months time. Should wetting recur, the dose may be increased to the previously lowest effective dose and maintained again for a significant period of continence before tapering is once again attempted.

Desmopressin may be given either intranasally or orally. Doses are given at bedtime and range from 10 to 40 micrograms nasally or 0.2 to 0.6 mg orally. If successful, desmopressin may be tapered in a fashion similar to that described for imipramine. In some instances desmopressin may also be used on a "prn" basis, as for example when a child is on a "sleepover" and, although recently continent, doesn't want to risk a relapse.

Individual or family psychotherapy is generally indicated when complications, as described earlier, have accrued to a severe degree. Psychotherapy alone, however, has not been shown to be an effective treatment for enuresis per se.

BIBLIOGRAPHY

Al-Waili NS. Carbamazepine to treat primary nocturnal enuresis: double-blind study. *European Journal of Medical Research* 2000;26:40-44.

Burke JR, Mizusawa Y, Chan A, et al. A comparison of amitriptyline, vasopressin and amitriptyline with vasopressin in nocturnal enuresis. *Pediatric Nephrology* 1995;9:438-440.

Kramer NR, Bonitati AE, Millman RP. Enuresis and obstructive sleep apnea in adults. *Chest* 1998;114:634-637.

Leebeek-Groenewegen A, Blom J, et al. Efficacy of desmopressin combined with alarm therapy for monosymptomatic nocturnal enuresis. *The Journal of Urology* 2001;166:2546-2548.

Mikkelsen EJ, Rapoport JL, Nee L, et al. Childhood enuresis. I. Sleep patterns and psychopathology. *Archives of General Psychiatry* 1980;37:1139-1144.

Natochin YV, Kuznetsova AA. Nocturnal enuresis: correction of renal function by desmopressin and diclofenac. *Pediatric Nephrology* 2000;14:42-47.

Neveus T, Stenberg A, Lackgren G, et al. Sleep of children with enuresis: a polysomnographic study. *Pediatrics* 1999;103:1193-1197.

Odeh M, Oliven A. Coma and seizures due to severe hyponatremia and water intoxication in an adult with intranasal desmopressin therapy for nocturnal enuresis. *Journal of Clinical Pharmacology* 2001;41:582-584.

Rapoport JL, Mikkelsen EJ, Zavadil A, et al. Childhood enuresis. II. Psychopathology, tricyclic concentration in plasma, and antienuretic effect. *Archives of General Psychiatry* 1980;37:1146-1152.

Sakamoto K, Blaivas JG. Adult onset nocturnal enuresis. *The Journal of Urology* 2001;165:1914-1917.

Schulman SL, Stokes A, Salzman PM. The efficacy and safety of oral desmopressin in children with primary nocturnal enuresis. *The Journal of Urology* 2001;166:2427-2431.

Sener F, Hasanoglu E, Soylemezoglu O. Desmopressin versus indomethacin in primary nocturnal enuresis and the role of prostaglandins. *Urology* 1998;52:878-881.

von Gontard A, Schaumburg H, Hollmann E, et al. The genetics of enuresis: a review. *The Journal of Urology* 2001;166:2438-2443.

IMPULSE CONTROL DISORDERS NOT CLASSIFIED ELSEWHERE

129   Intermittent Explosive Disorder (DSM-IV-TR #312.34)

Intermittent explosive disorder is, as the name suggests, characterized by recurrent episodes of aggressiveness in a patient whose personality and general functioning is not otherwise typified by impulsiveness, irritability, or generalized aggressiveness. After the episode, patients feel genuine regret or guilt and often complain that the "attacks" or "spells" are not "part" of them and that, although they wish to stop the attacks, they seem to have little or no control.

Intermittent explosive disorder has also been known as "episodic dyscontrol syndrome" and "explosive personality." It is more common in men than women, and, although precise figures are lacking, it appears to be a rare disorder.

ONSET

No premorbid behavioral abnormalities have been consistently demonstrated in these patients. The onset of the disorder is heralded by the first episode of aggressiveness, and this usually occurs between the late teenage years and the mid-twenties.

CLINICAL FEATURES

The episode itself may be ushered in by a sense of uneasiness. Soon thereafter, over minutes or longer, there is a sense of rising tension. The patient may then, despite efforts at restraint, erupt into aggressive behavior. Those around the patient may be assaulted, or the patient's wrath may be turned on furniture or other property. Attempts at restraining the patient are met with violent resistance. After a variable period, generally no more than an hour, the aggressiveness subsides spontaneously. The patient may appear spent, with often only a spotty memory for what happened. Remorse and guilt follow upon surveying the destruction.

These episodes may have no precipitating event at all; if one is present, it may appear absurdly trivial in light of the ensuing violence. One patient destroyed most of the furniture after spilling some coffee on a chair. Another one violently beat an elderly gentleman who happened to stand in the way on the sidewalk.

In between episodes these patients do not display any significant abnormalities.

COURSE

The natural course of intermittent explosive disorder has not been adequately studied. Clinical experience suggests that the frequency of the episodes varies widely among patients. Whether the episodes ever cease to occur, indicating a spontaneous remission, is not clear.

COMPLICATIONS

At the least, the occurrence of these episodes puts a strain on any relationship. In some cases social ostracism may occur; at worse the patient may be incarcerated.

ETIOLOGY

Patients with intermittent explosive disorder are more likely than controls to have "soft" findings on neurologic examination and nonspecific changes, such as focal or diffuse slowing, on EEGs; furthermore these patients are also more likely to display reactive hypoglycemia on glucose tolerance testing. Taken together, these findings are consistent with the notion that intermittent explosive disorder results from epileptoid activity within the limbic system, perhaps triggered by associated abnormalities such as hypoglycemia.

DIFFERENTIAL DIAGNOSIS

Patients with schizophrenia, especially paranoid schizophrenia, may display episodes of violence, and irritable manics may be continuously violent. "Anger attacks" may be seen in a depressive episode of major depression, and "rage attacks" may be seen in patients with Tourette's syndrome, especially those with a concurrent attention-deficit/hyperactivity disorder. In all these disorders, however, the accompanying signs and symptoms indicate the correct diagnosis.

Patients with antisocial or borderline personality disorder, or with conduct disorder, may episodically be violent. However, here, in addition to the accompanying symptoms of the personality disorder or the conduct disorder, are other features that distinguish these patients from those with intermittent explosive disorder. Specifically, in these disorders the aggressiveness is usually goal directed and "understandable." Furthermore, although the sociopath may say he is sorry, he has in fact no true regret.

In borderline personality disorder the intervals between episodes is characterized by irritability and impulsiveness rather than by the normal functioning seen in intermittent explosive disorder.

Episodic aggressiveness may also occur in pathologic intoxication and in certain individuals upon intoxication with phencyclidine, amphetamine, cocaine, or related substances. Here the history of antecedent substance use facilitates the diagnosis. Anabolic steroid abuse may also prompt aggressive behavior.

Delirium, dementia, mental retardation, and personality change may all be associated with disinhibition or a lack of self-restraint, which may be followed by violence on the most trivial of provocations.

Epilepsy may be associated with intermittent violence in one of two ways. First, although very rare, there are documented cases of directed violence occurring during complex partial seizures. Second, in a minority of patients with complex partial seizures secondary to temporal lobe lesions, episodes of impulsive violence may occur interictally.

Hypothalamic lesions, very rarely, may cause episodic violence.

Finally, intermittent explosive disorder may be feigned by a malingerer as part of an insanity plea.

TREATMENT

There are no well-controlled treatment studies for intermittent explosive disorder. Several agents, however, show promise. Propranolol, in doses of 400 to 640 mg/day, is perhaps the best studied. Lithium, carbamazepine, valproate, and phenytoin have also been reported effective.

Great caution must be used in prescribing benzodiazepines to these patients. These drugs have a disinhibiting effect and may indeed aggravate the patient's condition.

Alcohol and illicit drug use should be avoided.

BIBLIOGRAPHY

Bach-Y-Rita G, Lion JR, Climent C, et al. Episodic dyscontrol: a study of 130 violent patients. *The American Journal of Psychiatry* 1971; 127:1473-1478.

Budman CL, Bruun RD, Park KS, et al. Explosive outbursts in children with Tourette's disorder. *Journal of the American Academy of Child and Adolescent Psychiatry* 2000;39:1270-1276.

Drake ME, Hietter SA, Pakalnis A. EEG and evoked potentials in episodic-dyscontrol syndrome. *Neruopsychobiology* 1992;26:125-128.

Fava M, Rosenbaum JF, Pava JA, et al. Anger attacks in unipolar depression, Part I: Clinical correlates and response to fluoxetine treatment. *The American Journal of Psychiatry* 1993;150:1158-1163.

Jenkins SC, Maruta T. Therapeutic use of propranolol for intermittent explosive disorder. *Mayo Clinic Proceedings* 1987;62:204-214.

McElroy SL, Soutullo CA, Beckman DA, et al. DSM-IV intermittent explosive disorder: a report of 27 cases. *The Journal of Clinical Psychiatry* 1998;59:203-210.

Maletzky BM. The episodic dyscontrol syndrome. *Diseases of the Nervous System* 1973;34:178-185.

Mattes JA. Comparative effectiveness of carbamazepine and propranolol for rage outbursts. *The Journal of Neuropsychiatry and Clinical Neurosciences* 1990;2:159-164.

Olvera RL. Intermittent explosive disorder: epidemiology, diagnosis and management. *CNS Drugs* 2002;16:517-526.

Tonkonogy JM, Geller JL. Hypothalamic lesions and intermittent explosive disorder. *The Journal of Neuropsychiatry and Clinical Neurosciences* 1992;4:45-50.

Woermann FG, van Elst LT, Koepp MJ, et al. Reduction of frontal neocortical gray matter associated with affective aggression in patients with temporal lobe epilepsy: an objective voxel by voxel analysis of automatically segmented MRI. *Journal of Neurology, Neurosurgery, and Psychiatry* 2000;68:162-169.

130 Kleptomania (DSM-IV-TR #312.32)

The patient with kleptomania steals, not for gain, but rather to placate an irrational and irresistible urge to steal. Indeed, after the theft the patient often discards the stolen object or perhaps stores it in a closet.

Although thought to be rare, the actual prevalence of kleptomania is not known: less than 5% of all apprehended shoplifters, however, are affected. In clinical sample, females far outnumber males.

ONSET

Though kleptomania may begin any time from childhood to middle years, most patients fall ill in their late teens or early twenties.

CLINICAL FEATURES

The restless urge to steal may mount gradually over hours or a day or more, or may strike the patient suddenly while walking down the aisle of a store. The object eventually stolen may or may not be valuable, and in any case most patients generally have enough money to buy it.

Characteristically, patients have given little forethought to the theft, and though there may be some effort to avoid apprehension, most engage in little, if any, actual planning. Furthermore, patients always act alone; there are never any accomplices.

As the object is stolen and hurriedly stuffed into a pocket or purse, tension lyses, and patients experience a wave of relief or pleasure. Some throw the stolen object away shortly after leaving the store; others may take it home and hide it. Almost always, however, they feel a sense of guilt or anxious remorse, and some may despairingly resolve to never do it again. Most patients with kleptomania also have an affective disorder, most often major depression or, somewhat less commonly, bipolar disorder. Bulimia nervosa, obsessive-compulsive disorder, and alcohol abuse or alcoholism are also common.

COURSE

Kleptomania may pursue either a chronic course, with the frequency of thefts waxing and waning over time, or an episodic course, with long stretches of time marked by an absence of theft.

COMPLICATIONS

The humiliation and suffering of capture and punishment await any person with kleptomania.

ETIOLOGY

The fact that first degree relatives of patients are more likely than controls to have a mood disorder or obsessive-compulsive disorder is consistent with the notion that kleptomania is a variant of either a mood disorder or a member of the "obsessive-compulsive spectrum."

DIFFERENTIAL DIAGNOSIS

Ordinary theft, as may occur in conduct disorder and antisocial personality disorder, is distinguished by the presence of gain as a motive, the absence of an irresistible impulse, and the presence of planning and forethought. Ordinary thieves may also malinger and feign kleptomania to avoid criminal responsibility.

Thrill-seeking in young adolescents is distinguished by the motive. Here, what is sought is the thrill of "getting away" with something, rather than the relief of tension. Furthermore, the thrill-seeker often goes to the store in a group and may be acting on a "dare."

Patients with schizophrenia may steal in obedience to a voice commanding them to do so, and manic patients may steal because, as far as they are concerned, they own the store anyway.

Demented patients may forget they put something in their pocket, or fail to understand that they must pay before they leave the store. Patients with mental retardation may similarly fail to understand that they cannot have something without paying for it.

TREATMENT

Behavior therapy may be helpful in some cases.

Although there are no controlled studies of pharmacologic treatment of kleptomania, anecdotal reports and open studies suggest efficacy for SSRIs (especially fluoxetine and paroxetine), lithium, divalproex, topiramate, and also for naltrexone in doses of 100 to 150 mg.

BIBLIOGRAPHY

Dannon PN. Topiramate for the treatment of kleptomania: a case series and review of the literature. *Clinical Neuropharmacology* 2003;26:1-4.
Goldman MJ. Kleptomania: making sense of the nonsensical. *The American Journal of Psychiatry* 1991;148:986-996.
Grant JE, Kim SW. Clinical characteristics and associated psychopathology of 22 patients with kleptomania. *Comprehensive Psychiatry* 2002; 43:378-384.
Grant JE, Kim SW. An open-label study of naltrexone in the treatment of kleptomania. *The Journal of Clinical Psychiatry* 2002;63:349-356.
Lepkifker E, Dannon PN, Ziv R, et al. The treatment of kleptomania with serotonin reuptake inhibitors. *Clinical Neuropharmacology* 1999;22: 40-43.
McElroy SL, Pope HG, Hudson JI, et al. Kleptomania: a report of 20 cases. *The American Journal of Psychiatry* 1991;148:652-657.
Presta S, Marazzitis D, Dell'Osso L, et al. Kleptomania: clinical features and comorbidity in an Italian sample. *Comprehensive Psychiatry* 2002; 43:7-12.

131 Pyromania (DSM-IV-TR #312.33)

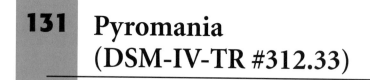

Pyromania is characterized by repeated fire setting. Unlike simple arson, however, there appears to be no motive for setting fires other than a fascination with fire. Pyromania is more common in males than females, and is a rare disorder: only perhaps 1% of all those who set fires have this disorder, while the rest have some understandable motive, such as revenge or financial gain.

ONSET

Onset is in childhood or teenage years.

CLINICAL FEATURES

Fascination with fires may manifest itself in a number of ways in addition to fire-setting itself. These patients often delight in watching fires and may regularly follow fire engines. Some may even end up as volunteer firefighters.

The fire setting itself is not impulsive; indeed often there is considerable forethought and planning. The sense of anticipation may be quite acute just before the fire, and pyromaniacs typically may be found in the crowd observing with delight their handiwork.

Pyromania rarely occurs in isolation, and most patients also suffer from either alcoholism or major depression.

COURSE

The frequency with which fires are set varies widely; the overall course is not known.

COMPLICATIONS

Arrest and incarceration may await the patient.

ETIOLOGY

Very little research has been done on pyromania per se, with almost all of the studies on fire setting dealing with individuals with either simple arson or one of the other disorders noted below, under "differential diagnosis."

DIFFERENTIAL DIAGNOSIS

Children are often fascinated by fires, and some may set fires in the backyard or on the sidewalk. This "normal" fascination with fire, however, is not strong, and major blazes do not occur except by accident.

Simple arson is suggested by the presence of a motive, such as revenge or financial gain, and may be seen in normal individuals or those with a conduct disorder or antisocial personality disorder.

Patients with a psychosis, as for example schizophrenia, may set fires on the basis of delusions or command hallucinations.

In patients with mental retardation or dementia fire setting may occur secondary to a lack of self-restraint, absent forethought, or simply by accident.

There are very rare case reports suggesting that setting fires may represent a means to self-induce a particular form of reflex epilepsy. Presumably, the sight of a fire triggers a simple partial seizure which manifests as a sense of pleasure, and patients, desirous of that pleasurable experience, may set fires to obtain it. Certainly, if there is a history of clear cut seizures, an EEG examination both with and without exposure to fire would be appropriate.

TREATMENT

There are no controlled treatment studies on pyromania; anecdotally both behavior therapy and cognitive behavior therapy have been successful.

BIBLIOGRAPHY

Barnett W, Spitzer M. Pathological fire setting 1951-1991: a review. *Medicine, Science, and the Law* 1994;34:4-20.

Geller JR. Firesetting in the adult psychiatric population. *Hospital & Community Psychiatry* 1987;38:501-506.

Lejoyeux M, Arbaretaz M, McLoughlin M, et al. Impulse control disorders and depression. *The Journal of Nervous and Mental Disease* 2002;190:312-314.

Milrod LM, Urion DK. Juvenile fire setting and the photoparoxysmal response. *Annals of Neurology* 1992;32:222-223.

Ritchie EC, Huff TG. Psychiatric aspects of arsonists. *Journal of Forensic Sciences* 1999;44:733-740.

132 Pathological Gambling (DSM-IV-TR #312.31)

Pathological gambling is characterized by a recurrent, compelling fascination with the prospect of gambling and winning. Driven by this prospect, patients spend ever-increasing amounts of time and money on gambling and continue to gamble despite ever-mounting losses. Neither financial ruin nor the loss of all personal standing can stop them; many eventually resort to fraud and theft to support their quest.

This disorder is more common in men than women and occurs in up to 3% of the adult population of the United States.

ONSET

In males the onset is often in adolescence; in females it tends to be delayed until early adult years.

The onset itself is often protracted over many years, with the frequency of gambling increasing insidiously. Occasionally, one may see an acute onset. Here the patient dates the onset of the gambling career to a chance "big win" that seemed to trigger off the drive to keep gambling, ever hoping for another big win.

CLINICAL FEATURES

For patients, gambling becomes the single most important motivating aspect of life. Former pursuits no longer interest these patients and may be neglected unless, of course, they can be brought into the service of further gambling. Over time, larger and larger bets are required to satisfy their restless urge; small wagers may be despised as the fascination with making a big win grows. These patients seem unable to walk away from a loss and call it quits; they have an incessant, heartbreaking hope that, given just "one more chance," they may be able to recoup all their losses. Indeed in the excitement of such a desperate hope, they may truly "bet the farm," staking their house or entire life savings on one roll of the dice.

Those who attempt to stop find themselves more or less powerless over the incessant craving for the excitement of the dare, the wager, and the risk. For most, the tension is unbearable, the desire irresistible. Loans from family and friends go unpaid; taxes are evaded. Theft, embezzlement, and fraud are not seen as unreasonable if they provide the money for more gambling. Bankruptcy, even the threat of imprisonment, fails to deter these patients.

These patients are often overconfident and extremely energetic. When not engaged in some "high stakes" endeavor, they tend to be bored and irritable. Losses may leave them depressed, but this generally gives way to the restless hope that the next bet will pay off.

Other disorders appear with greater frequency than would be expected by chance alone and include alcoholism, major depression and bipolar disorder.

COURSE

This is a chronic disorder that tends to pursue a waxing and waning course over long periods. For those who are able to bring a halt to their gambling, relapses are common.

COMPLICATIONS

Bankruptcy, divorce, and imprisonment are not uncommon as the gambling consumes ever-larger sums. Suicide, likewise, appears not uncommon.

ETIOLOGY

Pathological gambling is familial, and, among first-degree relatives of patients, in addition to finding an increased prevalence of pathologic gambling, one also finds an increased prevalence of alcoholism, major depression, and bipolar disorder.

Disturbances in dopaminergic and serotoninergic function appear to be present in pathological gambling. CSF levels of dopamine are decreased, and PET scanning has demonstrated either a reduced affinity or a reduced number of post-synaptic dopamine receptors within the striatum. With regard to serotonin, although CSF levels of its metabolite 5-HIAA appear normal, several pharmacologic challenge tests strongly suggest the presence of disturbances. Specifically, the prolactin response to low-dose intravenous clomipramine is blunted, whereas to intravenous mCPP it is enhanced; furthermore, mCPP infusion also induces an abnormal euphoria in pathological gamblers. Given the known role of dopamine in the hedonic response and of serotonin in impulsiveness, these findings are entirely consistent with the phenomenonology of the disorder.

DIFFERENTIAL DIAGNOSIS

The "social" gambler is distinguished from the patient by the fact that the social gambler can, and does, "walk away" from a loss. Unlike the pathologic gambler, the normal social gambler can prospectively set a maximum tolerated loss and can stop when that limit is reached.

Patients with antisocial personality disorder often gamble to excess and may steal to gamble further. However, here, unlike the pathologic gambler, the patient controls the gambling in a cold, calculating way. When the consequences begin to infringe on other activities, the sociopath, like the normal gambler, can walk away from it.

Manic patients may gamble away a fortune with breathtaking speed. Here, however, the gambling occurs only within the context of the manic episode; once that remits these patients are often filled with genuine remorse and are not interested in going back to the track.

Recently, it has become apparent that compulsive gambling may occur in a small minority of patients with Parkinson's disease when they are treated with levodopa.

TREATMENT

Both behavioral treatment with imaginal desensitization and cognitive-behavioral therapy have been successful. Among self-help groups, Gamblers Anonymous may also produce impressive results in those who comply with the program and maintain their attendance at meetings.

Double blinded studies have demonstrated an effectiveness for paroxetine and fluvoxamine; however, replication efforts failed to substantiate these findings. Naltrexone, 150-200 mg, also has some double-blind support. Single-blinded studies suggest an effectiveness for either lithium or divalproex.

If alcoholism or a mood disorder is present, it must be treated.

BIBLIOGRAPHY

Allcock CC. Pathological gambling. *The Australian and New Zealand Journal of Psychiatry* 1986;20:259-265.

Bergh C, Eklund T, Sodersten P, et al. Altered dopamine function in pathological gambling. *Psychological Medicine* 1997;27:473-475.

Blanco C, Petkova E, Ibanex A, et al. A pilot placebo-controlled study of fluvoxamine for pathological gambling. *Annals of Clinical Psychiatry* 2002;14:9-15.

Bolen DW, Boyd WH. Gambling and the gambler: a review and preliminary findings. *Archives of General Psychiatry* 1968;18:617-630.

Custer RL. Profile of the pathological gambler. *The Journal of Clinical Psychiatry* 1984;45(Suppl 12):35-38.

Grant JE, Kim SW, Potenza MN, et al. Paroxetine treatment of pathological gambling: a multi-centre randomized controlled trial. *International Clinical Psychopharmacology* 2003;18:243-249.

Kim SW, Grant JE, Adson DE, et al. Double-blind naltrexone and placebo comparison study in the treatment of pathological gambling. *Biological Psychiatry* 2001;49:914-921.

Kim SW, Grant JE, Adson DE, et al. A double-blind placebo-controlled study of the efficacy and safety of paroxetine in the treatment of pathological gambling. *The Journal of Clinical Psychiatry* 2002;63:501-507.

Ladouceur R, Sylvain C, Boutin C, et al. Cognitive treatment of pathological gambling. *The Journal of Nervous and Mental Disease* 2001;189:774-780.

MacCallum F, Blaszczynski A. Pathological gambling and comorbid substance use. *The Australian and New Zealand Journal of Psychiatry* 2002;63:411-415.

McConaghy N, Armstrong MS, Blaszczynski A, et al. Controlled comparison of aversive therapy and imaginal desensitization in compulsive gambling. *The British Journal of Psychiatry* 1983;142:366-372.

Molina JA, Sainz-Artiga MJ, Fraile A, et al. Pathologic gambling in Parkinson's disease: a behavioral manifestation of pharmacologic treatment? *Movement Disorders* 2000;15:869-872.

Pallanti S, Quercioli L, Sood E, et al. Lithium and valproate treatment of pathological gambling: a randomized single-blind study. *The Journal of Clinical Psychiatry* 2002;63:559-564.

Roy A, Adinoff B, Roehrich L, et al. Pathological gambling. A psychopathological study. *Archives of General Psychiatry* 1988;45:369-373.

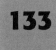

133 Trichotillomania (DSM-IV-TR #312.39)

Individuals with trichotillomania are recurrently overcome with the impulse to pull out their hair. Attempts to resist the impulse are followed by anxiety and an insupportable sense of tension. The resultant hair loss tends to be patchy and is most commonly found on the scalp. The lifetime prevalence of trichotillomania is not known with certainty, but it is probably no higher than 1%. Among adults it is far more common in females than males.

ONSET

Trichotillomania usually has an onset in late childhood or early teenage years.

CLINICAL FEATURES

The central symptom of trichotillomania is the irresistible urge to pull out one's hair. The patient almost always mounts a resistance to this urge, but shortly gives up in the face of mounting tension. Upon surrendering to the urge, most patients experience considerable relief; the subsequent hair pulling itself is often carried out in a deliberate, almost ritualized fashion. At times, especially when alone and bored, patients may begin pulling their hair with little or no sense of tension. Most patients deny hair pulling is painful; afterward, many mouth or eat the plucked hair; rarely, bezoars may form.

Most patients show hair loss on the scalp, yet a substantial minority have additional loss from the eyelashes, eyebrows, pubic or axillary hair, or beard. Hair loss may occur anywhere on the scalp but is most common at the vertex or occiput.

The resultant baldness is usually patchy; the patches themselves may be sharply demarcated or more often irregular and poorly demarcated. Observers have commented on the "moth-eaten" appearance of the scalp.

Most patients do their utmost to conceal the hair loss. Hairstyles are changed; hats and scarves become routine; wigs may be worn. Furthermore, if questioned about their baldness most patients deny that they pull their own hair.

Upon examination, one finds a mixture of normal hair and short, broken ones. The underlying scalp itself is not inflamed, and scarring is not evident. Biopsy specimens likewise fail to reveal any inflammation or scarring; growing "catagen" hairs are present. Often one observes dilatation of the follicular infundibula and the presence of keratin plugs.

Compared to the general population, patients with trichotillomania are more likely to have major depression or a borderline personality disorder; panic disorder, eating disorders, obsessive-compulsive disorder, and alcohol abuse or alcoholism may also be seen.

COURSE

Childhood onset cases tend to remit spontaneously by teenage years. Later onsets, by contrast, are generally associated with a chronic course which, itself, may take one of two patterns: in one, the frequency of hair pulling gradually waxes and wanes over the months, without any true remissions; in the other episodes characterized by more or less frequent hair pulling are separated by long intervals of remission.

COMPLICATIONS

Embarrassment is almost universal in trichotillomania; humiliation and depression occur, and some patients may give up jobs or relationships rather than endure the humiliation.

ETIOLOGY

Among first-degree relatives, there is a modestly, but statistically, significant increase in the frequency of trichotillomania; one also finds increased rates of depression, obsessive-compulsive disorder and substance use disorders. One MRI study noted a reduction in the size of the left putamen, but this has not been replicated; SPECT studies have shown various changes, but a discernible pattern has not as yet emerged.

DIFFERENTIAL DIAGNOSIS

Hair pulling per se does not indicate a diagnosis of trichotillomania. Most children and adolescents at times play with their hair and may even pull some out. Here, however, the hair pulling is limited; the urge, if present, is suppressible, and the hair loss is mild and does not result in patchy baldness.

Patients with mental retardation may pull out enough hair to create patches of baldness. However, in contrast to patients with trichotillomania, mentally retarded patients make little or no attempt to resist pulling out their hair and evidence neither embarrassment nor humiliation about their behavior.

Superficially, trichotillomania may appear similar to obsessive-compulsive disorder; indeed some patients may speak of a "compulsion" to pull their hair out. However, in obsessive-compulsive disorder, the compulsions are in the service of some other purpose; they are not an end in themselves. The patient who feels compelled to recurrently recheck to see if the door is locked does so not simply to touch the door but rather to calm the fear that the door has been left open. In contrast, the urge of the patient with trichotillomania to pull out hair is no more than that, with no further purpose to the hair pulling.

Patients with schizophrenia may root out great quantities of hair; however, the hair pulling is generally prompted by a delusion, for example, that the hair is poison or radioactive; or perhaps by a hallucination, a voice threatening the patient with torture should the hair not be removed.

A number of diseases may cause seemingly inexplicable hair loss. Patch hair loss may be seen in tinea capitis, systemic lupus erythematosus, secondary syphilis, and alopecia areata. These, conditions are distinguished from trichotillomania by the absence of normal, albeit broken, hairs in the affected areas and by the presence of inflammation on clinical examination or in biopsy specimens. Other disorders or conditions associated with hair loss often mentioned in the differential diagnosis include hypothyroidism, alopecia totalis, vitamin A intoxication, chronic lithium or valproate treatment and thallium poisoning; however, in all these cases the hair loss is typically generalized, in contrast to the patchy hair loss seen in trichotillomania.

TREATMENT

Clomipramine, 150-200 mg, is modestly more effective than placebo; fluoxetine, however, is not. Cognitive behavior therapy with habit reversal is quite effective, and is also superior to treatment with clomipramine.

BIBLIOGRAPHY

Bouwer C, Stein DJ. Trichobezoars in trichotillomania: case report and review of the literature. *Psychosomatic Medicine* 1998;60:658-660.

Christenson GA, Mackenzie TB, Mitchell JE. Characteristics of 60 adult chronic hair pullers. *The American Journal of Psychiatry* 1991;148:365-370.

du Toit PL, van Kradenburg J, Niehaus DJ, et al. Characteristics and phenomenology of hair-pulling: an exploration of subtypes. *Comprehensive Psychiatry* 2001;42:247-256.

Ninan PT, Rothbaum BO, Marsteller FA, et al. A placebo-controlled trial of cognitive-behavioral therapy and clomipramine in trichotillomania. *The Journal of Clinical Psychiatry* 2000;61:47-50.

O'Sullivan RL, Rauch SL, Breiter HC, et al. Reduced basal ganglia volumes in trichotillomania measured by morphometric magnetic resonance imaging. *Biological Psychiatry* 1997;42:39-45.

Schlosser S, Black DW, Blum N, et al. The demography, phenomenology, and family history of 22 persons with compulsive hair pulling. *Annals of Clinical Psychiatry* 1994;6:147-152.

Steichenwein SM, Thornby JI. A long-term, double-blind, placebo-controlled crossover trial of the efficacy of fluoxetine for trichotillomania. *The American Journal of Psychiatry* 1995;152:1192-1196.

Swedo SE, Leonard HL, Rapoport JL. A double-blind comparison of clomipramine and desipramine in the treatment of trichotillomania (hair pulling). *The New England Journal of Medicine* 1989;321:497-501.

Swedo SE, Rapoport JL, Leonard HL, et al. Regional cerebral glucose metabolism of women with trichotillomania. *Archives of General Psychiatry* 1991;48:828-833.

van Minnen A, Hoogduin KA, Keijsers GP, et al. Treatment of trichotillomania with behavioral therapy or fluoxetine: a randomized, waiting-list controlled study. *Archives of General Psychiatry* 2003;60:517-522.

PERSONALITY DISORDERS

134 Paranoid Personality Disorder (DSM-IV-TR #301.0)

The person with paranoid personality disorder is characteristically distrustful and on guard, quick to take offense and read malevolence into what others do, and prone to harbor deep, long-standing resentments. Some may literally withdraw into the protection of a hilltop fastness, whereas others may zealously take up causes against what they see as the source of evil. Many lead tensely quiet lives, left well enough alone by their neighbors who sense the danger in them.

Accurate prevalence figures are difficult to obtain; it may occur in from 0.5% to 2% of the population. It appears to be more common among males than females.

ONSET

The coalescence of paranoid traits appears to occur during adolescence.

CLINICAL FEATURES

As far as these people are concerned, most others are ill-intentioned or hostile; being suspicious and watchful then seems only natural, even prudent. Keenly observing those around them, these people are prone to see insult where none exists and quick to take offense where none is intended. A less than respectful greeting becomes an attack; a passerby who accidentally steps off the sidewalk onto the person's lawn is clearly testing the limits of his tolerance and forbearance.

Relations with neighbors or co-workers are generally tense and brittle. To others, these people appear to have a "chip on the shoulder." They question motives and intentions and are quick to feel betrayed. Grudges form, and these people may wait intently for their chance to exact some form of revenge. They may file lawsuits that are pursued with righteous tenacity.

Intimacy or cooperation are almost impossible for these people to achieve because for them every relationship seems to be one of either dominance or submission. They are keenly aware of rank and authority, and the closer they get to others the more important it becomes for them to be in the dominant position. Only around the clearly submissive can these people begin to relax, but even these relationships may not last long because they come to despise such abject weakness and refuse to associate with such weaklings any further.

At times these people may settle into a sort of truce with those around them. To the outside world they seem cold and humorless.

Left to themselves they may become preoccupied with machines, computers, or dossiers of various sorts. They may take great pride in their independence and self-sufficiency and look with disdain on those with weaker hearts who allow themselves to depend on others.

Such uneasy truces, at times, however, may be impossible for these people to maintain. Under great stress they may pass from having mere ideas of reference to actually developing transient delusions of persecution. What they perceive as insults and assaults can no longer be borne, and violence may occur.

COURSE

Paranoid personality disorder appears to be a chronic, lifelong condition.

COMPLICATIONS

These people rarely succeed in occupations that require any personal contact; likewise they rarely have friends or successful marriages.

Interestingly, however, the generally maladaptive nature of paranoid traits may become quite adaptive in certain situations, such as guerilla warfare.

ETIOLOGY

Paranoid personality disorder is over-represented among the first degree relatives of patients with schizophrenia, and it is suspected that the personality disorder exists as a "forme fruste" of paranoid schizophrenia.

DIFFERENTIAL DIAGNOSIS

The persecutory subtype of delusional disorder may resemble paranoid personality disorder; however, in delusional disorder delusions are chronic, whereas in paranoid personality disorder they are transient or may not occur at all. Furthermore, the patient with delusional disorder does not tend to display the constant vigilance and pervasive mistrust seen in personality disorder.

Paranoid schizophrenia may superficially mimic paranoid personality disorder; however, in schizophrenia one sees not only chronic delusions or hallucinations but also a greater or lesser degree of incoherence or illogical speech, characteristics that are not seen in paranoid personality disorder. It must be borne in mind, however, that in some cases paranoid personality traits may constitute a lengthy prodrome to schizophrenia; hence long-term diagnostic follow-up is in order.

Furthermore, in both paranoia and in paranoid schizophrenia, the onset tends to be in adult years, in contrast with the onset in teenage years in paranoid personality disorder.

Alcoholic paranoia is distinguished by its later age of onset, the associated alcoholism, and the chronicity of the delusions.

In borderline personality disorder one may see deep mistrust and anger; however, on close inspection, these people, in contrast to those with a paranoid personality disorder, desperately want a relationship.

TREATMENT

These patients rarely seek treatment themselves. They see nothing wrong with themselves and would interpret any suggestion that they seek treatment as an insult or as part of a movement to discredit them. A studied courtesy on the part of the physician may ease these patients somewhat. Low-dose antipsychotics may be helpful but it is critical to avoid side effects here as

patients with paranoid personality disorder rarely tolerate them. Should a patient respond to either haloperidol or risperidone, consideration may be given to using a long-acting intramuscular preparation.

BIBLIOGRAPHY

Dalkin T, Murphy P, Glazebrook C, et al. Premorbid personality in first-onset psychosis. *The British Journal of Psychiatry* 1994;164:202-207.

Kendler KS, McGuire M, Gruenberg AM, et al. The Roscommon Family Study. III. Schizophrenia-related personality disorders in relatives. *Archives of General Psychiatry* 1993;50:781-788.

Kendler KS, Gruenberg AM, Kinney DK. Independent diagnoses of adoptees and relatives as defined by DSM-III in the provincial and national samples of the Danish Adoption Study of Schizophrenia. *Archives of General Psychiatry* 1994;51:456-468.

Rodriguez Solano JJ, Gonzales De Chavez M. Premorbid personality disorders in schizophrenia. *Schizophrenia Research* 2000;44:137-144.

Shapiro D. *Neurotic styles.* New York, 1965, Basic Books.

Varma SL, Sharma I. Psychiatric morbidity in the first-degree relatives of schizophrenic patients. *The British Journal of Psychiatry* 1993;162: 672-678.

135 Schizoid Personality Disorder (DSM-IV-TR#301.20)

Schizoid personality disorder is marked by detachment, social isolation and emotional coldness. This is probably an uncommon disorder, and may be slightly more common in males.

ONSET

Schizoid traits typically appear in adolescence or late childhood.

CLINICAL FEATURES

Individuals with schizoid personality disorder are characteristically aloof, detached, and socially isolated. They take little or no pleasure in social relationships and experience little interest in being with others or having sexual relations with others. Lacking any desire or interest in relationships, and indeed being more comfortable by themselves, these patients are generally found engaged in solitary pursuits, often involving machines, computers or mechanical routines.

If forced into conversations or social activities, these individuals are typically awkward, socially inept and seemingly incapable of grasping the nuances or subtleties of normal social interchange.

Occasionally, if under great stress, individuals may experience delusions or hallucinations: these, however, are generally brief, lasting less than a day, and resolve spontaneously.

COURSE

Schizoid personality disorder is chronic.

COMPLICATIONS

These individuals are generally incapable of succeeding in any endeavor that requires emotional give and take, and thus may fail at any work that requires social interchange and also find themselves without any friends to help them during times of crisis.

ETIOLOGY

Schizoid personality disorder is more common among relatives of patients with schizophrenia or schizotypal personality disorder, and is often considered to be one of the "schizophrenia spectrum" disorders. Like schizophrenia, it is also associated with *in utero* malnutrition.

DIFFERENTIAL DIAGNOSIS

Distinguishing adults with Asperger's syndrome (described in the chapter on autism) from adults with schizoid personality disorder may be very difficult on clinical grounds. The age of onset, however, is distinctive: although patients with Asperger's syndrome may not come to clinical attention until they reach elementary school, a careful history will reveal an onset in very early childhood, long before the onset typical for schizoid personality disorder.

Schizotypal personality disorder is distinguished by the chronic presence of peculiarities or oddities of speech and behavior.

Paranoid personality disorder is distinguished by the presence of a pervasive suspiciousness and distrust.

Avoidant personality disorder, like schizoid personality disorder, is marked by social isolation; here, however, individuals desperately want a relationship, in contrast with schizoid individuals, who prefer the isolation.

Schizophrenia, with the exception of the simple subtype, is distinguished by the chronic presence of hallucinations, delusions or loosening of associations. The simple subtype is distinguished by its gradual downhill course, which contrasts with the stable course of schizoid personality disorder.

TREATMENT

These individuals generally do not do well in group therapy or individual therapy which involves interpretation or emotional interchange. Within the context of a calmly supportive doctor-patient relationship, however, they may respond to gentle suggestions regarding work or limited social exchanges. First generation neuroleptics are not helpful; whether second generation agents have anything to offer here is not clear.

BIBLIOGRAPHY

Cull A, Chick J, Wolff S. A consensual validation of schizoid personality in childhood and adult life. *The British Journal of Psychiatry* 1984;144:646-648.

Fulton M, Winokur G. A comparative study of paranoid and schizoid personality disorders. *The American Journal of Psychiatry* 1993;150:1363-1367.

Hoek HW, Susser E, Buck KA, et al. Schizoid personality disorder after prenatal exposure to famine. *The American Journal of Psychiatry* 1996;153:1637-1639.

Wolff S, Chick J. Schizoid personality disorder in childhood: a controlled follow-up study. *Psychological Medicine* 1980;10:85-100.

136 Schizotypal Personality Disorder (DSM-IV-TR #301.22)

Persons with schizotypal personality disorder are distant and aloof from others; their thoughts and behavior tend toward the peculiar, and others often view them as odd or eccentric. Schizotypal personality disorder is not rare and may indeed be present in up to 3% of the general population. It may be more common in males than females.

ONSET

Schizotypal traits may become evident in early adolescence or, at times, in childhood.

CLINICAL FEATURES

Although these people may not actively avoid contact with others, when they do find themselves in the company of others they remain set apart, unconnected, and aloof. At times, albeit with hesitation, they may express their opinions, and when they do, certain peculiarities become apparent. They may have mystical concerns or abstruse and inexplicable philosophic quandaries. Certain beliefs may be expressed with a guarded enthusiasm. They may have premonitions; their dreams may foretell the future; others may be aware of their abilities; and they may hear whisperings about themselves.

Rarely, however, does one find these people involved in a true conversation with give and take. For the most part, others are put off as much by their pedantic humorouslessness as by their eccentricities.

Occasionally, if under great stress, these persons may transiently become delusional. The delusion tends to be either persecutory or hypochondriacal. They may have to move because forces have gathered in the attic; they may consult their internist for bizarrely characterized aches and pains. After the stress has passed and the delusions have faded, these people may be embarrassed to admit that they ever thought that way.

COURSE

The course of this disorder appears to be chronic.

COMPLICATIONS

These people are rarely able to form intimate relationships, and work that requires social contact is generally not possible. When left alone they may be able to do simple tasks; however, any work requiring abstract thought is often confounded and sidetracked by the peculiarities of their thought.

ETIOLOGY

The notion that schizotypal personality disorder represents a forme fruste of schizophrenia is supported by multiple lines of evidence. To begin, the frequency of schizotypal personality disorder is increased in the first degree relatives of patients with schizophrenia, and the converse is also true, namely that the rate of schizophrenia is increased in the first degree relatives of patients with schizotypal personality disorder. Patients with schizotypal personality disorder also evidence the same disturbances of smooth pursuit eye movement as are seen in schizophrenia. Finally, one sees atrophy of structures on the left superior temporal gyrus in schizotypal personality disorder, similar to what is seen in schizophrenia.

DIFFERENTIAL DIAGNOSIS

Autism and Asperger's syndrome are distinguished by their onset in very early childhood.

A long prodrome to schizophrenia prospectively may be indistinguishable from a schizotypal personality disorder. The subsequent development of enduring psychotic symptoms, however, reveals the correct diagnosis. Further difficulties may arise in the case of simple schizophrenia, for in this subtype psychotic symptoms may be transient and minimal. The progressive deterioration in functioning seen in simple schizophrenia eventually distinguishes it from the more stable level of functioning seen in schizotypal personality disorder.

Some females with the fragile X syndrome, as described in that chapter, may display schizotypal traits.

Schizoid personality disorder is distinguished by the absence of peculiar beliefs, magical thinking, etc.

People with borderline personality disorder, like those with schizotypal personality disorder, may become psychotic under great stress; however, unlike those with schizotypal personality disorder, those with borderline personality disorder are typically more affective, with inappropriately severe anger, stormy relationships, and impulsivity.

TREATMENT

Within the context of a long-term supportive psychotherapeutic relationship, patients should be diplomatically directed toward work that demands little in the way of personal contact, individual initiative, or abstract thinking. Should the patient attempt an intimate relationship, contact with the patient's partner is in order to help correct the inevitable distortions that the patient will develop about the relationship.

In more severe cases, attendance at a day hospital may enable the patient to continue living independently.

Low doses of first or second generation antipsychotics may ameliorate some of the symptoms.

BIBLIOGRAPHY

Dickey CC, McCarthy RW, Voglmaier MM, et al. Smaller left Heschl's gyrus volume in patients with schizotypal personality disorder. *The American Journal of Psychiatry* 2002;159:1521-1527.

Goldberg SC, Schulz SC, Schulz PM, et al. Borderline and schizotypal personality disorders treated with low dose thiothixene vs placebo. *Archives of General Psychiatry* 1986;43:680-686.

Jacobsberg LB, Hymowitz P, Barasch A, et al. Symptoms of schizotypal personality disorder. *The American Journal of Psychiatry* 1986;143:1222-1227.

Kendler KS, Gardner CO. The risk for psychiatric disorders in relatives of schizophrenic and control probands: a comparison of three independent studies. *Psychological Medicine* 1997;27:411-419.

Siever LJ, Keefe R, Bernstein DP, et al. Eye tracking impairment in clinically identified patients with schizotypal personality disorder. *The American Journal of Psychiatry* 1990;147:740-745.

Siever LJ, Silverman JM, Horvath TB, et al. Increased morbid risk for schizophrenia-related disorders in relatives of schizotypal personality disordered patients. *Archives of General Psychiatry* 1990;47:634-640.

Sobesky WE, Hull CE, Hagerman RJ. Symptoms of schizotypal personality disorder in fragile X women. *Journal of the American Academy of Child and Adolescent Psychiatry* 1994;33:247-255.

137 Antisocial Personality Disorder (DSM-IV-TR #301.7)

Patients with antisocial personality disorder lack a full capacity to sympathize with or pity others; they tend to have no respect for the law or for the rights of others and seem relatively unfazed by the consequences that await them should they be caught. Thus unrestrained, they tend to do whatever they want; in extreme cases, other people are treated with no greater respect or affection than would be shown to an insect.

In the distant past, this disorder was known as "moral insanity," a name that hints at the fundamental aspect of this disorder. At times, "psychopathy" has been used as a synonym, but this term has been used synonymously for other disorders as well. A more enduring synonym is "sociopathy," from which is derived the useful sobriquet, the "sociopath."

Antisocial personality disorder is much more common in males than females and is much more prevalent among the transient populations of impoverished inner cities. From 3% to 5% of all American males have this disorder, in contrast to about 1% of females. As might be expected, over half of all prison inmates are found to have this disorder.

ONSET

The onset of this disorder is always in childhood. In boys a pattern of antisocial behavior is often apparent before the age of eight. In girls, the pattern may not become fully established until puberty.

The antisocial tendencies may appear insidiously, as when the child gradually commits more and more minor infractions, or at times dramatically, as when a child "senselessly" murders a playmate or a family member.

CLINICAL FEATURES

A peaceful, yet not oppressive, society rests upon the restraint that each person exercises over those urges and impulses that might lead to unnecessary harm to others. That restraint, in turn, rests on two things: on sympathy, affection, or love for others, which temper our impulses, and on respect for the law and social norms, or, failing respect, an effective fear of the consequences that await those who break these rules. To varying degrees, sociopaths lack these qualities and lack them to such a degree that they repeatedly, in most areas of their lives, fail to maintain their conduct in conformity with the rules.

Sociopaths lack any enduring sympathy or fellow-feeling. Although at times they may evidence some affection for others, such feelings pale rapidly when the other person is found to be in the way of the sociopath's wants. Sociopaths evidence a remarkable degree of selfishness and egocentricity; others are manipulated as if they had no more inherent value than a pawn on a chessboard, exploited when it serves the sociopath's purpose, discarded or sacrificed when no longer useful. Genuine shame, guilt, or remorse are foreign emotions in sociopaths; they may feign guilt when such an act serves to get others off their backs, yet once surveillance is lifted, guilt is again lacking.

Lacking any respect for the law or any compelling fear of consequences, sociopaths, when seized by impulse or temptation, are easily swept past the bounds set by law and custom. They are irritable with authority and seem comfortable when aggressive. If caught, they rarely admit to being at fault, and blame is cast on others—the police, judges, parents, or society at large. They have little recognition that most of those who are successful in life are so primarily because they do conform to social norms; rather, the sociopath sees the successful citizen as simply a better "con," as someone who was "smart" enough to "get away with it."

Although deficient in morality, sociopaths may otherwise evidence a high development of other faculties. Indeed they may show a fine and discriminating taste in food, music, literature, and the arts. Their feelings, insofar as they concern themselves, may be complex and highly developed; they may be remarkably intelligent. Such gifted sociopaths become expert at "conning" others; they may come across as caring, delightful, and personally attractive. So long as they get what they want, they seem immune to depression or anxiety. Some successful politicians have been sociopaths.

In practice, however, most sociopaths, like the rest of the population, have only a modicum of these gifts or endowments. Thus limited in their ability to deceive others, they come across, at best, as "slick" rather than cunning and as manipulative rather than deftly diplomatic. Unable to successfully pursue a Machiavellian course through life, they repeatedly come into open conflict with society, breaking laws and failing to live up to everyday responsibilities.

Telling the truth is a matter of convenience for sociopaths; if a lie would prove more useful, that is what is heard. This may progress to the point of using aliases or of lying in almost all situations. Being faithful in a relationship, whether marriage or not, is likewise a matter of convenience. If the partner no longer pleases him or commits the mistake of making too many demands, the sociopath may simply discard the relationship and move on to another. Marriages rarely last for more than a year. If children become a burden they may be neglected or even abandoned. Money that should properly go for food, clothing, or shelter is used for more immediate pleasures, such as gambling, alcohol, or drugs.

Financial obligations are disregarded as soon as they crimp the sociopath's lifestyle. Bills are left unpaid; debts are left outstanding; alimony and child support payments are way overdue.

The normal practice of staying at one job and living in one place is often too confining for sociopaths. Should it not suit them, they simply may not go to work; quitting one job after another or being fired for insubordination is common. Sociopaths may go for months or longer with no work and seem unconcerned. "Moving on" is a common theme. Some sociopaths travel from town to town and state to state; roots are not put down; being transient becomes a way of life.

Reckless, violent, and often cruel behavior is common. Those who get in the way may be assaulted; fights are very common. When others have what the sociopath wants, theft, fraud, and embezzlement are seen. Most sociopaths have a long history of arrests. Children and wives are beaten, and murder may be committed. Abuse of alcohol, cocaine, stimulants, opioids, and other substances is common, and when this occurs, whatever restraints or craftiness the sociopath had may disappear. Promiscuity is often found; some sociopaths boast of an incredible number of sexual partners. Female sociopaths often lack the foresight to use contraceptives, and multiple pregnancies are common. Suicide threats are often heard, and though at times suicide may occur, more often than not these patients do not seriously act on these threats, and they pass as soon as the sociopath's demands are met.

The expression of sociopathy is influenced by age, and the childhood history of adult sociopaths shows some typical features. As children, sociopaths often started fights and at times would use weapons. Often they acquired a "reputation" in the neighborhood, and other children were advised to keep away from them. Bullying or cruelty to younger or smaller playmates, and cruelty, often savage, to animals is common. Early sexual activity is common, often voluntary, sometimes not.

Overall, sociopathic boys and girls seem wild and undisciplined; punishment has little lasting effect on them, and they seem unmoved by kindness. They often simply run away when efforts are made to enforce conventional rules. Most are recurrently truant from school; indeed a history of satisfactory academic adjustment militates strongly against this diagnosis. Stealing and extortion are common; property may be destroyed just for the pleasure of it. Fire setting is common. Habitual lying for no purpose other than to escape deserved punishment or to get one's undeserved way is very common.

COURSE

Although sociopathic tendencies and attitudes are chronic and lifelong, the frequency of actual antisocial acts changes with time. Highest in late adolescence, the frequency gradually decreases, so the majority of patients seem to "burn out" by the age of 45. After that, the frequency of antisocial acts is quite low; some patients eventually become amusing raconteurs. Many, however, become hypochondriacally preoccupied with minor aches and pains.

COMPLICATIONS

Imprisonment is common; violent death is more common than in the general population. Promiscuity and use of intravenous drugs may lead to AIDS and other infectious diseases.

ETIOLOGY

Antisocial personality disorder is more common in the first-degree relatives of patients than of controls, and adoption studies have demonstrated a strong genetic influence. Although inheritance is clearly important, it is not as yet clear what is inherited; in this regard, however, it is of interest that the CSF level of 5-HIAA of newborns with a family history of antisocial personality disorder is lower than that of control newborns. There is also evidence supporting the notion that attention-deficit/hyperactivity disorder predisposes to the development of sociopathy.

It may be that sociopathy, as currently diagnosed, in fact represents several etiologically different disorders. For example, persons may have inherited an inability to empathize with others. Others, perhaps due to extreme hyperactivity, simply are unable to learn from experience and are unable to profit from either punishment or reward. Finally, there may be genetically normal children who are either not disciplined in early childhood or who are encouraged, subtly or otherwise, to engage in behavior forbidden to the rest of society.

DIFFERENTIAL DIAGNOSIS

A criminal record, no matter how long, does not of itself qualify a person for a diagnosis of antisocial personality disorder. In simple criminality, one finds either that the onset of criminal behavior was well beyond puberty, or that the antisocial behavior, unlike the case in sociopathy, fails to pervade all aspects of the person's life. In sociopathy, selfishness and exploitation are evident in the patient's relations with family, friends, and society at large. By contrast, the person with simple criminality may have normal, indeed exceptionally loving, relationships with family or children.

A teenager with simple adolescent rebelliousness differs from the teenage sociopath in that the rebellious teenager suffers from remorse and guilt. Indeed his morality, though at odds with that of his parents, may be quite concordant with that of other socially responsible adults.

By convention, those under the age of 18 are not given the diagnosis of antisocial personality disorder even though they have the signs and symptoms described earlier. Rather, the diagnosis of conduct disorder is given. The merit in this lies in the fact that in some of these adolescents the signs and symptoms remit before adult years.

Those with a narcissistic personality disorder are exploitative and manipulative, yet here, in contrast with antisocial personality disorder, the purpose is to feed their vanity and sense of glory, not simply to achieve financial gain. Indeed the narcissist may have a deep respect for law and custom and take pride in following them.

Patients with a borderline personality disorder are often impulse-ridden and, driven by those impulses, may commit antisocial acts. Here, however, in contrast to the sociopath, the borderline patient experiences affection, and suffers from conscience.

Patients with mental retardation may have a history of antisocial behavior dating back to childhood, yet here, in contrast with sociopathy, the patient simply lacks the cognitive ability to appreciate rules and consequences. The sociopath recognizes them, but simply chooses not to abide by them.

Patients with early-onset schizophrenia may commit numerous antisocial acts, yet here the behavior may be traced to command hallucinations or delusional beliefs. Manic patients, especially irritable manics, are notorious for their antisocial behavior. However, the antisocial behavior here is clearly episodic, being confined within the episodes of mania themselves.

Patients suffering from personality change, as described in that chapter, or a dementia may exhibit prominent, sustained, antisocial behavior. Here, in almost all circumstances, however, the premorbid history shows a nonsociopathic personality structure. Other useful clues include the often episodic explosiveness seen in secondary disorders of personality and the generalized intellectual decrement that accompanies the disinhibitions seen in dementia.

Differentiating alcoholism, cocaine addiction, or stimulant or opioid addiction from sociopathy may be very difficult. Lying, manipulation, and crime in the service of ensuring an uninterrupted supply of alcohol or drugs is quite common. In cases where the alcohol or substance use disorder began relatively late in life, the consequent late age of onset of antisocial behavior stands in contrast to the childhood onset seen in sociopathy. In cases where the substance use began very early in life, or where a reliable early history is not available, diagnostic certainty may not be possible until a long period of abstinence passes. If the antisocial phenomena clear up with abstinence, then sociopathy in all likelihood is not present. If, however, the antisocial behavior and attitudes persist into sobriety, then both diagnoses should be made.

TREATMENT

In general, sociopaths present for treatment only to escape consequences or because they are under court order. Once freed from these concerns, almost all drop out of treatment.

No evidence supports any long-term effectiveness of individual or family psychotherapy or for behavior therapy in antisocial personality disorder. Some evidence suggests that long-term stays in well-organized, strict, and tightly structured residential treatment centers may help. For those sociopaths who have alcoholism, intense involvement in Alcoholics Anonymous not only may help the alcoholism but also may be followed by a partial remission of the sociopathy.

When impulsiveness is prominent, lithium or carbamazepine may be useful. Whereas lithium does not alter the basic personality structure, its use, by reducing the intensity of the impulses, may be followed by a reduction in the frequency of antisocial acts. In the "cold blooded" or predatory type of sociopath, however, these medications are of no use.

Debate exists as to how to treat the sociopath who also evidences residual symptoms of childhood hyperactivity. Some clinicians recommend methylphenidate; however, the risk of abuse is so high among sociopaths that a more prudent choice would be bupropion or lithium.

By and large, unfortunately, sociopathy remains resistant to currently available treatments. For the dangerous sociopath, incarceration until the disorder "burns out" may be the only safe alternative.

BIBLIOGRAPHY

Black DW, Baumgard CH, Bell SE. A 16- to 45-year follow-up of 71 men with antisocial personality disorder. *Comprehensive Psychiatry* 1995;36:130-140.

Cadoret RJ, O'Gorman TW, Troughton E, et al. Alcoholism and antisocial personality. Interrelationships, genetic and environmental factors. *Archives of General Psychiatry* 1985;42:161-167.

Cadoret RJ, Troughton E, Bagford J, et al. Genetic and environmental factors in adoptee antisocial personality. *European Archives of Psychiatry and Neurologic Sciences* 1990;239:231-240.

Cleckley HM. *The mask of sanity,* St Louis, 1941, Mosby.

Constantino JN, Morris JA, Murphy DL. CSF 5-HIAA and family history of antisocial personality disorder in newborns. *The American Journal of Psychiatry* 1997;154:1771-1773.

Gerstley LJ, Alterman AI, McLellan AT, et al. Antisocial personality disorder in patients with substance abuse disorders: a problematic diagnosis? *The American Journal of Psychiatry* 1990;147:173-178.

Robins LN. Sturdy childhood predictors of adult antisocial behavior: replications from longitudinal studies. *Psychological Medicine* 1978; 8:611-622.

Shapiro D. *Neurotic styles,* New York, 1965, Basic Books.

Borderline Personality Disorder (DSM-IV-TR #301.83)

Patients with a borderline personality disorder have been aptly characterized as being "stably unstable." Their attitudes and feelings, both about themselves and others, are subject to dramatic, at times violent, change. Their relationships with others are intense and generally stormy; a clinging dependency may alternate with enraged attacks. Their histories often reveal a life of tumult and chaos.

The lifetime prevalence of borderline personality disorder is estimated at 2%; it is far more common in females than males.

ONSET

Symptoms are often apparent by early teenage years; by late teenage years the pattern of instability is generally set.

CLINICAL FEATURES

These patients experience a pervasive sense of loneliness and emptiness. They cannot count on feeling well; their mood may plummet unpredictably into despair, or they may be seized by an unreasoning irritability. Desperate to borrow some order and comfort from others, they fear abandonment, perhaps more than anything else. They do not tolerate being alone; weekends without an assurance of companionship may offer a terrifying prospect. Yet, at the same time, they are fearful of engulfment; lacking any stable sense of themselves they fear, in a very literal way, losing themselves in others, as if in joining with another they lose their own boundaries and dissolve into or become subsumed by the person they wish to be with.

These patients tend to have very strong feelings about others. Predictably, in turn, they tend to elicit comparably strong reactions from others. They tend to perceive others as either all good or as all bad. Others may be idealized, even worshipped. They are seen as a balm, a source of comfort and salvation. The relationship is seen as essential and vital to the patient's existence. Often the patient clings to the other person and fiercely resents any perceived threats to the relationship. They may have daydreams of a primitive, ideal, and exclusive relationship. However, should the patient feel rejected or abandoned, this loving adoration may be shattered and swept aside by a fierce rage. Suddenly, the other person is reviled and devalued. The other person is now seen as a pretense, a sham, as hollow and without substance. Curses may be hurled; at times the patient may exact revenge for being so unmercifully tricked.

Predictably, these patients rarely enjoy any stable relationships; others can rarely tolerate the intense and unpredictable changes in them. Idealization and adoration may be a seductive lure for some, but often the intense demandingness of the patient gives the other person pause. Such a pause is often taken as an abandonment or a threat of one, and then the other person may become subject to a torrent of abuse. Eventually, the relationship can no longer bear these extremes, and the patient once again becomes alone.

Thus alone, and unable to "fill the emptiness," these patients are often bitter, cynical, and sarcastic. Some may give up entirely in their quest for a relationship and set out to establish a structure of self-sufficiency. Inevitably, however, such an edifice is fragile, intensely brittle, and maintained only with enormous effort. Interestingly, many of these patients form strong attachments to "transitional objects," such as teddy bears, and indeed may bring them to the hospital.

When desperate, these patients may go to any extreme to fill the void. Intoxication may be sought, and alcohol is often the preferred intoxicant. Promiscuous behavior is common. At times the thrill of daredevil recklessness may be sought. They may be involved in high-speed car races, knife fights, or worse. Oblivion may be sought.

The thought of suicide is often a constant companion. In despair, they yearn for death as relief; when relatively calm, it may be viewed as a very rational alternative. Suicidal behavior is common. At times it may appear manipulative. Some patients have slashed their wrists and forearms so many times as to create a veritable "ladder" of scars. Relatively innocuous overdoses are common. At times, however, the intent is serious; shooting, hanging, and serious overdoses are not uncommon.

At times patients may mutilate themselves with no interest in killing themselves. When asked why they slashed or gouged themselves, they may have difficulty offering a reason. Some do it to relieve tension, whereas others use it as a way to inflict a feeling, to convince themselves that they are still in fact alive.

At times, certain patients may display psychotic symptoms. Voices may be heard and are generally critical; ideas or delusions of reference may occur and may be accompanied by guardedness. They may have an interest in the occult or superstitious matters; some patients come to hold these beliefs strongly. These psychotic symptoms may be quite brief and transient; in other instances, however, they may linger, waxing and waning for weeks or longer. Often these symptoms may be precipitated by extreme stress, most typically the fear of, or the actual fact of, abandonment.

Patients with a borderline personality disorder often have other disorders. Alcohol abuse or alcoholism are not uncommon; and the same holds true for dysthymia, major depression, and bipolar disorder. Panic attacks may occur. Likewise, bulimia nervosa may develop, and when it does, kleptomania is also often in evidence.

COURSE

Although this is a chronic disorder, most patients experience a diminution in the intensity of symptoms, especially impulsivity, as they reach middle years.

COMPLICATIONS

Predictably, these patients are often unable to sustain marriage or a career. Up to 10% may eventually commit suicide.

ETIOLOGY

Serotoninergic functioning appears to be disturbed in this disorder. For example, patients have an abnormal response to intravenous infusion of the serotonin agonist mCPP, and PET scanning has indicated deficient utilization of serotonin precursors in the cortex and striatum.

MRI studies have also yielded intriguing results. Structural MRI has demonstrated a subtle degree of atrophy in the hippocampus and amygdala, and functional MRI has demonstrated increased activity in the amygdala upon exposure to aversive pictures.

Patients with borderline personality disorder appear incapable of modulating affects, and the foregoing results are consistent with that: serotonin is known to be involved in the regulation of mood and impulsivity, and the amygdala is central to the experience of affect, in particular negative affect.

The genesis of these biochemical and structural changes is not as yet clear. Although borderline personality disorder is clearly familial, it is not clear whether this represents a genetic factor or the effects of a shared environment. There is no question that the childhood of these patients is marked by neglect and abuse, often sexual, and these early experiences could quite plausibly result in such a clinical picture. Until adoption studies are done, this question will remain unanswered.

DIFFERENTIAL DIAGNOSIS

Patients with histrionic personality disorder often exhibit dramatic changes, yet one sees a qualitative difference between these attention-seeking histrionics and the desperate stratagems of the borderline patient. The histrionic patient may be disappointed if the histrionics fail their purpose, but will otherwise persevere. In contrast, the borderline patient often feels desolate, utterly alone and empty, and unable to carry on.

Patients with narcissistic personality disorder may become enraged, albeit at times quietly and frostily, if others turn their backs. In the narcissistic patient, however, the issue is the loss of admiration, rather than the threat of desolate loneliness faced by the borderline patient.

Dysthymia, if of early onset, chronic, and characterized by irritability, may present in a fashion similar to borderline personality disorder. Here, however, the experience of the patient is one of depression, not emptiness, and one rarely sees the mercurial change in attitude so characteristic of a borderline personality disorder.

Likewise, cyclothymia, if of early onset, chronic, and characterized by irritability, may preclude the establishment of stable, enduring relationships. When depressed, these patients, as is the case with dysthymia, complain of depression and not emptiness. Unlike dysthymics, however, cyclothymics experience relatively abrupt changes in mood. Generally, however, these shifts into a heightened irritability occur spontaneously, rather than being the sequelae of abandonment.

Mild cases of schizophrenia may superficially resemble borderline personality disorder; however, close inquiry generally reveals the typical bizarreness and strangeness of schizophrenia that is lacking in borderline personality disorder, even when these patients are psychotic.

In the case of adolescent patients, the boundary between the "normal" tumult and rebelliousness of adolescence and an incipient borderline personality disorder may be obscure. Most teenagers, however, no matter what degree of turmoil they go through, do not experience a pervasive sense of loneliness and emptiness and continue to maintain friendships.

TREATMENT

These patients are among the most difficult treatment prospects faced by a psychiatrist. Even in the most skillful hands, progress at best evolves slowly and haltingly. Setbacks are the rule, and patients often become extraordinarily demanding, enraged, or suicidal. When a substance use disorder, such as alcoholism, is present, it is critical to treat this as little progress can be expected otherwise.

Most patients are seen in individual psychotherapy, typically with concurrent group treatment, and recent work suggests that one particular form of psychotherapy, dialectical behavior therapy, leads to a reduction in the frequency of suicidal or self-injurious behavior.

Definite structure and firm limit setting are required, for without these a deterioration of the patient's condition is almost inevitable. The times and lengths of appointments must be strictly adhered to; during the session a more than average amount of direction and support is required. Often firm limits must be placed on telephone calls; in addition, fees must be scrupulously collected.

Hospitalizations, which often occur subsequent to suicidal ideation or behavior, should be kept as short as possible and highly structured. The focus should be on practical planning and not on the deeper aspects of the patient's emotional life. Partial hospitalization, employing psychoanalytically-oriented psychotherapy, by contrast, appears to engender enduring improvement.

The tendency for borderline patients to see people either as all good or as all bad, by virtue of its effect on any developing relationship, often leaves those involved in the patient's care split into one of two camps. Not uncommonly clinical personnel in a hospital are split by the patient into those who are drawn to the patient and are inclined to "go the extra mile" and those who see the patient as manipulative and demanding and who recommend immediate "therapeutic" discharge. Often, these two clinical camps find themselves at war. Indeed when one finds a staff in civil war, often one finds the war began after a particular borderline patient was admitted.

Medications for borderline personality disorder per se play a relatively minor part in overall treatment. Certainly if a mood disorder is also present, then medications are very important, but in the absence of a concurrent disorder, a strong reliance cannot be placed on psychopharmacologic interventions. Traditionally, antipsychotics, antidepressants and mood stabilizers have been used, and double-blinded studies offer some support for this. Specifically, among the antipsychotics, both the first generation agent trifluoperazine and the second generation agent olanzapine provided global relief; the results of double-blinded studies of haloperidol, however, have been mixed. Regardless of which antipsychotic is used, low doses are appropriate. Of the antidepressants, fluoxetine is helpful in reducing anger, and fluvoxamine in dampening rapid mood shifts; the MAOIs tranylcypromine and phenelzine offer an overall benefit, but patients are rarely able to adhere to the required diet. Mood stabilizers, given the affective dysregulation in this disorder, seem a logical choice, and indeed divalproex was associated with a global improvement in one small study, which, however, was marred by a high drop-out rate. Carbamazepine was noted to offer global improvement in one study, but a replication effort showed no benefit. Finally, a recent study demonstrated global improvement with omega-3 fatty acids: this is an intriguing finding which, however, requires replication.

In planning the psychopharmacologic treatment of patients with borderline personality disorder, it is important, given the chronicity of this disorder, to take the long view: sequential treatment trials of one agent at a time, if possible, are ideal, with the goal of finding the best regimen for any given patient. Choosing among the various agents may reasonably be guided by the clinical picture: in patients consumed with anger, fluoxetine is reasonable; in those with frequent psychotic experiences, an antipsychotic may be in order; and, in those with prominent mood shifts and impulsivity, a mood stabilizer may be most appropriate to begin with. Importantly, benzodiazepines should generally not be prescribed, as they may further disinhibit patients.

BIBLIOGRAPHY

Bateman A, Fonagy P. Treatment of borderline personality disorder with psychoanalytically oriented partial hospitalization: an 18-month follow-up. *The American Journal of Psychiatry* 2001;158:36-42.

Cardasis W, Hochman JA, Silk KR. Transitional objects and borderline personality disorder. *The American Journal of Psychiatry* 1997;154: 250-255.

Cowdry RW, Gardner DL. Pharmacotherapy of borderline personality disorder. Alprazolam, carbamazepine, trifluoperazine, and tranylcypromine. *Archives of General Psychiatry* 1988;45:111-119.

de la Fuente JM, Lotstra F. A trial of carbamazepine in borderline personality disorder. *European Neuropsychopharmacology* 1994;4:479-486.

Driessen M, Herrmann J, Stahl K, et al. Magnetic resonance imaging volumes of the hippocampus and the amygdala in women with borderline personality disorder and early traumatization. *Archives of General Psychiatry* 2000;57:1115-1122.

Gunderson JG, Singer MT. Defining borderline patients: an overview. *The American Journal of Psychiatry* 1975;132:1-10.

Herpetz SC, Dietrich TM, Wenning B, et al. Evidence of abnormal amygdala functioning in borderline personality disorder: a functional MRI study. *Biological Psychiatry* 2001;50:292-298.

Hollander E, Allen A, Lopez RP, et al. A preliminary double-blind, placebo-controlled trial of divalproex sodium in borderline personality disorder. *The Journal of Clinical Psychiatry* 2001;62:199-203.

Leyton M, Okazawa H, Diksic M, et al. Brain regional alpha-[11C]methyl-L-tryptophan trapping in impulsive subjects with borderline personality disorder. *The American Journal of Psychiatry* 2001;158:775-782.

Paris J, Zweig-Frank H. A 27-year follow-up of patients with borderline personality disorder. *Comprehensive Psychiatry* 2001;42:482-487.

Rinne T, van den Brink W, Wouters L, et al. SSRI treatment of borderline personality disorder: a randomized, placebo-controlled clinical trial for female patients with borderline personality disorder. *The American Journal of Psychiatry* 2002;159:2048-2054.

Riso LP, Klein DN, Anderson RL, et al. A family study of outpatients with borderline personality disorder and no history of mood disorder. *Journal of Personality Disorders* 2000;14:208-217.

Salzman C, Wolfson AN, Schatzberg A, et al. Effect of fluoxetine on anger in symptomatic volunteers with borderline personality disorder. *Journal of Clinical Psychopharmacology* 1995;15:23-29.

Skodol AE, Gunderson JG, Pfohl B, et al. The borderline diagnosis I: psychopathology, comorbidity, and personality structure. *Biological Psychiatry* 2002;51:936-950.

Soloff PH, Cornelius J, George A, et al. Effect of phenlezine and haloperidol in borderline personality disorder. *Archives of General Psychiatry* 1993;50:377-385.

Stein DJ, Hollander E, DeCaria CM, et al. m-Chlorophenylpiperazine challenge in borderline personality disorder: relationship of neuroendocrine response, behavioral response, and clinical measures. *Biological Psychiatry* 1996;40:508-1513.

Stevenson J, Meares R, Comerford A. Diminished impulsivity in older patients with borderline personality disorder. *The American Journal of Psychiatry* 2003;160:165-166.

Verheul R, Van Den Bosch LM, Koeter MW, et al. Dialectical behavior therapy for women with borderline personality disorder: 12-month, randomized clinical trial in The Netherlands. *The British Journal of Psychiatry* 2003;182:135-140.

Zanarini MC, Frankenburg FR. Olanzapine treatment of female borderline personality disorder patients: a double-blind, placebo-controlled pilot study. *The Journal of Clinical Psychiatry* 2001;62:849-854.

Zanarini MC, Frankenburg FR. Omega-3 fatty acid treatment of women with borderline personality disorder: a double-blind, placebo-controlled pilot study. *The American Journal of Psychiatry* 2003;160:167-169.

139 Histrionic Personality Disorder (DSM-IV-TR #301.50)

People with a histrionic personality disorder are dramatic, exaggerated, and often colorful. They seek incessantly to involve others in their drama and to keep themselves the center of attention. Others are often put off and find these people shallow, insincere, and unconvincing.

Histrionic personality disorder used to be called "hysterical personality disorder"; however, this is an unfortunate term because the possession of a hystera is by no means a prerequisite for this disorder. Indeed, though it is more commonly diagnosed in females, it may be just as common among males.

The prevalence of histrionic personality disorder is on the order of 2% or 3%.

ONSET

Histrionic traits often become evident around puberty.

CLINICAL FEATURES

People with a histrionic personality disorder create an impression by their dress, speech, and behavior. Females tend to dress seductively, provocatively, even exhibitionistically; males tend toward the "macho" image with striking hairstyles, "tough" or revealing clothing, and often an excess of jewelry. The speech of these people is emotional and expressive and is often accompanied by broad or exaggerated gestures. Their exciting and melodramatic stories may at first be engaging; however, pinning these people down as to details is often impossible. In relating a pivotal event, such as the death of a loved one, such a person may not be able to get beyond saying "most horrible," or "I was crushed, just crushed." In observing these people the practical, mundane, day-to-day aspects of living seem to hold little attraction for them. They are, however, attracted to crises, drama, and tragic events, and, should one not be going on, their behavior often creates one.

These people tend to be highly emotional. Mere acquaintances are greeted as if they are long-lost friends; they may have tears and exclamations; the handshake is too strong, too "sincere" and heartfelt; the embrace is too close and too long. Temper is always a problem; should these people be thwarted, should they not get their way, they may become explosively angry or threatening, or, conversely, they may withdraw into a devastated pout that seems to beg for sympathy and understanding.

Friends and acquaintances often find themselves part of the drama. These people are attracted to causes, fads, and often seek to have others play a supporting role in their quests. Romantic entanglements are common. Females seem unable to stop flirting, and males may seem restlessly "on the make." Promiscuity, though not uncommon, is not universal. Although sexual dysfunction may be present (e.g., decreased libido, anorgasmia, erectile dysfunction) at times the sexual behavior of these people may not be at all abnormal. Relationships tend to be short lived and often stormy. These people tend to become bored with others; conversely, others may finally become fed up with the histrionics and leave.

Those with a histrionic personality disorder rarely can maintain a stable, enduring, and meaningful relationship with another. Eventually, others find them shallow, unsubstantial, and lacking in any honest emotion. Thus, no longer engaged, others often prefer to end the relationship, much as they might wish to turn off a bad soap opera on the television, even with nothing else to watch.

Conversion symptoms are not uncommon in these people. Females are at high risk for Briquet's syndrome (somatization disorder) and males for antisocial personality disorder. Both males and females are at high risk for alcoholism.

COURSE

Histrionic personality disorder is a chronic lifelong disorder, and, although symptoms are modulated by the aging process, it is not clear whether these people "burn out," as is the case with antisocial personality disorder.

COMPLICATIONS

Stable, gratifying marriages or friendships are exceptional, and most of these people go from one damaged relationship to another. Work may not suffer as much; indeed these people may "shine" in certain occupations such as acting or entertainment.

ETIOLOGY

Although this disorder tends to run in families, the basis for this aggregation is not known.

DIFFERENTIAL DIAGNOSIS

Histrionic traits may occur in a number of other personality disorders; however, in each case certain differential points exist that clarify the diagnosis. Narcissistic patients are often quite vain and seek to be center stage; however, they lack the emotionality seen in histrionic patients. Borderline patients may at times be flamboyant and exaggerated, but in contrast to histrionic patients they possess an enduring sense of uncertainty and emptiness. Antisocial patients often lead quite colorful lives; however, in contrast to histrionic patients they rarely become dependent on, or deeply attached to, any other people.

Briquet's syndrome, or somatization disorder, is typified by histrionics; however, here the drama centers on only one theme: the patient's concern about having multiple other symptoms and illnesses. By contrast, the drama of the histrionic person covers a wide range of subjects.

In atypical depression, the behavior of the patient may be almost indistinguishable from that of someone with a histrionic personality disorder. Clearly, if atypical depression pursued an episodic course, the history of a period of normal functioning would rule out the diagnosis of a histrionic personality disorder. However, if atypical depression is chronic and of early onset, the diagnostician must rely on the presence of "atypical" depressive signs, such as hypersomnia, hyperphagia, and a pervasive sense of leaden fatigue.

In cyclothymia, patients may live from one flamboyant crisis to another. Here, however, one sees pressured speech, racing thoughts, and truly heightened mood, all of which are not part of histrionic personality disorder.

TREATMENT

There are no controlled studies of the treatment of histrionic personality disorder; anecdotally, patients improve with psychoanalytically-oriented individual or group psychotherapy.

BIBLIOGRAPHY

Apt C, Hurlebert DF. The sexual attitudes, behavior and relationships of women with histrionic personality disorder. *Journal of Sex & Marital Therapy* 1994;20:125-133.

Lillienfield SO, Van Valkenburng C, Larntz K, et al. The relationship of histrionic personality disorder to antisocial personality disorder and somatization disorders. *The American Journal of Psychiatry* 1986;143:718-722.

Luisada PV, Pele R, Pittard EA. The hysterical personality in men. *The American Journal of Psychiatry* 1974;131:518-522.

Morison J. Histrionic personality disorder in women with somatization disorder. *Psychosomatics* 1989;30:433-437.

Nestadt G, Romanoski AJ, Chahal R, et al. An epidemiological study of histrionic personality disorder. *Psychological Medicine* 1990;20:413-422.

Shapiro D. *Neurotic styles,* New York, 1965, Basic Books.

Slavney PR, McHugh PR. The hysterical personality. *Archives of General Psychiatry* 1974;30:325-329.

140 Narcissistic Personality Disorder (DSM-IV-TR #301.81)

People with a narcissistic personality disorder see themselves as superior to others, regardless of their actual achievements in life. They feel entitled to admiration and expect that others will defer to their wishes. Relationships are valued only insofar as they enhance these people's self-esteem; they have little capacity for empathy with others or any true interest in the well-being of others.

These patients tend to be very sensitive to criticism, or even a hint of criticism. If humiliated, they may react with overt rage; more often, however, they mask their reaction with an attitude of lofty indifference, as if what others think actually makes no difference to them.

This personality disorder is uncommon, occurring in less than 1% of the general population; it is somewhat more common among males than females.

ONSET

Narcissistic traits may make their appearance in childhood; during adolescence they gradually coalesce into a stable symptom complex.

CLINICAL FEATURES

These patients have a lofty opinion of themselves; they see their accomplishments as admirable and often indulge in daydreams or fantasies of glory, power, or idealized love. Personal defects are not tolerated. Grooming, dress, and makeup capture large amounts of time and must be impeccably done. The grand gesture is preferred, and entrances and exits are preferably done with a flourish. These people regard themselves as omniscient and omnipotent; they rarely permit themselves to stoop to ask others for assistance.

These patients tend to gravitate toward those who, in one way or another, reflect their grandiose image of themselves. The company of other "ideal creatures" is often quite satisfactory, yet if any fault is found within these acquaintances, they are discarded as unworthy. Admirers are tolerated, perhaps even welcomed at times, but are quickly discarded should any criticism be offered. Others are exploited for what they can do for the narcissistic person; of themselves they seem to have little value.

These people do not have truly reciprocal relationships with others. They may be socially correct, even polite, yet they are perceived as frosty and distant. They seem to lack a capacity for empathy or intimacy. Should an acquaintance be in need, their only motive for offering help would be to demonstrate their own power. These people do not make "anonymous" gifts of time or money and are rarely willing to sacrifice anything of their own.

People with narcissistic personality disorder do not tolerate unfavorable comparison with others. Should another's achievements seem to shine more brightly, these people may become intensely envious, even enraged, and often attempt to belittle or devalue the accomplishments of others. Should this fail to salve their wounded self-esteem, they often seek revenge. Any degree of criticism seems to touch them to the mortal quick; a vicious counterattack may occur, or, if that appears unlikely to succeed, they may withdraw from the field with a cold regal disdain and contempt for their opponents.

Others often feel exploited and manipulated by a narcissistic person. They feel as if they are regarded as mere pawns in the narcissist's life and, often in short order, come to regard the narcissist as abrasive and arrogant.

COURSE

This disorder is chronic and lifelong; with age, however, the clinical picture may change. These people are often intolerant of the inevitable decline that comes with age and often develop lingering, mild depressive symptoms.

COMPLICATIONS

Social and occupational complications follow inevitably from the symptoms of this disorder. The inability to love another or to form a friendship leaves these people with a sense of loneliness and isolation. Work may or may not suffer. If the narcissistic person happens to be talented, then the drive for admiration and praise may lead to brilliant success. However, should the narcissist happen to have only a normal complement of abilities, the inability to ask for or accept help leaves the narcissist stumbling and failing to accomplish what others, who can work cooperatively, are able to do.

ETIOLOGY

Although theories abound, nothing is known with certainty regarding the etiology of narcissistic personality disorder.

DIFFERENTIAL DIAGNOSIS

Four other personality disorders may at times enter into the differential diagnosis: antisocial, histrionic, obsessive-compulsive, and borderline.

In antisocial personality disorder one often sees vanity and always sees a persistent exploitation of others. Here, however, the purpose of the exploitation is for financial or material gain. This contrasts with narcissistic personality disorder, wherein financial gain may not even be an issue, so long as the narcissist's sense of personal glory is enhanced.

Those with histrionic personality disorder are notoriously vain and anxious to be in the spotlight of attention. Here, however, one finds a willingness to depend on others and to become strongly emotionally involved with them. This contrasts with narcissistic personality disorder, wherein a cool distance is kept between the narcissist and others, the narcissist being no more involved with others than with a trinket, which is discarded without sentiment as soon as it loses its luster.

Those with obsessive-compulsive personality disorder often evidence an air of superiority and conduct themselves with condescension toward others. Here, however, the smug sense of superiority derives from a perceived adherence to a rigid code of conduct, which others most regrettably fall short of. In contrast, in narcissistic personality disorder the grandiose superiority seems to rest on nothing. One sees no smugness about narcissists; they counterattack, sometimes with viciousness, should a stone of criticism approach the fragile vessel of their self-esteem.

Those with borderline personality disorder may affect an air of regal indifference and often tend to either devalue or idealize others. Here, however, longer observation reveals intense and dramatic swings in their self-conception and mood. Furthermore, one finds an almost frighteningly intense yearning for relationships with others, as if the borderline wished to fuse with them. This contrasts with narcissistic personality disorder, wherein the narcissist's behavior remains remarkably stable over time and rarely indicates an interest in friendship or love.

TREATMENT

Patients with narcissistic personality disorder have been treated with individual psychotherapy, group psychotherapy, and family therapy, and each method has anecdotally been reported as successful. However, no controlled outcomes studies have been carried out.

Apart from treating intercurrent disorders, especially depression, pharmacologic treatment is of no avail.

BIBLIOGRAPHY

Akhtar S. Narcissistic personality disorder: descriptive features and differential diagnosis. *The Psychiatric Clinics of North America* 1989; 12: 505-529.

Gunderson JG, Ronningstam E. Differentiating narcissistic and antisocial personality disorders. *Journal of Personality Disorders* 2001;15: 103-109.

Gunderson JG, Ronningstam E, Bodkin A. The diagnostic interview for narcissistic patients. *Archives of General Psychiatry* 1990;47: 676-680.

Ronningstam E. Comparing three systems for diagnosing narcissistic personality disorders. *Psychiatry* 1988;51:300-311.

Ronningstam E, Gunderson J. Identifying criteria for narcissistic personality disorder. *The American Journal of Psychiatry* 1990;147:918-922.

141 Avoidant Personality Disorder (DSM-IV-TR #301.82)

Avoidant personality disorder is characterized by timidity, social awkwardness, and a pervasive sense of inadequacy and fear of criticism. The lifetime prevalence of this disorder is in the range of 0.5 to 1%, and it is equally common among males and females.

As noted below, there is some doubt as to whether avoidant personality disorder represents a disorder *sui generis*, or, rather, is merely a form of very early onset, severe social phobia of the generalized type.

ONSET

The onset may be either in adolescence or in childhood, and may be marked by undue shyness and timidity.

CLINICAL FEATURES

These individuals characteristically view themselves as socially inept and awkward, and although desirous, sometimes desperately so, for intimate relations, they are so fearful of embarrassing or humiliating themselves in social situations that they remain withdrawn and self-effacing. In situations where others offer strong reassurance of acceptance, these individuals may be willing to venture into a social setting, but once there they remain tense, inhibited, and unwilling to relax for fear of making a misstep or doing something embarrassing.

Tragically, the conviction that these individuals have that they will be criticized and rejected often becomes a self-fulfilling prophecy, as others, spotting their painful timidity, may either avoid them or hold them up to ridicule.

COURSE

This disorder, although chronic, may lessen in severity as patients age.

COMPLICATIONS

Patients have great difficulty sustaining relationships or functioning in work situations that require any sort of assertiveness.

ETIOLOGY

Although unproven, it is thought by many authorities that avoidant personality disorder is no different from a very early onset social phobia of the generalized type.

DIFFERENTIAL DIAGNOSIS

Distinguishing avoidant personality disorder from very early onset social phobia of the generalized type may not be possible, as this disorder may merely be, as noted above, a form of social phobia.

Schizoid personality disorder is distinguished by an absence of interest in social relations.

Dependent personality disorder is distinguished by the differential response to the presence of a supportive figure: whereas dependent types may flourish and become active under such an aegis, avoidant types remain timid and fearful.

Dysthymia is distinguished by pervasive fatigue, anhedonia, and other vegetative signs and symptoms.

TREATMENT

Social skills training, combined with cognitive behavioral therapy, appears to be helpful. Given the probable identity between avoidant personality disorder and generalized social phobia, it is reasonable to treat these patients pharmacologically in a fashion similar to that described in Chapter 86.

BIBLIOGRAPHY

Alden LE, Laposa JM, Taylor CT, et al. Avoidant personality disorder: current status and future directions. *Journal of Personality Disorders* 2002;16:1-29.

Baillie AJ, Lampe LA. Avoidant personality disorder: empirical support for DSM-IV revisions. *Journal of Personality Disorders* 1998;12:23-30.

Schneier FR, Spitzer RL, Gibbon M, et al. The relationship of social phobia subtypes and avoidant personality disorder. *Comprehensive Psychiatry* 1991;32:496-502.

van Velzen CJ, Emmelkamp PM, Scholing A. Generalized social phobia versus avoidant personality disorder: differences in psychopathology, personality traits, and social and occupational functioning. *Journal of Anxiety Disorders* 2000;14:395-411.

142 Obsessive-Compulsive Personality Disorder (DSM-IV-TR #301.4)

Persons with an obsessive-compulsive personality disorder are typically rigid and perfectionistic. Their lives are orderly and carefully controlled; they give undue attention to details, rules, and schedules. These people rarely display any emotion and seem to march through life with a stultifying, regimental thoroughness.

The name given to this personality disorder is perhaps unfortunate, as it suggests an intimate relationship with obsessive-compulsive disorder, whereas in fact these two disorders indeed may not be related. Synonyms for the personality disorder include "compulsive personality disorder" and "anankastic personality disorder."

Obsessive-compulsive personality disorder occurs in about 1% of the general population.

ONSET

Obsessive-compulsive traits are often apparent in adolescence; by late adolescence or early adult years the gradual coalescence into the disorder has usually occurred.

CLINICAL FEATURES

These people appear to be saturated with scruples; moral rectitude seems second nature. Their lives are scheduled and orderly; perfectionism and cleanliness characterize their behavior. Details demand incisive attention, and lists and timetables are extensively used. Emotions are handled with intense care; displays of emotion are avoided, and the person's affect is constricted and tight.

Decisions are extremely difficult to make; these people are generally unwilling to decide unless they are absolutely certain that their decision is the one and only correct one. Motives and arguments are incessantly weighed in the balance, and just as the person appears to be leaning toward one decision or the other, another countervailing argument tips the scales back into a paralyzing indecision. Once, however, a decision is made, there is no turning back, and the new course of action is followed with single-minded intensity.

These people are often stubborn. They resent and resist any attempts of others to control them. Demands are met with a rigid defiance, as if any sign of weakness or relaxation on the patient's part would mean the destruction of autonomy and integrity. They are often frugal and parsimonious, at times miserly and unwilling to give anything away.

The relationships that these people form are often strained, stilted, and tense. They apply their own inflexible standards to others and insist that things are done the "correct" way. Their work and family lives are often formal and rigidly conformist. They seek to exercise a tyranny of rectitude over others and may become enraged when others dare to stray from the selected path.

Dysthymia or major depression are not uncommon in these people; some may develop hypochondriasis.

COURSE

Although this is a chronic disorder, some appear to relax as they enter middle and later years.

COMPLICATIONS

In mild cases, few complications may occur. If these people find work that demands attention to detail and generally relieves them of the responsibility for independent decisions, they may do quite well occupationally. Likewise, if the spouse is submissive, one may see little overt marital friction.

When symptoms are more severe, however, this disorder may be incapacitating. Lost in detail and paralyzed by indecision, these people may not be able to take action or produce a completed piece of work. Potentially pleasurable occasions, such as vacations, are turned into chores.

ETIOLOGY

Obsessive-compulsive personality disorder tends to run in families, and these persons tend to be the oldest in their sibships. It is not clear, however, whether this personality disorder is secondary to rigid upbringing or to a congenitally determined temperamental style.

DIFFERENTIAL DIAGNOSIS

As noted earlier, obsessive-compulsive personality disorder must be clearly distinguished from obsessive-compulsive disorder. Although patients with obsessive-compulsive disorder may also have an obsessive-compulsive personality disorder, they are just as likely to have some other personality disorder, or no personality disorder at all. Patients with obsessive-compulsive disorder have true obsessions and true compulsions, symptoms that are not found in uncomplicated obsessive-compulsive personality disorder.

People with a narcissistic personality disorder are concerned with perfection and correctness; however, here the concern springs from their desire for adulation, in contrast with the person with obsessive-compulsive personality disorder whose desire for perfectionism has its roots in fear and guilt.

TREATMENT

In contrast with patients with other personality disorders, these patients may be aware of the suffering their behavior engenders and may seek treatment. Medications do not appear helpful. Although no controlled studies are available that demonstrate a favorable influence by psychotherapy, these patients are generally seen in individual or group psychotherapy.

BIBLIOGRAPHY

Baer L, Jenike MA, Ricciardi JN, et al. Standardized assessment of personality disorders in obsessive-compulsive disorder. *Archives of General Psychiatry* 1990;47:826-830.

Bejerot S, Ekselius L, von Knorring L. Comorbidity between obsessive-compulsive disorder (OCD) and personality disorders. *Acta Psychiatrica Scandinavica* 1998;97:398-402.

Black DW, Noyes R, Pfohl B, et al. Personality disorder in obsessive-compulsive volunteers, well comparison subjects and their first-degree relatives. *The American Journal of Psychiatry* 1993;150:1226-1232.

Shapiro D. *Neurotic styles.* New York, 1965, Basic Books.

Skodol AE, Gunderson JG, McGlashan TH, et al. Functional impairment in patients with schizotypal, borderline, avoidant, or obsessive-compulsive personality disorder. *The American Journal of Psychiatry* 2002;159:276-283.

143 Passive-Aggressive Personality Disorder

People with passive-aggressive personality disorder automatically, almost instinctively, see any demand, request, or expectation, no matter how fair or reasonable, as unwarranted, unjust, and excessive. They see themselves as unfairly burdened, singled out, put upon. They live in resentment toward those who make demands on them, yet do not become openly hostile or angry. Rather, by all manner of sabotage and covert action, they seek to bring those who make demands to frustration, failure, and dismay.

Recently, whether or not passive-aggressive personality disorder actually exists as a discrete, identifiable entity has been debated, and the subject has been relegated to an appendix in DSM-IV, where it is also called "negativistic personality disorder." Recent work, however, suggests that reports of this disorder's demise are perhaps exaggerated, and further research is clearly needed.

ONSET

History often reveals that adults with passive-aggressive personality disorder displayed these traits in childhood; by late adolescence the traits have usually gradually become entrenched.

CLINICAL FEATURES

Symptoms are most likely to appear in settings where demands are routinely made, for example in the workplace or, most especially, the military. These patients, though appearing sullen and resentful, do not openly protest when asked to do something; indeed they may appear quite compliant with their superiors' wishes. Later, however, they may complain to their fellow workers about how unfair and unreasonable these demands are. Practical hints from co-workers as to how to get the job done with the minimal amount of effort are often brushed aside.

The superficial nature of the compliance of these people is often apparent to those around them. Dawdling, foot dragging, and all manner of inefficiencies and minor mistakes are common. Passive-aggressive people may claim to have "forgotten" central items; multiple excuses are offered for slowness. If taken to task by higher authorities, they may vigorously protest their innocence; occasionally, resentment may leak out in bitter accusations about the injustice of the demands laid on them. The threat of dismissal or punishment fails of its purpose; these people often become more stubborn and may become argumentative. At times they may actively seek revenge, and literally throw a wrench into the works; they may experience a bitter satisfaction if they are fired; it proves to them that they were right.

In extreme cases, these people may come to resent the expectations inherent in the routine activities of daily living. Grooming, bathing, even dressing themselves may be experienced as unreasonably burdensome. Should a family member, perhaps offended by body odor, insist on a bath, passive-aggressive people may take to bed, with the covers pulled over their eyes, for days. They allow others to dress them or bathe them, yet they refuse to give in and do it themselves.

Alcohol abuse or alcoholism may occur; dysthymia or major depression may also be seen. Hypochondriacal complaints are not uncommon. Rarely, suicide may occur.

COURSE

Passive-aggressive personality disorder is chronic and may not "burn out" as do some other personality disorders.

COMPLICATIONS

Passive-aggressive people may be fired or denied promotion; military service may be marked by time in the stockade or by a less than honorable discharge. Households may go untended; some patients literally live in filth. Disgusted spouses eventually abandon them.

ETIOLOGY

Although theories abound, nothing is known for certain regarding the etiology of passive-aggressive personality disorder.

DIFFERENTIAL DIAGNOSIS

Passive-aggressive behavior may occur in almost anyone and may at times be appropriate. For example, among prisoners of war forced into slave labor, inefficiency and obstructionism are praised. The difference here is that the prisoner of war has a purpose that goes beyond merely frustrating demands. Given the opportunity, the prisoner of war may rise up in more overt rebellion and after release work effectively at peacetime pursuits. By contrast, the person with passive-aggressive personality disorder does not overtly rise up and never works efficiently, regardless of what rewards are offered.

Those with paranoid personality disorder may resent demands and refuse to follow through; however, they are much more open in their hostility than the passive-aggressive patient. Accusations may be openly made, and naked, overt threats may follow.

Negativism, as seen in catatonic schizophrenia, may present as a mulish resistance to any demands. Other signs, such as waxy flexibility, stupor, and the like, suggest, however, the correct diagnosis.

TREATMENT

Most passive-aggressive people do not seek treatment; those who do may see it only as a means whereby their complaints may be vindicated. Individual or group psychotherapy is generally offered; however, their passive-aggressive behavior in treatment is usually successful in frustrating all therapeutic efforts. Most drop out of treatment early.

No systematic medication trials have been carried out for this disorder.

BIBLIOGRAPHY

Schneider K. *Psychopathic personalities,* Springfield, 1958, Charles C. Thomas.

Small IF, Small JG, Alig VB, et al. Passive-aggressive personality disorder: a search for a syndrome. *The American Journal of Psychiatry* 1970;126:973-983.

Sprock J, Hunsucker L. Symptoms of prototypic patients with passive-aggressive personality disorder: DSM-IIIR versus DSMIV negativistic. *Comprehensive Psychiatry* 1998;39:287-295.

Vereycken J, Vertommen H, Corveleyn J. Authority conflicts and personality disorders. *Journal of Personality Disorders* 2002;16:41-51.

Weltzer S, Morey LC. Passive-aggressive personality disorder: the demise of a syndrome. *Psychiatry* 1999;62:49-59.

MEDICATION-INDUCED DISORDERS

144 Anticholinergic Delirium

In sufficient dosage, any drug with anticholinergic properties capable of crossing the blood-brain barrier may cause a delirium (see the box on this page); certain plants, at times consumed for their intoxicating effect, may also cause an anticholinergic delirium and these include jimson weed (*Datura stramomium*) and Angel's Trumpet (*Datura sauveulons*).

The very young and the very old appear to be particularly vulnerable; indeed in some cases anticholinergic ophthalmic preparations passing down the lacrimal duct and absorbed through the nasal mucosa have caused delirium. Anticholinergic drugs also often play a significant part in the development of "post-operative" delirium.

ONSET

Onset may vary from gradual to acute, depending on the rapidity with which the blood level rises.

CLINICAL FEATURES

Typically the patient is restless and may be excited or agitated. Confusion, poor short-term memory, and disorientation may follow, and visual hallucinations are common.

The mouth is dry, the vision blurred, and the skin is hot and dry. In severe cases the skin may be scarlet. The pulse is rapid, the pupils dilated, and, if the ambient temperature is high, the body temperature may rise. Urinary retention may occur. In severe cases, dysarthria and seizures may occur.

With even higher doses, coma may occur, followed by cardio-respiratory depression and death.

COURSE

In the natural course of events, if the patient survives, a full recovery is expected at a time consistent with the half-life of the offending agent. Upon recovery, one sees a variable degree of amnesia for the delirium.

COMPLICATIONS

The complications of delirium are as described in that chapter.

ETIOLOGY

Central effects of the anticholinergic agent plus paralysis of the peripheral parasympathetic system account for most symptoms.

DIFFERENTIAL DIAGNOSIS

Heat stroke is clinically similar to an anticholinergic delirium. Here, however, the temperature is higher, typically over 106 degrees Fahrenheit, and a history of significant exposure to anticholinergic agents is lacking. The differential at times, however, can be confusing, as anticholinergic agents predispose to heat strokes by reducing sweating. Clearly, if the ambient temperature is low, heat stroke can be ruled out. In a heat wave, however, when the dose of anticholinergic ingested is substantial, then one might be confronted with a mixture of both anticholinergic delirium and heat stroke.

TREATMENT

Efforts to prevent further absorption, such as gastric lavage and activated charcoal, are accompanied by general supportive care, including intravenous fluids and, if the temperature is elevated, cooling blankets and fanning. Seizures may be treated with intravenous lorazepam.

In emergent situations, physostigmine may be given in a dose of 0.5 to 2 mg intravenously, at a rate no faster than 1 mg/minute, every 5 to 10 minutes until the patient is out of danger. Given that the half-life of each of the offending anticholinergic agents is considerably longer than the half-life of physostigmine, repeat doses are generally required, initially every 30 to 60 minutes. A failure to respond to physostigmine essentially rules out the diagnosis of anticholinergic delirium.

Given that physostigmine may cause bradycardia, asystole and seizures, there is debate as to its indications in anticholinergic delirium. In mild cases, it is probably appropriate to simply

---

Drugs that May Cause an Anticholinergic Delirium

Tricyclic antidepressants*	Antiparkinsonian anticholinergics*
Antipsychotics* (especially	Benztropine
"low-potency" antipsychotics)	Trihexyphenidyl
Antihistamines	Biperidin
Diphenhydramine*	Belladona alkaloids
Hydroxyzine*	Atropine
	Scopalamine
	Hyoscyamine
	Homatropine

*Covered in the respective chapter.

provide supportive care while the offending agent "washes out"; furthermore it must be kept in mind that, in the case of tricyclic overdose, where arrhythmias are the main concern, physostigmine does not offer any protection from cardiac effects. In severe cases, however, where agitation or tachycardia are life-threatening, or where the temperature must be urgently brought down, the use of physostigmine may be justified. In such cases, it is appropriate to have the patient under cardiac monitoring while physostigmine is in use.

BIBLIOGRAPHY

Baldessarini RJ, Gelenberg AJ. Using physostigmine safely. *The American Journal of Psychiatry* 1979;136:1608-1609.

Beaver KM, Gavin TJ. Treatment of acute anticholinergic poisoning with physostigmine. *The American Journal of Emergency Medicine* 1998;16:505-507.

Brizer DA, Manning DW. Delirium induced by poisoning with anticholinergic agents. *The American Journal of Psychiatry* 1982;139:1343-1344.

Burns MJ, Linden CH, Graudins A, et al. A comparison of physostigmine and benzodiazepines for the treatment of anticholinergic poisoning. *Annals of Emergency Medicine* 2000;35:374-381.

Duvoisin RC, Katz R. Reversal of central anticholinergic syndrome in man by physostigmine. *Journal of American Medical Association* 1968; 206:1963-1695.

Dyer CB, Ashton CM, Teasdale TA. Postoperative delirium. A review of 80 primary data-collection studies. *Archives of Internal Medicine* 1995; 155:461-465.

EI-Yousef MK, Janowsky D, Davis JM, et al. Reversal of antiparkinsonian drug toxicity by physostigmine: a controlled study. *The American Journal of Psychiatry* 1973;130:141-145.

Hall RC, Popkin MK, McHenry LE. Angel's Trumpet psychosis: a central nervous system anticholinergic syndrome. *The American Journal of Psychiatry* 1977;134:312-314.

Han L, McCusker J, Cole M, et al. Use of medications with anticholinergic effect predicts clinical severity of delirium symptoms in older medical inpatients. *Archives of Internal Medicine* 2001;161:1099-1105.

Tune LE. Anticholinergic effects of medication in elderly patients. *The Journal of Clinical Psychiatry* 2001;62(Suppl 21):11-14.

Tune LE, Bylsma FW, Hilt DC. Anticholinergic delirium caused by topical homatropine ophthalmic solution: confirmation by anticholinergic radioreceptor assay in two cases. *The Journal of Neuropsychiatry and Clinical Neurosciences* 1992;4:197.

145 Cholinergic Rebound

The abrupt discontinuation of long-term treatment with agents possessing anticholinergic activity may be followed by a syndrome known as cholinergic rebound. A synonym for this is cholinergic overdrive.

This syndrome occurs in about 30% of such cases of abrupt discontinuation, and, as one of its symptoms may be depression, it is of great importance to psychiatric practice.

ONSET

The length of the interval between discontinuation of the drug and the onset of symptoms is determined by the half-life of the drug. In the case of most tricyclic antidepressants, which have half-lives of a little less than a day, cholinergic rebound typically occurs within 36 to 48 hours.

CLINICAL FEATURES

In its fully developed form, the syndrome is characterized by depressed mood, anxiety, insomnia, nausea and abdominal cramping, with or without vomiting and diarrhea.

COURSE

In untreated patients, symptoms gradually resolve over 1 to 3 days.

COMPLICATIONS

The main complication arises from misdiagnosis. If the depressed mood and insomnia are mistaken for a recurrence of depression, then antidepressant treatment may be needlessly restarted.

ETIOLOGY

Chronic treatment with drugs possessing anticholinergic properties causes an up-regulation of postsynaptic acetylcholine receptors. This occurs with anticholinergic antiparkinsonian drugs (such as benztropine), low-potency first-generation antipsychotics, clozapine and tricyclic antidepressants. When these agents are gradually tapered, enough time is available for down-regulation, but when they are abruptly discontinued the up-regulated receptors are "unmasked," and cholinergic "overdrive" occurs. Symptoms are similar to those seen with physostigmine infusion.

DIFFERENTIAL DIAGNOSIS

A relapse of a depressive episode may be distinguished from cholinergic rebound by the abruptness of onset. Depressive relapses, if they are going to occur, appear slowly, perhaps one or two weeks after discontinuation of the tricyclic; by contrast, cholinergic rebound appears rapidly, within days.

TREATMENT

The best treatment is prevention: drugs with anticholinergic properties should, if possible, be tapered gradually, at a rate of no more than one quarter of the daily dose per day. This rule also holds true when one is planning to immediately start a different drug that does not have anticholinergic effects. For example, if one were to switch from a tricyclic to fluoxetine, from a low-potency antipsychotic to a high-potency first-generation one, or from clozapine to an antipsychotic with low anticholinergic potential (e.g., olanzapine or risperidone) then the initial drug should be tapered gradually. By contrast, if one were switching from desipramine to nortriptyline, which have comparable anticholinergic effects, one would not need to taper the desipramine, but one would simply stop it and immediately start the nortriptyline.

In cases where cholinergic rebound does occur, some patients may elect to simply wait it out. For others, however, the symptoms are sufficiently distressing as to warrant treatment. If restarting the discontinued drug is not feasible, then one may give a small dose of benztropine, e.g., 1 or 2 mg. Once symptoms are controlled, a gradual tapering is then undertaken.

BIBLIOGRAPHY

Delassus-Guenault N, Jegouzo A, Odou P, et al. Clozapine-olanzapine: a potentially dangerous switch. A report of two cases. *Journal of Clinical Pharmacy and Therapeutics* 1999;24:191-195.

Dilsaver SC. Antidepressant withdrawal syndromes: phenomenology and pathophysiology. *Acta Psychiatrica Scandinavica* 1989;79:113-117.

Dilsaver SC, Feinberg M, Greden JF. Antidepressant withdrawal symptoms treated with anticholinergic agents. *The American Journal of Psychiatry* 1983;140:249-251.

Hirose S. Insomnia related to biperidin withdrawal in two schizophrenic patients. *International Clinical Psychopharmacology* 2000;15:357-359.

Wolfe RM. Antidepressant withdrawal reactions. *American Family Physician* 1997;56:455-462.

146 Serotonin Syndrome

The serotonin syndrome, characterized classically by delirium and myoclonus, is a potentially fatal complication arising from any pharmacologic maneuver which abruptly increases serotoninergic tone in the central nervous system.

ONSET

The onset occurs within hours or days of one of the pharmacologic maneuvers noted below.

CLINICAL FEATURES

The most common presentation is with a variable combination of delirium, agitation, tachycardia, diaphoresis, myoclonus and hyperreflexia. Other clinical features include shivering, coarse tremors and extensor plantar responses. In severe cases, one may see hyperthermia, seizures, rhabdomyolysis, renal failure, cardiac arrhythmias and disseminated intravascular coagulation.

COURSE

Although potentially fatal, most patients survive the syndrome, and, provided that serotoninergic tone is decreased (if only by discontinuation of the offending medications), symptoms undergo substantial resolution within anywhere from a day to a week.

COMPLICATIONS

In those who survive, full recovery occurs, generally without sequelae.

ETIOLOGY

This syndrome occurs secondary to any one of a large number of pharmacologic maneuvers, all of which have in common the effect of enhancing central nervous system serotoninergic tone. Table 146-1 lists various combinations of medicines that have been implicated in causing the syndrome. It must be emphasized that most of these combinations, in fact, are safely used, and that the incidence of the serotonin syndrome with them is very, very low. One exception to this reassuring note is the combination of an MAOI and either an SSRI or venlafaxine, combinations that are strongly associated with the serotonin syndrome and which should not be used.

Other combinations rarely associated with the serotonin syndrome include the following: MAOIs and either dextromethorphan or meperidine; an SSRI with pentazocine; an SSRI with levodopa; an SSRI with risperidone; an SSRI with lithium and olanzapine; and an SSRI with linezolid (a relatively new antibiotic useful in methicillin-resistant staphylococcal infections).

There are also rare reports of the serotonin syndrome occurring secondary to monotherapy with fluoxetine, venlafaxine and mirtazapine.

DIFFERENTIAL DIAGNOSIS

The occurrence of delirium in the setting of one of the pharmacologic maneuvers noted above should immediately suggest the diagnosis. Should the medication history be unknown, the combination of delirium and myoclonus may suggest hepatic encephalopathy, uremic encephalopathy, hyponatremia or hypomagnesemia, each of which may be checked for with appropriate laboratory testing.

The neuroleptic malignant syndrome is distinguished clinically by an absence of myoclonus and by the presence of rigidity; furthermore, whereas an elevated temperature may be seen in both the neuroleptic malignant syndrome and the serotonin syndrome, it occurs earlier in the evolution of the neuroleptic malignant syndrome.

TREATMENT

The offending medications must be discontinued, and the patient should be provided with vigorous supportive care. Cyproheptadine, a serotonin antagonist, should be given orally, by nasogastric tube if necessary, in a dose of 4 to 8 mg every two hours until the patient is out of danger or a maximum dose of 32 mg is reached. Most patients respond to one or two doses.

■TABLE 146-1. Medication Combinations Associated with the Serotonin Syndrome

	MAOI	SSRI	cmi	vlfx	tca	trypt	busp	mirt	suma	cbz	li	traz	bup
MAOI		X	X	X	X	X							
SSRI	X			X	X	X	X	X	X	X			
cmi	X					X							
vlfx	X										X		
tca	X	X											
trypt	X	X	X										
busp		X										X	
mirt		X											
suma		X									X		
cbz		X											
li				X					X				
traz							X						X
bup												X	

Key: MAOI, monoamine oxidase inhibitor; SSRI, selective serotonin reuptake inhibitor; cmi, clomipramine; vlfx, venlafaxine; tca, tricyclic; trypt, tryptophan; busp, buspirone; mirt, mirtazapine; suma, sumatriptan; cbz, carbamazepine; li, lithium; traz, trazodone; bup, bupropion.

BIBLIOGRAPHY

Avarello TP, Cottone S. Serotonin syndrome: a reported case. *Neurological Sciences* 2002;23(Suppl 2):55-56.

Bernard L, Stern R, Lew D, et al. Serotonin syndrome after concomitant treatment with linezolid and citalopram. *Clinical Infectious Diseases* 2003;26:1197.

Gardner DM, Lynd LD. Sumatriptan contraindications and the serotonin syndrome. *The Annals of Pharmacotherapy* 1998;32:33-38.

Graudins A, Stearman A, Chan B. Treatment of the serotonin syndrome with cyproheptadine. *The Journal of Emergency Medicine* 1998;16:615-619.

Haslett CD, Kumar S. Can olanzapine be implicated in causing the serotonin syndrome? *Psychiatry and Clinical Neruosciences* 2002;56:533-535.

Hernandez JL, Ramos FJ, Infante J, et al. Severe serotonin syndrome induced by mirtazapine monotherapy. *The Annals of Pharmacotherapy* 2002;36:641-643.

Karki SD, Masood GR. Combination risperidone and SSRI-induced serotonin syndrome. *The Annals of Pharmacotherapy* 2003;33:388-391.

Mason PJ, Morris VA, Balcezak TJ. Serotonin syndrome. Presentation of 2 cases and review of the literature. *Medicine* 2000;79:201-209.

Pan JJ, Shen WW. Serotonin syndrome induced by low-dose venlafaxine. *The Annals of Pharmacotherapy* 2003;37:209-211.

Sternbach H. The serotonin syndrome. *The American Journal of Psychiatry* 1991;148:705-713.

147 Neuroleptic Malignant Syndrome (DSM-IV-TR #333.92)

The neuroleptic malignant syndrome is a rare and potentially fatal syndrome, characterized primarily by delirium, fever, rigidity, and autonomic instability, that occurs secondary to an abrupt diminution in dopaminergic tone, either due to the use of a dopamine blocking agent, such as an antipsychotic (also known as a neuroleptic), or, much less commonly, to withdrawal of a dopaminergic agent, such as levodopa. This is a rare syndrome, and occurs in less than 1% of antipsychotic-treated patients.

ONSET

Although the neuroleptic malignant syndrome may occur at any age, most patients are young adults. In cases secondary to treatment with antipsychotics, the onset is usually within a day or two of either beginning treatment or significantly increasing the dose; the latency, however, between the institution of the dopamine blockade and the onset of the syndrome is wide, with cases occurring within from hours to weeks or even months. The first sign is usually some rigidity that is either accompanied, or shortly followed, by fever, with the full syndrome generally evolving over 1 to 3 days.

CLINICAL FEATURES

The fully developed syndrome is marked by delirium, fever, rigidity, and autonomic instability. Delirium may become profound, and may merge into stupor; catatonic signs are often also in evidence. Fever ranges up to 102 degrees Fahrenheit, and in some cases much higher. Rigidity is generalized and may be extreme; tremor is often present and is generally coarse, and lacking in any pill-rolling. Autonomic instability may manifest with tachycardia, labile blood pressure, pallor, and diaphoresis, which may be profound.

The majority of patients experience rhabdomyolysis with myoglobulinuria, which, in severe cases, may cause acute renal failure. Most patients likewise display an elevated CK, at times as high as 15,000, along with an elevated white blood cell count, often over 15,000. LDH, AST, and alkaline phosphatase may also be increased.

In severe cases, respiratory failure may occur, and this may be multifactorial in etiology. In some cases, muscular rigidity of the chest wall musculature may be so severe that breathing simply becomes impossible; in other cases one may find evidence of pulmonary emboli arising from deep vein thrombi or aspiration pneumonia. A dreaded complication is disseminated intravascular coagulation.

Although the occurrence of the full tetrad of delirium, fever, rigidity, and autonomic instability in the setting of an abrupt diminution of dopaminergic tone leaves little doubt as to the diagnosis, there is debate as to the definition of milder forms of the syndrome. For example, when second-generation antipsychotics are involved, rigidity is often relatively mild and indeed may be absent. Tentatively, and from a practical point of view, the occurrence of any two of the tetrad in the appropriate pharmacologic setting should at the least raise one's diagnostic index of suspicion.

COURSE

Mortality may range from 10% or 20%, with most deaths occurring secondary to respiratory failure. In those who survive, symptoms gradually abate, provided that dopaminergic status is normalized, over a week or two. As might be expected, if the neuroleptic malignant syndrome were secondary to a depot antipsychotic, such as haloperidol decanoate or fluphenazine decanoate, then the course would be much longer, stretching to weeks or a month or more. Exceptionally, rigidity or catatonic signs may persist for many months, even in cases where a depot antipsychotic had not been used.

COMPLICATIONS

Although most who survive recover completely, exceptions do occur. Severe hypoxia during respiratory failure may lead to an anoxic encephalopathy, and grossly elevated temperatures may leave patients demented or with cerebellar damage.

ETIOLOGY

As noted earlier, the neuroleptic malignant syndrome occurs secondary to an abrupt diminution of dopaminergic tone. In most cases this is due to treatment with an antipsychotic, generally a high potency first-generation agent, such as haloperidol. The syndrome, however, has also been seen with low-potency first-generation agents, such as chlorpromazine, and with second-generation agents, such as olanzapine, risperidone, quetiapine, or clozapine. Other dopamine blockers capable of causing the syndrome include metoclopramide and promethazine; amoxapine, a tricyclic antidepressant metabolized to loxapine, an antipsychotic, has also been implicated. Furthermore, it appears that concurrent treatment with lithium may increase the risk of developing the syndrome.

Dopaminergic tone may also undergo a profound diminution if chronic treatment with dopaminergic agents is suddenly stopped or the dose is significantly reduced, and this has been noted in patients treated with levodopa, amantadine, or bromocriptine; in one case a mere abrupt switch from bromocriptine to pergolide precipitated the syndrome. Recognition of the syndrome in this setting has been hampered by its name, in that clearly no "neuroleptic" has been involved. A better name, and one that might not stand in the way of accurate diagnosis, might be "hypodopaminergic malignant syndrome."

Although it is currently unclear why only a minority of patients subjected to the same pharmacologic manipulations go on to develop the syndrome, some evidence suggests that the presence of certain alleles of the DRD2 gene may create a predisposition to the syndrome.

Although the mechanism whereby this abrupt diminution of dopaminergic tone produces the syndrome is not known with certainty, it is strongly suspected that there is a corresponding profound disturbance of hypothalamic functioning, and indeed in one autopsied case, necrotic changes were present in both anterior and lateral hypothalamic nuclei.

DIFFERENTIAL DIAGNOSIS

Malignant hyperthermia is distinguished by its association with the use of succinylcholine or inhalation anesthetics. Another, not uncommon cause of hyperthermia and delirium, heat stroke, is suggested by its occurrence during a heat wave or with strenuous exercise in hot weather and also by the presence of hot, dry skin and the lack of rigidity, both in marked contrast to the diaphoresis and rigidity of the neuroleptic malignant syndrome.

Recently a syndrome very similar to that seen in the neuroleptic malignant syndrome has been reported secondary to abrupt withdrawal of long-term treatment with either intrathecal or oral baclofen. Whether this represents a distinct syndrome or not is as yet unclear; it is clear, though, that the syndrome resolves with reinstatement of baclofen or with treatment with another GABAergic agent, such as a benzodiazepine.

Patients with parkinsonism who become febrile, as for example with a pneumonia, may resemble those with the neuroleptic malignant syndrome; however, certain features allow for a differential. First, if the dose of the dopaminergic agent had not been decreased, the diagnosis of neuroleptic malignant syndrome is very unlikely; second, although parkinsonian rigidity may increase with intercurrent illnesses, it still retains its "pill-rolling" character, a feature absent in the neuroleptic malignant syndrome.

Severe intoxication with phencyclidine is distinguished by the absence of rigidity and by the presence of myoclonus and nystagmus.

Lethal catatonia (also known as Stauder's lethal catatonia) may present a clinical picture very similar to that of neuroleptic malignant syndrome. Helpful diagnostic points include the history of antecedent catatonic symptoms and especially the resolution of the syndrome with parenteral lorazepam.

St. Louis encephalitis may be distinguished by the presence of stiff neck, prominent tremor, and the relative absence of rigidity in addition to the absence of any of the pharmacologic manipulations described earlier.

TREATMENT

Given the high mortality rate, hospitalization is necessary, and in some cases treatment in an intensive care unit may be required. Intensive supportive care is indicated, with particular attention to fluid and electrolyte balance: adequate hydration must be insured to reduce the risk of acute renal failure when rhabdomyolysis occurs. An elevated temperature may be treated with a cooling blanket, and adequate respiratory support must always be close at hand.

Efforts should also be undertaken to restore dopaminergic tone. Antipsychotics and other dopamine blockers should be stopped, and if the syndrome were due to discontinuation of a dopaminergic agent, it should, if possible, be restarted. Although there are no controlled studies of the pharmacologic treatment of the neuroleptic malignant syndrome, two drugs have substantial anecdotal support. Bromocriptine may be given orally, by nasogastric tube if necessary, in doses of from 2.5 to 20 mg tid. A more rapidly active alternative is dantrolene given in a dose of 1-2 mg/kg/day intravenously, with repeat doses as needed to relieve rigidity. In some cases, both bromocriptine and dantrolene may be used concurrently. Recently, success has also been reported with subcutaneous apomorphine. Finally, ECT has been reported as dramatically successful after a few treatments, and this in patients resistant to pharmacologic treatment.

If the syndrome occurred secondary to the use of an antipsychotic for schizophrenia, an exacerbation of psychotic symptoms often requires retreatment after the neuroleptic malignant syndrome has cleared. Although there are case reports of successful retreatment with the same drug which caused the syndrome, it is probably prudent to choose a different antipsychotic (e.g., in cases secondary to a high-potency first-generation agent, one might consider a low-potency first-generation agent, such as chlorpromazine) and to titrate the dose up very slowly; in any case, one should withhold treatment until the neuroleptic malignant syndrome has been in complete remission for at least two weeks.

BIBLIOGRAPHY

Addonizio G, Susman VL, Roth SD. Neuroleptic malignant syndrome: review and analysis of 115 cases. *Biological Psychiatry* 1987;22:1004-1015.

Buckley PF, Hutchinson M. Neuroleptic malignant syndrome. *Journal of Neurology, Neurosurgery, and Psychiatry* 1995;58:271-273.

Caroff SN, Mann SC, Keck PE, et al. Residual catatonic state following neuroleptic malignant syndrome. *Journal of Clinical Psychopharmacology* 2000;20:257-259.

Castillo E, Rubin RT, Holsboer-Trachsler E. Clinical differentiation between lethal catatonia and neuroleptic malignant syndrome. *The American Journal of Psychiatry* 1989;146:324-328.

Coffey RJ, Edgar TS, Francisco GE, et al. Abrupt withdrawal from intra-thecal baclofen: recognition and treatment of a potentially life-threatening syndrome. *Archives of Physical Medicine and Rehabilitation* 2002;83:735-741.

Figa-Talamanca L, Gualandi C, Di Meo L, et al. Hyperthermia after discontinuance of levodopa and bromocriptine therapy: impaired dopamine receptors a possible cause. *Neurology* 1985;35:258-261.

Hermesh H, Aizenberg D, Weizman A, et al. Risk for definite neuroleptic malignant syndrome: a prospective study in 223 consecutive in-patients. *The British Journal of Psychiatry* 1992;161:254-257.

Horn E, Lach B, Lapierre Y, et al. Hypothalamic pathology in the neuroleptic malignant syndrome. *The American Journal of Psychiatry* 1988;145:617-620.

Koch M, Chandragirl S, Rizvi S, et al. Catatonic signs in neuroleptic malignant syndrome. *Comprehensive Psychiatry* 2000;41:73-75.

Lal V, Sardana V, Thussu A, et al. Cerebellar degeneration following neuroleptic malignant syndrome. *Postgraduate Medical Journal* 1997;73:735-736.

Mihara K, Kondo T, Suzuki A, et al. Relationship between functional dopamine D2 and D3 receptor gene polymorphisms and neuroleptic malignant syndrome. *American Journal of Medical Genetics* 117:57-60.

Pope HG, Aizley HG, Keck PE, et al. Neuroleptic malignant syndrome: long-term follow-up of 20 cases. *The Journal of Clinical Psychiatry* 1991;52:208-212.

Pope HG, Keck PE, McElroy SL. Frequency and presentation of neuroleptic malignant syndrome in a large psychiatric hospital. *The American Journal of Psychiatry* 1986;143:1227-1233.

Reimer J, Kuhlmann A, Muller T. Neuroleptic malignant-like syndrome after rapid switch from bromocriptine to pergolide. *Parkinsonism & Related Disorders* 2002;9:115-116.

Rosebush P, Stewart T. A prospective analysis of twenty-four episodes of neuroleptic malignant syndrome. *The American Journal of Psychiatry* 1989;146:717-725.

Sechi GP, Tanda F, Mutani R. Fatal hyperpyrexia after withdrawal of levodopa. *Neurology* 1984;34:249-251.

Trollor JN, Sachdev PS. Electroconvulsive treatment of neuroleptic malignant syndrome: a review and report of cases. *The Australian and New Zealand Journal of Psychiatry* 1999;33:650-659.

Tsutsumi Y, Yamamoto K, Matsuura S, et al. The treatment of neuroleptic malignant syndrome using dantrolene sodium. *Psychiatry and Clinical Neurosciences* 1998;52:433-438.

Turner MR, Gainsborough N. Neuroleptic malignant-like syndrome after abrupt withdrawal of baclofen. *Journal of Psychopharmacology* 2001;15:61-63.

Wang HC, Hsieh V. Treatment of neuroleptic malignant syndrome with subcutaneous apomorphine. *Movement Disorders* 2001;16:765-767.

148 Tardive Dyskinesia (DSM-IV-TR #333.82)

Tardive dyskinesia is a movement disorder occurring as a side effect after chronic use of antipsychotic drugs. In contrast to the more typical "extrapyramidal" side effects of these drugs, however, tardive dyskinesia does not remit promptly when the offending medicine is discontinued, but rather persists for prolonged periods and may be permanent.

The most typical form of tardive dyskinesia is the choreiform one, often with buccolingual-masticatory movements. Less commonly, one encounters dystonic and akathitic forms, and rarely one may see tics or pain. Although some researchers treat these latter forms as separate entities, this distinction appears unwarranted. Another nosologic dispute centers on the question as to whether any fundamental difference exists between those cases wherein the abnormal movements are permanent and those in which they remit spontaneously several months after the antipsychotic is stopped. Some researchers have referred to this latter group as having "withdrawal dyskinesia." However, in all likelihood tardive dyskinesia, like most disorders, varies in severity, and whereas some cases are permanent, others may undergo a spontaneous remission.

The overall prevalence of tardive dyskinesia in patients chronically treated with first generation antipsychotics is anywhere from

20 to 30%; the age-specific prevalence, however, rises with age, such that among the elderly 50% or more will be affected. The prevalence of tardive dyskinesia with the second-generation agents is far less.

ONSET

Although tardive dyskinesia has been reported after only a month of treatment with an antipsychotic, this is very rare. In general, at least 6 months are required, and in most cases 1 or more years must pass before the abnormal movements first appear. When the dose of the antipsychotic is generally held constant, the onset is quite gradual and insidious. On the other hand, if the drug is stopped, or the dose abruptly and substantially reduced, the tardive dyskinesia may be "unmasked," and the abnormal movements "surface" quite abruptly.

CLINICAL FEATURES

In the more common choreiform type of tardive dyskinesia, the abnormal movements are most commonly seen in the lower face, somewhat less so in the extremities, and much less so in the trunk. The tongue may repetitively and rhythmically thrust against the inside of the cheek, billowing it out, or protrude beyond the lips creating what has euphemistically been termed a "fly-catcher" tongue, as shown in Figure 148-1. The astute clinician, however, need not wait for such obvious tongue movements before suspecting the disorder, as vermicular movements of the tongue, evident on close inspection, often precede the thrusting. Lip smacking, puckering, and pouting are also common, as are involuntary chewing movements. Somewhat less commonly, one may also see frequent blinking or blepharospasm. Repetitive facial grimacing may also be seen.

Repetitive shoulder shrugging may occur, as may a restless "piano playing" movement of the fingers. Foot tapping may occur, and in some cases a rocking, axial, "to and fro" movement may be seen. Rarely, pelvic thrusting may occur. Occasionally, the diaphragm may be involved, producing irregular grunting respirations.

Occasionally, rather than a pure chorea, a choreoathetosis may occur.

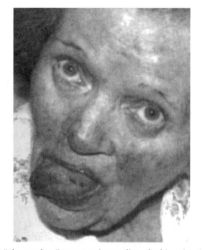

FIG. 148-1. "Fly-catcher" tongue in tardive dyskinesia. (From Parsons M. *Color atlas of clinical neurology*, ed 2, London, 1993, Wolfe.)

These choreiform movements wax and wane in severity throughout the day, and generally worsen with stress; they disappear with sleep. Some patients are able to voluntarily suppress them, but only for a brief period after which they recur. Typically, they are worsened by anticholinergic agents, such as benztropine. Interestingly, they become much worse should a depressive episode occur, and even more curiously, they tend to lessen and may even remit, albeit temporarily, during a manic episode.

The akathetic type of tardive dyskinesia is symptomatically very similar to the more typical akathisia seen early in treatment with antipsychotics. Patients complain of feeling restless, especially in their legs, and may "march in place." They may also have restless thoughts. In extreme cases, patients may complain that they feel like they could jump out of their skin.

The dystonic form of tardive dyskinesia is less frequently seen and may be more common in younger patients, especially males. Most commonly one sees cervical involvement (torticollis, retrocollis, anterocollis, lateralcollis) or cranial involvement with blepharospasm, facial grimacing or oculogyric crisis; less commonly the upper extremities or even the trunk may be involved.

Other, rare, manifestations of tardive dyskinesia include tics and pain. The condition of tardive tics is also referred to as "tardive tourettism" in recognition of the diagnostic confusion it may cause with Tourette's syndrome. Tardive pain is very rare, and is characterized by painful sensations in the oral or genital areas.

Although tardive dystonia, akathisia, tics, and pain may occur in isolation they typically occur in the setting of the more typical choreiform movements.

As noted earlier, tardive dyskinesia may be "unmasked" and first appear when the dose of the offending antipsychotic is reduced, or the drug is stopped. Conversely, if the dose of antipsychotic is increased, the abnormal movements may subside, becoming "masked" again. This relief, however, is only temporary in most cases, for with continued treatment with an antipsychotic, tardive dyskinesia may become more severe, and eventually in such cases the abnormal movements "surface" above the higher dose level.

Tardive psychosis, or, as it is more commonly known, "supersensitivity psychosis," may also be mentioned here. As described in Chapter 149, this is a very rare disorder characterized by the appearance of delusions and hallucinations occurring not because of an exacerbation of an underlying disorder but rather secondary to chronic dopamine blockade within the limbic system.

COURSE

The course of tardive dyskinesia has been most thoroughly studied with regard to the typical choreiform variety. In situations where the antipsychotic is continued after the abnormal movements emerge, in general one sees a gradual worsening up to a certain level, after which symptoms tend to wax and wane in severity but for the most part remain at a "plateau" of severity; in a small minority, however, there is a relentless progression in severity.

In cases where the antipsychotic is discontinued, initially there is an exacerbation of symptoms, corresponding to the "unmasking" referred to above. Subsequently, over the following weeks or months, at least some diminution of symptoms occurs, after which one of two courses may become evident. In perhaps a third of all cases, the abnormal movements continue to lessen and after many months, or a year or more, remit entirely. In others, however, they remain at a stable level of severity indefinitely. The elderly and those with more severe abnormal movements are more likely to display a chronic course.

COMPLICATIONS

Embarrassment and shame represent the most common complications. In extreme cases, patients may separate themselves entirely from others, leaving job and friends behind, becoming total recluses. Oral dyskinesias may also cause dental problems and dysarthria, and may predispose to aspiration.

ETIOLOGY

In the foregoing, only antipsychotics have been mentioned; however, any dopamine receptor blocker may cause tardive dyskinesia. Thus, in addition to the antipsychotics, cases have also occurred secondary to treatment with metoclopramide, prochlorperazine and to the antidepressant amoxapine, a drug which is normally metabolized to loxapine, an antipsychotic.

Although the etiology of tardive dyskinesia is not known with certainty, several risk factors have been identified, including treatment with first generation antipsychotics (especially high-potency agents), longer duration of treatment, a higher total lifetime antipsychotic burden in terms of milligrams, greater age, and female sex, with this latter factor being especially operative in postmenopausal females. Although second generation antipsychotics are far less likely to cause tardive dyskinesia than first generation agents, it must be borne in mind this syndrome has been reported secondary to clozapine, olanzapine, risperidone, quetiapine and ziprasidone.

The most commonly cited theory regarding the etiology of tardive dyskinesia posits an up-regulation of postsynaptic dopamine receptors within the basal ganglia secondary to chronic blockade, and PET scanning has indeed demonstrated increased metabolic activity in the globus pallidus and motor cortex. Attractive as this theory is, however, it does not explain several observations. First, based on this theory one would expect symptoms to remain stable unless the dopamine blockade was increased; in fact, however, as noted earlier, symptoms typically worsen despite the dose being kept the same. Second, given that the induced hyperdopaminergic state would exist throughout the basal ganglia one would not expect to see any clinical evidence of reduced dopaminergic tone; in fact, however, patients with the combination of tardive dyskinesia and antipsychotic-induced parkinsonism are not uncommon. Third, if up-regulation alone were the responsible mechanism, then one might reasonably expect all cases to eventually undergo a remission after antipsychotic discontinuation, in contrast with the actual state of affairs wherein most patients, though experiencing some improvement, remain chronically affected by abnormal movements. Given these observations, other mechanisms, acting perhaps in concert with an up-regulation of dopamine receptors, have been proposed, as for example disturbances in glutaminergic functioning and progressive glutamate-induced neurotoxicity.

DIFFERENTIAL DIAGNOSIS

In evaluating a patient with chronic chorea, dystonia, akathisia or tics the diagnosis of tardive dyskinesia is not considered unless the patient has been chronically treated with a dopamine-blocking agent. In cases where one of these abnormal involuntary movements do occur in the setting of chronic antipsychotic treatment, although tardive dyskinesia is high on the differential diagnosis, several other disorders must also be considered, as noted below.

Other choreiform disorders to consider include Huntington's disease, senile chorea, Wilson's disease, acquired hepato-cerebral degeneration, hyperthyroidism, systemic lupus erythematosus, Sydenham's chorea, chorea gravidarum and lesions of the striatum; chorea may also occur as an acute side-effect of various medications. Huntington's disease is suggested by the positive family history, and may be definitively diagnosed with genetic testing. Several clinical findings also favor a diagnosis of Huntington's disease. For example, the chorea of Huntington's disease is "flowing" and jumps, lightning-like, from one point of the body to another, rather than being rhythmic and repetitive as in tardive dyskinesia. Furthermore, in Huntington's disease one typically finds forehead chorea, a "milk-maid" grip, and a "dancing and prancing" gait, none of which are found in tardive dyskinesia. Senile chorea is distinguished by its late onset, in the seventh decade, and by an absence of tongue involvement. Wilson's disease is suggested by an onset from childhood to early adult years, by the presence of a Kayser-Fleischer ring, and by the appearance of other movement disorders, such as tremor. Given the fact that Wilson's disease is treatable, missing the diagnosis is tragic, and consequently any patient with a clinical presentation consistent with this disease should probably have copper studies. Acquired hepato-cerebral degeneration is suggested by the history of repeated episodes of hepatic encephalopathy and by the presence of the most common cause of such episodes, namely alcoholism. Sydenham's chorea is suggested by the history of other manifestations of rheumatic fever, and also by its self-limiting course, and chorea gravidarum enters the differential only when the patient is pregnant. Striatal lesions, such as infarcts or tumors, may cause chorea; however, here the chorea is and remains unilateral except in those very rare cases where bilateral striatal infarctions occur. Finally, medications capable of causing chorea include anticonvulsants (most commonly phenytoin; however, there are rare case reports implicating valproic acid and gabapentin), levodopa, oral contraceptives (especially in women with a history of Sydenham's chorea), stimulants (methylphenidate, pemoline, amphetamines and cocaine), and, rarely, lithium.

Dystonic disorders to consider include primary torsion dystonia (dystonia musculorum deformans), dopa-responsive dystonia, idiopathic cervical dystonia, Meige's syndrome, focal lesions of the basal ganglia or thalamus, and Wilson's disease; various medications may also cause dystonia as an acute side-effect. In all of these disorders, with the exception of Wilson's disease, one does not see chorea, in contrast to cases of tardive dystonia, which are generally accompanied by some chorea. Primary torsion dystonia and dopa-responsive dystonia are further suggested by their early age of onset, in childhood or adolescence, and by the onset of dystonia in the lower extremities, rather than, as in the case of tardive dystonia, the upper extremities. Idiopathic cervical dystonia is suggested by the often-present family history, but otherwise has clinical features quite similar to cases of tardive dystonia. Meige's syndrome is distinguished by the absence of other signs except blepharospasm, a pattern not seen in tardive dystonia, which involves other musculature, primarily on the neck. Differential considerations regarding focal lesions and Wilson's disease are the same as noted in the preceding paragraph. Drugs that, albeit rarely, may cause dystonia include levodopa, propranolol, gabapentin, MDMA (Ecstasy), cocaine, flunarazine, and cimetidine. Another class of drugs capable of causing dystonia, and in this case quite commonly so, are the antipsychotics. Here, however, one must clearly distinguish between an acute dystonia, which occurs shortly after initiating treatment or significantly increasing the dose, and tardive dystonia, which occurs only after chronic treatment, and which is "masked" if the dose is increased; another differential feature is the response to dose reduction, a maneuver followed by a diminution of dystonia when it is acute or, conversely, by an increase in the dystonia when it is of the tardive variety.

Akathisia may occur as a side-effect of various medications and as part of Parkinson's disease. Medications that rarely cause akathisia include the SSRIs and diltiazem; medications that commonly do include the antipsychotics. Here, however, as in the case of antipsychotic-induced dystonia, one must make a distinction between an acute akathisia and a tardive akathisia. Acute akathisia occurs within days or weeks of starting an antipsychotic, or significantly increasing the dose, and lessens with a dose decrease; by contrast tardive akathisia occurs only after chronic neuroleptic treatment, and worsens with a reduction in dose. Patients with Parkinson's disease are occasionally given antipsychotics, and in this case the history of the evolution of symptoms is critical: when akathisia is secondary to Parkinson's disease it is generally apparent early in the course, and long before the illness could have progressed to the point where neuroleptics were required for a levodopa-induced psychosis or for management of a Parkinson's disease dementia.

Tics may be seen with various drugs, such as stimulants, carbamazepine, or valproic acid, and here the temporal contiguity between the onset of tics and beginning the drug suggests the correct diagnosis. Tics, notoriously, also occur in Tourette's syndrome, and distinguishing Tourette's syndrome from "tardive tourettism" may be difficult in cases of Tourette's syndrome treated with antipsychotics wherein one sees a gradual increase in the severity of the tics. Certainly, if this increased severity of tics were accompanied by chorea, one would lean to a diagnosis of tardive dyskinesia. In doubtful cases, it may be appropriate in treating Tourette's disorder to switch from an antipsychotic to clonidine or, in adults, desipramine, with or without adjunctive clonazepam.

TREATMENT

The best "treatment" here is prevention, and antipsychotics should not be used chronically except for those disorders where they afford the only effective treatment. Additionally, in situations where their chronic use is indicated, the lowest effective dose should be used, and the patient should be routinely re-examined for evidence of tardive dyskinesia. Should such evidence occur, a decision must then be made balancing the risks of relapse against the risks of worsening of tardive dyskinesia.

If, on balance, discontinuing the antipsychotic appears safe, then the subsequent course is as described in that section. Pertinently, the sooner the antipsychotic is stopped after recognition of the tardive dyskinesia, the better the odds for a self-limiting course.

If the antipsychotic must be continued, or if the tardive dyskinesia persists long after the antipsychotic is stopped, then consideration might be given to treatment of the tardive dyskinesia itself. A number of preparations have demonstrated effectiveness in double-blinded studies, including tetrabenazine (not available in the United States), vitamin E (1200-1600 IU daily), clonidine (0.2 to 0.8 mg daily), vitamin B6 (400 mg/day), melatonin (in doses of 10 mg daily) and branched chain amino acids. Vitamin E has the most robust support: of 10 double-blinded studies, 8 were positive, one equivocal and one negative. Clonidine was effective in one out of two studies, as was melatonin, and vitamin B6 and branched chain amino acids each have backing of only one study. Given these findings, it seems appropriate to begin with vitamin E, allowing at least several weeks to judge the response. Many authors also advocate switching to one of the second-generation antipsychotics; however, there is as yet no evidence to suggest that this does anything other than "mask" the symptoms with a new dopamine blockade, with the risk that, under this mask, the tardive dyskinesia may worsen. In the situation where symptoms are severe and resistant to medical treatment, consideration may be given to ECT, which has, in a large number of case reports and series, been reported as very successful in otherwise treatment-resistant cases, regardless of whether or not the patient suffered from a mood disorder.

The tardive dystonia variant may respond to high dose anticholinergics, such as 20 mg of trihexyphenidyl; however, if choreiform movements are also present, these agents may worsen the chorea. In cases where the dystonia is quite localized, botulinum toxin, as used in other dystonic disorders, may be effective.

The tardive akathisia variant may respond favorably to propranolol; however, doses may have to be high.

In all cases, depression, if present, should be treated, as this results in some relief.

At one time, "drug holidays" were proposed as a way to reduce the risk of tardive dyskinesia by reducing the cumulative burden of dopamine blockade. This has been shown not to be the case; indeed "drug holidays" may make tardive dyskinesia more likely.

BIBLIOGRAPHY

Adler LA, Edson R, Lavori P, et al. Long-term treatment effects of vitamin E for tardive dyskinesia. *Biological Psychiatry* 1998;43:868-872.

Beasley CM, Deliva MA, Tamura RN, et al. Randomized double-blind comparison of the incidence of tardive dyskinesia in patients with schizophrenia during long-term treatment with olanzapine or haloperidol. *The British Journal of Psychiatry* 1999;174:23-30.

Bharucha KJ, Sethi KD. Tardive tourettism after exposure to neuroleptic therapy. *Movement Disorders* 1995;10:791-793.

Burke RE, Fahn S, Jankovic J, et al. Tardive dystonia: late onset and persistent dystonia caused by antipsychotic drugs. *Neurology* 1982;32: 1335-1346.

Chouinard G, Jones BD. Neuroleptic-induced supersensitivity psychosis: clinical and pharmacologic characteristics. *The American Journal of Psychiatry* 1980;137:16-21.

Dufresne RL, Wagner RL. Antipsychotic-withdrawal akathisia versus antipsychotic-induced akathisia: further evidence for the existence of tardive akathisia. *The Journal of Clinical Psychiatry* 1988;49:435-438.

Ford B, Greene P, Fahn S. Oral and genital tardive pain syndromes. *Neurology* 1994;44:2115-2119.

Granacher RP. Differential diagnosis of tardive dyskinesia: an overview. *The American Journal of Psychiatry* 1981;138:1288-1297.

Jeste DV, Potkin SG, Sinha S, et al. Tardive dyskinesia—reversible and persistent. *Archives of General Psychiatry* 1979;36:585-590.

Kent TA, Wilbur RD. Reserpine withdrawal psychosis: the possible role of denervation supersensitivity of receptors. *The Journal of Nervous and Mental Disease* 1982;170:502-504.

Kiriakakis V, Bhatia KP, Quinn NP, et al. The natural history of tardive dystonia. A long-term follow-up study of 107 cases. *Brain* 1998;121: 2053-2066.

Lerner V, Miodownik C, Kapstan A, et al. Vitamin B(6) in the treatment of tardive dyskinesia: a double-blind, placebo-controlled, crossover study. *The American Journal of Psychiatry* 2001;158:1511-1514.

Lu ML, Pan JJ, Teng HW, et al. Metoclopramide-induced supersensitivity psychosis. *The Annals of Pharmacotherapy* 2002;36:1387-1390.

Ondo WG, Hanna PA, Jankovic J. Tetrabenazine treatment for tardive dyskinesia: assessment by randomized videotape protocol. *The American Journal of Psychiatry* 1999;156:1279-1281.

Pahl JJ, Mazziotta JC, Bartzokis G, et al. Positron-emission tomography in tardive dyskinesia. *The Journal of Neuropsychiatry and Clinical Neurosciences* 1995;7:457-465.

Richardson MA, Bevans ML, Weber JG, et al. Branched chain amino acids decrease tardive dyskinesia symptoms. *Psychopharmacology* 1999;143:358-364.

Sachdev P. Clinical characteristics of 15 patients with tardive dystonia. *The American Journal of Psychiatry* 1993;150:498-500.

Sachdev P, Loneragan C. Intravenous benztropine and propranolol challenges in tardive akathisia. *Psychopharmacology* 1993;113:119-122.

Sewell DD, Kodsi AB, Caligiun MP, et al. Metoclopramide and tardive dyskinesia. *Biological Psychiatry* 1994;36:630-632.

Shamir E, Barak Y, Shalman I, et al. Melatonin treatment for tardive dyskinesia: a double-blind, placebo-controlled, crossover study. *Archives of General Psychiatry* 2001;58:1049-1052.

Steiner W, Laporta M, Chouinard G. Neuroleptic-induced supersensitivity psychosis in patients with bipolar affective disorder. *Acta Psychiatrica Scandinavica* 1990;81:437-440.

Tripodianakis J, Markianos M. Clonidine trial in tardive dyskinesia. Therapeutic response, MHPG, and plasma DBH. *Pharmacopsychiatry* 1986;19:365-367.

van Harten PN, Hoek HW, Matroos GE, et al. Intermittent neuroleptic treatment and risk for tardive dyskinesia: Curacao Extrapyramidal Syndromes Study III. *The American Journal of Psychiatry* 1998;155:565-567.

Weinberger DR, Bigelow LB, Klein ST, et al. Drug withdrawal in chronic schizophrenic patients: in search of neuroleptic-induced supersensitivity psychosis. *Journal of Clinical Psychopharmacology* 1981;1:120-123.

Woerner MG, Alvir JM, Saltz BL, et al. Prospective study of tardive dyskinesia in the elderly: rates and risk factors. *The American Journal of Psychiatry* 1998;155:1521-1528.

Yassa R, Nair NP. A 10-year follow-up study of tardive dyskinesia. *Acta Psychiatrica Scandinavica* 1992;86:262-266.

149 Supersensitivity Psychosis

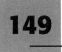

Supersensitivity psychosis, also known as tardive psychosis, is a rare, and late-appearing, side effect of chronic treatment with antipsychotics.

ONSET

After a year or more of treatment with an antipsychotic, the psychosis emerges: this emergence may, if the antipsychotic is continued at the same dose, be gradual, or, if the dose were substantially reduced, or the medication discontinued, abrupt.

CLINICAL FEATURES

The psychosis is characterized by delusions and hallucinations similar to those seen in schizophrenia. These symptoms may or may not be accompanied by a tardive dyskinesia.

COURSE

With discontinuation of the antipsychotic, symptoms very gradually decrease in severity: although remissions do occur, it is not clear what percentage of cases remit and what percentage persist in a chronic fashion.

COMPLICATIONS

These are similar to those outlined in the chapter on secondary psychosis.

ETIOLOGY

Although the etiology is unknown, it is speculated that with chronic treatment with dopamine-blocking antipsychotics there is an up-regulation of post-synaptic dopamine receptors in the limbic system: this supersensitivity in turn leads to a hyper-dopaminergic state within the limbic system which in turn produces the psychosis. Although almost all reported cases have occurred secondary to antipsychotics, cases have also been reported due to chronic treatment with the non-antipsychotic dopamine-blocking drug metoclopramide.

The presumed analogy between supersensitivity psychosis and tardive dyskinesia accounts for the alternative name for this condition, tardive psychosis.

As noted below, most cases occur in patients with schizophrenia, and this led some authors to doubt whether a supersensitivity psychosis existed at all: it was thought that any psychotic symptoms occurring in such patients were, rather than representing a new disorder, namely supersensitivity psychosis, merely indicators of an exacerbation of the schizophrenia itself. These criticisms were initially difficult to refute, but the subsequent occurrence of a psychosis in patients who did not have schizophrenia but who had undergone long-term antipsychotic treatment for depression provides strong support for its existence.

DIFFERENTIAL DIAGNOSIS

The emergence of a psychosis in the setting of a reduction of dose or discontinuation of chronic antipsychotic treatment should prompt consideration of this diagnosis.

As most patients chronically treated with antipsychotics have schizophrenia, the main differential for supersensitivity psychosis is an exacerbation of the underlying disorder for which the antipsychotic was being used. One helpful differential point lies in the mode of onset of psychotic symptoms subsequent to dose reduction or discontinuation of the antipsychotic. In cases of schizophrenia where patients have been doing well, with little or no symptoms, relapses, if they do occur, come on gradually with dose reduction: by contrast, supersensitivity psychosis appears fairly abruptly.

In patients with mood disorders who have been chronically treated with an antipsychotic and who develop a psychosis with dose reduction or discontinuation of the antipsychotic, a helpful differential point is whether or not the psychotic symptoms appear in the context of a prominent relapse of mood symptoms: if the psychotic symptoms do occur in the setting of a relapse of mania or depression, then one may not need to invoke an additional diagnosis to explain them; if, however, the psychotic symptoms appeared in the setting of euthymia, then the underlying mood disorder could not be used to account for them and a diagnosis of supersensitivity psychosis is more likely.

TREATMENT

The best treatment, on analogy with tardive dyskinesia, is prevention, and antipsychotics should probably not be used chronically for conditions that respond to other agents.

Should a supersensitivity psychosis occur, it may be treated symptomatically by increasing the dose of the antipsychotic: whether or not, in such cases, the psychosis will eventually re-emerge, as may occur with tardive dyskinesia, is not clear. It is also not clear if approaches effective in tardive dyskinesia, such as vitamin E, would be effective here.

BIBLIOGRAPHY

Chouinard G. Severe cases of neuroleptic-induced supersensitivity psychosis. Diagnostic criteria for the disorder and its treatment. *Schizophrenia Research* 1991;21-33.

Kirkpatrick B, Alphs L, Buchanen RW. The concept of supersensitivity psychosis. *The Journal of Nervous and Mental Disease* 1992;180: 265-270.

Lu ML, Pan JJ, Teng HW, et al. Metoclopramide-induced supersensitivity psychosis. *The Annals of Pharmacotherapy* 2002;36:1387-1390.

Steiner W, Laporta M, Chouinard G. Neuroleptic-induced supersensitivity psychosis in patients with bipolar affective disorder. *Acta Psychiatrica Scandinavica* 1990;81:437-440.

150 Rabbit Syndrome

The rabbit syndrome is an uncommon movement disorder that occurs as a side effect of chronic antipsychotic treatment, being seen in approximately 4% of patients treated with antipsychotics. Although most cases have occurred secondary to first generation agents, there are reports of the syndrome occurring secondary to the second generation agent risperidone.

ONSET

The onset is gradual, occurring after months or years of treatment with an antipsychotic.

CLINICAL FEATURES

The syndrome presents as a rhythmic rest tremor of the jaw, at a frequency and amplitude such that the appearance is for all the world that of a rabbit chewing. Importantly, there is no associated rigidity or bradykinesia, nor is there evidence of tremor anywhere else.

COURSE

With continued treatment with an antipsychotic, the tremor gradually becomes more pronounced; with discontinuation of the medication, the tremor, over weeks or months, gradually decreases in amplitude and in most cases remits; however, the proportion of cases which remain chronic is not known.

COMPLICATIONS

Chewing may become very difficult, and poorly chewed food may be aspirated; speech becomes tremulous and eventually dysarthric.

ETIOLOGY

As noted earlier, the rabbit syndrome occurs as a side effect of antipsychotics; however, its relation to other side effects, such as parkinsonism and tardive dyskinesia, is not clear.

DIFFERENTIAL DIAGNOSIS

Essential tremor can produce a tremor of the chin; however, it is generally more rapid than that seen in a chewing movement and is almost always preceded by tremor in the hands.

Parkinsonism may also produce a jaw tremor; however, in parkinsonism, this jaw tremor is almost always preceded by other parkinsonian symptoms, such as a rest tremor of the hands, rigidity, bradykinesia, flexion posture and the like.

Tardive dyskinesia may be considered, but in tardive dyskinesia abnormal movements are exacerbated by treatment with antiparkinsonian anticholinergic agents, which stands in contrast to the rabbit syndrome, which, as noted below, is relieved by them.

TREATMENT

Discontinuation of the antipsychotic is, as noted earlier, followed by a gradual, and more or less complete, remission. If treatment with an antipsychotic, however, is essential, or if the tremor does not clear completely with discontinuation, then an antiparkinsonian agent, such as benztropine, may be used.

BIBLIOGRAPHY

Deshmukh DK, Joshi VS, Agarwal MR. Rabbit syndrome—a rare complication of long-term neuroleptic medication. *The British Journal of Psychiatry* 1990;157:293.

Hoy JS, Alexander B. Rabbit syndrome secondary to risperidone. *Pharmacotherapy* 2002;22:513-515.

Todd R, Lippmann S, Manshadi M, et al. Recognition and treatment of the rabbit syndrome, an uncommon complication of neuroleptic therapies. *The American Journal of Psychiatry* 1983;140:1519-1520.

Wada Y, Yamaguchi N. The rabbit syndrome and antiparkinsonian medication in schizophrenic patients. *Neuropsychobiology* 1992; 25:149-152.

Yassa R, Lal S. Prevalence of the rabbit syndrome. *The American Journal of Psychiatry* 1986;143:656-657.

MALINGERING AND FACTITIOUS ILLNESS

151 Malingering (DSM-IV-TR #V65.2)

Malingerers intentionally and purposefully feign illness to achieve some recognizable goal. They may wish to get drugs, win a lawsuit, or avoid work or military service. At times the deceit of the malingerer may be readily apparent to the physician; however, medically sophisticated malingerers have been known to deceive even the best of diagnosticians.

Some malingerers may limit their dissembling simply to voicing complaints. Others may take advantage of an actual illness and embellish and exaggerate their symptoms out of all proportion to the severity of the underlying disease. Some may go so far as to actually stage an accident, and then go on to exaggerate any symptoms that may subsequently develop. Falsification of medical records may also occur.

Neurologic, psychiatric, and rheumatic illnesses are often chosen as models. Malingerers may complain of headache, paresthesias, weakness, whiplash, or pain of any sort. Those accused of crimes may feign amnesia or complain of voices that they say made them do it. Depression may be feigned in hopes of obtaining disability payments. Low back pain is a favorite complaint for malingerers.

Several features may serve to alert the physician to the possibility of malingering. First, look for obvious gains to patients should they be certified as ill, for example those who specifically request narcotics for pain or those seeking to win a personal injury lawsuit. Second, be alert to any discrepancies between the patient's complaints and what is known about the laws of anatomy and pathophysiology. As is described in the chapter on conversion disorder, often here too one finds that the patient's complaints "violate" these laws. Third, look carefully at cases where the patient is either unwilling to accept a justifiably good prognosis or is uncooperative with treatment. Finally, keep in mind that patients with an antisocial personality disorder are just as likely to lie as to tell the truth.

In suspect cases, collateral history should always be obtained from others who know the patient well, and this should be done before the patient has a chance to talk with them. When someone complains of constantly incapacitating back pain and the spouse reports how well the patient plays volleyball, the diagnostic evaluation is essentially over. Laboratory testing, if relevant, should always be performed, but often patients feign illness wherein laboratory testing is generally noncontributory.

A peculiar example of malingering is what is known as Ganser's syndrome. This is seen for the most part in prisoners awaiting either trial or sentencing. Also known as the "nonsense syndrome,"

it is characterized by the appearance of nonsense responses to questions. Typically, the patient appears dazed and confused, and responds to questions with answers that are always somewhat off the mark and past the point. For example, if the patient is asked to add 5 plus 3, he may respond "7"; with coaching he may offer other "guesses," such as 6 or 9, or any other number except the correct one. Or if asked where he is, the jailed prisoner may say he is in the locked ward of a hospital. Visual and auditory hallucinations may be described. Confused and disoriented as these patients may appear, they are nevertheless capable of finding their way around the jail and of doing those things that are necessary to maintain a minimum level of comfort in jail or prison. All in all, these patients act out the "popular" conception of insanity to escape trial or punishment. Once the trial has occurred or punishment has been imposed, the "insanity" often clears up quickly.

One should be sure not to misdiagnose a case of schizophrenia as Ganser's syndrome. At times patients with schizophrenia may not have their antipsychotics continued after being jailed and may become floridly psychotic a few days later. A similar fate may await alcoholics who develop delirium tremens after imprisonment separates them from alcohol.

Malingering should be distinguished from a conversion symptom. In both instances a variance occurs between the patient's complaints and what is known about the laws of anatomy and pathophysiology. In malingering the goal is apparent, whereas in the patient with a conversion symptom, any recognizable "goal" may be lacking. Furthermore, the patient with a conversion symptom is at the mercy of that symptom and may be incapacitated by it, whereas the malingerer can turn the symptom on and off at will.

Factitious illness may represent a subset of malingering and is a little more difficult to recognize because the goal of the dissimulation is something most normal people would not entertain, namely the sick role itself.

What the physician should do once certain that the patient is malingering is debatable. Some patients may be "reachable," and a frank but nonjudgmental discussion may be helpful. Others, heavily invested in their lies, should be told the simple truth, that they are not sick, and politely sent on their way. Whatever approach is taken, the physician must not attempt to placate the patient. To tell a malingerer that, yes, they might be sick, or to prescribe medication, is simply to reinforce and reward lying, and this is a disservice to anyone.

BIBLIOGRAPHY

Bash IY, Alpert M. The determination of malingering. *Annals of the New York Academy of Sciences* 1980;347:86-99.

LoPiccolo CJ, Goodkin K, Baldewicz TT. Current issues in the diagnosis and management of malingering. *Annals of Medicine* 1999;31:166-174.

Resnick PJ. Defrocking the fraud: the detection of malingering. *The Israel Journal of Psychiatry and Related Sciences* 1993;30:93-101.

Sigal M, Altmark D, Alfici S, et al. Ganser syndrome: a review of 15 cases. *Comprehensive Psychiatry* 1992;33:134-138.

Swanson DA. Malingering and associated syndromes. *Psychiatric Medicine* 1984;2:287-293.

Tsoi WF. The Ganser syndrome in Singapore. A report on ten cases. *The British Journal of Psychiatry* 1973;123;567-572.

Whitlock FA. The Ganser syndrome. *The British Journal of Psychiatry* 1967;113:19-29.

152 Factitious Illness (factitious disorders, DSM-IV-TR #300.16, 300.19)

When illness is feigned, one may or may not be able to discern a more or less understandable motive. When one can, for example when someone complains of a "bad back" to escape the draft, such feigning is referred to as "malingering." When one cannot find a motive—indeed when it appears that the only possible motive could be the desire to be a patient in the hospital—one speaks of a "factitious illness."

Typically the patient presenting at the emergency room with a factitious illness has a personality disorder with prominent borderline, masochistic, and at times antisocial traits. Often they also have had some exposure to medicine and hospitals, having worked as aides, physical therapists, and the like. The frequency with which hospitalization is sought varies widely. On the one hand, admission may be quite sporadic and occur only at times of great stress. On the other hand, however, there are some whose lives are consumed by these un-needed hospital stays. One variety of this severe pattern is known as "Munchausen's syndrome," named after the famous German baron who traveled from city to city, telling fascinating tales about himself. Patients with Munchausen's syndrome, in addition to wandering and being hospitalized in numerous different cities, often also display what is known as "pseudologia fantastica," or a capacity for spinning out elaborate tales, at times intermixed with some actual facts, which listeners often find, sometimes despite themselves, intriguing and fascinating.

Typically, the factitial patient presents at the emergency room with an often very convincing history suggestive of a serious disease process. The chief complaint may be of hemoptysis or perhaps of chest pain suggestive of unstable angina. Thermometers may be warmed to simulate a fever, and some have been known to inject themselves with feces to produce a fever. Furosemide may be taken to produce hypokalemia, insulin to produce hypoglycemia, or thyroid hormone to produce hyperthyroidism. Seizures may be reported, and some may bite their tongue to produce a more convincing picture. Once admitted, they may make frequent demands for narcotics, and staff members are often split and played off one against the other. Diagnostic tests are welcomed, even demanded, and as the tests become ever more invasive and dangerous, the patient, seemingly paradoxically, becomes more content. Eventually the physician becomes suspicious. One may see too many old surgical scars; the abdomen may look like a surgical battleground, and evidence of old craniotomies and numerous cutdowns may be seen. Requests to contact family members, friends, or previous physicians are denied, and despite the gravity of the patient's complaints, no visitors arrive. As more and more tests come back negative, the complaints may change. Chest pain may fail to recur, but severe abdominal pain may take its place. The "fever" may subside as the nursing staff comes to observe the patient throughout the encounter with a thermometer, yet hematuria may unexpectedly appear after the patient pricks his finger and drops blood into the urine sample. Eventually, confronted with the physician's almost certain conclusion that there is "nothing wrong," the factitial patient typically becomes angry, accuses the staff of incompetence, and leaves the hospital against medical advice.

Occasionally, one may also encounter factitious psychiatric illness. Patients may complain of voices and visions or of deep despair and may report severe suicidal ideation. Although such people readily gain admission, the factitial nature of their complaints rarely holds up to the scrutiny of an experienced psychiatrist or psychiatric nurse. The complaints either fail to match any known disorder, or they change in ways that are simply not possible. Confronted with these impressions, the factitial patient also demands discharge; however, at times a wrist may be cut or a noose may be fashioned to convince the physician of the reality of the complaints.

A particularly loathsome variation on factitious illness is the use of a "proxy." Here, a parent may force anticoagulants, diuretics, or other agents on a child and use the results as a ticket for the child's admission. Suspicion may be aroused when one notes a certain satisfaction, even contentment, on the parent's part as the child is subjected to ever more invasive diagnostic procedures.

Factitial patients may be distinguished from those with hypochondriasis, Briquet's syndrome, or conversion disorder not only by their deliberate simulation of illness but also by their insistence on hospitalization and their ready submission to potentially dangerous procedures. Those with these other disorders, although believing themselves to be ill, do not pursue the proof of that with such blatant disregard for their own safety.

Managing the factitial patient in the hospital is almost impossible. Often the best one can do is to recognize the simulation for what it is as soon as possible and avoid doing any harm with invasive tests. Psychotherapy is generally rejected by the factitial patient, and admission to a psychiatric ward is generally contraindicated because it might serve to increase the patient's repertoire of symptoms. After discharge the factitial patient typically resumes a peripatetic existence, going from hospital to hospital, ever-changing cities, states, or even countries to avoid becoming known.

BIBLIOGRAPHY

Aduan RP, Fauci AS, Dale DC, et al. Factitious fever and self-induced infection: a report of 32 cases and review of the literature. *Annals of Internal Medicine* 1979;90:230-242.

Asher R. Munchausen's syndrome. *Lancet* 1951;1:339-341.

Bhugra D. Psychiatric Munchausen's syndrome. Literature review with case reports. *Acta Psychiatrica Scandinavica* 1988;77:497-503.

Feldman MD, Rosenquist PB, Bond JP. Concurrent factitious disorder and factitious disorder by proxy. Double Jeopardy. *General Hospital Psychiatry* 1997;19:24-28.

Folks DG. Munchausen's syndrome and other factitious disorders. *Neurologic Clinics* 1995;13:267-281.

Hay GG. Feigned psychosis: a review of the simulation of mental illness. *The British Journal of Psychiatry* 1983;143:8-10.

Pope HG, Jonas JM, Jones B. Factitious psychosis: phenomenology, family history, and long-term outcome of nine patients. *The American Journal of Psychiatry* 1982;139:1480-1483.

Popli AP, Masand PS, Dewan MJ. Factitious disorders with psychological symptoms. *The Journal of Clinical Psychiatry* 1992;53:315-318.

Reich P, Gottfried LA. Factitious disorders in a teaching hospital. *Annals of Internal Medicine* 1983;99:240-247.

Skau K, Mouridsen SE. Munchausen syndrome by proxy: a review. *Acta Paediatrica* 1995;84:977-982.

Wallach J. Laboratory diagnosis of factitious disorders. *Archives of Internal Medicine* 1994;154:1690-1696.

SUICIDAL AND VIOLENT BEHAVIOR

153 Suicidal Behavior

Suicidal ideation is common, with a lifetime prevalence of about 10%; suicide attempts, however, are much less common, with a lifetime prevalence of only 0.3%, and completed suicide is rarer still, occurring in about 0.012%.

For the clinician, one of the most difficult tasks is gauging the risk of a suicide attempt or a completed suicide among those with suicidal ideation. Overreacting leads to too many hospitalizations, with all their disruptiveness; underreacting, however, may be a fatal error. Although certain risk factors for suicide attempts and completed suicide exist, as described below, it must be borne in mind that they provide only the roughest of guidelines.

RISK FACTORS

In gauging the risk of attempted or completed suicide among adults with suicidal ideation, factors to consider include age, race, religious affiliation, sex, the presence or absence of strong personal bonds, the presence or absence of recent significant losses, concurrent psychiatric or general medical illnesses, any history of prior attempts, the patient's current mental status and certain other aspects of the patient's recent behavior, and, finally, the intended means of suicide.

Younger patients, that is to say those under 45, are more likely to make an attempt than are older patients, especially those over 60, who are more likely to commit suicide.

Blacks, at least in the United States, are more likely to make attempts, in contrast to whites, who are more likely to succeed; American Indians, however, have an even higher rate.

Certain religious faiths, such as Roman Catholicism or Judaism, strongly prohibit suicide and make completed suicide unlikely; by contrast, most Protestant faiths, lacking such a strong prohibition, are less likely to constitute a restraining influence. The mitigating effect of Roman Catholicism and Judaism, of course, depends on the depth of the patient's belief: for those lacking a strong faith, simple membership in the denomination has no influence on the risk of completed suicide.

Females are more likely to attempt suicide, and males to complete it, and this is true for all ages.

The presence of strong personal bonds of friendship or affection argue for an attempt; by contrast, those who live in isolation or are estranged from those they were once close to are at higher risk for completed suicide.

Recent losses, such as divorce, relocation and leaving behind all that was familiar and dear, or the death of a loved one, all increase the risk of completed suicide.

Certain psychiatric or general medical illnesses also increase the risk of completed suicide. Important among the psychiatric illnesses are depression (either of major depression or bipolar disorder), a mixed-manic episode, alcoholism, schizophrenia and borderline personality disorder.

The suffering of depression, when coupled with its attendant pessimism and hopelessness, often reduces the patient to a position where suicide seems not only desirable but also often logical. Agitation increases the risk, and the risk is further compounded when guilt demands the ultimate punishment, and even higher still when delusions of guilt occur. Paradoxically, the listlessness and anergia of severe depression may protect the patient: suicide simply requires too much energy. Consequently, the risk is greatest when the depressed patient is first beginning to improve and has regained some energy but not any hope or optimism.

Mixed manic episodes constitute a fertile ground for completed suicide, as they are characterized by intense dysphoria and despair combined with more than a sufficient amount of energy to act with violence on suicidal impulses.

Alcoholics who are actively drinking or who have just recently become sober constitute a group that accounts for many suicides, and this is especially the case when there is a concurrent depression. The despair, self-pity, and fierce resentment felt by most such drinkers is fertile ground for self-destruction.

Schizophrenia increases the risk, and, in contrast with most other illnesses, the risk is higher among the relatively young who are early on in the course of the illness than it is among those who are older and who have "burnt out." Good education and high ambition also increase the risk in schizophrenia; the absolute inability to live up to earlier goals creates a barren sense of hopelessness for the patient with schizophrenia. Auditory hallucinations that command patients to kill themselves may also play a role; however, they may not be as important as was once thought.

Although borderline personality disorder is notorious for suicidal behavior (with some patients' histories containing literally dozens of admissions for suicide attempts), a not insignificant minority, perhaps 5%, actually do die at their own hands.

In addition to these psychiatric illnesses, certain general medical illnesses, generally those associated with long-term suffering and an overall bleak prognosis, also increase the risk of completed suicide. Notable among these are cancer, chronic renal failure with hemodialysis, AIDS, multiple sclerosis and Huntington's disease. Furthermore, and for reasons yet obscure, epilepsy characterized by complex partial seizures also increases the risk of death by suicide.

A history of suicide attempts may also increase the risk of completed suicide; however, this holds true only if the prior attempt occurred within a specific period of time. Initially, in the period immediately following an attempt, the risk is generally low. Over the subsequent 1 or 2 years it remains higher and then tends to drop down; patients whose prior attempts were 2 or more years in the past tend to be at not much greater risk than those who have never made an attempt.

The current mental status and certain other aspects of the patient's recent behavior may also help in gauging the risks. An intractable sense of hopelessness places the patient at a higher risk; conversely, a flicker of hope, no matter how dim, may allow the patient to endure current suffering. Those who give away their valuables, finalize their will, or make similar arrangements may be indicating that their mind is made up. Another indication that a depressed patient has settled on suicide as a way out is a sudden and unexpected brightening of mood. Some, having arrived at a decision that will finally provide relief, may almost seem cheerful as they prepare their death.

The intended means of suicide also affects the risk of completion. A patient who plans to use a highly lethal method in a situation that would make discovery and rescue most unlikely is at greater risk for death than the patient whose method is relatively innocuous and who plans the deed in circumstances that at times almost ensure discovery and rescue. For example, patients who plan to hang themselves in unfrequented woods are at greater risk than patients who contemplate an overdose of over-the-counter sleeping tablets while lying in bed with their bed-partner. One should, however, ask the patient what was expected from the method, for some may underestimate or overestimate lethality. For example, some may believe that fluoxetine is as lethal as a tricyclic antidepressant; conversely, others may be completely unaware of the high lethality of acetaminophen.

Using the foregoing risk factors to gauge the risk of attempted or completed suicide is not straightforward. Although reasonably certain judgments may be made in cases where patients fall at the "extremes" of risk, there is an enormous gray area, which, unfortunately, contains most patients with suicidal ideation. Lest one despair of making any estimate of risk, however, consider the following "extreme" examples. First, consider the case of a 68-year-old white protestant male who is referred by his internist after he told the internist that he was thinking of killing himself. History revealed that the patient had no children and no close friends, and that his wife had died eight months earlier. Subsequently he'd become depressed, had lost weight, sleep, energy and all capacity to enjoy things, and four months before seeing his internist he'd taken an overdose of codeine. The patient's past medical history was remarkable for lung cancer, currently in remission with ongoing chemotherapy. During the interview the patient reported he'd given up all hope of ever getting better and that he'd actually felt a little better since deciding to kill himself, and had finalized his will; he had bought a gun and planned to drive to a deserted field and shoot himself in the head. Clearly, such a patient is at very high risk, and should be immediately hospitalized.

On the other "extreme" of risk, consider the case of a 25-year-old black married, devoutly Catholic female who lived at home with her husband and children and who came to the interview at the urging of her friends. History revealed that for the past three months the patient, though not experiencing any recent losses, and in otherwise good health, had become depressed with some loss of sleep, difficulty concentrating, fatigue and an overall sense that life wasn't as enjoyable as it once had been. Although she'd never thought of suicide before and had certainly never made an attempt, she found herself occasionally thinking about suicide since becoming depressed, and had told her closest friends, who promptly encouraged her to get help. During the interview, the patient, though depressed, still had some hope that things might get better; when asked whether she'd actually thought about how she might kill herself, she confessed that she'd imagined taking some over-the-counter sleeping pills and then lying down next to her sleeping husband, and waiting for the pills to work. In this case, the risk of completed suicide is low, and such a patient may reasonably be treated on an outpatient basis.

Certainly, most patients do not fall at these extremes, and with regard to this vast majority which exist in the gray zone of risk assessment, making an estimate as to risk is difficult and anxiety-provoking. Faced with such a difficult clinical problem, many clinicians would like to be able to turn to an algorithm or computer program to assist them in estimating the risk. Unfortunately, however, and despite occasional claims to the contrary, none of these methods have been shown to be reliable, and hence clinical judgment, however inadequate it may feel, must be relied on.

Understandably, clinicians have also hoped that laboratory tests may provide some help, and, although certainly nothing is ready for clinical use, there is some hope that reliable testing may be available in the future. There is strong evidence that serotoninergic functioning is markedly disturbed in those who commit suicide. CSF levels of 5-HIAA, a metabolite of serotonin, are reduced in such patients, whereas the number of 5-HT2A receptors on platelets, which serve as models for neurons, is increased. Although obtaining CSF for the purpose of estimating the risk of suicide is probably not practical, obtaining platelets is routine, and it is conceivable that measuring the density of 5-HT2A receptors on platelets could become another method for estimating the risk of suicide.

TREATMENT

If the risk of suicide is judged to be relatively low, outpatient treatment may be appropriate. Prescriptions for any potentially lethal drugs should be restricted to a nonlethal amount, and the physician must watch for any evidence of "stockpiling." In this vein, if an antidepressant is indicated, one with a low lethality in overdose should be considered, for example an SSRI. Firearms should be disposed of or turned over to others for safekeeping, frequent outpatient sessions should be scheduled, and patients should be instructed to call if they feel unable to control themselves. If the risk is high, the patient should be admitted, preferably to a locked ward; involuntary confinement may be required. Patients should be thoroughly searched for any potential means of destruction, such as pills, knives, rope, and the like. Frequent, direct observation is required, and in some cases continuous observation is indicated. Stockpiling should be carefully guarded against: even a highly skilled nurse may not be able to detect "cheeking" if the patient is clever and determined enough. Given this, liquid concentrates or suspensions may be preferable to tablets.

Concurrent psychiatric and general medical conditions should be aggressively treated, and in this regard it is worthy of note that, in patients with bipolar disorder, lithium greatly reduces the long-term risk of suicide and clozapine reduces the risk of suicide attempts in those with schizophrenia.

BIBLIOGRAPHY

Appleby L. Suicide in psychiatric patients: risk and prevention. *The British Journal of Psychiatry* 1992;161:749-758.

Barraclough B, Bunch J, Nelson B, et al. A hundred cases of suicide: clinical aspects. *The British Journal of Psychiatry* 1974;125:355-373.

Borg SE, Stahl M. Predication of suicide; a prospective study of suicides and controls among psychiatric patients. *Acta Psychiatrica Scandinavica* 1982;65:221-232.

Cheng AT. Mental illness and suicide. A case-control study in east Taiwan. *Archives of General Psychiatry* 1995;52:594-603.

Henriksson MM, Aro HM, Marttunen MJ, et al. Mental disorders and comorbidity in suicide. *The American Journal of Psychiatry* 1993;150:935-940.

Meltzer HY, Alphs L, Green AI, et al. Clozapine treatment for suicidality in schizophrenia. *Archives of General Psychiatry* 2003;60:82-91.

Michel K. Suicide risk factors: a comparison of suicide attempters with suicide completers. *The British Journal of Psychiatry* 1987;150:78-82.

Murphy GE. Clinical identification of suicidal risk. *Archives of General Psychiatry* 1972;27:356-359.

Nierenberg AA, Gray SM, Grandin LD. Mood disorders and suicide. *The Journal of Clinical Psychiatry* 2001;62(Suppl 25):27-30.

Nordstrom P, Samuelsson M, Asberg M. Survival analysis of suicide risk after attempted suicide. *Acta Psychiatrica Scandinavica* 1995;91:336-340.

Pandey GN. Altered serotonin function in suicide. Evidence from platelet and neuroendocrine studies. *Annals of the New York Academy of Sciences* 1997;836:182-200.

Roy A. Risk factors for suicide in psychiatric patients. *Archives of General Psychiatry* 1982;39:1089-1095.

Tondo L, Baldassarini RJ. Reduced suicide risk during lithium maintenance treatment. *The Journal of Clinical Psychiatry* 2000;61(Suppl 9):97-104.

154   Violent Behavior

In considering violence, it is useful to differentiate between premeditated violence and impulsive (or "affective") violence. Premeditated violence may be seen in antisocial personality disorder; however, such cold-blooded, "predatory," acts are relatively uncommon. Much more frequently violence occurs in the heat of the moment, arising in the fertile soil of anger, irritability or rage.

Although research has not as yet yielded a full picture of the biology of impulsive violence, several findings do appear to be robust. First, it is clear that this form of violence runs in families, and although much of this may be accounted for by being raised in an atmosphere of abuse and violence, family, twin, and, tellingly, adoption studies also suggest a strong genetic component. Second, lesions within the limbic system, particularly the hypothalamus, may cause rage and aggressive behavior. Finally, CSF studies have repeatedly demonstrated decreased levels of 5-HIAA, a metabolite of serotonin, and platelet studies have demonstrated a reduced number of imipramine binding sites. Taken together, these findings are consistent with the notion that impulsive violence arises in the setting of serotoninergic dysfunction within the limbic system, in particular the hypothalamus, and that this dysfunction, in some cases, may be inherited.

Although predicting who is likely to engage in impulsive violence is difficult, certain risk factors are helpful.

RISK FACTORS

Risk factors for impulsive violence may be divided into those relating to demographics, the patient's psychiatric diagnosis, past history of violence, and, most importantly, the patient's current mental status.

Demographically, young adult males are most likely to be violent, in contrast with females of any age and with older males.

Certain illnesses, dealt with below, are associated with violent behavior, and of all these the two most important are mania and paranoid schizophrenia.

Mania of the irritable type, whether seen in bipolar disorder or schizoaffective disorder, is characterized by a short fuse and a very high temper, and if patients' demands are unmet or their purposes thwarted, they frequently erupt into a furious aggression.

Paranoid schizophrenia leaves patients on guard and suspicious, and such patients, if pressed or agitated, may "counter-attack" in what they see as fully justified self-defense.

Delusional disorder, like paranoid schizophrenia, may also be characterized by violence occurring on the basis of delusions. A patient with the erotomanic subtype of delusional disorder may assault the significant others of those with whom the patient feels erotically involved; a patient with the jealous subtype may assault a lover believed to have been faithless and cheating; and a patient with the persecutory subtype may, like the patient with paranoid schizophrenia, turn in self-defense on the imagined persecutors.

Catatonic schizophrenia, uncommonly seen these days, may be associated with "senseless" and unpredictable violence as patients abruptly emerge from a catatonic stupor into an excited catatonic state.

Various personality disorders may also be associated with violence, including paranoid personality disorder, antisocial personality disorder and borderline personality disorder. Patients with paranoid personality disorder, though chronically on guard and distrustful of others, are generally able to restrain themselves unless unusually provoked, as for example may occur when such patients are brought involuntarily to the hospital. Antisocial personality disorder may, as noted above, be associated with premeditated violence, and predicting this, of course, depends on becoming privy to the patient's plans. Sociopaths may also engage in impulsive violence, and this is generally predictable on the basis of how agitated they become when their plans or desires are thwarted. Borderline personality disorder is characterized by impulsivity and irritability, and when these patients feel abandoned or betrayed they may lash out at those they once depended on.

Patients with significant cognitive deficits, as may be seen in delirium, dementia or mental retardation, may lack both the ability to understand their present situation and to exercise self-restraint, leaving them prone to agitation or aggression. Delirious patients, especially those with a "noisy" delirium, may, in their confusion, misinterpret the efforts of nursing personnel as dangerous and assault the nurses in self-defense. Demented patients may likewise disastrously misinterpret others' efforts and may also become irritable and irascible when, because of their dementia, they are unable to cope with situations, such as finding things at home or in a store, that used to be routine. Mentally retarded patients may, in concert with their developmental age, fight with caretakers who deny them the food or amusements they wish to enjoy.

Personality change, especially of the frontal lobe type, may be characterized by "disinhibition" wherein, with the dissolution of self-restraint, patients do what they want to do, and take what they want to take, and become aggressive with those who stand in their way.

Various intoxications may be associated with violence. The "mean drunk" is a common sight in any emergency room, and patients with phencyclidine intoxication may unpredictably erupt with severe violence. Intoxication with stimulants, as for example cocaine, may cause delusions of persecution which, in turn, may induce the patient to attack the supposed persecutors.

Withdrawal from certain substances, notably heroin and cocaine, may be associated with a craving so strong that patients may kill to obtain their next dose.

Intermittent explosive disorder manifests with paroxysms of explosive, destructive anger, and these may occur either spontaneously or in response to relatively trivial provocations.

Finally, violence may be associated with complex partial seizures. Most of the time, such violence is only seen post-ictally, and only when staff attempt to restrain the confused patient. Very rarely, spontaneous, directed violence may occur during the seizure itself: for many years the occurrence of such events was doubted; however, there are well-documented case reports of video-EEG documented ictal violence.

A past history of violent behavior may be helpful, especially if the current situation mirrors one in the past wherein the patient did become violent. Another historical variable to consider is whether or not the patient had ever been cruel to animals: for reasons yet obscure, those patients who as children tortured cats or dogs are especially likely to behave violently as adults.

Finally, and most importantly, one should attend to the patient's current mental status. Hostility, irritability and progressively escalating agitation are all significant storm warnings, and when such patients have singled out a target and have a weapon at hand, whether it be a knife, gun, piece of furniture or simply balled fists, the likelihood of violence is very high. Indeed, when an experienced nurse reports that a patient is about to "go off," rapid intervention is generally required.

Utilizing these risk factors may or may not require considerable clinical judgment. Some cases are clear: for example a young man with paranoid schizophrenia who had backed himself into a corner and was ever more angrily threatening to kill anyone who came close is someone who requires immediate intervention. Most cases, however, are not so obvious; for example, many a "mean drunk" will calm down if simply left alone, perhaps in a private room.

TREATMENT

In situations where violence appears imminent, several interventions may be considered, including talking with the patient, medications and seclusion, with or without restraints.

Verbal interventions should generally be tried unless the patient has already "blown" or is just "on the edge," provided, of course, that the patient is capable of engaging in discussion: psychosis, cognitive deficits and some intoxications may make any attempts at verbal intervention futile. In the case of patients who are more or less still in control, an interview with a physician who is calm in voice, manner and posture, and who is able to speak with the patient without anxiety, authoritarianism or supercilliousness, may yield dramatic benefits. The setting for such interviews varies with the patient's condition. Those who seem in relatively good control may be seen in an office, with the door closed, whereas in the case of patients who are closer to "losing it," the door should be left open, and consideration should be given to having a guard in the hallway, but out of view. Regardless of whether the door is open or closed, the interview area should be cleared of potential weapons, such as scissors, and the physician should remove ties, necklaces and earrings; further, it is preferable that both the physician and patient be seated, and that both have unobstructed access to the door. If an office is not available and the patient must be seen in a public area, always attempt to remove the interview as far as possible from the view of others in order to avoid putting the patient into a situation where violence is necessary to "save face."

Medications useful in the face of violence include antipsychotics and benzodiazepines, as described in the chapter on rapid pharmacologic treatment of agitation.

Seclusion, with or without restraints, may be required when patients have lost control. In some cases, seclusion alone, with the attendant reduction in stimulation, may eventually prove effective; in other cases, restraints are required. One mustn't be shy about using restraints: despite the current fashion to do away with them, they may be life saving, especially in cases of mania, psychosis or delirium.

If the patient is not already hospitalized, this should generally be accomplished unless the underlying cause of the violence, e.g., alcohol intoxication, is expected to resolve in less than a day: in such cases, patients may generally be treated in the emergency room.

Once the threat of imminent violence is past, it is critical to ensure that any underlying disorder is rapidly treated, as described in their respective chapters. In addition to any available disorder-specific treatments, consideration may also be given to one of several medicines, each of which appears effective in reducing impulsive violence, often across diagnostic categories. Divalproex, lithium and carbamazepine are each effective, and may be utilized in a manner similar to that for the treatment of mania. Propranolol, often in high dose (if tolerated, up to from 240 to 640 mg daily) or nadolol (120 mg/day) are both effective in reducing violence in schizophrenia and dementia, and low dose risperidone (e.g., 0.5 to 2 mg daily) may also reduce aggression associated with dementia.

Finally, in the United States, if the intended victim is known, the clinician is legally bound to inform not only that person but also the police in whose jurisdiction the patient is and the police in whose jurisdiction the intended victim is.

BIBLIOGRAPHY

Elliott FA. Violence. The neurologic contribution: an overview. *Archives of Neurology* 1992;49:595-603.

Fava M. Psychopharmacologic treatment of pathologic aggression. *The Psychiatric Clinics of North America* 1997;20:427-451.

Felthous AR, Kellert SR. Childhood cruelty to animals and later aggression against people: a review. *The American Journal of Psychiatry* 1987; 144:710-717.

Lee R, Coccaro E. The neuropsychopharmacology of criminality and aggression. *Canadian Journal of Psychiatry* 2001;46:35-44.

Lindenmayer JP, Kotsaftis A. Use of sodium valproate in violent and aggressive behaviors: a critical review. *The Journal of Clinical Psychiatry* 2000;61:123-128.

Meltzer JE. Underlying mechanisms of psychosis and aggression in patients with Alzheimer's disease. *The Journal of Clinical Psychiatry* 2001; 62(Suppl 21):23-25.

Ratey JJ, Sorgi P, O'Driscoll GA, et al. Nadolol to treat aggression and psychiatric symptomatology in chronic psychiatric inpatients: a double-blind, placebo-controlled study. *The Journal of Clinical Psychiatry* 1992;53:41-46.

Sheard MH. Lithium in the treatment of aggression. *The Journal of Nervous and Mental Disease* 1975;160:108-118.

DELIRIUM, DEMENTIA, AND OTHER SECONDARY SYNDROMES

155 Delirium (DSM-IV-TR #293.0)

Delirium is a syndrome of many different causes characterized by confusion and loss of short-term memory. This syndrome has various synonyms, all of which tend to emphasize different facets of the clinical picture. They include encephalopathy, acute organic brain syndrome, acute confusional state, and, less commonly, acute toxic psychosis.

In most cases delirium exists on a continuum between alertness and stupor. The diseases that are capable of causing delirium do so by compromising, on a global basis, cerebral functioning, and when the disease is severe enough and the compromise sufficiently great, stupor, and eventually coma, may supervene.

As might be expected, the prevalence of delirium is highest among those most likely to have one or more of the diseases that are capable of causing such global compromise of cerebral function. Thus among patients on a general medical-surgical ward, the prevalence ranges from 10 to 30%; however, among elderly inpatients it may rise to as high as 40%.

ONSET

Delirium may occur at any age; however, it tends to be most common among the elderly and the very young. The onset is generally relatively acute; however, in some cases a subacute onset lasting days or weeks may be seen.

CLINICAL FEATURES

The hallmark of delirium is confusion, or, as it also has been called, clouding of the sensorium. Patients may appear somewhat dazed and unclear about their surroundings. They have difficulty perceiving correctly what goes on around them, and one may have difficulty capturing and holding their attention—they tend to drift off. Short-term memory is poor, and patients tend to lose grasp of what happened only minutes before; disorientation to time and place are common accompanying features.

Delusions and illusions or hallucinations may occur. Cracks in the ceiling may seem to be alive and moving; the ringing of a telephone is a fire alarm. Hallucinations tend to be visual: the family is gathered about the bed; animals burrow under the blankets; an angel hovers outside the window. They may hear sounds or muffled whispers; a voice may announce the patient's death or impending execution. Delusions tend to be of the persecutory type and are rarely systematized. The syringe is filled with poison; the

hospital is an elaborate prison; the physicians wish only to experiment on the patient.

The patient's speech may be circumstantial, tangential, or incoherent. Though not universal, a classic sign is carphologia, wherein the patient repetitively and aimlessly picks at the sheets or bed clothes. Sleep reversal may occur.

Upon formal mental status testing, in addition to confusion, one finds a degree of disorientation to time and/or place, an inability to recall all of three words after 5 minutes, and a decreased attention span, as measured by testing the digit span.

The overall behavior of the delirious patient may tend either toward agitation or quietude. Patients with an overactive or "noisy" delirium may be unable to stay in bed; they may climb over the bed rails, pull out intravenous lines and attempt to escape out the window. Those with delusions of persecution may refuse all care and even may attack those who try to take care of them. Frightening hallucinations may leave the patient terrified and screaming.

On the other hand, patients with a "quiet" or underactive delirium may not draw any clinical attention at all. They may lie listless and uncomplaining and do whatever they are told. All the while, however, they may have no sense of what is going on around them or why they are where they are.

Typically, though not universally, the symptoms of delirium tend to fluctuate over time. "Sundowning" is often seen as the patient's confusion worsens with the coming of night. In some cases, especially in the morning, patients may display a "lucid interval" wherein they appear quite clear and alert. Such morning lucid intervals may mislead diagnosticians as they make morning rounds.

Upon recovery from the delirium, patients have at best a patchy recall for the experience.

COURSE

The course of delirium is determined by the course of the underlying disease and by the effectiveness of any treatment given for that disease. In some cases recovery is prompt and complete, as for example when the delirium of hypoglycemia is promptly corrected by a glucose infusion. In other cases delirium may subside to leave the patient with a dementia. For example, a large ischemic cerebral infarction, with prominent surrounding edema, may cause a delirium which then subsides as the edema resolves, only to leave the patient with a dementia related to the loss of cerebral tissue.

With some diseases one may find patients with a chronic dementia with "superimposed" episodes of delirium. Multiple sclerosis is an example. Here a multiplicity of old, mature plaques may leave the patient demented; however, as new areas of inflammation appear, delirium may ensue that resolves as the inflammation subsides.

COMPLICATIONS

With a "quiet" delirium, patients may have no complications at all. In an agitated, "noisy" delirium, however, patients may be unable to cooperate with their care. Medicines may be refused, premature extubations may occur, and patients may fall and injure themselves as they attempt to flee.

ETIOLOGY

As noted earlier, delirium stems from a global disturbance in cerebral functioning. This disturbance may result from a truly "global" cause, for example when hypoglycemia deprives every neuron of its necessary supply of glucose. On the other hand, at times a localized lesion may exert "distant" effects, thus causing global compromise. An example would be a mass lesion that causes herniation, or perhaps a lesion strategically placed in a structure that in turn has "global" connections, for example an infarction of the thalamus. Table 155-1 lists most causes of delirium; almost all of these are covered in detail in their respective chapters.

When, after a thorough history and physical, the cause of the delirium is not apparent, one should "screen" for some of the more common causes with the following tests: CBC, sodium, potassium, calcium, glucose, BUN, creatinine, bilirubin, ammonia, and liver enzymes. A urine drug screen for illicit drugs may also be ordered in selected cases. If these are unrevealing or if one suspects a mass lesion, a CT or, preferably, MRI scan of the head may be obtained. EEGs are generally not necessary, unless one suspects complex partial status epilepticus. Arterial blood gases are obtained whenever one suspects respiratory failure.

Any given delirium may have multiple etiologies. Common examples include the alcoholic with a combination of delirium tremens and Wernicke's encephalopathy, and "post-operative" delirium. This last entity is seen in a substantial minority of patients post-operatively and is generally related to multiple factors, including medications (particularly those with anticholinergic effect), metabolic disturbances, hypoxia, decreased cerebral perfusion due to myocardial ischemia, and various infectious processes. Also, certain phenomena, although innocuous in young, healthy individuals, may be quite capable of producing delirium in the elderly or those with other illnesses. For example, dextromethorphan, taken with impunity by adults, may, in an elderly patient, cause considerable confusion. A temporal correlation between starting or increasing the dose of a drug and the occurrence of delirium should arouse suspicion.

DIFFERENTIAL DIAGNOSIS

Dementia is distinguished from delirium by the absence of confusion.

At the height of a manic episode (i.e., stage III mania), patients may become confused and disoriented; such symptoms, however, are a natural part of the mania and do not indicate a separate syndrome. The same holds true for a patient with stuporous

■**TABLE 155-1.** Causes of Delirium

Substance Intoxication
cannabis
phencyclidine
inhalants
stimulants (including cocaine)
methanol

Substance Withdrawal
alcohol (delirium tremens)
sedative-hypnotics

Medication Induced
anticholinergics
serotonin syndrome
neuroleptic malignant syndrome
lithium
levodopa
bromocriptine
amantadine
baclofen
prednisone
digoxin
cimetidine
theophylline
beta-blockers
isoniazid

Seizures
complex partial seizures
petit mal seizures
post-ictal state (after complex partial or grand mal seizures)

Heredodegenerative Disorders
diffuse Lewy body dementia
Alzheimer's disease (terminally)

Vascular Disorders
multi-infarct dementia
large or strategically placed infarctions (e.g., thalamic)
lacunar dementia
Binswanger's disease
polyarteritis nodosa
cranial arteritis
granulomatous angiitis
hypertensive encephalopathy
Behcet's syndrome

Immune-Related Disorders
limbic encephalitis
systemic lupus erythematosus
Hashimoto's encephalopathy

Brain Injury
carbon monoxide poisoning
subdural hematoma
delayed radiation encephalopathy
delayed post-anoxic encephalopathy

Mass Lesions and Hydrocephalus
brain tumor
brain abscess
acute hydrocephalus

Endocrinologic Disorders
Cushing's syndrome
adrenocortical insufficiency
hyperthyroidism ("thyroid storm")

Heavy Metal Poisoning
lead
thallium
arsenic

Vitamin Deficiency
Wernicke's encephalopathy (thiamine)
pellagra (niacin)

Infectious Disorders Directly Involving the Central Nervous System
neurosyphilis
tuberculosis
subacute measles encephalitis
infectious mononucleosis
mumps
acute viral meningoencephalitis
zoster
herpes simplex encephalitis
HIV
cytomegalovirus encephalopathy
mycoses
toxoplasmosis

Metabolic Disorders
dehydration
hyperglycemia
hypoglycemia
hypernatremia
hyponatremia
hypokalemia
hypermagnesemia
hypomagnesemia
hypercalcemia
hypocalcemia
uremia
dialysis dysequilibrium syndrome
hepatic encephalopathy
hepatic porphyria
respiratory failure

Others
high fever
severe hypotension (e.g., as in shock or grossly reduced cardiac output due to congestive heart failure, infarction or arrythmia)
severe anemia
infectious processes that do not directly involve the central nervous system (e.g., sepsis, pneumonia, or, in the elderly, even trivial infections, such as a urinary tract infection)
disseminated intravascular coagulation
thrombotic thombocytopenic purpura
Sydenham's chorea
chorea gravidarum

catatonic schizophrenia or a patient with undifferentiated schizophrenia in the midst of a severe exacerbation.

TREATMENT

Concurrent with pursuing symptomatic treatment as outlined below, discovering the cause of the delirium and treating that cause are essential.

Efforts should be made to help patients remain in contact with their surroundings. Large clocks and calendars are kept in full view, as are familiar pictures. The importance of having a window in the room cannot be overstated. At night the room should be quiet and bed rails kept up; a call button should be close at hand and a night light left on. In some cases around-the-clock attendance by sitters or family members (presuming there is not intense conflict within the family) may be helpful. Nursing procedures that can be delayed until daylight hours should be.

For patients with a "quiet" delirium, the foregoing symptomatic measures may suffice. Additional measures, however, are often required for the agitated, "noisy" patient. Antipsychotics constitute the mainstay of symptomatic pharmacologic treatment of delirium; however, it should be noted that there has been, remarkably, only one double-blinded study of their use in delirium. In this study of delirium in patients hospitalized with AIDS, both haloperidol and chlorpromazine were more effective than placebo. Of these two, chlorpromazine is not in common use, whereas haloperidol has become a standard. Haloperidol may be given in a dose of from 0.5 to 5 mg im, or 1 to 10 mg po, with repeat doses every hour if given intramuscularly or every two hours when given po, with the size of the repeat dose adjusted according to the patient's response. Treatment is continued until the patient is manageable and out of danger, limiting side effects occur or a maximum dose of 50 mg is reached. Once acute treatment has been effective, the patient may be continued on a regular daily dose roughly equivalent to three-quarters of the total dose needed during acute treatment, with provision for prn doses should there be a significant "breakthrough" of symptoms. Once the underlying cause of the delirium has resolved, the dose of the antipsychotic may be tapered over two or three days and then discontinued. Second-generation antipsychotics, such as risperidone, olanzapine, quetiapine, and ziprasidone, are also used in the treatment of delirium, and anecdotally have been successful; if risperidone is used, the ratio of risperidone dose to oral haloperidol dose is roughly 1:4.

Lorazepam or other benzodiazepines have no place in the treatment of delirium with the important exception of alcohol or sedative-hypnotic withdrawal. Small doses of lorazepam (e.g., 0.5 to 1.0 mg) may, however, be used at night to promote sleep.

At times, around-the-clock nursing care may be required; furthermore, restraints, either soft or leather, may likewise be required, and one should not hesitate in ordering them when the patient's delirious behavior becomes dangerous.

BIBLIOGRAPHY

Breitbart W, Marotta R, Platt MM, et al. A double-blind trial of haloperidol, chlorpromazine, and lorazepam in the treatment of delirium in hospitalized AIDS patients. *The American Journal of Psychiatry* 1996;153:231-237.

Lipowski ZJ. Transient cognitive disorders (delirium, acute confusional states) in the elderly. *The American Journal of Psychiatry* 1983;140:1426-1436.

Lipowski ZJ. Delirium (acute confusional state). *The Journal of American Medical Association* 1987;258:1789-1792.

Lipowski ZJ. Delirium in the elderly patient. *The New England Journal of Medicine* 1989;320:578-582.

Meagher DJ, O'Hanlon D, O'Mahony E, et al. Relationship between symptoms and motoric subtype of delirium. *The Journal of Neuropsychiatry and Clinical Neurosciences* 2000;12:51-56.

Roche V. Southwestern Internal Medicine Conference. Etiology and management of delirium. *The American Journal of the Medical Sciences* 2003;325:20-30.

Trzepacz PT. The neuropathogenesis of delirium: a need to focus our research. *Psychosomatics* 1994;35:374-391.

Winawer N. Postoperative delirium. *The Medical Clinics of North America* 2001;85:1229-1239.

156 Dementia (DSM-IV-TR #290.40-290.44, 294.10, 294.11, 294.8)

Dementia is a syndrome of multiple different etiologies characterized by a global decrement in cognitive functioning occurring in a clear sensorium. Though not confused, patients have difficulty with short-term memory and, to a relatively lesser degree, long-term memory. Intellectual abilities are likewise impaired. The ability to think abstractly fails, and patients become more and more concrete; relatively simple calculations are now beyond their grasp, and the ability to exercise "good judgment" in complex situations is lost.

In the past, dementia was also known as "chronic organic brain syndrome." Given, however, that not all dementias are necessarily chronic and irreversible, this term might best be dropped from our lexicon.

As most of the more common diseases that cause dementia occur in the elderly, the prevalence of dementia shows a striking association with age. Whereas anywhere from 5% to 10% of the entire population over the age of 65 is demented, at least 30% of the population over 80 is so affected.

ONSET

Both age and mode of onset are determined by the underlying disease. The onset may be acute (e.g., after head trauma) or insidious (e.g., with a slowly growing brain tumor). Furthermore, the onset may either be in early years (e.g., with adrenoleukodystrophy) or in later years (e.g., Alzheimer's disease).

CLINICAL FEATURES

The loss of short-term memory may manifest in a variety of ways. Patients may forget where they put their keys; they may forget to turn off the stove or lock the doors at night. Deficits in long-term memory, which are always less severe than short-term memory losses, may become apparent when patients are unable to find their way home or forget where their grown children live. Short-term memory is formally tested by asking patients to recall three unrelated objects after 5 minutes; long-term memory is assessed by asking them to name the last four Presidents or to recall significant facts from their own distant personal history, such as where they went to school or when their parents died.

A deficiency in abstract thinking often becomes evident when the patient is faced with a new and complex task or situation. For example, the retired accountant may not be able to figure out and properly complete a new tax form, or a former champion chess player may be beaten again and again by relative novices. Abstract thinking may be formally tested by asking the patient to find similarities between apples and oranges or pencils and typewriters. Patients may also be asked to explain what old proverbs mean to them. The demented patient may be unable to see any similarity between a pencil and a typewriter and may give a "concrete" response to a proverb. For example, if asked what "don't cry over spilled milk" means, the demented patient may reply "well, it's already spilled."

The loss of calculating ability may become evident when the patient tries to make change or perhaps fails in balancing the checkbook. Formal testing is accomplished by asking the patient to perform simple addition and subtraction, and, if successful, to then attempt serial 7's by subtracting 7 from 100 and then 7 from the remainder, and so forth.

The loss of good judgment is often what first calls the patient to clinical attention. Subtleties are lost on the patient, and complex social situations may be approached with unaccustomed crudeness. A statesman might swear at a colleague, rather than use a "diplomatic" approach; an elderly retiree may begin propositioning teenagers. Manners and social graces are lost: food may be ravenously eaten; patients may indulge in crude jokes and overly boisterous laughter at parties. Grooming, dress, and hygiene often suffer. Patients may neglect to shave; makeup is applied haphazardly; crumbs of food are left on the shirt front.

Along with decay of good judgment, one often sees a "personality change." In some cases maladaptive personality traits become more prominent; a conscientious patient may become extremely rigid and cruelly critical; a circumspect patient may become suspicious and guarded. In other cases the personality may seem to change entirely: a prudish patient may become flirtatious and seductive; a happy-go-lucky patient may become irritable and demanding.

At times the deficits in abstracting ability or calculation may first become evident in what is known as an acute "catastrophic reaction." This may occur when patients, in facing a task that they had always been able to accomplish before, find that task completely beyond their ability to grasp. A typical example would be a checkout line in a store, when the patient, completely unable to manage the financial transaction, becomes extremely agitated. Such catastrophic reactions reflect the patient's enforced awareness of their deficits.

Often, hallucinations and delusions occur. The hallucinations may be either visual or, less commonly, auditory. Patients may see dead relatives or perhaps animals or complex scenes. Music and voices may be heard, or at times only creakings, footfalls, or sirens. A very common delusion is the belief that something has been stolen. Typically the patient puts something away and then, forgetting where it is and unable to find it, may accuse others of having stolen it. Another common delusion involves jealousy, and the patient may accuse the spouse of having an affair. Finally, one may encounter the "phantom boarder syndrome" wherein the patient believes that someone is hiding somewhere, perhaps in the attic or basement.

Other symptoms and signs, such as apraxia, agnosia, and aphasia, may or may not occur, depending on the underlying cause of the dementia.

COURSE

The course is determined by the underlying cause and may be either static or progressive. For example, the traumatic dementia following severe head injury tends to be "static," with symptoms generally remaining the same over the years. Conversely, Alzheimer's disease causes a relentlessly progressive dementia.

Although in the natural course of events almost all of the dementias are chronic, in some cases treatment may effect a remission. This may occur, for example, with treatment of hypothyroidism or hypovitaminosis B_{12}. In cases with structural damage, however, such as infarcts, a full remission is not possible.

Regardless of whether the course is static or progressive, patients with dementia are prone to the development of delirium during intercurrent illnesses. Urinary tract infections, attacks of bronchitis, and mild degrees of dehydration, all of which might have passed without complication before the dementia, now often cause a superimposed delirium. Thus the course of dementia may be "punctuated" by recurrent deliria.

COMPLICATIONS

Patients may wander away from home, perhaps only to become lost, but perhaps also out into a busy street. Some may insist on driving or using hazardous machinery long after they have lost the ability to do so. Those who insist on handling their finances and business affairs may become bankrupt.

In more advanced cases, patients are prone to decubiti, falls and fractures, dehydration, and the like.

ETIOLOGY

The box on p. 285 lists most of the important causes of dementia. Of all these, the most common cause of dementia is Alzheimer's disease; other common causes include certain of the vascular dementias (e.g., multi-infarct dementia, lacunar dementia, Binswanger's disease), alcoholic dementia, diffuse Lewy body disease, advanced Parkinson's disease, various tumors, normal pressure hydrocephalus, subdural hematoma, and, especially among younger adults, AIDS. Although only 10% or less of all cases of dementia are due to potentially fully reversible causes, one should nevertheless diligently search for these, with special attention to Wilson's disease, Hashimoto's encephalopathy, systemic lupus erythematosus, subdural hematoma, certain tumors (e.g., meningiomas or low-grade gliomas), normal pressure hydrocephalus, hyper- or hypothyroidism, and either vitamin B_{12} or folate deficiency.

When, after a thorough history and physical examination, the cause is not clear, instituting a "screen" of laboratory tests is

Causes of Dementia

SUBSTANCE RELATED
Inhalants
Alcoholic dementia
Methanol intoxication
Marchiafava-Bignami disease

HEREDODEGENERATIVE DISORDERS
Alzheimer's disease
Pick's disease
Parkinson's disease
Diffuse Lewy body disease
Huntington's disease
Wilson's disease
Progressive supranuclear palsy
Multiple system atrophy
Myotonic dystrophy
Amytrophic lateral sclerosis
Cerebrotendinous xanthomatosis
Adrenoleukodystrophy
Metachromatic leukodystrophy
Hallervorden-Spatz disease

VASCULAR DISORDERS
Multiinfarct dementia
Lacunar dementia
Binswanger's disease
Polyarteritis nodosa
Cranial arteritis
Granulomatous angiitis
Hypertensive encephalopathy
CADASIL
Cerebral amyloid angiopathy
Wegener's granulomatosis

IMMUNE-MEDIATED DISORDERS
Limbic encephalitis
Multiple sclerosis
Hashimoto's encephalopathy
Systemic lupus erythematosus
Sarcoidosis

BRAIN INJURY
Postanoxic dementia
Delayed postanoxic encephalopathy
Traumatic dementia
Subdural hematoma
Dementia pugilistica
Delayed radiation encephalopathy

MASS LESIONS AND HYDROCEPHALUS
Brain tumor
Brain abscess
Hydrocephalus
Normal-pressure hydrocephalus

ENDOCRINOLOGIC DISORDERS
Hyperthyroidism (apathetic type)
Hypothyroidism

METAL POISONING
Lead encephalopathy
Manganese dementia
Thallium poisoning
Arsenic poisoning
Mercury poisoning
Dialysis dementia

VITAMIN DEFICIENCIES
Pellagra
Vitamin B_{12} deficiency
Folic acid deficiency

INFECTIOUS AND RELATED DISORDERS
Neurosyphilis
Tuberculosis
Lyme dementia
Whipple's disease
Progressive rubella panencephalitis
Subacute sclerosing panencephalitis
Encephalitis lethargica
Creutzfeldt-Jakob disease
AIDS dementia
Progressive multifocal leuko-encephalopathy
Cytomegalovirus encephalopathy
Mycoses

Toxoplasmosis

METABOLIC DISORDERS
Hypoglycemia
Hypocalcemic encephalopathy
Acquired hepatocerebral degeneration

may be given to a second level screen with an EEG and lumbar puncture. If a lumbar puncture is performed, the following are routinely ordered: total protein, glucose, cell count and differential, VDRL, HIV antibodies, myelin basic protein, oligoclonal bands, IgG level, India ink preparation, gram stain and routine culture and sensitivity. A simultaneous blood glucose and serum protein electrophoresis should also be obtained. Other CSF studies (e.g., PCR assay for tuberculosis, fungal cultures) are ordered as indicated.

DIFFERENTIAL DIAGNOSIS

Among children mental retardation may be distinguished from dementia by the course. In mental retardation cognitive development increases only up to a point (at the most to about a sixth-grade level), then "flattens out," without any decrement. By contrast, in dementia, cognitive ability undergoes a definite falling off. Occasionally, as in Down's syndrome, the same disease may cause both mental retardation and a dementia.

"Benign senescent forgetfulness" is the term applied to the mild degree of memory loss that is a normal part of aging. Unfortunately, given a person with a recent slight loss of memory, one cannot definitively tell, prospectively, whether the memory loss will remain mild or progress and be joined by other cognitive losses. Thus only long-term follow-up can reliably distinguish between benign senescent forgetfulness and a very gradually progressive dementia.

Delirium is distinguished from dementia primarily by the presence of confusion. At times, however, certain diseases can cause both delirium and dementia. A common example is multiinfarct dementia, wherein each fresh infarct creates a delirium, which in turn gradually clears along with the peri-lesional edema, leaving the patient, however, one "step" further down into dementia. Another important example is diffuse Lewy body disease, wherein delirium typically occurs early on in the course of the dementia.

Depression, especially in the elderly, may cause at times profound cognitive deficits. This "dementia syndrome of depression" (or, as it has also been called, "pseudodementia") is suggested by a history of depressive episodes, the presence of typical "vegetative" signs (e.g., insomnia, weight loss) and by the patient's tendency to give up trying on being asked difficult mental status questions. In doubtful cases, a "diagnosis by treatment response" to an antidepressant may be justified; however, one must keep in mind that the cognitive deficits of any given elderly patient may be due not only to depression but also to some other process, such as Alzheimer's disease.

Amnesia, as may occur in Korsakoff's syndrome, may superficially resemble dementia. However, in these cases only memory is lost; abstracting and calculating abilities are retained.

TREATMENT

The first task is to arrive at an accurate diagnosis of the causative disease and then, if any specific treatment is available, to institute it. Concurrent with this, symptomatic measures, if required, may be instituted.

The demands placed on patients should be reduced commensurate with their reduced cognitive abilities. Weapons should be removed and, eventually, patients will have to surrender the car keys, credit cards and the checkbook. Guardianship may be required.

prudent. Among adults the vast majority of cases are identified by one of the following: MRI scan with enhancement, ANA, ESR, thyroid profile with TSH, B12 and folate levels (or, for enhanced sensitivity, homocysteine and methylmalonic acid levels), calcium, HIV and FTA-ABS (neither an RPR nor a VDRL are adequate for testing for neurosyphilis as both may be normal in such cases). If Wilson's disease is suspected, copper and ceruloplasmin levels are obtained, and if Hashimoto's encephalopathy seems likely, anti-thyroid antibodies. If this first "screen" is negative, consideration

Familiar routine and surroundings should be maintained for as long as possible. A move from a lifetime home to a retirement apartment may be catastrophic for patients who are unable to remember and familiarize themselves with new surroundings. Night-lights are a necessity, and for patients who wander, locking doors and even windows may be necessary.

If hospitalization or institutionalization is required, certain measures can reduce the risk of a catastrophic reaction. The patient's room should have a window, a large calendar (marked off day by day), and a large clock, preferably a digital one. Familiar photographs and personal items (even furniture, if possible) should be brought, and arrangements should be made for delivery of the patient's local newspaper. Visits from family and friends should generally be encouraged.

At times, institutionalization may be avoided by the use of home sitters, visiting nurses, "Meals on Wheels," and adult day-care centers.

Symptomatic pharmacologic treatment of dementia may be required for agitation or aggression, delusions or hallucinations, depression and insomnia.

Agitation or aggression may be treated with antipsychotics, antiepileptic drugs, or trazodone. Both low-dose risperidone and haloperidol (i.e., 0.5 to 1.5 mg) are effective, but risperidone is better tolerated. Carbamazepine in low doses (yielding blood levels at the low end of the "therapeutic range") is helpful, and there is some indication that divalproex may also be effective. Trazodone, in doses of 50 to 250 mg, was found equivalent to haloperidol in one study. Choosing among these agents is difficult, as there are few comparison studies. Certainly, if there were concurrent delusions or hallucinations, an antipsychotic would be a reasonable first choice; however, these agents must be used with extreme care in cases of diffuse Lewy body disease, given the risk of severe antipsychotic-induced parkinsonism. Initial doses should be low, and titration should be gradual, and this is especially the case with carbamazepine and trazodone, given the risk of hypotension and falls.

Delusions or hallucinations generally respond to risperidone; however, in the case of diffuse Lewy body disease, there is now evidence that rivastigmine, a cholinesterase inhibitor, may also be effective.

Depression may be treated with an SSRI, such as citalopram; if a tricyclic is deemed preferable, consideration may be given to nortriptyline.

Insomnia may be treated with low dose lorazepam or zolpidem.

Certain dementing disorders have specific treatments (e.g., cholinesterase inhibitors for Alzheimer's disease) and these are specified in the appropriate chapter.

All medication regimens should be kept as simple as possible, with the lowest number of pills and the least number of dosings per day possible.

Proper glasses, hearing aids and dentures, if needed, are essential. Quad canes and walkers should be encouraged, and wheelchairs avoided if at all possible. Rigorous internal medical follow-up is required in all cases, and it must be borne in mind that seemingly trivial disorders, such as urinary tract infections, may cause significant agitation in elderly demented patients.

BIBLIOGRAPHY

Arnold SE, Kumar A. Reversible dementias. *The Medical Clinics of North America* 1993;77:215-230.

Brodaty A, Ames D, Snowdon J, et al. A randomized, placebo-controlled trial of risperidone for the treatment of aggression, agitation, and psychosis of dementia. *The Journal of Clinical Psychiatry* 2003;64:134-143.

Corey-Bloom J, Thal LJ, Galasko D, et al. Diagnosis and evaluation of dementia. *Neurology* 1995;45:211-218.

De Deyn PP, Rabheru K, Rasmussen A, et al. A randomized trial of risperidone, placebo, and haloperidol for behavioral symptoms of dementia. *Neurology* 1999;53:946-955.

Gustafson L. Clinical classification of dementia conditions. *Acta Neurologica Scandinavica* 1992;85(suppl 139):16-20.

Nyth AL, Gottfries CG, Lyby K, et al. A controlled multicenter clinical study of citalopram and placebo in elderly depressed patients with and without concomitant dementia. *Acta Psychiatrica Scandinavica* 1992;86:138-145.

Porsteinsson AP, Tariot PN, Erb R, et al. Placebo-controlled study of divalproex for agitation in dementia. *The American Journal of Geriatric Psychiatry* 2001;9:58-66.

Sultzer DL, Gray KF, Gunay I, et al. A double-blind comparison of trazodone and haloperidol for treatment of agitation in patients with dementia. *The American Journal of Geriatric Psychiatry* 1997;5:60-69.

Tariot PN, Erb R, Podgorski CA, et al. Efficacy and tolerability of carbamazepine for agitation and aggression in dementia. *The American Journal of Psychiatry* 1998;155:54-61.

Vicosio BA. Dementia: when is it not Alzheimer's disease? *The American Journal of the Medical Sciences* 2002;324:84-95.

157   Amnesia

Memory may be either "procedural" or "declarative." Procedural memory refers to the ability to remember how to do something, as for example how to ride a bicycle or play a piano. Declarative memory, in contrast, refers to the ability to remember facts or events, such as who the last three presidents were or what happened earlier in the day: the remembrance of facts is known as "semantic" memory, and that of events, "episodic" memory.

In clinical practice, the most important kind of amnesia deals with declarative memory of the episodic type, and this is the type of amnesia covered in this chapter. Episodic amnesia may be further usefully divided into anterograde and retrograde forms. Anterograde amnesia is said to be present when patients are unable to form new memories on an ongoing basis, and is tested for on the mental status exam by giving patients three words, and then, five minutes later, asking them to recall them: when anterograde amnesia is present, patients find they have no memory of them. Retrograde amnesia is said to be present when patients are unable to summon up memories they once had. For example, patients who, prior to the onset of the amnesia, had no difficulty recalling what happened a month earlier will, once the retrograde amnesia has set in, be unable to recall those events.

ONSET

The onset may vary from acute to gradual, depending on the underlying cause.

CLINICAL FEATURES

Most, but not all, cases of amnesia are characterized by a combination of anterograde and retrograde elements, with the anterograde element being most profound. In evaluating such patients, one finds that they are generally unable to recall events which occurred subsequent to the onset of the amnesia, including events that transpire during the interview itself. Thus, if the amnesia began a week earlier, patients are unable to recall events since then, and are also unable to recall the physician's name (assuming the physician had not been met before the onset of the amnesia) or the three words given on the mental status examination after the passage of five minutes. Moment-to-moment memory, however, is maintained, and patients may have a normal digit span and be able to follow a conversation. The retrograde aspect of the amnesia becomes apparent when the physician asks questions about what happened prior to the onset of the amnesia. Here, the patient's difficulty in recalling events prior to the onset of the amnesia typically exhibits a "temporal gradient" wherein recall is poorest for events relatively close to the onset of the amnesia, better, but still spotty, for events further back in the past, and generally good for events in the distant past.

Amnesias may be either chronic (as may occur in Korsakoff's syndrome) or transient, as for example in transient global amnesia. In transient cases, the clinical picture changes radically once patients recover. Subsequent to recovery, the retrograde amnesia either clears entirely or shrinks substantially, and patients are once again able to recall events that occurred up to the onset of the amnesia. They are also able to form new memories, and hence can recall events that have happened since the amnesia remitted and, of course, are now able to recall three words given to them during a mental status examination. They cannot, however, recall events that transpired during the amnesia, and it is as if, in looking back in time, patients experience a blank in their sequential recollections, a blank which corresponds to the time when the amnesia was in effect.

As noted, although most cases of amnesia have both anterograde and retrograde components, there are exceptions characterized by pure retrograde amnesia: here, although patients have no difficulty in recalling events that occurred subsequent to the onset of the retrograde amnesia, they are unable to recall events from the past.

COURSE

As noted earlier, amnesia may be either chronic or transient, depending on the underlying cause.

COMPLICATIONS

When anterograde amnesia is present, as is generally the case, some degree of supervision is required. When amnesia is transient, it may constitute little more than an inconvenience, with patients simply being observed in a safe environment until the amnesia remits. When chronic, however, amnesia is disabling, and institutional care may be required in severe cases.

ETIOLOGY

The various causes of amnesia are listed in Table 157-1. These are divided into two groups, namely those characterized by a combination of anterograde and retrograde components, which is by far the most common, and then those characterized by pure retrograde amnesia, which are very rare. The amnesias with both an anterograde and a retrograde component are further subdivided into those which are chronic, such as Korsakoff's syndrome (as often seen in alcoholism), and those which are transient, and remit spontaneously, as for example transient global amnesia.

With the exception of dissociative amnesia, the etiology of which is not known, all of the other causes involve damage or dysfunction of certain specific parts of the central nervous system.

Amnesias characterized by a combination of anterograde and retrograde components almost always involve bilateral lesions in the circuit of Papez. This circuit begins in the mammillary body of the hypothalamus and involves, successively, the mammillothalamic tract, anterior nucleus of the thalamus, cingulate cortex, cingulum, subicular cortex of the temporal lobe, hippocampus and, finally, the fornix, which, after leaving the hippocampus, connects back to the mammillary body, thus completing the circuit.

Pure retrograde amnesia has been noted in rare cases of trauma or encephalitis damaging the temporal pole bilaterally.

DIFFERENTIAL DIAGNOSIS

Delirium and dementia, although typically presenting with at least some defect in memory, are distinguished from the amnestic disorders by the presence of other cognitive deficits, such as confusion and deficient abstracting or calculating ability.

Depression, as may be seen in major depression or bipolar disorder, may be associated with great difficulty in memory; however, the diagnosis is suggested by the presence of depressed mood and vegetative symptoms and also by patients' response to questions during the mental status examination: upon being asked to recall the three words given five minutes earlier, patients with amnesia will generally try hard, whereas patients with depression, fatigued by the effort to do anything, generally give up, uttering a weary "I can't."

■**TABLE 157-1.** Causes of Amnesia

Anterograde with a variably extensive retrograde component
  Chronic
    Korsakoff's syndrome
    Infarction or tumor involving any structure in the circuit of Papez
    Limbic encephalitis
    Prodrome to Alzheimer's or Pick's disease
    Traumatic brain injury
    Cerebral anoxia
    Herpes simplex encephalitis
    Status epilepticus
  Transient
    Transient global amnesia
    Alcoholic blackouts
    Pure epileptic amnesia
    Concussion
    Transient ischemic attacks
    Dissociative amnesia
Pure retrograde
  Traumatic brain injury
  Herpes simplex encephalitis
  Dissociative amnesia

Benign senescent forgetfulness is a condition characterized by very mild anterograde and retrograde amnesia in the elderly, and is generally considered a normal part of ageing. This diagnosis, however, must always be tentative, as, with time and extended follow-up, the amnesia may worsen and become clinically significant, eventually revealing itself as a prodrome to Alzheimer's disease.

TREATMENT

Treatment is directed at the underlying cause. Supervision is required when anterograde amnesia is ongoing, and some patients may require institutionalization. In chronic cases, consideration may be given to certain mnenomic devices, such as lists and "memory boards" to help the patient keep track of events.

BIBLIOGRAPHY

Benson DF, Geschwind N. Shrinking retrograde amnesia. *Journal of Neurology, Neurosurgery, and Psychiatry* 1967;30:539-544.

Colchester A, Kingsley D, Lasserson D, et al. Structural MRI volumetric analysis in patients with organic amnesia, 1: methods and comparative findings across diagnostic groups. *Journal of Neurology, Neurosurgery, and Psychiatry* 2001;71:13-22.

Kopelman MD, Lasserson D, Kingsley D, et al. Structural MRI volumetric analysis in patients with organic amnesia, 2: correlations with anterograde memory and executive tests in 40 patients. *Journal of Neurology, Neurosurgery, and Psychiatry* 2001;71:23-28.

Seltzer B, Benson DF. The temporal pattern of retrograde amnesia in Korsakoff's disease. *Neurology* 1974;24:527-530.

Spiers HJ, Maguire EA, Burgess N. Hippocampal amnesia. *Neurocase* 2001;7:357-382.

158 Personality Change (personality change due to a general medical condition, DSM-IV-TR #310.1)

An apparently unaccountable change in a patient's personality may signify the presence of any of a variety of diseases affecting the brain. In some cases such a change in personality may be the only symptom, whereas in others it may only be a prodrome to a far more global expression of brain disease, such as dementia.

Synonyms include "personality change due to a general medical condition," "secondary personality disorder," and "organic personality syndrome."

ONSET

The age and mode of onset are determined by the underlying cause. A brain tumor may cause an insidiously progressive personality change; on the other hand, a personality change following a stroke may come on fairly acutely and then remain static.

CLINICAL FEATURES

The personality change itself may be characterized by either an aggravation of previously relatively minor personality traits or by the appearance of traits previously foreign to the patient. For example, a previously outgoing, if slightly penny-pinching person may gradually become miserly and unwilling to go out, or a previously staid, almost prudish person may begin to show an indiscreet sexual interest in young teenagers. At times the changes may be quite dramatic. Unprovoked anger and aggressiveness, persecutory ideas, impulsivity, lability, or gross indifference may occur.

Two specific kinds of personality change, namely the frontal lobe syndrome and the interictal personality syndrome (also known as the Geschwind syndrome), are discussed in their respective chapters.

Regardless of the kind of personality change, those around the patient often comment that "he is not himself anymore." Indeed this complaint may be what leads family members to bring the patient to medical attention.

COURSE

The course is determined by the underlying disease.

COMPLICATIONS

Personality change may impair the patient's ability to relate to family, friends, and co-workers, resulting in divorce, job termination, or legal difficulties.

ETIOLOGY

Personality change may result from a variety of conditions, as listed in Table 158-1, each of which is covered in more detail in its own chapter.

DIFFERENTIAL DIAGNOSIS

Personality change is distinguished from a personality disorder by the course. A personality disorder has its onset in teenage years or earlier and represents not so much a change as a coalescence of traits already present in childhood. By contrast a "personality change" signifies a break with an already established character structure. Personality disorders never have an onset in adult life, whereas a personality change, as might be expected from the etiologies noted above, usually occurs in adult years or later.

Dementia is distinguished from personality change by deficits in memory, abstracting abilities, and the like.

Schizophrenia may present with a long prodromal personality change. Telltale mannerisms and behavior often hint at the correct diagnosis.

■TABLE 158-1. Conditions Associated with a Personality Change

Epileptic Disorders
Interictal personality syndrome

Heredodegenerative Disorders
Alzheimer's disease
Pick's disease
Amyotrophic lateral sclerosis
Huntington's disease
Wilson's disease
Myotonic muscular dystrophy

Vascular Disorders
Infarction (esp. of frontal lobe, temporal lobe, basal ganglia, or thalamus)
Multi-infarct dementia
Lacunar dementia

Immune-Related Disorders
Limbic encephalitis
Multiple sclerosis

Brain Injury
Closed head injury
Subdural hematoma

Mass Lesions and Hydrocephalus
Tumors (esp. of frontal or temporal lobes)
Normal pressure hydrocephalus

Metal Poisoning
Lead
Mercury
Manganese

Vitamin Deficiency
B12 deficiency

Infectious and Related Disorders
Neurosyphilis
Post-viral encephalitis
Creutzfeldt-Jakob disease
AIDS

TREATMENT

Concurrent with symptomatic treatment, one must diagnose and, if possible, treat the underlying cause.

Typically, some form of supervision is required; guardianship may be indicated. Lability, impulsivity or aggressiveness may be treated with a mood stabilizer such as lithium, divalproex or carbamazepine; propranolol in high doses (up to 640 mg) may also be useful for aggressiveness.

The treatment of the frontal lobe syndrome and the interictal personality syndrome are as described in those chapters.

BIBLIOGRAPHY

Aitken L, Simpson S, Burns A. Personality change in dementia. *International Psychogeriatrics* 1999;11:263-271.

Brooks DN, McKinlay W. Personality and behavioral change after severe blunt head injury—a relative's view. *Journal of Neurology, Neurosurgery, and Psychiatry* 1983;46:336-344.

Max JE, Robertson BA, Lansing AE. The phenomenology of personality change due to traumatic brain injury in children and adolescents. *The Journal of Neuropsychiatry and Clinical Neurosciences* 2001;13:161-170.

Pelegrin Valero C, Gomez Hernanadez R, Munoz Cespedes JM, et al. Nosologic aspects of personality change due to head trauma. *Revista de Neurologia* 2001;32:681-687.

Tsai SJ, Hsiao YH. Secondary personality change in psychiatric in-patients. *Psychiatry and Clinical Neurosciences* 1999;53:433-435.

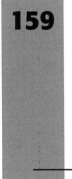

159 Secondary Psychosis (psychotic disorder due to a general medical condition, DSM-IV-TR #293.81-293.82; substance-induced psychotic disorder, DSM-IV-TR #291.3, 291.5, 292.11, 292.12)

The most common causes of psychosis are one of the primary, or idiopathic, psychotic disorders, such as schizophrenia, schizoaffective disorder and delusional disorder. Psychosis, however, may also occur secondary to a large number of general medical conditions, substances of abuse or medications, and one of the most important tasks for the clinician is to differentiate between primary and secondary psychoses, and, when a secondary one is present, to address, if possible, the underlying cause in the hopes of definitively relieving the patient's psychosis.

ONSET

The underlying cause determines both the age and mode of onset of the psychosis.

CLINICAL FEATURES

Patients may have delusions, or hallucinations, or both. Although any kind of delusion is possible, delusions of persecution or reference are perhaps most common. Hallucinations, likewise, may be of any type, including auditory, visual, tactile, olfactory and gustatory, but in general auditory and visual hallucinations are most common. Importantly, patients with a secondary psychosis are not confused, and have intact orientation and memory; furthermore, when hallucinations are present, these patients lack insight into their pathologic nature and believe that their hallucinatory experience is as "real" as any other experience.

COURSE

The course is determined by the underlying cause. Secondary psychoses may be either self-limited, as for example a psychosis secondary to cocaine intoxication, which resolves gradually as the cocaine washes out, or chronic, as in the case of inter-ictal psychoses.

COMPLICATIONS

At the least, psychosis is a distracting experience; at worst, patients who act on their delusions, or in reaction to hallucinations, may engage in the most regrettable of behaviors.

ETIOLOGY

Table 159-1 lists the major causes of secondary psychosis, including substances, medications and various general medical conditions.

With this table in mind, the cause of the psychosis may generally be determined. With regard to substances of abuse, the psychosis with amphetamines, cocaine, hallucinogens, phencyclidine and cannabis always has its inception during intoxication, which immediately suggests the diagnosis, which, in turn, is confirmed by a positive drug screen, and, importantly, by a resolution of the psychosis with abstinence. Alcoholics may develop either alcoholic paranoia, characterized by delusions of persecution, or alcohol hallucinosis, characterized by auditory hallucinations, and although these disorders may persist for very long periods into sobriety, they always have their onset within the context of chronic, severe, active alcoholism. Anabolic steroids may cause a psychosis, and this etiology is suggested by the "bulked up" appearance of the patient, accompanied, in males, by acne, testicular atrophy and a low serum testosterone level.

With regard to medication-induced psychosis, one generally looks for a connection between the onset of the psychosis and either the initiation of a drug or a significant increase in dose. Of the medications listed in the table, dopaminergic agents, such as levodopa and bromocriptine, and sympathomimetics, such as phenylpropanolamine and phenylephrine, are by far the most common offenders; only very rarely is psychosis seen with bupropion, fluoxetine or disulfiram. The psychosis that may rarely occur in association with baclofen is unusual, in that it only occurs after chronic use of baclofen, and then only as a withdrawal phenomenon, after the baclofen is abruptly discontinued. The psychosis seen with antipsychotics is also unusual in that it occurs only after chronic use: this "supersensitivity psychosis" is rare, and is generally seen in association with tardive dyskinesia, thus prompting the alternative name of "tardive psychosis."

With regard to psychoses secondary to general medical conditions, it is useful, from a clinical point of view, to divide these medical conditions into those with more or less specific associated features and those which generally lack such features.

In the case of general medical conditions with specific features, the table lists, in parentheses, the specific features which, though

■**TABLE 159-1.** Causes of Secondary Psychosis
Substances of abuse:
amphetamines
cocaine
hallucinogens
phencyclidine
cannabis
alcohol (alcohol hallucinosis and alcoholic paranoia)
anabolic steroids
Medications:
dopaminergic drugs
sympathomimetics
bupropion
fluoxetine
disulfiram
baclofen (upon discontinuation)
antipsychotics (supersensitivity, or "tardive," psychosis)
Secondary to general medical conditions with specific features:
associated with epilepsy
ictal psychosis
post-ictal psychosis
psychosis of forced normalization
chronic inter-ictal psychosis
associated with "encephalitic" features (fever, headache)
herpes simplex encephalitis
infectious mononucleosis
encephalitis lethargica
post-encephalitic psychosis
post-head trauma
Huntington's disease (chorea)
Sydenham's chorea (chorea)
chorea gravidarum (chorea)
manganism (parkinsonism)
Creutzfeldt-Jakob disease (esp. the "new-variant" type) (ataxia, myoclonus)
Hashimoto's encephalopathy (myoclonus)
Wilson's disease (various abnormal involuntary movements)
AIDS (thrush, *Pneumocystis* pneumonia)
systemic lupus erythematosus (arthralgia, rash, pleurisy, pericarditis)
hyperthyroidism (tremor, tachycardia)
hypothyroidism (cold intolerance, voice change, constipation, myxedema)
Cushing's syndrome ("Cushingoid" habitus, e.g., "moon" facies)
adrenocortical insufficiency (abdominal complaints and dizziness)
hepatic porphyria (abdominal pain)
Secondary to general medical conditions without specific features:
cerebral tumors
cerebral infarction
multiple sclerosis
neurosyphilis
vitamin B$_{12}$ deficiency

not invariable, are generally present. Most of these are fairly self-evident, and do not require further elaboration. Those associated with a history of epilepsy or with encephalitic features, however, merit some further discussion. "Epileptic psychoses" come in four varieties. Ictal psychoses are, in fact, simple partial seizures manifesting as delusions or hallucinations and, like any seizure, these are of paroxysmal onset. Post-ictal psychoses, appearing after a more or less lengthy "lucid" interval following a flurry of complex partial seizures, are immediately suggested by the preceding complex partial seizure, and are distinguished from the common post-ictal delirium on two counts, first that the delirium occurs immediately, without a "lucid" interval, and, second, that the delirium is characterized by confusion, a sign not seen in the post-ictal psychosis. The next two epileptic psychoses are, as a group, distinguished by their appearance "inter-ictally," that is to say at some time distant from a seizure. The psychosis of forced normalization is a rare disorder which appears, paradoxically, when anticonvulsants have been perfectly effective, not only in abolishing seizures, but in completely "normalizing" the EEG. The diagnosis here may be confirmed by simply "backing off" on the anticonvulsants to allow for the emergence of some inter-ictal epileptiform discharges on the EEG and then observing the patient to see if the psychosis resolves spontaneously. Finally, the chronic inter-ictal psychosis, which may be relatively common, is seen only in patients with chronic, poorly controlled epilepsy (with either complex partial or grand mal seizures): this psychosis, which is of gradual onset, otherwise, from a clinical point of view, appears almost identical to the psychosis seen in paranoid schizophrenia.

Encephalitic features, such as fever, headache, and perhaps lethargy, when accompanying a psychosis of acute onset, should always prompt immediate consideration of herpes simplex encephalitis: one would not, given its treatability, wish to miss this diagnosis.

In the case of general medical conditions without specific features, the most important to consider are cerebral tumors, particularly of the frontal or temporal lobes. Although these may initially present solely with a psychosis, in all cases other signs and symptoms, such as headache, aphasia, hemiparesis or seizures, eventually supervene, thus suggesting the correct diagnosis. Cerebral infarctions, particularly of the frontal, parietal or temporal lobes, may also present with psychosis; here, however, in addition to "neighborhood" signs and symptoms, such as hemiparesis, aphasia or neglect, it is the acute onset, over hours, which immediately suggests the diagnosis. Multiple sclerosis is characterized by evidence of cerebral lesions "disseminated in time and space," and a careful history and neurological examination, by revealing these, will suggest the diagnosis. Neurosyphilis remains the "Great Imitator." Although most patients will have other evidence of the disease, such as Argyll Robertson pupils, tremor, or seizures, there are cases wherein psychosis constituted the sole clinical expression of the disease. Vitamin B_{12} deficiency may also rank as an "Imitator": although most patients will have either a macrocytic anemia or sensory polyneuropathy, there are documented cases of psychosis representing the only clinical expression of the disease.

In most cases, the history and neurologic examination will greatly narrow the number of possible causes, and thus laboratory testing serves primarily as a confirmatory measure. Occasionally, however, although one strongly suspects that a patient's psychosis is secondary, the history and neurologic examination are unrevealing, and in such cases a "laboratory screen," such as is listed in Table 159-2, is appropriate. With such a screen, well over 90% of cases may be accurately diagnosed. Importantly, one must not rely on a "screen" to the neglect of a thorough history and examination; further, even when the history and examination do not pinpoint a diagnosis, often one comes away with some suspicions, and it is these suspicions which should guide one's selections of tests from the table.

DIFFERENTIAL DIAGNOSIS

Both delirium and dementia may be accompanied by hallucinations and delusions; however, these syndromes are immediately distinguished from psychosis by the presence of confusion or cognitive deficits, such as disorientation or defective memory.

Once delirium and dementia have been ruled out, the chief differential task is to distinguish between a secondary psychosis and one of the primary psychoses, namely schizophrenia, schizoaffective disorder and delusional disorder. Although there are no

■**TABLE 159-2.** A Laboratory Screen for Causes of Secondary Psychosis

Urine and serum drug screen (substances of abuse)
HIV (AIDS)
FTA-ABS (neurosyphilis)
ANA (systemic lupus erythematosus)
antithyroid antibodies (Hashimoto's encephalopathy)
B12 level (or, for greater sensitivity, methylmalonic and homocysteine levels) (B12 deficiency)
thyroid profile with TSH (hyperthyroidism, hypothyroidism)
cortisol level (Cushing's syndrome)
copper and ceruloplasmin levels (Wilson's disease)
MRI of head with enhancement (encephalitis, tumors, infarctions, multiple sclerosis)
EEG (epileptic psychoses, Creutzfeldt-Jakob disease)

hard and fast rules here, certain guidelines are helpful. First, consider the mode and age of onset. The primary psychoses are generally of gradual onset in adolescent or early adult years; although some of the secondary psychoses may have a similar mode and age of onset, most of the secondary psychoses are of either acute onset (i.e., over hours or days) or have an onset in later years. Consequently, either an acute onset or a late age of onset of psychosis suggests a secondary cause. Next, look closely for any signs or symptoms which are atypical for the primary psychoses, but which may be seen in secondary cases, such as seizures, abnormal involuntary movements (e.g., chorea, myoclonus, parkinsonism), or focal signs (e.g., hemiparesis, aphasia, neglect).

TREATMENT

Treatment is directed at the underlying cause, and in many cases successful treatment of the underlying disorder will be followed by a remission of the psychosis. In cases where the underlying cause is untreatable, or wherein the psychosis persists beyond otherwise successful treatment of the underlying cause, consideration may be given to symptomatic treatment with an antipsychotic. Overall, as pointed out in the chapter on schizophrenia, the second generation agents, such as risperidone, are generally better tolerated; however, if a first generation agent is deemed appropriate, haloperidol may be used. In any case, it is generally appropriate to "start low and go slow" with dosage titration, keeping in mind that many, but certainly not all, secondary psychoses will respond to relatively low doses, e.g., 1 to 3 mg of risperidone.

BIBLIOGRAPHY

Boutros NN, Bowers MB. Chronic substance-induced psychotic disorders: state of the literature. *The Journal of Neuropsychiatry and Clinical Neurosciences* 1996;8:262-269.

Dilsaver SC. Differentiating organic from functional psychosis. *American Family Physician* 1992;45:1173-1180.

Evans DL, Edelsohn GA, Golden RN. Organic psychosis without anemia or spinal cord symptoms in patients with vitamin B12 deficiency. *The American Journal of Psychiatry* 1983;140:218-221.

Little JT, Sunderland T. Psychosis secondary to encephalitis and encephalopathies. *Seminars in Clinical Neuropsychiatry* 1998;3:4-11.

Rosenthal RN, Miner CR. Differential diagnosis of substance-induced psychosis and schizophrenia in patients with substance use disorders. *Schizophrenia Bulletin* 1997;23:187-193.

Catatonia occurs in one of two forms: *stuporous catatonia* and *excited catatonia*. Stuporous catatonia is by far the most common form, and is characterized by immobility, mutism and a large number of other symptoms, as described below. Excited catatonia, in contrast with the stuporous form, is characterized by a bizarre, purposeless and frenzied hyperactivity.

ONSET

The onset is determined by the underlying cause and may range from acute to subacute.

CLINICAL FEATURES

Stuporous catatonia, in addition to immobility and mutism, is also characterized by a peculiar muscular rigidity known as waxy flexibility, negativism (or, less commonly, its opposite, automatic obedience), echopraxia or echolalia, and posturing.

The immobility of stuporous catatonia may persist for hours or days, with little, if any, changes in the patient's position. Some may lie in bed, perhaps with the legs rigidly extended and adducted; others may curl up into a ball. The eyes may or may not be open; if open, patients often stare fixedly ahead. Patients may not move even to relieve themselves and the bed may become fouled with urine and feces; in some cases, food placed in the mouth is not swallowed, and aspiration may occur. Importantly, despite even a profound degree of immobility, patients remain alert, as evidenced by the fact that, upon recovery, they often display an astonishingly accurate recall of what was said around them.

Mutism may or may not be complete; in some cases patients may at times utter incomprehensible phrases.

Waxy flexibility, also known as cerea flexibalitas and catalepsy, represents the combination of generalized lead-pipe rigidity and a tendency for patients' limbs to remain, in the absence of any instructions to do so, in any position they are placed in. Bedside testing for this is readily accomplished in one of two ways. First, in taking a patient's pulse, hold the patient's arm up while you do so and then, when finished, simply remove your hand, saying nothing: if waxy flexibility is present, the patient's arm may remain elevated. A second method may be utilized if the patient's head is on a pillow. Again, without saying anything, simply gently slide the pillow out from under the patient's head: if waxy flexibility is present, the head will remain aloft, in the same position, as if on a "psychological pillow."

Negativism represents a mulish tendency to resist whatever is asked, and may be either passive or active. In passive negativism, patients simply do not comply with requests or commands, even if compliance would clearly be to their advantage. Thus, patients may not bathe if taken to the bath, and may not eat if food is placed in front of them. Active negativism goes further, in that here patients do the opposite of what is asked, even if in doing so they place themselves in danger: if asked to come through a doorway into a room, they may back up, or if asked to avoid touching a hot stove, they may place a hand upon it. Importantly, this negativism does not represent mere stubbornness

or contrariness; to the contrary, the negativistic behavior seems instinctual, and to occur outside of any conscious control.

Automatic obedience represents the opposite of negativism, in that here patients do whatever is asked of them, or whatever the situation seems to demand. This is not mere agreeableness, for patients act more in a robotic or automaton-like fashion. If placed at a table with food on it, they will eat, even if not asked to, or if asked to submit to a painful maneuver they would mechanically go through with it, unless asked to stop.

Echopraxia and echolalia represent a kind of automatic obedience in that patients, without being asked to, automatically mimic what the physician either does or says. Thus, if echopraxia is present, the patient may look at a watch if the physician does, or, if echolalia is present, rigidly and immediately repeat what the physician said.

Posturing is characterized by a tendency of patients to automatically and spontaneously assume more or less bizarre postures or positions: one patient lifted a leg, and stood, stork-like, for hours; another squatted with arms held out in a cruciform position and head bowed tightly to the chest, holding this position, again, for hours.

Excited catatonia, as noted earlier, is characterized by bizarre, purposeless and frenzied hyperactivity. Isolated and uninvolved with others, patients may gesticulate, march in place or declaim incomprehensible phrases; in some cases verbigeration may occur, wherein speech becomes loud, rapid, bizarre and senseless. In severe cases, excited catatonia may merge into Stauder's lethal catatonia, also known as malignant catatonia. Here, as the excitation increases, fever, tachycardia and hypotension supervene, and in some cases death may follow.

In some cases, particularly when the catatonia is due to schizophrenia, the stuporous and excited forms of catatonia may alternate in the same patient. Thus, after lying immobile in a catatonic stupor for weeks or even months, a patient may suddenly become agitated, rise up in a frenzy of purposeless behavior and perhaps assault someone, only then to sink back into a stupor.

COURSE

This is determined by the underlying cause, and ranges from brief and transient, as may occur with ictal catatonia, to chronic or even lifelong, as may occur in schizophrenia.

COMPLICATIONS

Stuporous catatonics are prone to aspiration, dehydration, malnutrition and decubitus ulcers. Excited catatonics may unintentionally injure themselves, and are also, as noted above, at risk for death if lethal catatonia supervenes.

ETIOLOGY

In addition to schizophrenia and mood disorders, a large number of general medical conditions or medications may also be at fault, as listed in Table 160-1.

Stuporous Catatonia
Depressive episodes of major depression or bipolar disorder
Manic episodes of bipolar disorder
Epilepsy
    Ictal catatonia
    Postictal psychosis
    Psychosis of forced normalization
    Chronic interictal psychosis
Encephalitis
    Herpes simplex encephalitis
    Encephalitis lethargica
Focal lesions, especially of the medial or inferior aspects of the frontal lobes
Medications
    Antipsychotics
    Disulfiram
    During benzodiazepine withdrawal
Miscellaneous causes
    Hepatic encephalopathy
    Limbic encephalitis
    Systemic lupus erythematosus
    Stage III Lyme disease
    Subacute sclerosing panencephalitis
    Wilson's disease
Excited Catatonia
    Viral encephalitis

DIFFERENTIAL DIAGNOSIS

Stuporous catatonia must be distinguished from akinetic mutism and from stupor of other causes. Akinetic mutes, though immobile and mute, are lacking in waxy flexibility, negativism and the other symptoms described above. Stupor of other causes is readily distinguished by the fact that in stuporous catatonia patients remain alert, in stark contrast to the somnolence seen in stupor.

Excited catatonia may be distinguished from mania by close attention to the absence or presence of purpose and involvement with others during the activity. Excited catatonics, as noted earlier, are isolated and uninvolved with others: indeed they may confine themselves to a closet or under the bed where they continue to gesticulate and declaim. By contrast, the manic, no matter how fragmented, retains an interest in others and wants to be involved.

The neuroleptic malignant syndrome may be distinguished from lethal catatonia on several counts. First, lethal catatonia always evolves out of a typical excited catatonic state and represents, in essence, an intensification of the preceding excitation. The neuroleptic malignant syndrome, however, may arise out of clinical conditions other than excited catatonia, provided of course that there had been an abrupt diminution of dopaminergic tone. Given, however, that patients with excited catatonia are often prescribed antipsychotics, this guideline is not infallible. In such a case, one must look to the clinical picture: in lethal catatonia, rigidity is not found, whereas it is a cardinal feature of the neuroleptic malignant syndrome; furthermore, whereas in lethal catatonia fever arises in the setting of mounting excitation, in the neuroleptic malignant syndrome it occurs in the setting of increasing rigidity and immobility.

TREATMENT

Treatment is directed at the underlying cause. Should emergent treatment be required, lorazepam given parenterally in a dose of 2 mg is generally effective. Should lorazepam be ineffective and the patient's condition is life threatening, ECT may be utilized.

BIBLIOGRAPHY

Bush G, Fink M, Petrides G, et al. Catatonia. II. Treatment with lorazepam and electroconvulsive therapy. *Acta Psychiatrica Scandinavica* 1996;93:137-143.

Castillo E, Rubin RT, Holsboer-Trachsler E. Clinical differentiation between lethal catatonia and neuroleptic malignant syndrome. *The American Journal of Psychiatry* 1989;146:324-328.

Lim J, Yagnik P, Schraeder P, et al. Ictal catatonia as a manifestation of nonconvulsive status epilepticus. *Journal of Neurology, Neurosurgery, and Psychiatry* 1986;49:833-836.

Rosebush PI, Mazurek MF. Catatonia after benzodiazepine withdrawal. *Journal of Clinical Psychopharmacology* 1996;16:315-319.

Singerman B, Raheja R. Malignant catatonia—a continuing reality. *Annals of Clinical Psychiatry* 1994;6:259-266.

Taylor MA, Abrams R. Catatonia: prevalence and importance in the manic phase of manic-depressive illness. *Archives of General Psychiatry* 1977;34:1223-1225.

Taylor MA, Fink M. Catatonia in psychiatric classification: a home of its own. *The American Journal of Psychiatry* 2003;160:1233-1241.

161 Secondary Depression (mood disorder due to a general medical condition, with depressive features, DSM-IV-TR #293.83; substance-induced mood disorder with depressive features, DSM-IV-TR #291.89, 292.84)

Although clinically significant depression is most commonly caused by one of the primary, or idiopathic, mood disorders, such as major depression, it must be borne in mind that depression may also occur secondary to general medical conditions, such as Cushing's syndrome, or secondary to medications, such as prednisone, or substances of abuse, as may be seen in alcoholism.

A clear distinction must be drawn between the term "secondary depression," as used here, and "secondary depression," as used in some research literature. In the research literature a depressive illness is considered "secondary" if it is preceded by another psychiatric illness, regardless of whether the two are etiologically linked. By contrast, "secondary" as used here implies a direct etiologic link between the depressive symptoms and the disease, medication or drug underlying them.

ONSET

The age and mode of onset are determined by the underlying cause. In general, when depression occurs secondary to medications, the onset is relatively abrupt.

CLINICAL FEATURES

In all cases, a depressed, irritable or dysphoric mood is present, and in most cases one or more vegetative symptoms may be present, such as loss of interest, fatigue, difficulty with concentration and memory, and appetite and sleep changes.

COURSE

The course is determined by the course of the underlying disease, and may range from very brief, as for example with ictal depressions, to extraordinarily prolonged, as may be seen in untreated hypothyroidism.

COMPLICATIONS

Complications seen are similar to those described in the chapter on major depression.

ETIOLOGY

Various causes of secondary depression are listed in Table 161-1: of these, the most common are medications and substances of abuse. Of medications, corticosteroids (especially prednisone) and interferons are the most common offenders; the others in the list are less likely as causes of secondary depression, and before assigning an etiologic role to any of them one would want to see an especially strong correlation between starting the medication or increasing the dose and the onset of the depression. Cholinergic rebound, as explained in that chapter, occurs when patients abruptly discontinue long term treatment with anticholinergic agents, such as benztropine. Of the substances of abuse, alcoholism is a very common cause of depression, and this depression may persist into sobriety for up to a month or more. Withdrawal from stimulants such as amphetamines or cocaine may be associated with a profound depression, which, however, typically remits within several weeks. Anabolic steroid withdrawal may also cause depression, which may last anywhere from weeks to months before undergoing a spontaneous remission. Of the general medical conditions capable of causing depression, several deserve further discussion. Cushing's syndrome and hypothyroidism are particularly common causes; hyperthyroidism, while typically associated with anxiety, may, especially in the elderly, present as "apathetic" hyperthyroidism with prominent depressive features. Of the vascular disorders, cerebral infarctions near the left frontal pole are a common cause, and these depressions may persist for a year or more. Among the neurodegenerative disorders, Alzheimer's disease causes depression in a significant minority, as do Parkinson's and Huntington's disease and diffuse Lewy body disease. Patients

■ TABLE 161-1. Causes of Secondary Depression

Medications
corticosteroids (e.g., prednisone) or ACTH
interferon alpha or beta
propranolol
clonidine
reserpine
alpha-methyldopa
nifedipine
oral contraceptives
pimozide
metoclopramide
cimetidine
ranitidine
clomiphene
tamoxifen
isotretinoin
"cholinergic rebound"

Substances of Abuse
alcohol
stimulant withdrawal
anabolic steroid withdrawal

General Medical Conditions
Endocrinologic disorders
   Cushing's syndrome
   adrenocortical insufficiency
   hypothyroidism
   hyperthyroidism
Vascular disorders
   cerebral infarction, especially near left frontal pole
   multi-infarct dementia
   Binswanger's disease
Neurodegenerative disorders
   Alzheimer's disease
   Parkinson's disease
   Huntington's disease
   diffuse Lewy body disease
Associated with epilepsy
   ictal depression
   inter-ictal depression
Other disorders
   multiple sclerosis
   traumatic brain injury
   obstructive sleep apnea
   pancreatic cancer
   limbic encephalitis
   systemic lupus erythematosus
   Creutzfeldt-Jakob disease, especially the "new variant" type
   neurosyphilis
   Lyme disease
   hypercalcemia
   hypocalcemia
   vitamin B_{12} deficiency
   pellagra

with epilepsy may experience simple partial seizures manifest by affective symptoms alone, and this is immediately suggested by the paroxysmal onset and brief duration of the depression. These ictal depressions, however, are rare; by contrast, up to one-third of patients with chronic complex partial seizures may experience enduring inter-ictal depressive symptoms.

DIFFERENTIAL DIAGNOSIS

A depressive episode, occurring as part of one of the primary mood disorders, such as major depression or bipolar disorder, may be difficult to distinguish from a secondary depression. Certain features atypical for primary mood disorders, however, may suggest the correct diagnosis. For example, hyperacute onsets (over a few days) are very unusual for a primary mood disorder but not at all unusual for depressions occurring secondary to medications. Additionally, one may look for symptoms that are atypical for a primary mood disorder. For example, if a depressed patient complains of hair loss and voice change, the diagnosis of an affective disorder should be withheld until thyroid function testing is completed and found to be normal. Finally, whenever a patient who carries a diagnosis of a primary mood disorder fails to respond to otherwise adequate treatment, the diagnostician should look closely for evidence of a secondary cause.

In some cases one of the etiologic factors described above may have precipitated, or "triggered," a depressive episode in a patient so predisposed, rather than having caused it per se. Consider, for example, a patient with major depression, with a past history of numerous episodes of depression, who became severely depressed 2 days after starting metoclopramide, with symptoms almost identical to those of prior episodes. Here the correct diagnosis would not be secondary depression but rather major depression, with the current episode being precipitated by the medication.

Normal depression or grief in the face of a debilitating or life-threatening illness must not be confused with depression that is directly caused by that disease. For example, consider a patient with multiple sclerosis whose plaques are totally confined to the spinal cord; paraplegic and incontinent, the patient becomes disconsolate and demoralized. Contrast this patient with another patient with multiple sclerosis whose plaques are confined to the limbic system. Here no motor or sensory defects are present, but the patient may develop a profound depression directly caused by limbic plaques. Whenever a patient has an illness capable of directly affecting the central nervous system and the depressive symptoms seem out of proportion to other symptoms, a tentative diagnosis of a secondary depression is merited.

Akinesia secondary to antipsychotics may simulate a depression. However, in akinesia one typically does not see a depressed mood. Though akinetic patients may appear slowed down and may indeed complain of sluggish thoughts, they generally do not complain of feeling depressed.

TREATMENT

If possible, the cause is treated. If this is not possible or is ineffective, then one may treat the patient with an antidepressant. In general, SSRIs are preferable, given their favorable side effect profile, and of the SSRIs, escitalopram is probably the best choice, given that it has the fewest potential drug-drug interactions. An exception to this rule might be in Parkinson's disease or diffuse Lewy body disease, as SSRIs may, in some cases, exacerbate parkinsonism. Tricyclic antidepressants have also been used, and of the tricyclics, nortriptyline is the safest and has the best track record in the treatment of secondary depressions; indeed, it may be superior to SSRIs in the treatment of depression secondary to frontal infarctions. Escitalopram may be started at 5 or 10 mg, and increased to 20 mg if necessary; nortriptyline should be started at a low dose, say 10 mg, and increased gradually, with the aim of obtaining a blood level within the therapeutic "window": given the possibility of arrhythmias, a pre-treatment EKG and periodic monitoring are appropriate.

Methylphenidate has been used in elderly patients whose secondary depressions are marked by apathy and psychomotor retardation. Although there are no comparative studies between methylphenidate and antidepressants in secondary depression, methylphenidate, by virtue of its rapidity of onset, may be preferable when depression is life threatening. Methylphenidate may be initiated at 5 or 10 mg daily, with similar daily dose adjustments until the patient improves, limiting side effects occur, or a maximum dose of approximately 60 mg is reached.

BIBLIOGRAPHY

Brookes G, Crawford P. The associations between epilepsy and depressive illness in secondary care. *Seizure* 2002;11:353-355.

Levin HS, Goldstein FC, MacKenzie EJ. Depression as a secondary condition following mild and moderate traumatic brain injury. *Seminars in Clinical Neuropsychiatry* 1997;2:207-215.

Lipsey JR, Robinson RG, Pearlson GD, et al. Nortriptyline treatment for post-stroke depression: a double-blind trial. *Lancet* 1984;1:297-300.

Masand P, Pickett P, Murray GB. Psychostimulants for secondary depression in medical illness. *Psychosomatics* 1991;32:203-208.

Patton SB, Love EJ. Can drugs cause depression? A review of the evidence. *Journal of Psychiatry & Neuroscience* 1993;18:92-102.

Roy A. Aetiology of secondary depression in male alcoholics. *The British Journal of Psychiatry* 1996;169:753-757.

Starkstein SE, Robinson RG, Price TR. Comparison of patients with and without poststroke major depression matched for size and location of lesion. *Archives of General Psychiatry* 1988;45:247-252.

162 Secondary Mania (mood disorder due to a general medical condition with manic features, DSM-IV-TR #293.83; substance-induced mood disorder with manic features, DSM-IV-TR #292.84)

Although most cases of mania occur as part of one of the primary mood disorders, such as bipolar disorder, mania may also occur secondary to various general medical conditions, such as multiple sclerosis, to certain medications, such as prednisone, or to the use of certain substances of abuse, such as cocaine or anabolic steroids.

ONSET

The age of onset of secondary mania is determined by the underlying cause, and the same is true of the mode of onset, which may range from gradual, as with a tumor, to acute, over several days, as may occur with high-dose prednisone.

CLINICAL FEATURES

The mood is heightened and may be either irritable, or, somewhat less commonly, euphoric, or mixed. Other possible symptoms include hyperactivity, increased energy, and pressured speech.

COURSE

The course is determined by the underlying cause.

COMPLICATIONS

Complications are similar to those described for mania in the chapter on bipolar disorder.

ETIOLOGY

The different causes of secondary mania are listed in Table 162-1. Cerebral infarction, closed head injury and hemodialysis are all fairly obvious. With regard to infarctions, mania has little localizing value, as it has been seen with infarction of the mesencephalon, thalamus, anterior limb of the internal capsule, caudate nucleus and either the gray or subjacent white matter of the frontal, temporal or parietal lobes: mania may, however, have lateralizing value as the vast majority of cases occurred with lesions on the right side. Both of the endocrinologic disorders capable of causing mania have distinctive features, as noted in the table, and distinctive features are also found in other disorders, such as chorea in Huntington's disease, Sydenham's chorea and chorea gravidarum, and the combination of delirium, myoclonus and asterixis in hepatic or uremic encephalopathy. Multiple sclerosis is a notorious cause of mania, and here one typically finds a large burden of

plaques within the cerebrum, rather than the cord. Alzheimer's disease, neurosyphilis and Creutzfeldt-Jakob disease are all suggested by the appearance of mania in the setting of dementia. Ictal mania, representing a simple partial seizure manifesting solely with a mood change, is immediately suggested by its paroxysmal onset, and post-ictal mania by a preceding flurry of complex partial seizures, from which the mania is separated by a brief "lucid" interval. Tumors, lupus erythematosus and vitamin B12 deficiency are all very rare causes of secondary mania.

Of the medications capable of causing mania, by far the two most common offenders are prednisone and levodopa. In the case of prednisone, fully three-quarters of patients who take high doses (80 or more mg daily) will develop some degree of mania.

■ TABLE 162-1. Causes of Secondary Mania

General medical conditions
    cerebral infarction
    closed head injury
    hemodialysis
    Cushing's syndrome ("Cushingoid" habitus)
    thyrotoxicosis (proptosis, tremor, tachycardia)
    Huntington's disease (chorea)
    Sydenham's chorea (chorea)
    chorea gravidarum (chorea)
    hepatic encephalopathy (delirium, asterixis, myoclonus)
    uremia (delirium, asterixis, myoclonus)
    multiple sclerosis
    Alzheimer's disease
    neurosyphilis
    Creutzfeldt-Jakob disease
    ictal mania
    post-ictal mania
    cerebral tumors
    systemic lupus erythematosus
    vitamin B12 deficiency
Medications
    corticosteroids (e.g., prednisone) or ACTH
    levodopa
    zidovudine
    oral contraceptives
    procyclidine
    propafenone
    diltiazem
    buspirone
    phenytoin
    baclofen discontinuation
    methyldopa discontinuation
    reserpine discontinuation
Substances of abuse
    stimulants (cocaine, amphetamines)
    hallucinogens
    anabolic steroids

Although levodopa-induced mania is not as common, occurring in only up to 10% of patients, the resulting euphoria may be so profound that some patients have escalated their dosage well beyond what is required for the control of parkinsonism. The other medications in the list are much less likely to cause mania, and before one would attribute any given case of mania to one of them, one would want to see a particularly strong connection between the mania and either starting or increasing the dose of the medicine in question. Of interest, in the case of baclofen, methyldopa and reserpine, mania occurs not upon initiation of treatment but only when, after long-term treatment, the medicine is abruptly discontinued.

Substances of abuse capable of causing mania include stimulants, wherein mania occurs as part of the intoxication, hallucinogens, wherein mania may, rarely, occur as a sequela to intoxication, and the anabolic steroids. The mania occurring with chronic use of anabolic steroids may be particularly severe, and is more often characterized by irritability than euphoria.

DIFFERENTIAL DIAGNOSIS

Given that most cases of mania occur as part of a primary mood disorder, namely bipolar disorder, the first step in the work of differential diagnosis is to be alert to certain features, which, as they are atypical for bipolar disorder, suggest the presence of a secondary cause.

First, consider the age of onset of the mania, and, if there were earlier episodes, the age of onset of the first one. Bipolar disorder typically has an onset in the teens or early twenties, and in almost all cases the first episode occurs before the age of 50. Thus, if the onset is past the age of 50, one should suspect a secondary cause. Next, search for any signs which are atypical for bipolar mania, such as a Cushingoid habitus, proptosis, abnormal involuntary movements (e.g., chorea, asterixis, myoclonus), dementia or seizures. Finally, consider whether or not the mania was preceded by any conditions known to be capable of causing secondary mania, such as significant head trauma, hemodialysis, and various medications and substances of abuse.

A further consideration in the differential diagnosis of bipolar mania from secondary mania involves those cases of bipolar disorder wherein a medication (such as levodopa or prednisone) or a substance of abuse (such as a stimulant) precipitates a fresh episode of mania in a patient with bipolar disorder. Although some authors advise considering these episodes as secondary, it seems more appropriate to not add another diagnosis but just to note that the patient has bipolar disorder and that the current episode of mania happened to be precipitated by the medication or drug.

TREATMENT

Treatment is directed at the underlying cause. If this is not correctable or if the manic symptoms demand immediate treatment, then one may proceed in a manner similar to that described for the acute treatment of mania in the chapter on bipolar disorder. Lithium, divalproex or carbamazepine may be used, and, if the patient also has, or is at risk for, seizures, using divalproex or carbamazepine makes good sense. Should adjunctive treatment be required, the protocol outlined in the chapter on Rapid Pharmacologic Treatment of Agitation may be followed. Once the mania has been brought under control, continuation treatment should be maintained until the underlying cause of the secondary mania has been controlled.

In some cases, one may also wish to consider preventive treatment with a mood stabilizer when a patient with a known history of secondary mania is about to encounter the same precipitant that caused an earlier episode. A good example of this is the patient who requires intermittent courses of high dose prednisone, as may occur in rheumatoid arthritis or multiple sclerosis. In these cases, preventive treatment with lithium or divalproex has been shown to be effective.

BIBLIOGRAPHY

Cummings JL, Mendez MF. Secondary mania with focal cerebrovascular lesions. *The American Journal of Psychiatry* 1984;141:1084-1087.
Falk WE, Mahnke MD, Poskanzer MD. Lithium prophylaxis of corticotropin-induced psychosis. *Journal of the American Medical Association* 1979;241:1011-1012.
Jorge RE, Robinson RG, Starkstein SE, et al. Secondary mania following traumatic brain injury. *The American Journal of Psychiatry* 1993;150:916-921.
Krauthammer C, Klerman GL. Secondary mania: manic syndromes associated with antecedent physical illness or drugs. *Archives of General Psychiatry* 1978;35:1333-1339.
Kulisevsky J, Berthier ML, Pujol J. Hemiballismus and secondary mania following a right thalamic infarction. *Neurology* 1993;43:1422-1424.
Lee S, Chun CC, Wing YK, et al. Mania secondary to thyrotoxicosis. *The British Journal of Psychiatry* 1991;159:712-713.
Nizamie SH, Nizamie A, Borde M, et al. Mania following head injury: case reports and neuropsychological findings. *Acta Psychiatrica Scandinavica* 1988;77:637-639.
Patten SB, Klein GM, Lussier C, et al. Organic mania induced by phenytoin: a case report. *Canadian Journal of Psychiatry* 1989;34:827-828.
Peet M, Peters S. Drug-induced mania. *Drug Safety* 1995;12:146-153.
Starkstein SE, Boston JD, Robinson RGG. Mechanisms of mania after brain injury: 12 case reports and review of the literature. *The Journal of Nervous and Mental Disease* 1988;176:87-100.
Starkstein SE, Mayberg HS, Berthier ML, et al. Mania after brain injury: neuroradiological and metabolic findings. *Annals of Neurology* 1990;27:652-659.
Starkstein SE, Pearlson GD, Boston J, et al. Mania after brain injury: a controlled study of causative factors. *Archives of Neurology* 1987;44:1069-1073.
Stasiek C, Zetin M. Organic manic disorders. *Psychosomatics* 1985;26:394.

163 Secondary Anxiety (anxiety disorder due to a general medical condition, DSM-IV-TR #293.89; substance-induced anxiety disorder, DSM-IV-TR #292.89)

Anxiety may occur as part of one of the primary anxiety disorders, such as generalized anxiety disorder or panic disorder, or may appear secondary to a general medical condition, such as hyperthyroidism, as a side effect to a medication such as an antidepressant, or in association with the use of a substance of abuse, such as caffeine.

ONSET

The onset is determined by the underlying cause.

CLINICAL FEATURES

Secondary anxiety may occur either in a persistent, more or less chronic form, or may present in discrete episodes or attacks.

In cases of chronic secondary anxiety, patients complain of unremitting anxiety or tension generally associated with such autonomic symptoms as shakiness, tremor, and palpitations.

In cases where secondary anxiety occurs in discrete episodes, the symptomatology is similar to that described for a panic attack, as noted in the chapter on panic disorder.

COURSE

The course is determined by the underlying cause.

COMPLICATIONS

Complications are similar to those described either for generalized anxiety disorder or panic disorder.

ETIOLOGY

The possible causes of chronic secondary anxiety are noted in Table 163-1. Hyperthyroidism is suggested by heat intolerance, prominent diaphoresis and proptosis; hypocalcemia may or may not be accompanied by tetany or Trousseau's or Chvostek's signs. Chronic obstructive pulmonary disease (COPD) and congestive heart failure (CHF) are immediately suggested by the prominent dyspnea, and anxiety as a sequela to severe traumatic brain injury or stroke is suggested by the strong temporal correlation between these events and the onset of the persistent anxiety; of note, with regard to stroke, it appears that infarctions of the left frontal lobe are most likely to cause chronic anxiety. A strong temporal correlation between the onset of anxiety and the initiation or dose increase of any of the medicines listed in the table also suggests a causal link; in the case of chronic use of clonidine or of

anticholinergics, the anxiety appears as a kind of "rebound" after abrupt discontinuation of either of these. Of the substances of abuse, withdrawal from alcohol or sedative-hypnotics may be difficult to diagnose, as most alcoholics or sedative-hypnotic addicts simply do not admit their substance use, and are much more likely to complain of "nerves." Nicotine withdrawal, however, is more readily diagnosed, as patients are often much more open about their smoking.

The possible causes of discrete episodes of secondary anxiety are noted in Table 163-2. Attacks occurring in Parkinson's disease may be quite disabling and are seen during the "off" period in patients treated with levodopa. Simple partial seizures, rarely, may manifest with anxiety alone, and are suggested by their paroxysmal onset, over seconds or a minute. Hypoglycemia should be suspected when anxiety attacks occur in patients on oral anti-diabetic agents or insulin, or are confined to the post-prandial period. Paroxysmal atrial tachycardia is suggested by the almost instantaneous onset of tachycardia, often is a second or less, by the prominence of the tachycardia relative to other symptoms and by the ability of the Valsalva maneuver to terminate the attack. Angina or myocardial infarction is suggested by the occurrence of the anxiety attack in a patient with multiple risk factors for coronary artery disease and by the concurrent experience of dyspnea and chest pain: although chest pain may also occur in patients with panic disorder, it is far more likely to be seen in patients with angina or a myocardial infarction. Pulmonary embolism is suggested by prominent dyspnea, and may be suspected in patients with thrombophlebitis or

■ **TABLE 163-1.** Causes of Chronic Secondary Anxiety

Due to a General Medical Condition
   hyperthyroidism
   hypocalcemia
   chronic obstructive pulmonary disease
   congestive heart failure
   post traumatic brain injury
   post-stroke
As a Side-Effect to a Medication
   sympathomimetics
   theophylline
   caffeine
   yohimbine
   antidepressants (tricyclics, monoamine-oxidase inhibitors, SSRIs, bupropion)
   clonidine withdrawal
   anticholinergic withdrawal
In Association with Substances of Abuse
   alcohol withdrawal
   sedative-hypnotic withdrawal
   nicotine withdrawal

■**TABLE 163-2.** Causes of Discrete Episodes of Secondary Anxiety

Due to a General Medical Condition
  Parkinson's disease
  simple partial seizure
  hypoglycemia
  paroxysmal atrial tachycardia
  angina or myocardial infarction
  pulmonary embolism
  asthmatic attack
  hyperventilation
  pheochromocytoma
  mastocytosis
As a Side-Effect to a Medication
  sympathomimetics
Substance Intoxication
  caffeine
  stimulants (amphetamines, cocaine)
  cannabis
  hallucinogens

those who have undergone prolonged immobilization. Asthma and hyperventilation are also suggested by the prominence of dyspnea, and, in the case of asthma, wheezing. Pheochromocytoma is marked by prominent headache and hypertension, and mastocytosis by generalized flushing during the attack. Anxiety occurring secondary to any of the medications and substances or substances of abuse listed in the table is generally of gradual onset, and thus does not raise the question of a discrete attack; in some instances, however, if the dose is high enough and absorption is sufficiently rapid, an actual attack may occur.

TREATMENT

Treatment is directed at the underlying cause. In cases of chronic secondary anxiety, if such treatment is ineffective or not possible, one may consider utilizing a benzodiazepine such as diazepam or chlordiazepoxide beginning with daily doses of 5-10 or 25-50 mg, respectively. In patients with significant hepatic impairment, lorazepam, starting in doses of 1 to 3 mg, is a reasonable alternative.

BIBLIOGRAPHY

Cameron OG. The differential diagnosis of anxiety: psychiatric and medical disorders. *The Psychiatric Clinics of North America* 1985; 8:3-23.

MacKenzie TB, Popkin MK. Organic anxiety syndrome. *The American Journal of Psychiatry* 1983;140:342-344.

Schuckit MA. Anxiety related to medical disease. *The Journal of Clinical Psychiatry* 1983;44:31-37.

Stoudemire A. Epidemiology and psychopharmacology of anxiety in medical patients. *The Journal of Clinical Psychiatry* 1996;57(Suppl 7):64-75.

164   Frontal Lobe Syndrome

Bilateral, or occasionally unilateral, damage to the prefrontal or orbitofrontal area may cause the fairly distinctive frontal lobe syndrome. Indeed some properly situated tumors may present with this syndrome alone, lacking any of the more "traditional" localizing signs, such as motor aphasia or hemiplegia.

ONSET

The onset is determined by the underlying cause and ranges from quite gradual, as may be seen with a meningioma, to acute, as when a simultaneous infarction of the regions subserved by both anterior cerebral arteries occurs.

CLINICAL FEATURES

The frontal lobe syndrome is characterized by varying combinations of disinhibition, affective changes (euphoria, irritability or depression), perseveration, difficulties in planning ahead and making decisions, and abulia.

With disinhibition, attention to social nuances, good manners, or customary morality is lost. Patients may eat with gluttony, grooming and dress may suffer, and sexual indiscretions may become prominent, with exhibitionism, unwelcomed sexual advances, or public masturbation.

When euphoria occurs, it tends to be silly and non-infectious; patients may become facetious, inappropriately jocular, and are often given to simple, silly puns (witzelsucht). Irritability is less common, but some patients may fly into a rage when frustrated. Depression, likewise, is less common than euphoria.

Perseveration often involves simple tasks, and patients may spend long periods of time opening and closing books or buttoning and unbuttoning shirts.

Difficulties in planning ahead may put patients at great financial or personal risk: unable to see looming disaster, they may engage in unwise investments or personal relationships. Complex situations may be beyond their cognitive grasp, and such patients may be unable to see their way through to decisions.

Abulia is also commonly seen. Here the patient may appear apathetic and lacking in spontaneity; rarely is initiative taken, and some patients may sit for hours untroubled by their complete inactivity.

Although most patients have a combination of these features, the location of the lesion may influence their relative prominence. Thus, lesions in the orbitofrontal area are more likely to cause disinhibition and affective changes, with right-sided lesions being associated with euphoria and left-sided lesions with depression. Dorsolateral frontal lesions, by contrast, are more associated with perseveration and cognitive changes.

Many patients with a frontal lobe syndrome may also display certain "pathologic" reflexes, such as the snout, rooting, palmomental, and grasping or groping reflexes. Gegenhalten, or an increasing lead-pipe rigidity with repeated extension and flexion of the limb, may also be seen, as may apraxia of gait. Incontinence of urine and feces may occur.

COURSE

The course of frontal lobe syndrome is determined by the underlying cause.

COMPLICATIONS

Work, except that which is rote, suffers; family members are alienated, and legal consequences may accrue until the correct diagnosis is made.

ETIOLOGY

The frontal lobe exists in a functional circuit, with projections successively connecting the frontal lobe with the caudate nucleus, lenticular nucleus and thalamus, which eventually projects back to the frontal lobe itself. As might be expected, the frontal lobe syndrome, although most commonly occurring secondary to lesions directly affecting the frontal lobes, has also been seen with lesions of any of the other structures in this circuit. Although in the vast majority of cases bilateral involvement is present, there are documented cases of the frontal lobe syndrome occurring secondary to unilateral lesions of the frontal lobe, caudate or thalamus.

Frontal lobe syndrome may occur secondary to a variety of causes (see the box on this page).

DIFFERENTIAL DIAGNOSIS

Abulia, especially when accompanied by some depressive symptoms, may suggest a diagnosis of a depressive episode either of major depression or bipolar disorder. The indifference and lack of spontaneity seen in the frontal lobe syndrome, however, contrasts with the painfully weighted-down experience of the depressed patient.

If euphoria occurs, a diagnosis of mania may be suggested. The euphoria seen in frontal lobe syndrome, however, is shallow and lacks the "infectious" quality seen in mania; furthermore, one rarely sees pressured speech or activity in the frontal lobe syndrome.

TREATMENT

Pending successful treatment of the underlying cause, close supervision at home or, if that is not possible, admission to a secure facility may be required. If treatment of the underlying cause is either unsuccessful or not possible, empirically based pharmacologic treatment may be justified. Antidepressants may be used for depression and antipsychotics for disinhibition. Propranolol may be helpful if rage attacks occur, as described in the chapter on intermittent explosive disorder.

Causes of the Frontal Lobe Syndrome

Alzheimer's disease*	Rupture of aneurysm of anterior communicating artery
Pick's disease*	Brain tumors*
Frontotemporal dementia*	Brain abscess*
Progressive supranuclear palsy*	Orbitofrontal contusion
Amyotrophic lateral sclerosis*	Remote effect of lesions in dorsomedial nucleus of the thalamus and of the globus pallidus
Lacunar dementia*	
Various frontal lesions	
Infarcts in the territory of the anterior cerebral artery	

*See the respective chapter.

BIBLIOGRAPHY

Adie WJ, Critchley M. Forced grasping and groping. *Brain* 1927;50:142.

Avery TL. Seven cases of frontal tumor with psychiatric presentation. *British Journal of Psychiatry* 1971;119:19.

Frazier CH. Tumor involving the frontal lobe alone: a symptomatic survey of 105 verified cases. *Archives of Neurology and Psychiatry* 1936;35:525.

Greene KA, Marciano EF, Dickman CA, et al. Anterior communicating artery aneurysm paraparesis syndrome: clinical manifestations and pathologic correlates. *Neurology* 1995;45:45.

Mesulam MM. Frontal cortex and behavior. *Annals of Neurology* 1986; 19:320.

Penfield W, Evans J. The frontal lobes in man: a clinical study of maximum removals. *Brain* 1935;58:115.

Strub RL. Frontal lobe syndrome in a patient with bilateral globus pallidus lesions. *Archives of Neurology* 1989;46:1024.

Williamson RT. On the symptomatology of gross lesions (tumors and abscesses) involving the prefrontal region of the brain. *Brain* 1896;19:346.

165 Utilization Behavior

Utilization behavior, also known as the "environmental dependency syndrome," is an uncommon syndrome occurring secondary to frontal or thalamic lesions, wherein patients involuntarily make use of, or utilize, whatever happens to be in view.

ONSET

The onset may be fairly acute, as for example after an infarction of the frontal lobe, or gradual, as may occur with a slowly growing frontal tumor.

CLINICAL FEATURES

Patients appear, in a sense, to have lost their autonomy as they become "dependent" on the environment in that they feel compelled to "utilize" whatever objects might be at hand. For example, a patient in an examining room might, upon seeing a tongue depressor, pick it up and attempt to examine the physician's oral cavity; or, another patient, upon seeing a bed, might feel compelled to get into it and pull the covers up. Importantly, such patients utilize these objects without being asked to, and typically persist in their behavior even if told to stop. If asked why they are acting as they do, most will reply to the effect that they "had" to.

COURSE

This is determined by the nature of the underlying lesion; in the case of infarctions, gradual recovery is the rule.

COMPLICATIONS

The compulsive utilization of objects might clearly derail other projects, and could also prove socially embarrassing.

ETIOLOGY

Utilization behavior is most commonly seen with unilateral or bilateral lesions of the frontal lobes, generally in their inferior portions; cases have also been reported with unilateral or bilateral thalamic lesions.

DIFFERENTIAL DIAGNOSIS

Forced grasping or groping is distinguished by the fact that here, once the patient has grasped an object, nothing is done with it except to hold on. The alien hand syndrome, although characterized by complex behavior on the part of the involved hand, is distinguished by the presence of "intermanual conflict" wherein the left hand acts at cross-purposes with the right hand; by contrast, in utilization behavior, both hands work together, toward the same purpose.

Echolalia and echopraxia are easily distinguished by the fact that they represent an imitation of what the physician says or does: by contrast, in utilization behavior, the physician does nothing at all but observe.

In delirium patients often pick up and use objects near at hand; however, here one finds confusion in contrast with the clear sensorium seen with utilization behavior.

TREATMENT

Treatment is directed at the underlying cause; supervision may be required to protect the patient from utilizing potentially dangerous objects, such as machines.

BIBLIOGRAPHY

Eslinger PJ, Warner GC, Grattan LM, et al. "Frontal lobe" utilization behavior associated with paramedian thalamic infarction. *Neurology* 1991;41:450-452.

Hashimoto R, Yoshida M, Tanaka Y. Utilization behavior after right thalamic infarction. *European Neurology* 1995;35:58-62.

Ishihara K, Nishino H, Maki T, et al. Utilization behavior as a white matter disconnection syndrome. *Cortex* 2002;38:379-387.

Lhermitte F. Human anatomy and the frontal lobes. Part II: Patient behavior in complex and social situations: the "environmental dependency syndrome." *Annals of Neurology* 1986;19:335-343.

Lhermitte F, Pillon B, Serdaru M. Human anatomy and the frontal lobes. Part I: Imitation and utilization behavior: a neuropsychological study of 75 patients. *Annals of Neurology* 1986;19:326-334.

Bilateral interruption of corticobulbar fibers anywhere along their course from the cortex to the bulbar nuclei may cause the syndrome of pseudobulbar palsy, which, in its fully developed form, is characterized by pathological laughing and crying, dysarthria, dysphagia and a shuffling gait.

ONSET

The age of onset reflects the age of onset of the various disorders that may cause pseudobulbar palsy, as discussed under Etiology.

CLINICAL FEATURES

Pathological laughing and crying, or, as it is also called, "emotional incontinence," is characterized by outbursts of laughter or crying, which typically occur upon the most trivial of precipitants, and which are not accompanied by any concurrent sense of mirth or sadness. Patients may be exasperated by the experience, not only because they don't feel the corresponding emotion but also because they are unable to control the emotional display. One patient laughed uncontrollably whenever an observer approached the bedside; another wept copiously when the bed sheets were changed. The synonym for this phenomenon, "emotional incontinence," hints at the uncontrollability of the emotional output and at the distress it causes the patient. Figure 166-1 illustrates an episode of pathological laughter.

Speech becomes dysarthric. It is monotone, slurred, and at times explosive. The patient may seem to run out of breath and may have to pause several times to complete the sentence.

Dysphagia results from deficits in both chewing and swallowing. Food may simply lie in the mouth and patients may have to push it back with their fingers. Impairment in swallowing may lead to regurgitation of food into the nose or to aspiration.

The gait is often stiff and shuffling, and patients are prone to falls.

Upon neurologic examination, further evidence of damage to corticobulbar tracts is provided by hyperactive jaw jerk and gag reflexes, and by an inability to protrude the tongue on command. Given that the nearby corticospinal tracts are also often involved, one may also find increased deep tendon reflexes and positive Babinski signs.

COURSE

The course of this syndrome reflects the course of the underlying disease.

COMPLICATIONS

The emotional incontinence may be particularly distressing to family or friends, who may take offense at the emotional display, and aspiration may be life threatening.

ETIOLOGY

Interruption of the corticobulbar fibers may occur in the cortex, centrum semiovale, internal capsule or brainstem, and may be due to any of a large number of lesions, as noted in Table 166-1.

Vascular disorders are the most common cause of pseudobulbar palsy, and classically, in the case of cortical infarctions, one finds a history of unilateral infarction in the past, followed by a new infarction on the opposite side, and the appearance of the syndrome. Of the neurodegenerative causes, amyotrophic lateral sclerosis is a common cause, but the syndrome is only seen when bulbar involvement occurs: when the disease is confined to the cord, the syndrome does not occur. Of the other causes, closed head injury and MS are common offenders.

DIFFERENTIAL DIAGNOSIS

Pathologic laughing or crying may be mistaken for emotional lability; however, the absence of any corresponding mirth or sadness suggests the correct diagnosis. Affectless laughter may also be seen in schizophrenia; however, here the symptom is always accompanied by other "negative" symptoms, phenomena that are not seen in pseudobulbar palsy.

TREATMENT

Double-blinded studies have demonstrated the effectiveness of amitriptyline (in doses of from 50 to 75 mg), nortriptyline (in doses of 50 to 100 mg) and citalopram (in doses of 10 to 20 mg),

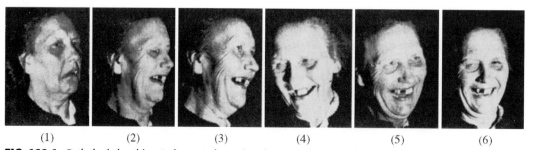

(1) (2) (3) (4) (5) (6)

FIG. 166-1. Pathologic laughing. In frame 1 the patient is at rest; frames 2 through 6 show her laughing, despite the fact that she was attempting to stop and did not feel at all happy. (From Vinken PJ, Bruyn GW. *Handbook of clinical neurology*, Vol 45 (revised 1), New York, 1985, Elsevier.)

and open studies have suggested effectiveness for fluoxetine, paroxetine and fluvoxamine. Although weeks may be required for a response, some patients will show dramatic improvement over a matter of days. If amitriptyline or nortriptyline are used, the dose should be gradually titrated up, with careful regard for hypotension and anticholinergic side-effects; in the case of nortriptyline, it may also be prudent to check blood levels in the case of non-response to see if the patient's level is within the "therapeutic window." Citalopram, given its favorable side-effect profile and its general lack of drug-drug interactions, may be the preferred agent, at least to start with.

Aspiration must be guarded against, and the underlying disease, if possible, treated.

BIBLIOGRAPHY

Anderson G, Vestergaard K, Riis J. Citalopram for poststroke pathological crying. *Lancet* 1993;342:837-839.

Dichgans M, Mayer M, Uttner I, et al. The phenotypic spectrum of CADASIL: clinical findings in 102 cases. *Annals of Neurology* 1998;44:731-739.

Gallagher JP. Pathologic laughter and crying in ALS: a search for their origin. *Acta Neurologica Scandinavica* 1989;80:114-117.

Karp BI, Laureno R. Pontine and extrapontine myelinolysis: a neurologic disorder following rapid correction of hyponatremia. *Medicine* 1993;72:359-373.

Lieberman A, Benson DF. Control of emotional expression in pseudobulbar palsy. A personal experience. *Archives of Neurology* 1977;34:717-719.

Robinson RG, Parikh RM, Lipsey JR, et al. Pathological laughing and crying following stroke: validation of a measurement scale and a double-blind treatment study. *The American Journal of Psychiatry* 1993;150:286-293.

Schiffer RB, Herndon RM, Rudick RA. Treatment of pathologic laughing and weeping with amitriptyline. *The New England Journal of Medicine* 1985;312:1480-1482.

Zeilig G, Drubach DA, Katz-Zeilig M, et al. Pathological laughter and crying with closed traumatic brain injury. *Brain Injury* 1996;10:591-597.

167 Klüver-Bucy Syndrome

After subjecting monkeys to bilateral temporal lobectomies, Drs. Klüver and Bucy, in 1939, reported the emergence of a peculiar behavioral syndrome, which eventually was named after them. The terminology used by Klüver and Bucy was idiosyncratic, and, perhaps in part because of this, there has been persistent uncertainty as to the definition of the syndrome in humans. Many authors, however, speak of the following characteristics: emotional placidity, "hypermetamorphosis," "hyperorality," "psychic blindness" and hypersexuality. The syndrome itself has high localizing value, as in all cases one finds bilateral damage or dysfunction of the temporal lobes.

ONSET

The onset ranges from paroxysmal, as in the case of a complex partial seizure, to subacute, as during recovery from a closed head injury, to gradual and insidious, as may occur in Pick's disease.

CLINICAL FEATURES

Although overall placid and emotionally docile, patients nevertheless seem drawn to come into contact with whatever is nearby, whether it be another person or an inanimate object; furthermore, in the midst of this "hypermetamorphic" behavior, patients typically put whatever they find to their mouths, whether edible or not, where they lick, taste or eat it. During such "hyperoral" behavior, patients may eat toilet paper, styrofoam cups or drink their own urine, and if food happens to be at hand they may display a remarkable gluttony, sometimes with equally remarkable weight gain. This indiscriminate mouthing of objects is but one manifestation of their "psychic blindness" wherein they appear to have a peculiar kind of agnosia such that they fail to avoid toxic or dangerous objects or situations. The hypersexuality of these patients evidences the same indiscriminateness: patients may make sexual advances to anyone, of any age, sex or station, or they may simply masturbate without regard for where they are or whom they're with.

COURSE

The course is determined in large part by the underlying cause. Ictal cases, of course, remit fully and spontaneously after minutes, whereas cases occurring on the basis of a neurodegenerative disorder, such as Pick's disease, are chronic; in other cases, as for example after herpes simplex encephalitis or closed head injury, there may be some gradual improvement over many months.

COMPLICATIONS

The bizarre nature of these symptoms generally renders the patient incapable of participating with others at work or at home.

■**TABLE 167-1.** Causes of the Klüver-Bucy Syndrome

With clear precipitants
    post-closed head injury or bilateral temporal contusions
    post-herpes simplex viral encephalitis
    post-status epilepticus
    bilateral temporal lobectomy
    late-delayed radiation encephalopathy
Gradual onset
    Pick's disease
    Fronto-temporal dementia
    Alzheimer's disease
    Huntington's disease
Associated with epilepsy
    ictal
    post-ictal

ETIOLOGY

The various disorders capable of causing dysfunction or damage to the temporal lobes bilaterally, and thus capable of causing the Klüver-Bucy syndrome, are listed in Table 167-1.

Of the obvious precipitants capable of causing the syndrome, head injury is one of the most common causes, and in the case of closed head injury, patients may "emerge" from an apallic state directly into the Klüver-Bucy syndrome. Of the neurodegenerative disorders capable of causing a Klüver-Bucy syndrome of gradual onset, both Pick's disease and fronto-temporal dementia, which preferentially and early affect the temporal lobes, may actually present with the syndrome; by contrast, when the syndrome appears in Alzheimer's or Huntington's disease, it is usually only after the disease is far advanced and patients are already demented. Ictal Klüver-Bucy syndrome has been noted during complex partial seizures, and the syndrome may also be seen as a variant of the post-ictal psychosis, being preceded by a "flurry" of seizures and separated from the last of this "flurry" by a "lucid" interval.

DIFFERENTIAL DIAGNOSIS

In its fully developed form, this syndrome is almost unmistakable. The diagnosis of partial forms after readily recognizable precipitants, such as head injury or viral encephalitis, is also generally apparent.

Should Pick's disease or fronto-temporal dementia present with a partial Klüver-Bucy syndrome, the bizarre hyperorality and hypersexuality might suggest schizophrenia, but in the syndrome one does not see the hallucinations and delusions which typify schizophrenia.

TREATMENT

There are no blinded studies of the treatment of Klüver-Bucy syndrome. Anecdotally, both haloperidol and SSRIs have been noted to reduce hypermetamorphosis and hypersexuality, and leuprolide has been used successfully for the hypersexuality.

BIBLIOGRAPHY

Hart RP, Kwentus JA, Frazier RB, et al. Natural history of Klüver-Bucy syndrome after treated herpes encephalitis. *Southern Medical Journal* 1986;79:1376-1378.

Janati A. Klüver-Bucy syndrome in Huntington's chorea. *The Journal of Nervous and Mental Disease* 1985;173:632-635.

Klüver H, Bucy PC. Preliminary analysis of functions of the temporal lobes in monkeys. *Archives of Neurology and Psychiatry* 1939;42:979-1000.

Lam LC, Chiu HF. Klüver-Bucy syndrome in a patient with nasopharyngeal carcinoma: a late complication of radiation brain injury. *Journal of Geriatric Psychiatry and Neurology* 1997;10:111-113.

Lilly R, Cummings JL, Benson F, et al. The human Klüver-Bucy syndrome. *Neurology* 1983;33:1141-1145.

Nakada T, Lee H, Kwee IL, et al. Epileptic Klüver-Bucy syndrome: case report. *The Journal of Clinical Psychiatry* 1984;45:87-88.

Ott BR. Leuprolide treatment of sexual aggression in a patient with dementia and the Klüver-Bucy syndrome. *Clinical Neuropharmacology* 1995;18:443-447.

Slaughter J, Bobo W, Childers MK. Selective serotonin reuptake inhibitor treatment of post-traumatic Klüver-Bucy syndrome. *Brain Injury* 1999;13:59-62.

168 Alien Hand Syndrome

The alien hand syndrome represents one of the most extraordinary and remarkable phenomena seen in clinical practice. Here, the patient find that one of the hands, almost invariably the left one, begins to act autonomously, and to engage in purposeful and complex behavior that is at definite cross-purposes with what the patient consciously wills and intends to do with the right hand. For example, in one case a patient wished to button his shirt and began to do so with his right hand; soon thereafter, the left hand, despite the patient's intentions, followed along, unbuttoning the buttons that had just been fastened by the right hand. Or, in another example, a patient, while frying a steak, flipped it over with her right hand. Immediately thereafter, the left hand flipped the steak back.

This syndrome was first described by Kurt Goldstein in 1908, and fleshed out by Akelaitis in a 1941 article in the *American Journal of Psychiatry* about patients who had undergone section of the corpus callosum for control of intractable epilepsy. Akelaitis named it "diagonistic dyspraxia," but this name never gained currency, and the current name is derived from an article by Brion and Jedynak in a 1972 issue of the *Revue Neurologique*, where the authors spoke of *le signe de la main étrangère*. Akelaitis' original observation of an association of the syndrome with lesions of the corpus callosum, however, has held true, in that almost all cases involve damage of one sort or another to the corpus callosum.

ONSET

The onset is determined by the underlying cause, and may range from acute, as when the corpus callosum undergoes infarction, or gradual, as in the case of tumors of the same structure.

CLINICAL FEATURES

As illustrated by the examples above, the cardinal feature of the alien hand syndrome is complex behavior of the left hand which is at definite cross-purposes with what the patient wishes and wills to do with the right hand. In addition to the examples already given, this "inter-manual conflict" may play out in a variety of other ways. One patient, wanting to drink a cup of coffee, pulled the cup toward himself with this right hand, only to find that the left hand pushed it back away. Another patient, wishing to get some clothes out of a drawer, opened the drawer with his right hand, upon which the left hand began to push it closed. Finally, there are rare reports of murderous alien hands. In one case, after suffering a callosal infarction, the patient found her left hand unbuttoning her gown, crushing cups on her tray, fighting with her right hand as she tried to pick up a telephone to make a call, and, finally, attempting to choke her.

Importantly, patients experience the behavior of the left hand as alien, autonomous and independent of them. They may speak of the left hand as being disobedient, or may speak to it as if it were another person.

COURSE

The course is determined by the underlying cause.

COMPLICATIONS

The behavior of the alien hand may significantly interfere with routine activities of daily living, and may impair patients' abilities to cooperate with rehabilitation programs.

ETIOLOGY

As indicated above, the vast majority of cases occur secondary to lesions of the corpus callosum, and the alien hand syndrome may be considered one of the callosal disconnection syndromes. Lesions include surgical section, infarction, hemorrhage and tumors. Exceptions to this rule are rare, but have included biparietal infarctions and infarction of the medial aspect of the frontal and parietal cortices. There is also one definite case of the alien hand syndrome occurring in Creutzfeldt-Jakob disease.

Cortico-basal ganglionic degeneration is typically listed as one of the causes of the alien hand syndrome; however, a close reading of the published reports reveals only "alien hand-like" behaviors, such as levitation and forced groping.

Activity in the right hemisphere is normally controlled by the "eloquent" left hemisphere, but with section of the corpus callosum, the anatomic bridge which allows for this control is destroyed and the right hemisphere now is able to act autonomously. This autonomous activity, in turn, is manifested in the behavior of the left hand. In a sense, with both hemispheres acting independently, a "two minds" situation has been created, with the conflict between them evident in the "inter-manual" conflict of the two hands.

DIFFERENTIAL DIAGNOSIS

The alien hand syndrome must be differentiated from apraxia, the "levitation phenomenon" and forced groping.

The apraxic left hand is simply clumsy and unable to execute complex activities; here any "conflict" between the left and right hands merely represents an inability of the left hand to "cooperate": there is no evidence of the left hand acting at cross purpose.

The levitation phenomenon is seen with parietal lobe injuries. Here the left hand involuntarily levitates, but does nothing more than hang in space. The lack of complex behavior of the levitated hand distinguishes it from an alien hand.

Forced groping is most commonly confused with the alien hand syndrome, but a careful examination of the behavior of the groping left hand will allow a correct differential. In forced groping, the affected hand will involuntarily reach out and grope for objects that come into view, and, if contact is made with an object, grab onto it and not let go. One patient found that whenever he walked through a doorway his left hand would reach out for the doorknob, grab it and not let go, requiring the patient to stop and, with his right hand, pry the left hand off the knob. Note here, however, that the behavior of the left hand, once it has found its object, remains simple and confined to merely grasping and hanging on. This is in marked contrast to the behavior of an alien hand which, once in contact with an object, will do something complex with it. Thus, whereas a groping hand might reach out to grasp a spatula, it would not do anything further with it, in contrast with the alien hand which might use it to turn some food over in the frying pan. The failure to distinguish between a groping hand and an alien hand has led to considerable nosologic confusion; some authors have even proposed that there are "two" alien hand syndromes: one is "callosal" and corresponds to the description in this book whereas the other is "frontal." This purported "frontal" alien hand syndrome, upon close reading of the clinical examples, is nothing other than forced groping.

TREATMENT

Treatment is directed at the underlying condition. In some cases, patients may have to immobilize the alien hand with a wrist restraint or render it less problematic by putting a mitten on it.

BIBLIOGRAPHY

Akelaitis AJ. Psychobiological studies following section of the corpus callosum. *The American Journal of Psychiatry* 1941;97:1147-1157.

Bogen JE. The callosal syndrome. In: Heilman KM, Valnestein E (eds). *Clinical neuropsychology*, 2nd ed. New York, 1985, Oxford University Press.

Brion S, Jedynak CP. Troubles de transport interhemispherique: a propos de trois observations de tumeurs du corps calleux. *Revue Neurologique* 1972;126:257-266.

Feinberg TE, Schindler K, Flanagan NG, et al. Two alien hand syndromes. *Neurology* 1992;42:19-24.

Geschwind DH, Iacoboni M, Mega MS, et al. Alien hand syndrome: interhemispheric motor disconnection due to a lesion in the midbody of the corpus callosum. *Neurology* 1995;45:802-808.

Goldstein K. Sur Lehre der motorischen Apraxia. *Monatschrift fur Psychologie und Neurologie* 1908;11:169-187.

Ong Hai BG, Odderson IR. Involuntary masturbation as a manifestation of stroke-related alien hand syndrome. *American Journal of Physical Medicine & Rehabilitation* 2000;79:395-398.

Suwanwela NC, Leelacheavsit N. Isolated corpus callosal infarction secondary to pericallosal artery disease presenting as alien hand syndrome. *Journal of Neurology, Neurosurgery, and Psychiatry* 2002;72:533-536.

Tanaka Y, Yoshida A, Kawahata N, et al. Diagonistic dyspraxia: clinical characteristics, responsible lesions and possible underlying mechanism. *Brain* 1996;119:859-874.

An elevated temperature, if sufficiently high, may directly cause a delirium. Although the temperature "threshold" at which delirium occurs varies among different patients, almost all patients with a temperature over 106° F (41.1° C) will become delirious.

Under normal circumstances, body temperature is kept within a narrow range by various mechanisms, all of which operate in concert under the control of the hypothalamus. Within the anterior hypothalamus there is a thermoregulatory center which constantly samples the temperature of the blood circulating through the hypothalamus, compares that to a "set-point," and then, depending on whether the body temperature is above or below the set-point, activates, much like a thermostat, either heat-dissipating or heat-generating and conservatory measures. Heat dissipation is accomplished largely via cutaneous vasodilatation and sweating, and heat generation and conservation by the muscular activity of shivering and by vasoconstriction.

Elevations of body temperature may occur via either a resetting of the hypothalamic set-point or one of several other mechanisms, including increased heat generation (e.g., running a marathon), increased ambient temperature (as in a "heat wave"), or a failure of normal heat-dissipating mechanisms, as, for example, may occur when drugs with anticholinergic properties inhibit sweating.

When temperature elevation occurs due to a resetting of the hypothalamic set-point, one speaks of fever, or, as it used to be called, pyrexia. The most common mechanism whereby the set-point is elevated, thereby producing a fever, involves molecules known as "pyrogens." Pyrogens may be either exogenous or endogenous: exogenous pyrogens include portions of infectious agents, such as bacteria or viruses; these exogenous pyrogens in turn stimulate monocytes and macrophages to produce endogenous pyrogens, such as interleukin-1, interleukin-6 and tumor necrosis factor-alpha. Endogenous pyrogens then stimulate the production of prostaglandins within the anterior hypothalamus which reset the set-point higher: the effect is much like simply setting a thermostat higher, and the body's heat-generating and conservatory mechanisms are brought into play.

Temperature elevation due to mechanisms other than a resetting of the hypothalamic set-point is referred to as "hyperthermia." Familiar clinical examples of this include malignant hyperthermia, heat stroke, the neuroleptic malignant syndrome and severe intoxication with cocaine, amphetamines, MDMA ("Ecstasy") or phencyclidine.

In evaluating a patient with increased temperature, it is critical to determine whether the elevation represents fever or hyperthermia, as the diagnostic evaluations and treatment approaches, as noted below, are different. The clinical setting provides the strongest clue. Certainly if the patient had an obvious infectious process known to commonly cause fever, such as pneumonia, one would lean toward a diagnosis of fever; conversely, if the patient was taking an anticholinergic drug, or if the skin, though hot, was dry, or if the patient were found in an un-air conditioned apartment during a heat wave, then hyperthermia would be more likely. Another clue involves the actual temperature itself. It appears that the maximum setting of the hypothalamic set-point is around 106 degrees F, or 41.1 degrees C: consequently, fevers, that is to say temperature elevations secondary to resetting of the set-point, generally never rise beyond 106 degrees F; temperatures above 106 degrees F almost represent hyperthermia, and indicate a non-infectious mechanism, such as heat stroke.

In determining whether a patient with an elevated temperature has either a fever or hyperthermia, it must be kept in mind that although "pure" cases of fever or hyperthermia are the rule, "mixed" cases may also be seen. A common example of such a mixed case would be an elderly patient with fever due to pneumonia and with hyperthermia due to the administration of an anticholinergic agent, such as benztropine.

Finally, one very rare cause of hyperthermia bears mentioning. Damage to the anterior hypothalamus, as may occur with tumors or after rupture of an anterior communicating artery aneurysm, may cause profound, even fatal, temperature elevations.

ONSET

The onset of the delirium may be acute or subacute, depending on the rapidity with which the temperature rises.

CLINICAL FEATURES

Initially patients are restless, at times anxious and irritable. Sleep is disturbed, and vivid nightmares may occur.

As the temperature rises further, confusion and disorientation appear and most patients begin to experience hallucinations. Although auditory hallucinations may occur, visual ones are much more characteristic. The bed rail may be seen as a bar on a cell; the stethoscope hanging from the physician's neck may appear as a noose. Fantastic scenes may occur; an entourage of figures and persons may troop through the sick room.

With further rises, restlessness and confusion increase and drowsiness eventually appears. In time the patient may simply lie in bed, mumbling incoherently, picking at the sheets.

Eventually, if the temperature rises high enough coma occurs (and this is generally almost always the case at 107° F [41.7° C] or higher), and death may follow.

Importantly, given that rectal temperature is higher than oral temperature by about 0.7 degrees F or 0.4 degrees C, it is critical, in order to follow a patient's course, to always use the same method, whether it be oral or rectal; furthermore, neither axillary nor tympanic temperatures should be utilized, as they are inaccurate. Automated oral temperature probes are also to be avoided, as they are notorious for under-estimating the actual temperature.

COURSE

The course of the delirium parallels that of the elevated temperature and remits as the temperature falls. In general the patient recovers completely; however, when temperature elevations of 107 degrees F or higher are sustained for hours, patients, if they survive, may be left with evidence of cerebellar dysfunction, or, less commonly, with a dementia.

COMPLICATIONS

The complications of delirium are as described in that chapter. Seizures may occur, especially in epileptics and young children.

ETIOLOGY

Reversible neuronal dysfunction occurs as the temperature rises, and patients with pre-existing cerebral disease, as for example Alzheimer's disease, are more likely to develop a delirium. Once the temperature passes beyond 106 degrees F neuronal death begins, and in this regard the cerebellum appears most susceptible.

DIFFERENTIAL DIAGNOSIS

Diseases that not only cause fever but also directly affect the brain must be excluded. Examples include viral encephalitides and cerebral abscess.

TREATMENT

Regardless of whether the patient has fever or hyperthermia, the underlying cause, if possible, should be treated. In the case of fever, one may also be given antipyretics such as aspirin, non-steroidal antiinflammatory agents or acetaminophen. Importantly, as these agents all work by interfering with pyrogen-induced prostaglandin production, they are not effective in hyperthermia. Other symptomatic measures that are useful for both fever and for hyperthermia include measures to reduce heat generation and enhance heat dissipation, such as bed rest, unclothed, in an air-conditioned room, continual fanning, cool water sponge baths and cooling blankets: in severe cases, ice-water baths, infusion of room-temperature saline or gastric or colonic lavage with iced-saline, may be considered.

For severe agitation, parenteral lorazepam may be used as described in the chapter on rapid treatment. Antipsychotics, especially the phenothiazines, are generally contraindicated for two reasons. First, they may inactivate the hypothalamic thermoregulatory mechanism, producing a state or "poikilothermia" with a failure of normal sweating and vasodilatation. Second, they may, via their anticholinergic effects, also reduce sweating.

BIBLIOGRAPHY

Aldemir M, Ozen S, Kara IH, et al. Predisposing factors for delirium in the surgical intensive care unit. *Critical Care* 2001;5:265-270.

Ebaugh FG, Barnacle CH, Ewalt JR. Delirious episodes associated with artificial fever: a study of 200 cases. *The American Journal of Psychiatry* 1936;16:191-217.

Ebaugh FG, Barnacle CH, Ewalt JR. Psychiatric aspects of artificial fever therapy. *Archives of Neurology and Psychiatry* 1938;39:1203-1212.

Francis J, Martin D, Kapoor WN. A prospective study of delirium in hospitalized elderly. *The Journal of the American Medical Association* 1990;263:1097-1101.

Wexler RK. Evaluation and treatment of heat-related illnesses. *American Family Physician* 2002;65:2307-2314.

Yaqub B, Al Deeb S. Heat strokes: aetiopathogenesis, neurological characteristics, treatment and outcome. *Journal of the Neurological Sciences* 1998;156:144-151.

PARTIAL SEIZURES, EPILEPSY, AND RELATED DISORDERS

170 Simple and Complex Partial Seizures

Partial seizures are of paroxysmal onset, and generally last on the order of minutes. These seizures are further divided into two types, namely simple and complex, with the distinction between them resting on whether or not there is any disturbance of consciousness during the seizure and any amnesia for it postictally, during simple partial seizures patients remain alert and clear, and after the seizure they are able to fully recall the events of the seizure itself; by contrast, during complex partial seizures there is some disturbance or defect of consciousness, ranging from a sense of "fuzziness" to profound confusion, and, postictally, there is always some degree of amnesia for the events that transpired during the ictus. The symptomatology seen during a partial seizure is extraordinarily varied, reflecting, in large part, the variability in location of the seizure focus. For example, simple partial seizures arising from foci in the motor cortex may present with clonic twitching of a hand, whereas those arising from foci in the temporal lobe may present with hallucinations or with panic. Although complex partial seizures always, as noted below under etiology, reflect epileptic activity in the temporal lobes, the symptomatology here may also be quite varied, ranging from lip-smacking in the setting of profound confusion to singing and dancing in a state of relatively preserved consciousness.

ONSET

The age of onset is determined by the underlying cause of the seizure, and may range from childhood to old age. Childhood and adolescent onset cases often occur secondary to neuronal migration disorders or mesial temporal sclerosis, whereas adult onset cases more often indicate the presence of mass lesions, such as tumors, or head trauma or cortical infarction.

CLINICAL FEATURES

Simple partial seizures may present with motor signs, somato sensory or special sensory symptoms, autonomic symptoms or signs, or with psychic symptoms. Motor symptoms typically consist of clonic or tonic activity beginning in the fingers or hands, face, or feet, which may remain localized or may spread in a "Jacksonian" march to adjacent body areas, as for example from the fingers to the hand, arm and finally to the face. Very rarely, there may be bilateral motor activity without any defect of consciousness at all, and this may be seen with foci in the supplementary motor area on the mesial surface of the frontal lobe. Occasionally, one may also see an "inhibitory" simple partial seizure with motor symptoms, wherein, rather than motor activity,

one sees an ictal paralysis. Such an inhibitory seizure, which is an ictal event, must be distinguished from a postictal "Todd's paralysis" which may follow upon the end of a typical motor seizure.

Somatosensory or special sensory symptoms consist of hallucinations, which may be tactile, visual, auditory or gustatory. Tactile hallucinations typically consist of parasthesiae, numbness, sensations of warmth or cold, or, uncommonly, pain. Interestingly, these tactile hallucinations may also undergo a "march," with, for example, parasthesiae beginning in the fingers, then marching to the hand, and up the forearm and arm. Visual hallucinations tend to be simple, often consisting of geometric forms. Auditory hallucinations also tend to be simple, and patients may hear buzzing or ringing noises. Olfactory hallucinations tend to be unpleasant, as for example of something rotten, or burning. Gustatory hallucinations also tend to be unpleasant; classically there may be the taste of a "copper penny."

Autonomic symptoms classically involve a sense of something "rising" from the epigastrium; there may also be abdominal cramping or diarrhea.

Psychic symptoms are of greatest interest to psychiatry, and are extraordinarily varied. There may be déjà vu or jamais vu, forced thoughts, macropsia or micropsia, hyperacusis or hypoacusis, depersonalization, anxiety (to the point of panic), depression and euphoria. Patients may experience sexual arousal and even orgasm, and some may find themselves involuntarily laughing or crying, without any corresponding sense of mirth or sadness. Complex visual or auditory hallucinations may also occur: some patients may vividly hallucinate a scene, as if watching a movie, and others may hear voices or singing. Very rarely, simple partial seizures may present as paroxysmal, brief delusions: one patient experienced an ictal Capgras phenomenon whereas another, during the seizure, was convinced that his body was under the direct control of outside forces.

Complex partial seizures are always accompanied by some clouding or defect of consciousness. Some patients appear quite confused and perplexed; others are more "in touch" and may respond to simple requests, walk about without bumping into things, and in some cases patients may, to superficial observation, seem quite alert and responsive. The behavior seen during a complex partial seizure ranges from simple automatisms to very complex behavior. With profound confusion, one generally sees simple automatisms such as lip smacking, fumbling with clothing or sheets, looking around or walking aimlessly. Complex behavior ranges from pelvic thrusting to driving a car, disrobing or dancing. Rarely, patients may become violent. Although ictal violence most commonly occurs when an attempt is made to restrain a patient who is walking about or trying to get out of bed, there are rare cases, with video-EEG documentation, of patients engaging in unprovoked attacks on others during the seizure. Regardless of the duration or symptomatology of a complex partial seizure, most patients, subsequent to the termination of the seizure, experience some degree of dysphoria, confusion, fatigue, or somnolence. Furthermore, all patients have a variable degree of amnesia for the events of the partial complex seizure proper.

Although a scalp EEG and an MRI scan of the head are standard parts of the work-up for any patient with partial seizures, it must be borne in mind that both may be normal, even in cases of indubitable epilepsy. In the case of simple partial seizures, the interictal EEG is often normal, and even an ictal EEG may be normal; with complex partial seizures, both interictal and ictal EEGs are more often abnormal, but even here if the focus is at some distance from the surface, as for example on the mesial surface of the temporal lobe, the scalp EEG may remain normal even when depth EEGs reveal ongoing paroxysmal activity.

COURSE

The course of the partial seizure per se, as noted above, is generally quite brief, lasting on the order of two to three minutes. Partial status epilepticus, however, may occur, with interesting results. In the case of simple partial status epilepticus, clonic motor activity may persist for months or even years, and cases of ictal anxiety or depression lasting weeks, albeit rare, have been reported. Complex partial status epilepticus is even more intriguing: patients may travel long distances, and, rarely, psychosis, with delusions and bizarre behavior, have occurred and persisted for days.

The course in terms of seizure recurrence and frequency is in large part determined by the underlying cause, and varies quite widely.

COMPLICATIONS

Simple partial seizures generally have few complications, although motor or inhibitory seizures may have consequences depending on what the patient is doing at the time.

In the case of complex partial seizures, accidents may occur should the patient be driving, swimming, and the like. Recurrent complex partial seizures may also be followed by the development of a chronic interictal psychosis or the interictal personality syndrome.

ETIOLOGY

In almost all cases of partial seizures there is an anatomical abnormality or "epileptogenic focus." In the case of simple partial seizures, the spread of paroxysmal electrical activity from this focus is generally quite limited: there may be some, as in the case of a clinical "march," but for the most part the reach of the epileptic activity is limited; furthermore, the symptomatology of the seizure reflects fairly well the location of the focus, with motor symptoms suggesting the motor cortex, visual symptoms the occipital cortex, etc. With complex partial seizures, however, the situation is more complex. It appears that in order for the full clinical expression of a complex partial seizure to occur, both temporal lobes must be involved. This is not to say that there must be a focus in both lobes, because in most cases the epileptic activity simply spreads from one temporal lobe to the other, as for example via the corpus

callosum. Furthermore, although both temporal lobes must be involved, the actual focus in some cases is not in either temporal lobe, but is at some distance. For example, a focus in the frontal lobe may fire and the activity may then propagate to the ipsilateral temporal lobe via the uncinate fasciculus, thence spreading via the corpus callosum to the contralateral temporal lobe.

The nature of the epileptogenic focus varies widely. As noted earlier, the age of onset of the seizure may provide a clue, with childhood and adolescent onset cases often occurring secondary to mesial temporal sclerosis or a neuronal migration disorder. Other causes of relatively early-onset seizures include certain congenital disorders, such as Sturge-Weber syndrome, tuberous sclerosis, von Recklinghausen's disease and autism. Although mesial temporal sclerosis or neuronal migration disorders may also cause adult onset cases, one must consider other causes in adults, including tumors, vascular malformations, cortical infarction, head trauma, metabolic derangements (e.g., hypoglycemia, hypocalcemia, hypomagnesemia), withdrawal from alcohol or sedative-hypnotics, and various medications, including tricyclic antidepressants, bupropion, antipsychotics (especially clozapine). In instances where partial seizures are clearly precipitated by a metabolic derangement, withdrawal or a medication, one must still assume that there is a localized anatomic abnormality, and search for it: a common example here is the patient with alcohol withdrawal and head trauma in the distant past, which left a cortical scar.

DIFFERENTIAL DIAGNOSIS

Both simple and complex partial seizures must be differentiated from other seizure types. In the case of simple partial seizures, this is fairly straightforward, if one keeps in mind the distinctive feature of simple partial seizures, namely the preservation of full consciousness and recall. Complex partial seizures, petit mal ("absence") seizures, and grand mal (generalized tonic-clonic seizures) seizures all are accompanied by a greater or lesser degree of disturbance of consciousness and amnesia postictally; indeed there is only one other seizure type, namely atonic (or "astatic") seizures which may occur in the setting of intact consciousness. These atonic seizures typically consist of a generalized and abrupt loss of motor tone with a similarly abrupt fall, a characteristic that has led to another synonym, namely "drop attacks." Atonic seizures, however, are uncommon and generally only occur in the setting of uncontrolled epilepsy characterized in turn by the chronic and frequent recurrence of complex partial seizures.

Complex partial seizures must be distinguished from petit mal seizures and amnestic seizures. Petit mal seizures occur without an aura and are typically very brief, lasting on the order of ten seconds. The symptomatology of the seizure, in most cases, is fairly unelaborate, and often consists of a blank stare and brief interruption of all ongoing activity; although there may be some very simple motor accompaniments, such as bilateral eyelid fluttering or a few automatisms, such as lip smacking, overall patients just appear to be momentarily "absent." The offset of the seizure is very abrupt and there is no postictal confusion or fatigue; indeed, patients often appear to simply "snap to." Although the frequency of these seizures can vary widely, typically they occur multiple times a day. Complex partial seizures, in contrast, are often preceded by an aura, typically accompanied by a greater number and more elaborate automatisms, last longer, on the order of minutes, and are generally followed by some postictal confusion. Amnestic seizures are characterized solely by a brief period, generally lasting minutes, of anterograde amnesia. During the amnestic seizure itself, patients behave absolutely normally and are fully conscious and clear; after the seizure, however, they have no recall of what happened or what they did while the seizure was ongoing. Complex partial seizures are similar, in that there is also an inability to recall what happened during the seizure; however, during complex partial seizures there is also some disturbance of consciousness, and it is this feature which distinguishes them from amnestic seizures.

Simple partial seizures must also be distinguished from aurae to complex partial or grand mal seizures; however, this is really more a matter of terminology than anything else. As noted earlier, in all cases of partial epilepsy there is an anatomical epileptogenic focus, and, in a very literal sense, it is the extent of the spread or propagation of electrical activity from this focus that determines the kind of seizure one sees: if the spread is minimal, a simple partial seizure is manifested; if the spread eventually involves both temporal lobes, a complex partial seizure occurs; and finally, if the spread is generalized a grand mal seizure results. Consider then, a patient with a focus in the motor cortex of the precentral gyrus. If the spread is confined to the motor cortex, then one may see only some clonic activity of the hand and speaks of a simple partial seizure. If, however, after a few seconds, the electrical activity propagates to the ipsilateral and immediately to the contralateral temporal lobe, the clinical picture is different: first, one sees the clonic activity of the hand but this motor activity after a few seconds is then followed by a complex partial seizure with confusion and automatisms. In this second case, rather than calling the clonic motor activity of the hand a simple partial seizure, it is referred to as an aura to the complex partial seizure. Although one might just as accurately say that a simple partial seizure was followed by a complex partial one, the use of the term "aura" is hallowed by time and tradition, and is unlikely to disappear.

Simple and complex partial seizures must also be distinguished from a number of other non-epileptic but episodic disorders which have a more or less paroxysmal onset. With regard to simple partial seizures some mimics include transient ischemic attacks and migraine. Transient ischemic attacks are suggested by their occurrence in the setting of vascular risk factors and also by their onset, which is generally over seconds or minutes, rather than being truly paroxysmal. Migraine aurae are suggested by the following headache, and although some patients with migraine may occasionally experience an aura alone, not followed by a headache, one can always find a history of the same aura being followed by the typical headache. Panic attacks, as may be seen in panic disorder, may be difficult to distinguish from simple partial seizures manifesting with anxiety alone: differential clues include the finding, during the history, of other, more obvious, seizure types (e.g., complex partial or grand mal seizures) and by the truly paroxysmal onset of the seizure which contrasts with panic attacks, which may take minutes to crescendo. With regard to complex partial seizures, one must consider various parasomnias, intermittent explosive disorder and dissociative fugue. Complex partial seizures may arise during sleep, and in such cases parasomnias, such as somnambulism, REM sleep behavior disorder or night terrors must be considered. Given that it is very rare for complex partial seizures to occur only nocturnally, one should look for a history of seizures occurring during waking hours; in doubtful cases, polysomnography may be required. Intermittent explosive disorder may be considered, and in some cases the differential may be so difficult that a "diagnosis by treatment response" to an antiepileptic drug is justified. Dissociative fugue is distinguished not only by the preservation of consciousness but also by the fact that many dissociative fugue patients assume a new identity, a phenomenon never seen in complex partial seizures.

Finally, partial seizures may be mimicked by "pseudoseizures." These "psychogenic" seizures may be seen in conversion disorder, Briquet's syndrome, malingering and factitious illness, and, depending on the medial sophistication of the individual, may be very difficult to distinguish from a partial seizure. The occurrence of bona fide seizures in the history may not be a reliable diagnostic sign, as many patients with epilepsy will also, at times, display pseudoseizures. Ictal EEGs are helpful, but it must be borne in mind that a negative ictal EEG, while suggestive of a pseudoseizure, is not conclusive evidence, given that during a simple partial seizure the EEG may be normal. Placebo induction, though held as unethical by some, may be considered, and although there are rare case reports of electrographically verified seizures occurring with placebo, most events induced by placebo are, in fact, pseudoseizures. When the differential question is whether the patient is having a pseudoseizure or a complex partial seizure, a prolactin level should be obtained about 15 minutes after the event, and a neuron-specific enolase level from 24 to 48 hours after the event. With pseudoseizures, these are generally normal, but with complex partial seizures one or both may generally be elevated.

TREATMENT

When recurrent seizures are anticipated, it is reasonable to begin an antiepileptic drug. Of the multiple antiepileptic drugs available, the following are clearly effective as monotherapy for partial seizures: phenytoin, carbamazepine, lamotrigine, divalproex, oxcarbazepine and gabapentin; topiramate may be, but some of the data are conflicting. The choice among these should be guided not only by the results of double-blinded comparator studies but also the patient's past experience, if any, with them, and the burden of anticipated side effects. Comparator studies are few and far between: it appears that phenytoin and carbamazepine are generally equally effective. Carbamazepine and lamotrigine appear equally effective, and carbamazepine may have a therapeutic edge over divalproex. Given the similarities between carbamazepine and oxcarbazepine one might expect oxcarbazepine to also have an edge here also, but that has not been demonstrated. With regard to side-effects, most of these drugs are generally well tolerated; among them, however, oxcarbazepine and gabapentin stand out as having a low burden of side-effects; topiramate, should it pan out as effective monotherapy, is especially attractive given its tendency to cause weight loss. Other antiepileptic drugs, including levetiracetam, tiagabine and zonisamide, have not as yet demonstrated effectiveness as monotherapy.

Should the first trial of monotherapy fail, one might consider trying another drug in a second, or even third, monotherapy trial. In cases where monotherapy will clearly be unsatisfactory, one should consider combination treatment with two antiepileptic drugs. In this regard, any two of the monotherapy agents may be combined or one may add levetiracetam, tiagabine or zonisamide. There are multiple drug-drug interactions possible with most of these combinations, as discussed in their respective chapters, and these must be closely watched for: levetiracetam is an exception, and appears to lack any interaction with other antiepileptic drugs; gabapentin is also favorable in this regard, with the only interaction noted being with the seldom used antiepileptic drug felbamate. Triple combinations, although sometimes effective, are generally to be avoided, given the multitude of sometimes severe pharmacodynamic and pharmacokinetic interactions possible.

When optimum anti-epileptic drug therapy fails to provide seizure control, one must decide whether to live with a less than perfect result or consider surgery. Although traditionally surgery has been considered a last resort, many authorities now urge early consideration, rather than allowing patients to live with severe, uncontrolled epilepsy for years and risk the development of mirror foci, with a worsening of the epilepsy, or the occurrence of an interictal psychosis or interictal personality syndrome.

Precipitating factors, such as metabolic disturbances (particularly hypoglycemia), alcohol, drug use, sleep apnea and insomnia, should be addressed and corrected. In the case of complex partial seizures or when simple partial seizures occasionally undergo secondary generalization to grand mal seizures, driving, swimming, or operating potentially dangerous machinery should be forbidden until patients are seizure-free for at least six months.

BIBLIOGRAPHY

Chadwick DW, Anhut H, Greiner MJ, et al. A double-blind trial of gabapentin monotherapy for newly diagnosed partial seizures. International gabapentin monotherapy study group 945-77. *Neurology* 1998;51:1282-1288.

Currie S, Heathfield KWG, Henson RA, et al. Clinical course and prognosis of temporal lobe epilepsy: a survey. *Brain* 1971;97:173-190.

Devinsky O, Kelley K, Porter RJ, et al. Clinical and electroencephalographic features of simple partial seizures. *Neurology* 1988;38:1347-1352.

Gilliam FG, Veloso F, Bomhof MA, et al. A dose-comparison trial of topiramate as monotherapy in recently diagnosed partial epilepsy. *Neurology* 2003;60:196-202.

Henriksen GF. Status epilepticus partialis with fear as clinical expression: report of a case and EEG findings. *Epilepsia* 1973;14:39-46.

King DW, Marsan CA. Clinical features and ictal patterns in epileptic patients with EEG temporal lobe foci. *Annals of Neurology* 1971;2:138-141.

Mattson RH, Cramer JA, Collins JF, et al. Comparison of carbamazepine, phenobarbital, phenytoin and primidone in partial and secondarily generalized tonic-clonic seizures. *The New England Journal of Medicine* 1985;313:145-151.

Mattson RH, Cramer JA, Collins JF. A comparison of valproate with carbamazepine for the treatment of complex partial seizures and secondarily generalized tonic-clonic seizures in adults. The Department of Veteran's Affairs Epilepsy Cooperative Study No. 264 Group. *The New England Journal of Medicine* 1992;327:765-771.

Mayeux R, Alexander MP, Benson DF, et al. Poriomania. *Neurology* 1979;29:1616-1619.

Mosewich RK, So EL. A clinical approach to the classification of seizures and epileptic syndromes. *Mayo Clinic Proceedings* 1996;71:405-414.

Schacter SC, Vazquez B, Fisher RS, et al. Oxcarbazepine: double-blind, randomized, placebo-controlled, monotherapy trial for partial seizures. *Neurology* 1999;52:732-777.

Theodore WH, Porter RJ, Penry JK. Complex partial seizures: clinical characteristics and differential diagnosis. *Neurology* 1983;33:1115-1121.

Williams D. The structure of emotions reflected in epileptic experiences. *Brain* 1956;79:29-67.

171 Postictal Psychosis

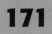

Following a cluster of grand mal or complex partial seizures, a minority of patients, after a lucid interval, will develop a transitory postictal psychosis. In epilepsy overall, the prevalence of this is about 4%; in those with medically intractable epilepsy, however, the prevalence rises to as high as 18%.

ONSET

Although cases have occurred after only a year of epilepsy, in most instances the first postictal psychosis does not occur until the epilepsy has persisted for a decade or more.

Typically, after recovering from the last of a cluster of seizures, patients enjoy a lucid interval lasting for from hours to a week or more, following which the psychosis appears acutely.

CLINICAL FEATURES

Typically, patients experience delusions, generally of persecution, accompanied by hallucinations, which tend to be auditory; a minority may also have loosened associations or mannerisms, and in rare instances stuporous catatonia may be seen. Mood changes may accompany the delusions and hallucinations, and although these tend to be depressive, manic symptomatology has also been noted. Critically, there is generally no confusion, disorientation or memory loss: the sensorium remains clear.

The EEG is either normal or shows mild diffuse slowing: there is no ictal activity.

COURSE

In most instances the psychosis spontaneously remits within a few days; there is a wide range here, however, from merely hours up to three months.

Recurrences of postictal psychosis after subsequent seizures are seen in a little over one-half of patients, and with each recurrence the duration of the psychosis lengthens until, in rare instances and with recurrent seizures, the psychoses merge to create a chronic psychosis.

COMPLICATIONS

The complications of postictal psychosis, in general, are as described in the chapter on secondary psychosis. Notably, these patients are less likely to be compliant with their antiepileptic medications, thus setting the stage for more seizures.

ETIOLOGY

Although the etiology of postictal psychosis is not known, depth EEG recordings make it clear that the psychosis does not result from ictal activity. SPECT studies have revealed increased metabolic activity bilaterally in the temporal and frontal cortices; however, the mechanism underlying this is not clear.

MRI studies have demonstrated an association between mesial temporal sclerosis and postictal psychosis; furthermore, among patients with hippocampal atrophy those with a relatively preserved anterior portion of the hippocampus are also more likely to become psychotic.

DIFFERENTIAL DIAGNOSIS

Postictal delirium is distinguished on two counts. First, in the case of postictal delirium, there is no lucid interval following the seizure. Second, postictal delirium is marked by confusion and disorientation, findings absent in postictal psychosis.

TREATMENT

Aggressive attempts at seizure control are necessary, and if this is not possible, consideration should be given to neurosurgical intervention.

When the psychosis endangers the patient or others, or interferes with medical care, patients may be treated with a

neuroleptic. Although haloperidol has traditionally been used in doses of from 5 to 10 mg daily, risperidone, in doses of from 2 to 4 mg, is probably a better choice, given its overall better tolerability. Importantly, given the course of the disorder, chronic treatment is almost never required, and thus an attempt to taper the neuroleptic should be made after patients have been free of psychosis for a matter of days.

BIBLIOGRAPHY

Brielmann RS, Kalnins RM, Hopwood MJ, et al. TLE patients with postictal psychosis: mesial dysplasia and anterior hippocampal preservation. *Neurology* 2000;55:1027-1030.

Devinsky O, Abramson H, Alper K, et al. Postictal psychosis: a case control series of 20 patients and 150 controls. *Epilepsy Research* 1995;20:247-253.

Leutmezer F, Podreka I, Asenbaum S, et al. Postictal psychosis in temporal lobe epilepsy. *Epilepsia* 2003;44:582-590.

Liu HC, Chen CH, Yeh IJ, et al. Characteristics of postictal psychosis in a psychiatric center. *Psychiatry and Clinical Neurosciences* 2001;55: 635-639.

So NK, Savard G, Andermann F, et al. Acute postictal psychosis: a stereo EEG study. *Epilepsia* 1990;31:188-193.

172 Psychosis of Forced Normalization

The psychosis of forced normalization was first described by Landolt in 1953. He described a series of epileptic patients who became psychotic after antiepileptic drugs had both "normalized" their EEGs and controlled their seizure disorder. A synonym for this disorder is "alternative psychosis," a name which speaks to the notion that the clinical condition alternates between uncontrolled seizures and an abnormal EEG on the one hand, and, on the other, successful treatment with a normal EEG and the appearance of a psychosis.

This is probably a rare condition.

ONSET

The onset is fairly acute, occurring within days of effective seizure control and normalization of the EEG.

CLINICAL FEATURES

Auditory hallucinations, delusions, incoherence and catatonic features have been noted. Importantly, confusion is either absent or minimal.

The EEG is normal, or near normal, in stark contrast to "pre-normalization" EEGs which show abundant interictal epileptiform spikes.

COURSE

Although the clinical impression is that the psychosis generally remits within days to weeks, reliable data are lacking. It does appear that with the recurrence of seizures or epileptiform spikes that the psychosis promptly remits.

COMPLICATIONS

These are as described in the chapter on secondary psychosis: some patients may effectively "treat" their psychosis by becoming noncompliant with antiepileptic drugs and having a seizure.

ETIOLOGY

Although the psychosis is clearly related in some fashion to effective suppression of epileptic activity, the underlying mechanism is not known. One study found that among patients with medically refractory complex partial seizures the psychosis of forced normalization was associated with an early onset of seizures, below the age of 10.

DIFFERENTIAL DIAGNOSIS

Ictal psychoses are distinguished by their paroxysmal onset and ictal activity on the EEG. Postictal psychoses are differentiated by their appearance just after a seizure. Chronic interictal psychoses are distinguished by their appearance in the setting of uncontrolled epilepsy.

TREATMENT

In most reports, neuroleptics have been given, generally haloperidol, with variable results. Some authors have advocated reducing doses of antiepileptic drugs to allow for the reappearance of epileptiform spikes or an occasional seizure.

BIBLIOGRAPHY

Kanemoto J, Takeuchi J, Kawasaki J, et al. Characteristics of temporal lobe epilepsy, with special reference to psychotic episodes. *Neurology* 1996;47:1199-1203.

Landolt H. Some clinical electroencephalographic correlations in epileptic psychoses (twilight states). *Electroencephalography and Clinical Neurophysiology* 1953;5:121.

Landolt H. Serial electroencephalographic investigations during psychotic episodes in epileptic patients and during schizophrenic attacks. In: de Haas, HML (ed), *Lectures on epilepsy*. London, 1958, Elsevier.

Pakainis A, Drake ME, John K, et al. Forced normalization. Acute psychosis after seizure control in seven patients. *Archives of Neurology* 1987;44:289-292.

Stevens JR. Psychiatric implications of psychomotor epilepsy. *Archives of General Psychiatry* 1966;14:461-471.

Yamamoto T, Pipo JR, Akaboshi S, et al. Forced normalization induced by ethosuximide therapy in a patient with intractable myoclonic epilepsy. *Brain & Development* 2001;23:62-64.

173 Chronic Interictal Psychosis

Approximately 6% of patients with epilepsy will develop a chronic psychosis that, phenomenologically, appears very similar to the psychosis seen in schizophrenia. Indeed, the chronic interictal psychosis has been characterized as a phenocopy or "mock up" of schizophrenia and has been studied in the hopes of finding clues to the etiology of schizophrenia itself.

ONSET

The onset of the psychosis ranges from gradual to subacute, and occurs after patients have suffered from uncontrolled epilepsy for from 10 to 23 years.

CLINICAL FEATURES

The psychosis, as noted above, is quite similar to that seen in schizophrenia. Thus, most patients have delusions, which may be of persecution, grandeur or reference; hallucinations are very common, and generally auditory in nature, and a minority of patients may also have catatonic features. Importantly, although some patients have confusion, this is generally mild and does not constitute a prominent part of the overall clinical picture.

COURSE

Although some patients may experience gradual improvement, remissions appear very uncommon and most patients experience a chronic course.

COMPLICATIONS

The complications are similar to those described for schizophrenia.

ETIOLOGY

The chronic interictal psychosis occurs in the setting of chronic epilepsy, and appears to be more common in those with complex partial seizures, left-sided epileptogenic foci and mesial temporal sclerosis on the left. Furthermore, patients with congenital lesions, such as cortical dysplasia, are at higher risk than those with acquired lesions, such as tumors.

Overall, the evidence is consistent with the idea that the psychosis occurs secondary to seizure-induced neural reorganization in the left temporal lobe, especially its mesial aspects, with an increased vulnerability conferred by the presence of congenital cortical dysplasia.

DIFFERENTIAL DIAGNOSIS

The differential of psychosis occurring in patients with epilepsy includes, in addition to chronic interictal psychosis, ictal psychosis, postictal psychosis and the psychosis of forced normalization. Ictal psychoses are distinguished by their paroxysmal onset, over seconds, and relative brevity. Postictal psychoses are suggested by the brief lucid interval that separates them from a preceding seizure. The psychosis of forced normalization is distinguished from a chronic interictal psychosis by its association with final achievement of not only complete seizure control but also of "normalization" of the EEG.

The chronic interictal psychosis must also be distinguished from schizophrenia. Epilepsy and schizophrenia are both relatively common disorders, and their co-occurrence in the same patient is not unlikely. Certainly, if the psychosis began before the epilepsy did, or had an onset within the first few years of epilepsy, a diagnosis of chronic interictal psychosis is unlikely. Conversely, if the psychosis had an onset that was both ten or more years after the onset of the epilepsy and fell within the sixth or later decades of life, the diagnosis of schizophrenia becomes unlikely.

TREATMENT

The best treatment is prevention, and the possibility of development of a chronic interictal psychosis should be a strong incentive for aggressive antiepileptic treatment.

Antipsychotics, traditionally haloperidol in doses of from 5 to 10 mg daily, are often used, with mixed results. Risperidone, given its overall better tolerability, may also be considered, in doses of from 2 to 6 mg.

Once the chronic interictal psychosis has set in, successful treatment of the epilepsy, whether with antiepileptic drugs or surgery, may or may not be followed by a gradual remission of the psychosis.

BIBLIOGRAPHY

Maier M, Mellers J, Toone B, et al. Schizophrenia, temporal lobe epilepsy and psychosis: an in vivo magnetic resonance spectroscopy and imaging study of the hippocampus/amygdala complex. *Psychological Medicine* 2000;30:571-581.

Mendez MF, Grau R, Doss RC, et al. Schizophrenia in epilepsy: seizure and psychosis variables. *Neurology* 1993;43:1073-1077.

Reutens DC, Savard G, Andermann F, et al. Results of surgical treatment in temporal lobe epilepsy with chronic psychosis. *Brain* 1997;120:1929-1936.

Roberts GW, Done DJ, Bruton C, et al. A "mock up" of schizophrenia: temporal lobe epilepsy and schizophrenia-like psychosis. *Biological Psychiatry* 1990;28:127-143.

Sherwin I, Peron-Magnan P, Bancaud J, et al. Prevalence of psychosis in epilepsy as a function of the laterality of the epileptogenic lesion. *Archives of Neurology* 1982;39:621-625.

174 Interictal Personality Syndrome

The interictal personality syndrome, also known as the Geschwind Syndrome or the temporal lobe epilepsy personality syndrome, represents a personality change occurring in the context of epilepsy with chronically recurrent complex partial seizures. This is a controversial entity: some authors either doubt its existence or consider it very rare, whereas others believe it is common.

ONSET

The onset of the personality change is very gradual and insidious, occurring after years of uncontrolled complex partial seizures.

CLINICAL FEATURES

Classically, the personality change is characterized by "viscosity," religious or philosophical preoccupations, and hyposexuality.

Viscosity, or, as it is also known, "stickiness," is characterized by an inability on the patient's part to break away from a train of thought or a certain emotion, with thoughts and emotions plodding on and adhering to one another in a sort of "viscous" mass. Speech is verbose and circumstantial, and patients may engage in hypergraphia, writing seemingly interminably long letters or reports, filled with ramblings and inessential details. Emotions tend to persist long past any inciting event, and patients may seem "stuck" in them. In some cases this viscosity manifests in other ways: some patients, upon shaking the physician's hand at the end of an interview, will simply hang on well past any goodbyes, requiring the physician to actively disengage his or her hand.

Religious, philosophical, ethical and metaphysical concerns are common in this personality change. Patients may be preoccupied with abstruse matters, and their conversation and writings reflect this.

Hyposexuality is manifest primarily by a loss of libido.

COURSE

Once established, this personality change is chronic.

COMPLICATIONS

Work and personal relations may suffer, and some patients may become isolated.

ETIOLOGY

It is suspected that recurrent epileptic activity in the temporal lobes leads to a neural reorganization of the limbic system, resulting in the personality change.

DIFFERENTIAL DIAGNOSIS

The chronic interictal psychosis is distinguished by delusions and hallucinations, phenomena which are not part of the interictal personality syndrome.

Temporal lobe tumors may cause both complex partial seizures and, by virtue of ongoing and progressive destruction of the temporal lobe, a personality change.

TREATMENT

There is no known treatment.

BIBLIOGRAPHY

Bear DM, Fedio P. Quantitative analysis of interictal behavior in temporal lobe epilepsy. *Archives of Neurology* 1977;34:454-467.

Benson DF. The Geschwind Syndrome. *Advances in Neurology* 1991;55:411-421.

Blumer D. Evidence supporting the temporal lobe epilepsy personality syndrome. *Neurology* 1999;53(Suppl 2):9-12.

Devinsky O, Najjar S. Evidence against the existence of a temporal lobe epilepsy personality syndrome. *Neurology* 1999;53(Suppl 2):13-25.

Geschwind N. Interictal behavioral changes in epilepsy. *Epilepsia* 1983;24(Suppl 1):23-30.

Waxman SG, Geschwind N. The interictal behavior syndrome of temporal lobe epilepsy. *Archives of General Psychiatry* 1975;32:1580-1586.

175 Alzheimer's Disease (dementia of the Alzheimer's type, DSM-IV-TR #294.10, 294.11)

Alzheimer's disease, also known as "dementia of the Alzheimer's type," is the most common cause of dementia, accounting for slightly less than one half of all cases. The prevalence of Alzheimer's disease increases with aging, from 5% of the entire population aged 65 or more to 20% of the entire population aged 80 or more. Alzheimer's disease is slightly more common among women than men.

The typical neuropathology of this disease was first described by Alois Alzheimer, a colleague of Kraepelin's. In the past this disease was known as either "presenile dementia," or "senile dementia," depending on whether the onset was before or after the age of 65. Recent evidence strongly suggests, however, that such a distinction is unwarranted, and although these terms are still seen in the literature, one should probably abandon them in favor of the more inclusive eponym of "Alzheimer's disease." Of some historical note is the fact that this eponym itself comes to us courtesy of Kraepelin, who encouraged the reluctant Alzheimer to lend his name to his discovery.

ONSET

Although Alzheimer's disease may occur at almost any age, the onset typically occurs after the age of 50, with an ever-increasing number of cases appearing in ensuing years. An onset in early adult years, though unusual, may be seen, and, although extraordinarily rare, childhood onset cases have also been reported.

The onset itself is generally quite gradual and insidious. A gradual decline in short-term memory or a progressive change in the patient's personality may occur. By contrast, however, the actual event that brings the patient to medical attention may be acute and at times catastrophic. For example, if the patient leaves an adult lifelong home and moves to a new neighborhood, the memory defect may preclude orientation to the new surroundings, and the patient may be found wandering the streets, trying to find "home." Or a heretofore modest and moralistic patient may, after a personality deterioration spanning many years, be arrested for masturbating in front of some neighborhood children.

Less commonly, Alzheimer's disease may present as an isolated progressively worsening dysphasia or, less commonly, dyspraxia.

CLINICAL FEATURES

In most cases the earliest signs are, as noted, either a memory loss or a personality change.

The memory loss is initially of the short-term variety. Patients become "forgetful" and are unable to find their keys or their wallets. In time the ability to recall hitherto well-known facts about the past becomes progressively impaired. Typically, this "blanket" of retrograde amnesia initially covers more recent events say of the past few months or years. With time, however, the blanket extends progressively farther back, even into childhood. The names of grandchildren may be forgotten, then of one's own children. Women may eventually begin to introduce themselves by their maiden names, having forgotten the fact that they were married.

With memory loss, disorientation occurs, first to time and then to place. Often, it is a matter of patients localizing themselves just ahead of the advancing blanket of amnesia. If hospitalized, patients may insist they are at home, perhaps years earlier. With time and progression of the disease, some patients, when asked their current address and age, may give the address of their childhood home and an appropriate age. Eventually, all orientation may be lost, even to century and to country.

The personality change, though non-specific, tends to be characterized by a certain coarsening of patients' behavior: they take less interest in others; and more and more become focused only on those matters of immediate selfish concern: car, house, clothing, and food. Other patients may undergo an exaggeration of a preexisting trait, as occurs when frugal patients become stingy and moralistic ones, accusatory and defaming. Occasionally, rather than an accentuation of an old personality trait, a new one may emerge, such as heightened sexual interest, at times leading to great indiscretion, with hasty marriages or involvement with children.

Psychiatric symptomatology is very common, and may include depression, euphoria, psychosis or agitation.

Depressive symptoms are less common, occurring in perhaps a quarter of all patients. Appetite, weight, and energy may fail, increased tension and agitation may be seen, and insomnia may be severe. Mood congruent delusions are not uncommon here. Patients may become convinced that they are impoverished or that their organs are shriveled up. Some may wander at night, unable to sleep, bewailing their fate.

Euphoria is less common, occurring in less than 10%; in general, rather than a full manic syndrome, one typically sees a mere bland euphoria or a tendency to overtalkativeness.

Psychosis, with hallucinations or delusions, or both, is seen in about one-quarter of patients, and is one of the most common reasons for institutionalization. Visual hallucinations are more common than auditory ones. Patients may hallucinate complex scenes and activities that may be variously amusing or terrifying, or they may hear voices or whisperings. Delusions generally have a persecutory theme: patients may believe things are stolen, or the food or medicine poisoned; some may believe that an intruder (the "phantom boarder") lurks somewhere in the house, or that imposters have taken over the bodies of family members.

Agitation becomes progressively more common with disease progression, and may occur concomitant with psychotic symptoms or independently.

In time most patients eventually display certain elementary "cortical" signs, such as aphasia and apraxia. Spasticity, which is rare throughout most of the course, may eventually occur, and patients may eventually become incontinent, bedridden, and contracted. Occasionally, late in the disease, seizures or myoclonus may occur.

MRI or CT scanning shows varying degrees of generalized cortical atrophy (Figure 175-1). The EEG typically shows generalized slowing. Although routine CSF studies are normal, recent work indicates that Alzheimer's disease may be distinguished by an increased amount of total or phosphorylated tau protein. At present, however, the only truly definitive method for making the diagnosis is a brain biopsy, a procedure which is rarely undertaken.

Alzheimer's disease occurs frequently in patients with Down's syndrome. The concurrence of Alzheimer's disease and Parkinson's disease or Binswanger's disease is not uncommon.

COURSE

Although an occasional patient may experience a temporary plateau of symptoms, for most the disease is relentlessly progressive with death occurring, often from an intercurrent infection

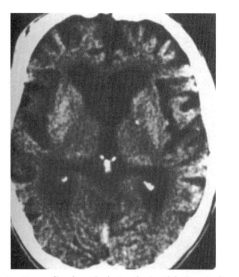

FIG. 175-1. Generalized cortical atrophy in Alzheimer's disease. (From Osborn AG, Winthrop S. *Diagnostic neuroradiology*, St. Louis, 1994, Mosby.)

such as pneumonia, within 5 to 7 years. The range, however, is wide, with some patients succumbing in less than a year and others surviving for up to 20 years. Those with an early onset, before the age of 65, tend to have a more rapid progression of the disease.

COMPLICATIONS

Complications are as described in the chapter on dementia. The devastation wreaked by this disease in the life of the patient and in the lives of those close to the patient is perhaps unparalleled by any other illness.

ETIOLOGY

In most cases the brain shows generalized, symmetric atrophy, with the frontal and temporal lobes being most severely affected. The precentral and postcentral gyri are often relatively spared. Exceptions, however, do occur, and some brains, though burdened with great numbers of neurofibrillary tangles and senile plaques, may display little or no atrophy.

The distinctive microscopic features are senile plaques (also known as neuritic plaques) and neurofibrillary tangles.

Senile plaques, which may be incredibly numerous, are composed of intermingled neuritic processes and glial cells, with a central core of amyloid. The beta-amyloid protein of the amyloid core is derived from the amyloid precursor protein, which is coded for by a gene on chromosome 21.

Neurofibrillary tangles consist of paired helical filaments found within the cell body, which are composed primarily of hyperphosphorylated tau protein.

Neuronal loss occurs, and the intensity of this process parallels the pattern of atrophy.

In general, senile plaques and neurofibrillary tangles first appear in the hippocampus, amygdala, parahippocampal gyrus, and the temporal gyri. Exceptions, however, do occur. For example, in rare cases the initial locus may be in the parietal lobe. Most gray areas of the brain are eventually affected, with the relative exception of the thalamus and the basal ganglia. The nucleus basalis of Meynert and certain brainstem nuclei, including the serotoninergic superior central nucleus and the noradrenergic locus ceruleus, are typically also affected.

The loss of cells in the nucleus basalis of Meynert is of particular importance. The overwhelming majority of cholinergic neurons originate from this nucleus, and as cell dropout proceeds here, a parallel decrease in the activity of presynaptic choline acetyltransferase in the hippocampus and the cerebral cortex occurs. In turn, a good correlation exists between the level of cognitive decline, particularly memory loss, and the decline in choline acetyltransferase activity. A similar correlation between the severity of the dementia and the burden of neurofibrillary tangles is also seen, particularly in the temporal neocortex. In a similar vein, a correlation exists between the presence of degenerative changes (e.g., neurofibrillary tangles) in the superior central nucleus and the locus ceruleus and the occurrence of depressive symptoms.

In perhaps 5% of cases, Alzheimer's disease is inherited on an autosomal dominant basis, with mutations in the genes for the amyloid precursor protein on chromosome 21, presenilin 1 on chromosome 14 and presenilin 2 on chromosome 1.

The heritability of the remaining cases is currently unclear. Some investigators consider them to be "sporadic" and presumably caused by environmental factors, whereas others believe that almost all of these cases are familial, with their "sporadic" nature explained by the death of parents before they reached the age of highest risk for the onset of Alzheimer's disease.

Recently an association has been demonstrated between the presence of the epsilon 4 allele of apolipoprotein E and the occurrence of both familial and "sporadic" cases of Alzheimer's disease. This allele is present in anywhere from 7% to 30% of normals, but may be found in as many as 50% of patients with Alzheimer's disease. Although clearly a "risk factor," genotyping for apolipoprotein E, at present, is not useful for diagnostic purposes.

DIFFERENTIAL DIAGNOSIS

The normal, albeit slight, loss of memory that accompanies aging, often known as "benign senescent forgetfulness," may be particularly difficult to differentiate from early Alzheimer's disease. The finding of cortical atrophy on CT or MRI scanning may not be helpful, as this is a common finding in otherwise healthy persons over the age of 60. In such cases the diagnosis may have to await prolonged clinical observation.

Other diseases capable of causing a chronically progressive dementia of gradual or insidious onset include Binswanger's disease, the lacunar state, normal pressure hydrocephalus, cerebral amyloid angiopathy (in the pre-hemorrhagic period), diffuse Lewy body disease, Pick's disease and frontotemporal dementia. With the exception of diffuse Lewy body disease, Pick's disease and frontotemporal dementia most of these are readily identified with an MRI scan. Diffuse Lewy body disease is suggested by the relatively early occurrence of confusion and either spontaneous or antipsychotic-induced parkinsonism. Pick's disease and frontotemporal dementia are suggested by a prominent personality change with, at least initially, little or no memory loss: classically one sees elements of either or both of the frontal lobe syndrome and the Klüver-Bucy syndrome.

Alcoholic dementia may also have a gradual course, but here the presence of chronic, active alcoholism is almost impossible to miss.

Other possibilities include hypothyroidism, vitamin B12 deficiency, neurosyphilis and Creutzfeldt-Jakob disease. The first three are readily determined by appropriate lab testing and Creutzfeldt-Jakob disease is suggested by its relatively rapid course and by the early occurrence of myoclonus.

A depressive episode, as part of a major depression or bipolar disorder, if of insidious onset, may resemble early Alzheimer's disease. A history of previous episodes of depression, the presence of typical vegetative symptoms, and an apathetic response to the mental status questions all suggest depression. In some cases, however, a definite diagnosis may not be possible, and in such cases a "diagnosis by treatment response" to an antidepressant may be in order.

TREATMENT

Although a "magic bullet" for Alzheimer's disease has clearly not as yet been found, certain medicines offer modest benefit, and these may be conveniently divided into three classes, according as to whether they may prevent the development of the disease, retard its progression once it has set in, or offer some symptomatic relief.

Chronic treatment with ibuprofen may reduce the risk of Alzheimer's disease. Given the dangers of long-term NSAID use, this should probably be reserved for those with a strong family history, or perhaps for individuals homozygous for the epsilon 4 allele of apolipoprotein E.

Both vitamin E and selegiline, in total daily doses of 2000 IU and 10 mg, respectively, may each retard the progression of the disease, and given its benign side-effect profile, it may be reasonable to offer vitamin E to all patients.

Symptomatic treatments may be divided according to whether they are intended to improve memory, depression, psychosis or agitation.

Drugs capable of improving memory include the cholinesterase inhibitors donepezil, galantamine, rivastigmine and metrifonate; tacrine, given its hepatotoxicity, is rarely used. Another agent which improves memory is the NMDA antagonist memantine. As there are no head-to-head comparisons of the various cholinesterase inhibitors or between a cholinesterase inhibitor and memantine, most clinicians will stick with the agent they have the most experience with, namely donepezil. Although most of the patients studied with these cholinesterase inhibitors and memantine had mild to moderate disease, recent work suggests that even those with severe disease may benefit. Details regarding each of these agents may be found in their respective chapters.

Depression may improve with an SSRI (e.g., sertraline), and psychosis with low doses of olanzapine (5-10 mg) or haloperidol (2-3 mg). Agitation may also respond to either olanzapine or haloperidol, and in patients resistant to these medications one may consider carbamazepine, in doses of roughly 400 mg daily.

The general treatment of dementia is as outlined in that chapter; eventually most patients will require institutional care.

BIBLIOGRAPHY

Bennett DA, Wilson RS, Schneider JA, et al. Apolipoprotein E epsilon4 allele, AD pathology, and the clinical expression of Alzheimer's disease. *Neurology* 2003;60:246-252.

Bierer LM, Hoff PR, Purohit DP, et al. Neocortical neurofibrillary tangles correlate with dementia severity in Alzheimer's disease. *Archives of Neurology* 1995;52:81-88.

Buerger K, Zinkowski R, Teipel SJ, et al. Differential diagnosis of Alzheimer disease with cerebrospinal fluid levels of tau protein phosphorylated at threonine 231. *Archives of Neurology* 2002;59:1267-1272.

Devanand DP, Marder K, Michaels KS, et al. A randomized, placebo-controlled dose-comparison trial of haloperidol for psychosis and disruptive behaviors in Alzheimer's disease. *The American Journal of Psychiatry* 1998;155:1512-1520.

Feldman H, Gauthier S, Hecker J, et al. A 24-week, randomized, double-blind study of donepezil in moderate to severe Alzheimer's disease. *Neurology* 2001;57:613-620.

Filip V, Kolibas E. Selegiline in the treatment of Alzheimer's disease: a long-term randomized placebo-controlled trial. Czech and Slovak Senile Dementia of Alzheimer Type Study Group. *Journal of Psychiatry & Neuroscience* 1999;24:234-243.

in t'Veld BA, Ruitenberg A, Hofman A, et al. Nonsteroidal antiinflammatory drugs and the risk of Alzheimer's disease. *The New England Journal of Medicine* 2001;345:1515-1521.

Janssen JC, Beck JA, Campbell TA, et al. Early onset familial Alzheimer's disease: mutation frequency in 31 families. *Neurology* 2003;60: 235-239.

Lyketsos CG, Sheppard JM, Steele CD, et al. Randomized, placebo-controlled, double-blind clinical trial of sertraline in the treatment of depression complicating Alzheimer's disease: initial results from the Depression in Alzheimer's Disease study. *The American Journal of Psychiatry* 2000;157:1686-1689.

Mohs, RC, Breitner JCS, Silverman JM, et al. Alzheimer's disease: morbid risk among first-degree relatives approximates 50% by 90 years of age. *Archives of General Psychiatry* 1987;44:405-408.

Olin JT, Fox LS, Pawluczyk S, et al. A pilot randomized trial of carbamazepine for behavioral symptoms in treatment-resistant outpatients with Alzheimer disease. *The American Journal of Geriatric Psychiatry* 2001;9:400-405.

Raskind MA, Cyrus PA, Ruzicka BB, et al. The effects of metrifonate on the cognitive, behavioral, and functional performance of Alzheimer's disease patients. Metrifonate Study Group. *The Journal of Clinical Psychiatry* 1999;60:318-325.

Resiberg B, Doody R, Stoffler A, et al. Memantine in moderate-to-severe Alzheimer's disease. *The New England Journal of Medicine* 2003; 348:1333-1341.

Rockwood K, Mintzer J, Truyen L, et al. Effects of a flexible galantamine dose in Alzheimer's disease: a randomized, controlled trial. *Journal of Neurology, Neurosurgery, and Psychiatry* 2001;71:589-595.

Rosler M, Anand R, Cicin-Sain A, et al. Efficacy and safety of rivastigmine in patients with Alzheimer's disease: international randomized controlled trial. *British Medical Journal* 1999;318:633-638.

Sano M, Ernesto C, Thomas RG, et al. A controlled trial of selegiline, alpha-tocopherol, or both as treatment for Alzheimer's disease. The Alzheimer's Disease Cooperative Study. *The New England Journal of Medicine* 1997;336:1216-1222.

Street JS, Clark WS, Gannon KS, et al. Olanzapine treatment of psychotic and behavioral symptoms in patients with Alzheimer disease in nursing care facilities: a double-blind, randomized, placebo-controlled trial. The HGEU Study Group. *Archives of General Psychiatry* 2000;57:968-976.

Watkins PB, Zimmerman HJ, Knapp MJ, et al. Hepatotoxic effects of tacrine administration in patients with Alzheimer's disease. *The Journal of the American Medical Association* 1994;271:992-998.

176 Pick's Disease

Pick's disease, first described in 1892 by the neuropsychiatrist Arnold Pick, is a rare cause of dementia, which is distinguished from many other dementing diseases by its tendency to present with a personality change, which in turn has elements of both the frontal lobe and Klüver-Bucy syndromes. This disease is also known as "lobar atrophy," a name derived from the distinctive, at times knife-like, atrophy of the temporal and frontal lobes.

ONSET

The onset is gradual, and although most patients fall ill in their fifties or sixties, onsets as early as 21 years of age have been reported. The onset itself, as just noted, is generally characterized by a personality change, described below.

CLINICAL FEATURES

Classically, patients manifest such "frontal lobe" signs as disinhibition along with elements of the Klüver-Bucy syndrome, such as hypermetamorphosis, hypersexuality and hyperorality, with at times pronounced gluttony. Importantly, although most patients eventually evidence such cognitive deficits as poor short-term memory, deficient calculations, and concreteness, these typically appear only after the personality change has been well-established. Over time, in addition to dementia, patients also typically develop an aphasia, often of the motor, or expressive, type; furthermore, seizures may also occur late in the course.

Rarely, aphasia may be prominent early on and, very rarely, Pick's disease may present with aphasia, in which case one speaks of the syndrome of "primary progressive aphasia."

CT or MRI scans typically reveal pronounced atrophy of the frontal or anterior portions of the temporal lobes, or both.

COURSE

The course is one of relentless progression to a profound degree of dementia. The outcome is universally fatal, with death occurring in from 3 to 10 years, generally secondary to an intercurrent illness, such as pneumonia.

COMPLICATIONS

Complications are as described in the chapter on dementia.

ETIOLOGY

Grossly, one finds, as noted earlier, pronounced atrophy of the frontal and temporal lobes, with, classically, a "knife-like" appearance, as demonstrated in Figure 176-1. Interestingly, in the case of the temporal lobe, the posterior two-thirds of the superior temporal gyrus tends to be relatively spared. Microscopically, there is widespread neuronal loss and gliosis, and both Pick cells and Pick bodies are seen: Pick cells are ballooned neurons with central chromatolysis; Pick bodies are argentophilic intracytosplasmic inclusions, which represent aggregations of straight, or at times twisted, tau neurofilaments.

Although most cases are sporadic, autosomal dominant transmission has been noted, and in these cases mutations in the tau gene have been identified.

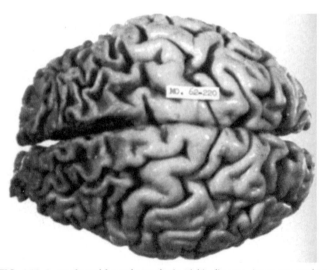

FIG. 176-1. Profound frontal atrophy in Pick's disease. (From Haymaker W. *Bing's local diagnosis in neurological disease*, ed 15, St. Louis, 1969, Mosby.)

DIFFERENTIAL DIAGNOSIS

Pick's disease is distinguished from Alzheimer's disease by the early appearance of a personality change, and its persistence for a prolonged period in the absence of amnesia or other cognitive deficits. Fronto-temporal dementia may be difficult to distinguish on clinical grounds; however, MRI scanning may be helpful here, as the atrophy of fronto-temporal dementia, although preferentially affecting the frontal and temporal lobes, rarely assumes the "knife-like" character seen in classic Pick's disease.

TREATMENT

There is no specific treatment for Pick's disease; the treatment of the frontal lobe syndrome, the Klüver-Bucy syndrome and of dementia in general is discussed in the respective chapters.

BIBLIOGRAPHY

Binetti G, Locascio JJ, Corkin S, et al. Differences between Pick disease and Alzheimer disease in clinical appearance and rate of cognitive decline. *Archives of Neurology* 2000;57:225-232.

Cummings JL, Duchen LW. Klüver-Bucy syndrome in Pick disease: clinical and pathologic correlations. *Neurology* 1981;31:415-421.

Mendez MF, Selwood A, Mastri AR, et al. Pick's disease versus Alzheimer's disease: a comparison of clinical characteristics. *Neurology* 1993; 43:289-292.

Pickering-Brown S, Baker M, Yen SH, et al. Pick's disease is associated with mutations in the tau gene. *Annals of Neurology* 2000;48: 859-867.

Zhukareva V, Mann D, Pickering-Brown S, et al. Sporadic Pick's disease: a tauopathy characterized by a spectrum of pathological tau isoforms in gray and white matter. *Annals of Neurology* 2002;51: 730-739.

177 Frontotemporal Dementia

The definition of frontotemporal dementia is not settled. Some authorities conceive of it as a syndrome encompassing all degenerative disorders affecting primarily the frontal and temporal lobes, and thus include Pick's disease, those cases of amyotrophic lateral sclerosis with dementia and prominent frontal lobe degeneration, and a group of other, more recently described diseases such as "dementia lacking distinctive histologic features (DLDH)" and "frontotemporal dementia and parkinsonism linked to chromosome 17 (FTDP-17)." Other authorities reserve the term for this group of newly described disorders, and this is the way it is conceived of in this book.

Given the unsettled definition of frontotemporal dementia, however, the reader is cautioned to carefully evaluate any papers on this subject to be sure of how the authors define the term.

Frontotemporal dementia is common, and may account for up to 20% of all cases of dementia with an onset before the age of 65.

ONSET

The onset is insidious and usually occurs between the ages of 40 and 65.

CLINICAL FEATURES

A personality change generally constitutes the initial symptom, and this may have features of either the frontal lobe syndrome or the Klüver-Bucy syndrome, depending on whether the burden of the disease process falls first on the frontal or the temporal lobe.

In "frontal variant" frontotemporal dementia, one may see disinhibition and socially inappropriate behavior such as sexual indiscretions, coarse behavior and gluttonous eating; grooming and dress may also suffer. Mood changes may appear and may tend toward either depression, or somewhat less commonly a bland euphoria; anxiety and irritability may also occur. Abulia may occur, and patients may fail to engage in any spontaneous activity. Primitive reflexes, such as forced grasping or groping, may be found, and some patients may become incontinent of bladder and bowel.

In "temporal variant" frontotemporal dementia hyperorality, hypersexuality and ritualistic behavior may occur. Hyperorality is manifest by a tendency of patients to put almost anything into their mouths, whether it is edible or not; where food is involved there may be a remarkable gluttony, sometimes with marked preferences for sweets. Hypersexual behavior may include indiscriminate sexual advances, regardless of the other person's age or sex, or public masturbation. Ritualistic behavior often has a compulsive character to it as patients perseveratively hoard, count or rearrange objects.

Although the personality change seen in frontotemporal dementia may initially strongly favor either the frontal or temporal variant, eventually most patients have features of both. Delusions or hallucinations may occur, and are eventually seen in up to one-quarter of patients.

Importantly, memory is generally intact early on in the course of the disease and, again early on, one generally does not see evidence of apraxia or difficulty with calculations. Eventually, however, memory loss does appear; further, many patients, again late in the course, may evidence a degree of aphasia, often of the motor variety. Mild parkinsonian features may be seen in some cases.

MRI scanning generally reveals at least a degree of frontal and anterior temporal atrophy; however, this generally does not assume the "knife-like" pattern seen in Pick's disease.

For some of the familial cases, genetic testing is available.

COURSE

The course is one of gradual deterioration, with death within 1 to 25 years; at the end most patients are mute and akinetic.

COMPLICATIONS

The complications are similar to those described in the chapters on dementia, the frontal lobe syndrome and the Klüver-Bucy syndrome.

ETIOLOGY

Half or more of all cases are familial and exhibit an autosomal dominant pattern of inheritance. Some of these familial cases (such as frontotemporal dementia and parkinsonism linked to chromosome 17) are characterized by mutations in the tau gene on chromosome 17 and display tau positive neuronal inclusions; others, also linked to chromosome 17 (such as hereditary dysphasic disinhibition dementia), are marked by an absence of tau protein.

Sporadic cases also occur, most notably a disorder known as dementia lacking distinctive histologic features: here one finds spongiform change in the frontal cortex along with an absence of tau protein.

DIFFERENTIAL DIAGNOSIS

Pick's disease, on clinical grounds, may be indistinguishable from frontotemporal dementia: one differential clue, however, is the presence of "knife-like" atrophy of the frontal and anterior temporal lobes which is characteristic of Pick's disease but rare in frontotemporal dementia.

Amyotrophic lateral sclerosis may present with a dementia with prominent frontal lobe features; however, the concurrent or eventual appearance of fasciculations serves to indicate the correct diagnosis.

Alzheimer's disease is suggested by the early, and prominent, memory loss.

TREATMENT

The overall treatment of dementia is as described in that chapter; specific approaches for the frontal lobe syndrome and the Klüver-Bucy syndrome are likewise described in those chapters.

Open studies have suggested that SSRIs, such as paroxetine, may ameliorate some aspects of the personality change.

BIBLIOGRAPHY

Goedert M, Ghetti B, Spillantini MG. Tau gene mutations in fronto-temporal dementia and parkinsonism linked to chromosome 17 (FTDP-17). Their relevance for understanding the neurodegenerative process. *Annals of the New York Academy of Sciences* 2000;920: 74-83.

Janssen JC, Warrington EK, Morris HR, et al. Clinical features of frontotemporal dementia due to intronic tau 10 (+16) mutation. *Neurology* 2002;58:1161-1168.

Knopman DS, Mastri AR, Frey WH, et al. Dementia lacking distinctive histologic features: a common non-Alzheimer degenerative dementia. *Neurology* 1990;40:251-256.

Lantos PL, Cairns NJ, Khan MN, et al. Neuropathologic variation in frontotemporal dementia due to the intronic tau 1 (+16) mutation. *Neurology* 2002;58:1169-1175.

Lendon CL, Lynch T, Norton J, et al. Hereditary dysphasic disinihibition dementia: a frontotemporal dementia linked to 17q21-22. *Neurology* 1998;50:1546-1555.

Pasquier F, Petit H. Frontotemporal dementia: its rediscovery. *European Neurology* 1997;38:1-6.

Snowden JS, Neary D, Mann DM. Frontotemporal dementia. *The British Journal of Psychiatry* 2002;180:140-143.

Swartz JR, Miller BL, Lesser IM, et al. Frontotemporal dementia: treatment response to serotonin selective reuptake inhibitors. *The Journal of Clinical Psychiatry* 1997;58:212-216.

Zhukareva V, Vogelsberg-Ragaglia V, Van Deerlin VM, et al. Loss of brain tau defines sporadic and familial tauopathies with frontotemporal dementia. *Annals of Neurology* 2001;49:165-175.

178 Parkinson's Disease

Parkinson's disease, also known as paralysis agitans, shaking palsy, or "idiopathic parkinsonism," is characterized in most cases by a triad of tremor, rigidity, and bradykinesia. In about one-third of all cases, dementia eventually appears, and depression of variable severity may be seen in about one-fifth of all patients.

Parkinson's disease is a relatively common illness, having a lifetime prevalence of about 0.25% among the general population. It is somewhat more common among males than females.

ONSET

The onset is gradual and insidious and generally occurs in the fifties or early sixties. Later onsets are seen, as are earlier ones. Young adults may be affected, and very rarely a juvenile form is encountered. The first obvious symptom, usually occurring in only one arm or leg, is often either tremor or rigidity. Patients also complain of a sense of slowness or a loss of dexterity.

The premorbid personality structure may be marked by rigidity, moralism, conscientiousness, and an aversion to taking risks.

CLINICAL FEATURES

The evolution of symptoms is gradual; often they spread to the other limb on the same side, and eventually to all four limbs. In its fully developed state, Parkinson's disease stamps the patient with a clinical picture that once seen is readily recognized.

The patient stands in a stooped "flexion" posture; the arms are partially flexed, the knees slightly bent. Two patients with a typical appearance are in Figure 178-1. A rhythmic three to seven cycle/second tremor, present at rest, is typically seen in the hands, where it presents the classic "pill-rolling" appearance. It may also be seen in the lips or the chin. Postural instability is present. If patients are lightly pushed on the chest, their backward walk is unable to keep pace with the center of gravity as they topple over

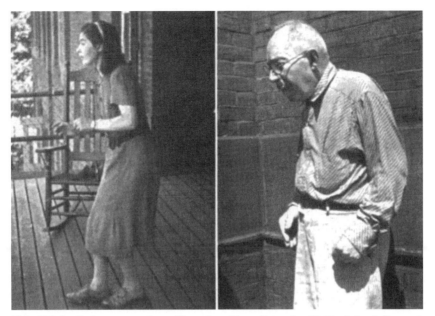

FIG. 178-1. Flexion posture in parkinsonism. (From Haymaker W. *Bing's local diagnosis in neurological diseases,* St. Louis, 1969, Mosby.)

backward; this "retropulsion" is mirrored by the phenomenon of "propulsion" that follows when patients are lightly pushed on the back.

Rigidity is eventually present in all four limbs. Although typically cogwheeling in character, some patients may have only lead-pipe rigidity.

In walking, patients exhibit the classic "marche a petit pas" as they shuffle along with small steps. In some cases, there may be festination, wherein the patient, though seeming to hurry along, takes ever smaller steps, and seems progressively closer to toppling over forward, as if the steps cannot keep up with the bent-forward torso.

"Masked facies" are typically present, along with a reduced frequency of spontaneous blinking, giving the patient a vacant, blank look. Drooling is common.

Speech is hypophonic and is often monotone and lacking in inflection. At times, the patient may repeat the same word or sound again and again. Gestures and body language are lost.

Bradykinesia is evident as the patient attempts to carry out a task; at times the patient may appear to move as if encased in molasses. Buttoning a shirt may take 15 minutes; dressing completely may take hours. A very important variation of bradykinesia is bradyphrenia. Here the patient's thoughts are slowed down; problems that were once thought through in moments may now require minutes or longer. This is not due to confusion or to poor concentration, but rather to a thickened slowing of the march of thought.

Some patients may also evidence what is known as "freezing," wherein, despite generally being "on" and able to walk, they suddenly find themselves "frozen" in place and unable to set in motion a willed act, such as taking a step. This freezing often occurs at a threshold of some sort, such as a doorway, and, curiously, may be relieved by proper visual cues. For example, if sequential, transversely oriented, stretches of opaque tape, spaced about one foot-pace apart, are placed on the hallway floor in front of patients, the "freeze" may suddenly lyse; interestingly, the same effect may at times be produced if the patient simply imagines such markers in front of them.

Handwriting eventually deteriorates into a scratchy micrographia.

The dementia seen in Parkinson's disease tends to be relatively mild and is generally not characterized by dysphasia or dyspraxia.

The depression occurring in Parkinson's disease is symptomatically quite similar to that seen in dysthymia or major depression. Interestingly, no correlation is seen between the severity of the depressive symptoms and the severity of the motor symptoms.

In addition to depression, about one-quarter of patients will also eventually experience anxiety attacks, which, in the vast majority of cases, occur only during a "wearing off" period of immobility as the effects of a previous dose of levodopa abate.

COURSE

Although the rate of progression is quite variable, over three quarters of patients will be severely disabled within 15 years of the onset of symptoms. Although not lethal per se, Parkinson's disease predisposes to such potentially lethal conditions as pneumonia or decubiti.

COMPLICATIONS

Motor symptoms may impose severe restrictions on even simple activities of daily living. The complications of dementia, depression, or panic attacks are as described respectively in those chapters.

ETIOLOGY

The substantia nigra shows a substantial loss of neurons; indeed over 60% must be lost before the typical motor symptoms occur. Remaining cells generally contain Lewy bodies, which are eosinophilic cytoplasmic inclusions.

Neuronal loss and Lewy body formation are also seen in the locus ceruleus and the serotoninergic superior central nucleus. A correlation is seen between the fall in CSF 5-hydroxyindoleacetic acid and the presence of depressive symptoms.

The dementia seen in Parkinson's disease appears related to the presence of Lewy bodies in either the cerebral cortex or the nucleus basalis of Meynert.

Parkinson's disease is probably a result of both genetic and environmental influences. Familial cases clearly exist, and robust evidence from PET scanning shows nigrostriatal pathology in the clinically unaffected monozygotic and dizygotic twins of patients with Parkinson's disease. Conversely, an association exists between Parkinson's disease and a history of drinking well water in childhood.

DIFFERENTIAL DIAGNOSIS

The phenomenon of parkinsonism is not confined to Parkinson's disease, and may play a prominent part in a host of other disorders.

Diffuse Lewy body disease is suggested by the early appearance of dementia and by the presence of episodes of confusion.

Progressive supranuclear palsy is distinguished by axial rigidity, rather than flexion, by an absence of tremor, by frequent, unexplained falls early in the course of the illness, and by the appearance of a supranuclear ophthalmoplegia for downward gaze.

Multiple system atrophy is suggested by ataxia and by prominent autonomic signs, such as impotence, urinary incontinence or retention, and orthostatic syncope.

Arteriosclerotic parkinsonism (also known as "vascular parkinsonism") is suggested by an absence of tremor and by the presence of evidence of damage to the corticospinal and corticobulbar tracts, such as hyperreflexia, Babinski signs and pseudobulbar palsy; such patients may also exhibit a "magnetic" gait, wherein their feet seem "stuck" to the floor.

Dementia pugilistica is suggested by the history of repeated head trauma and the presence of ataxia and dysarthria, signs which prompted the common name for this disorder, namely the "punch drunk syndrome."

Fahr's syndrome, though at times accompanied by ataxia or intention tremor, may present with parkinsonism alone, and in such cases the diagnosis may rest on finding calcification in the basal ganglia.

Corticobasal-ganglionic degeneration is suggested by the strikingly asymmetric nature of the parkinsonian rigidity and by the presence of apraxia and "cortical" sensory loss on the involved side, and by myoclonus.

Finally, one must never forget the most common cause of parkinsonism, namely that seen as a side-effect of antipsychotic drugs.

TREATMENT

Various pharmacologic agents are available for the treatment of the motor aspects of Parkinson's disease, including selegiline, direct-acting dopaminergic agents, levodopa (with or without carbidopa and/or entacapone), amantadine and anticholinergic agents. With the exception of selegiline and entacapone, wherein most patients are treated with the same dose, pharmacologic management typically requires multiple dosage adjustments. In general, these should be undertaken cautiously, one drug at a time, utilizing small dosage increments and giving adequate time to assess the effect of any change.

Selegiline, at doses of 10 mg or less daily, is a selective monoamine-oxidase inhibitor, which provides very modest symptomatic relief of motor symptoms, and which may also, although this is very controversial, perhaps retard the overall progression of the disease.

Direct-acting dopaminergic agents include carbergoline, pramipexole, ropinirole, pergolide, and bromocriptine. Bromocriptine, the first of these agents to come into clinical use, appears somewhat less effective than the others. Of these agents, cabergoline may be preferable, given that its long half-life allows for once-daily dosing.

Levodopa, almost always used with the aromatic L-amino acid decarboxylase inhibitor carbidopa as a combination levodopa/carbidopa preparation, is substantially more effective than the direct-acting dopaminergic agents, and because of this many clinicians advocate its use from the beginning in all patients. Unfortunately, however, over time most patients treated with levodopa develop troubling motor fluctuations. These motor fluctuations occur in a variety of forms, the two most common of which are an end-of-dose "wearing off" of effect and peak-dose dyskinesias. There is also a suggestion, though this is very controversial, that the use of levodopa may actually hasten the progression of the disease. One way to deal with motor fluctuations is to add entacapone, which is a peripheral catechol-O-methyltransferase inhibitor: in most cases, this will prolong the effect of a dose of levodopa and also allow for a dose reduction, which, in turn, will be followed by a reduction in any peak-dose dyskinesia. Another method for dealing with motor fluctuations is, if one is not already being used, to add a direct-acting dopaminergic agent: this will both provide some protection during the nadir of dopa levels between doses, thus reducing the severity of any wearing off, and, by allowing for a dose reduction of the levodopa, also reduce the severity of any peak-dose dyskinesias.

Amantadine exerts several effects of interest with regard to Parkinson's disease. First, as an indirect and a direct dopaminergic agent, it serves to relieve some of the motor symptoms; however, in this regard it is less effective than either the direct-acting dopaminergic agents, such as cabergoline, or levodopa itself. It is also an NMDA antagonist, and via this mechanism it appears to reduce the peak-dose dyskinesias seen with levodopa.

Anticholinergics, such as trihexyphenidyl and benztropine, although effective against motor symptoms, especially tremor, have so many side-effects that they are rarely used.

Keeping these facts in mind about these various agents, a therapeutic strategy may be developed, which differs depending on how advanced the patient's motor symptoms are when first seen.

In mild disease, it is reasonable to begin with selegiline alone, or with a combination of selegiline and a direct-acting dopaminergic agent. In most cases, this will provide acceptable control for years; eventually, however, it will be necessary to add levodopa/carbidopa, and when this does occur, it is reasonable to add entacapone shortly thereafter.

When, on first evaluation, patients have moderate or severe disease, it is appropriate to begin levodopa/carbidopa, adding entacapone and a direct-acting dopaminergic agent soon thereafter.

In levodopa-treated patients with significant motor fluctuations, despite optimum concurrent treatment with entacapone and a direct-acting dopaminergic agent, one may "space out" the total daily dose of levodopa/carbidopa from the standard thrice-daily regimen to up to six doses per day. This maneuver not only serves to blunt the nadir of dopa levels between dosages, and thus reduce the wearing off effect, but also, by allowing a reduction in each individual levodopa dose, will reduce the severity of the peak-dose dyskinesias. When dyskinesias prove disabling despite this strategy, one may add amantadine.

Eventually, despite optimum medical treatment, many patients will become completely disabled. In such cases, one may consider deep brain stimulation of either the subthalamic nucleus or the pars interna of the globus pallidus. In emergency cases, one should also consider ECT. ECT has been shown, in double-blinded studies, to relieve the motor symptoms of Parkinson's disease regardless of whether patients are depressed or not, and to do so at times in a dramatically effective way. As such, ECT may be life saving, and although repeat treatments may be required to maintain the benefit, this is a small price to pay to keep patients alive and mobile pending surgery, or, if that is not an option, as an ongoing measure.

When dementia occurs, one may add donepezil in a dose of from 5 to 10 mg daily. Although, theoretically, this medication, by increasing cholinergic tone, might be expected to worsen motor symptomatology, in practice this does not appear to occur.

Hallucinations or delusions may occur as a side-effect to direct-acting dopaminergic drugs or levodopa, or as part of a dementia. When they occur as a side-effect, dose reduction may be helpful; when dose reduction is not feasible, or when they appear as part of the dementia, an antipsychotic may be added. First-generation antipsychotics tend to aggravate motor symptoms and are often avoided because of this. Of the second-generation drugs, two have been shown, in double-blinded studies, to relieve psychotic symptoms without worsening motor symptoms, namely risperidone and clozapine. Remarkably, in the case of clozapine, motor symptoms, rather than worsening, actually improve somewhat. Both drugs are given in low doses (e.g., 1-2 mg of risperidone and 6.25-50 mg of clozapine); as to the choice between them, risperidone may be preferable, given the risk of agranulocytosis with clozapine and the necessity for ongoing CBCs.

Depression is typically treated with an antidepressant, either a tricyclic or an SSRI. There has been, however, only one positive double-blinded study of antidepressant treatment in Parkinson's disease, and that found nortriptyline to be superior to placebo. When nortriptyline is ineffective, or poorly tolerated, one may consider an SSRI: although SSRIs occasionally worsen motor symptoms in certain patients, overall they are well tolerated.

Panic attacks, as noted earlier, are for the most part confined to "wearing-off" periods, and in these cases, the first approach should be to avoid these by adding entacapone and a direct-acting dopaminergic agent, if they are not already in place, and by increasing the frequency with which levodopa/carbidopa is given during waking hours. In cases where these measures are ineffective, some clinicians have added clonazepam or an antidepressant; however, there are no blinded studies to offer guidance here.

BIBLIOGRAPHY

Aarsland D, Laake K, Larsen JP, et al. Donepezil for cognitive impairment in Parkinson's disease: a randomized controlled study. *Journal of Neurology, Neurosurgery, and Psychiatry* 2002;72:708-712.

Andersen J, Aabro E, Gulmann N, et al. Anti-depressive treatment in Parkinson's disease. A controlled trial of the effect of nortriptyline in patients with Parkinson's disease treated with L-DOPA. *Acta Neurologica Scandinavica* 1980;62:210-219.

Andersen K, Balldin J, Gottfries CG, et al. A double-blind evaluation of electroconvulsive therapy in Parkinson's disease with "on-off" phenomenon. *Acta Neurologica Scandinavica* 1987;76:191-199.

Apaydin H, Ahlskog JE, Parisi JE, et al. Parkinson disease neuropathology: later-developing dementia and loss of the levodopa response. *Archives of Neurology* 2002;59:102-112.

Burn DJ, Mark MH, Playford ED, et al. Parkinson's disease in twins studied with 18F-dopa and positron emission tomography. *Neurology* 1992;42:1894-1900.

Colosimo C, Albanese A, Hughes AJ, et al. Some specific clinical features differentiate multiple system atrophy (striatonigral variety) from Parkinson's disease. *Archives of Neurology* 1995;52:294-298.

Ellis T, Cudkowicz ME, Sexton PM, et al. Clozapine and risperidone treatment of psychosis in Parkinson's disease. *The Journal of Neuropsychiatry and Clinical Neurosciences* 2000;12:364-369.

Holthoff VA, Vieregge P, Kessler J, et al. Discordant twins with Parkinson's disease: positron emission tomography and early signs of impaired cognitive circuits. *Annals of Neurology* 1994;36:176-182.

Lazzarini AM, Myers RH, Zimmerman TR, et al. A clinical genetic study of Parkinson's disease: evidence for dominant transmission. *Neurology* 1994;44:499-506.

Poewe WH, Deuschl G, Gordin A. Efficacy and safety of entacapone in Parkinson's disease patients with suboptimal levodopa response: a 6-month randomized placebo-controlled double-blind study in Germany and Austria (Celomen study). *Acta Neurologica Scandinavica* 2002;105:245-255.

Rinne UK, Bracco F, Chouza C, et al. Carbergoline in the treatment of early Parkinson's disease: results of the first year of treatment in a double-blind comparison of cabergoline and levodopa. The PKDS009 Collaborative Study Group. *Neurology* 1997;48:363-368.

Shoulson I, Oakes D, Fahn S, et al. Impact of sustained deprenyl (selegiline) in levodopa-treated Parkinson's disease: a randomized placebo-controlled extension of the deprenyl and tocopherol antioxidative therapy of parkinsonism trial. *Annals of Neurology* 2002;51:604-612.

Vazquez A, Jimenez-Jimenez FJ, Garcia-Ruiz P, et al. "Panic attacks" in Parkinson's disease. A long-term complication of levodopa therapy. *Acta Neurologica Scandinavica* 1993;87:14-18.

Verhagen Metman L, Del Dotto P, van den Munckhof P, et al. Amantadine as treatment for dyskinesias and motor fluctuations in Parkinson's disease. *Neurology* 1998;50:1323-1326.

179 Diffuse Lewy Body Disease

Diffuse Lewy body disease, also known as "Lewy body dementia," "senile dementia of the Lewy body type," or "cortical Lewy body disease," ranks, at least in autopsy studies, as the second most common cause of dementia, right after Alzheimer's disease. As the name implies, it is characterized pathologically by the presence of Lewy bodies diffusely spread throughout the cortex; clinically it may present in one of three ways, with dementia, concurrent dementia and parkinsonism or with parkinsonism alone.

ONSET

The onset of symptoms is gradual, often in the seventh or eighth decades.

CLINICAL FEATURES

When the disease presents with dementia one may see, in addition to typical cognitive deficits in memory, calculating and abstracting abilities, a distinctive day-to-day fluctuation in the severity of these cognitive deficits, with exacerbations accompanied by confusion. Furthermore, hallucinations, more often visual than auditory, or delusions, often of persecution, typically accompany the dementia, either from the outset or after a period of time spanning up to several years. Finally, these patients also display a pronounced sensitivity to antipsychotics, with a tendency to develop severe parkinsonism.

When the disease presents with dementia and parkinsonism, a notable feature is the relative mildness of the parkinsonian signs and symptoms relative to the severity of the dementia; furthermore, one also sees the same antipsychotic sensitivity, with a pronounced and at times dramatic worsening of the parkinsonism upon administration of an antipsychotic.

When the disease presents with parkinsonism alone, there may be few distinctive features. However, and generally within a year, a dementia appears, which may in turn soon come to dominate the overall clinical picture.

Other features that may appear over time include myoclonus and varying degrees of aphasia, apraxia and agnosia. There is also an interesting association with REM sleep behavior disorder, in that a substantial minority of patients with REM sleep behavior disorder will eventually develop diffuse Lewy body disease.

COURSE

The course is chronic and gradually progressive, with death within one to 20 years, with most patients succumbing within 12 to 13 years.

COMPLICATIONS

Complications are as described in the chapter on dementia.

ETIOLOGY

A mild degree of cortical atrophy is seen; microscopically there is neuronal loss, and, in surviving neurons, Lewy bodies, throughout the cerebral cortex, and in the nucleus basalis of Meynert, substantia nigra, locus ceruleus and pedunculopontine nucleus.

DIFFERENTIAL DIAGNOSIS

When the disease presents with dementia, Alzheimer's disease may be considered; however, the day-to-day fluctuations and the pronounced antipsychotic sensitivity suggest the correct diagnosis.

A presentation with concurrent dementia and parkinsonism is fairly distinctive, although diagnostic consideration may be given to arteriosclerotic parkinsonism or Fahr's syndrome.

When diffuse Lewy body disease presents with parkinsonism alone, it may be very difficult to distinguish from Parkinson's disease, and one may have to wait for the emergence of a dementia to make the differential: in diffuse Lewy body disease, dementia typically occurs relatively soon after the onset of parkinsonism, generally within a year or so, in contrast with Parkinson's disease, wherein dementia, should it occur at all, appears only after the parkinsonism has been well-established for many years.

TREATMENT

Although there is no cure for diffuse Lewy body disease, symptomatic treatments for the dementia and parkinsonism are available.

Dementia, and any accompanying psychotic symptoms, may be partially relieved by rivastigmine in doses of from 6 to 12 mg daily. Should hallucinations or delusions persist to an unacceptable degree, or should agitation be extreme, one may consider an antipsychotic; however, extreme caution is in order here, given the pronounced antipsychotic sensitivity seen in this disease. Although there are no blinded studies of antipsychotic treatment in diffuse Lewy body disease, one might, reasoning by analogy from Parkinson's disease, consider risperidone.

Parkinsonism, if severe enough to require treatment, responds well to levodopa/carbidopa; it is not clear whether direct-acting dopaminergic agents are as effective in diffuse Lewy body disease as they are in Parkinson's disease.

BIBLIOGRAPHY

Bryne EJ, Lennox G, Lowe J, et al. Diffuse Lewy body disease: clinical features in 15 cases. *Journal of Neurology, Neurosurgery, and Psychiatry* 1989;52:709-717.

Gibb WRG, Luthert PJ, Janota I, et al. Cortical Lewy body dementia: clinical features and classification. *Journal of Neurology, Neurosurgery, and Psychiatry* 1989;52:185-192.

Hely MA, Reid WG, Halliday GM, et al. Diffuse Lewy body disease: clinical features in nine cases without coexistent Alzheimer's disease. *Journal of Neurology, Neurosurgery, and Psychiatry* 1996;60:531-538.

Louis ED, Goldman JE, Powers JM, et al. Parkinsonian features of eight pathologically diagnosed cases of diffuse Lewy body disease. *Movement Disorders* 1995;10:188-194.

Louis ED, Klatka LA, Liu Y, et al. Comparison of extrapyramidal features in 31 pathologically confirmed cases of diffuse Lewy body disease and 34 pathologically confirmed cases of Parkinson's disease. *Neurology* 1997;48:376-380.

McKeith IG, Fairbairn A, Perry R, et al. Neuroleptic sensitivity in patients with senile dementia of the Lewy body type. *British Medical Journal* 1992;305:673-678.

McKeith I, Del Ser T, Spano P, et al. Efficacy of rivastigmine in dementia with Lewy bodies: a randomized, double-blind, placebo-controlled study. *Lancet* 2000;356:2031-2036.

Turner RS, D'Amato CJ, Chervin RD, et al. The pathology of REM sleep behavior disorder with comorbid Lewy body dementia. *Neurology* 2000;55:1730-1732.

Wesnes KA, McKeith IG, Ferrara R, et al. Effects of rivastigmine on cognitive function in dementia with Lewy bodies: a randomized placebo-controlled international study using the cognitive drug research computerized assessment system. *Dementia and Geriatric Cognitive Disorders* 2002;13:183-192.

180 Cortico-basal Ganglionic Degeneration

Cortico-basal ganglionic degeneration, also known as corticobasal ganglionic degeneration or corticobasal degeneration, is a rare disorder characterized classically by a strikingly asymmetric parkinsonism, which is typically accompanied by a dementia.

ONSET

The onset is gradual, usually sometime in the seventh decade.

CLINICAL FEATURES

As noted, the classic presentation is with parkinsonism, typically akinetic-rigid in character, which typically begins in one upper extremity and remains asymmetric for years. The parkinsonism is often accompanied by a dystonia, and, in the affected limb, cortical sensory loss and apraxia are common; late in the course of the disease, myoclonus may appear. Dementia occurs in the majority, and although classically it is described as only occurring well after the parkinsonism has set in, recent work suggests that, in a large number of cases, the dementia may precede the movement disorder. Depression may also occur.

The alien hand syndrome is said to be classic for cortico-basal ganglionic degeneration; however, a close reading of the case reports indicates that, rather than an alien hand, these patients have either the levitation phenomenon or forced grasping or groping.

MRI scanning reveals asymmetric cortical atrophy, generally involving the parietal and frontal lobes contralateral to the involved limb.

COURSE

Over time the parkinsonism finally does become bilateral, and in some cases mild cerebellar signs or a supranuclear ophthalmoplegia may appear; death generally comes after 6 to 10 years.

COMPLICATIONS

The complications of cortico-basal ganglionic degeneration are similar to those described in the chapters on dementia and Parkinson's disease.

ETIOLOGY

Although most cases are sporadic, an autosomal dominant pattern may occur and such cases have been linked to chromosome 17q.

Macroscopically, early on one sees unilateral atrophy of the parietal lobe and the posterior portion of the ipsilateral frontal lobe; over time, the temporal lobe and anterior portions of the frontal lobe become involved and contralateral atrophy also occurs. Microscopically, there is neuronal loss and gliosis, not only in these areas but also in the basal ganglia and substantia nigra. Surviving neurons are often swollen and achromatic and contain tau neurofilaments.

DIFFERENTIAL DIAGNOSIS

Parkinson's disease is distinguished by the more rapid appearance of bilateral involvement and by the absence of apraxia and myoclonus.

Multiple system atrophy is distinguished by the presence of autonomic insufficiency, with urinary incontinence or retention, or erectile dysfunction.

Progressive supranuclear palsy is distinguished by its onset with symmetrical parkinsonism.

TREATMENT

The general treatment of dementia is as described in that chapter; if antipsychotics are required care must be taken to not aggravate the parkinsonism. The parkinsonism itself generally does not respond well to levodopa; clonazepam may be used if myoclonus is troublesome.

BIBLIOGRAPHY

Bergeron C, Pollanen MS, Weyer L, et al. Unusual clinical presentations of cortico-basal ganglionic degeneration. *Annals of Neurology* 1996;40:893-900.

Grimes DA, Lange AE, Bergeron CB. Dementia as the most common presentation of cortico-basal ganglionic degeneration. *Neurology* 1999;53:1969-1974.

Massman PJ, Kreiter KT, Jankovic J, et al. Neuropsychological functioning in cortico-basal ganglionic degeneration: differentiation from Alzheimer's disease. *Neurology* 1996;46:720-726.

Riley DE, Lang AE, Lewis A, et al. Cortico-basal ganglionic degeneration. *Neurology* 1990;40:1203-1212.

Wenning GK, Litvan I, Jankovic J, et al. Natural history and survival of 14 patients with corticobasal degeneration confirmed at postmortem examination. *Journal of Neurology, Neurosurgery, and Psychiatry* 1998;64:184-189.

Huntington's disease, also known as Huntington's chorea or chorea major, is an autosomally dominant inherited disease characterized by the insidious onset, and subsequent relentless progression, of a combination of chorea and dementia. Although the lifetime prevalence is not high (0.008 to 0.004% in whites, and only a third as much in blacks and one-tenth as much in Japanese), these patients are commonly seen in clinic and hospital.

ONSET

The onset is extremely insidious, and typically occurs in the late thirties, with a wide range, extending from childhood to the eighth decade. Although the initial symptomatology may consist of either chorea or a dementia, eventually all patients, if they live long enough, will develop both.

Chorea may manifest initially as clumsiness, restlessness or a tendency to drop things from the hands. The dementia of Huntington's disease typically presents with a personality change, often with poor judgment and impulsivity.

CLINICAL FEATURES

Chorea often first appears in the face or upper limbs but eventually progresses to the trunk and legs. One may see grimacing, shrugging of the forehead, and jerking of the head; shoulder shrugging and purposeless hand movements are seen. In shaking the patient's hand, one may note the classic "milkmaid grip," wherein the patient's grasping of the examiner's hand feels as if the patient were milking a cow. Early in the course of the disease the patient often attempts to disguise the chorea by merging the abnormal movements with purposeful ones; the motion of an arm initially flung up in a choreic jerk may then be purposefully continued and directed to the head, as if to smooth the hair back.

Typically the choreiform movements jump from one area to another, sometimes with lightning-like fluidity. They are typically worse with stress of any sort and disappear in sleep.

The word "chorea" means "the dance" in Latin and is an apt name, in light of the characteristic gait displayed by these patients. Some observers have characterized it as "stuttering" or "halting," but perhaps the most descriptive phrase is a "dancing and prancing" gait.

Eventually the chorea becomes so severe that voluntary activity is not possible, and simple activities such as eating or dressing become impossible. Dysarthria may occur; however, aphasia is not seen. Dysphagia may occur, and choking may be fatal. Terminally, seizures may occur. In some cases, after many years of illness the chorea may gradually fade, to be replaced by an equally disabling rigid akinetic state. Eventually, patients become bedridden; most die of an intercurrent infection, often a pneumonia.

Apart from the chorea, the physical examination is generally unremarkable. Sensation remains normal; however, one may occasionally see hypotonicity, increased deep tendon reflexes, and rarely an extensor plantar response. One classic sign, in itself a kind of chorea, is an inability to maintain the tongue protruded past the lips.

The dementia of Huntington's disease, as noted earlier, often presents with a personality change, which may be the most distressing part of the dementia for the family. Patients lose interest in former things and may become slovenly in their dress and grooming; irritability, demandingness, and impulsivity are common and personal judgment becomes poor. Interestingly, although some patients recognize that they are ill and attempt to cooperate with those who try to help them, many stoutly deny that anything is wrong. The depth of this denial is at times astounding: patients whose chorea is so severe as to preclude ambulation may continue to insist that nothing is wrong.

Delusions are a relatively common accompaniment of the dementia, and these are often of a persecutory type. Well-formed visual hallucinations may occur; auditory hallucinations appear less common. Depressed mood, fatigue, anorexia, and insomnia may appear; rarely one may see euphoria with pressure of speech and of activity.

An unusual form of Huntington's disease, the "Westphal variant," may appear in patients with childhood onset. Here, rather than chorea, patients display an akinetic rigid state. Dementia is present, and seizures occur with some frequency.

Routine analysis of urine, blood, and cerebrospinal fluid is normal. Electroencephalogram may show diffuse abnormalities, often generalized slowing, but is not diagnostic. CT or MRI scanning eventually reveals a degree of cortical atrophy and, due to atrophy of the caudate, a characteristic dilation of the anterior horns of the lateral ventricle, giving them the classic "butterfly" configuration, as shown in the CT scan in Figure 181-1. Early in the course of otherwise definite Huntington's disease, however, CT and MRI scans may be normal.

Genetic testing is now readily available, and should generally be ordered first whenever there is a reasonable clinical suspicion of the disease, as a positive test obviates the need for other investigations, such as MRI scanning.

COURSE

Huntington's disease is relentlessly progressive; most patients die within 10 to 30 years after onset, with an average life expectancy of

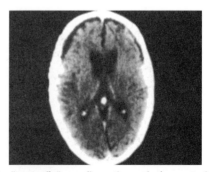

FIG. 181-1. "Butterfly" configuration of the anterior horns in Huntington's disease. (From Perkin GD, Hochberg FH, Miller DC. *Atlas of clinical neurology*, ed 2, London, 1993, Wolfe.)

about 15 years. The Westphal variant, described earlier, tends to be more rapidly progressive, with an average life expectancy of about 10 years. Conversely, those with a late onset may experience a more gradual progression of symptoms.

COMPLICATIONS

Most patients experience embarrassment over their chorea; not uncommonly, the chorea and dysarthria of Huntington's disease may lead to false arrests for public intoxication. With progression of the dementia, the ability to sustain one's occupational and family roles is lost; additionally the chorea interferes to a progressively greater degree with any manual activity. Eventually, patients lose their jobs, and many are divorced. Suicide is not uncommon.

ETIOLOGY

Huntington's disease is a fully penetrant, autosomal dominant disease due to an expansion of a CAG trinucleotide repeat in the *huntingtin* gene on chromosome 4: normally there are from 10 to 29 repeats but in Huntington's disease anywhere from 36 to 121 repeats may be found. Spontaneous mutations do occur, but are very rare, and, provided that the family tree is complete, one may trace the disease back for generations upon generations.

Macroscopically, there is widespread but generally mild cortical atrophy, most pronounced in the frontal and parietal lobes. The caudate and putamen demonstrate considerable atrophy, as shown in Figure 181-2, the globus pallidus less so. Microscopically, there is neuronal loss in the caudate and putamen, and less so in the globus pallidus. Neuronal loss is also seen in the cerebral cortex.

In the caudate nucleus and putamen, the medium-sized spiny neurons bear the brunt of the atrophic process; however, eventually almost all cells are lost. In cases of near total cell loss in the caudate, one sees clinically the terminal akinetic rigid state.

DIFFERENTIAL DIAGNOSIS

Whenever one encounters a case of gradually progressive chorea of insidious onset in an adult, genetic testing for Huntington's disease should probably be obtained. If it is negative, then one should

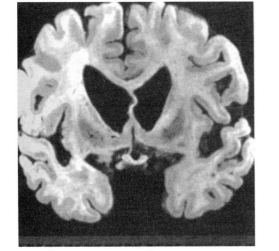

FIG. 181-2. Striatal atrophy in Huntington's disease. (From Kissane JM, ed. *Anderson's pathology*, ed 9, St. Louis, 1990, Mosby.)

check for Wilson's disease, dentatorubropallidoluysian atrophy and neuroacanthocytosis with, respectively, copper studies, genetic testing, and three "wet preps" to determine whether or not acanthocytes are present. With later onsets, in the seventh or eighth decade, one may also consider senile chorea, which remains a "rule out" diagnosis after other diagnostic possibilities have been eliminated.

Another differential to consider is schizophrenia. As noted earlier, Huntington's disease may present with a dementia, and in some of these cases, psychotic symptoms may appear quite early on, and may indeed dominate the clinical picture. Such patients, then, might bear a resemblance to patients with schizophrenia who had also developed tardive dyskinesia of the classic choreiform type. Some clues to the differential rest on the nature of the chorea: in Huntington's disease, choreiform movements are non-repetitive and extremely variable and fleeting, now appearing on one part of the body and moments later at another, in a different form; by contrast in tardive dyskinesia the choreiform movements are often repetitive and tend to recur in the same spot. Furthermore, in Huntington's disease one often sees forehead chorea and a "dancing and prancing" gait, phenomena not found in tardive dyskinesia.

TREATMENT

Antipsychotics constitute the traditional mainstay of treatment for both chorea and for psychotic symptoms. Haloperidol is most widely used, in doses generally of from 2 to 10 mg daily: when it is used, akathisia should be carefully watched for and treatment with propranolol or benztropine may be required. Second generation agents, such as olanzapine and risperidone, have also been used with success, and carry a lower liability of extrapyramidal side effects. A recent addition to the armamentarium against chorea in Huntington's disease is amantadine, often in high dose of 200 mg bid.

Depressive symptoms may be treated with SSRIs, such as fluoxetine or sertraline, or a tricyclic, such as nortriptyline.

Predicting which patient will respond to what regimen is very difficult in this disease, and not uncommonly one must try several agents before finding one which offers some relief.

Treating Huntington's disease can be a heart-rending experience. Patients, well aware of the dismal prognosis, often end up like George Huntington's original patients did, isolated from the society of their fellows and simply waiting to die. Many are desperate to try any potentially curative regime, and given the hopeless prognosis, it is reasonable to discuss any possibilities with them. In this regard, neural transplantation may be considered, and is offered on a research basis at some centers. A more readily available treatment, however, consists of highly unsaturated fatty acids, such as the ethyl ester of eicosapentaenoic acid: in two double-blinded studies, listed in the bibliography, these halted the progression of the disease. Whether these astounding results will be replicated remains to be seen.

All clinically unaffected relatives should be offered genetic testing. Extensive counseling must be available if results are positive. Most affected individuals question whether they should have children themselves; in such cases, the availability of vasectomy or tubal ligation should be noted.

BIBLIOGRAPHY

Barr AN, Fischer JH, Koller WC, et al. Serum haloperidol concentrations and choreiform movements in Huntington's disease. *Neurology* 1988;38:84-88.

Bonnelli RM, Mahnert FA, Niederwieser G. Olanzapine for Huntington's disease: an open label study. *Clinical Neuropharmacology* 2002;25:263-265.

Campbell AMG, Corner B, Norman RM, et al. The rigid form of Huntington's disease. *Journal of Neurology, Neurosurgery, and Psychiatry* 1965;24:71-77.

Kremer B, Goldberg P, Andrew SE, et al. A world-wide study of the Huntington's disease mutation: the sensitivity and specificity of measuring CAG repeats. *The New England Journal of Medicine* 1994;330:1401-1406.

Puri BK, Bydder GM, Counsell SJ, et al. MRI and neuropsychological improvement in Huntington disease following ethyl-EPA treatment. *Neuroreport* 2002;13:123-126.

Ranen NG, Lipsey JR, Treisman G, et al. Sertraline in the treatment of severe aggressiveness in Huntington's disease. *The Journal of Neuropsychiatry and Clinical Neurosciences* 1996;8:338-340.

Vaddadi KS, Soosai E, Chiu E, et al. A randomized, placebo-controlled, double blind study of treatment of Huntington's disease with unsaturated fatty acids. *Neuroreport* 2002;13:29-33.

Verhagen Metman L, Morris MJ, Farmer C, et al. Huntington's disease: a randomized, controlled trial using the NMDA-antagonist amantadine. *Neurology* 2002;59:694-699.

182 Neuroacanthocytosis

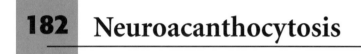

Neuroacanthocytosis, also known as chorea-acanthocytosis, is a rare, autosomal recessive disorder characterized by chorea, dementia, and an excessive percentage of acanthocytic red blood cells.

ONSET

The onset is insidious, and generally in the fourth or fifth decade.

CLINICAL FEATURES

Chorea is generally the first symptom, and this may be joined by other abnormal involuntary movements such as dystonia, tics or, less commonly, a mild parkinsonism. Over time, a dementia or personality change is seen in over one-half of all patients; other symptoms include seizures and a peripheral sensorimotor polyneuropathy. A classic and distinctive, yet uncommon, symptom is involuntary mutilating lip or tongue biting.

CT or MRI scanning may reveal atrophy of the striatum.

Peripheral blood smears demonstrate greater than 10% acanthocytes. Given the possibility of false negatives, at least three "wet preps" are required.

The creatine kinase (CK) level is elevated in the majority of cases.

COURSE

Neuroacanthocytosis is gradually progressive, leading to death on average 14 years later.

COMPLICATIONS

The complications of dementia or personality change are as described in those chapters; chorea or dystonia may become disabling.

ETIOLOGY

As noted earlier, this is an autosomal recessive condition, and it occurs secondary to any of a large number of mutations in the CHAC gene on chromosome 9q21. There is considerable phenotypic heterogeneity in affected families.

Macroscopically, there is atrophy of the caudate, putamen and globus pallidus; microscopically neuronal loss and gliosis are seen not only in these structures but also in the substantia nigra.

DIFFERENTIAL DIAGNOSIS

Huntington's disease is suggested by its autosomal dominant mode of inheritance and by an absence of dystonia, tics and acanthocytosis.

The McLeod phenotype may faithfully mimic neuroacanthocytosis, even to the point of comprising acanthocytosis. The McLeod phenotype, however, is an X-linked disorder, and testing will demonstrate the presence of the red cell Kell antigen.

TREATMENT

The general treatment of dementia and personality change is as described in those chapters; chorea may be treated with an antipsychotic.

BIBLIOGRAPHY

Danek A, Rubio JP, Rampoldi L, et al. McLeod neuroacanthocytosis: genotype and phenotype. *Annals of Neurology* 2001;50:755-764.

Dobson-Stone C, Danek A, Rampoldi L, et al. Mutational spectrum of the CHAC gene in patients with chorea-acanthocytosis. *European Journal of Human Genetics* 2002;10:773-781.

Hardie RJ, Pullon HW, Harding AE, et al. Neuroacanthocytosis. A clinical, haemotological and pathological study of 19 cases. *Brain* 1991;114:13-49.

Kartsounis LD, Hardie RJ. The pattern of cognitive impairments in neuroacanthocytosis. A frontosubcortical dementia. *Archives of Neurology* 1996;53:77-80.

Rinne JO, Daniel SE, Scaravilli F, et al. The neuropathological features of neuroacanthocytosis. *Movement Disorders* 1994;9:297-304.

Wilson's disease, also known as hepatolenticular degeneration, is an autosomally recessively inherited disease characterized by copper deposition in the liver and brain, most prominently in the basal ganglia and the cortex. The estimated prevalence is about 3 in 100,000, and although it is probably equally common in females as in males, males appear to outnumber females in clinic populations.

ONSET

The onset of symptoms is insidious and may occur anywhere from between the ages of 5 and 50. The majority of patients, however, present some time between late childhood and early adult years. The presentation itself may be characterized by abnormal movements, personality change or psychosis, dementia or a hepatitis.

CLINICAL FEATURES

Abnormal movements seen in Wilson's disease include dystonia, chorea, tremor or parkinsonism. Dystonia may affect the neck, producing a toricollis, the upper or lower extremities, or the face, whereby a fixed, vacuous smile may be produced; oculogyric crises may also be seen. Chorea may involve the upper or lower extremities, as may tremor: classically, but infrequently, one sees a "wing-beating" tremor, wherein the upper extremities oscillate up and down, mimicking the beating wings of a frightened bird. Parkinsonism in Wilson's disease is typically characterized by rigidity of the extremities, accompanied at times by bradykinesia. Occasionally one may see cerebellar signs, such as dysarthria, clumsiness and intention tremor.

The personality change of Wilson's disease often manifests with lability, disinhibition and, at times, bizarre behavior.

Psychosis in Wilson's disease may be characterized by hallucinations, both auditory and visual, delusions, and Schneiderian First Rank Symptoms: it is of interest that one of Wilson's first patients presented with a psychosis, without any other symptomatology whatsoever.

The dementia of Wilson's disease has no distinguishing characteristics.

Hepatic inflammation may cause malaise, fever and abdominal pain, and an elevation of serum transaminases.

Regardless of whether patients first experience abnormal movements, personality change, psychosis or dementia, eventually, with disease progression, almost all patients develop a "mixed" picture, involving all of these phenomena.

Other clinical features include the Kayser-Fleischer ring and a Coombs-negative hemolytic anemia. The Kayser-Fleischer ring consists of a golden-brown discoloration of the corneal limbus due to deposition of copper in Descemet's membrane, which may be visible to the naked eye or require slit-lamp examination. Although the overwhelming majority of patients have a Kayser-Fleischer ring, there have been cases of indubitable Wilson's disease which lacked it. Anemia may occur when an overwhelming burden of copper "spills over" from the liver into the systemic circulation.

Serum ceruloplasmin and copper levels are both low, but the free copper level is elevated, as is the 24-hour urinary excretion of copper. Liver biopsy reliably reveals increased copper levels.

MRI scanning may reveal a degree of cortical atrophy along with bilaterally symmetric increased signal intensity on T2-weighted scans in the basal ganglia (as illustrated in Figure 183-1), the thalami, the mesencephalon and the pons.

COURSE

Although temporary partial remissions may occur, the overall course of the disease is one of relentless progression unto death. In some, especially those with fulminant hepatic involvement, death may occur in a matter of months; others may live for decades. On the average, however, most patients die within 5 to 10 years of the onset of symptoms.

COMPLICATIONS

The complications, by and large, are as described in the chapters on personality change, psychosis and dementia. Hepatic involvement, if severe, may precipitate an hepatic encephalopathy.

ETIOLOGY

Wilson's disease, as noted, is inherited in an autosomal recessive fashion, and is due, in turn, to any one of over a hundred different mutations in the gene for the copper-transporting ATPase, *ATP7B*, found on the long arm of chromosome 13.

Normally, copper is absorbed through the intestines, and is eventually bound to ceruloplasmin in the liver, after which it

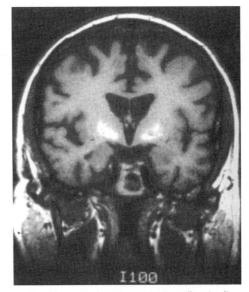

FIG. 183-1. Basal ganglia hyperintensity in Wilson's disease. (From Perkin GD, Hochberg FH, Miller DC. *Atlas of clinical neurology*, ed 2, London, 1993, Wolfe.)

undergoes biliary excretion. When ceruloplasmin is defective, biliary excretion is reduced and hepatic copper levels rise, with an eventual overflow into the systemic circulation. Copper deposition within the liver leads to hepatitis, and within the brain to the various neuropsychiatric symptoms noted earlier. Neuronal loss occurs, and in advanced cases there may be spongiosus or actual cavitation. In general, the basal ganglia are most severely affected (more so the putamen than the caudate or globus pallidus), followed by the thalami, frontal cortex, midbrain (particularly the substantia nigra and the red nucleus), pons and cerebellum.

DIFFERENTIAL DIAGNOSIS

In evaluating a child, adolescent or young adult with abnormal movements, personality change, psychosis or dementia, one should consider, in addition to Wilson's disease, schizophrenia, Huntington's disease, metachromatic leukodsytrophy, Hallervorden-Spatz disease, and cerebral tumors, especially of the temporal or frontal lobes. In practice, and given the treatability of Wilson's disease, it is appropriate to consider copper studies in any patient of this age, with compatible symptomatology, whose illness cannot be clearly accounted for on the basis of some other disease.

TREATMENT

All patients, whether symptomatic or not, should receive one of the various medications available that reduce copper burden. D-penicillamine chelates copper and hastens its urinary excretion, and although it is the most established treatment, it has numerous and sometimes severe side-effects; furthermore, in a substantial minority of patients, penicillamine treatment may be followed by an exacerbation of symptoms, which may be very severe. Other chelating agents include trientine and ammonium tetrathiomolybdate. Although trientine is much better tolerated than penicillamine, it is somewhat less effective. Tetrathiomolybdate appears as effective as penicillamine and does not carry the risk of early symptom evaluation, but, in the United States, is currently available only at certain research centers. A final option is oral zinc, which is very well tolerated: zinc induces the synthesis of intestinal metallothionene, which in turn has a high affinity for copper, thus preventing its absorption. Zinc, however, appears somewhat less effective than the chelating agents, and must not be given with them, as it will substitute for copper, and thus obviate their effect. Although the optimum approach has not as yet been agreed upon, it appears that zinc may be appropriate for presymptomatic patients; for symptomatic patients, however, a chelating agent is probably required and here there is much controversy. Some authors recommend penicillamine, whereas others, impressed by penicillamine's side-effects and its potential for worsening neuropsychiatric symptomatology, argue for trientine or tetrathiomolybdate. The clinical response to treatment with a chelating agent is slow, and improvement may not be seen for four to six months, with up to two years required for maximal improvement. The eventual degree of improvement varies with clinical severity before treatment. Patients with mild symptoms may experience essentially complete remission; those with more severe symptoms continue to experience some disability. Regardless of whether complete remission is achieved, treatment with chelating agents should be continued for the life of the patient.

At one point, reducing copper intake by avoiding copper-rich foods (e.g., shellfish, legumes, nuts, grains, coffee, chocolate, and organ meats) was recommended; however, this appears only minimally effective and cannot substitute for medical treatment.

In cases of fulminant hepatitis or in cases with neurologic or hepatic disease unresponsive to chelation treatment, liver transplantation may be considered. After successful transplantation neurologic improvement is gradual but may be substantial.

Symptomatic treatment of personality change, psychosis or dementia may proceed as outlined in those chapters. Given that most patients have at least a degree of hepatic failure, dosage adjustments of routine medications are generally required.

All of the patient's siblings should be tested for Wilson's disease with serum copper and ceruloplasmin levels and 24-hour urinary copper level; in doubtful cases, liver biopsy should be strongly considered.

BIBLIOGRAPHY

Brewer GJ, Yuzbasiyan-Gurkan V, Johnson V, et al. Treatment of Wilson's disease with zinc XII: dose regimen requirements. *The American Journal of the Medical Sciences* 1993;305:199-202.

Brewer GJ, Hedera P, Kluin KJ, et al. Treatment of Wilson disease with ammonium tetrathiomolybdate: III. Initial therapy in a total of 55 neurologically affected patients and follow-up with zinc therapy. *Archives of Neurology* 2003;60:379-385.

Dahlman T, Hartvig P, Lofholm M, et al. Long-term treatment of Wilson's disease with triethylene tetramine dihydrochloride (trientine). *Quarterly Journal of Medicine* 1995;88:609-616.

Demirkiran M, Jankovic J, Lewis RA, et al. Neurologic presentation of Wilson disease without Kayser-Fleischer rings. *Neurology* 1996;46:1040-1043.

Dening TR, Berrios GE. Wilson's disease: psychiatric symptoms in one hundred and ninety-five cases. *Archives of General Psychiatry* 1989;46:1126-1134.

Glass JD, Reich SG, DeLong MR. Wilson's disease: development of neurological disease after beginning penicillamine therapy. *Archives of Neurology* 1990;47:595-596.

McDonald LV, Lake CR. Psychosis in an adolescent patient with Wilson's disease: effects of chelation therapy. *Psychosomatic Medicine* 1995;57:202-204.

Roh JK, Lee TG, Wie BE, et al. Initial and follow-up brain MRI findings and correlation with the clinical course in Wilson's disease. *Neurology* 1994;44:1064-1068.

Saatci I, Topcu M, Baltaoglu FF, et al. Cranial MR findings in Wilson's disease. *Acta Radiologica* 1997;38:250-258.

Shah AB, Chernov I, Zhang HT, et al. Identification and analysis of mutations in the Wilson disease gene (ATPB7): population frequencies, genotype-phenotype correlation, and functional analyses. *American Journal of Human Genetics* 1997;61:317-328.

Starosta-Rubinstein S, Young AB, Kluin K, et al. Clinical assessment of 31 patients with Wilson's disease: correlation with structural changes on magnetic resonance imaging. *Archives of Neurology* 1987;44:365-370.

Stracciari A, Tempestini A, Borghi A, et al. Effect of liver transplantation on neurological manifestations in Wilson disease. *Archives of Neurology* 2000;57:384-386.

Svetel M, Sternic N, Pejovic S, et al. Penicillamine-induced lethal status dystonicus in a patient with Wilson's disease. *Movement Disorders* 2001;16:568-569.

Walshe JM, Yealland N. Wilson's disease: the problem of delayed diagnosis. *Journal of Neurology, Neurosurgery, and Psychiatry* 1992;55:692-696.

Wilson SAK. Progressive lenticular degeneration: a familial nervous disease associated with cirrhosis of the liver. *Brain* 1912;34:295-509.

Progressive supranuclear palsy, also known as the Steele-Richardson-Olszewski syndrome, is a rare disorder that may be slightly more common in males than females and is characterized classically by postural instability with falls, atypical parkinsonism, supranuclear ophthalmoplegia and dementia.

ONSET

The onset is gradual and insidious, occurring generally in the sixth through eighth decades, and in most cases is marked by an unsteady gait or unexplained falls.

CLINICAL FEATURES

Patients tend to walk with a broad-based gait and small, shuffling steps, and may fall for no apparent reason. Over time, an atypical parkinsonian picture emerges, characterized by the symmetrical onset of a rigid-akinetic state. Unlike classic parkinsonism, however, these patients generally do not have tremor, and, rather than presenting with a stooped, "flexion" posture, they typically display some axial dystonia, and to be quite upright, with their heads held up in extension. Dystonic rigidity may also be seen in the face, and this may be accompanied by a reduced frequency of blinking, such that patients may seem to have an "astonished" facial expression. A typical patient is illustrated in Figure 184-1. Within the first few years, most, but not all, patients will exhibit the classic and distinctive feature of this disease, namely supranuclear ophthalmoplegia. Here, there is a partial paralysis of voluntary vertical gaze, affecting primarily downward gaze, such that patients may have great difficulty in walking downstairs. The supranuclear origin of this paralysis is indicated by the full range of extraocular movements with the doll's head maneuver.

Dementia eventually supervenes in about one-half of all patients, and, in addition to deficits in memory, orientation and calculations, there are often also elements of a frontal lobe syndrome. "Cortical" signs, such as aphasia, apraxia or agnosia, are generally absent.

Other features seen in a minority of patients with advanced disease include seizures and pseudobulbar palsy, with emotional incontinence, dysarthria and dysphagia.

MRI scanning typically reveals atrophy of the midbrain, along with some modest cerebral cortical atrophy, most prominently in the frontal lobes and anterior portions of the temporal lobes.

COURSE

The overall duration of the disease ranges from 2 to 25 years, with most patients dying in from six to nine years, generally of an intercurrent pneumonia.

COMPLICATIONS

The complications of dementia are as described in that chapter; the gait disorder is often particularly disabling.

ETIOLOGY

Microscopically, one finds widespread neuronal loss and astrocytosis, most particularly in the midbrain (including the tectum, periaqueductal gray, locus ceruleus, raphe nuclei, red nucleus and substantia nigra), globus pallidus, subthalamic nucleus, thalamus (particularly the parafascicular and centre median nuclei), cerebellar dentate nuclei and the frontal and temporal cortices. Progressive supranuclear palsy is one of the "tauopathies" and in surviving neurons there are neurofibrillary tangles, dissimilar from those seen in Alzheimer's disease.

Although some familial cases, consistent with autosomal dominant inheritance, have been reported, most cases are sporadic. Nevertheless, genetic factors do play a role, as almost all patients will have a specific, normally occurring tau genotype: it appears that this genotype confers a "susceptibility" to some, as yet unknown, other factor.

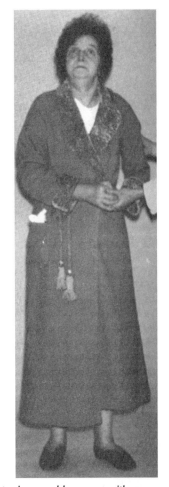

FIG. 184-1. Sixty-six-year-old woman with progressive supranuclear palsy. (From Parsons M. *Color atlas of clinical neurology*, ed 2, London, 1993, Wolfe.)

DIFFERENTIAL DIAGNOSIS

In distinguishing progressive supranuclear palsy from other parkinsonian conditions, two features are very distinctive, namely the early onset, within the first year, of postural instability and unexplained falls, and, second, the appearance of supranuclear ophthalmoplegia at any point.

Parkinson's disease is further distinguished by the asymmetric onset of rigidity, which is often accompanied by tremor and by a flexion, rather than extension posture. Diffuse Lewy body disease is marked by the early onset of dementia, often accompanied by confusion. Corticobasal-ganglionic degeneration is suggested by an asymmetric onset of rigidity and also by the presence of "cortical" signs such as apraxia and, classically, the alien hand syndrome. Multiple system atrophy of the striato-nigral type is marked by ataxia or autonomic insufficiency (impotence, postural dizziness, urinary incontinence), signs generally not seen in progressive supranuclear palsy. Arteriosclerotic, or vascular, parkinsonism may be very difficult to distinguish clinically from progressive supranuclear palsy, but is suggested by such "long tract" signs as hyperreflexia and extensor plantar responses. In doubtful cases, MRI scanning will reveal multiple lacunar infarctions.

TREATMENT

Although certain medications may offer some relief of the parkinsonism, the effect is generally very modest, and not sustained; furthermore, these patients tend to be very sensitive to medications, and even with low doses may develop confusion or hallucinations. Medications that have been used with some limited success include levodopa, amitriptyline (in doses of 25 to 75 mg), and idazoxan, which is not available in the United States. Donepezil is not helpful for the dementia, and may worsen the parkinsonism.

Overall care is supportive, with an emphasis on preservation of mobility and ambulation; tube feeding may eventually be required.

BIBLIOGRAPHY

Birdi S, Rajput AH, Fenton M, et al. Progressive supranuclear palsy diagnosis and confounding features: report on 16 autopsied cases. *Movement Disorders* 2002;17:1255-1264.

Collins SJ, Ahlskop JE, Parisi JE, et al. Progressive supranuclear palsy: neuropathologically based diagnostic clinical criteria. *Journal of Neurology, Neurosurgery, and Psychiatry* 1995;58:167-173.

Daniel SE, de Bruin VMS, Lees AJ. The clinical and pathological spectrum of Steele-Richardson-Olszewski syndrome (progressive supranuclear palsy): a reappraisal. *Brain* 1995;118:759-770.

de Yebenes JG, Sarasa JL, Daniel SE, et al. Familial progressive supranuclear palsy: description of a pedigree and review of the literature. *Brain* 1995;118:1095-1103.

Engel PA. Treatment of progressive supranuclear palsy with amitriptyline: therapeutic and toxic effects. *Journal of the American Geriatrics Society* 1996;44:1072-1074.

Ghika J, Tennis M, Hoffman E, et al. Idazoxan treatment in progressive supranuclear palsy. *Neurology* 1991;41:986-991.

Golbe LI, Davis PH, Schoenberg BS, et al. Prevalence and natural history of progressive supranuclear palsy. *Neurology* 1988;38:1031-1034.

Higgins JJ, Adler RL, Loveless JM. Mutational analysis of the tau gene in progressive supranuclear palsy. *Neurology* 1999;53:1421-1424.

Kompoliti K, Goetz CG, Litvan I, et al. Pharmacological treatment in progressive supranuclear palsy. *Archives of Neurology* 1998;55:1099-1102.

Litvan I, Mangone CA, McKee A, et al. Natural history of progressive supranuclear palsy (Steele-Richardson-Olszewski syndrome) and clinical predictors of survival: a clinicopathological study. *Journal of Neurology, Neurosurgery, and Psychiatry* 1996;60:615-620.

Litvan I, Campbell G, Mangone CA, et al. Which clinical features differentiate progressive supranuclear palsy (Steele-Richardson-Olszewski syndrome) from related disorders? A clinicopathological study. *Brain* 1997;120:65-74.

Litvan I, Phipps M, Pharr VL, et al. Randomized placebo-controlled trial of donepezil in patients with progressive supranuclear palsy. *Neurology* 2001;57:467-473.

Maher ER, Lees AJ. The clinical features and natural history of the Steele-Richardson-Olszewski syndrome (progressive supranuclear palsy). *Neurology* 1986;36:1005-1008.

Morris HR, Gibbs G, Katzenschlager R, et al. Pathological, clinical and genetic heterogeneity in progressive supranuclear palsy. *Brain* 2002;125:969-975.

Newman GC. Treatment of progressive supranuclear palsy with tricyclic antidepressant. *Neurology* 1985;35:1189-1193.

Nygaard TG, Duvoisin RC, Manocha M, et al. Seizures in progressive supranuclear palsy. *Neurology* 1989;39:138-140.

Steele JC. Progressive supranuclear palsy. *Brain* 1972;95:693-704.

Steele JC, Richardson JC, Olszewski J. Progressive supranuclear palsy: a heterogenous degeneration involving the brainstem, basal ganglia and cerebellum, with vertical gaze and pseudobulbar palsy, vertical dystonia and dementia. *Archives of Neurology* 1964;10:333-359.

185 Multiple System Atrophy

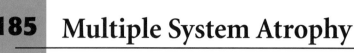

Multiple system atrophy is a sporadic disorder characterized by varying admixtures of parkinsonism, ataxia and autonomic failure. Although the prevalence of this disorder is not known with certainty, it may be more common than thought, as many cases go misdiagnosed as Parkinson's disease.

ONSET

The onset is insidious and may occur at any time from the fifth through the eighth decades.

CLINICAL FEATURES

Multiple system atrophy may present with any one of three subtypes, including the striatonigral variant, olivopontocerebellar variant and the Shy-Drager variant.

The striatonigral variant is characterized by a parkinsonism similar to that seen in Parkinson's disease with the exception that tremor is unusual: thus, patients with the striatonigral variant typically have a flexion posture (which may be extreme) and rigidity. Other symptoms may accompany this parkinsonism, including hyperreflexia, extensor plantar responses, supranuclear ophthalmoplegia for downward gaze, and myoclonus (which is generally subtle and confined to the hands).

The olivopontocerebellar variant is characterized by ataxia, dysarthria and scanning speech; in some cases reflex myoclonus may appear.

The Shy-Drager variant is characterized by autonomic insufficiency, with orthostatic hypotension, urinary incontinence or retention, and erectile dysfunction.

Although these variants may present in "pure" form, this is very uncommon, and in most cases, some evidence of all three types will be found. For example, a patient with the striatonigral variant may, in addition to prominent parkinsonism, also have some subtle ataxia.

Dementia occurs in a minority of patients with multiple system atrophy, and is often accompanied by elements of a frontal lobe syndrome. There are very rare case reports of this disorder presenting with dementia.

Interestingly, there is a strong association between multiple system atrophy and REM sleep behavior disorder; indeed, it appears that the majority of patients with the striatonigral variant may be so affected and that in these cases the REM sleep behavior disorder may precede the parkinsonism by years or even decades.

MRI scanning in the striatonigral variant may reveal decreased signal intensity in the putamen with an accompanying "rim" of increased signal on T2-weighted scans on the lateral border of the putamen, and may also reveal a distinctive "hot cross bun" sign in the pons, with linear areas of increased signal intensity on T2-weighted scans resembling the markings on the top of a hot cross bun. In the olivopontocerebellar variant, atrophy of the pons and cerebellum may be seen.

COURSE

Multiple system atrophy is gradually progressive, with a mean survival of from 8 to 10 years.

COMPLICATIONS

The complications of dementia are as described in that chapter; parkinsonism and ataxia may confine patients to wheelchair or bed, and a significant minority will eventually develop laryngeal stridor.

ETIOLOGY

Pathologically, there is atrophy of the putamen, inferior olives, cerebellum and pontine nuclei. Microscopically, cell loss and astrocytosis are seen not only in these structures but also in the substantia nigra, locus ceruleus and intermediolateral gray of the spinal cord. These findings vary in prominence among the different subtypes; however, all cases exhibit the unifying pathologic feature of the disease, namely cytoplasmic inclusions within oligodendroglia.

The etiology of these changes is not known; as noted earlier, this is a sporadic disorder which does not appear to be inherited in any fashion.

DIFFERENTIAL DIAGNOSIS

The striatonigral variant is often, as noted above, misdiagnosed as Parkinson's disease. Features which help to distinguish multiple system atrophy include a poor response to treatment with levodopa, ataxia, orthostatic hypotension greater than expected for Parkinson's disease, and urinary incontinence, urinary retention, or erectile dysfunction.

The olivopontocerebellar variant is distinguished from spinocerebellar ataxia by the lack of a family history and by the presence of parkinsonism and autonomic insufficiency.

TREATMENT

Parkinsonism may be treated with levodopa, as described in the chapter on Parkinson's disease, but the response is either poor or short-lived. Orthostatic hypotension may respond to fludrocortisone and urinary incontinence to anticholinergics. If sildenafil is used for erectile dysfunction, great caution must be used as these patients are particularly prone to severe hypotension with sildenafil. Laryngeal stridor may respond to CPAP but tracheostomy may be required.

The treatment of dementia is as described in that chapter; if antipsychotics are used, great care should be taken to avoid exacerbating parkinsonism or orthostatic hypotension.

BIBLIOGRAPHY

Bhattacharya K, Saadia D, Eisenkraft B, et al. Brain magnetic resonance imaging in multiple-system atrophy and Parkinson disease: a diagnostic algorithm. *Archives of Neurology* 2002;59:835-842.

Sakakibara R, Hattori T, Uchiyama T, et al. Urinary dysfunction and orthostatic hypotension in multiple system atrophy: which is the more common and earlier manifestation? *Journal of Neurology, Neurosurgery, and Psychiatry* 2000;68:65-69.

Watanabe H, Saito Y, Terao S, et al. Progression and prognosis in multiple system atrophy: an analysis of 230 Japanese patients. *Brain* 2002; 125:1070-1083.

Wenning GK, Braune S. Multiple system atrophy: pathophysiology and management. *CNS Drugs* 2001;15:839-852.

Wenning GK, Ben-Shlomo Y, Hughes A, et al. What clinical features are most useful to distinguish definite multiple system atrophy from Parkinson's disease? *Journal of Neurology, Neurosurgery, and Psychiatry* 2000;68:434-440.

Spinocerebellar ataxia (SCA), also known as autosomal dominant cerebellar ataxia, is an uncommon, dominantly inherited disorder characterized by a slowly progressive cerebellar ataxia which may rarely be accompanied by either a dementia or a psychosis.

Before proceeding, remarks are in order regarding the nomenclature of this disorder. Originally, the name was autosomal dominant cerebellar ataxia, or ADCA, in deference to the cardinal features of the disorder, namely its autosomal dominant mode of inheritance and its primary clinical expression in a slowly progressive cerebellar ataxia. ADCA was further subdivided into types I, II and III depending primarily on the presence or absence of certain associated clinical features. With the discovery of the genetic basis of the disorder, however, it became apparent that there was considerable genetic and phenotypic heterogeneity, and that the type I, type II and type III classificatory system failed to "cleave" nature at the genetic "joints." Consequently, this name has fallen into disfavor, and has been largely replaced by the name given to the genes in question, spinocerebellar ataxia, or *SCA*.

ONSET

The onset is insidious and, although generally occurring in early to middle adult years, may be seen anywhere from childhood to senescence. The first symptom, in almost all cases, is ataxia.

CLINICAL FEATURES

The dominant feature clinically is a cerebellar ataxia, which is often accompanied by dysarthria and nystagmus. Over time, other features may accrue, but these are generally not prominent and for the most part play only a minor role in the overall clinical picture; they may include one or more of the following: decreased vibratory sense, hyperreflexia, extensor plantar responses, muscle atrophy, fasciculations, tremor, titubation, parkinsonism, supranuclear ophthalmoplegia, dystonia, chorea and pigmentary retinopathy.

Dementia, though uncommon, may appear after many years. Psychosis is even rarer, and appears to run in certain families.

MRI scanning may reveal atrophy of the inferior olives, pons or cerebellum.

Genetic testing is available, and should be performed.

COURSE

The disease is gradually progressive, with death in from 15 to 30 years.

COMPLICATIONS

Ataxia eventually necessitates the use of a wheelchair; the complications of dementia and secondary psychosis are as outlined in those chapters.

ETIOLOGY

Multiple different genetic loci have been identified (spanning *SCA1* to *SCA14*) on multiple different chromosomes.

At autopsy, in addition to atrophy of the inferior olives, pons and cerebellum, there may also be atrophy of Clarke's column, the spinocerebellar tracts, substantia nigra, globus pallidus, subthalamic nucleus and cerebral cortex.

DIFFERENTIAL DIAGNOSIS

Multiple system atrophy of the olivopontocerebellar type is distinguished by an absence of a family history and by the presence of evidence of autonomic failure, such as postural dizziness, urinary incontinence or erectile dysfunction.

Friedrich's ataxia is suggested by the autosomal recessive pattern of inheritance and an early age of onset.

Dentatorubropallidoluysian atrophy is considered by many to be one of the spinocerebellar ataxias; however, given its distinctive clinical features (such as early onset dementia, prominent chorea or parkinsonism, and myoclonus), it is treated, in this book, in its own chapter.

Gerstmann-Straussler-Scheinker disease may be clinically indistinguishable from ADCA.

Other disorders that may present in adult years with a gradually progressive ataxia include alcoholic cerebellar degeneration, vitamin B12 deficiency, hypothyroidism and neurosyphilis.

TREATMENT

In some families, amantadine may reduce the severity of ataxia; the treatment of dementia and of secondary psychosis is as described in those chapters.

Genetic testing may be offered to family members.

BIBLIOGRAPHY

Burk K, Globas C, Bosch S, et al. Cognitive deficits in spinocerebellar ataxia 2. *Brain* 1999;122:769-777.

Goizet C, Lesca G, Durr A, et al. Presymptomatic testing in Huntington's disease and autosomal dominant cerebellar ataxias. *Neurology* 2002;59:1330-1336.

Ishikawa A, Yamada M, Makino K, et al. Dementia and delirium in 4 patients with Machado-Joseph disease. *Archives of Neurology* 2002;59:1804-1808.

Lee WY, Jin DK, Oh MR, et al. Frequency analysis and clinical characterization of spinocerebellar ataxia types 1, 2, 3, 6, and 7 in Korean patients. *Archives of Neurology* 2003;60:858-863.

Schols L, Amoiridis G, Buttner T, et al. Autosomal dominant cerebellar ataxia: phenotypic differences in genetically defined subtypes? *Annals of Neurology* 1997;42:924-932.

Twels R, Yencyitsomanus PT, Sirinavin C, et al. Autosomal dominant cerebellar ataxia with dementia: evidence for a fourth disease locus. *Human Molecular Genetics* 1994;3:177-180.

Dentatorubropallidoluysian Atrophy

Dentatorubropallidoluysian atrophy is a rare, autosomal dominantly inherited disorder typically characterized, in adults, by slowly progressive dementia, ataxia and chorea. The somewhat cumbersome name of this disorder is derived from those structures most affected by the disease process, namely the dentate nucleus, nucleus rubor (red nucleus), globus pallidus and corpus luysii (subthalamic nucleus).

Some authorities include dentatorubropallidoluysian atrophy under the rubric of the spinocerebellar ataxias; however, given that its clinical presentation is quite different from these, it is presented separately in this book.

ONSET

The onset is gradual, and may occur either in childhood or adult years, with the clinical presentation being heavily influenced by the age of onset.

CLINICAL FEATURES

Childhood onset cases are characterized by myoclonus, dementia and ataxia.

Adult onset cases typically present with one or more of dementia, chorea and ataxia; eventually most cases come to display all three features. Other features, present in a minority, may include psychosis, seizures, parkinsonism or dystonia.

MRI scanning may reveal brainstem or cerebellar atrophy, and genetic testing is available.

COURSE

Although clearly gradually progressive, the overall course of dentatorubropallidoluysian atrophy has not been well delineated.

COMPLICATIONS

The complications of dementia and of secondary psychosis are as described in those chapters.

ETIOLOGY

As noted earlier, this is an autosomal dominant condition, and it represents a mutation in the gene for atrophin 1 on chromosome 12. Importantly, there is generally considerable phenotypic heterogeneity within the same family.

Neuronal loss and gliosis are found not only in the cerebellar dentate nucleus, red nucleus, globus pallidus and subthalamic nucleus but also the inferior olives, substantia nigra, striatum, thalamus and cerebral cortex.

DIFFERENTIAL DIAGNOSIS

In adults, when dementia, psychosis and chorea are prominent, Huntington's disease may be suspected, and where ataxia is prominent, one of the classic spinocerebellar ataxias often enters the differential. In such cases, the diagnosis may rest on genetic testing.

TREATMENT

The general treatment of dementia is as described in that chapter. In cases similar to Huntington's disease, it would not be unreasonable to consider treatments that are effective in that disorder.

Genetic testing should be offered to family members.

BIBLIOGRAPHY

Adachi N, Arima K, Asada T, et al. Dentatorubro-pallidoluysian atrophy (DRPLA) presenting with psychosis. *The Journal of Neuropsychiatry and Clinical Neurosciences* 2001;13:258-260.

Licht DJ, Lynch DR. Juvenile dentatorubral-pallidoluysian atrophy: new clinical features. *Pediatric Neurology* 2002;26:51-54.

Munoz E, Mila M, Sanchez A, et al. Dentatorubropallidoluysian atrophy in a Spanish family: a clinical, radiological, pathological, and genetic study. *Journal of Neurology, Neurosurgery, and Psychiatry* 1999; 67:811-814.

Warner TT, Lennox GG, Janota I, et al. Autosomal-dominant dentatorubropallidoluysian atrophy in the United Kingdom. *Movement Disorders* 1994;9:289-296.

Warner TT, Williams LD, Walker RW, et al. A clinical and molecular genetic study of dentatorubropallidoluysian atrophy in four European families. *Annals of Neurology* 1995;37:452-459.

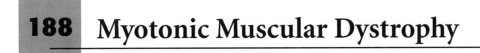

188 Myotonic Muscular Dystrophy

Myotonic muscular dystrophy, also known as myotonia dystrophica or myotonia atrophica, is a not uncommon hereditary disorder, with a lifetime prevalence of about 5 per 100,000, occurring in both males and females. In addition to myotonia and weakness, and other typical signs, patients may develop a dementia and may also, although this is controversial, exhibit a specific personality pattern.

ONSET

The onset is gradual and insidious and may be noted anywhere from adolescence up to 50 years of age. In most cases symptoms become discernible between the late teenage years and the late twenties.

CLINICAL FEATURES

The cardinal symptoms of myotonic muscular dystrophy are myotonia and weakness. Typically, this is primarily distal in distribution, and more evident in the upper than the lower extremities. Other typical symptoms include a distinctive appearance characterized by frontal baldness, ptosis, and wasting of the facial and neck musculature (shown in Figure 188-1), cataracts, sensorineuronal deafness, and gonadal failure, producing testicular atrophy and impotence in men and menstrual irregularity in women. Cardiac abnormalities may occur and include A-V block, fascicular block, intraventricular conduction delay and ventricular arrhythmias. A cardiomyopathy, which may present as congestive failure, is less common.

Mild cognitive impairment is common, and in some cases a dementia may supervene. The personality of these patients has variously been characterized by suspiciousness, guardedness and avoidance.

Hypersomnia may occur, and in some patients this may be one of the most distressing symptoms.

MRI scanning may reveal cortical atrophy, ventricular enlargement, and numerous areas of increased signal intensity in the white matter.

The children of females with myotonic dystrophy may suffer from a congenital form of myotonic dystrophy that tends to be severe and to be accompanied by mental retardation.

Genetic testing is available.

COURSE

The illness is progressive, and although those with mild cases and later onsets may have a normal life span, those with severe cases or early onsets tend to die early, often of respiratory or cardiovascular disease.

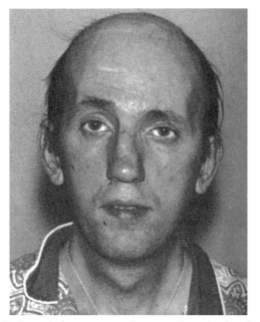

FIG. 188-1. Typical appearance in myotonic muscular dystrophy. (From Parsons M. *Color atlas of clinical neurology*, ed 2, London, 1993, Wolfe.)

COMPLICATIONS

The complications of dementia are as described in that chapter.

ETIOLOGY

Myotonic muscular dystrophy is inherited in an autosomal dominant pattern with almost 100% penetrance but quite variable expression. The gene in question, *DMPK*, is on chromosome 19 and codes for a protein kinase, and the genetic abnormality consists of an expansion of a normally occurring CTG triplet. This expansion can enlarge with succeeding generations, thus accounting for the phenomenon of anticipation, wherein the disease worsens in succeeding generations. The fundamental defect appears to affect the cellular membrane; the precise biochemical nature of this defect, however, is not known. Neuronal heterotopias, or collections of displaced neurons, have been noted in the cerebrum of some patients. Cell loss in the dorsal raphe and superior central nuclei of the upper brainstem has been noted in some patients, particularly those with hypersomnia.

DIFFERENTIAL DIAGNOSIS

Myotonia congenita is distinguished by an absence of weakness and the other typical symptoms seen in myotonia dystrophica. The PROMM syndrome (proximal myotonic myopathy) is distinguished by proximal rather than distal limb atrophy, the absence of dementia, and the presence of myalgia.

TREATMENT

There is no specific treatment for the disorder. Both modafinil and methylphenidate may relieve hypersomnolence. Various medications may relieve myotonia (phenytoin, disopyramide, procainamide and nifedipine), but, as myotonia, per se, is generally of little concern, these medications are rarely warranted, especially in light of their potential cardiac effects.

Yearly EKGs are in order, and should there be evidence of a significant arrhythmia, 24-hour monitoring is indicated. In some cases cardiac pacing may be required. These patients are prone to develop respiratory failure during anesthesia; consequently surgery must be undertaken with great care. Hearing aids may be required, as may cataract surgery.

No specific treatment is available for dementia; general measures are as outlined in that chapter.

Genetic counseling should be offered, and given the highly variable expression of the disease, it may be appropriate to offer genetic testing to apparently unaffected relatives.

BIBLIOGRAPHY

Abe K, Fujimura H, Toyooka K, et al. Involvement of the central nervous system in myotonic dystrophy. *Journal of the Neurological Sciences* 1994;127:179-185.

Batten FE, Gibb HP. Myotonia atrophica. *Brain* 1909;32:187-196.

Delaporte C. Personality patterns in patients with myotonic dystrophy. *Archives of Neurology* 1998;55:635-640.

Finlay M. A comparative study of disopyramide and procainamide in the treatment of myotonia in myotonic dystrophy. *Journal of Neurology, Neurosurgery, and Psychiatry* 1982;45:461-463.

Grant R, Sutton DL, Behan PO, et al. Nifedipine in the treatment of myotonia in myotonic dystrophy. *Journal of Neurology, Neurosurgery, and Psychiatry* 1987;50:199-206.

Huber SJ, Kissel JT, Shuttleworth EC, et al. Magnetic resonance imaging and clinical correlates of intellectual impairment in myotonic dystrophy. *Archives of Neurology* 1989;46:536-540.

MacDonald JR, Hill JD, Tarnopolsky MA. Modafinil reduces excessive somnolence and enhances mood in patients with myotonic dystrophy. *Neurology* 2002;59:1876-1880.

Mathieu J, Allard P, Potvin L, et al. A 10-year study of mortality in a cohort of patients with myotonic dystrophy. *Neurology* 1999;52:1658-1662.

Perini GI, Menegazzo E, Ermani M, et al. Cognitive impairment and (CTG)n expansion in myotonic dystrophy patients. *Biological Psychiatry* 1999;46:425-431.

Ricker K, Koch MC, Lehmann-Horn F, et al. Proximal myotonic myopathy: clinical features of a multisystem disorder similar to myotonic muscular dystrophy. *Archives of Neurology* 1995;52:25-31.

Shelbourne P, Davies J, Buxton J, et al. Direct diagnosis of myotonic dystrophy with a disease-specific DNA marker. *The New England Journal of Medicine* 1993;328:471-475.

van der Meche FG, Bogaard JM, van der Sluys JC, et al. Daytime sleep in myotonic dystrophy is not caused by sleep apnoea. *Journal of Neurology, Neurosurgery, and Psychiatry* 1994;57:626-628.

189 Amyotrophic Lateral Sclerosis

Although most patients with amyotrophic lateral sclerosis (ALS) (also known as "Lou Gehrig's disease") exhibit only the typical evidence of upper and lower motor neuron disease, a small minority, perhaps 10%, will also have a dementia.

Amyotrophic lateral sclerosis itself is more common among males than females and has a lifetime prevalence of about 4 to 6 per 100,000.

ONSET

Onset is unusual before the forties, and the prevalence rises with increasing age. The onset itself is typically gradual and insidious.

CLINICAL FEATURES

Although in most cases the dementia occurs only after more typical signs of amyotrophic lateral scelrosis are in evidence, occasionally dementia may be the presenting sign of the disease. The dementia itself often has elements of a frontal lobe syndrome, and in rare cases the frontal lobe symptoms may initially dominate the clinical picture.

Typical signs indicate involvement, as noted below, of both upper and lower motor neurons. When the corticobulbar tracts and bulbar nuclei are involved, one sees pseudobulbar palsy and atrophy and fasciculations of the tongue. When the corticospinal and anterior horn motor nuclei are involved, one sees spasticity with weakness, atrophy and fasciculations. Typically the hands are first involved, and early wasting in the hand muscles is demonstrated in Figure 189-1.

COURSE

In almost all cases, amyotrophic lateral sclerosis is relentlessly progressive, with the majority of patients succumbing within 3 years.

COMPLICATIONS

The complications of dementia are as described in that chapter; they are, however, overshadowed by the disability imposed by progressive weakness.

ETIOLOGY

In demented patients, neuronal loss and gliosis are present in the frontal and, to a lesser degree, temporal cortices. Typically, one also finds neuronal loss in the precentral gyrus, with atrophy of the

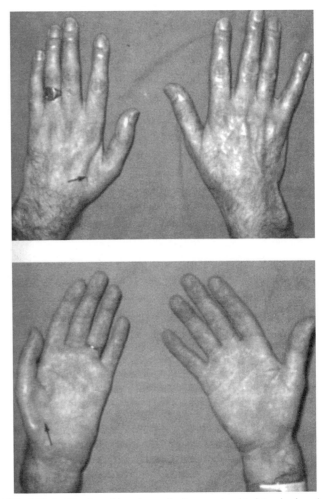

FIG. 189-1. Wasting of hand muscles in amyotrophic lateral sclerosis. (From Parsons M. *Color atlas of clinical neurology,* London, 1993, Wolfe.)

corticobulbar and corticospinal tracts and atrophy of their target neurons in the bulbar nuclei (especially the hypoglossal nucleus and dorsal motor nucleus of the vagus nerve) and anterior horn nuclei.

Almost all cases are sporadic; in the United States only about 5% are inherited in an autosomal dominant fashion. Although the actual cause of the degeneration is not known, a disturbance in excitotoxin functioning is suspected.

DIFFERENTIAL DIAGNOSIS

In those rare cases where amyotrophic lateral sclerosis presents with a dementia, consideration may be given to Pick's disease and to frontotemporal dementia; the eventual appearance of typical upper and lower motor neuron signs, however, indicates the correct diagnosis.

Rarely, an amyotrophic lateral sclerosis-like syndrome may be seen in lead or mercury poisoning or as a paraneoplastic syndrome in association with plasma cell dyscrasias or lung or renal cancer.

TREATMENT

The general treatment of dementia is as outlined in that chapter. Although no specific treatment for amyotrophic lateral sclerosis itself is available, much can be done to ease the suffering.

Riluzole may prolong life by a matter of months, but does not appreciably improve the quality of life.

Eventually, respiratory failure threatens, and patients have to decide between a trachestomy with ventilation or palliative care.

BIBLIOGRAPHY

Brownell B, Oppenheimer DR, Hughes JT. The central nervous system in motor neuron disease. *Journal of Neurology, Neurosurgery, and Psychiatry* 1970;33:338-357.

Cavalleri F, De Renzi E. Amyotrophic lateral sclerosis with dementia. *Acta Neurologica Scandinavica* 1994;89:391-394.

Ferrer I, Roig C, Espino A, et al. Dementia of the frontal lobe type and motor neuron disease: a Golgi study of the frontal cortex. *Journal of Neurology, Neurosurgery, and Psychiatry* 1991;54:932-934.

Gallagher JP. Pathologic laughter and crying in ALS: a search for their origin. *Acta Neurologica Scandinavica* 1989;80:114-117.

Horoupian DS, Thai L, Katzman R, et al. Dementia and motor neuron disease: morphometric, biochemical, and Golgi studies. *Annals of Neurology* 1984;16:305-313.

Neary D, Snowden JS, Mann DMA, et al. Frontal lobe dementia and motor neuron disease. *Journal of Neurology, Neurosurgery, and Psychiatry* 1990;53:23-32.

Peavy GM, Herzog AG, Rubin NP, et al. Neuropsychological aspects of dementia of motor neuron disease: a report of two cases. *Neurology* 1992;42:1004-1008.

190   Cerebrotendinous Xanthomatosis

Cerebrotendinous xanthomatosis is a rare, recessively inherited disorder that often causes dementia. Although also known as Van Bogaert's disease, cholestanolosis, or cholestanol storage disease, the name "cerebrotendinous xanthomatosis" is particularly felicitous as it draws attention to the concurrent appearance of xanthomas in the brain and in tendons, with tendinous involvement giving rise to one of the virtually pathognomonic signs of the disease, namely Achilles tendon enlargement.

ONSET

Onset is very gradual, and although it may occur anywhere from infancy to middle years, most patients become symptomatic in late childhood or early teenage years.

CLINICAL FEATURES

Fully developed, classic, cases are characterized by dementia, ataxia, spasticity, a peripheral sensorimotor polyneuropathy, Achilles tendon enlargement (as illustrated in Figure 190-1) and chronic, intractable diarrhea. Although the disease itself may present with any one of these features, history generally reveals that the first evidence of the disease was either juvenile cataracts or intractable diarrhea. Importantly, the overall evolution of the clinical picture is very gradual, with symptoms and signs gradually accruing over many years or even decades.

The EEG may show diffuse slowing. CT scanning typically reveals diffuse lucencies in the cerebral and cerebellar white matter,

whereas MRI scanning reveals increased signal intensity on T2-weighted scans in the same area; MRI scanning also typically reveals increased signal intensity on T2-weighted scans in the cerebellar dentate nuclei.

Serum cholestanol levels are grossly increased; cholesterol levels, however, are normal or decreased. Genetic testing is available.

COURSE

This is a very gradually progressive disorder: those with an early age of onset and severe symptoms generally succumb within 10 to 20 years, whereas those with later onsets and mild symptoms may live a normal lifespan.

COMPLICATIONS

The complications of dementia are as outlined in that chapter.

ETIOLOGY

A defect in bile acid synthesis occurs secondary to a mutation in the gene for sterol 27-hydroxylase, *CYP27*, located on the long arm of chromosome 2. Secondary to decreased activity of this enzyme, cholestanol levels are increased and cholestanol deposition occurs in the cerebrum, cerebellum, peripheral nerves, cornea and tendons. Widespread demyelinization is present in the brain, and in some cases actual xanthomas may form.

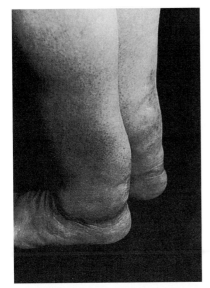

FIG. 190-1. Gross enlargement of the Achilles tendon due to xanthomatous deposits. (From Vinken PJ, Bruyn GW. *Handbook of clinical neurology*, Vol 66 (rev 22), New York, 1996, Elsevier.)

DIFFERENTIAL DIAGNOSIS

Whenever dementia occurs in the setting of juvenile cataracts, tendon enlargement or chronic diarrhea, cerebrotendinous xanthomatosis should be very high on the differential diagnosis.

Dementia occurring in the setting of ataxia may also be seen in metachromatic leukodystrophy, inhalant dependence, and, in adults, spinocerebellar ataxia and multiple system atrophy.

TREATMENT

Chenodeoxycholic acid, in a dose of approximately 750 mg daily, dramatically reduces cholestanol levels and is generally followed by an arrest of disease progression and, in many, at least partial remission. When the response to chenodeoxycholic acid is not as robust as hoped, the addition of either pravastatin, 10 mg daily, or simvastatin, 40 mg daily, may be beneficial; importantly, however,

neither of these agents, if given in isolation, is effective in this disease.

First-degree relatives should be offered genetic testing to detect heterozygotes and presymptomatic homozygotes.

BIBLIOGRAPHY

Bencze KS, Vande Polder DR, Prockop LD. Magnetic resonance imaging of the brain and spinal cord in cerebrotendinous xanthomatosis. *Journal of Neurology, Neurosurgery, and Psychiatry* 1990;53:166-167.

Berginer VM, Salenb G, Shefer S. Long-term treatment of cerebrotendinous xanthomatosis with chenodeoxycholic acid. *The New England Journal of Medicine* 1984;311:1649-1652.

Berginer VM, Berginer J, Korczyn AD, et al. Magnetic resonance imaging in cerebrotendinous xanthomatosis: a prospective clinical and radiologic study. *Journal of the Neurological Sciences* 1994;122:102-108.

Canelas HM, Quintao ECR, Scaff M, et al. Cerebrotendinous xanthomatosis: clinical and laboratory study of two cases. *Acta Neurologica Scandinavica* 1983;67:305-311.

De Stefano N, Dotti MT, Mortilla M, et al. Magnetic resonance imaging and spectroscopic changes in brains of patients with cerebrotendinous xanthomatosis. *Brain* 2001;124:121-131.

Farpour H, Mahloudji M. Familial cerebrotendinous xanthomatosis: report of a new family and review of the literature. *Archives of Neurology* 1975;32:223-225.

Meiner V, Meiner Z, Reshef A, et al. Cerebrotendinous xanthomatosis: molecular diagnosis enables presymptomatic detection of a treatable disease. *Neurology* 1994;44:288-290.

Nakamura T, Matsuzawa Y, Takemura K, et al. Combined treatment with chenodeoxycholic acid and pravastatin improves plasma cholestanol levels associated with marked regression of tendon xanthomas in cerebrotendinous xanthomatosis. *Metabolism* 1991;40:741-746.

Soffer D, Benharroch D, Berginer V. The neuropathology of cerebrotendinous xanthomatosis revisited: a case report and a review of the literature. *Acta Neuropathologica* 1995;90:213-220.

Verrips A, Wevers RA, Van Engelen BG, et al. Effect of simvastatin in addition to chenodeoxycholic acid in patients with cerebrotendinous xanthomatosis. *Metabolism* 1999;48:233-238.

Verrips A, Hoefsloot LH, Steenbergen GC, et al. Clinical and molecular genetic characteristics of patients with cerebrotendinous xanthomatosis. *Brain* 2000;123:908-919.

Verrips A, van Engelen BG, Wevers RA, et al. Presence of diarrhea and absence of tendon xanthomas in patients with cerebrotendinous xanthomatosis. *Archives of Neurology* 2000;57:520-524.

191 Adrenoleukodystrophy

Adrenoleukodystrophy is a rare, X-linked disorder characterized pathologically by the accumulation of very long chain fatty acids variously in the brain, spinal cord and adrenal glands, leading to a clinical picture that may include any or all of dementia, spasticity or adrenal failure.

ONSET

Although most patients fall ill in either childhood or adolescence, adult onset cases may also occur.

CLINICAL FEATURES

Childhood and adolescent-onset adrenoleukodystrophy typically presents with a personality change followed by dementia, which is accompanied by either a hemianopia or cortical blindness and eventually by spasticity.

Adult onset cases are typified by spinal cord involvement, generally resulting in a spastic paraparesis. Occasionally, however, adults may present with cerebral involvement, either with a dementia, or, rarely, a psychosis.

Seizures may eventually appear in about one-fifth of patients with cerebral involvement; although very long chain fatty acids also accumulate in peripheral nerves, clinical evidence of a polyneuropathy is scant.

Adrenocortical insufficiency may be so mild as to cause few symptoms; in other cases, however, one sees typical features such as anorexia, nausea, vomiting, diarrhea, and abdominal pain. Melanoderma, commonly found in skin folds, may also be present.

The EEG in cases with cerebral involvement typically shows bilaterally symmetric slowing, which is initially seen in the occipital region and gradually spreads forward.

CT scans often show bilateral lucencies in the occipital lobes that gradually spread anteriorly. Contrast enhancement is often seen at the advancing border of the lucent area, as shown in Figure 191-1. MRI scans display increased signal intensity on T2-weighted images in the same areas.

The cerebrospinal fluid often contains elevated protein.

With adrenal involvement one may see hypokalemia, decreased cortisol levels and increased ACTH levels.

The diagnosis is made by demonstrating elevated levels of very long chain fatty acids in cultured skin fibroblasts or in plasma.

Although most female carriers are asymptomatic, a minority may show mild evidence of the disease.

COURSE

In childhood-onset cases the disease is relentlessly progressive, and in a matter of years patients are left blind, demented and bed-bound; death usually occurs within three to five years.

In adult-onset cases, progression is much slower, and in some instances there may be partial remissions.

COMPLICATIONS

Complications are as described in the chapter on dementia.

ETIOLOGY

Any of a large number of mutations may occur in the *ALD* gene on the X chromosome, resulting in defective function of a peroxisomal membrane-associated protein and the accumulation of very long-chain fatty acids in the white matter of the brain or spinal cord, peripheral nerves and the adrenal cortex.

Cerebral demyelinization occurs initially in the occipital lobes, and gradually advances into the parietal and temporal lobes; the U-fibers are generally spared, as is the gray matter. An inflammatory response is seen at the boundary between the advancing demyelinization and normal white matter; behind this boundary, white matter is replaced by gliotic tissue.

DIFFERENTIAL DIAGNOSIS

In children, metachromatic leukodystrophy is suggested by ataxia, and subacute sclerosing panencephalitis by myoclonus.

In adults, MRI findings may suggest a diagnosis of progressive multiple sclerosis.

TREATMENT

Reducing dietary intake of very long-chain fatty acids is not helpful. "Lorenzo's oil," though capable of reducing the levels of very long-chain fatty acids, does not lead to clinical improvement.

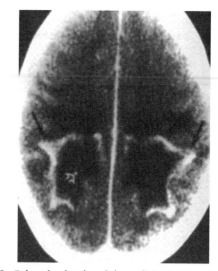

FIG. 191-1. Enhancing border of demyelinization in adrenoleukodystrophy. (From Osborn AG. *Diagnostic neuroradiology*, St. Louis, 1994, Mosby.)

Bone marrow stem-cell transplantation, if undertaken very early in the course of the disease, may halt its progression and, in some cases, be followed by partial remission.

Steroid replacement therapy may or may not be required.

Female relatives should be offered testing for very long-chain fatty acid levels.

BIBLIOGRAPHY

Coria F, Garcia-Viejo MA, Delgado JA, et al. Diagnosis of X-adrenoleukodystrophy phenotypic variants. *Acta Neurologica Scandinavica* 1993;87:499-502.

Farrell DF, Hamilston SR, Knauss TA, et al. X-linked adrenoleukodystrophy: adult cerebral variant. *Neurology* 1993;43:1518-1522.

Garside S, Rosebush PI, Levinson AJ, et al. Late-onset adrenoleukodystrophy associated with long-standing psychiatric symptoms. *The Journal of Clinical Psychiatry* 1999;60:460-468.

Moser HW, Moser AE, Singh I, et al. Adrenoleukodystrophy: survey of 303 cases: biochemistry, diagnosis, and therapy. *Annals of Neurology* 1984;16:628-641.

Schaumburg HH, Powers JM, Raine CS, et al. Adrenoleukodystrophy: a clinical and pathological study of 17 cases. *Archives of Neurology* 1975;32:577-591.

Shapiro E, Krivit W, Lockman L, et al. Long-term effect of bone-marrow transplantation for childhood-onset cerebral X-linked adrenoleukodystrophy. *Lancet* 2000;356:713-718.

van Geel RM, Assies J, Haverkort EB, et al. Progression of abnormalities in adrenomyeloneuropathy and neurologically asymptomatic X-linked adrenoleukodystrophy despite treatment with "Lorenzo's oil." *Journal of Neurology, Neurosurgery, and Psychiatry* 1999;67:290-299.

van Geel BM, Bezman L, Loes DJ, et al. Evolution of phenotypes in adult male patients with X-linked adrenoleukodystrophy. *Annals of Neurology* 2001;49:186-194.

Metachromatic leukodystrophy, first described by Alois Alzheimer, is a rare, autosomal recessively inherited disorder characterized by a deficiency of arylsulfatase A activity and an accumulation of its substrate, sulfatides, within multiple organs, including the brain, leading, in some adolescent- or adult-onset cases, to dementia or psychosis.

ONSET

Three forms are recognized, depending on the age of onset: late infantile, within the first two years of life; juvenile between the ages of 5 and early adolescence; and adult onset at any time from adolescence to the seventh decade. Regardless of the age of onset, the mode of onset is very gradual.

CLINICAL FEATURES

The late infantile form is characterized by weakness, hypotonia and seizures.

Juvenile onset cases typically present with personality change and dementia, which may be accompanied by ataxia, peripheral neuropathy and long-tract signs, such as extensor plantar responses.

The adult onset form may have a variety of presentations, including psychosis, personality change or dementia. The psychosis seen in metachromatic leukodystrophy is characterized by auditory hallucinations and bizarre delusions: importantly, such a psychosis may constitute the only evidence of the disease for years. The personality change may have certain elements of the frontal lobe syndrome, with a neglect of personal affairs, disinhibited and socially inappropriate behavior and irritability. The dementia, likewise, often has "frontal lobe" features. Regardless of which presentation occurs, most, but not all, patients, sooner or later, also develop ataxia, a peripheral neuropathy or spasticity; in a minority, seizures may also occur.

In most cases, diagnostic imaging will reveal evidence of diffuse white matter disease, manifesting as radiolucent areas on CT scanning and diffusely increased signal intensity on T2-weighted MRI scanning, as illustrated in Figure 192-1. Exceptions, however, occur, and in some cases, rather than diffuse changes, there may be bilaterally symmetric areas of lucency or increased signal intensity in the frontal and parietal lobes. Eventually, with disease progression and further destruction of white matter, extensive ventricular dilatation is seen, leaving, in some cases, only a thin rim of white matter, corresponding to the U-fibers, between the ventricles and the overlying cortex.

Nerve conduction studies almost always reveal slowing.

An often mentioned, but rarely seen, finding in metachromatic leukodystrophy is nonfilling of the gallbladder upon cholecystography, secondary to infiltration of the gallbladder by sulfatides.

The diagnosis is confirmed by finding reduced leukocyte arylsulfatase A activity and a corresponding increased sulfatide content in urinary sediment or on sural nerve biopsy.

The phenomenon of metachromasia, from which this disorder gets its name, may be seen in a variety of tissues. Both cresyl violet and toluidine blue undergo a chromatic metamorphosis, turning from violet or blue to brown or golden brown when applied to affected cells, as may be found in the urinary sediment or in the sural nerve.

COURSE

This disease is eventually fatal. Death comes within 2 to 10 years in the late infantile and juvenile forms, whereas in adult onset cases a terminal state may not be reached for 15 or more years.

COMPLICATIONS

The complications of psychosis or dementia are as described in those chapters.

ETIOLOGY

Normally, arylsulfatase A catabolizes sulfatides. In metachromatic leukodystrophy an autosomally recessively inherited defect in the activity of arylsulfatase A exists secondary to any of a large number of different mutations in the responsible gene on chromosome 22, resulting in a widespread accumulation of sulfatides, most importantly in the central and peripheral nervous system, the gallbladder epithelium, and renal epithelium. The excessive amount of these positively charged sulfatides, by reorienting the negatively charged molecules of cresyl violet or toluidine blue, gives rise to the metachromasia.

The accumulation of sulfatides leads to a widespread degeneration of the myelin sheath both centrally and peripherally. The entire white matter of the brain and cord are affected, with, in the brain, a relative sparing of the U-fibers.

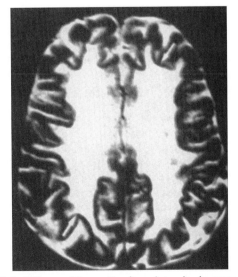

FIG. 192-1. Diffuse white matter hyperintensity in metachromatic leukodystrophy. (From Osborn AG. *Diagnostic neuroradiology*, St. Louis, 1994, Mosby.)

DIFFERENTIAL DIAGNOSIS

Adrenoleukodystrophy may be distinguished by hemianopia or cortical blindness, and subacute sclerosing panencephalitis by myoclonus. Among adults, schizophrenia may enter the differential when metachromatic leukodystrophy presents with psychosis: here, the finding of a peripheral neuropathy, ataxia or long-tract signs argues against schizophrenia and may prompt an MRI scan which, in turn, will reveal the white matter signs.

In making the diagnosis of metachromatic leukodystrophy it is important, in doubtful cases, to demonstrate not only reduced leukocyte arylsulfatase A activity but also an accumulaton of sulfatides in tissue samples. This is because there is a condition known as "pseudodeficiency" of arylsulfatase A wherein, despite a laboratory finding of reduced arylsulfatase A activity, there is, in fact, no accumulation of sulfatides.

TREATMENT

Antipsychotics may be required for psychotic symptoms, and anticonvulsants for seizures. Bone marrow transplantation may retard progression but does not alter the eventual outcome.

BIBLIOGRAPHY

Alves D, Pires MM, Guimaraes A, et al. Four cases of late onset meta-chromatic leukodystrophy in a family: clinical, biochemical and neuropathological studies. *Journal of Neurology, Neurosurgery, and Psychiatry* 1986;49:1417-1422.

Berger J, Loschl B, Bernheimer H, et al. Occurrence, distribution, and phenotype of arylsulfatase A mutations in patients with metachromatic dystrophy. *American Journal of Medical Genetics* 1997;69:335-340.

Betts TA, Smith WT, Kelly RE. Adult metachromatic leukodystrophy (sulphatide lipidosis) simulating acute schizophrenia: report of a case. *Neurology* 1968;18:1140-1142.

Finelli PF. Metachromatic leukodystrophy manifesting as a schizophrenic disorder: computed tomographic correlation. *Annals of Neurology* 1985;18:94-95.

Hageman ATM, Gabreels FJM, de Jong JGN, et al. Clinical symptoms of adult metachromatic leukodystrophy and arylsulfatase A pseudodeficiency. *Archives of Neurology* 1995;52:408-413.

Hyde TM, Ziegler JC, Weinberger DR. Psychiatric disturbances in metachromatic leukodystrophy. Insights into the neurobiology of psychosis. *Archives of Neurology* 1992;49:401-406.

Manowitz P, Kling A, Kohn H. Clinical course of metachromatic leukodystrophy presenting as schizophrenia. A report of two living cases in siblings. *The Journal of Nervous and Mental Disease* 1978;166:500-506.

Reider-Grosswasser I, Bornstein N. CT and MRI in late-onset metachromatic leucodystrophy. *Acta Neurologica Scandinavica* 1987;75:64-69.

Skomer C, Stears J, Austin J. Metachromatic leukodystrophy (MLD). XV. Adult MLD with focal lesions by computed tomography. *Archives of Neurology* 1983;40:354-355.

193 Hallervorden-Spatz Disease

Hallervorden-Spatz disease is a rare recessively inherited disorder occurring due to mutations in the gene for pantothenate kinase on chromosome 20, which presents with varied combinations of dementia and abnormal movements, most particularly dystonia.

There is controversy over the name of this disorder. Although no one disputes that it was discovered by Drs. Hallervorden and Spatz, concern has been expressed about honoring them with an eponym, given their participation in the highly unethical scientific investigations that were undertaken in Germany during the Nazi era. Whether an alternative name, such as "pantothenate kinase-associated degeneration," will gain currency is not as yet clear; for the time being then, and in the interests of clear communication among physicians, the current eponym will be used in this book.

ONSET

The onset is insidious, and although most cases manifest in childhood or adolescence, adult onset cases do occur.

CLINICAL FEATURES

The clinical picture is in part determined by the age of onset. Childhood or adolescent onset cases typically present with a slowly progressive dystonic rigidity, prominent in both the extremities and the face. Although this may initially be unilateral, as illustrated in Figure 193-1, bilateral involvement eventually occurs. Dementia follows the onset of the dystonia.

Adult onset cases may present with parkinsonism, dystonia, athetosis, chorea or dementia: eventually, over time and with progression of the disease, most patients end up with a combination of an extrapyramidal syndrome and dementia. In some cases, depression may figure prominently early in the course of the disease.

Abnormalities found on MRI scanning are highly distinctive and may be present before any clinical evidence of the disease. Typically, in the globus pallidus bilaterally there is, on T2-weighted images, decreased signal intensity in the lateral portion combined with increased signal intensity in the medial portion, yielding the striking "eye of the tiger" sign.

COURSE

The illness progressively worsens, with death occurring in from 10 to 15 years.

COMPLICATIONS

The complications of dementia are as described in that chapter.

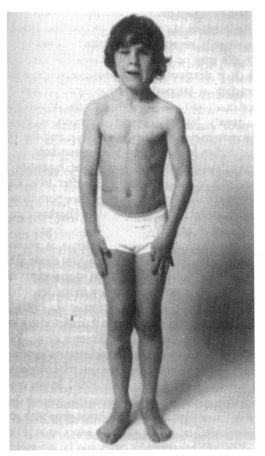

FIG. 193-1. Facial and upper extremity dystonic rigidity in Hallervorden-Spatz disease. (From Swaiman KF, ed. *Pediatric neurology: principles and practice*, vol 1, ed 2, St. Louis, 1994, Mosby.)

prominent in the globus pallidus, it also occurs in the pars reticulata of the substantia nigra and in the cerebral cortex.

DIFFERENTIAL DIAGNOSIS

In children and adolescents, the prominent dystonia may suggest Wilson's disease, dopa-responsive dystonia and primary torsion dystonia. Adult onset cases, when characterized by dementia and abnormal movements, may suggest Wilson's disease or corticobasal-ganglionic degeneration. In some cases, the differential may rest on finding the distinctive "eye of the tiger" sign on MRI scanning.

TREATMENT

Although there are no blinded treatment studies, empirical trials with standard agents for the various abnormal movements are probably justified; some cases with prominent dystonia have been helped by thalamotomy.

BIBLIOGRAPHY

Angellini L, Nardocci N, Rumi V, et al. Hallervorden-Spatz disease: clinical and MRI study of 11 cases diagnosed in life. *Journal of Neurology* 1992;239:417-425.

Cooper GE, Rizzo M, Jones RD. Adult-onset Hallervorden-Spatz syndrome presenting as cortical dementia. *Alzheimer Disease and Associated Disorders* 2000;14:120-126.

Dooling EC, Schoene WC, Richardson EP. Hallervorden-Spatz syndrome. *Archives of Neurology* 1974;30:70-83.

Grimes DA, Lange AE, Bergeron C. Late adult onset chorea with typical pathology of Hallervorden-Spatz syndrome. *Journal of Neurology, Neurosurgery, and Psychiatry* 2000;69:392-395.

Hayflick SJ, Westaway SK, Levinson B, et al. Genetic, clinical, and radiographic delineation of Hallervorden-Spatz syndrome. *The New England Journal of Medicine* 2003;348:33-40.

Jankovic J, Kirkpatrick JB, Blomquist KA, et al. Late-onset Hallervorden-Spatz disease presenting as familial parkinsonism. *Neurology* 1985;35:227-234.

Morphy MA, Feldman JA, Kilburn G. Hallervorden-Spatz disease in a psychiatric setting. *The Journal of Clinical Psychiatry* 1989;50:66-68.

Shevell MI, Peiffer J. Julius Hallervorden's wartime activities: implications for science under dictatorship. *Pediatric Neurology* 2001;25:162-165.

Zhou B, Westaway SK, Levinson B, et al. A novel pantothenate kinase gene (*PANK2*) is defective in Hallervorden-Spatz syndrome. *Nature Genetics* 2001;28:345-349.

ETIOLOGY

As noted earlier, this recessively inherited disorder occurs secondary to mutations in the gene, *PANK2*, located on chromosome 20, leading to reduced activity of pantothenate kinase.

Macroscopically, the globus pallidus is atrophic, and exhibits a rust-brown discoloration. Microscopically, one sees neuronal loss, axonal spheroids and iron deposition, and although this is most

194 Von Recklinghausen's Disease

Von Recklinghausen's disease, also known as neurofibromatosis type I or "peripheral" neurofibromatosis, is a genetic disorder characterized by the appearance of café-au-lait spots and multiple neurofibromas. The neurofibromas may arise from the peripheral nerves or from the cranial nerves, either from their central or peripheral portions.

This is a not uncommon disorder, with a prevalence of perhaps 1 in 3000. It is equally common among males and females.

Astrocytomas and meningiomas, along with multiple other types of tumors, may be found in association with von Recklinghausen's disease. Mental retardation occurs in a small minority, and other children may have developmental disabilities or hyperactivity.

ONSET

Café-au-lait spots are present at birth and tend to become more prominent throughout adolescence. The neurofibromas, although occasionally apparent in infancy, are more likely to become apparent in early adolescence and to enlarge in early adult years. Other tumors, such as astrocytomas or meningiomas, may develop from late childhood into adult years.

CLINICAL FEATURES

Café-au-lait spots and Lisch nodules of the iris are universally present in adults, and axillary freckles may also be seen. The peripheral neurofibromas, which may occur anywhere, are most common on the trunk. They range in size from a grain of sand up to a walnut or larger. Some patients have only a few; in other cases there may literally be thousands. They may be sessile or polypoid; occasionally plexiform neurofibromas are seen that may grow to become enormous and extremely disfiguring. Neurofibromas may be painful to strong touch; occasionally, neuralgic pains may occur. Figure 194-1 shows a 12-year-old patient with both café-au-lait spots and truncal neurofibromas.

Neurofibromas occurring on the central portions of the peripheral nerves or on the cranial nerves may compress adjacent structures, such as the cord or the brain stem.

Anywhere from 5% to 10% of patients may be mentally retarded, and a higher percentage have one or more of the developmental disabilities, such as dyslexia. There is also a higher than expected prevalence of attention deficit/hyperactivity. Skeletal abnormalities, especially kyphoscoliosis, occur in a minority.

Astrocytomas and meningiomas are not uncommon and present with otherwise typical symptoms. Optic gliomas may occur in up to a quarter of all patients. Hamartomas of the hypothalamus are occasionally seen and may lead to premature puberty. Extracranial tumors, such as pheochromocytomas, leukemia, and Wilms' tumor, also have been noted. Occasionally the peripheral neurofibromas themselves may enlarge with sarcomatous change, and this may be heralded by an increasing pain. Seizures may occur in a minority of patients.

MRI scanning generally reveals scattered areas of increased signal intensity on T2-weighted scans, most particularly in the globus pallidus, cerebellar white matter, internal capsule and cerebral white matter. Although controversial, there may be an association between the number of these areas and the presence of cognitive deficits. Interestingly, as patients age into adult years, the number and size of these areas actually decrease.

COURSE

After a period of progression during adolescence, the course of the peripheral neurofibromas is often marked by long periods of quiescence in adulthood, often lasting many years. Renewed growth, however, may occur during pregnancy or with use of oral contraceptive agents, or, in either sex, may occur unpredictably.

Von Recklinghausen's disease is generally not fatal; should death occur, it is usually due to the occurrence of one of the other tumors noted above.

COMPLICATIONS

Embarrassment and shame are in direct proportion to the visibility of the disfiguring lesions. The complications of mental retardation, developmental disabilities, and hyperactivity are as described in their respective chapters.

ETIOLOGY

As much as one half of all cases may be due to spontaneous mutations. In the rest, von Recklinghausen's disease is inherited as an autosomal dominant trait with almost complete penetrance but with great variability in clinical expression even within the same family. The gene is located on chromosome 17 and codes for a protein named neurofibromin. In some cases signs and symptoms may be so mild as to escape detection, and this may account for the apparent "skipping" of generations.

The neurofibromas themselves are apparently derived from Schwann cells and contiguous fibroblasts.

In some cases one also finds scattered glial nodules, neuronal heterotopias or white matter spongiotic changes, and these lesions

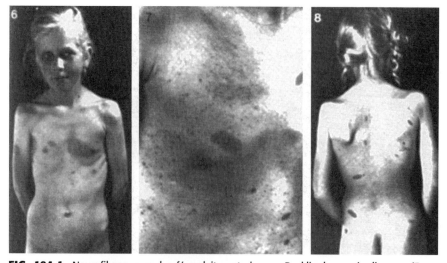

FIG. 194-1. Neurofibromas and café-au-lait spots in von Recklinghausen's disease. (From Weidemann HR, Kunze J, Dibbern H. *Atlas of clinical syndromes: a visual aid to diagnosis,* ed 2, London, 1992, Wolfe.)

may account for the areas of increased signal intensity seen on MRI scanning.

DIFFERENTIAL DIAGNOSIS

The diagnosis is self-evident when large numbers of neurofibromas are present. In cases where these are lacking or undetectable, cutaneous manifestations are extremely valuable diagnostic signs. Axillary freckling is almost pathognomonic. Café-au-lait spots may occur in normal individuals; however, the presence of six or more spots reliably indicates the presence of von Recklinghausen's disease.

Neurofibromatosis type II is a rare disorder with a prevalence of about one in a million. It is genetically distinct from von Recklinghausen's disease, or neurofibromatosis type I, and is inherited in an autosomal dominant pattern with the gene being located on chromosome 22. Often called "central" neurofibromatosis, this disorder is characterized by the development of bilateral acoustic neuromas. Meningiomas may also occur. Cutaneous manifestations are sparse and may be totally absent.

TREATMENT

Since excision of peripheral neurofibromas may predispose to sarcomatous change, such treatment should be reserved for unacceptably disfiguring lesions. Central neurofibromas likewise do not require removal unless they compress other tissues. Other tumors are treated in the usual fashion.

Developmental disabilities, attention-deficit/hyperactivity, and mental retardation are treated as outlined in those chapters.

Genetic counseling should be offered; given the variability of clinical expression possible within the same family, patients with minimal symptoms should be warned of the possibility that a child may be severely affected.

BIBLIOGRAPHY

DiMario FJ, Ramsby G. Magnetic resonance imaging lesion analysis in neurofibromatosis type 1. *Archives of Neurology* 1998;55:500-505.

DiPaolo DP, Zimmerman RA, Rorke LB, et al. Neurofibromatosis type I: pathologic substrate of high-signal-intensity foci in the brain. *Radiology* 1995;195:721-724.

Huson SN, Harper PS, Compston DAS. Von Recklinghausen neurofibromatosis: a clinical and population study in south-east Wales. *Brain* 1988;111:1355-1381.

Legius E, Descheemaeker MJ, Steyaert A, et al. Neurofibromatosis type 1 in childhood: correlation of MRI findings with intelligence. *Journal of Neurology, Neurosurgery, and Psychiatry* 1995;59:638-640.

North K, Joy P, Yuille D, et al. Specific learning disability in children with neurofibromatosis type 1: significance of MRI abnormalities. *Neurology* 1994;44:878-883.

Rosman NP, Pearce J. The brain in multiple neurofibromatosis (von Recklinghausen's disease): a suggested neuropathological basis for the associated mental defect. *Brain* 1967;90:829-837.

195 Multi-infarct Dementia

Multiple large cortical or subcortical infarcts may cause a dementia that is associated with multiple "focal" signs, such as aphasia or hemiplegia, and, classically, with a "stepwise" downhill course. Although accurate prevalence figures are not available, this is probably a common cause of dementia in the elderly.

A word of caution may be in order here regarding nomenclature. Of the vascular conditions capable of causing a dementia, three stand out as being relatively common. First, there may be multiple, relatively large, ischemic infarctions in either cortical or subcortical areas, due primarily to large vessel disease. Second, there may be multiple small subcortical "lacunar" infarctions, due to small vessel disease. Third, and finally, there may be widespread rarefaction and demyelinization of the cerebral white matter, again due to small vessel disease. The dementias caused by these three different conditions have received various names, and it is critical, in reading the literature, to closely examine the definition used by the authors. In this book, the first condition is referred to as "multi-infarct dementia," the second as "lacunar dementia" and the third as "Binswanger's disease."

ONSET

The onset is typically in the fifties or sixties and in many cases there is a history of typical "strokes" with various presentations, such as aphasia, apraxia, hemiplegia and the like. The actual onset of the dementia may be abrupt, if there is a large, strategically placed infarction, or more fluctuating and gradual, if the dementia rests on the serial occurrence of several smaller, and less strategically placed, infarctions.

CLINICAL FEATURES

Although some patients may present with an otherwise unremarkable dementia, with typical deficits in short-term memory, abstracting ability, orientation, and the like, in many cases the dementia is marked by depression, agitation, hallucinations and delusions. Depression may be heavily tinged with irritability, and agitation at times may be severe. Hallucinations are generally visual, and delusions tend to be either of persecution or misidentification.

Upon examination, other evidence of focal lesions is found, including varying degrees of hemiplegia, hemianopia, aphasia, apraxia, neglect and the like. Late in the course, pseudobulbar palsy, as described in that chapter, may appear, and seizures may likewise occur.

Because most cases are secondary to arteriosclerosis, general examination typically reveals hypertension and signs of arteriosclerosis, such as bruits, reduced pulses, and so forth. However, one should also be alert to the possible presence of signs of rare causes of multi-infarct dementia, such as polyarteritis nodosa, systemic lupus erythematosus, and the like.

MRI or CT scanning generally reveals evidence of multiple cortical infarcts, as demonstrated in the CT scan shown in Figure 195-1.

COURSE

As noted earlier, the classic course of multi-infarct dementia is one of stepwise deterioration. With each fresh lesion, an abrupt deterioration occurs, after which, as there is some neuronal recovery from the insult, one may see partial improvement with a new plateau being maintained until the next lesion forces the patient down yet another "step." Many patients, however, rather than a clear-cut "stepwise" course, may evidence a more gradual deterioration.

Intercurrent delirium is common in multi-infarct dementia. In patients with a "stepwise" course, each "step" down may be characterized by a delirium, which in turn reflects the effects of peri-infarction edema. Furthermore, these patients, having lost most of their cerebral "reserve," are prone to develop delirium in the face of what, in other patients, would be trivial insults, as for example bronchitis or various over-the-counter medications.

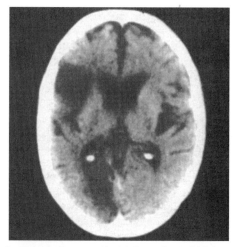

FIG. 195-1. Multiple large cortical infarcts in multi-infarct dementia. (From Perkin GD, Hochberg FH, Miller DC. *Atlas of clinical neurology*, ed 2, London, 1993, Wolfe.)

The duration of the disease ranges from months to decades. At the end, the patient's condition may have deteriorated to the point of requiring total care. Death often occurs due to either a large cerebral lesion or to some other sequela of arteriosclerosis, such as a myocardial infarction.

COMPLICATIONS

The complications of multi-infarct dementia, in general, are as discussed in the chapter on dementia. The pronounced affective changes, especially irritability, often necessitate hospitalization.

ETIOLOGY

At autopsy, there is evidence of multiple, scattered, and generally bilateral infarctions or intra-cerebral hemorrhages. Occasionally, only a few large lesions may occur, and even more rarely there may be only one "strategic" lesion, as for example a large infarction in the hippocampus and related structures.

In the vast majority of cases, lesions are secondary to arteriosclerosis or to emboli, originating from either the heart or large vessels. "Watershed" infarctions, occurring at the critical juncture of two or more arterial systems during episodes of hypotension, may be more common than is currently appreciated.

Far less common causes of infarcts include systemic lupus erythematosus, polyarteritis nodosa, cranial arteritis, migraine, vasculitis secondary to cocaine or amphetamines, meningovascular neurosyphilis, tuberculous meningitis, thrombocytopenic purpura, and hypercoagulable or hyperviscosity syndromes.

Mention should be made at this point of a "static" form of multi-infarct dementia, which may occur as a single event. Some causes of such acute-onset, multifocal and bilateral lesions are as follows: hypertensive encephalopathy, disseminated intravascular coagulation, and multifocal arterial spasm in subarachnoid hemorrhage. In such cases, unless one sees a recurrence of the underlying condition, the course of the dementia is stable and not stepwise as described above.

DIFFERENTIAL DIAGNOSIS

The early appearance of focal signs serves to differentiate multi-infarct dementia from Alzheimer's disease; it must be borne in mind, however, that many patients have a "mixed" dementia, with contributions not only from multiple infarcts but also Alzheimer's disease. Furthermore, it is not uncommon to see individual patients with a mixture of vascular pathology, including not only large infarctions but also lacunes and diffuse white matter disease.

Importantly, finding one or more infarcts in a demented patient does not necessarily mean that a patient's dementia is of the multi-infarct type. Indeed most stroke patients are not demented. However, the probability of dementia increases if there are numerous bilateral strokes involving more or less strategic areas, such as the frontal, parietal, or temporal lobes. Conversely, if the patient had only one stroke in a "non-strategic" area, such as the occipital lobe, one would be hard pressed to attribute a dementia in such a patient to a stroke.

TREATMENT

The general therapy of the demented patient is as described in that chapter. Antidepressants may be useful when depression is pervasive. Owing to the risk of watershed infarction, agents liable to cause hypotension are to be avoided, and in this regard an SSRI, such as citalopram or escitalopram, is a reasonable choice. Antipsychotics may help reduce confusion, delusions, irritability, and lability; again, agents liable to produce hypotension are in general to be avoided. Haloperidol or risperidone, in low doses, are reasonable first choices. There is suggestive evidence that memantine and donepezil may be helpful, and either one may be worthy of trial.

Concurrent with symptomatic treatment, the underlying cause should be treated, and consideration should be given to the use of clopidogrel or a combination of aspirin and dipyridamole.

BIBLIOGRAPHY

Binetti G, Bianchetti A, Padovani A, et al. Delusions in Alzheimer's disease and multi-infarct dementia. *Acta Neurologica Scandinavica* 1993;88:5-9.

Erkinjuntti T, Haltia M, Palo J, et al. Accuracy of the clinical diagnosis of vascular dementia: a prospective clinical and post-mortem neuropathological study. *Journal of Neurology, Neurosurgery, and Psychiatry* 1988;51:1037-1044.

Gorelick PB, Chatterjee A, Patel D, et al. Cranial computed tomographic observations in multi-infarct dementia. A controlled study. *Stroke* 1992;23:804-811.

Huletter C, Nochlin D, McKeel D, et al. Clinical-neuropathological findings in multi-infarct dementia: a report of six autopsied cases. *Neurology* 1997;48:668-672.

Jayakumar PN, Taly AB, Shanmugam V, et al. Multi-infarct dementia: a computed tomographic study. *Acta Neurologica Scandinavica* 1989;73:292-295.

Meyer JS, Chowdhury MH, Xu G, et al. Donepezil treatment of vascular dementia. *Annals of the New York Academy of Sciences* 2002;977:482-486.

Ladurna G, Iliff LD, Lechner H. Clinical factors associated with dementia in ischemic stroke. *Journal of Neurology, Neurosurgery, and Psychiatry* 1982;45:97-101.

Orgogozo JM, Rigaud AS, Stoffler A, et al. Efficacy and safety of memantine in patients with mild to moderate vascular dementia: a randomized, placebo-controlled trial (MMM 300). *Stroke* 2002;33:1834-1839.

Wilcock G, Mobius HJ, Stoffler A. A double-blind, placebo-controlled multicentre study of memantine in mid to moderate vascular dementia (MMM 500). *International Clinical Psychopharmacology* 2002;17:297-305.

The lacunar state is characterized by the presence of multiple bilateral cystic infarctions scattered in the cerebral white matter, basal ganglia, internal capsule, thalamus, and brain stem. If these cystic lesions, or lacunae, are sufficiently numerous and properly situated, then the lacunar state will give rise to a dementia.

The prevalence and sex ratio of lacunar dementia are unknown. The clinical impression, however, is that it is not rare.

ONSET

The onset appears to be gradual and appears to occur in the fifties or sixties.

CLINICAL FEATURES

In general the dementia is of the "frontal lobe" type with symptoms such as apathy, lack of initiative, and forgetfulness. Affective lability may occur, as may episodes of confusion. Associated findings include urinary incontinence and a grasp reflex.

Before the onset of the dementia, and persisting concurrent with it, one may find one or more of the "lacunar syndromes," including dysarthria-clumsy hand, ataxic hemiparesis, pure motor hemiplegia, and pure sensory stroke.

As further lacunar infarctions occur, pseudobulbar palsy, as described in that chapter, occurs quite commonly.

CT scanning is only about one-half as sensitive as routine T1- and T2-weighted MRI scanning; in the case of MRI scanning, gadolinium enhancement may indicate which lacunes are "fresh"; however, diffusion-weighted scanning is far more sensitive in this regard.

COURSE

Lacunar dementia is a progressive condition, and although most patients display a more or less gradual worsening, in some there may be a "step-wise" course, with a relatively abrupt deterioration corresponding to a fresh lacunar infarction.

COMPLICATIONS

Complications are as described in the chapters on dementia and on pseudobulbar palsy.

ETIOLOGY

Lacunae, which, as noted earlier, are found in the cerebral white matter, basal ganglia, internal capsule, thalamus, and brain stem, are small fluid-filled cysts ranging in size from 2 to 20 mm. The specimen shown in Figure 196-1 demonstrates multiple lacunae in the basal ganglia and centrum semiovale. These are presumed to represent infarctions in the territories of small penetrating vessels secondary to lipohyalinosis or arteriosclerotic changes in those vessels or, in a minority of cases, to emboli. In general, dementia does not appear until perhaps a dozen or more lacunae have accumulated; however, one may, at times, see a dementia after only one or a few lacunar infarctions, provided these are in "strategic" areas, such as the thalamus.

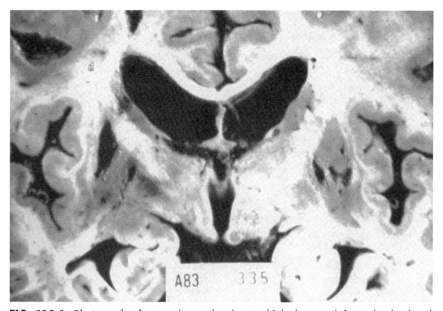

FIG. 196-1. Photograph of a specimen showing multiple lacunar infarcts in the basal ganglia and centrum semiovale. (From Nelson JS, Parisi JE, Schochet SS. *Principles and practice of neuropathology*, St. Louis, 1993, Mosby.)

DIFFERENTIAL DIAGNOSIS

The early presence of the focal deficits of the "lacunar syndromes," noted earlier, and, if present, a "step-wise" course, differentiate lacunar dementia from Alzheimer's disease, normal pressure hydrocephalus and Binswanger's disease. Multi-infarct dementia, on clinical grounds, may be difficult to distinguish, and the differential may rest on MRI scanning. Furthermore, it must be borne in mind that many patients with lacunes will also have other vascular lesions, such as the large cortical infarctions seen in multi-infarct dementia and the demyelinization of Binswanger's disease.

TREATMENT

The general treatment of dementia is as outlined in that chapter. Antidepressants may be useful for depression, antipsychotics for confusion or delusions and hallucinations. Agents likely to cause hypotension and reduce flow in the penetrating arterioles are to be avoided. Consequently, if an antidepressant is required, an SSRI or nortriptyline may be chosen, and if an antipsychotic is required, an agent such as haloperidol or one of the second-generation antipsychotics should be considered. Conditions predisposing to vascular disease, such as diabetes mellitus, hyperlipidemia and hypertension, should be controlled, and it is prudent to add either enteric-coated aspirin, an aspirin/dipyridamole combination or clopidogrel.

BIBLIOGRAPHY

Fukuda H, Kobayashi S, Okada K, et al. Frontal white matter lesions and dementia in lacunar infarction. *Stroke* 1990;21:1143-1149.

Ishii N, Nishihara Y, Imamura T. Why do frontal lobe symptoms predominate in vascular dementia with lacunes? *Neurology* 1986;36:340-345.

Katz DI, Alexander MP, Mandell AM. Dementia following strokes in the mesencephalon and diencephalon. *Archives of Neurology* 1987;44: 1127-1133.

Lindgren A, Staaf G, Geijer B, et al. Clinical lacunar syndromes as predictors of lacunar infarcts. A comparison of acute clinical lacunar syndromes and findings on diffusion-weighted MRI. *Acta Neurologica Scandinavica* 2000;101:128-134.

Loeb C, Gandolfo C, Croce R, et al. Dementia associated with lacunar infarction. *Stroke* 1992;23:1225-1229.

Regli L, Regli F, Maeder P, et al. Magnetic resonance imaging with gadolinium contrast agent in small deep (lacunar) cerebral infarcts. *Archives of Neurology* 1993;50:175-180.

Stapf C, Hofmeister C, Hartmann A, et al. Predictive value of clinical lacunar syndromes for lacunar infarcts on magnetic resonance imaging. *Acta Neurologica Scandinavica* 2000;101:13-18.

Weisberg LA. Lacunar infarcts. *Archives of Neurology* 1982;39:37.

Wolfe N, Linn R, Babikian VL, et al. Frontal system impairment following multiple lacunar infarcts. *Archives of Neurology* 1990;47:129-132.

197 Binswanger's Disease

Binswanger's disease, first described by Otto Binswanger in 1894, is characterized pathologically by a wide-spread arteriolopathy and bilateral areas of demyelinization in the centrum semiovale, and clinically by a gradually progressive dementia. Methodologic difficulties have precluded reliable estimates as to sex ratio or prevalence; however, it is probably not as rare as has been reported.

Binswanger's disease is also known as subcortical arteriosclerotic encephalopathy, chronic progressive subcortical encephalopathy, or encephalitis subcorticalis chronica progressiva.

ONSET

The onset is gradual and insidious, usually occurring in the fifties and sixties.

CLINICAL FEATURES

When patients finally come to medical attention, the clinical picture is generally characterized by forgetfulness, inattention, concrete thinking, and often a certain degree of depression. In more advanced cases one may see disorientation, a degree of confusion, at times delusions that are often persecutory, and hallucinations that tend to be visual. Agitation may occasionally be seen.

On examination minor focal deficits may or may not be present. An extensor plantar response or asymmetric deep tendon reflexes may be observed. Rarely, however, one may find a notable hemiplegia or a pronounced aphasia. In advanced cases, pseudobulbar palsy, as described in that chapter, may occur.

CT scans may reveal periventricular lucencies in the centrum semiovale. T2-weighted MRI scanning is far more sensitive, revealing multiple bilateral patchy areas of increased signal intensity in the same area, as shown in Figure 197-1.

COURSE

Although in most cases dementia is relentlessly progressive, in some cases temporary "plateaus" may occur.

COMPLICATIONS

Complications are as described in the chapter on dementia.

ETIOLOGY

At autopsy, examination of the centrum semiovale reveals numerous areas of demyelinization with varying degrees of gliosis; occasionally, cystic areas may also be seen. There is usually a degree of ventricular dilation. The cortical gray matter is spared. Lacunar infarcts, as described in the chapter on lacunar dementia, occasionally may be seen, and, less commonly, large cortical infarctions may also be present.

Examination of the vasculature reveals lipohyalinosis of the small penetrating arterioles. The larger vessels at the base of the brain may or may not display atherosclerotic changes.

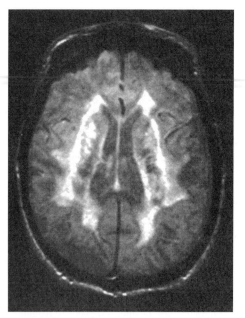

FIG. 197-1. Multiple, patchy, confluent areas of increased signal intensity in Binswanger's disease. (From Perkin GD, Hochberg FH, Miller DC. *Atlas of clinical neurology*, ed 2, London, 1993, Wolfe.)

Currently, demyelinization is thought to be secondary to arteriolar insufficiency, causing partial infarctions. The cause of the arteriolopathy, however, is not exactly clear; although most patients with Binswanger's disease are hypertensive, identical changes may be seen in normotensive patients.

DIFFERENTIAL DIAGNOSIS

The slow and gradually progressive course of Binswanger's disease often suggests Alzheimer's disease, and at times differentiating the two may be difficult. The appearance of minor focal signs relatively early in the course suggests Binswanger's disease, as would the appearance of a typical leukoencephalopathy on MRI scanning. Such a finding, however, is also typical of cerebral amyloid angiopathy, and the critical differential diagnosis between these two conditions is discussed further in that chapter.

Normal pressure hydrocephalus may mimic Binswanger's disease. Here, however, the early onset of apraxia of gait and of urinary incontinence, coupled with a prominent degree of ventricular enlargement, would serve to suggest the correct diagnosis.

Symmetric periventricular hyperintensity or ventricular "capping" on MRI scanning is not suggestive of Binswanger's disease and may indeed have little or no clinical significance. Furthermore, one may normally find a few small, scattered areas of increased signal intensity in the centrum semiovale of elderly nondemented patients.

TREATMENT

Treatment is similar to that described for lacunar dementia.

BIBLIOGRAPHY

Bennet DA, Wilson RS, Gilley DW, et al. Clinical diagnosis of Binswanger's disease. *Journal of Neurology, Neurosurgery, and Psychiatry* 1990; 53:961-965.

Bogucki A, Janczewska E, Koszewska I, et al. Evaluation of dementia in subcortical arteriosclerotic encephalopathy (Binswanger's disease). *European Archives of Psychiatry and Clinical Neuroscience* 1991;241: 91-97.

Caplan LR, Schoene WC. Clinical features of subcortical arteriosclerotic encephalopathy (Binswanger's disease). *Neurology* 1978;28: 1206-1215.

Kinkel WR, Jacobs L, Polachini I, et al. Subcortical arteriosclerotic encephalopathy (Binswanger's disease). Computed tomographic, nuclear magnetic resonance, and clinical correlations. *Archives of Neurology* 1985;42:951-959.

Lin JX, Tomimoto H, Akiguchi I, et al. Vascular cell components of the medullary arteries in Binswanger's disease brains: a morphometric and immunoelectron microscopic study. *Stroke* 2000;31:1838-1842.

Loizou LA, Kendall BE, Marshall J. Subcortical arteriosclerotic encephalopathy: a clinical and radiological investigation. *Journal of Neurology, Neurosurgery, and Psychiatry* 1981;44:294-304.

Revesz T, Hawkins CP, du Boulay EP, et al. Pathological findings correlated with magnetic resonance imaging in subcortical arteriosclerotic encephalopathy (Binswanger's disease). *Journal of Neurology, Neurosurgery, and Psychiatry* 1989;52:1337-1344.

Roman GC. Senile dementia of the Binswanger type: a vascular form of dementia in the elderly. *The Journal of the American Medical Association* 1987;258:1782-1788.

Rosenberg GA, Cornfield M, Stovring J, et al. Subcortical arteriosclerotic encephalopathy (Binswanger's disease): computerized tomography. *Neurology* 1979;29:1102-1106.

Tomonaga M, Yamanouchi H, Tohgi H, et al. Clinicopathologic study of progressive subcortical vascular encephalopathy (Binswanger type) in the elderly. *Journal of the American Geriatrics Society* 1982;30: 524-529.

198 Polyarteritis Nodosa

Polyarteritis nodosa, or, as it is sometimes called, periarteritis nodosa, is a rare disorder characterized by a widespread, segmental, necrotizing panarteritis principally involving medium and small arteries. Almost any organ, except the lung, may be damaged by numerous areas of infarction in the territory supplied by the affected artery. The central nervous system is affected in about one quarter of the cases, presenting often as either a delirium or dementia.

ONSET

Although the disease may occur at any age, most patients fall ill in their late forties. The onset itself may range from gradual and insidious to acute.

CLINICAL FEATURES

As a rule, by the time central nervous system involvement becomes clinically apparent, the patient is already ill with either constitutional symptoms, such as fever, malaise, or weight loss, or symptoms referable to other organs, most commonly the kidneys, gastrointestinal tract, or musculoskeletal system.

Dementia or delirium may occur, and these do not appear to have any distinctive clinical features. Other common symptoms referable to the central nervous system include headaches, seizures, and localizing signs, such as hemiplegia, depending on the location of the infarct. Occasionally, subarachnoid hemorrhage may occur.

Significant renal disease may lead to severe hypertension, possibly with a hypertensive encephalopathy, or to renal failure, with a uremic encephalopathy.

Peripheral nervous system involvement may present as a sensorimotor mononeuritis multiplex that in time may evolve into a somewhat asymmetric polyneuropathy.

Anemia may occur secondary to gastrointestinal blood loss or as an "anemia of chronic disease." Leukocytosis is seen, often over 20,000; eosinophilia generally is not seen. The erythrocyte sedimentation rate is generally elevated. If the kidneys are affected, hematuria and proteinuria may be found. One may see a false positive VDRL.

The EEG may show diffuse slowing, or, if a large infarct has occurred, localized slowing may be seen. CT and MRI scanning may reveal multiple infarcts. The cerebrospinal fluid is usually unremarkable unless a subarachnoid hemorrhage has occurred. Arteriography may reveal multiple aneurysmal dilatations. Definitive diagnosis is made by biopsy of affected tissue, often muscle, peripheral nerve, or testis.

COURSE

Although spontaneous remissions do occur, they are rare, and in most cases there is a relentless or even fulminant progression to death, with only 10 to 20% of patients still alive after five years.

COMPLICATIONS

Complications are as described in the chapters on dementia and on delirium.

ETIOLOGY

With the exception of those serving the lungs, almost any medium or small artery may become inflamed. The intima may proliferate, leading to thrombosis and infarction, or nodular fibrosis may occur, thus giving affected arteries a "nodose" character. The muscular layer may become sufficiently weakened that aneurysms form, which are then liable to rupture.

Within the brain, multiple infarcts and hemorrhages are found scattered throughout the cortex, white matter, basal ganglia, and brain stem. Although large arteries are generally not involved, involvement of the middle cerebral and basilar arteries has been reported.

The cause of this widespread arteritis is not known; however, an immune mechanism is strongly suspected. This appears especially to be the case when polyarteritis nodosa is associated with hepatitis B antigenemia, wherein immune complex deposition has been noted on affected arteries.

DIFFERENTIAL DIAGNOSIS

The diagnosis of polyarteritis nodosa is often entertained when a patient presents with a febrile multisystem illness. Systemic lupus erythematosus may be differentiated by serologic testing; Wegener's granulomatosis is distinguished by involvement of the upper respiratory tract and the sinuses.

TREATMENT

Prednisone, in a dose of 40 to 60 mg/day, may afford symptomatic relief and, when combined with cyclophosphamide, has been reported to induce remission.

BIBLIOGRAPHY

Ford RG, Siekert RG. Central nervous system manifestations of periarteritis nodosa. *Neurology* 1965;15:114-122.

Nadeau SE. Neurologic manifestations of systemic vasculitis. *Neurologic Clinics* 2002;20:123-150.

Oran I, Memis A, Parildar M, et al. Multiple intracranial aneurysms in polyarteritis nodosa: MRI and angiography. *Neuroradiology* 1999;41: 436-439.

Provenzale JM, Allen NB. Neuroradiologic findings in polyarteritis nodosa. *American Journal of Neuroradiology* 1996;17:1119-1126.

Takahashi JC, Sakai N, Iihara K, et al. Subarachnoid hemorrhage from a ruptured anterior cerebral artery aneurysm caused by polyarteritis nodosa. Case Report. *Journal of Neurosurgery* 2002;96:132-134.

199 Cranial Arteritis

Cranial arteritis, also known as temporal arteritis or giant cell arteritis, is a condition characterized by inflammation of certain large, principally cranial, arteries producing symptoms in keeping with the vascular territories involved. Most commonly, the superficial temporal artery is involved; however, other branches of the external carotid artery may be affected, including the occipital and facial arteries, as may branches of the internal carotid artery, most especially the ophthalmic artery; other arteries involved less often are the vertebral arteries and the coronary arteries.

Although headache, visual loss, and constitutional symptoms are by far the most common symptoms of cranial arteritis, some 5% to 10% of patients also develop cerebral infarction.

This is a relatively uncommon disorder that is seen primarily in caucasians, especially those of Nordic descent.

ONSET

Onset before the age of 50 is rare, and the prevalence rises with increasing age. The onset itself may be gradual or subacute.

CLINICAL FEATURES

Cranial arteritis typically presents with a temporal headache in the setting of constitutional symptoms, such as malaise, anorexia, fatigue and low-grade fever. The headache is generally unilateral, and the underlying temporal artery may be tender and inflamed. More posteriorly located headaches may occur if the superficial occipital artery is affected. Involvement of the facial artery may lead to jaw "claudication" wherein jaw pain occurs with chewing. When the ophthalmic artery is involved, visual loss or blindness may occur.

Most patients will also have an associated polymyalgia rheumaticia, with diffuse muscle aching and stiffness, most marked in the neck and shoulders.

Involvement of the posterior, middle or anterior cerebral arteries, or the vertebral arteries, or their branches may cause ischemia or infarction, with the production of a delirium or a dementia.

Although exceptions occur, the erythrocyte sedimentation rate is generally elevated over 50 mm/minute (Westergren), often to 100 or higher. Mild anemia may be evident and a mild elevation of alkaline phosphatase may be seen. The inflamed superficial arteries may or may not be tender or nodular, and the pulses may be increased or absent.

Biopsy of an affected artery is diagnostic. However, given the segmental nature of these lesions, multiple biopsies may be required.

COURSE

Cranial arteritis usually undergoes a spontaneous remission in anywhere from several months up to 3 years.

COMPLICATIONS

The onset of blindness may be sudden.

The complications of delirium or of dementia are as described in those chapters.

ETIOLOGY

Involved arteries show a granulomatous panarteritis with giant cell involvement. Thrombi may occur, and emboli may be generated. The cause of the inflammation is not known; however, an autoimmune process is suspected.

DIFFERENTIAL DIAGNOSIS

In addition to other causes of stroke, consideration is given to polyarteritis nodosa, granulomatous angiitis, and systemic lupus erythematosus.

TREATMENT

Evidence of involvement of the internal carotid, vertebral or coronary arteries demands emergent treatment with prednisone, in doses of 60 mg. After symptoms have been brought under control, and the sedimentation rate has fallen, tapering may be cautiously attempted.

BIBLIOGRAPHY

Caselli RJ. Giant cell (temporal) arteritis: a treatable cause of multi-infarct dementia. *Neurology* 1990;40:753-755.

Caselli RJ, Hunder GG. Giant cell (temporal) arteritis. *Neurologic Clinics* 1997;15:893-902.

Caselli RJ, Hunder GG, Whisnant JP. Neurologic disease in biopsy proven giant cell (temporal) arteritis. *Neurology* 1988;38:378-391.

Shenberger KN, Meharg JG, Lane CD. Temporal arteritis presenting as ataxia and dementia. *Postgraduate Medicine* 1981;69:246-249.

Granulomatous angiitis, also known as primary angiitis of the central nervous system, is a rare disorder characterized pathologically by a vasculitis confined to the central nervous system, and clinically by headache and either delirium or dementia.

ONSET

Most patients are in their 30's or 40's, and symptoms evolve subacutely, generally over a few weeks time.

CLINICAL FEATURES

Classically, patients present with a cognitive change, either delirium or dementia, in the setting of prominent headache. Seizures are common, and some patients may have gradually evolving focal deficits, such as hemiplegia.

The peripheral white blood cell count and erythrocyte sedimentation rate are typically within normal limits. MRI scanning may be normal, or may reveal bilateral, but asymmetric, areas of increased signal intensity on T2-weighted scans within the cerebrum or cerebellum. Angiography likewise may or may not be abnormal, and in those cases where it is abnormal, it may or may not disclose classical vasculitic "beading." Lumbar puncture may reveal an elevated protein and a lymphocytic pleocytosis with a normal glucose. Brain biopsy, including both brain parenchyma and leptomeningeal tissue, is the diagnostic "gold standard," but it must be borne in mind that in some cases the biopsy may "miss" affected tissue.

COURSE

Untreated, progressive deterioration occurs in almost all cases, with a fatal outcome within months. Some survive only days; others may live for 2 or more years.

COMPLICATIONS

The complications of delirium or dementia are as described in those chapters.

ETIOLOGY

As the name implies, a widespread granulomatous angiitis affects small leptomeningeal and small- or medium-sized parenchymal vessels. Multiple small areas of infarction occur, primarily in the cerebrum, affecting both gray and white matter, but also at times in the cerebellar cortex, in the superficial aspects of the brain stem, and, rarely, in the cord. In severe cases the subarachnoid space may be filled with exudate.

The cause of the angiitis is not known; an autoimmune mechanism is suspected, perhaps triggered by a viral infection.

DIFFERENTIAL DIAGNOSIS

Although prominent headache in a delirious patient may suggest this diagnosis, granulomatous angiitis often enters the differential only when all other diagnostic possibilities have been ruled out or appear very unlikely. When granulomatous angiitis is considered a reasonable possibility, it is generally appropriate to proceed to biopsy.

TREATMENT

The general treatment of delirium and of dementia is discussed in the respective chapters. A combination of cyclophosphamide and corticosteroids may retard the progression of the disease, and in some cases effect a remission.

BIBLIOGRAPHY

Abu-Shakra M, Khraishi M, Grossman H, et al. Primary angiitis of the CNS diagnosed by angiography. *Quarterly Journal of Medicine* 1994;87:351-358.

Alhalabi M, Moore PM. Serial angiography in isolated angiitis of the central nervous system. *Neurology* 1994;44:1221-1226.

Calabrese LH, Mallek JA. Primary angiitis of the central nervous system. Report of 8 new cases, review of the literature and proposal for diagnostic criteria. *Medicine* 1988;67:20-39.

Hughes JT, Brownell B. Granulomatous giant cell angiitis of the central nervous system. *Neurology* 1966;16:293.

Kolodny EH, Rebeiz JJ, Caveness VS, et al. Granulomatous angiitis of the central nervous system. *Archives of Neurology* 1968;19:510-524.

Koo EH, Massey EW. Granulomatous angiitis of the central nervous system: protean manifestations and response to treatment. *Journal of Neurology, Neurosurgery, and Psychiatry* 1988;51:1126-1133.

Moore PM. Diagnosis and management of isolated angiitis of the central nervous system. *Neurology* 1989;39:167-173.

Singh S, Soloman T, Chacko G, et al. Primary angiitis of the central nervous system: an ante-mortem diagnosis. *Journal of Postgraduate Medicine* 2000;46:272-274.

201 Hypertensive Encephalopathy

Severe hypertension, regardless of cause, may cause an encephalopathy that can be fatal if untreated.

ONSET

The age of onset is determined by the underlying cause of the hypertension; most patients are middle-aged. The onset of the encephalopathy itself is generally fairly acute, evolving over days.

CLINICAL FEATURES

The blood pressure is severely and generally acutely elevated, with diastolics sometimes over 130 or 140 mmHg.

Typically patients develop a delirium and experience headache and nausea and vomiting; bilateral visual blurring or blindness is common and seizures may occur. On examination, in addition to the elevated blood pressure, one may see retinal hemorrhages or papilledema, and occasionally there may be focal findings such as aphasia or hemiplegia.

Acute renal and cardiac failure may occur, and if the pressure remains elevated, coma may supervene.

MRI scanning typically reveals bilateral areas of increased signal intensity on T2-weighted scans in the posterior white matter, affecting primarily the occipital and parietal lobes. CT scanning may reveal radiolucencies in the same areas, but is less sensitive than MRI scanning.

COMPLICATIONS

Hypertensive encephalopathy is a potentially fatal condition; among those who survive there may be evidence of cerebral infarction, and if these are sufficiently numerous and strategically placed, the patient may be left with a multi-infarct dementia.

The complications of delirium are as described in that chapter.

ETIOLOGY

As blood pressure rises above a critical level, cerebral vessel autoregulation fails, with extravasation of fluid into surrounding tissues; petechial hemorrhages may also occur and in some cases vessels may undergo fibrinoid necrosis with infarction of downstream tissues.

DIFFERENTIAL DIAGNOSIS

A grossly elevated diastolic pressure, of itself, is not sufficient for a diagnosis of hypertensive encephalopathy. Indeed, in patients with chronic and gradually worsening hypertension, disastolics of over 130 may be tolerated without immediate clinical sequelae. Thus, before making the diagnosis of hypertensive encephalopathy, one must see evidence of "target organ" damage, which, in the case of the brain, consists of delirium, visual changes, and the like.

Uremic encephalopathy tends to be of more gradual onset, and the BUN in uremia is almost always over 100 mg/dl.

Intracerebral hemorrhage, perhaps occurring secondary to hypertension, may present in a similar fashion, but the diagnosis is readily made with MRI or CT scanning.

TREATMENT

Hypertensive encephalopathy represents a medical emergency, and the pressure must be lowered within the hour. Normotensive levels are not the immediate goal; the pressure should be lowered only to the point at which symptoms clear, generally at diastolics between 110 and 120 mmHg. Overly rapid correction may lead to watershed infarctions. Once the danger has passed, normotensive levels may be sought over the next few days.

Intravenous sodium nitroprusside is the agent of choice; intravenous labetalol or diazoxide are alternatives. In less urgent situations, or where intravenous access is not available, intramuscular hydralazine may be given, in a dose of from 10 to 20 mg every 30 minutes until the pressure is acceptably controlled.

Seizures may be controlled with intravenous lorazepam.

BIBLIOGRAPHY

Chester EM, Agamanolis DP, Banker BQ, et al. Hypertensive encephalopathy: a clinicopathologic study of twenty cases. *Neurology* 1978;28:928-939.

Hauser RA, Lacey DM, Knight MR. Hypertensive encephalopathy: magnetic resonance imaging demonstration of reversible cortical and white matter lesions. *Archives of Neurology* 1988;45:1078-1083.

Healton EB, Brust JC, Feinfeld DA, et al. Hypertensive encephalopathy and the neurologic manifestations of malignant hypertension. *Neurology* 1982;32:127-132.

Schwartz RB, Jones KM, Kalina P, et al. Hypertensive encephalopathy: findings on CT, MR imaging, and SPECT imaging in 14 cases. *American Journal of Roentgenology* 1992;159:379-383.

Schwartz RB, Mulkern RV, Gudbjartsson H, et al. Diffusion-weighted MR imaging in hypertensive encephalopathy: clues to pathogenesis. *American Journal of Neuroradiology* 1998;19:859-862.

Cerebral amyloid angiopathy, also known as congophilic angiopathy or congophilic amyloid angiopathy, is being increasingly recognized as a cause of dementia with or without accompanying lobar intracerebral hemorrhages.

ONSET

The average age of onset is in the sixties, and patients may present with either a gradually progressive dementia or with one or more lobar hemorrhages.

CLINICAL FEATURES

The gradually progressive dementia is, of itself, non-specific, but may be accompanied by minor, and often transient, focal deficits, or by partial seizures.

Lobar intracerebral hemorrhages present with headache, vomiting, and a focal deficit, such as hemiplegia or aphasia, consistent with the location of the hemorrhage; when the hemorrhage is relatively large, delirium, stupor or coma may occur.

When dementia is present, MRI scanning will reveal a widespread leukoencephalopathy and, in many cases, small foci of decreased signal intensity, indicative of old petechial hemorrhages. CT or MRI scanning will, of course, also reveal any old, or fresh, lobar hemorrhages, as illustrated in Figure 202-1.

COURSE

Dementia, if present, gradually worsens, and the intracerebral hemorrhages tend to recur.

COMPLICATIONS

The complications of dementia are as described in that chapter.

ETIOLOGY

Amyloid deposition occurs in the walls of small and medium-sized cortical arteries and arterioles, resulting in fibrinoid degeneration with the formation of microaneurysms; such affected vessels are "congophilic," staining well with Congo red dye, thus accounting for one of the names of this disease. White matter within the areas of distribution of these arteries undergoes rarefaction and demyelinization, and, with minor rupture of microaneurysms, petechial hemorrhages may occur. With rupture of larger vessels, lobar hemorrhages appear.

It appears that the dementia of this disorder is caused by the widespread leukoencephalopathy, and that the petechial hemorrhages, acutely, account for transient focal deficits, and chronically serve as foci for partial seizures.

Although the great majority of cases of cerebral amyloid angiopathy are sporadic, two autosomal dominant forms have been identified, namely the Dutch and the Icelandic types of "hereditary cerebral hemorrhage with amyloidosis."

Importantly, this condition is not related to systemic amyloidosis, whether of the primary or secondary type.

DIFFERENTIAL DIAGNOSIS

The combination of a slowly progressive dementia with a lobar intracerebral hemorrhage is suggestive, and if there are two or

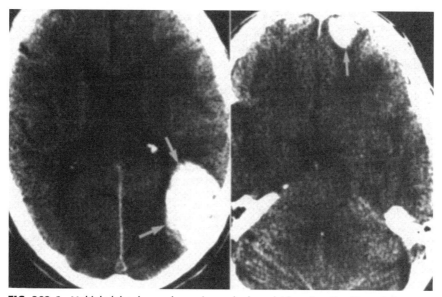

FIG. 202-1. Multiple lobar hemorrhages in cerebral amyloid angiopathy. (From Osborn AG. *Diagnostic neuroradiology*, St. Louis, 1994, Mosby.)

more hemorrhages, the diagnosis is almost certain. Importantly, it must be stressed that only lobar hemorrhages are of diagnostic import here: deep subcortical hemorrhages, as for example in the putamen, are generally not related to cerebral amyloid angiopathy and hence the presence of such deep intracerebral hemorrhages does not argue for this diagnosis.

Although cerebral biopsy, perhaps obtained during evacuation of a hemorrhage, is required for a definite diagnosis, the occurrence of two or more lobar intracerebral hemorrhages in a patient over the age of 55, in the absence of other causes, such as head trauma, vascular malformations, blood dyscrasias, or excessive anticoagulation, is so distinctive that biopsy, from a clinical point of view, may not be necessary.

In cases where patients have not as yet had their first intracerebral hemorrhage, and thus present solely with a gradually progressive dementia, MRI findings will also suggest Binswanger's disease: in such cases, the finding of evidence for multiple old petechial hemorrhages will argue for a diagnosis of cerebral amyloid angiopathy. This is a critical differential to make, because aspirin, which is appropriate for patients with Binswanger's disease, is relatively contraindicated in cerebral amyloid angiopathy.

TREATMENT

There is no known treatment that will halt the deposition of amyloid. Given the presence of microaneurysms and the ever-present risk of hemorrhage, heparin, warfarin, tissue plasminogen activator and aspirin are all relatively contraindicated. The general treatment of dementia is discussed in that chapter.

BIBLIOGRAPHY

Cosgrove GR, LeBlanc R, Meagher-Villemure K, et al. Cerebral amyloid angiopathy. *Neurology* 1985;35:625-631.

Gilles C, Brucher JM, Khoubesserian P, et al. Cerebral amyloid angiopathy as a cause of multiple intracerebral hemorrhages. *Neurology* 1984; 34:730-735.

Good CD, Ng VW, Clifton A, et al. Amyloid angiopathy causing widespread miliary hemorrhages within the brain evident on MRI. *Neuroradiology* 1998;40:308-311.

Greenberg SM, Vonsattel JP, Stakes JW, et al. The clinical spectrum of cerebral amyloid angiopathy: presentations without lobar hemorrhage. *Neurology* 1993:43:2073-2079.

Knudsen KA, Rosand J, Karluk D, et al. Clinical diagnosis of cerebral amyloid angiopathy: validation of the Boston criteria. *Neurology* 2001;56:537-539.

Pendlebury WW, Iole ED, Tracy RP, et al. Intracerebral hemorrhage related to cerebral amyloid angiopathy and t-PA treatment. *Annals of Neurology* 1991;29:210-213.

Yoshimura M, Yamanmouchi H, Kuzuhara S, et al. Dementia in cerebral amyloid angiopathy: a clinicopathological study. *Journal of Neurology* 1992;239:441-450.

203 Wegener's Granulomatosis

Wegener's granulomatosis is an uncommon disease characterized by a systemic necrotizing granulomatous vasculitis, affecting most prominently the respiratory tract and kidney, but also, in from one quarter to one half of all cases, the central and/or peripheral nervous system.

ONSET

Although the range of age of onset is fairly wide, most patients fall ill in their thirties or forties.

CLINICAL FEATURES

Over 90% of patients exhibit symptoms referable to the respiratory tract, and the disease most commonly presents with upper respiratory symptoms, such as otitis media, epistaxis, or rhinorrhea. Involvement of the nasal septum may lead to its collapse, as shown in Figure 203-1. Pulmonary infiltrates may be asymptomatic or may present with cough or hemoptysis.

Glomerulonephritis eventually occurs in over three quarters of all patients and may present with proteinuria and microscopic hematuria.

When the nervous system is involved the most common symptom is a peripheral neuropathy, either a polyneuropathy or a mononeuropathy multiplex. Cranial neuropathies may also occur, and in a smaller minority there may be a dementia, strokes or seizures. Localized granulomatous infiltrations of the hypothalamus may lead to diabetes insipidus.

Proptosis secondary to an extension of the granulomatous process into the orbit from an adjacent sinus may occur; occasionally the granulomatous process may extend directly into the temporal lobe.

MRI scanning may reveal dural thickening and enhancement, areas of old infarction, or granulomas. Analysis of the cerebrospinal fluid may reveal an elevated total protein and a lymphocytic pleocytosis.

The erythrocyte sedimentation rate is elevated, and leukocytosis may be evident. Although the rheumatoid factor may be positive, the ANA is negative. Over 90% of patients will have elevated levels of ANCA (anti-neutrophil cytoplasmic antibody) of either the "c-ANCA" or "p-ANCA" type. Although this finding is fairly specific for Wegener's granulomatosis, definitive diagnosis requires biopsy, from the respiratory tract or the kidneys.

COURSE

Symptoms are progressive, and once significant renal involvement occurs, death usually follows within months.

COMPLICATIONS

Complications are as described in the chapter on dementia.

past: for some, this may mean only events of the previous few hours, but for others the period of retrograde amnesia may stretch back years. Concurrent with this inability to remember what happened recently, patients are also unable to store in memory present, ongoing events. Most patients, although not confused, are bewildered as they look around and cannot recall how they came to be where they are, and most will repeatedly, and sometimes agitatedly, ask what the matter is or what is going on.

Formal mental status examination, if conducted during the episode itself, reveals disorientation to place and time (but not to person), normal digit span, inability to recall the names of three unrelated objects after 5 minutes, and inability to recall events of the relatively recent past.

The episode generally lasts anywhere from 4 to 18 hours, averaging about six hours, and, rather than remitting suddenly, tends to fade gradually.

After the episode remits the retrograde amnesia is lost, and patients are once again able to recall events up to the start of the episode. However, although patients also once again become able to keep track of where they are and the like, they remain forever unable to recall what happened during the episode; it remains a fixed "island" of amnesia.

COURSE

Typically, only one episode occurs; recurrences are seen in only a minority of patients, generally after an interval of 2 or 3 years.

COMPLICATIONS

Long-term complications appear almost nil. Most patients are more or less incapacitated during the attack; however, some may be able to carry on complex, over-learned behaviors, such as playing a musical instrument.

ETIOLOGY

SPECT studies have revealed hypoperfusion in the mesial temporal structures, and diffusion-weighted MRI reveals increased signal intensity, consistent with cellular edema, in the mesial temporal structures on the left. Although it is thus clear that dysfunction of mesial temporal, or related, structures is involved in transient global amnesia, the mechanism underlying this dysfunction is not clear. Migrainous, vascular and epileptic mechanisms have all been proposed, and each have some support. There is clearly an association between migraine and transient global amnesia, and proponents of this mechanism suggest that the temporal dysfunction occurs secondary to spreading depression of Lãeo. Transient ischemia could also cause this dysfunction, and proponents of this mechanism suggest, in effect, that transient global amnesia represents a TIA. The problem with this theory is that patients with transient global amnesia generally have few vascular risk factors and do not experience typical TIA's any more frequently than controls; one interesting finding, though, that might salvage the vascular theory, is that patients with transient global amnesia are more likely to have an incompetent internal jugular valve than are controls and more likely to experience venous reflux in the jugular system during a Valsalva maneuver. Given that transient global amnesia often follows upon activities that include a Valsalva-type maneuver, the idea that venous congestion in mesial temporal

structures could be at the base of transient global amnesia becomes attractive. The final proposed mechanism, namely that transient global amnesia represents a kind of partial seizure, though on the surface attractive, pales when one considers that these patients are no more likely to have typical partial or grand mal seizures than are controls and that the episode itself, rather than having an abrupt offset, as is typical of an epileptic event, resolves gradually.

DIFFERENTIAL DIAGNOSIS

In addition to transient global amnesia, there are only a few disorders capable of causing episodic amnesia, and these include alcoholic blackouts, "pure epileptic amnesia," transient ischemic attacks and the "localized" type of dissociative amnesia. Alcoholic blackouts are distinguished by the presence of intoxication and by the fact that patients in a blackout generally are not aware of it, and rarely ask the kind of bewildered questions seen in an episode of transient global amnesia. Pure epileptic amnesia is suggested by abrupt onset and abrupt offset, by its tendency to recurrence and by a history of other, more obvious, seizure types. Transient ischemic attacks may be suggested by the concurrence of other symptoms reflecting ischemia in other areas: for example, decreased flow in the posterior cerebral artery, in addition to causing ischemia in the mesial temporal lobe, might also cause ischemia in the mesial occipital lobe, thus adding an hemianopia to the amnesia. Other, suggestive, clues would be the presence of numerous vascular risk factors, and the onset, which, rather than being sudden, over seconds, may evolve over many minutes. Dissociative amnesia of the "localized" type is suggested by the youth of the patient and by the fact that patients with dissociative amnesia typically do not repeatedly ask what the matter is.

TREATMENT

Reassurance and close observation during the episode itself is generally sufficient for acute treatment. As might be expected given the uncertainty over etiology, there is controversy regarding the best preventive treatment. Some authors recommend only watchful waiting, others, who favor either a migrainous or epileptic basis, recommend divalproex, whereas those who believe that transient global amnesia represents ischemia recommend enteric coated aspirin. Clearly, if the episode were related to a Valsalva-type manuever, it would be appropriate to adopt strategies that would avoid an increase in intra-thoracic pressure.

BIBLIOGRAPHY

Byer JA, Crowley WJ. Musical performance during transient global amnesia. *Neurology* 1980;30:80-82.

Fisher CM. Transient global amnesia: precipitating activities and other observations. *Archives of Neurology* 1982;39:605-608.

Heathfield K, Croft P, Swash M. The syndrome of transient global amnesia. *Brain* 1973;96:729-736.

Hodges JR, Warlow CP. The aetiology of transient global amnesia. A care-control study of 114 cases with prospective follow-up. *Brain* 1990;113:639-657.

Kushner MJ, Hauser WA. Transient global amnesia: a case-control study. *Annals of Neurology* 1985;18:684-695.

Maalikjy Akkawi N, Agosti C, Anzola GP, et al. Transient global amnesia: a clinical and sonographic study. *European Neurology* 2003;49:67-71.

Melo TP, Ferro JM, Ferro H. Transient global amnesia: a case control study. *Brain* 1992;115:261-270.

Miller JW, Petersen RC, Metter EJ. Transient global amnesia: clinical characteristics and prognosis. *Neurology* 1987;37:733-737.

Sander D, Winbeck K, Etgen T, et al. Disturbance of venous flow patterns in patients with transient global amnesia. *Lancet* 2000;356: 1982-1984.

Strupp M, Bruning R, Wu RH, et al. Diffusion-weighted MRI in transient global amnesia: elevated signal intensity in the left mesial temporal lobe in 7 of 10 patients. *Annals of Neurology* 1998;43:164-170.

Zorzon M, Antonutti L, Mase G, et al. Transient global amnesia and transient ischemic attack: natural history, vascular risk factors, and associated conditions. *Stroke* 1995;26:1536-1542.

IMMUNE-MEDIATED DISORDERS

206 Limbic Encephalitis

Limbic encephalitis, first described by Brierly et al. in 1960, is one of the "paraneoplastic" syndromes and, in all likelihood, occurs secondary to an autoimmune assault on limbic structures triggered by a remote cancer, which, in most cases, is a small cell lung cancer. Although this is a rare disorder, occurring in less than 1% of patients with lung cancer, it is nevertheless important to recognize, as it may be the first evidence of an underlying malignancy. The term "paraneoplastic dementia" has been used as a synonym; however, this may not be appropriate given the fact that although limbic encephalitis can cause a dementia, it also can, and often does, cause other syndromes, such as delirium or psychosis.

ONSET

The onset of symptoms is gradual, spanning many weeks.

CLINICAL FEATURES

Limbic encephalitis may present with delirium, personality change, psychosis, or partial seizures, with or without secondary generalization. Other, less common, presentations include dementia, amnesia, somnolence or catatonia. With progression, a mixed picture may emerge, consisting of a combination of any or all of the foregoing.

The electroencephalogram is abnormal in about three-quarters of cases, showing slowing or epileptiform abnormalities or both, generally in the temporal areas.

MRI scanning, especially early in the course, is more often normal than not; with progression, however, one may see increased signal intensity in the mesial temporal areas on T2-weighted scans.

Anti-neuronal antibodies are generally, but not always, present in the serum. Anti-Hu (also known as type 1 anti-neuronal antibody, or ANNA-1) is most commonly seen with limbic encephalitis, and is strongly associated with small cell lung cancer. Other anti-neuronal antibodies include anti-Ri (ANNA-2), which is associated with opsoclonus-myoclonus, and anti-Yo, associated with cerebellar degeneration. Recently discovered antibodies include anti-Ma, associated with breast cancer, anti-Ma2, with testicular cancer, and anti-amphiphysin, which may be seen with a variety of tumor types. Most labs also have a "paraneoplastic profile" available, and when one suspects a limbic encephalitis but cannot determine the kind of underlying malignancy, ordering a "profile" is prudent, rather than ordering only one or two specific antibodies.

The cerebrospinal fluid may be either normal or show a mild lymphocytic pleocytosis or an elevated total protein.

Patients with a limbic encephalitis may have other paraneoplastic syndromes including subacute cerebellar degeneration,

brain stem encephalitis (with varying combinations of oculomotor pareses, nystagmus, dysphagia and dysarthria), myelitis, opsoclonus-myoclonus, and peripheral polyneuropathy.

COURSE

The course of limbic encephalitis is quite variable. In most cases it appears that there is a gradual worsening over weeks or months, followed by a relatively stable period which, however, may be interrupted by exacerbations. Rarely, there may be a remission, regardless of whether the underlying tumor is treated or not; in most cases, however, death is the final result, with this eventuality being reached anywhere from months to many years after the onset.

COMPLICATIONS

The complications of delirium, personality change, secondary psychosis and dementia are as described in those chapters.

ETIOLOGY

In most cases limbic structures display neuronal loss with lymphocytic infiltration, typically in a perivascular distribution. These changes tend to be most prominent in the medial temporal lobe, affecting primarily the hippocampus and the amygdala, and in all likelihood result from an autoimmune attack upon these tissues. The most common underlying malignancy is a small cell lung cancer; other types include non-small cell lung cancers and cancers of the thymus, breast, testicle, ovary and colon, and Hodgkin's disease. Importantly, as testicular cancers are very difficult to detect, it is appropriate to consider a testicular ultrasound for men with a limbic encephalitis in whom no cause can be found.

DIFFERENTIAL DIAGNOSIS

Once it has been established that the encephalopathy is occurring in the context of a primary cancer situated outside the nervous system, other disorders should be ruled out before making a definitive diagnosis of limbic encephalitis. These include metastatic disease, an endocrinologic syndrome secondary to tumor-mediated hormonal changes (e.g., Cushing's syndrome, hypercalcemia, hypoglycemia, or hyponatremia), and opportunistic infections such as cytomegalovirus, herpes simplex, or progressive multi-focal leukoencephalopathy.

Furthermore, if anticancer treatment has begun, especially cranial irradiation, side effects to that treatment must be considered.

TREATMENT

Some degree of improvement may or may not be seen with treatment of the primary cancer. Some patients have improved with prednisone; however, this is unpredictable. The treatment of delirium, personality change, secondary psychosis and dementia is as described in those chapters. Seizures are often very difficult to control.

BIBLIOGRAPHY

Antoine J, Honnorat J, Anterion CT, et al. Limbic encephalitis and immunological perturbations in two patients with thymoma. *Journal of Neurology, Neurosurgery, and Psychiatry* 1995;58:706-710.

Antoine JC, Absi L, Honnorat J, et al. Antiamphiphysin antibodies are associated with various paraneoplastic neurological syndromes and tumors. *Archives of Neurology* 1999;56:172-177.

Bakheit AMO, Kennedy PGE, Behan PO. Paraneoplastic limbic encephalitis: clinico-pathological correlations. *Journal of Neurology, Neurosurgery, and Psychiatry* 1990;53:1084-1088.

Brierley JB, Corsellis JAN, Hierons R, et al. Subacute encephalitis of later adult life mainly affecting the limbic area. *Brain* 1960;83:357-368.

Corsellis JAN, Goldberg GJ, Norton AR. "Limbic encephalitis" and its association with carcinoma. *Brain* 1968;91:481-496.

Deodhare S, O'Connor P, Ghazarian D, et al. Paraneoplastic limbic encephalitis in Hodgkin's disease. *The Canadian Journal of Neurological Sciences* 1996;23:138-140.

Glaser GH, Pincus JH. Limbic encephalitis. *The Journal of Nervous and Mental Disease* 1969;149:59-67.

Graus F, Keime-Guilbert F, Rene R, et al. Anti-Hu-associated paraneoplastic encephalomyelitis: analysis of 200 patients. *Brain* 2001;124:1138-1148.

Gultekin SH, Rosenfeld MR, Voltz R, et al. Paraneoplastic limbic encephalitis: neurological symptoms, immunological findings and tumour association in 50 patients. *Brain* 2000;123:1481-1494.

Tandon R, Walden R, Falcon S. Catatonia as a manifestation of paraneoplastic encephalopathy. *The Journal of Clinical Psychiatry* 1988;49:121-122.

Tsukamoto T, Mochizuki R, Mochizuki H, et al. Paraneoplastic cerebellar degeneration and limbic encephalitis in a patient with adenocarcinoma of the colon. *Journal of Neurology, Neurosurgery, and Psychiatry* 1993;56:713-716.

Voltz R, Gultekin SH, Rosenfeld MR, et al. A serologic marker of paraneoplastic limbic and brain-stem encephalitis in patients with testicular cancer. *The New England Journal of Medicine* 1999;340:1788-1795.

207 Multiple Sclerosis

Clinically, multiple sclerosis is characterized by the evolution of a variety of signs and symptoms indicating the presence of lesions within different parts of the central nervous system. Pathologically, one finds an ever-increasing burden of plaques scattered throughout the central nervous system, generally within the white matter. This dissemination of lesions over space and time represents the diagnostic hallmark of multiple sclerosis. In a minority of patients, appropriately situated plaques may cause depression, euphoria, dementia or psychosis.

ONSET

Most patients fall ill in their twenties or thirties. The range of onset, however, is wide, with rare onsets occurring in childhood or after the age of 60.

The initial symptoms may be so mild and evanescent that they pass unnoticed. Common presenting symptoms include transient weakness, generally of the lower extremities, paresthesiae, and retrobulbar neuritis.

CLINICAL FEATURES

Psychiatric symptomatology occurs in a minority of patients and is most often seen later in the course of the disease.

Clinically significant depressive symptomatology develops in about one-quarter of all patients, and although in some cases this depression is of the "reactive" type in the face of a devastating disease, it is clear, as noted below under "etiology," that depression also occurs as a direct result of plaque formation in the brain.

A "bland" euphoria, without any accompanying pressure of speech or hyperactivity, is not uncommon, and, in a very small minority, one may see a full manic syndrome.

Dementia eventually occurs in the majority of patients. Although dementia may constitute the presentation of multiple sclerosis, this is very rare, and in most cases dementia only appears after the disease is very far advanced.

Psychosis, with delusions and hallucinations, is uncommon; very rarely it may constitute the presentation of the disease.

Other, more common, symptoms include spasticity, retrobulbar neuritis, incontinence, constipation, ataxia, dysarthria, scanning speech, intention tremor, nystagmus, paresthesiae, impotence, decreased libido, anorgasmia, and pain. Acute pain may occur as trigeminal neuralgia, Lhermitte's sign, or painful tic-like extremity dysesthesiae. Fatigue is a very common symptom and may at times be severe. Pseudobulbar palsy with prominent emotional incontinence occurs in about one-tenth of patients, but usually is not seen until the disease is far advanced. Less common symptoms include seizures, tinnitus, vertigo, hemifacial spasm, and facial myokymia. Internuclear ophthalmoplegia, although not common in multiple sclerosis, is by contrast extremely rare in any other disease and thus constitutes an important diagnostic clue.

MRI scanning has become an extremely important diagnostic tool as it demonstrates white matter lesions in over 90% of patients; indeed it very often demonstrates asymptomatic lesions. Gadolinium enhancement discloses which plaques are undergoing active inflammation. Figure 207-1A shows multiple bilateral lesions on a T2-weighted scan, typical of multiple sclerosis; Figure 207-1B is a T1-weighted image of the same area with gadolinium enhancement demonstrating that only two of the plaques seen in A

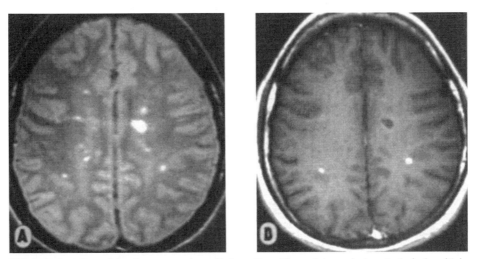

FIG. 207-1. *A*, T2-weighted scan reveals multiple scattered hyper-intense lesions typical of multiple sclerosis. *B*, A scan of the same patient with gadolinium enhancement indicates which lesions are active. (From Kucharczyk W, ed. *MRI: central nervous system,* New York, 1990, Gower.)

are active. CT scanning is far less sensitive, even with double-contrast enhancement.

Evoked potentials, whether visual, somatosensory, or brain stem auditory, were once used to demonstrate lesions in the respective white matter tracts; however, with the advent of MRI scanning these tests have fallen into disuse in the workup of patients with suspected multiple sclerosis.

The cerebrospinal fluid is abnormal in almost all patients during periods of active disease. Findings, in order of decreasing frequency, include oligoclonal bands, elevated gamma globulin or elevated IgG index, mild mononuclear pleocytosis, mildly elevated total protein, and the presence of myelin basic protein.

COURSE

The majority of patients experience a relapsing and remitting course. Episodes of symptoms may come on acutely within minutes or hours, or perhaps over days, persist for weeks, months, or longer, and then gradually undergo a remission. The remission, however, is rarely complete, and most patients have residual symptoms. The interval between episodes is extremely variable, ranging from months to over 20 years. The next episode may consist of either a reappearance of symptoms that had remitted, an exacerbation of residual symptoms, or completely new symptoms. Over time and with repeated episodes, the residuals become increasingly severe and disabling.

In a minority of cases exhibiting typical relapses and remissions, perhaps one-tenth, the overall course may undergo a malignant evolution into one characterized by relentless progression: such patients are said to have a "secondary" progressive course. In an even smaller minority of cases, the disease may exhibit a "primary" progressive course, and display a relentless progression from the very start.

Although those with a chronic progressive course or those with frequent relapses tend to have a poorer prognosis, predicting with certainty the course for any given individual patient is very difficult.

Multiple sclerosis is rarely fatal per se. Most patients die of intercurrent diseases such as urinary tract infections, pneumonia, or decubiti, generally after about 35 years. Exceptions occur,

however. Some may live out a normal life span and die of some disease unrelated to the multiple sclerosis. Conversely, some may experience a fulminant course, often accompanied by delirium, with death occurring within weeks.

Pregnancy itself does not reliably alter the course of the disease one way or the other; however, it appears that exacerbations may be more likely during the first 3 months postpartum. Exacerbations may also be precipitated by extreme fatigue or an infectious illness, such as a viral upper respiratory infection.

Increased body temperature, as may occur in the summer or in a hot bath, reliably worsens symptoms.

COMPLICATIONS

Euphoria generally causes little difficulty; however, mania may require hospitalization. Depression or irritability may impair the patient's ability to cooperate with treatment or carry on with daily activities. The complications of dementia are as described in that chapter. Complications of delusions or hallucinations vary according to the specific content of these experiences.

Other symptoms may eventually leave the patient bed-bound or wheelchair-bound, incontinent, and perhaps in pain.

ETIOLOGY

Plaques may occur anywhere within the central nervous system and range in size from less than a millimeter to, in extreme cases, several centimeters. Although the overwhelming majority are confined to the white matter, small plaques may occasionally be seen in gray matter. Acutely the plaque displays perivascular inflammation, loss of oligodendrocytes, and demyelinization. Axon cylinders themselves are generally spared but not always. Surrounding the acute plaque is an often large area of edema. As the inflammation and edema subside, any symptoms referable to the plaque also begin to undergo at least a partial resolution. A chronic, non-inflamed plaque consists of axons and a glial scar and accounts for the residual symptoms seen after the acute attack. Occasionally, in severe cases, the inflammation may be so profound as to leave a chronic cyst in its wake. With repeated disease exacerbation, new plaques are added and older ones enlarged.

As noted earlier, although the depression of multiple sclerosis may have "reactive" elements, similar to depression seen in other debilitating diseases, it also appears to occur as a direct result of plaque formation. For example, patients with primarily cord involvement, though severely impaired, are less likely to develop depression than are patients whose plaques reside primarily within the cerebrum. Furthermore, among cases with cerebral involvement, depression is more likely to occur when the plaques are located either in the white matter of the right temporal lobe or in the arcuate fasciculus on the left.

Dementia is associated with an increasing burden of cerebral plaques, especially within the corona radiata, insula and hippocampus.

Although the cause of the inflammation is not known, several lines of evidence support the hypothesis that multiple sclerosis represents an autoimmune disorder triggered by a relatively common viral infection of childhood in genetically susceptible people.

The incidence of multiple sclerosis rises dramatically and sequentially from the general population to first-degree relatives, then to dizygotic twins, and eventually to monozygotic twins, wherein estimates of concordance range anywhere from 25% to 40%, if one relies on clinical diagnosis, and up to 70%, if one accepts MRI evidence. Also, as one might expect, significant linkage exists between this disease and certain HLA haplotypes.

The evidence for an infectious agent acting on a fertile genetic background includes the finding of increasing prevalence with higher latitudes, and the existence of certain epidemics of multiple sclerosis, notably in the Faroe Islands after World War II. Two facts support the notion that the critical exposure to the infectious agent must occur in childhood. First, the concordance rate among spouses is no higher than among the general population. Second, if persons from a temperate climate emigrate from this high-risk area to a low-risk tropical area after the age of 15, they would still be at greater risk than those native to the tropical area.

The identity of this presumed infectious agent is not as yet known. Measles has been suspected, given that patients with multiple sclerosis have higher antibody titers than the general population to this virus, but as yet no infectious agent has been found guilty.

The evidence for an immune response rests not only on the finding of oligoclonal bands and increased IgG in the cerebrospinal fluid, but also on alterations in T cell population. The absolute and relative numbers of suppressor T cells fall just before an exacerbation. Furthermore, the number of helper T cells appears to rise during exacerbations.

DIFFERENTIAL DIAGNOSIS

Other diseases affecting the central nervous system and capable of producing a relapsing and remitting course include Behcet's syndrome, polyarteritis nodosa and systemic lupus erythematosus. All of these diseases, however, are, rather than being confined to the nervous system, systemic in nature and produce symptoms referable to other organ systems, such as the skin, joints, kidneys or gastrointestinal tract. Multi-infarct dementia or the lacunar state might enter into the differential, but here MRI scanning will immediately allow a correct differential.

When patients are seen during the first episode of illness, a confident differential between multiple sclerosis and acute disseminated encephalomyelitis may not be possible. One clue, however, may be provided by MRI scanning. Acute disseminated encephalomyelitis is a monophasic event, and consequently, all the plaques visualized on T2-weighted scans should also undergo gadolinium enhancement. By contrast, in at least some cases of multiple sclerosis, the first episode of demyelinization may have escaped clinical detection, and in such cases the only evidence of that episode would be an old, "burnt-out" plaque, which does not enhance. Consequently in such cases, one would, on gadolinium enhanced T1-weighted scans, find areas of decreased signal intensity which did not enhance, as would be expected with an inactive plaque. Of course, this diagnostic aide would be absent in cases of multiple sclerosis where there had been no prior episodes of demyelinization, and in these cases watchful waiting may be required to make the differential.

The differential diagnosis of conversion disorder is as discussed in that chapter. Although Briquet's syndrome, or somatization disorder, is often listed in the differential diagnosis of multiple sclerosis, the fact that in Briquet's syndrome the symptoms are referable to a number of different organ systems distinguishes it from multiple sclerosis, which is confined to one organ system, the central nervous system.

The finding of oligoclonal bands, elevated IgG, or myelin basic protein is not specific to multiple sclerosis and may be seen in other conditions, such as neurosyphilis, Lyme dementia, Behcet's syndrome, and sarcoidosis.

TREATMENT

Acute attacks may be treated with corticosteroids, and although there is controversy over the best regimen, many authors recommend intravenous high dose methylprednisolone (e.g., 250 mg IV q 6h) for three days, followed by oral prednisone, 60 mg daily for five days, with the dose then tapered in 10 mg increments over the next 10 days. Such treatment may induce a transient mania, and in cases where there is a history of this during prior steroid-treated episodes, lithium may be given on a preventive basis. Treatments capable of reducing the frequency of relapses include interferon beta-1a (as either a subcutaneous preparation, given three times weekly ["Rebif"], or an intramuscular preparation given once weekly ["Avonex"]), interferon beta-1b ("Betaseron"), or glatiramer (formerly known as copolymer ["Copaxone"]). These agents offer modest benefit, and, in the case of interferons, neutralizing antibodies may occur. Of note, interferon beta-1b may be more effective than weekly injections of interferon beta-1a, and, of all the interferons, interferon beta-1b is the only one shown to be effective in patients with a secondary progressive course. Unfortunately, it appears that interferon beta-1b is also the most likely to induce neutralizing antibodies.

Immunosuppressants, such as mitoxantrone, azathioprine and cyclophosphamide, may be helpful; however, their toxicity often outweighs any benefit.

Depression may be treated with antidepressants, such as SSRIs. Euphoria, if bland, rarely requires treatment; should mania occur, however, a mood stabilizer, such as lithium, divalproex or carbamazepine, may be used, and in this regard, given the effectiveness of carbamazepine in neuropathic pain, it may be preferable. The overall treatment of dementia, secondary psychosis and pseudobulbar palsy is as outlined in those chapters. If fatigue is problematic, amantadine, in a dose of 100 mg bid, may be helpful; pemoline may also be helpful, but may not be as effective as amantadine, and given its potential hepatotoxicity, this agent has fallen into disfavor. Baclofen may be used for spasticity, and recent work suggests that gabapentin is also useful in this regard.

BIBLIOGRAPHY

Barnes D, Hughes RA, Morris RW, et al. Randomized trial of oral and intravenous methylprednisolone in acute relapses of multiple sclerosis. *Lancet* 1997;349:902-906.

Berg D, Supprian T, Thomas J, et al. Lesion pattern in patients with multiple sclerosis and depression. *Multiple Sclerosis* 2000;6:156-162.

Bergin JD. Rapidly progressing dementia in disseminated sclerosis. *Journal of Neurology, Neurosurgery, and Psychiatry* 1957;20:285-292.

Comi G, Fillippi M, Wolinsky JS. European/Canadian multicenter, double-blind, randomized, placebo-controlled study of the effects of glatiramer acetate on magnetic-resonance imaging-measured disease activity and burden in patients with relapsing multiple sclerosis. *Annals of Neurology* 2001;49:290-297.

Cottrell SS, Wilson SAK. The affective symptomatology of disseminated sclerosis. *Journal of Neurology and Psychopathology* 1926;7:1-30.

Cutter NC, Scott DD, Johnson JC, et al. Gabapentin effect on spasticity in multiple sclerosis: a placebo-controlled, randomized trial. *Archives of Physical Medicine and Rehabilitation* 2000;81:164-169.

Durelli L, Verdun E, Barbero P, et al. Every-other-day interferon beta-1b versus once-weekly interferon beta-1a for multiple sclerosis: results of a 2-year prospective randomized multicenter study (INCOMIN). *Lancet* 2002;359:1453-1460.

European Study Group on interferon beta-1b in secondary progressive MS. Placebo-controlled multicentre randomized trial of interferon beta-1b in treatment of secondary progressive multiple sclerosis. *Lancet* 1998;352:1491-1497.

Falk WE, Mahnke MW, Poskanzer DC. Lithium prophylaxis of corticotropin-induced psychosis. *The Journal of the American Medical Association* 1979;241:1011-1012.

Feinstein A, Feinstein K, Gray T, et al. Prevalence and neurobehavioral correlates of pathological laughing and crying in multiple sclerosis. *Archives of Neurology* 1997;54:1116-1121.

Fontaine B, Seilhean D, Tourbah A, et al. Dementia in two histologically confirmed cases of multiple sclerosis: one case with isolated dementia and one case associated with psychiatric symptoms. *Journal of Neurology, Neurosurgery, and Psychiatry* 1994;57:353-359.

Franklin GM, Nelson LM, Filley CM, et al. Cognitive loss in multiple sclerosis: case reports and review of the literature. *Archives of Neurology* 1989;46:162-167.

Hulter BM, Lundberg PO. Sexual function in women with advanced multiple sclerosis. *Journal of Neurology, Neurosurgery, and Psychiatry* 1995;59:83-86.

Krupp LB, Coyle PJ, Doscher C, et al. Fatigue therapy in multiple sclerosis: results of a double-blind, randomized, parallel trial of amantadine, pemoline, and placebo. *Neurology* 1995;45:1956-1961.

Pine DS, Douglas CJ, Charles E, et al. Patients with multiple sclerosis presenting to psychiatric hospitals. *The Journal of Clinical Psychiatry* 1995;56:297-306.

PRISMS Study Group. Randomized double-blind placebo-controlled study of interferon beta-1a in relapsing/remitting multiple sclerosis. *Lancet* 1998;352:1498-1504.

Rabins PV, Brooks BR, O'Donnell P, et al. Structural brain correlates of emotional disorder in multiple sclerosis. *Brain* 1986;109:585-597.

Tsolaki M, Drevelegas A, Karachristianou S, et al. Correlation of dementia, neuropsychological and MRI findings in multiple sclerosis. *Dementia* 1994;5:48-52.

Whitlock FA, Siskind MM. Depression as a major symptom of multiple sclerosis. *Journal of Neurology, Neurosurgery, and Psychiatry* 1980;43:861-865.

Zorzon M, de Masi R, Nasuelli D, et al. Depression and anxiety in multiple sclerosis. A clinical and MRI study in 95 subjects. *Journal of Neurology* 2001;248:416-421.

208 Systemic Lupus Erythematosus

Systemic lupus erythematosus is an autoimmune disorder characterized by the presence of autoantibodies directed toward various organs, including the brain and cerebral vessels: anti-neuronal antibodies may directly attack neurons, and when vessels are damaged by antibodies, there may be infarctions.

Cerebral lupus may manifest with psychosis, mood changes (either depression, or, much less commonly, hypomania), delirium or dementia, and indeed more than half of all patients with lupus will develop one or more of these symptoms at some time during the illness.

Lupus is far more common among females than males and among blacks than whites. The lifetime prevalence for lupus among black females is about 0.4%.

ONSET

Although lupus can appear at almost any age, including among the elderly, the majority of patients fall ill sometime between puberty and 40 years of age. The onset itself ranges from gradual to acute.

CLINICAL FEATURES

Cerebral lupus rarely occurs in isolation. The overwhelming majority of these patients also experience other symptoms, such as arthralgia, rashes, constitutional symptoms (fatigue, fever, or weight loss), pleurisy, pericarditis, nephritis, and various cytopenias (anemia, often of chronic disease, leukopenia, or thrombocytopenia). A malar, "butterfly" rash, as shown in Figure 208-1, occurs in over one-half of all patients.

In cerebral lupus characterized by psychosis, patients may experience delusions, often of persecution, along with hallucinations, which may be either visual or auditory. Mood changes generally consist of depressive symptoms, although hypomanic ones have also been observed. Delirium or dementia may appear, and in many cases there is a "mixed" picture, with episodes of delirium occurring on a background of dementia.

Other symptoms of cerebral lupus, roughly in order of descending frequency, include seizures, focal deficits, such as hemiplegia, cerebellar symptoms, increased intracranial pressure, and abnormal involuntary movements such as dystonia, hemiballism, and, most especially, chorea. Optic neuritis and transverse

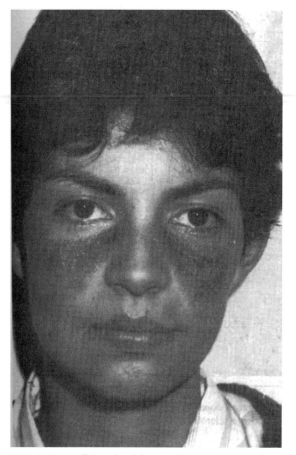

FIG. 208-1. "Butterfly" rash of lupus. (From Stein JH, ed. *Internal medicine,* St. Louis, 1994, Mosby.)

myelitis may also occur. Many cases of cerebral lupus are also accompanied by either a peripheral polyneuropathy or a mononeuritis multiplex.

MRI scanning may be normal, despite clinically obvious central nervous system involvement, and this appears to be most often the case when the clinical manifestations, such as psychosis, depression, delirium, grand mal seizures or dementia, are due to a diffuse assault upon neurons by antineuronal antibodies. In other cases, especially those with focal findings, MRI scanning may reveal relatively small areas of increased signal intensity on T2-weighted scans, corresponding to small vessel disease or, in the case of large vessel disease, there may be large areas of increased signal intensity in the area of distribution of the large cerebral vessels.

The cerebrospinal fluid may be normal or may show an increased protein or, less commonly, a mild lymphocytic pleocytosis. In cases characterized by a direct assault upon neurons by antineuronal antibodies, the IgG index is elevated and oligoclonal bands may be found, as may antineuronal antibodies.

The serum ANA is positive in over 95% of cases, and the serum VDRL may be falsely positive. Since the ANA test lacks specificity, a positive result is followed up by a more specific test, such as anti-double-stranded DNA or anti-Sm. In cases characterized by psychosis, depression, delirium, grand mal seizures or dementia, the serum antiribosomal P antibody level is also often elevated. In cases characterized by small or large vessel disease, the serum anti-phospholipid antibody level is generally elevated, and such patients, clinically, are also likely to have livedo reticularis.

COURSE

Although lupus tends to be a chronic disease, symptoms generally wax and wane over long periods of time, with partial, and at times complete, albeit temporary, remissions. Death may occur, usually secondary to renal failure or to some intercurrent infection.

COMPLICATIONS

The complications of secondary psychosis, depression or mania, or of delirium or dementia are as described in those chapters.

ETIOLOGY

Systemic lupus erythematosus represents an autoimmune disorder occurring in genetically susceptible individuals, and is characterized by autoantibodies to various tissues, which produce their damage either directly, or through activation of the complement system.

The central nervous system may be affected via any of a variety of mechanisms. Neurons may undergo direct attack by antineuronal antibodies, and this mechanism appears to underlie most cases of psychosis, depression, delirium and dementia. Small vessels may also be the target of antibodies producing a vasculitis with small infarctions; infarction in the area of distribution of large vessels may also occur, with the large cerebral vessels themselves undergoing occlusion due to a vasculitic process, thrombus formation, early atherosclerosis or emboli from Libman-Sacks endocarditis. These infarctions, whether due to small or large vessel disease, appear to underlie the focal findings seen in lupus, for example hemiplegia, and may also, if sufficiently numerous, cause a multi-infarct dementia.

Importantly, in addition to these "direct" effects of lupus upon the brain, there may also be other factors in play, including bacterial, fungal or tubercular infections, side effects to steroids, and malignant hypertension.

DIFFERENTIAL DIAGNOSIS

Polyarteritis nodosa, sarcoidosis, and, in older patients, cranial arteritis may all mimic cerebral lupus to a certain degree, and it is good practice to check an ANA whenever patients manifest neuropsychiatric symptomatology in the setting of a systemic disorder characterized by constitutional symptoms, arthralgia or rash.

Procainamide, hydralazine, and, less commonly, alpha-methyldopa may all induce a lupus-like syndrome. A host of other drugs, including chlorpromazine, carbamazepine, phenytoin, and primidone, have also been rarely implicated. Cerebral symptoms are unusual in drug-induced lupus. In doubtful cases, antibody profiles may help distinguish drug-induced from naturally occurring lupus. Although all patients with drug-induced lupus have ANA antibodies, few have antibodies to double-stranded DNA or to the Sm antigen. Conversely, patients with drug-induced lupus typically do have antihistone antibodies, whereas these are less common in patients with naturally occurring lupus. Despite the rare association of chlorpromazine, carbamazepine, and phenytoin with drug-induced lupus, these agents are not contraindicated in naturally occurring lupus.

A very important differential for affective changes is treatment with steroids itself. In addition, patients immunosuppressed by steroids, azathioprine, or cyclophosphamide are at risk for opportunistic CNS infections.

TREATMENT

Cerebral lupus is generally considered an indication for aggressive treatment. Oral prednisone may be given in doses of approximately 60 mg daily, and then tapered either to discontinuation or to the lowest dose capable of controlling symptoms; in severe cases it may be appropriate to begin treatment with intravenous methylprednisolone, 250 mg IV q 6h for a matter of days, to rapidly bring symptoms under control, after which a switch may be made to oral prednisone. Concurrent treatment with an immunosuppressant, such as cyclophosphamide or azathioprine, may also be required.

Symptomatic treatment of secondary psychosis, depression or mania, or of delirium or dementia, is discussed in those chapters.

BIBLIOGRAPHY

Asherson RA, Mercey D, Phillips G, et al. Recurrent stroke and multi-infarct dementia in systemic lupus erythematosus: association with antiphospholipid antibodies. *Annals of the Rheumatic Diseases* 1987;46:605-611.

Bennett R, Hughes CRV, Bywaters EGL. Neuropsychiatric problems in systemic lupus erythematosus. *British Medical Journal* 1972;4:342-345.

Bluestein HG, Williams GW, Steiberg AD. Cerebrospinal fluid antibodies to neuronal cells: association with neuropsychiatric manifestations of systemic lupus erythematosus. *The American Journal of Medicine* 1981;70:240-246.

Dennis MS, Byrne EJ, Bendall P. Neuropsychiatric systemic lupus erythematosus in elderly people: a case series. *Journal of Neurology, Neurosurgery, and Psychiatry* 1992;55:1157-1161.

Feinglass EJ, Arnett FC, Dorsch CA. Neuropsychiatric manifestations of systemic lupus erythematosus: diagnosis, clinical spectrum, and relationship to other features of the disease. *Medicine* 1976;55:323-329.

Isshi K, Hirohata S. Differential roles of the anti-ribosomal P antibody and antineuronal antibody in the pathogenesis of central nervous system involvement in systemic lupus erythematosus. *Arthritis and Rheumatism* 1998;41:1819-1827.

Johnson RT, Richardson EP. The neurological manifestations of systemic lupus erythematosus. *Medicine* 1968;47:337-369.

Mitsias P, Levine SR. Large cerebral vessel occlusive disease in systemic lupus erythematosus. *Neurology* 1994;44:385-393.

O'Connor JF, Musher DM. Central nervous system involvement in systemic lupus erythematosus. *Archives of Neurology* 1966;14:157-164.

Sailer M, Burchert W, Ehrenheim C, et al. Positron emission tomography and magnetic resonance imaging for cerebral involvement in patients with systemic lupus erythematosus. *Journal of Neurology* 1997; 244: 186-193.

Schneebaum AB, Singleton JD, West SG, et al. Association of psychiatric manifestations with antibodies to ribosomal P proteins in systemic lupus erythematosus. *The American Journal of Medicine* 1991;90:54-62.

West SG, Emien W, Wener MH, et al. Neuropsychiatric lupus erythematosus: a 10-year prospective study on the value of diagnostic tests. *The American Journal of Medicine* 1995;99:153-163.

Wong KL, Woo EK, Yu YL, et al. Neurological manifestations of systemic lupus erythematosus: a prospective study. *Quarterly Journal of Medicine* 1991;81:857-870.

209 Hashimoto's Encephalopathy

Hashimoto's encephalopathy is an autoimmune disorder that is characterized by delirium, dementia or psychosis, and which is related, in an as yet unknown way, to Hashimoto's thyroiditis. The encephalopathy appears to be an uncommon disorder, and is more frequent in females than males.

ONSET

The onset may occur anywhere from childhood to old age, and may be subacute, as is seen when it presents with a delirium, or gradual, when dementia constitutes the presentation.

CLINICAL FEATURES

The delirium of Hashimoto's encephalopathy is characterized by confusion, myoclonus, partial or grand mal seizures, and, rarely, chorea. In some cases there may also be stroke-like episodes with focal findings, such as aphasia. The EEG is abnormal in most cases, with generalized slowing, frontal rhythmic slow activity, triphasic waves or periodic sharp complexes. MRI scanning may display increased signal intensity on T2-weighted scans in the white matter, and, in those cases characterized by stroke-like episodes, subcortical infarctions may be visualized.

The dementia of Hashimoto's encephalopathy, like the delirium, is generally accompanied by myoclonus; however, months may pass between the onset of the dementia and the appearance of myoclonus.

In addition to delirium and dementia, Hashimoto's encephalopathy may, rarely, present with a psychosis.

Antithyroid antibodies are present and both antithyroid peroxidase (formerly known as antimicrosomal antibody) and antithyroglobulin antibodies should be sought. The TSH may be normal or elevated, and the free T4 may be either reduced or within normal limits. Importantly, there is no correlation between the appearance of delirium and dementia and thyroid status.

COURSE

The delirium typically follows a relapsing and remitting course.

The overall course of the dementia is not known.

In one case report, the psychosis was relapsing and remitting.

COMPLICATIONS

The complications of delirium, dementia and secondary psychosis are as described in those chapters.

ETIOLOGY

Although Hashimoto's thyroiditis and Hashimoto's encephalopathy are clearly related, the connection between them, as noted earlier, is not clear. Although antithyroid antibodies are present in both disorders, and are probably responsible for thyroid damage in

Hashimoto's thyroiditis, it appears that other, as yet unknown, antibodies underlie the autoimmune assault on the cerebrum in Hashimoto's encephalopathy.

The pathology of Hashimoto's encephalopathy is characterized by both a vasculitis and a widespread leukoencephalopathy.

DIFFERENTIAL DIAGNOSIS

Hashimoto's encephalopathy must be distinguished from other disorders capable of causing myoclonus. When Hashimoto's encephalopathy presents with delirium, these include hyponatremia, hypomagnesemia, hepatic encephalopathy and uremic encephalopathy; when it presents with dementia, Creutzfeldt-Jakob disease must be considered; and when it presents with psychosis, intoxication with phencyclidine or dopaminergic agents must be ruled out.

TREATMENT

Prednisone is generally very effective; in resistant cases immunosuppresents such as azathioprine may be required.

The symptomatic treatment of delirium, dementia and secondary psychosis is as discussed in those chapters.

BIBLIOGRAPHY

Bohnen NI, Parnell KJ, Harper CM. Reversible MRI findings in a patient with Hashimoto's encephalopathy. *Neurology* 1997;49:246-247.

Henchey R, Cibula J, Helveston W, et al. Electroencephalographic findings in Hashimoto's encephalopathy. *Neurology* 1995;45:977-981.

Kothbauer-Margreiter I, Sturzenegger M, et al. Encephalopathy associated with Hashimoto thyroiditis: diagnosis and treatment. *Journal of Neurology* 1996;243:585-593.

Shaw PJ, Walls TJ, Newman PK, et al. Hashimoto's encephalopathy: a steroid-responsive disorder associated with high anti-thyroid antibody titers—report of 5 cases. *Neurology* 1991;41:228-233.

Taurin G, Golfier V, Pinel JF, et al. Choreic syndrome due to Hashimoto's encephalopathy. *Movement Disorders* 2002;17:1091-1092.

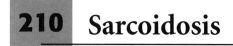

210 Sarcoidosis

Sarcoidosis is an uncommon systemic disorder characterized by the occurrence of sarcoid granulomas in various organs: neurosarcoidosis, with involvement of the central or peripheral nervous systems, is seen in about 5% of cases.

Sarcoidosis appears equally common among males and females; it appears with increased frequency among northern Europeans and among blacks in North America.

ONSET

The onset may be either acute or gradual, and tends to occur in the twenties or thirties.

CLINICAL FEATURES

Although sarcoidosis may be protean in its manifestations, certain common presentations deserve note. Perhaps 90% of patients have pulmonary involvement, which may manifest clinically with symptoms such as dyspnea or cough, or may be asymptomatic and discovered only when a chest x-ray reveals bilateral hilar lymphadenopathy or a characteristic reticulonodular pattern. Other symptoms include erythema nodosum, lupus pernio, uveitis, lymphadenopathy, arthropathy, and parotid gland enlargement. Hepatic involvement may occur in almost three quarters of all patients; however, hepatic failure is rare. Hypercalcemia occurs in a minority of patients, and some of these patients may go on to develop nephrocalcinosis and renal failure.

Neurosarcoidosis may be characterized by involvement of the brain, cranial nerves or peripheral nerves. Cerebral involvement may manifest with a personality change (often with features of the frontal lobe syndrome), amnesia, dementia, delirium, seizures

(either partial or grand mal), or, very rarely, psychosis; in addition, the hypothalamus and, less commonly, the pituitary are also commonly involved, and patients may develop hypersomnolence, hyperphagia, diabetes insipidus or galactorrhea. Of the cranial nerves, the facial nerve is most often involved, and here the peripheral facial palsy may be either unilateral or bilateral; the optic nerve or chiasm is also often involved, and patients may present with blindness or field defects. Peripheral nerve involvement may be characterized by either a mononeuritis multiplex or a polyneuropathy.

Other evidence of central nervous system involvement includes obstructive hydrocephalus and cerebral infarctions.

MRI scanning is far more sensitive than CT scanning, and granulomatous changes typically show up as areas of increased signal intensity on T2-weighted scans. On gadolinium-enhanced T1-weighted scans these areas typically enhance (as illustrated in Figure 210-1); furthermore, one may also see enhancement of the meninges.

Analysis of the cerebrospinal fluid may reveal elevated protein, decreased sugar, and a pleocytosis, predominantly lymphocytic. The IgG index may be increased, and in some cases there may also be oligoclonal bands.

The serum angiotensin-converting enzyme level is elevated in over half the patients with sarcoidosis.

Definitive diagnosis is made by a biopsy of an affected area, generally the lung.

COURSE

The course is variable: spontaneous remission may be seen after many months in up to one-half of cases, whereas in the rest one sees

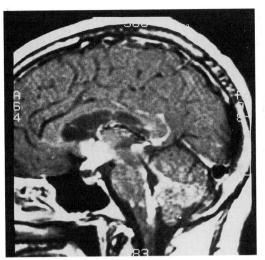

FIG. 210-1. Enhancing lesions of the hypothalamus and pituitary in a patient with sarcoidosis. (From Vinken PJ, Bruyn GW. *Handbook of clinical neurology*, vol 71 (revised 27), New York, 1998, Elsevier.)

either a pattern of relapses and remissions or a chronic progression. Acute onset cases tend to have the most favorable prognosis.

COMPLICATIONS

Complications of personality change, amnesia, dementia, delirium and psychosis are as described in the respective chapters.

ETIOLOGY

In neurosarcoidosis multiple granulomas are found in the cerebrum and leptomeninges. With regard to cerebral involvement, although granulomas may be found anywhere in the brain, there is a predilection for the hypothalamus. Leptomeningeal involvement, although seen over the convexities, is more common at the base of the brain, where cranial nerves may be entrapped.

The granulomas are almost always noncaseating and typically contain lymphocytes and giant cells. The granulomas themselves result from an enhanced helper T cell response directed toward the involved tissues; in turn monocytes and macrophages are attracted, and a granuloma is formed. The precise cause of the enhanced T cell response, however, is not known.

DIFFERENTIAL DIAGNOSIS

The diagnosis of neurosarcoidosis is often suspected when there is evidence of central or peripheral nervous system involvement in the clinical setting of typical pulmonary disease. Such a clue,

however, may not always be present early on, and in such cases the diagnosis would require a high index of suspicion; over time, however, almost all cases of neurosarcoidosis eventually show typical pulmonary changes, thus suggesting the correct diagnosis.

Other disorders which may enter the differential diagnosis include tuberculosis, meningovascular syphilis and multiple sclerosis.

Very rarely a dementia or delirium in a patient with sarcoidosis, rather than indicating the presence of granulomas in the central nervous system, may be secondary to hepatic or renal failure.

TREATMENT

Treatment with prednisone often is followed by a reduction in the size of granulomas and clinical improvement; it does not, however, alter the natural course of the disease and should be reserved until symptoms become troubling; in cases where steroids are ineffective or not tolerated, methotrexate may be helpful. Diabetes insipidus may require treatment with desmopressin; anterior pituitary failure may require other hormonal replacement therapy. Hydrocephalus may require shunting, and solitary masses may rarely have to be removed. Seizures may generally be controlled with phenytoin or carbamazepine. The general treatment of dementia is as outlined in that chapter.

BIBLIOGRAPHY

Chapelon C, Ziza JM, Pietter JC, et al. Neurosarcoidosis: signs, course and treatment in 35 confirmed cases. *Medicine* 1990;69:261-276.

Cordingley G, Navarro C, Brust JCM, et al. Sarcoidosis presenting as senile dementia. *Neurology* 1981;31:1148-1151.

Douglas AC, Maloney AFJ. Sarcoidosis of the central nervous system. *Journal of Neurology, Neurosurgery, and Psychiatry* 1973;36:1024-1033.

Jefferson M. Sarcoidosis of the nervous system. *Brain* 1957;80:540-556.

Luke RA, Stern BJ, Krumholz A, et al. Neurosarcoidosis: the long-term clinical course. *Neurology* 1987;37:461-463.

Oksanen V. Neurosarcoidosis: clinical presentations and course in 50 patients. *Acta Neurologica Scandinavica* 1986;73:283-290.

Pentland B, Mitchell JD, Cull RE, et al. Central nervous system sarcoidosis. *Quarterly Journal of Medicine* 1985;56:457-465.

Sabaawi M, Gutierrez-Nunez J, Fragala MR. Neurosarcoidosis presenting as schizophreniform disorder. *International Journal of Psychiatry in Medicine* 1992;22:269-274.

Scott TF. Neurosarcoidosis: progress and clinical aspects. *Neurology* 1993;43:8-12.

Sharma OP. Neurosarcoidosis: a personal perspective based on the study of 37 patients. *Chest* 1997;112:220-228.

Stern BJ, Krumholz A, Johns C, et al. Sarcoidosis and its neurological manifestations. *Archives of Neurology* 1985;42:909-917.

Stuart CA, Neelon FA, Lebovitz HE. Hypothalamic insufficiency: the cause of hypopituitarism in sarcoidosis. *Annals of Internal Medicine* 1978;88:589-594.

211 Postanoxic Encephalopathy

Global interruption of oxygen supply to the brain, whether due to deficient oxygenation or to grossly reduced blood flow, if prolonged for 5 minutes or more, causes a coma, often leaving patients who survive with varying degrees of permanent residual damage.

Such global anoxia may result from the following: drowning, strangulation, respiratory arrest or severe respiratory depression, cardiac arrest, ventricular fibrillation, shock, and carbon monoxide poisoning.

ONSET

Among those who survive and who awaken from coma, some may be left in a persistent vegetative state, others may emerge into a chronic dementia, whereas others may eventually experience a more or less complete recovery.

CLINICAL FEATURES

The dementia of postanoxic encephalopathy is of variable severity and may or may not be accompanied by delusions or hallucinations or restlessness; occasionally, rather than a dementia, one may see an amnesia with both anterograde and retrograde components. Focal signs, such as cortical blindness, visual agnosia, apraxia or aphasia, may occur, as may seizures and abnormal movements. Typically, in the case of abnormal movements, there is a latency between recovery of consciousness and their onset, lasting anywhere from weeks to months, or, exceptionally, years. Parkinsonism may occur, and this is often accompanied by dystonia; dystonia may also occur by itself, and tends to be generalized. Action myoclonus may also be seen.

MRI or CT scanning may demonstrate ventricular enlargement, laminar cortical necrosis (as illustrated in Figure 211-1), and, in those cases with parkinsonism or dystonia, lesions within the basal ganglia.

COURSE

Some improvement in the dementia may be seen in the first few months, after which the course is static. In the case of parkinsonism and dystonia, there may be a gradual progression over many years.

COMPLICATIONS

The complications of dementia are noted in the chapter on dementia. In a minority of cases, patients, after a period of stability, may go on to develop a delayed postanoxic leukoencephalopathy, as described in that chapter.

ETIOLOGY

The gray matter is more susceptible to anoxic injury than is the white matter, and, in the gray matter, the occipital and parietal cortices are more susceptible than are the frontal and temporal cortices. Within the cortex, one may see either the classic pattern of laminar cortical necrosis or evidence of scattered, multifocal damage. Within the temporal lobe the hippocampus may also suffer significant necrosis. Other gray matter often involved include the basal ganglia, cerebellar cortex and thalamus.

DIFFERENTIAL DIAGNOSIS

Delayed postanoxic encephalopathy is distinguished by the latent interval between the recovery from coma and the onset of symptoms.

TREATMENT

As there is no specific treatment for the dementia itself, management is symptomatic, as described in the chapter on dementia. With regard to restlessness, single-blinded and open case studies suggest benefit from risperidone (in low doses of 1 mg or less), amitriptyline and levodopa/carbidopa. Levodopa and direct-acting

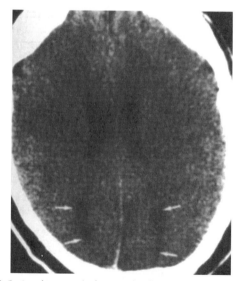

FIG. 211-1. Laminar cortical necrosis demonstrated on a CT scan. (From Osborn AG. *Diagnostic neuroradiology,* St. Louis, 1994, Mosby.)

dopaminergic agents have also, anecdotally, been successful in relieving the parkinsonism and dystonia. Action myoclonus has traditionally been treated with clonazepam, often in relatively high doses of 6 mg or more daily; case reports also suggest effectiveness for valproic acid and for levetiracetam.

BIBLIOGRAPHY

Bhatt MH, Obeso JA, Marsden CD. Time course of postanoxic akinetic-rigid and dystonic syndromes. *Neurology* 1993;43:314-317.

Chadwick D, Jenner P, Harris R, et al. Manipulation of brain serotonin in the treatment of myoclonus. *Lancet* 1975;2:434-435.

Debette S, Kozlowski O, Steinling M, et al. Levodopa and bromocriptine in hypoxic brain injury. *Journal of Neurology* 2002;249:1678-1682.

Krauss GL, Bergin A, Kramer RE, et al. Suppression of post-hypoxic and post-encephalitic myoclonus with levetiracetam. *Neurology* 2001;56: 411-412.

Kuoppamaki M, Bhatia KP, Quinn N. Progressive delayed-onset dystonia after cerebral anoxic insult in adults. *Movement Disorders* 2002;17: 1345-1349.

Rollinson RD, Gilligan BS. Postanoxic action myoclonus (Lance-Adams syndrome) responding to valproate. *Archives of Neurology* 1979;36: 44-45.

Silver BV, Collins L, Zidek KA. Risperidone treatment of motor restlessness following anoxic brain injury. *Brain Injury* 2003;17:237-244.

Szlabowicz JW, Stewart JT. Amitriptyline treatment of agitation associated with anoxic encephalopathy. *Archives of Physical Medicine and Rehabilitation* 1990;71:612-613.

212 Carbon Monoxide Poisoning

Carbon monoxide poisoning may be accidental or through suicidal intent; in the latter case typically either a hose is hooked to the exhaust on a car and then directed into the closed car where the patient sits, or the car is placed in a tightly sealed garage, where the patient awaits the end.

ONSET

The symptoms of poisoning may evolve gradually, or in some cases patients may abruptly worsen, slipping into a coma within moments.

CLINICAL FEATURES

Although it is customary to relate symptoms to the percent of carboxyhemoglobin in the blood, this relationship is rough at best, and decisions as to treatment are often better based on symptoms rather than on the carboxyhemoglobin level. Table 212-1 lists possible symptoms, and the carboxyhemoglobin levels they are traditionally associated with. The appearance of delirium, no matter how mild, represents a critical threshold regarding treatment, as noted below.

The classically described "cherry red" color of the lips, nails, and sometimes skin is rarely seen; indeed patients tend to be cyanotic.

COURSE

In cases where coma does not occur, recovery is usually complete. Those who do become comatose, however, upon awakening may be left with deficits, and the longer the coma the more likely this is to occur.

COMPLICATIONS

Deficits following coma may include a postanoxic encephalopathy, as described in that chapter. Rarely, after an interval of apparent recovery from coma, patients may develop a delayed postanoxic leukoencephalopathy, as described in that chapter.

Patients who have survived carbon monoxide poisoning may also, after a delay of weeks or longer, develop either parkinsonism or chorea: in the case of parkinsonism, one may see gradual progression, potentially to a severe akinetic-rigid syndrome. Other, rare, delayed sequelae include abulia and vocal and motor tics.

ETIOLOGY

Carbon monoxide binds very strongly with hemoglobin, thus displacing oxygen, leading to tissue hypoxia. It also impairs cellular respiration by binding to mitochondrial cytochrome oxidase.

DIFFERENTIAL DIAGNOSIS

The history usually makes the diagnosis straightforward; the possibility of a concomitant drug overdose must be borne in mind.

TREATMENT

The goal of acute treatment is to eliminate carbon monoxide as soon as possible. In the presence of room air, carbon monoxide has a half-life of from four to six hours; with 100% oxygen the half-life falls to about one hour and with hyperbaric 100% oxygen to

■TABLE 212-1. Symptoms of Carbon Monoxide Poisoning

Carboxyhemoglobin Level (%)	Symptoms
10 to 30	Headache
	Mild delirium
30 to 40	Increased headache
	Worsened delirium
	Nausea and vomiting
40 to 50	Stupor
	Faintness
	Ataxia
	Possible cyanosis
50 to 60	Coma
	Convulsions
> 60	Death

one-half hour or less. In patients with very mild symptoms and low carboxyhemoglobin levels, 100% oxygen at one atmospheric pressure might be sufficient; however, whenever delirium or more severe symptoms are present, it is imperative to begin hyperbaric treatment as soon as possible: recent work has made it clear that early institution of hyperbaric treatment dramatically reduces the risk of such complications as parkinsonism. In all cases, bed rest is indicated until recovery is complete.

BIBLIOGRAPHY

Davou P, Rondot P, Marion MH, et al. Severe chorea after acute carbon monoxide poisoning. *Journal of Neurology, Neurosurgery, and Psychiatry* 1986;49:206-208.

Finck PA. Exposure to carbon monoxide: review of the literature and 567 autopsies. *Military Medicine* 1966;131:1513-1519.

Lee MS, Marsden CD. Neurological sequelae following carbon monoxide poisoning: clinical course and outcome according to the clinical types and brain computed tomography scan findings. *Movement Disorders* 1994;9:550-558.

Lugaresi A, Montagna P, Merreale A, et al. "Psychic akinesia" following carbon monoxide poisoning. *European Neurology* 1990;30:167-169.

Pulst SM, Walshe TM, Romero JA. Carbon monoxide poisoning with features of Gilles de la Tourette's syndrome. *Archives of Neurology* 1983;40:443-444.

Weaver LK, Hopkins RO, Chan KJ, et al. Hyperbaric oxygen for acute carbon monoxide poisoning. *The New England Journal of Medicine* 2002;347:1057-1067.

213 Delayed Postanoxic Leukoencephalopathy

After recovering from the acute effects of a global anoxic insult, some patients, regardless of whether or not they were left with a postanoxic encephalopathy upon initial recovery from the anoxic insult, may go on to develop a delayed postanoxic leukoencephalopathy. This dreaded, albeit delayed, complication of global anoxia is seen in only 2 or 3% of patients and is characterized by either a delirium or a movement disorder, or both.

ONSET

In all cases, the history reveals a preceding episode of global cerebral anoxia with coma, or, occasionally, merely delirium. After experiencing a variable degree of recovery, patients then enjoy an interval of stable functioning ranging from two days to two months, with an average of three weeks, after which symptoms appear, generally in an acute fashion, over one or two days.

CLINICAL FEATURES

Typically, patients present with a delirium which is marked by apathy or irritability, and may progress to mutism. Incontinence is common, and on examination one may find hyperreflexia and Babinski signs. A movement disorder may accompany the delirium, or occur independently, and generally consists of parkinsonism or, in a smaller percentage, dystonia or chorea. In cases where the movement disorder occurs in isolation, the latent interval between the global anoxic insult and the onset of the movement disorder may be quite long, sometimes up to a half-year, or even longer.

CT or MRI scanning may show areas of demyelination in the white matter, primarily in the frontal lobes. In cases characterized by a movement disorder, lesions may also be seen in the basal ganglia, primarily the globus pallidus.

COURSE

In a small minority of cases, the leukoencephalopathy is relentlessly progressive and patients become comatose and may die. In the great majority, however, the prognosis is favorable, with perhaps three-quarters of patients experiencing a more or less complete recovery over 6 to 12 months time; in the remainder, one sees a residual dementia. The course of the movement disorder appears less favorable: it appears that in most cases the abnormal movements are chronic, whereas in some they actually undergo a slow progression.

COMPLICATIONS

The complications of delirium are as described in that chapter.

ETIOLOGY

The initial anoxic insult may be secondary to drowning, strangulation, respiratory arrest or severe respiratory depression, cardiac arrest, ventricular fibrillation, shock, or carbon monoxide poisoning. At autopsy, generally massive, diffuse, symmetric demyelination of the white matter is evident, with the gray matter being relatively spared. Although the mechanism underlying this delayed demyelination is not known, it is strongly suspected to occur secondary to an autoimmune onslaught triggered by cellular damage occurring during the initial anoxic insult.

DIFFERENTIAL DIAGNOSIS

The clinical differentiation between postanoxic encephalopathy and delayed postanoxic leukoencephalopathy rests primarily on the course. Postanoxic encephalopathy is evident shortly after recovery from coma, whereas in the delayed postanoxic leukoencephalopathy there is a "lucid" interval between recovery from coma and the onset of symptoms.

TREATMENT

Although there are no controlled studies, a case may be made, given the suspected mechanism underlying the demyelination, for a course of methylprednisolone, followed by prednisone, similar to that recommended for multiple sclerosis. The general treatment of delirium is as described in that chapter; the optimum treatment for any movement disorder is not clear.

BIBLIOGRAPHY

Choi IS. Delayed neurologic sequelae in carbon monoxide intoxication. *Archives of Neurology* 1983;40:433-435.

Choi IS. Parkinsonism after carbon monoxide poisoning. *European Neurology* 2002;48:30-33.

Dooling EC, Richardson EP. Delayed encephalopathy after strangling. *Archives of Neurology* 1976;33:196-199.

Inagaki T, Ishino H, Seno H, et al. A long-term follow-up study of serial magnetic resonance images in patients with delayed encephalopathy after acute carbon monoxide poisoning. *Psychiatry and Clinical Neurosciences* 1997;51:421-423.

Kobayashi K, Isaki K, Fukutani Y, et al. CT findings of the interval form of carbon monoxide poisoning compared with neuropathological findings. *European Neurology* 1984;23:34-43.

Min SK. A brain syndrome associated with delayed neuropsychiatric sequelae following acute carbon monoxide intoxication. *Acta Psychiatrica Scandinavica* 1986;73:80-86.

Norris CR, Trench JM, Hook R. Delayed carbon monoxide encephalopathy: clinical and research implications. *The Journal of Clinical Psychiatry* 1982;43:294-295.

Plum F, Posner JB, Hain RF. Delayed neurological deterioration after anoxia. *Archives of Internal Medicine* 1962;110:56-63.

214 Traumatic Brain Injury

Head trauma may be usefully classified according to the mechanism whereby the brain is injured: missile wounds, which are relatively uncommon in civilian life; crush injuries, wherein the stationary head is struck, as might happen when a car falls off its jack striking the garage mechanic working beneath it; and, most commonly, acceleration-deceleration injuries. Acceleration-deceleration injury most frequently occurs in motor vehicle accidents; for example, when a rapidly moving car strikes an abutment and the freely moving head comes to a violent instant deceleration on the dashboard. Actual contact, however, need not occur, and significant acceleration-deceleration injury may occur with a violent whiplash: all that is necessary is that the cranium stop and the still-moving gelatinous brain violently come to a halt against the inside of the vault, thus injuring itself.

The extent of brain damage after head injury is not necessarily related to the presence or absence of a fracture. Certainly, if a comminuted compound fracture occurred and fragments of bone lacerated the brain and came to a rest deeply embedded in the parenchyma, this would be most significant. However, severe, even fatal, brain damage may occur without any damage to the cranium at all.

In a missile injury, sequelae are naturally related to the path of the missile and the structures destroyed in that path. Although distant tissue may be damaged by an expanding pressure wave, some patients may make a remarkable recovery.

In a crush injury the parenchyma underlying the point of impact is contused and perhaps lacerated.

In acceleration-deceleration injuries, structures that extend for some length, such as axons, capillaries, and penetrating arterioles, are subject to enormous shearing and torsional strain and consequently undergo various degrees of damage or actual rupture. A condition known as diffuse axonal injury, or DAI, results whenever widespread demyelinization or axonal rupture occurs. Capillaries may also be ruptured, leading to petechial hemorrhages, and ruptured arterioles may produce intracerebral hematomas. In addition to DAI, such violent acceleration or deceleration may also cause lacerations of the parenchyma or contusions.

As missile and crush injuries are relatively uncommon in normal civilian life, they are not considered further here. The rest of this chapter focuses on the clinically far more important category of acceleration-deceleration injuries, often referred to as "closed-head" cases. These occur primarily in motor vehicle, motorcycle, and bicycle accidents and are most common among males in their late teens or early twenties.

ONSET

Diffuse axonal injury occurs immediately subsequent to the acceleration-deceleration trauma, and renders patients unconscious. With extensive DAI, the patient never awakens, and death ensues shortly. In somewhat less severe cases the patient may remain in a coma for a relatively prolonged period, only to awaken into a "vegetative state" that persists until death by some intercurrent illness. Those with lesser degrees of DAI experience a shorter period of coma, after which they awaken into a delirium which gradually clears and is replaced by a personality change, dementia, or both.

CLINICAL FEATURES

The personality change is typically characterized by irritability and moodiness, and there may be violent outbursts; much less commonly, there may be facetiousness and a shallow euphoria.

The dementia is of variable severity, and is often marked by inattentiveness, difficulty with concentration, and poor memory; typically there is also an amnesia for the trauma itself, and there is a fair correlation between the extent of the amnesia surrounding the trauma and the overall severity of the DAI. The patient may also experience headache, dizziness, and tinnitus.

On examination, one may see focal signs, reflecting areas of more severe damage, as in hemorrhage or severe contusion. Cranial nerve palsies, seizures, and varying degrees of aphasia or hemiparesis may be seen.

In a small minority, DAI may also manifest as depression or mania.

MRI scanning is superior to CT scanning for defining the underlying damage. Acutely, hematomas, contusions, and areas of small petechial hemorrhage may be visualized; chronically, one sees a degree of cortical atrophy coupled with varying degrees of glial scarring and leukomalacia.

COURSE

In most cases one sees some degree of gradual improvement. Although this is most marked over the first half year, improvement may continue for up to a year and a half or sometimes longer. Eventually, however, the clinical picture stabilizes and remains static for the remainder of the patient's life.

COMPLICATIONS

Complications are as described in the chapters on dementia, personality change, and secondary depression or mania.

ETIOLOGY

The shearing forces created by the acceleration or the deceleration typically cause axonal damage and petechial hemorrhages in the corpus callosum and the dorso-lateral quadrants of the mesencephalon. More widespread axonal damage typically occurs at the junction of gray and white matter. Hematomas secondary to shorn arterioles typically occur in the white matter of the frontal or temporal lobes but also may be seen in the deep gray structures. Contusions and lacerations are typically located on the undersurface of the frontal and temporal lobes.

Chronically, one sees cortical atrophy and ventricular enlargement. Diffuse microglial scars are present at the sites of axonal injury in addition to the residuals from any hematomas, lacerations, or contusions.

DIFFERENTIAL DIAGNOSIS

As noted earlier, the patient with a traumatic brain injury typically experiences gradual improvement. Consequently, any worsening of the clinical picture suggests an intercurrent disorder, such as a subdural hematoma, hydrocephalus (which may be due to shearing and scarring of the aqueduct or, if subarachnoid hemorrhage had occurred, to impaired outflow of cerebrospinal fluid at the arachnoid villi), ischemic infarctions secondary to posttraumatic thrombosis of the middle cerebral or posterior cerebral arteries (a rare occurrence), traumatic pneumocephalus (if a fracture

occurred at the base), and, in cases of compound fracture, an intracranial abscess. One other cause of "delayed" deterioration is an intracerebral hematoma, which, though secondary to arteriolar damage at the time of injury, may be delayed in its onset for up to a week and a half.

The postconcussion syndrome is distinguished by the absence of significant impairment of memory and concentration. It may be noted, however, that some speculate that, just as diffuse axonal injury must exist on a continuum of severity, so too would its clinical expression, ranging from death, to dementia, down to a most minimal clinical disturbance, which indeed may be the postconcussion syndrome.

Dementia pugilistica is clearly distinguished by its course. Patients with traumatic dementia improve over time, whereas patients with dementia pugilistica show a progressive downhill course.

TREATMENT

The general treatment of personality change is considered in that chapter; in cases characterized by violent outbursts, propranolol, in high doses of from 240-600 mg daily, may be helpful.

The general treatment of dementia is outlined in that chapter; in addition, amantadine, in doses of 100 mg bid, may improve cognitive functioning.

BIBLIOGRAPHY

Adams JH, Graham DI, Murray LS, et al. Diffuse axonal injury due to nonmissile head injury in humans: an analysis of 45 cases. *Annals of Neurology* 1982;12:557-563.

Blumbergs PC, Jones NR, North JB. Diffuse axonal injury in head trauma. *Journal of Neurology, Neurosurgery, and Psychiatry* 1989;52:838-841.

Meythaler JM, Brunner RC, Johnson A, et al. Amantadine to improve neurorecovery in traumatic brain injury-associated diffuse axonal injury: a pilot double-blind randomized trial. *The Journal of Head Trauma Rehabilitation* 2002;17:300-313.

Oppenheimer DR. Microscopic lesions in the brain following head injury. *Journal of Neurology, Neurosurgery, and Psychiatry* 1968;31:229-236.

Parizel PM, Ozsarlak Van Goethem JW, van den Hauwe L, et al. Imaging findings in diffuse axonal injury after closed head trauma. *European Radiology* 1998;8:960-965.

Strich SJ. Diffuse degeneration of the cerebral white matter in severe dementia following head injury. *Journal of Neurology, Neurosurgery, and Psychiatry* 1956;19:163-185.

215 Postconcussion Syndrome (postconcussional disorder)

A concussion is a brief loss of consciousness, generally lasting no more than a few minutes, following either a blow to the head or, less commonly, sudden acceleration or deceleration, as may occur in a car accident. Although most concussion patients recover rapidly and completely, a minority go on to develop the postconcussion syndrome.

Patients with this syndrome, also known as "postconcussional disorder," experience headache, difficulty with concentration and memory, fatigue, dizziness, and various admixtures of irritability, depression, and anxiety. Interestingly, only a modest correlation appears to exist between the severity of the injury and the development of these symptoms.

ONSET

Although the postconcussion syndrome may occur at any age, it is decidedly uncommon among children. The syndrome itself usually appears within a day of the concussion itself.

CLINICAL FEATURES

Headache tends to be severe and may be either constant or paroxysmal. Loud noises, coughing, sneezing, or stress may exacerbate it, and it may be characterized as either dull or throbbing.

Difficulty with concentration and memory may be most disturbing to the patient. Patients may complain that they are no longer able to complete tasks that before the concussion presented no difficulty. Fatigue may be either constant or evident only when patients attempt to exert themselves.

The dizziness may be either a lightheadedness or vertigo. When vertigo is present, it may be exacerbated or precipitated by changes in position or sudden movements.

Irritability is a prominent symptom, and patients may have great difficulty controlling their temper. Depression and, less commonly, anxiety may be complained of, and some patients may experience severe insomnia.

Other symptoms occasionally seen include photophobia, hyperacusis, and hyperhidrosis, which at times may be severe.

Many patients report that alcohol, even in small amounts, reliably exacerbates their symptoms.

COURSE

Symptoms improve gradually, and complete recovery generally occurs in a matter of months. In some cases remission may occur within weeks, whereas in others gradual improvement may continue for up to 3 years. Symptoms persisting beyond 3 years tend to be chronically stable.

COMPLICATIONS

Most patients experience at least some difficulty in completing their work, and friction with family members or coworkers is not uncommon.

ETIOLOGY

The pathology of postconcussion syndrome is not known. However, some suspect that a mild degree of diffuse axonal injury induced by shear and torsion during the head trauma may underlie the symptoms.

DIFFERENTIAL DIAGNOSIS

Dementia seen after traumatic brain injury is distinguished by the presence of pronounced cognitive deficits.

Other sequelae to head trauma may produce symptoms similar to those seen in postconcussion syndrome. These include subdural hematoma, contusion or laceration, and hydrocephalus.

Posttraumatic stress disorder is distinguished by the involuntary reexperiencing of the event in dreams, waking thoughts, and the like.

Malingering may occur after a concussion, especially in cases of lawsuits. In many cases only prolonged observation beyond the resolution of the lawsuit resolves the diagnostic question.

Conversion symptoms may occur after head trauma; the diagnostic approach here is as outlined in the chapter on conversion disorder.

TREATMENT

Reassurance is critical. Patients should be fully informed regarding the good prognosis and should be encouraged to resume their normal duties progressively, as their symptoms gradually subside. Non-opioid analgesics are indicated for headache, and antihistamines may partially relieve the dizziness. Antidepressants may help relieve irritability, depression, and insomnia. Alcohol should be forbidden until recovery is complete.

BIBLIOGRAPHY

Bohnen N, Twijnstra A, Wijnen G, et al. Tolerance for light and sound of patients with persistent post-concussional symptoms 6 months after mild head injury. *Journal of Neurology* 1991;238:443-446.

Chen SH, Kareken DA, Fasteneau PS, et al. A study of persistent postconcussion symptoms in mild head trauma using positron emission tomography. *Journal of Neurology, Neurosurgery, and Psychiatry* 2003;74:326-332.

Symonds C. Concussion and its sequelae. *Lancet* 1962;1:1-5.

Watson MR, Fenton GW, McClelland RJ, et al. The post-concussional state: neurophysiological aspects. *The British Journal of Psychiatry* 1995;167:514-521.

216 Subacute and Chronic Subdural Hematoma

Head trauma, which especially in the elderly need not be severe, may result in an accumulation of blood between the dura and the arachnoid. These subdural hematomas vary in their time of onset and may be acute, occurring within hours, subacute, presenting within two or three weeks of the trauma, or chronic, with the onset of symptoms delayed for weeks, months, or even years. Subacute subdural hematomas may present with delirium, and chronic subdural hematomas may cause a dementia. This chapter deals only with subacute and chronic subdural hematomas. Acute subdural hematomas tend to be clinically obvious, presenting often within hours of severe trauma as a neurosurgical emergency, with stupor, focal signs, seizures, or herniation.

The annual incidence of chronic subdural hematoma in the general adult population is somewhat over 0.001%. Among those over 70, however, the incidence rises to above 0.007%. Overall, subdural hematomas are more likely to occur in males than females.

ONSET

Subacute subdural hematomas tend to present fairly rapidly, and generally one notes that the patient is obviously ill. Chronic subdural hematomas, however, often present gradually and insidiously.

CLINICAL FEATURES

Subacute subdural hematomas tend to present with drowsiness and delirium, and symptoms may fluctuate for days. Focal signs often occur, and in time uncal herniation with stupor, coma, and death may occur. In up to a quarter of patients with subacute subdural hematomas, the hematomas are bilateral.

Chronic subdural hematomas may be caused by trivial head injury. Indeed anywhere from one quarter to one half of these patients cannot recall the responsible trauma. After a latent interval of weeks, months, or more, patients typically develop a dementia that is often accompanied by headache; a personality change may also occur, and, rarely, the presentation may be with depression. Focal signs may or may not be present; indeed even large hematomas may fail to cause them. If focal signs do occur, hemiparesis is perhaps the most common. Rarely, seizures or papilledema may be seen. So-called false localizing signs may occur when uncal herniation compresses the contralateral cerebral peduncle or posterior cerebral artery, producing homolateral hemiparesis or homonymous hemianopsia, respectively. As with subacute subdural hematomas, chronic subdural hematomas are commonly bilateral.

On both CT and MRI images, the subdural hematoma presents as a mass, generally over the frontal or parietal convexity, with a concave medial border. On the unenhanced CT scan, the mass is initially hyperdense; however, after a week or two, as the blood degrades, the mass may become "isodense" with the underlying cortex. After several weeks, however, when most of the blood has been resorbed leaving a proteinaceous fluid, the mass becomes relatively radiolucent. In Figure 216-1 a subacute subdural hematoma is isodense with the underlying brain but is distinguished by the faint line of enhancement at the boundary between it and the brain beneath it. By contrast the chronic subdural hematoma depicted in Figure 216-2 is now quite lucent relative to the underlying brain and easily distinguishable from it.

On T1-weighted MRI scans the signal intensity of the mass initially falls between that of cerebrospinal fluid and the cortex. By 1 or 2 weeks the intensity is quite bright, and after 3 weeks or so the hematomas become relatively "isointense" with the underlying cortex. Rebleeding into a hematoma may occur and would alter the appearance according to the age of the rebleed.

COURSE

Subacute subdural hematomas tend to evolve over a matter of weeks and may progress to coma and death or undergo stabilization, after which there may be either gradual improvement, representing resorption of the hematoma, or a chronic course.

Chronic subdural hematomas may undergo gradual progression or may stabilize.

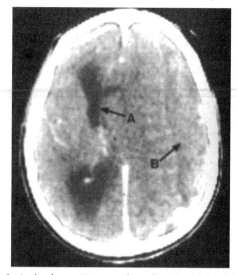

FIG. 216-1. An isodense CT scan of a subacute subdural hematoma. (From Parsons M. *Color atlas of clinical neurology*, ed 2, London, 1993, Wolfe.)

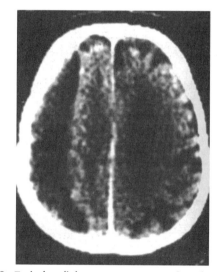

FIG. 216-2. Typical radiolucent appearance of a chronic subdural hematoma. (From Parsons M. *Color atlas of clinical neurology*, ed 2, London, 1993, Wolfe.)

COMPLICATIONS

Complications are as described in the chapters on delirium and dementia.

ETIOLOGY

In contrast to acute subdural hematoma, which may result from arterial bleeding, subacute and chronic subdural hematomas generally follow upon rupture of the bridging veins between the cortex and the dura. Meeting little resistance, the blood gradually dissects through the subdural space over the convexity, forming a large but relatively thin mass. In some cases spread may also occur to the interhemispheric fissure or along the tentorium. Coagulation occurs, and within a week or two substantial hemolysis has converted much of the clot into a relatively clear fluid.

By the third week fibroblasts from the inner surface of the dura have begun to form a new membrane, thus encapsulating the hematoma. Small hematomas may become completely fibrosed; larger ones remain as fluid-filled capsules. Over time the encapsulated hematoma tends to expand, and, as noted earlier, evidence of rebleeding may be seen on CT or MRI scanning. Eventually the membrane may become calcified. Symptoms occur secondary to compression of the underlying parenchyma and to brain shifts, which may result in herniation.

Subdural hematomas are more common among the elderly, alcoholics, patients with blood dyscrasias, and those taking anticoagulants.

DIFFERENTIAL DIAGNOSIS

Any expanding mass lesion may mimic a chronic subdural hematoma. Subdural hygromas (resulting from an escape of subarachnoid fluid through a tear in the arachnoid up into the subdural space) may be indistinguishable from a chronic subdural hematoma.

TREATMENT

Evacuation or drainage is generally required for subacute subdural hematomas, and, in the case of chronic subdural hematomas accompanied by dementia, these procedures may allow for a considerable restoration of cognitive abilities. The general treatment of dementia and delirium is as described in the respective chapters.

BIBLIOGRAPHY

Annegers JF, Hauser WA, Coan SP, et al. A population-based study of seizures after traumatic brain injuries. *The New England Journal of Medicine* 1998;338:20-24.

Black DW. Mental changes resulting from subdural hematoma. *The British Journal of Psychiatry* 1984;145:200-203.

Cameron MN. Chronic subdural hematoma: a review of one hundred and fourteen cases. *Journal of Neurology, Neurosurgery, and Psychiatry* 1978;41:834-839.

Ishikawa E, Yanaka K, Sugimoto K, et al. Reversible dementia in patients with chronic subdural hematomas. *Journal of Neurosurgery* 2002; 96:680-683.

217 Dementia Pugilistica

Dementia pugilistica is a distinct syndrome that develops secondary to repeated blows to the head and is characterized by dementia, ataxia, and parkinsonism. This syndrome is also known as the "punch drunk syndrome," "punch drunkenness," or "chronic traumatic encephalopathy."

Dementia pugilistica is found not only in boxers but also among jockeys who repeatedly fall from horses. The prevalence of dementia pugilistica among boxers is not known; however, it may be substantial. Although dementia pugilistica heretofore has been found exclusively in males, the number of female jockeys makes the eventual appearance of dementia pugilistica among females inevitable.

ONSET

The onset of symptoms is gradual, and occurs anywhere from 5 to 40 years after there has been an accumulation of a sufficient number of significant blows to the head, which, in professional boxers, is generally seen after a dozen fights. Although some boxers will still be active when symptoms appear, most will have long since retired from the ring.

CLINICAL FEATURES

The dementia progresses gradually and does not appear to have any distinguishing features, with the possible exception of an undue amount of irritability. Ataxia and dysarthria may be present, and the similarity of the clinical picture to that seen in alcohol intoxication has prompted the colloquial name for this disorder, the "punch drunk" syndrome. Parkinsonism may also appear, and may be disabling.

MRI scanning generally displays cerebral atrophy and a large cavum septi pellucidi.

COURSE

This is a chronic condition, and symptoms may either undergo a relentless, gradual progression, or eventually "plateau off," leaving behind a static clinical picture.

COMPLICATIONS

Complications are as described in the chapter on dementia.

ETIOLOGY

The cerebral cortex is atrophied, and in most cases there is a large cavum septi pellucidi, as illustrated in Figure 217-1; atrophy is also typically present in the corpus callosum and fornix. Microscopically, there are widespread neurofibrillary tangles and senile plaques. Although the tangles are almost identical to those seen in Alzheimer's disease, the plaques are not and have a diffuse, rather than a discrete, morphology. Cell loss is noted in the locus ceruleus and in the substantia nigra; however, there are no Lewy bodies. The cerebellar cortex is also atrophied, and Purkinje cells are reduced in number.

The mechanism whereby repeated blows to the head produces these pathologic changes is not known.

DIFFERENTIAL DIAGNOSIS

Normal pressure hydrocephalus may develop many years after a traumatic subarachnoid hemorrhage, and may be characterized by dementia and gait disturbance; here, however, one does not find parkinsonism.

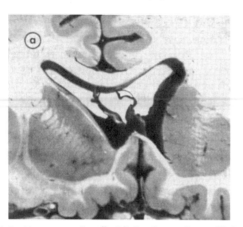

FIG. 217-1. Cavum septi pellucidi in dementia pugilistica. (From Roberts GW, Leigh PN, Wienberger DR. *Neuropsychiatric disorders,* Singapore, 1993, Mosby Europe.)

Chronic subdural hematoma may likewise present long after head trauma; however, here lateralizing signs, such as hemiplegia, may be present. Furthermore, cerebellar and parkinsonian signs are also lacking.

TREATMENT

The overall treatment of dementia is as described in that chapter. When irritability is prominent, propranolol, in high doses of 240 mg or more, may be helpful. Parkinsonism may respond to levodopa/carbidopa or direct-acting dopaminergics. If boxing itself cannot be banned, the use of head gear and larger gloves may reduce the risk of dementia pugilistica.

BIBLIOGRAPHY

Bogdanoff B, Natter HM. Incidence of cavum septum pellucidum in adults: a sign of boxer's encephalopathy. *Neurology* 1989;39:991-992.

Corsellis JAN. Boxing and the brain. *British Medical Journal* 1989;298: 105-109.

Corsellis JAN, Bruton CJ, Freeman-Browne D. The aftermath of boxing. *Psychological Medicine* 1973;3:270-303.

Critchley M. Medical aspects of boxing, particularly from a neurological standpoint. *British Medical Journal* 1957;1:357-366.

Harvey PKP, Davis JN. Traumatic encephalopathy in a young boxer. *Lancet* 1974;2:928-929.

Jordan BD. Neurologic aspects of boxing. *Archives of Neurology* 1987; 44:453-459.

Martland HS. Punch drunk. *Journal of the American Medical Association* 1928;91:1103-1107.

Roberts GW. Immunocytochemistry of neurofibrillary tangles in dementia pugilistica and Alzheimer's disease: evidence for a common genesis. *Lancet* 1988;2:1456-1458.

Roberts GW, Allsop D, Bruton C. The occult aftermath of boxing. *Journal of Neurology, Neurosurgery, and Psychiatry* 1990;53:373-378.

Schmidt ML, Zhukareva V, Newell KL, et al. Tau isoform and phosphorylation state in dementia pugilistica recapitulate Alzheimer's disease. *Acta Neuropathologica* 2001;101:518-524.

218 Radiation Encephalopathy

After irradiation of the brain, three different forms of radiation encephalopathy may occur: acute, early-delayed, and late-delayed. Acute radiation encephalopathy is a fairly common, but transient, complication of cerebral irradiation, and consists of drowsiness, headache and nausea, and, in a small minority, seizures. This acute form of radiation encephalopathy tends to occur toward the end of, or just after, a course of irradiation, and generally responds to a brief course of steroids. Of more concern are the early- and late-delayed forms of radiation encephalopathy, and these are discussed here.

ONSET

Early-delayed radiation encephalopathy appears subacutely anywhere from one and one-half to four months after a course of radiation; by contrast, late-delayed radiation encephalopathy has a gradual, even insidious, onset, and occurs anywhere from 6 to 24 months after radiation treatment; in some cases the delay may be much longer, up to years or even decades.

CLINICAL FEATURES

The clinical symptomatology of both early- and late-delayed radiation encephalopathy is strongly influenced by whether the original irradiation was focal, as for example for a brain tumor, or whole-brain, as might be performed for prophylaxis in patients with leukemia.

Delayed radiation encephalopathies following focal irradiation tend to present in a fashion similar to that of an expanding mass lesion, and this is the case regardless of whether the encephalopathy is of the early- or late-delayed type.

Encephalopathies following whole-brain irradiation, by contrast, differ in their symptomatology according to whether they are of the early- or late-delayed type. Early-delayed radiation encephalopathy following whole-brain radiation may be characterized by delirium, drowsiness, headache, nausea, and, occasionally, fever. Late-delayed radiation encephalopathy following whole brain irradiation presents with dementia, which, over time, is often accompanied by ataxia and incontinence.

MRI scanning shows areas of increased signal intensity on T2-weighted scans in both early- and late-delayed radiation encephalopathy, which, as might be expected, is focal in cases following focal irradiation, and diffuse, throughout the white matter, in cases following whole-brain irradiation, as illustrated in Figure 218-1. In cases following whole-brain irradiation, there is also often cortical atrophy and ventricular dilatation.

In cases where large cerebral vessels were exposed, one may also see delayed cerebral infarctions due to a radiation-induced vasculitis.

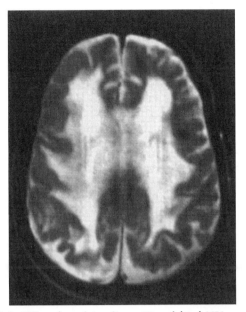

FIG. 218-1. Diffuse hyperintensity on T2-weighted MRI scan in centrum semiovale of a patient with delayed radiation encephalopathy secondary to whole brain irradiation. (From Yock DH. *Imaging of CNS disease: a CT and MR teaching file*, ed 2, St. Louis, 1991, Mosby.)

Other variants include somnolence or hyperphagia when the hypothalamus was irradiated, and hypothyroidism or adrenocortical insufficiency if the pituitary was exposed.

In passing, one should also note that irradiation, in addition to producing the above described syndromes, may also, albeit very rarely, cause actual de novo formation of meningiomas or gliomas.

COURSE

Early-delayed radiation encephalopathy tends to be self-limited, with symptoms generally resolving within six to eight weeks. By contrast, late-delayed radiation encephalopathy is generally progressive over the years, and may result in death.

COMPLICATIONS

Complications are as described in the chapters on delirium and dementia.

ETIOLOGY

Although the risks of a delayed encephalopathy increase with increasing doses of radiation, such encephalopathies are not uncommonly seen after "safe" doses.

In the case of early-delayed radiation encephalopathy, one sees a degree of demyelinization. In late-delayed radiation encephalopathy, in addition to demyelinization, there is also a small-vessel vasculopathy with proliferation of the vascular endothelium with subsequent ischemic changes, which may be severe.

DIFFERENTIAL DIAGNOSIS

Although the history of irradiation is highly suggestive, diagnostic problems may arise in cases following focal irradiation, where the signs and symptoms could be compatible with either a delayed encephalopathy or a recurrence of the tumor. In cases where symptoms arise within months after irradiation, watchful waiting may resolve the diagnostic question: a resolution of symptoms indicates an early-delayed encephalopathy, whereas their progression is more consistent with tumor recurrence. When, however, symptoms occur only after a year of more has passed since irradiation, watchful waiting is generally not helpful, given that late-delayed radiation encephalopathy, like a tumor, is generally progressive. MRI scanning may likewise be of little help, given that both conditions may produce similar MRI images. PET or SPECT scanning, however, may resolve the issue, given that tumors are metabolically active, whereas areas of delayed radiation encephalopathy are not. In doubtful cases, biopsy may be required.

TREATMENT

In early delayed radiation encephalopathy, prednisone or dexamethasone may hasten remission.

In late delayed radiation encephalopathy secondary to localized irradiation, excision of the damaged area may be required; in other cases of localized irradiation and in cases of late delayed radiation encephalopathy secondary to whole brain irradiation, anticoagulation may halt or delay progression.

The general treatment of delirium and dementia is as outlined in the respective chapters.

BIBLIOGRAPHY

DeAngelis LM, Delattre JY, Posner JB. Radiation-induced dementia in patients cured of brain metastases. *Neurology* 1989;39:789-796.

Duffey P, Chari G, Cartlidge NE, et al. Progressive deterioration of intellect and motor function occurring several decades after cranial irradiation. A new facet in the clinical spectrum of radiation encephalopathy. *Archives of Neurology* 1996;53:814-818.

Glantz MJ, Burger PC, Friedman AH, et al. Treatment of radiation-induced nervous system injury with heparin and warfarin. *Neurology* 1994;44:2020-2027.

Kaufman M, Swartz BE, Mandelkern M, et al. Diagnosis of delayed cerebral radiation necrosis following proton beam therapy. *Archives of Neurology* 1990;47:474-476.

Lam KS, Tse VK, Wang C, et al. Effects of cranial irradiation in hypothalamic-pituitary function—a 5-year longitudinal study in patients with nasopharyngeal carcinoma. *Quarterly Journal of Medicine* 1991;78:165-176.

Morris JGL, Grattan-Smith P, Panegyres PK, et al. Delayed cerebral radiation necrosis. *Quarterly Journal of Medicine* 1994;87:119-129.

Rottenberg DA, Chernik NL, Teck MDF, et al. Cerebral necrosis following radiotherapy of extracranial neoplasms. *Annals of Neurology* 1977;1:339.

219 Brain Tumors

Depending on location and rate of growth, brain tumors are capable of producing a seemingly innumerable variety of signs and symptoms. A thorough discussion of these tumors lies outside the scope of this book. The focus of the ensuing discussion is on their capacity to cause dementia and related syndromes.

Most brain tumors are primary central nervous system neoplasms; metastases account for only about a fifth of all tumors. Of the primary brain tumors, the most common are gliomas, including glioblastoma multiforme, astrocytomas, oligodendrogliomas, and ependymomas. The next most common primary brain tumor is a meningioma. Primary central nervous system lymphoma, once decidedly rare, is now seen with some frequency among those with AIDS and those treated with immunosuppressants.

Metastases tend to be multiple and, in rough order of decreasing frequency, have as their source the lung, breast, gastrointestinal tract, kidney, prostate, and thyroid. Melanoma and choriocarcinoma, though not common malignancies, not uncommonly metastasize to the brain.

ONSET

Although brain tumors may occur at any age, the peak incidence tends to be in middle and late middle age. Highly malignant tumors, such as glioblastoma multiforme and metastases, tend to present fairly acutely, perhaps over several months. By contrast, meningiomas, astrocytomas, oligodendrogliomas, and ependymomas may present very gradually over many months or even years.

CLINICAL FEATURES

Tumors situated in the frontal lobes or the rostral portion of the corpus callosum are particularly prone to cause dementia, which indeed may be the only symptom of the tumor for a long time. One also often sees a personality change, typically a frontal lobe syndrome.

Tumors of the temporal lobe may cause delirium, psychosis, or a personality change.

Tumors of the thalamus are rare, but may present with dementia.

Elevated intracranial pressure, often due to peri-tumoral edema, may occur. Although this is classically associated with headache, nausea and vomiting, and papilledema, in some patients the most prominent symptom of elevated intracranial pressure may be a personality change or a dementia, which is marked by drowsiness and slowed thinking.

Partial seizures, with or without secondary generalization, are common.

Enhanced CT or, preferably, enhanced MRI scanning is the most important diagnostic test. Biopsy is often required for a definitive diagnosis of the type of tumor. When a metastatic tumor is suspected and there is no obvious primary, it is appropriate to consider chest x-ray or chest CT, mammography, stool for occult blood and so forth.

COURSE

In general, the clinical condition of the patient tends to gradually worsen, with the overall pace being determined by the aggressiveness of the underlying tumor. Some tumors, such as a glioblastoma multiforme, cause a rapid deterioration, with death within a year or two, whereas others, such as low-grade astrocytomas or meningiomas, may be compatible with very long survival.

Exceptionally, there may be an acute exacerbation, and this may be seen in cases where there is hemorrhage into the tumor (as may occur with glioblastoma multiforme or metastatic tumors), compression of a major artery with subsequent stroke, or acute obstruction of cerebrospinal fluid outflow producing acute hydrocephalus.

COMPLICATIONS

Complications of dementia, delirium, personality change and secondary psychosis are as described in those chapters.

ETIOLOGY

Although a genetic factor may play a role in some tumors, the etiology of most primary brain tumors is unknown.

DIFFERENTIAL DIAGNOSIS

The differential diagnosis of dementia is as discussed in that chapter. Slowly growing tumors may cause a clinical picture similar in some degrees to Alzheimer's disease, subdural hematoma, normal pressure hydrocephalus, or Binswanger's disease.

TREATMENT

Therapy is dictated by the nature of the tumor and its location and may include any or all of surgical excision, radiation therapy, and chemotherapy.

Steroids are often effective in reducing edema and in lowering intracranial pressure.

If radiation is used, then one must be alert to the development of a delayed radiation encephalopathy, as described in that chapter.

BIBLIOGRAPHY

Black PM. Brain tumors (first of two parts). *The New England Journal of Medicine* 1991;324:1471.

Black PM. Brain tumors (second of two parts). *The New England Journal of Medicine* 1991;324:1555.

Cole G. Intracranial space-occupying masses in mental hospital patients: necropsy study. *Journal of Neurology, Neurosurgery, and Psychiatry* 1978;41:73.

Cunha UG. An investigation of dementia among elderly outpatients. *Acta Psychiatrica Scandinavica* 1990;82:261-263.

Delattre JY, Krol G, Thaler HT, et al. Distribution of brain metastases. *Archives of Neurology* 1988;45:741-744.

Filley CM, Kleinschmidt-DeMasters BK. Neurobehavioral presentations of brain neoplasms. *The Western Journal of Medicine* 1995;163: 19-25.

Galasko D, Kwo-On-Yuen PF, Thai L. Intracranial mass lesions associated with late-life psychosis and depression. *The Psychiatric Clinics of North America* 1988;11:151-166.

Hunter R, Blackwood W, Bull JWD. Three cases of frontal meningiomas presenting psychiatrically. *British Medical Journal* 1968;3:9.

Patchell RA. Brain metastases. *Neurologic Clinics of North America* 1991; 9:817.

Schwartz RB. Neuroradiology of brain tumors. *Neurologic Clinics of North America* 1995;13:723.

Shapiro WR. Brain tumors. *Seminars in Oncology* 1986;13:1.

220   Brain Abscess

Brain abscesses may occur secondary to trauma (a missile wound), to localized spread (from otitis media), or to hematogenous spread (from bronchiectasis or endocarditis). The clinical presentation is generally acute, and delirium is typically part of the clinical picture.

Brain abscesses are relatively rare, and males appear to be more likely affected than females.

ONSET

Brain abscesses may occur at any age; however, children, adolescents, and young adults are most commonly affected.

The actual onset typically occurs over a few days or weeks.

CLINICAL FEATURES

Abscesses may be single or multiple. Those secondary to local spread tend to be single; those secondary to hematogenous spread tend to be multiple. Abscesses tend to occur in the white matter and may be found, in order of decreasing frequency, in the temporal, frontal, parietal, and occipital lobes.

Headache and delirium are common symptoms; focal signs are also common and reflect the location of the abscess or abscesses. Generalized and, less commonly, focal seizures may occur. Increased intracranial pressure eventually occurs in the majority of patients and leads to increasing headache with nausea and vomiting. Papilledema may or may not be seen. An abrupt worsening of the clinical picture may signal rupture of the abscess into the ventricles or into the subarachnoid space.

Fever, leukocytosis, and an elevated sedimentation rate are present in less than half of the patients, and in these patients such signs may be only intermittent. Their presence generally indicates continued activity in the original source of the infection; such evidence of inflammation may also occur during the stage of cerebritis, before encapsulation has occurred.

The EEG typically shows a slow wave focus. Lumbar puncture is generally contraindicated.

MRI or CT scanning, both with enhancement, should be done in every case, as the image thus produced is often diagnostic. MRI scanning is superior to CT scanning. Figure 220-1 is of a gadolinium-enhanced T1-weighted MRI scan demonstrating enhancing capsules around a primary and an adjacent "daughter" abscess.

COURSE

Untreated, cerebral abscess is generally fatal, and patients may die within days to weeks of the onset. In rare cases the abscess, in the natural course of events, may undergo complete fibrosis with a halt in the progression of symptoms.

COMPLICATIONS

Complications of delirium are as described in that chapter.

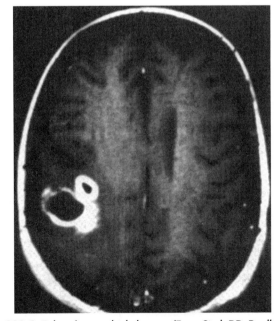

FIG. 220-1. Enhancing cerebral abscess. (From Stark DD, Bradley WG. *Magnetic resonance imaging,* vol 1, ed 2, St. Louis, 1992, Mosby.)

Of those patients who survive, perhaps over 50% develop seizures within a year. Residual focal deficits are also common.

ETIOLOGY

The most common infectious sources are the middle ear and the paranasal sinuses; infectious material may also be introduced by penetrating injury, such as a bullet, or a depressed skull fracture, and occasionally after neurosurgery. Metastatic spread occurs through a bacteremia or septicemia from foci such as bronchiectasis, lung abscess, empyema, dental abscesses, or endocarditis. Congenital heart disease is a common cause in children. Bacteremia secondary to intravenous drug abuse may also cause a brain abscess.

The initial lesion is a localized cerebritis. Over a few days, necrosis begins to occur, and within 2 weeks a fibrous capsule begins to form. The abscess itself may be spherical or oval and may be multiloculated. Surrounding edema is common and may be severe. If the patient survives long enough, the fibrous capsule may become quite thick and tough.

The responsible organism may be a bacterium, yeast, fungus, or parasite. In patients with AIDS, the most likely cause is toxoplasmosis, which is described in its own chapter.

DIFFERENTIAL DIAGNOSIS

When fever and leukocytosis are absent, a brain tumor is often considered. When these signs of infection are present, however, one may consider a subdural empyema or an encephalitis, especially herpes simplex encephalitis.

The presence of an infectious source is a strong diagnostic clue; however, since in perhaps a fifth of all cases the source of a brain abscess may never be found, the absence of an infectious source should never rule out the diagnosis.

Blood cultures are obtained in all cases, and potential sources of infection are investigated and, if possible, cultured.

TREATMENT

Delirium may be symptomatically treated as outlined in that chapter. Antiepileptic drugs, such as phenytoin or carbamazepine, are generally administered and, given the risk of seizures, may be continued chronically.

Antibiotics are given, the choice being determined by the presumed organism. In some cases, particularly those caught during the stage of cerebritis, antibiotics or antihelminthics alone may effect a cure. In all cases, however, immediate neurosurgical consultation must be obtained.

BIBLIOGRAPHY

Beller AJ, Sahar A, Praiss I. Brain abscess: review of 89 cases over a period of 30 years. *Journal of Neurology, Neurosurgery, and Psychiatry* 1973;36:757-768.

Berg B, Franklin G, Cuneo R, et al. Non-surgical cure of brain abscess: early diagnosis and follow-up with computerized tomography. *Annals of Neurology* 1978;3:474.

Calfee DP, Wispelwey B. Brain abscess. *Seminars in Neurology* 2000; 20:353-360.

Jefferson AA, Keogh AJ. Intracranial abscesses: a review of treated patients over 20 years. *Quarterly Journal of Medicine* 1977;46:389-400.

Lu CH, Chang WN, Lin YC, et al. Bacterial brain abscess: microbiological features, epidemiological trends and therapeutic outcomes. *Quarterly Journal of Medicine* 2002;95:501-509.

Rosenblum D, Ehrlich V. Brain abscess and psychosis as a complication of a halo orthosis. *Archives of Physical Medicine and Rehabilitation* 1995;76:865-867.

221 Hydrocephalus

Hydrocephalus is characterized by an enlargement of the cerebral ventricles secondary to increased pressure of the cerebrospinal fluid. Hydrocephalus may be usefully divided into two types, noncommunicating and communicating, depending on whether or not the communication between the ventricular system and the subarachnoid space is compromised.

Noncommunicating hydrocephalus may be secondary to obstruction at any of the following levels: the foramen of Monro, the aqueduct of Sylvius, or the exit foramina of Magendie and Luschka. Meningeal scarring is often responsible for obstruction at the exit foramina, and tumors for more proximal obstructions.

In communicating hydrocephalus, the obstruction is often found at the arachnoid villi, as may occur after a subarachnoid hemorrhage.

Hydrocephalus may be divided further into chronic and acute forms, depending on how rapidly the pressure of the cerebrospinal fluid rises. Chronic forms often present with dementia, whereas the acute form constitutes an emergency because it often rapidly produces coma and death.

The following discussion is confined to hydrocephalus occurring in adult years; childhood onset cases lie outside the scope of this book.

ONSET

Chronic hydrocephalus often presents gradually and insidiously, whereas the presentation of acute hydrocephalus may evolve over days, or even an hour or less.

CLINICAL FEATURES

Chronic hydrocephalus, as noted, typically presents with a dementia, and this dementia is generally marked by forgetfulness, apathy and a generalized slowing of thought and activity. The gait is unsteady and urinary incontinence is often seen; on examination there may be hyper-reflexia and extensor plantar responses. Of interest, there also appears to be an association between stenosis of the aqueduct of Sylvius and a chronic psychosis.

Acute hydrocephalus typically presents as a catastrophic clinical event, with headache, stupor and vomiting. Depending on the rapidity with which the intracranial pressure rises, there may or may not be papilledema. Coma and death may rapidly ensue.

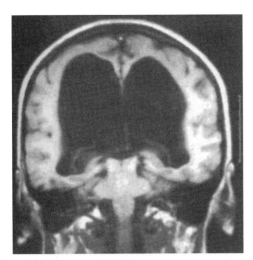

FIG. 221-1. Chronic hydrocephalus. (From Yock DH. *Imaging of CNS disease: a CT and MR teaching file*, ed 2, St. Louis, 1991, Mosby.)

Although both CT and MRI scanning are adequate to demonstrate the ventricular enlargement, MRI scanning is far more accurate in pinpointing the cause of the hydrocephalus. Figure 221-1 shows a coronal T1-weighted MRI scan of chronic hydrocephalus in an adult secondary to stenosis of the aqueduct of Sylvius.

COURSE

In chronic hydrocephalus, symptoms tend to worsen progressively as the increased cerebrospinal fluid pressure leads to ever-greater ventricular enlargement. In most cases, however, a new equilibrium is eventually reached and the "active" hydrocephalus becomes "arrested" with no further increase in ventricular size, and a lack of any further progression of symptoms.

Acute hydrocephalus, as noted earlier, is rapidly progressive and generally fatal.

COMPLICATIONS

The complications of dementia are as described in that chapter.

ETIOLOGY

As noted earlier, hydrocephalus may be either non-communicating or communicating. Non-communicating hydrocephalus may occur secondary to tumors blocking the foramen of Monro or third ventricle, atresia or inflammation of the aqueduct of Sylvius, or compression of the aqueduct by a nearby tumor, or to scarring of the foramina of Magendie or Luschka, as may occur after meningitis or a subarachnoid bleed. Communicating hydrocephalus may occur secondary to an over-production of cerebrospinal fluid, as with a papilloma of the choroid plexus or to impaired egress of the cerebrospinal fluid through the arachnoid granulations into the subdural sinuses, as may occur after

subarachnoid hemorrhage or occlusion of the granulations by tumor cells. Normal pressure hydrocephalus, a specific form of communicating hydrocephalus, is discussed in the next chapter.

Chronic hydrocephalus may be either non-communicating or communicating; in cases of chronic hydrocephalus of the non-communicating type, the obstruction is always partial. Acute hydrocephalus is generally of the non-communicating type, and here the obstruction is more or less complete, thus accounting for the very rapid rise in intracranial pressure.

DIFFERENTIAL DIAGNOSIS

Clinically, chronic hydrocephalus may mimic Alzheimer's or Binswanger's disease, and the differential often rests on whether neuroimaging demonstrates ventricular enlargement or not. Importantly, however, finding ventricular enlargement on CT or MRI scanning does not necessary imply an increased intracranial pressure, as it may merely represent a "hydrocephalus ex vacuo": here, atrophy of the cerebral cortex, as may occur with normal ageing or in certain degenerative conditions, leaves behind an enlarged ventricular space without any increase in pressure at all. The distinction between "true" hydrocephalus, with increased intracranial pressure, and "hydrocephalus ex vacuo" is based on two findings. First, if the degree of ventricular enlargement is disproportionately great compared with the degree of sulcal widening, then one may presume increased intracranial pressure. Second, if on T2-weighted MRI scanning there is substantial increased signal intensity surrounding the lateral ventricles, as would occur with transependymal extravasation of fluid, then the likelihood of increased pressure is also greater.

TREATMENT

Various shunting procedures are available and neurosurgical consultation is indicated in all cases, regardless of the duration of the chronic hydrocephalus: even long-standing cases may respond to shunting. The overall treatment of dementia is as discussed in that chapter.

Acute hydrocephalus is a neurosurgical emergency.

BIBLIOGRAPHY

Gustafson L, Hagberg B. Recovery in hydrocephalic dementia after shunt operation. *Journal of Neurology, Neurosurgery, and Psychiatry* 1978;41:940-947.

Harrison MJG, Robert CM, Uttley D. Benign aqueductal stenosis in adults. *Journal of Neurology, Neurosurgery, and Psychiatry* 1974;37:1322-1328.

Mataro M, Poca MA, Sahuquillo J, et al. Cognitive changes after cerebrospinal fluid shunting in young adults with spina bifida and assumed arrested hydrocephalus. *Journal of Neurology, Neurosurgery, and Psychiatry* 2000;68:615-621.

Nag TK, Falconer MA. Non-tumoral stenosis of the aqueduct in adults. *British Medical Journal* 1966;2:1168-1170.

Roberts JK, Trimble MR, Robertson M. Schizophrenic psychosis associated with aqueductal stenosis in adults. *Journal of Neurology, Neurosurgery, and Psychiatry* 1983;46:892-898.

Normal pressure hydrocephalus is a form of chronic communicating hydrocephalus wherein the cerebrospinal fluid pressure is either normal or only intermittently increased, and then only to a mild degree. Classically, this disorder presents with a triad of dementia, apraxia of gait, and urinary incontinence or urgency. It is a rare disorder and more common in males than females.

ONSET

The onset of symptoms is gradual and insidious and generally occurs in middle or older years.

CLINICAL FEATURES

The dementia is characterized by forgetfulness, slowness of thought and action, and indifference. Rarely, the clinical picture may be dominated by depression, personality change, or, even more rarely, mania.

The apraxic gait of these patients is somewhat stiff-legged and may appear broad-based or shuffling. The gait has a hesitancy about it, as if the feet were "glued to the floor," or as if the "clutch is slipping."

Urinary incontinence is typically listed as the third classic sign of normal pressure hydrocephalus; however, this may be only intermittent and then not noted, or, rather than incontinence, the patient may experience only urgency.

On examination there is hyperreflexia, and the plantar responses may be extensor; the grasp and snout reflexes may also be present. There is no papilledema.

The cerebrospinal fluid opening pressure is generally normal or only mildly elevated. Prolonged monitoring, however, often demonstrates transient increases, often at night during sleep. The cerebrospinal fluid is otherwise normal; in particular the protein is not elevated.

CT or MRI scanning shows enlargement of the lateral and third ventricles, and often of the fourth ventricle. Periventricular lucency on CT scanning or periventricular hyperintensity on T2-weighted MRI scanning may be seen secondary to transependymal fluid shifts. Figure 222-1 demonstrates ventricular enlargement in an elderly man with normal pressure hydrocephalus; Figure 222-2 is a CT scan of the same patient taken after shunting and resolution of his symptoms.

The electroencephalogram may be normal or show diffuse nonspecific slowing.

COURSE

Most cases evidence a gradual progression of symptoms. Eventually the patient may become unable to stand and may be mute and withdrawn. In many cases this progression of hydrocephalus eventually arrests.

COMPLICATIONS

Complications are as described in the chapter on dementia.

ETIOLOGY

As noted earlier, normal pressure hydrocephalus is a form of chronic communicating hydrocephalus, and it is presumed to be due to an impairment in the normal egress of cerebrospinal fluid out through the arachnoid granulations into the subdural venous sinuses. The cause of this impaired outflow is not clear: although some cases appear to have followed subarachnoid hemorrhage, in most cases there is no obvious cause and the autopsy is unrevealing. Given the unknown etiology of normal pressure hydrocephalus, some authors have also referred to it as idiopathic chronic communicating hydrocephalus.

The mechanism whereby the hydrocephalus produces symptoms is probably related to stretching the long axonal fibers that run in a periventricular course around the lateral ventricles themselves.

DIFFERENTIAL DIAGNOSIS

The differential diagnosis is as discussed in the preceding chapter on hydrocephalus.

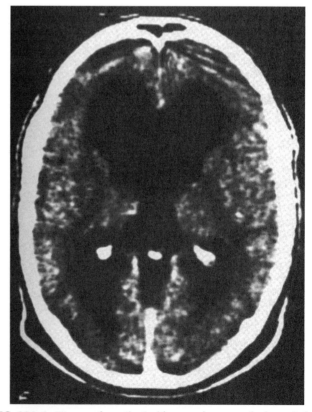

FIG. 222-1. CT scan of a patient with normal pressure hydrocephalus. (From Leech RW, Brunback RA. *Hydrocephalus: current clinical concepts*, St. Louis, 1991, Mosby.)

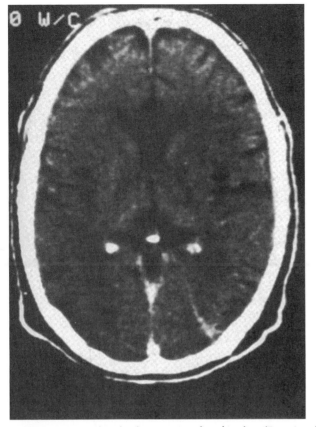

FIG. 222-2. Same patient in Figure 222-1 after shunting. (From Leech RW, Brunback RA. *Hydrocephalus: current clinical concepts*, St. Louis, 1991, Mosby.)

TREATMENT

A shunting procedure should be considered in all cases. In many institutions the decision as to whether or not to shunt is based on the results of the CSF tap test. In this test anywhere from 20 to 30 ml of CSF is withdrawn via lumbar puncture, with videotapes being made of the patient's gait before and after the "tap": a substantial improvement in gait generally predicts an overall good response to shunting.

The overall treatment of dementia is as described in that chapter.

BIBLIOGRAPHY

Adams RD, Fisher CM, Hakim S, et al. Symptomatic occult hydrocephalus with "normal" cerebrospinal fluid pressure. *The New England Journal of Medicine* 1965;273:117-126.

Bech-Azeddine R, Waldemar G, Knudson GM, et al. Idiopathic normal-pressure hydrocephalus: evaluation and findings in a multidisciplinary memory clinic. *European Journal of Neurology* 2001;8:601-611.

Crowell RM, Tew JM, Mark VH. Aggressive dementia associated with normal pressure hydrocephalus. *Neurology* 1973;23:461-464.

Hill ME, Lougheed WM, Barnett HJM. A treatable form of dementia due to normal pressure, communicating hydrocephalus. *Canadian Medical Association Journal* 1967;97:1309-1311.

Kwentus JA, Hart RP. Normal pressure hydrocephalus presenting as mania. *The Journal of Nervous and Mental Disease* 1987;175:500-502.

Rosen H, Swigar ME. Depression and normal pressure hydrocephalus. A dilemma in neuropsychiatric differential diagnosis. *The Journal of Nervous and Mental Disease* 1976;163:35-40.

Sand T, Bovim G, Grimse R, et al. Idiopathic normal pressure hydrocephalus: the CSF tap test may predict the clinical response to shunting. *Acta Neurologica Scandinavica* 1994;89:311-316.

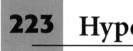
223 Hyperthyroidism

Hyperthyroidism, which is much more common among females than males, results from an excessive elevation of free thyroxine levels or, rarely, solely from an elevation of free triiodothyronine levels. The most common causes are Graves' disease, toxic multinodular goiter, or a thyroiditis, most commonly Hashimoto's thyroiditis.

ONSET

Graves' disease tends to have a gradual onset in the twenties or thirties, multinodular goiter appears in the elderly, and Hashimoto's thyroiditis in early adult or middle years.

CLINICAL FEATURES

Typically, patients are apprehensive, and, although fatigued and tired, they are often restless and unable to sit still. They may complain of diaphoresis and heat intolerance, an increased frequency of bowel movements, and weight loss despite an increased appetite and an increased food intake. On examination one generally finds tachycardia, widened palpebral fissures (as illustrated in Figure 223-1), a fine tremor and generalized hyperreflexia. Women may complain of menstrual irregularities and men may experience erectile dysfunction. A proximal myopathy, affecting primarily the pelvic musculature, is not uncommon, and, rarely, chorea may appear.

Although anxiety is classically associated with hyperthyroidism, depressive symptoms are more common, being seen in anywhere from one-quarter to one-half of all patients. Rarely one may see a mania or hypomania, and even more rarely there may be a psychosis.

Thyroid storm is a dreaded complication of hyperthyroidism. Typically, a patient with untreated hyperthyroidism undergoes a significant stress, such as surgery, an infection, or some other acute illness, and then rapidly experiences a severe exacerbation of all the typical symptoms noted above. Fever often appears and in a small minority seizures occur; untreated, delirium often supervenes, and this may progress to stupor and coma.

Apathetic hyperthyroidism, generally seen only in the elderly, represents an atypical variant of hyperthyroidism and is characterized, as the name suggests, by apathy, which is often accompanied by lethargy. Remarkably, the "autonomic" symptoms of typical hyperthyroidism are for the most part absent, and one generally does not see diaphoresis, tremor or hyperreflexia. Tachycardia, however, is seen in apathetic hyperthyroidism, and many patients will also have atrial fibrillation and "high output" heart failure. Cognitive deficits are not uncommon in this form of hyperthyroidism and in some cases a dementia may occur.

In most cases of hyperthyroidism, the free thyroxine level is elevated; an exception occurs in "T3 thyrotoxicosis," and whenever the clinical picture is compatible with hyperthyroidism but the free thyroxine level is normal, one should order a free T3 level. The thyroid-stimulating hormone level is either normal or low in cases of primary thyroid disease; in the rare instances of hypothalamic or pituitary hyperthyroidism, the TSH level is increased.

COURSE

Given the chronic course of most of the underlying etiologies, most cases of hyperthyroidism are likewise chronic; an exception to this is Hashimoto's thyroiditis which, in most cases, is self-remitting and may, depending on the amount of inflammatory damage inflicted on the thyroid gland, be followed by hypothyroidism.

COMPLICATIONS

The complications of secondary anxiety, depression and psychosis, and of dementia and delirium, are as described in the respective chapters.

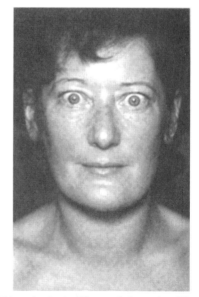

FIG. 223-1. Widened palpebral fissures in hyperthyroidism. (From Hall R, Evered DC. *Color atlas of endocrinology*, ed 2, London, 1990, Wolfe.)

ETIOLOGY

The most common cause of hyperthyroidism is Graves' disease, followed by multinodular goiter and Hashimoto's thyroiditis. Other causes include toxic solitary adenoma and thyrotoxicosis factitia.

DIFFERENTIAL DIAGNOSIS

A depressive episode of major depression or bipolar disorder may come to mind; however, the presence of weight loss in the face of an increased appetite, rather than the decreased appetite, argues against it. In cases of apathetic hyperthyroidism, however, appetite may not be increased, and given the importance of not missing this diagnosis, it is reasonable, in all cases of geriatric depression, to check thyroid function.

Generalized anxiety disorder also is often considered, and in some instances only thyroid function testing will resolve the issue. One clue, however, can be gathered simply by shaking the patient's hand: in both disorders, the palm is usually diaphoretic; however, in generalized anxiety disorder the palm is cold, whereas in hyperthyroidism, one feels a warm palm.

Alcohol withdrawal is distinguished by its acute onset and by the history of excessive alcohol use.

Hashimoto's encephalopathy should be considered in hyperthyroid patients with psychosis, delirium or dementia, when these syndromes fail to resolve with normalization of the free thyroxine level, or when they appear disproportionately severe relative to the level of elevation of the free thyroxine index. In considering this differential, one must keep in mind the distinction between Hashimoto's thyroiditis and Hashimoto's encephalopathy. Both disorders are characterized by an autoimmune response; in Hashimoto's thyroiditis this is directed primarily at the thyroid gland, whereas in Hashimoto's encephalopathy it is directed at the cerebral cortex. Although these two disorders can, and do, occur in isolation, it is not rare to find both disorders in the same patient: in such a case the autoimmune attack on the thyroid causes hyperthyroidism, whereas the autoimmune attack on the cerebral cortex may cause psychosis, delirium or dementia. In such an instance treatment of the hyperthyroidism may not be followed by a complete resolution of the neuropsychiatric symptomatology, and in such cases steroid treatment may be required. Diagnostic clues to the existence of Hashimoto's encephalopathy include seizures and, most importantly, myoclonus.

Before leaving this discussion of differential diagnosis, further words regarding apathetic hyperthyroidism may be in order. Given the lack of prominent autonomic symptomatology, making this diagnosis requires a high index of suspicion, and clinical findings which should raise one's suspicion include atrial fibrillation and unexplained tachycardia.

TREATMENT

If required, most autonomic symptoms may be rapidly controlled with propranolol, 20 to 40 mg every 4 to 6 hours, provided there are no contraindications, such as COPD or asthma. This should not, however, be used alone, and thyroid synthesis should be reduced by using either methimazole or propylthiouracil. Once thyroid hormone levels have been normalized, consideration may be given to treatments such as radioactive iodine or subtotal thyroidectomy.

Thyroid storm, given its high mortality rate, is a medical emergency and transfer to an ICU is appropriate in most cases.

BIBLIOGRAPHY

Arnold BM, Casal G, Higgins HP. Apathetic thyrotoxicosis. *Canadian Medical Association Journal* 1974;111:957-958.

Brenner I. Apathetic hyperthyroidism. *The Journal of Clinical Psychiatry* 1978;39:479-480.

Dayan CM. Interpretation of thyroid function tests. *Lancet* 2001;357: 619-624.

Fukui T, Hasegawa Y, Takenaka H. Hyperthyroid dementia: clinicoradiological findings and response to treatment. *Journal of the Neurological Sciences* 2001;184:81-88.

Lahey FH. Non-activated (apathetic) type of hyperthyroidism. *The New England Journal of Medicine* 1931;204:747-748.

Martin FI, Deam DR. Hyperthyroidism in elderly hospitalized patients. Clinical features and treatment outcomes. *The Medical Journal of Australia* 1996;164:200-203.

Palacios A, Cohen MA, Cobbs R. Apathetic hyperthyroidism in middle age. *International Journal of Psychiatry in Medicine* 1991;21:393-400.

Peake RL. Recurrent apathetic hyperthyroidism. *Archives of Internal Medicine* 1981;141:258-260.

Taylor JW. Depression in thyrotoxicosis. *The American Journal of Psychiatry* 1975;132:552-553.

Thomas FB, Mazzaferri EL, Skillmann TG. Apathetic thyrotoxicosis: a distinctive clinical and laboratory entity. *Annals of Internal Medicine* 1970;72:679-685.

Trivalle C, Doucet J, Chassagne P, et al. Differences in the signs and symptoms of hyperthyroidism in older and younger patients. *Journal of the American Geriatrics Society* 1996;44:50-53.

Trzepacz PT, McCue M, Klein I, et al. A psychiatric and neuropsychological study of patients with untreated Graves' disease. *General Hospital Psychiatry* 1988;10:49-55.

Weetman AP. Grave's disease. *The New England Journal of Medicine* 2000;343:1236-1248.

224 Hypothyroidism

Hypothyroidism typically causes a distinctive dullness and slowing of thought that, when severe, may progress to a dementia; depression may also be seen, and, rarely, patients may become psychotic. Hypothyroidism, when severe, is traditionally referred to as "myxedema," and in cases where psychosis does occur, one may speak of "myxedema madness."

Hypothyroidism is relatively common among adults, occurring in about 1.4% of females and about 0.1% of males. The vast majority of cases are secondary to Hashimoto's thyroiditis, thyroidectomy, or radioactive iodine treatment; it is also not uncommon to see hypothyroidism occur in patients who have abruptly discontinued long-term treatment with thyroid supplementation.

ONSET

The onset is determined by the underlying cause. Those cases caused by Hashimoto's thyroiditis occur gradually in the late thirties or early forties, whereas those secondary to thyroidectomy may occur relatively soon postoperatively, sometimes within as few as 2 or 3 weeks.

CLINICAL FEATURES

Typically, speech and action become slowed and retarded. Minutes may pass before the patient answers a question, and loosening one button may require a full minute. Initiative is diminished; memory seems fogged, and patients have difficulty comprehending what is said to them. In severe cases a lethargic, withdrawn dementia may occur.

Depression occurs in a substantial minority of patients, and this may be accompanied by anxiety, irritability and querulousness.

Psychosis, or "myxedema madness," is typically characterized by delusions of persecution; less commonly, patients may experience hallucinations that tend to be either auditory or visual, or, much less commonly, olfactory or gustatory.

Common accompanying symptoms include a voice change, with deepening and hoarseness, cold intolerance, hair loss and weight gain. Partial deafness may occur and males may experience erectile dysfunction and women may have menorrhagia.

The skin becomes myxedematous. Particularly on the face, the dorsal surfaces of the hands and feet, and in the supraclavicular fossae, the skin is dry and displays a boggy, nonpitting puffiness. Figure 224-1 shows a woman with nonpitting edematous changes of the face. Bradycardia and hypotension are common; hypothermia may be present, and a variable degree of pericardial effusion is not uncommon. Deep tendon reflexes may be reduced; characteristically the ankle jerk is "hung up" with a very slow relaxation phase. Vibratory sense is reduced; rarely, one may see a facial palsy or cerebellar ataxia.

Myxedematous infiltration may cause a carpal or tarsal tunnel syndrome; infiltration of the tongue and pharynx may lead to obstructive sleep apnea.

The free thyroxine level is reduced; thyroid-stimulating hormone (TSH) is increased in primary hypothyroidism and decreased in secondary or tertiary hypothyroidism. Hyponatremia

may occur, and may be part of the syndrome of inappropriate ADH (antidiuretic hormone) secretion. The EEG demonstrates diffuse slowing. Low voltage may be seen on the ECG, and cardiomegaly on the chest x-ray.

Hypothyroidism occurring in utero or in early infancy may cause cretinism, with mental retardation and short stature. The facial appearance is characterized by a short broad nose and a dull, phlegmatic expression. When hypothyroidism occurs in older children, linear growth and intellectual development slow and may come to a standstill.

Before leaving this discussion of clinical features, some words about "subclinical" primary hypothyroidism are in order. Here, although the free thyroxine level is still within normal limits, the TSH is mildly elevated. Such a combination of laboratory findings indicates that although the free thyroxine level may be still within the broadly defined limits of normal, it is below the normal for the patient in question, as indicated by the elevated TSH. Although such patients may not have any symptoms referable to this, the finding is nevertheless very significant, and for two reasons. First, such findings may indicate that the patient is in the very early stages of primary hypothyroidism and that, with time, the free thyroxine level will fall far enough such that the typical symptoms of hypothyroidism, noted above, will appear. Second, even if the free thyroxine level does not fall further, this minimally depressed level will, in cases where patients are suffering from major depression or bipolar disorder, blunt the response to antidepressants or mood stabilizers.

COURSE

The clinical course is determined by the underlying cause and parallels, in general, the changes in thyroid hormone levels. In some cases there is a relentless progression to a potentially fatal "myxedema coma" characterized by stupor or coma, hypothermia,

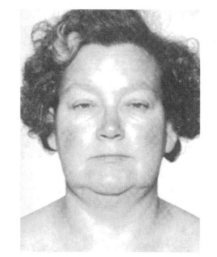

FIG. 224-1. Myxedema. (From Hall R, Evered DC. *Color atlas of endocrinology*, ed 2, London, 1990, Wolfe.)

■**TABLE 224-1.** Causes of Hypothyroidism

	Primary	Secondary	Tertiary
Site of lesion	Thyroid gland	Pituitary	Hypothalamus
Free T4	Decreased	Decreased	Decreased
TSH	Increased	Decreased	Decreased
Response to TRH	Blunted	Blunted	Augmented
Examples	Hashimoto's thyroiditis, radioactive iodine treatment or thyroidectomy, iodine deficiency, lithium	Pituitary tumor or apoplexy	Tumor, infarction, or granuloma of hypothalamus; carbamazepine

bradycardia, respiratory depression, and, in a substantial minority, seizures.

COMPLICATIONS

The complications of dementia, secondary depression and secondary psychosis are as described in those chapters.

ETIOLOGY

As outlined in Table 224-1, hypothyroidism may be "primary," "secondary," or "tertiary." In primary hypothyroidism, which is by far the most common form, the thyroid itself is damaged; in secondary hypothyroidism, which is far less common, the pituitary is damaged; and in tertiary hypothyroidism, which is very rare, the lesion is situated in the hypothalamus.

DIFFERENTIAL DIAGNOSIS

The syndromes of dementia, depression and psychosis have multiple etiologies, as discussed in their respective chapters. Their occurrence secondary to hypothyroidism is often suggested by the slowing, lethargy and myxedematous appearance characteristic of these patients.

In cases of primary hypothyroidism caused by Hashimoto's thyroiditis, neuropsychiatric symptomatology may occur not only secondary to hypothyroidism per se but also due to Hashimoto's encephalopathy or to other autoimmune disorders associated with Hashimoto's thyroiditis, such as systemic lupus erythematosus, pernicious anemia, Addison's disease, and autoimmune destruction of the parathyroid glands with resultant hypocalcemia.

Adrenocortical insufficiency may also occur in cases of secondary hypothyroidism wherein pituitary corticotrophs have been destroyed.

TREATMENT

Treatment with once-daily thyroxine is generally curative. If the hypothyroidism is of relatively recent onset and the patient is neither elderly nor in poor health, one may begin with 0.05 mg and then increase the dose every week or two in 0.05 mg increments until the patient has reached a full replacement dose. In patients with long-standing hypothyroidism, in the elderly, or in those with poor health, particularly those with cardiovascular disease, treatment is begun with 0.0125 or 0.025 mg and increased in increments of 0.0125 or 0.025 mg every 4 to 8 weeks with careful monitoring of the clinical status, free thyroxine and TSH. For most

otherwise healthy adult females, 0.075 to 0.1 mg constitutes a full replacement dose; for males the range is 0.1 to 0.15 mg; elderly patients, however, may require only 0.075 mg or less. Once patients have been stabilized on an appropriate dose of thyroxine, it may be appropriate to consider treatment with a combination of thyroxine and triiodothyronine. Recent work has suggested that such combinations may lead to better overall functioning than treatment with thyroxine alone. If such a course of treatment is desired, one may reduce the dose of thyroxine by 0.05 mg and concurrently add 0.125 mg of triiodothyronine.

Importantly, in monitoring TSH levels, it must be borne in mind that in cases of long-standing primary hypothyroidism there may be such considerable hypertrophy of pituitary thyrotroph cells that four to eight weeks may be required for the TSH level to fall after a replacement dose has been reached.

Myxedema coma is a medical emergency and generally requires admission to an intensive care unit; intravenous thyroxine, in doses of 0.3 to 0.5 mg, is often required along with vigorous supportive care. Given that treatment of a hypothyroid patient with a sedative drug may precipitate myxedema coma, these agents should be avoided.

BIBLIOGRAPHY

Asher R. Myxoedematous madness. *British Medical Journal* 1949;22: 555-562.

Bunevicius R, Kazanavicius G, Zalinkevicius R, et al. Effects of thyroxine as compared with thyroxine plus triiodothyronine in patients with hypothyroidism. *The New England Journal of Medicine* 1999;340: 424-429.

Dugbarty AT. Neurocognitive aspects of hypothyroidism. *Archives of Internal Medicine* 1998;158:1413-1418.

Granet RB, Kalman TP. Hypothyroidism and psychosis: a case illustration of the diagnostic dilemma in psychiatry. *The Journal of Clinical Psychiatry* 1978;39:260-263.

Kleiner J, Altshuler L, Hendrick V, et al. Lithium-induced subclinical hypothyroidism: review of the literature and guidelines for treatment. *The Journal of Clinical Psychiatry* 1999;60:249-255.

Larson EB, Reifler BV, Featherstone HJ, et al. Dementia in elderly outpatients: a prospective study. *Annals of Internal Medicine* 1984;100: 417-423.

Logothetis J. Psychotic behavior as the initial indicator of adult myxedema. *The Journal of Nervous and Mental Disease* 1963;136:561-568.

Nickel SM, Frame B. Neurologic manifestations of myxedema. *Neurology* 1958;8:511-517.

Whybrow PC, Prange AJ, Treadway CR. Mental changes accompanying thyroid gland dysfunction. *Archives of General Psychiatry* 1969;20: 48-63.

Woeber KA. Update on the management of hyperthyroidism and hypothyroidism. *Archives of Internal Medicine* 2000;160:1067-1071.

Cushing's syndrome results from either sustained administration of high-dose exogenous corticosteroids, such as prednisone, or from excessive cortisol secretion by the adrenal cortex, which in turn may occur via a number of different mechanisms. Normally, corticotrophin-releasing hormone (CRH), produced in the hypothalamus, stimulates the pituitary gland to produce adrenocorticotrophic hormone (ACTH), which in turn stimulates the adrenal gland to produce cortisol. Excessive production of CRH by the hypothalamus, excessive production of ACTH due to a pituitary adenoma and excessive cortisol production by an adrenal adenoma or carcinoma are all possible mechanisms; another is the "ectopic ACTH syndrome" wherein a tumor, such as a small cell lung cancer, produces ACTH. Traditionally, the term "Cushing's disease" is reserved for those cases of Cushing's syndrome secondary to a pituitary adenoma.

At least one-half of patients with Cushing's syndrome have depressive or manic symptoms; delirium, psychosis and dementia may also occur but are far less common. In patients treated with prednisone, the incidence of these neuropsychiatric disturbances varies with the dose, from negligible at about 10 mg/day to about 20% or more in those taking 80 mg/day or more.

ONSET

The age of onset is determined by the underlying etiology. Cushing's disease itself tends to develop in adult years. The mode of onset likewise depends on the etiology. Cushing's disease may be of very gradual onset, over years. Cushing's syndrome secondary to ectopic ACTH may develop over several months, and a Cushing's syndrome secondary to prednisone administration may occur within days.

CLINICAL FEATURES

For unclear reasons, manic or hypomanic symptoms are generally seen only when Cushing's syndrome is secondary to exogenous steroid administration. When the syndrome occurs secondary to other causes, depressive symptoms are far more common.

Depression may be characterized by irritability, depressed mood, fatigue, decreased libido, poor memory or concentration, and psychomotor change, more commonly anxiety or agitation than retardation. Insomnia may also occur. Suicidal ideation is not uncommon, and up to 10% of these patients may make a suicide attempt.

Manic or hypomanic symptoms include euphoria or at times irritability, grandiosity, hyperactivity and hypertalkativeness, and a decreased need for sleep.

At times a "mixed" affective picture may occur, with alternating or intermingling manic and depressive symptoms.

Delirium, which may or may not occur in the context of mood changes, is seen in only about 1% of patients; both psychosis and dementia are very rare.

With chronically sustained administration of high dose corticosteroids or endogenous hypercortisolemia, a number of changes typically occur. Of these changes the most distinctive are those which go to make up the "Cushingoid habitus," which includes the following: a plethoric, "moon" facies (Figure 225-1, both before and after treatment); obesity, which is often truncal; violaceous abdominal striae (Figure 225-2); acne; and, in women, hirsutism. Other changes include myopathy, hypertension, easy bruisability, diabetes mellitus and amenorrhea; rarely, pseudotumor cerebri may occur. These findings are very diagnostically suggestive; however, it must be borne in mind that mood changes may occur very early on, especially in the case of corticosteroid treatment,

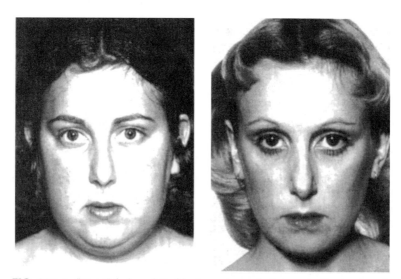

FIG. 225-1. "Moon" facies of Cushing's syndrome before and after treatment. (From Hall R, Evered DC. *Color atlas of endocrinology*, ed 2, London, 1990, Wolfe.)

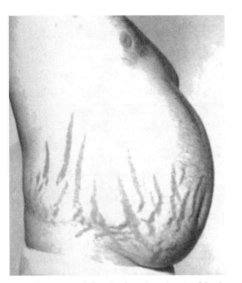

FIG. 225-2. Violaceous abdominal striae in Cushing's syndrome. (From Hall R, Evered DC. *Color atlas of endocrinology*, ed 2, London, 1990, Wolfe.)

long before these physiologic changes have had a chance to occur. Further, in cases of adrenal cancer, one may see wasting rather than obesity.

Diagnostic laboratory testing is discussed below, under "etiology."

COURSE

The course is determined by the underlying etiology.

COMPLICATIONS

Complications are as described in the chapters on secondary depression, secondary mania, delirium, secondary psychosis and dementia.

ETIOLOGY

Whenever Cushing's syndrome is suspected and the patient is not receiving exogenous corticosteroids, the first step is to determine whether or not, in fact, hypercortisolemia is present. Although an 8:00 A.M. serum cortisol level may be informative, this may, given the pulsatile nature of cortisol secretion, be falsely negative: a far more sensitive test is a 24 hour urine for free cortisol. If the 24 hour free cortisol level is elevated, the next step is to determine whether this excessive production of cortisol by the adrenal gland is ACTH independent, which would suggest an adrenal adenoma or carcinoma, or ACTH dependent, as might be seen with hypothalamic or pituitary disease or in the "ectopic ACTH syndrome." A simple way to determine this is to check an 8:00 A.M. cortisol and ACTH level: if the cortisol is increased but the ACTH is low, then one must suspect an adrenal tumor which is producing cortisol autonomously and independently of any stimulation by ACTH. If the ACTH level is high, the next step is to determine whether the source of the ACTH is the pituitary gland or an "ectopic" source, such as a small cell lung cancer (other sources include cancer of the thyroid, thymus, pancreas or ovaries and a pheochromocytoma). To accomplish this one performs the "high dose" dexamethasone test: here dexamethasone is given in a dose of 2 mg po q 6h for two days and on the second day a 24 hour urine for free cortisol

is collected. Pituitary adenomas retain some degree of normal suppressibility, and in the presence of such high levels of dexamethasone, the production of ACTH by the pituitary adenoma will fall with a resultant fall in the 24 hour urine free cortisol level. Malignancies producing "ectopic" ACTH, however, are not suppressible, and in such cases the 24 hour urine free cortisol remains elevated. An alternative to the high-dose dexamethasone test is the CRH stimulation test. Here, after obtaining two baseline ACTH levels 30 and 15 minutes before the test, one gives 1 microgram/kg of ovine CRH (corticorelin) i.v. over 60 seconds and then collects three ACTH levels at 15, 30, and 60 minutes subsequently. Since pituitary adenomas remain responsive to CRH, one will see a rise in ACTH level here; in contrast, "ectopic" sources of ACTH are not responsive to CRH and hence the ACTH levels will not rise.

If testing suggests an adrenal adenoma or carcinoma, then CT scanning of the abdomen is in order. If an ectopic source of ACTH is suspected, then appropriate testing, such as CT scanning of the lung, should be pursued. If a pituitary adenoma is suspected, then MRI scanning of the head with gadolinium enhancement is performed. Importantly, although MRI scanning picks up most macroadenomas, it is only about 50% sensitive for microadenomas; consequently, if the clinical picture strongly suggests a pituitary adenoma but MRI is negative, then one should consider bilateral sampling of the inferior petrosal sinuses for ACTH. Although this is a technically difficult test to perform, and may require referral to a specialized center, it may be very informative, revealing an elevated ACTH level in the sinus draining the side of the pituitary that harbors the microadenoma.

In practice, most cases of Cushing's syndrome are due either to exogenous corticosteroid administration or to a pituitary adenoma; a minority occur secondary to ectopic ACTH production and in a very small minority one finds an adrenal tumor. Finally, there are very rare cases of Cushing's syndrome secondary to hypothalamic overproduction of CRH.

DIFFERENTIAL DIAGNOSIS

In patients receiving exogenous steroids who develop depressive or manic symptoms the question arises as to whether these symptoms are secondary to the steroids or to the disease being treated by the steroids. This dilemma may occur, for example, with systemic lupus erythematosus, multiple sclerosis, or in brain tumor patients. In cases where changes in mental status precede steroid administration, the decision may be relatively straightforward. However, when symptoms follow steroid use, the only way to decide might be to alter the steroid dose. If the dose is increased and symptoms decrease, then the symptoms were most likely caused by the underlying disease, and vice versa. A similar approach may be made by lowering the dose.

When exogenous steroids are not being used, the concurrent appearance of depression or mania and a typical Cushingoid habitus strongly suggests Cushing's syndrome.

Finally, when a delirium occurs in a patient with known Cushing's syndrome, one must consider hypertensive encephalopathy or severe hyperglycemia before assuming that the delirium is secondary to the hypercortisolemia per se.

TREATMENT

Treatment of Cushing's syndrome is directed at the underlying cause and involves discontinuation or dose reduction of exogenous steroids or surgical treatment of pituitary adenomas, "ectopic"

ACTH-producing tumors, and adrenal tumors. When such surgery is not effective or is contraindicated, one may consider bilateral adrenalectomy or a "chemical" adrenalectomy by administering daily oral doses of one of the enzyme inhibitors metyrapone or ketoconazole; in such cases, however, one typically has to provide a daily maintenance dose of exogenous corticosteroid and one must watch closely for the development of Nelson's syndrome, with the appearance of an ACTH-secreting pituitary tumor and generalized hyperpigmentation.

Symptomatic treatment of manic symptoms with lithium, and depressive ones with antidepressants, may be required. Lithium, sometimes used prophylactically, has allowed patients to receive high-dose prednisone and not be troubled by manic symptoms. Antipsychotics may be used for the symptomatic treatment of delirium or, in the case of manic symptoms, until the lithium becomes effective.

BIBLIOGRAPHY

Jeffcoate WJ, Silverstone JT, Edwards CR, et al. Psychiatric manifestations of Cushing's syndrome: response to lowering of plasma cortisol. *Quarterly Journal of Medicine* 1979;148:465-472.

Johnson J. Schizophrenia and Cushing's syndrome cured by adrenalectomy. *Psychological Medicine* 1975;5:165-168.

Kelly WF. Psychiatric aspects of Cushing's syndrome. *Quarterly Journal of Medicine* 1996;89:543-551.

Kelly WF, Checkley SA, Bender DA, et al. Cushing's syndrome and depression—a prospective study of 26 patients. *The British Journal of Psychiatry* 1983;142:16-19.

Nieman LK. Diagnostic tests for Cushing's syndrome. *Annals of the New York Academy of Sciences* 2002;970:112-118.

Orth DN. Cushing's syndrome. *The New England Journal of Medicine* 1995;332:791-803.

Sonino N, Fava GA. Psychiatric disorders associated with Cushing's syndrome. *CNS Drugs* 2001;15:361-373.

Spillane JD. Nervous and mental disorders in Cushing's syndrome. *Brain* 1951;74:72-94.

226 Adrenocortical Insufficiency

Adrenocortical insufficiency may be either primary, caused by destruction of the gland itself, or secondary, caused by a lack of adrenocorticotropic hormone (ACTH) in either pituitary or hypothalamic failure.

Adrenocortical insufficiency may also be characterized as chronic or acute. Chronic cases may be either primary (e.g., those caused by gradual destruction of the gland by an autoimmune process) or secondary (e.g., due to a slow growing pituitary tumor). Similarly, acute cases may be either primary (e.g., in hemorrhagic infarction of the adrenal glands during septicemia) or secondary (e.g., with pituitary apoplexy). Often one also sees a chronic case undergo acute exacerbation; a common example is a patient with long-standing, very mild symptoms caused by gradual autoimmune destruction of the gland who undergoes a major stress, such as surgery, precipitating a crisis of adrenocortical failure.

The term "Addison's disease" has been used either to refer to all cases of primary adrenocortical insufficiency or to only those caused by an autoimmune destruction of the gland. Given this unfortunate lack of definitional clarity, this eponym is not used further here.

Adrenocortical insufficiency is a rare disorder. Acute adrenocortical insufficiency almost never escapes medical attention; the patient is obviously and severely ill. Chronic adrenocortical insufficiency, however, may escape detection, as it presents with symptoms such as fatigue that may be all too readily dismissed.

ONSET

Chronic cases may present gradually and insidiously over months to a year or more. This is typical of primary autoimmune adrenocortical insufficiency, which generally has an onset in early to middle adult years.

Acute cases can present in a fulminant fashion in as little as hours.

CLINICAL FEATURES

Chronic adrenocortical insufficiency typically presents with depressed mood, irritability, apathy, fatigue, and weakness. Concentration may be poor, and insomnia may occur. Almost all patients lose their appetite and lose some weight. Eventually, one sees prominent hypotension and postural dizziness, along with gastrointestinal complaints such as nausea, vomiting, constipation, or diarrhea. In severe cases a mild delirium may eventually supervene, and rarely a psychosis may occur. The blood glucose is often low, and if dehydration has occurred, the BUN is elevated. In primary cases wherein destruction of the adrenal cortex reduces levels not only of corticosteroids but also of mineralocorticosteroids, such as aldosterone, one also sees a mild degree of hyperkalemia and hyponatremia. Since aldosterone production is not completely dependent on ACTH secretion, these electrolyte disturbances are not seen in cases of secondary adrenocortical insufficiency. Another very important symptom seen in primary, but not secondary, chronic cases of adrenocortical insufficiency is hyperpigmentation.

Acute adrenocortical insufficiency presents with severe nausea, vomiting, and abdominal pain, with a rapidly falling blood pressure and eventual hypovolemic shock. Delirium develops and is rapidly followed by stupor and coma.

Primary and secondary adrenocortical insufficiency may be distinguished with laboratory testing, as outlined in Table 226-1.

COURSE

Untreated, most cases of chronic primary adrenocortical insufficiency are fatal usually within 2 years. Acute adrenocortical insufficiency is an acutely life-threatening medical emergency.

■TABLE 226-1. Endocrinologic Testing in Adrenocortical Insufficiency

	Primary	Secondary
Site of lesion	Adrenal gland	Pituitary or hypothalamic lesions, or pituitary suppression by exogenous steroids
Cortisol level	Reduced	Reduced
ACTH level	Increased	Reduced
Cortisol response to exogenous ACTH	Blunted	Enhanced

COMPLICATIONS

The complications of secondary depression, delirium and secondary psychosis are as described in those chapters.

ETIOLOGY

The most common cause of primary adrenocortical insufficiency is idiopathic autoimmune destruction of the gland. Other endocrine glands may also be independently targeted by the same autoimmune process that attacks the adrenals, and one should look for evidence of Hashimoto's thyroiditis, pernicious anemia, hypoparathyroidism with hypocalcemia, diabetes mellitus, and vitiligo. The association between Hashimoto's thyroiditis and adrenocortical insufficiency must be kept in mind, as the administration of thyroid hormone to a patient with hypothyroidism who also has chronic untreated adrenocortical insufficiency may provoke an "Addisonian crisis" with acute adrenocortical insufficiency and death.

Other causes of primary adrenocortical insufficiency include tuberculosis, cytomegalovirus infection (as may occur in AIDS), sarcoidosis, metastatic disease, amyloidosis, and, in acute cases, hemorrhagic necrosis (as may occur in septicemia or during overvigorous anticoagulation).

The most common cause of secondary adrenocortical insufficiency is rapid discontinuation of long-term steroid treatment. Any patient taking supraphysiologic doses of a steroid (e.g., 10 mg or more of prednisone a day) for more than a month suffers some degree of adrenocortical atrophy with a subsequent inability to meet physiologic demands when exogenous steroids are discontinued. Other causes of secondary adrenocortical insufficiency include pituitary apoplexy, pituitary tumors or granulomas, and, rarely, hypothalamic lesions.

DIFFERENTIAL DIAGNOSIS

Dysthymia, or a depressive episode of gradual onset, may be very difficult to distinguish from chronic adrenocortical insufficiency. A relative prominence of weakness and fatigue may alert one to an adrenal cause; the presence of nausea, vomiting, diarrhea, and, most importantly, postural dizziness would be additional clues. Certainly the triad of hyperkalemia, hyponatremia, and hypoglycemia would suggest a diagnosis of primary autoimmune chronic adrenocortical insufficiency.

Anorexia nervosa may likewise present with a clinical picture similar to chronic adrenocortical insufficiency. Here, however, one sees emaciation, the "pursuit of thinness," and, rather than hyperkalemia, one finds, if anything, hypokalemia.

TREATMENT

Glucocorticoids such as prednisone are required for both primary and secondary cases, and the dosage requirements may increase during times of stress. In primary cases, in which the adrenal cortex is destroyed, a mineralocorticoid such as fludrocortisone is also required.

Acute adrenocortical insufficiency, as noted above, is a medical emergency, requiring intravenous glucocorticoids, intravenous fluids, and intensive supportive care.

BIBLIOGRAPHY

Cleghorn RA. Adrenal cortical insufficiency: psychological and neurological observations. *Canadian Medical Association Journal* 1951;65:449-454.

Engel GL, Margolin SG. Neuropsychiatric disturbances in Addison's disease and the role of impaired carbohydrate metabolism in the production of cerebral functions. *Archives of Neurology and Psychiatry* 1941;45:881-884.

Lever EG, Stansfeld SA. Addison's disease, psychosis, and the syndrome of inappropriate secretion of antidiuretic hormone. *The British Journal of Psychiatry* 1983;143:406-410.

McFarland HR. Addison's disease and related psychoses. *Comprehensive Psychiatry* 1963;4:90-95.

Russel GA, Coulter JB, Isherwood DM, et al. Autoimmune Addison's disease and thyrotoxic thyroiditis presenting as encephalopathy in twins. *Archives of Disease in Childhood* 1991;66:350-352.

Varadaraj R, Cooper AJ. Addison's disease presenting with psychiatric features. *The American Journal of Psychiatry* 1986;143:553-554.

227 Lead Encephalopathy

■

Toxic levels of lead may accumulate in a variety of ways. Children with pica may eat lead-based paint chips. Welders, or workers at lead smelters or battery factories, may suffer occupational exposure, and drinkers who consume "moonshine" whiskey made with the help of old car radiators may ingest large amounts of lead. Other, less common sources include retained bullets, certain "alternative" medicines and lead-glazed pottery. Leaded gasoline used to be a major source, both to those who lived in traffic-congested areas and to those who inhaled gasoline fumes, but since lead additives were banned, this problem has essentially disappeared.

A sudden assumption of a massive burden of lead, as may occur in severe cases of pica, may produce an acute lead encephalopathy manifesting with a delirium. Conversely, chronic low-level exposure leads to an insidiously developing chronic lead encephalopathy, also known as "plumbism," manifesting primarily with dementia.

ONSET

Acute lead encephalopathy tends to evolve over several days, whereas chronic lead encephalopathy develops gradually and insidiously over a long period of time.

CLINICAL FEATURES

Acute lead encephalopathy, both in children and adults, presents with a delirium marked by confusion, insomnia, nightmares, emotional lability, and excitation, which may be quite severe; in some cases delusions and hallucinations also appear. Typically there is abdominal pain, vomiting and diarrhea, and classically the patient complains of a metallic taste. Convulsions, ataxia and other abnormal movements may be present. Hemolysis may occur, as may acute renal failure.

Chronic lead encephalopathy in children generally presents with cognitive deficits that may be very mild, manifest by only a drop of a few IQ points, or may be severe enough to constitute a dementia. There is also a strong association between lead exposure in children and the development of symptoms consistent with a diagnosis of attention-deficit/hyperactivity disorder. Convulsions may occur and may be particularly difficult to control.

Chronic lead encephalopathy in adults typically presents with a personality change and a dementia of variable severity. Patients may also complain of colicky abdominal pain, diarrhea or constipation, and a metallic taste. There may be a mild anemia, marked by basophilic stippling, and, less commonly, an interstitial nephritis; hyperuricemia and gout may also occur. With inorganic, but not organic, lead poisoning, one sees a symmetric motor polyneuropathy presenting classically with wrist or, less commonly, foot drop.

Blood lead levels of 80 microgram/dL or more are associated with an acute presentation, whereas lower levels, of 10 or 20 microgram/dL, if chronically maintained, are associated with a chronic encephalopathy. In both adults and children, "lead lines" may be seen at the border between the tooth and gingiva, and, in patients exposed in childhood, similar lead lines may be seen on x-rays of the long bones.

COURSE

Acute lead encephalopathy runs a rapid course with a mortality as high as 25% within a matter of days. Those who survive an acute attack are often left with dementia, seizures or spasticity.

Chronic lead encephalopathy gradually progresses until exposure ceases; subsequently there is very little spontaneous regression of symptoms already present.

COMPLICATIONS

Complications of delirium and of dementia are as described in those chapters.

ETIOLOGY

In acute lead encephalopathy, cerebral edema and widespread capillary dilatation are present.

In chronic lead encephalopathy one sees a degree of cortical atrophy and ventricular dilatation with widespread neuronal loss.

DIFFERENTIAL DIAGNOSIS

The appearance of a delirium or a dementia in the setting of abdominal complaints is highly suggestive of lead encephalopathy. Acute lead encephalopathy, with delirium, may be mimicked by porphyria or intoxication with other heavy metals, such as thallium or arsenic. Chronic lead encephalopathy, with dementia, may be mimicked by pellagra or Whipple's disease. If the abdominal complaints are overlooked, then the differential becomes very wide. Another, very important clue in the diagnosis of chronic lead encephalopathy in adults is a peripheral motor polyneuropathy.

TREATMENT

Acute lead encephalopathy is a medical emergency and requires hospitalization, often in an ICU, and mannitol or steroids may be required to control increased intracerebral pressure. Acute lead encephalopathy is an indication for aggressive treatment with a chelating agent; in cases of chronic lead encephalopathy there is some controversy as to how effective chelation is. Several chelating agents are available, including dimercarpol, penicillamine, calcium disodium edetate, and a new agent which may be given orally, dimercaptosuccinic acid.

The general treatment of delirium and dementia are as described in those chapters.

BIBLIOGRAPHY

Baghurst PA, McMichael AJ, Wigg NR, et al. Environmental exposure to lead and children's intelligence at the age of seven years—the Port Pirie Cohort Study. *The New England Journal of Medicine* 1992;327: 1279-1284.

Ballestra DJ. Adult chronic lead intoxication. A clinical review. *Archives of Internal Medicine* 1991;151:1718-1720.

Fisher AA, Le Couteur DG. Lead poisoning from complementary and alternative medicine in multiple sclerosis. *Journal of Neurology, Neurosurgery, and Psychiatry* 2000;69:687-689.

Jenkins CD, Mellins RB. Lead poisoning in children: a study of forty-six cases. *Archives of Neurology and Psychiatry* 1957;77:70-78.

Lifshitz M, Hashkanazi R, Phillip M. The effect of 2,3 dimercaptosuccinic acid in the treatment of lead poisoning in adults. *Annals of Medicine* 1997;29:83-85.

Matte TD, Proops D, Palazuelos E, et al. Acute high-dose lead exposure from beverage contaminated by traditional Mexican pottery. *Lancet* 1994;344:1064.

Needleman HL, Schell A, Ballinger D, et al. The long-term effects of exposure to low doses of lead in childhood. An 11-year follow-up report. *The New England Journal of Medicine* 1990;322:83-88.

Whitfield CL, Ch'ied LT, Whitehead JD. Lead encephalopathy in adults. *The American Journal of Medicine* 1972;52:289-298.

228 Manganism

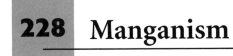

Chronic exposure to manganese may be followed by the development of a personality change, an atypical parkinsonism, and, less commonly, a dementia or psychosis. Although such exposure is generally restricted to manganese miners or to those who work in steel or battery factories, cases have also occurred among those who drank contaminated well water, and, rarely, in patients undergoing total parenteral nutrition.

ONSET

The onset is typically gradual.

CLINICAL FEATURES

The personality change is characterized by asthenia, fatigue, irritability, emotional lability and a peculiar tendency to laugh, often for no particular reason. Insomnia or somnolence may accompany these changes.

Parkinsonism may precede or follow the personality change and is characterized by bradykinesia, rigidity and postural instability with a tendency to fall backward; tremor is usually absent. The main atypical feature of this parkinsonism is the presence of dystonia, and patients may experience torticollis or a peculiar dystonic gait, characterized by toe-walking. This gait may at times be accompanied by flexion of the elbows, creating the classic "cock-walk," wherein the overall picture is reminiscent of the strutting of a rooster.

Dementia, when it occurs, is marked by a prominent amnestic component.

The psychosis of manganism, also known as "manganese madness," is characterized by hallucinations, delusions and excitation.

MRI scanning may reveal increased signal intensity on T1-weighted scanning in the globus pallidus.

Manganese levels are increased in the serum, hair, or in a 24-hour urine sample.

COURSE

With continued exposure, the clinical picture gradually worsens. With separation from manganese one may see gradual improvement, a static picture, or, in a substantial minority, a worsening of symptoms for many years, up to a decade or more.

COMPLICATIONS

The complications of personality change, dementia or secondary psychosis are as described in those chapters.

ETIOLOGY

Neuronal loss and gliosis, although widespread, is most prominent in the globus pallidus.

DIFFERENTIAL DIAGNOSIS

The combination of parkinsonism and personality change or dementia may suggest Parkinson's disease, diffuse Lewy body disease, multiple system atrophy, dementia pugilistica or arteriosclerotic parkinsonism; however, none of these is strongly marked by dystonia. A dystonic parkinsonism may, however, be seen in corticobasal ganglionic degeneration, progressive supranuclear palsy and late-onset Hallervorden-Spatz disease.

TREATMENT

Calcium versenate may remove manganese and if administered early enough may effect a substantial remission. Carbidopa/levodopa is generally not effective in relieving parkinsonian symptoms; as there are exceptions to this rule, however, a trial may be justified.

The general treatment of personality change, dementia and secondary psychosis is as outlined in those chapters. If antipsychotics are required, caution is necessary to prevent worsening the extrapyramidal symptoms, and second generation agents, such as quetiapine or olanzapine, may be preferable.

BIBLIOGRAPHY

Abd El Naby S, Hassanein M. Neuropsychiatric manifestations of chronic manganese poisoning. *Journal of Neurology, Neurosurgery, and Psychiatry* 1965;28:282-288.

Calne DB, Chu NS, Huang CC, et al. Manganism and idiopathic parkinsonism: similarities and differences. *Neurology* 1994;44:1583-1586.

Cook DG, Fahn S, Brairt KA. Chronic manganese intoxication. *Archives of Neurology* 1974;30:59-64.

Huang CC, Chu NS, Lu CS, et al. Long-term progression in chronic manganism: ten years of follow-up. *Neurology* 1998;50:698-700.

Lee JW. Manganese intoxication. *Archives of Neurology* 2000;57:597-599.

Lu CS, Huang CC, Chu NS, et al. Levodopa failure in chronic manganism. *Neurology* 1994;44:1600-1602.

Nagatomo S, Umehara F, Hanada K, et al. Manganese intoxication during total parenteral nutrition: report of two cases and review of the literature. *Journal of the Neurological Sciences* 1999;162:102-105.

Yamada M, Ohno S, Okayasyu I, et al. Chronic manganese poisoning: a neuropathological study with determination of manganese distribution in the brain. *Acta Neuropathologica* 1986;70:273-278.

229   Thallium Poisoning

Although thallium may be absorbed through the lungs or skin, such industrial exposure is rare, and most cases of poisoning occur secondary to ingestion, with either homicidal or suicidal intent.

ONSET

The onset may be either acute or gradual, depending on the acuteness of the exposure.

CLINICAL FEATURES

Acute poisoning typically evolves over a day, with vomiting, abdominal pain and diarrhea, which may be bloody. Shortly thereafter, a delirium appears which is typically accompanied by an often painful peripheral sensorimotor polyneuropathy; grand mal seizures may also occur as may a cranial neuropathy with diplopia or facial weakness. Alopecia, a very characteristic symptom, often begins at the same time and may be complete within 3 weeks. The motor neuropathy may be very severe, progressing, in some cases, to quadriparesis.

Chronic poisoning presents with alopecia, dementia and a sensorimotor polyneuropathy. Optic neuritis may also occur as may abdominal symptoms.

Thallium may be detected in serum and, more reliably, in a 24-hour urine sample. In cases of chronic poisoning, it may also be detected in hair.

COURSE

Acute cases are fatal about 10% of the time; those who survive experience a gradual improvement over the coming months, which may be complete or may leave behind a residual dementia. Chronic cases likewise show a variable degree of recovery over many months time.

COMPLICATIONS

The complications of delirium and dementia are as described in those chapters.

ETIOLOGY

In acute cases, there is widespread cerebral edema, often with petechial hemorrhages. In chronic cases, one sees widespread axonal damage in the cerebral hemispheres, accompanied by widespread neuronal loss, not only in the cortex but also prominently in the thalamus and basal ganglia.

DIFFERENTIAL DIAGNOSIS

The combination of alopecia, delirium or dementia, and a painful sensorimotor polyneuropathy is virtually specific; if alopecia is late in developing, a diagnosis of arsenic poisoning might be considered.

TREATMENT

If ingestion has been recent, gastric lavage, followed by activated charcoal, is in order. Thallium undergoes entero-hepatic recirculation, and oral Prussian blue, which binds thallium in the gut, should be given. Both hemodialysis and forced diuresis are also effective, and all measures should be continued until maximal recovery has occurred. The general treatment of delirium and of dementia are as described in those chapters.

BIBLIOGRAPHY

Atsmon J, Taliansky E, Landau M, et al. Thallium poisoning in Israel. *The American Journal of Medicine* 2000;320:327-330.

Bank WJ, Pleasure DE, Suzuki K, et al. Thallium poisoning. *Archives of Neurology* 1972;26:456-464.

Cavanaugh JB, Fuller NH, Johnson HRM, et al. The effects of thallium salts, with particular reference to the nervous system changes. *Quarterly Journal of Medicine* 1974;43:293-319.

Desenclos JC, Wilder MH, Coppenger GW, et al. Thallium poisoning: an outbreak in Florida, 1988. *Southern Medical Journal* 1992;85:1203-1206.

Moore D, House I, Dixon A. Thallium poisoning. Diagnosis may be elusive but alopecia is the clue. *British Medical Journal* 1993;306:1527-1529.

Reed D, Crawley J, Faro SN, et al. Thallotoxicosis. *Journal of the American Medical Association* 1963;183:516-522.

Thompson C, Dent J, Saxby P. Effects of thallium poisoning on intellectual function. *The British Journal of Psychiatry* 1988;153:396-399.

Wainwright AP, Kox WJ, House IM, et al. Clinical features and therapy of acute thallium poisoning. *Quarterly Journal of Medicine* 1988;69:939-944.

230 Arsenic Poisoning

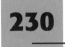

Although elemental arsenic is not toxic to the central nervous system, the ingestion of pentavalent or trivalent arsenic may cause a delirium or dementia. Such salts are found in some weed and rat killers and occasionally contaminate beer or moonshine whiskey. Occupational exposure, although rare, still at times occurs, and arsenic may at times be used in suicide or homicide attempts.

ONSET

Upon sudden exposure to large amounts, toxic signs occur acutely; chronic low-level exposure, however, produces a gradual onset.

CLINICAL FEATURES

Acute toxicity is manifested by abdominal pain, diarrhea, delirium, and, classically, the odor of garlic on the breath; within one to three weeks a sensorimotor peripheral polyneuropathy appears, which may be severe. Some cases are also characterized by grand mal seizures, and cardiac, renal and bone marrow toxicity may also occur.

Chronic exposure may cause both a dementia and a polyneuropathy; gastrointestinal symptoms are not a prominent feature and may be absent. Skin pigmentation and hyperkeratosis may be seen, and a mild degree of alopecia may occur.

Arsenic may be detected in a 24-hour urine sample and, provided that at least several weeks have elapsed since exposure, also in the hair and nails.

COURSE

Acute arsenic poisoning may be fatal. Those who survive have a variable degree of recovery over about a year. Some may be left with a degree of dementia or polyneuropathy.

COMPLICATIONS

Complications of delirium and of dementia are as described in those chapters.

ETIOLOGY

Acute intoxication may cause widespread petechial hemorrhages within the brain.

DIFFERENTIAL DIAGNOSIS

Thallium poisoning may be distinguished by the prominent alopecia.

TREATMENT

Acute poisoning is treated by gastric lavage and repeated saline enemas. In both acute and chronic cases treatment with a chelating agent, such as DMSA or DMPS, is indicated. The general treatment of delirium and of dementia is as described in those chapters.

BIBLIOGRAPHY

Campbell JP, Alvarez JA. Acute arsenic intoxication. *American Family Physician* 1989;40:93-97.

Freeman JW, Couch JR. Prolonged encephalopathy with arsenic poisoning. *Neurology* 1978;28:853-855.

Gerhardt RE, Crecelius EA, Hudson JB. Moonshine-related arsenic poisoning. *Archives of Internal Medicine* 1980;140:211-213.

Hutton JT, Christians BL. Sources, symptoms, and signs of arsenic poisoning. *The Journal of Family Practice* 1983;17:423-426.

Massey EW, Wold D, Heyman A. Arsenic: homicidal intoxication. *Southern Medical Journal* 1984;77:848-851.

Moore DF, O'Callaghan CA, Berlyne G, et al. Acute arsenic poisoning: absence of polyneuropathy after treatment with 2,3-dimercapto-propanesulphonate (DMPS). *Journal of Neurology, Neurosurgery, and Psychiatry* 1994;57:1133-1135.

Three forms of mercury are potentially toxic to humans: elemental mercury, organic mercury (methyl mercury or ethyl mercury), and salts of mercury, in which mercury may be either mercurous (monovalent) or mercuric (divalent).

Elemental mercury at room temperature is a liquid, and as such is not particularly toxic when swallowed, as it is very poorly absorbed from the gastrointestinal tract. However, with mild warming or with shaking, elemental mercury readily vaporizes into a lipophilic monoatomic form that, when inhaled, is rapidly and completely absorbed. It then readily crosses the blood-brain barrier and is taken up by neurons, inside of which it is oxidized and becomes toxic. Exposure to elemental mercury vapor occurs primarily among those using mercury in industry and among miners.

Organic mercury poisoning is generally accidental. Perhaps the most notorious example occurred in Minamata, Japan, where fishing waters had been contaminated with mercury in industrial waste. The mercury was converted to methyl mercury by microorganisms, and eventually concentrated in the fish eaten by the local inhabitants, resulting in severe brain damage. In another epidemic seeds treated with organic mercury as a fungicide, and intended only for planting, were mistakenly eaten as food. Among the organic mercury compounds, only methyl and ethyl mercury are generally toxic, and methyl mercury is the more toxic of the two. Methyl mercury is readily and almost completely absorbed from the gastrointestinal tract, easily crosses the blood-brain barrier, and is concentrated in neurons.

Mercury salts are used in the manufacture of plastics, fungicides, and electronics, and in nineteenth century England were used in felt manufacture, wherein chronic exposure by hatmakers led to the "mad hatter" syndrome made famous by Lewis Carroll in *Alice's Adventures in Wonderland.*

Although central nervous system toxicity tends to be more severe with either elemental mercury vapor or methyl mercury than with mercury salts, if a sufficient amount of mercury, regardless of its form, gains entry into the central nervous system, neuronal death and damage occur, leaving the patient, at worst, with dementia, ataxia, blindness, and tremor.

ONSET

The onset ranges from acute to gradual, depending on the nature of the exposure.

CLINICAL FEATURES

Acute exposure to organic mercury vapor causes pulmonary symptoms, with cough, dyspnea and an interstitial pneumonia. Acute exposure to organic mercury may cause nausea, vomiting and either diarrhea or constipation. Acute exposure to mercury salts causes more severe abdominal symptoms, with severe pain.

In those cases of acute exposure where patients survive, and in cases of gradual exposure, one may see a personality change and a dementia. The personality change is known as "erethism" and is characterized by emotional lability, nervousness, shyness, insomnia, forgetfulness and impaired concentration. With more severe exposure a dementia may occur. Accompanying symptoms include a peripheral polyneuropathy with prominent paresthesias, ataxia and dysarthria, more or less severe scotomas and constriction of visual fields, choreoathetosis, hearing loss, and a generalized tremor that may be quite severe, affecting even the lips and the tongue.

Mercury is also toxic to the kidneys, and especially in the case of mercury salts renal failure may occur.

In mercury poisoning, blood levels are generally above 3.6 microgram/dL, but the correlation between blood levels and clinical symptoms is at best rough.

In cases marked by erethism or dementia, MRI scanning may show atrophy of the cerebral cortex, most prominently in the calcarine cortex and the post-central area, and in the cerebellar cortex and the cerebellar vermis.

COURSE

In cases where the brain's burden of mercury is relatively mild, recovery may be nearly complete; however, when the burden is high and symptoms severe the illness is generally chronic.

COMPLICATIONS

Complications of personality change and of dementia are as described in those chapters.

ETIOLOGY

Mercury binds to sulfhydryl groups on various enzymes, thereby rendering them inactive and leading to cellular dysfunction or death. Within the brain, atrophic changes are seen in the calcarine cortex, cerebellum, and to a lesser degree in the parietal, frontal, and temporal lobes. In severe cases the entire cerebral cortex may be involved.

DIFFERENTIAL DIAGNOSIS

When the history of exposure is available, one has little trouble in diagnosis. When not available, the presence of tremors, paresthesias, and ataxia may suggest the correct diagnosis.

TREATMENT

With acute poisoning by organic mercury or mercury salts gastric lavage and activated charcoal are in order. In chronic cases, chelation therapy is indicated.

The general treatment of personality change and of dementia are as described in those chapters.

BIBLIOGRAPHY

Cinca I, Dumitrescu I, Omaca P, et al. Accidental ethyl mercury poisoning with nervous system, skeletal muscle, and myocardium injury. *Journal of Neurology, Neurosurgery, and Psychiatry* 1980;43:143-149.

Hay WJ, Richards AG, McMenemey WH, et al. Organic mercurial encephalopathy. *Journal of Neurology, Neurosurgery, and Psychiatry* 1963;26:199-202.

Korogi Y, Takahashi M, Okajima T, et al. MR findings in Minamata disease—organic mercury poisoning. *Journal of Magnetic Resonance Imaging* 1998;8:308-316.

O'Carroll RE, Masterton G, Dougall N, et al. The neuropsychiatric sequelae of mercury poisoning: the mad hatter's disease revisited. *The British Journal of Psychiatry* 1995;167:95-98.

Rustam H, Hamri T. Methyl mercury poisoning in Iraq: a neurological study. *Brain* 1974;97:499-510.

Tokuomi H, Uchino M, Imamura S, et al. Minamata disease (organic mercury poisoning): neuroradiologic and electrophysiologic studies. *Neurology* 1982;32:1369-1375.

Vroom FQ, Greer M. Mercury vapor intoxication. *Brain* 1972;95:305-318.

232 Dialysis Dementia

In the past, chronic hemodialysis with aluminum-containing dialysate was a not uncommon cause of dementia and death. With the reduction of aluminum concentrations in the dialysate, this disorder, in severe form, is vanishing. Milder forms, however, may still be seen.

ONSET

The onset is gradual and generally follows upon several years of chronic hemodialysis. Children seem especially vulnerable.

CLINICAL FEATURES

Typically, patients present with a peculiar expressive aphasia characterized by stuttering. With progression, the aphasia worsens and is joined by myoclonus, seizures and dementia. Rarely, the clinical picture may be marked by a psychosis or by mania.

The serum aluminum level is generally over 200 microgram/L.

The EEG typically shows bilateral spike and wave complexes on a background of diffuse, but frontally predominant, slowing.

COURSE

Untreated, the disorder is progressive, with an average survival of only six to seven months.

COMPLICATIONS

Complications are as described in the chapter on dementia.

ETIOLOGY

Neuronal loss is evident in the cerebral cortex, and in severe cases there may be laminar spongiform change. Aluminum levels are markedly elevated.

The source of the aluminum appears to be tap water used to make the dialysate. Some communities have naturally high aluminum levels in their water supply, and others add aluminum compounds during processing. Aluminum-containing antacids may also play a role.

DIFFERENTIAL DIAGNOSIS

Thiamine deficiency is not uncommon in chronic dialysis patients, and treatment with thiamine is probably warranted in cases which appear at all atypical for dialysis dementia. Other disorders, not uncommon in patients on dialysis, which are capable of causing a dementia include intracerebral hemorrhage, subdural hematoma and multiple ischemic infarcts.

TREATMENT

The maintenance of aluminum levels in the dialysate at or below 15 µg/L is mandatory, and patients on dialysis or those with uremia should avoid any medication containing aluminum.

Deferoxamine complexes with aluminum and should be considered.

Diazepam may reduce myoclonus but does not influence the overall course of the disease.

BIBLIOGRAPHY

Burks JS, Alfrey AC, Huddlestone J, et al. A fatal encephalopathy in chronic hemodialysis patients. *Lancet* 1976;1:764-768.

Chokroverty S, Bruetman E, Berger V, et al. Progressive dialytic encephalopathy. *Journal of Neurology, Neurosurgery, and Psychiatry* 1976;39:411-419.

Chui HC, Damasia AR. Progressive dialysis encephalopathy ("dialysis dementia"). *Journal of Neurology* 1980;222:145-157.

Davison AM, Walker GS, Oli H, et al. Water supply aluminium concentration, dialysis dementia, and effect of reverse-osmosis water treatment. *Lancet* 1982;2:785-787.

Hughes JR, Schreeder MT. EEG in dialysis encephalopathy. *Neurology* 1980;30:1148-1154.

Hung SC, Hung SH, Tarng DC, et al. Thiamine deficiency and unexplained encephalopathy in hemodialysis and peritoneal dialysis patients. *American Journal of Kidney Diseases* 2001;38:941-947.

Jack RA, Rivers-Bulkeley NT, Rabin PL. Secondary mania as a presentation of progressive dialysis encephalopathy. *The Journal of Nervous and Mental Disease* 1983;171:193-195.

Jagadha V, Deck JH, Halliday WC. Wernicke's encephalopathy in patients on peritoneal dialysis or hemodialysis. *Annals of Neurology* 1987; 21:78-84.

Lederman RJ, Henry CE. Progressive dialysis encephalopathy. *Annals of Neurology* 1978;4:199-204.

Makurkar SD, Dhar SK, Salta R, et al. Dialysis dementia. *Lancet* 1973;1:1412.

Snider WD, DeMaria AA, Mann JD. Diazepam and dialysis encephalopathy. *Neurology* 1979;29:414-415.

233 Pellagra

Niacin, also known as nicotinic acid or vitamin B_3, is a water-soluble B vitamin found in liver, yeast, poultry, fish, and meat. A related compound, niacinamide (also known as nicotinamide or nicotinic acid amide), may substitute for it. Another source of niacin is tryptophan, a small percentage of which is converted endogenously into niacin.

Niacin deficiency causes pellagra, which may occur either acutely in an "encephalopathic" form or gradually; the gradual onset cases are characterized by the classic "3 D's" of dementia, dermatitis and diarrhea.

ONSET

The acute, "encephalopathic" form evolves over days or a week; the gradual onset form, by contrast, develops insidiously over months or longer.

CLINICAL FEATURES

The acute, "encephalopathic" form is characterized by delirium, dysarthria, generalized cogwheel rigidity and myoclonus.

The gradual onset form, when fully developed, is characterized by the "3 D's." The dementia may present with depression, anxiety, and insomnia. Eventually, memory fails, and hallucinations and delusions may appear. In advanced cases ataxia and spasticity may appear, as well as parkinsonism, seizures and a polyneuropathy. The dermatitis is characterized initially by erythematous lesions in sun-exposed areas: eventually the skin becomes rough and hyperpigmented. The diarrhea may be severe and may be blood-tinged. Importantly, only about one-quarter of cases of pellagra present with the full triad, with the remainder presenting with only one or two of the "D's"; thus a patient may present with dementia alone.

Although the niacin blood level is generally low, this is not a reliable guide. A more reliable index of niacin deficiency is the measurement of one of its metabolites, N-methylniacinamide, in the urine. A low level of this metabolite reliably indicates niacin deficiency.

COURSE

The acute form is rapidly progressive, and coma and death may occur within weeks. The chronic form pursues a gradually progressive course, with death in a matter of years.

COMPLICATIONS

Complications of delirium and dementia are as described in those chapters.

ETIOLOGY

Niacin deficiency most commonly occurs due to dietary deficiency of niacin. The gradual onset form used to be common in the southeastern United States, where corn was a dietary staple among many people. As corn both lacks tryptophan and contains niacin only in a bound, biologically less available form, these people eventually became niacin deficient. Since flour was "enriched" with niacin in 1939, however, pellagra has almost disappeared in the United States; cases, however, still occur in malnourished alcoholics, and, less commonly, in other disorders associated with malnutrition such as Crohn's disease, anorexia nervosa or subsequent to extensive bowel resection.

Although most cases of pellagra do occur secondary to dietary deficiency or malabsorption, occasionally cases occur in conditions where the normal endogenous conversion of tryptophan to niacin is, for one reason or another, impaired. One example is in cases of carcinoid wherein the gross overutilization of endogenous tryptophan by the tumor leaves less available for conversion to niacin. Another mechanism is found in patients taking isoniazid. The normal enzymatic conversion of tryptophan to niacin is dependent on the "active" form of vitamin B_6; isoniazid inhibits conversion of B_6 to the active form, and hence less tryptophan can be converted into niacin.

Within the central nervous system, widespread chromatolysis and neuronal loss is seen in the cerebral cortex, basal ganglia and dentate nucleus of the cerebellum.

DIFFERENTIAL DIAGNOSIS

The acute, encephalopathic form occurring in a chronic alcoholic may be confused with Wernicke's encephalopathy or Marchiafava-Bignami disease. The prominent rigidity, however, is a clue to the correct diagnosis.

The gradual onset form is difficult to miss when the "3 D's" are present; however, as noted earlier most cases of gradual onset pellagra present with only one or two of the "D's," and the full picture may not emerge for many months. Consequently, a high index of suspicion is necessary, and pellagra should be considered in any malnourished patient who develops a dementia.

TREATMENT

Niacin may be given orally in doses of 300 to 1000 mg daily; should side effects to niacin be unacceptable, niacinamide may be given in doses of 400 to 600 mg daily. In severe cases or when patients are unable to take oral medications, niacinamide may be given intravenously.

The response to treatment is at times dramatic; once recovered, patients may be maintained on 50 to 100 mg of niacin daily. A balanced diet and robust supplementation of other vitamins, particularly thiamine, are also indicated.

In cases secondary to isoniazid, the administration of vitamin B_6 supplements in doses of 50 mg daily is generally sufficient; in some cases, however, only discontinuation of the isoniazid will allow for recovery.

BIBLIOGRAPHY

Burke GJ, Hiangabeza T. Isoniazid-induced pellagra in a patient on vitamin B supplement. *South African Medical Journal* 1977;51:719.

Hardwick SW. Pellagra in psychiatric patients: twelve recent cases. *Lancet* 1943;2:43-45.

Ishii N, Nishihara Y. Pellagra among chronic alcoholics: clinical and pathological study of 20 necropsy cases. *Journal of Neurology, Neurosurgery, and Psychiatry* 1981;44:209-215.

Ishii N, Nishihara Y. Pellagra encephalopathy among tuberculosis patients: its relation to isoniazid therapy. *Journal of Neurology, Neurosurgery, and Psychiatry* 1985;48:628-634.

Rapoport MJ. Pellagra in a patient with anorexia nervosa. *Archives of Dermatology* 1985;121:255-257.

Serdaru M, Hausser-Hauw C, Laplane D, et al. The clinical spectrum of alcoholic pellagra encephalopathy. A retrospective study of 22 cases studied pathologically. *Brain* 1988;111:829-842.

Spivak JL, Jackson DL. Pellagra: an analysis of 18 patients and a review of the literature. *Johns Hopkins Medical Journal* 1977;140:295-309.

Zaki I, Millard L. Pellagra complicating Crohn's disease. *Postgraduate Medical Journal* 1995;71:496-497.

234 Vitamin B₁₂ Deficiency

■

Vitamin B_{12} deficiency may lead to demyelinization within either the cerebrum or the spinal cord and peripheral nerves, and to defective hematopoiesis, with a macrocytic, or megaloblastic, anemia.

Vitamin B_{12}, or cobalamin, is produced only by certain bacteria. Humans obtain their supply indirectly by eating liver, other organ meats, beef, pork, milk, and eggs or directly by eating legumes contaminated with B_{12}-producing bacteria. Within the stomach, cobalamin binds to gastric R binder; this complex is then digested by pancreatic enzymes in the duodenum, and the liberated cobalamin is then bound to intrinsic factor, a glycoprotein secreted by the gastric parietal cells. The cobalamin-intrinsic factor complex passes to the ileum where it is bound to a receptor on the cell wall and absorbed. Inside the ileal cell, cobalamin is released from intrinsic factor and then bound to a carrier protein, transcobalamin II, and this cobalamin-transcobalamin II complex is secreted by the cell into the circulation. Storage of cobalamin occurs prominently in the liver.

Of the many causes of B_{12} deficiency noted under Etiology, by far the most common is pernicious anemia, wherein autoimmune destruction of gastric parietal cells leads to a deficiency of intrinsic factor and consequent deficient absorption of vitamin B_{12}. Clinically apparent B_{12} deficiency, which occurs equally among males and females, is currently rare, owing to the widespread use of parenteral vitamin B_{12}.

ONSET

The age of onset is determined by the underlying cause. Pernicious anemia generally occurs around the age of 50, but the range is wide, anywhere from 20 to 70. Owing to large stores of cobalamin in the liver, years may pass before the serum vitamin B_{12} level drops sufficiently to cause symptoms. Once a critical level has been passed, however, the symptoms may develop fairly rapidly, over months or weeks. Exposure to nitrous oxide, as may be used in dental anesthesia, may precipitate symptoms in patients with borderline low B_{12} levels, and in such cases the onset may be more acute.

CLINICAL FEATURES

Cerebral involvement may manifest with dementia, depression, or, rarely, with either mania or psychosis. Dementia is the most common manifestation of cerebral involvement, and may be complicated by delusions and hallucinations. When B_{12} deficiency manifests with psychosis, one speaks of "megaloblastic madness."

Spinal cord and peripheral nerve involvement generally go hand in hand. Pathologically, one sees demyelinization in the peripheral sensory nerves and in the posterior columns and lateral corticospinal tracts. Clinically, in fully developed cases, there is a loss of vibratory sense in the lower extremities, ataxia, a positive Romberg test, spastic weakness, extensor plantar responses, and either hyperreflexia or, if the sensory neuropathy is severe, hyporeflexia. Patients may complain of numbness and tingling in the lower extremities, and incontinence may occur.

MRI scanning reveals patchy areas of increased signal intensity on T2-weighted scans in the centrum semiovale, preferentially in the frontal lobes.

The electroencephalogram generally shows diffuse slowing. The cerebrospinal fluid is generally unremarkable; however, a slightly elevated total protein has been reported.

The anemia of B_{12} deficiency, as indicated earlier, is characterized by macrocytosis, and in some cases one sees only macrocytosis, without an accompanying anemia.

The serum B_{12} level is generally low; however, a much more sensitive test for intracellular B_{12} deficiency is the measurement of serum methylmalonic acid and homocysteine levels.

It must be stressed that cerebral involvement may occur in the absence of cord involvement and in the absence of anemia or macrocytosis; indeed in perhaps one-third of all cases of B_{12} deficiency with cerebral involvement the red blood cell indices are normal.

COURSE

Most cases of B_{12} deficiency are progressive, and patients generally die of some intercurrent illness in a matter of a few years.

COMPLICATIONS

The complications of dementia and of secondary depression, psychosis or mania are as described in those chapters.

ETIOLOGY

As noted earlier, the most common cause of B_{12} deficiency is pernicious anemia. This disease is characterized by the presence of anti-parietal cell antibodies, leading to the destruction of the gastric parietal cells and a loss of intrinsic factor. Importantly, patients with pernicious anemia may also have antibodies against the thyroid and the adrenal cortex, with either Hashimoto's thyroiditis or adrenocortical insufficiency. Other causes include strict vegetarianism or severe malnutrition, total or partial gastrectomy, inherited abnormalities of the R binder or of intrinsic factor, pancreatitis, steatorrhea or malabsorption of any cause, tapeworms, bacterial overgrowth (as may occur after a Billroth II operation), ileal disease (e.g., Crohn's disease), ileal resection, inherited abnormalities in the formation of the transcobalamin II-cobalamin complex, or inherited abnormalities in the intracellular metabolism of cobalamin. It also appears that treatment with omeprazole may decrease absorption of B_{12}, and such treatment could, conceivably, precipitate symptoms in patients with borderline low levels. Finally, there is also an association between AIDS and B_{12} deficiency.

The Schilling test may help determine the cause of the B_{12} deficiency. In the first stage of the Schilling test patients are given an intramuscular injection of 1000 mcg of cyanocobalamin, after which radiolabelled B_{12} is taken orally; a 24-hour urine is then collected and the amount of radiolabelled B_{12} in the urine is determined. If the urinary radioactive B_{12} level is low, then one may assume that B_{12} is not, for one reason or another, being absorbed via the ilium. If the urinary radioactive B_{12} level is normal, however, then one may assume an abnormality in "post-ileal" handling of B_{12}, as may occur with inherited abnormalities of the transcobalamin II-cobalamin complex. In cases where this "first stage" of the Schilling test is positive, then one proceeds to the second stage in an attempt to determine why B_{12} is not being absorbed through the ilium. In this second stage the patient is given oral radiolabelled vitamin B_{12} in combination with hog-derived intrinsic factor, and another 24 hour urine is collected. If this 24 hour urine level of radioactive B_{12} is normal, then one may assume that the patient has a deficiency of endogenously produced intrinsic factor, as seen in pernicious anemia or with gastrectomy. If, however, the 24 hour urine radioactive B_{12} level is low, then one must look for one of the other causes listed above.

In current practice, the Schilling test is rarely done. If one suspects pernicious anemia, it is more expedient to simply order anti-parietal cell and anti-intrinsic factor antibody levels, and if these are normal then one moves on to a consideration of the other possible causes.

Pathologically, there is demyelinization, and, in severe cases, axonal loss, in the centrum semiovale, posterior columns, lateral corticospinal tracts and peripheral sensory nerves.

DIFFERENTIAL DIAGNOSIS

Multiple sclerosis, which may also cause demyelinization in the cerebrum and cord, is high on the differential which, in turn, may rest solely on the determination of methylmalonic acid and homocysteine levels.

Folic acid deficiency may almost perfectly mimic vitamin B_{12} deficiency but is distinguished by the fact that although in folate deficiency the homocysteine level is increased, the methylmalonic acid level is normal.

Although the presence of macrocytosis in a patient with dementia, depression, mania or psychosis is a valuable diagnostic clue, it must be remembered that the red blood cell indices may be normal in these cases. Consequently, when the cause of one of these syndromes is not clear, a determination of methylmalonic acid and homocysteine levels should be considered.

TREATMENT

Vitamin B_{12} is given as cyanocobalamin. Although there is controversy regarding the best regimen, a prudent approach would be to give 1000 micrograms intramuscularly daily for a week, then weekly for four weeks, then monthly thereafter until maximal recovery has occurred. If the cause has been remedied, injections may then cease; however, as in most cases the underlying cause is not treatable, most patients require life-long treatment. Recent work has also suggested that cyanocobalamin given orally, in doses of 1 to 2 mg daily, may be as effective as cyanocobalamin given parenterally.

After patients have been treated for at least two weeks, folic acid, 2 mg orally daily, should be added. Folic acid must not be given earlier than this, as in such cases it may lead to an exacerbation of symptoms. Potassium levels should occasionally be checked, as hypokalemia may develop early in the course of treatment with B_{12}.

Improvement may not occur for months, and up to $1\frac{1}{2}$ years may be required before maximum improvement is seen. If treatment is begun early, before axonal loss has occurred, full recovery may be expected; however, if symptoms have been present for months, irreversible damage may already have occurred, and the recovery will not be complete.

BIBLIOGRAPHY

Evans DL, Edelsohn GA, Golden RN. Organic psychosis without anemia or spinal cord symptoms in patients with vitamin B_{12} deficiency. *The American Journal of Psychiatry* 1983;140:218-221.

Fraser TN. Cerebral manifestations of Addisonian pernicious anemia. *Lancet* 1960;2:458-459.

Goggans FC. A case of mania secondary to vitamin B12 deficiency. *The American Journal of Psychiatry* 1984;141:300-301.

Healton EB, Savage DG, Brust JCM, et al. Neurologic aspects of cobalamin deficiency. *Medicine* 1991;70:229-245.

Herzlich BC, Schiano TD. Reversal of apparent AIDS dementia complex following treatment with vitamin B12. *Journal of Internal Medicine* 1993;233:495-497.

Jefferson JW. The case of the numb testicles. *Diseases of the Nervous System* 1977;38:749-751.

Kuzminski AM, Del Giacco EJ, Allen RH, et al. Effective treatment of cobalamin deficiency with oral cobalamin. *Blood* 1998;92: 1191-1198.

Lerner V, Kanevsky M. Acute dementia with delirium due to vitamin B12 deficiency: a case report. *International Journal of Psychiatry in Medicine* 2002;32:215-220.

Lindenbaum J, Healton EB, Savage DG, et al. Neuropsychiatric disorders caused by cobalamin deficiency in the absence of anemia or macrocytosis. *The New England Journal of Medicine* 1988;318:1720-1728.

Marcuard SP, Albernaz L, Khazanie PG. Omeprazole therapy causes malabsorption of cyanocobalamin (vitamin B12). *Annals of Internal Medicine* 1994;120:211-215.

Rajan S, Wallace JI, Brodkin KI, et al. Response of elevated methylmalonic acid to three doses of oral cobalamin in older adults. *Journal of the American Geriatrics Society* 2002;50:1789-1795.

Ravakhah K, West BC. Case report: subacute combined degeneration of the spinal cord from folate deficiency. *The American Journal of the Medical Sciences* 1995;310:214-216.

Shorvon SD, Carney MWP, Chanarin I, et al. The neuropsychiatry of megaloblastic anemia. *British Medical Journal* 1980;281:1036-1038.

235 Folic Acid Deficiency

Folic acid, a critical ingredient in the synthesis of DNA, is found in abundance in fresh green vegetables, some fruits, yeast, kidney, and liver. Once absorbed through the proximal small intestine, folic acid undergoes enterohepatic recirculation, with a relatively small amount being stored in the liver. With folic acid deficiency there may be a macrocytic anemia, and, rarely, involvement of the cerebrum or the spinal cord and peripheral nerves.

ONSET

Given the limited hepatic storage, folic acid levels fall below normal within three months of the onset of dietary deficiency.

CLINICAL FEATURES

With involvement of the cerebrum, spinal cord, and peripheral nerves, a clinical picture emerges that is remarkably similar to that seen with vitamin B_{12} deficiency. As with B_{12} deficiency, a dementia may occur and this may or may not be accompanied by decreased vibratory sense in the lower extremities, ataxia, a positive Romberg test, and paraplegia with extensor plantar responses and either hyperreflexia or hyporeflexia.

Serum folic acid levels provide only a rough estimate of tissue levels, which are reflected more accurately by a red blood cell folate level. An even more sensitive test is the plasma homocysteine level, which is elevated in folate deficiency.

COURSE

This appears to be chronic.

COMPLICATIONS

The complications of dementia are as described in that chapter.

ETIOLOGY

The most common cause of folic acid deficiency is a diet lacking in the folate-rich foods described above; chronic alcoholics are particularly prone to develop such a deficiency. Intestinal disease, such as sprue, may also lead to malabsorption of folic acid.

Oral contraceptives, pyrimethamine, trimethoprim, pentamadine, cholestyramine, and, most notably, certain anticonvulsants have all been associated with folic acid deficiency. Phenytoin, primidone, and phenobarbital are the most commonly implicated. Increased requirements also deplete folic acid stores, and this may be seen in hyperthyroidism, pregnancy, lactation, and during the reticulocytosis following B_{12} replacement in cases of vitamin B_{12} deficiency. Folic acid may also be lost during hemodialysis.

DIFFERENTIAL DIAGNOSIS

As noted earlier, folic acid deficiency may produce an illness almost identical to that seen in vitamin B_{12} deficiency, and the differential may rest on determining both homocysteine and methylmalonic acid levels. In folic acid deficiency, the homocysteine level is increased but the methylmalonic acid level is normal; by contrast in vitamin B_{12} deficiency, both values are increased. The differential between folic acid deficiency and vitamin B_{12} deficiency is a critical one because if folic acid is given to patients with B_{12} deficiency before B_{12} stores are repleted, the damage to the central and peripheral nervous systems may increase.

TREATMENT

Parenteral treatment is almost never required, even in intestinal disease. A dose of 1 or 2 mg orally daily is usually sufficient. If the deficiency is secondary to an anticonvulsant, seizure control occasionally may be partially lost with folic acid treatment, requiring an adjustment in the antiepileptic regimen.

BIBLIOGRAPHY

Pincus JH, Reynolds EH, Glaser GH. Subacute combined system degeneration with folate deficiency. *Journal of the American Medical Association* 1972;221:496-497.

Ravakhah K, West BC. Case report: subacute combined degeneration of the spinal cord from folate deficiency. *The American Journal of the Medical Sciences* 1995;310:214-216.

Reynolds EH, Rothfeld P, Pincus JH. Neurological disease associated with folate deficiency. *British Medical Journal* 1973;2:398-400.

Strachan RW, Henderson JG. Dementia and folate deficiency. *Quarterly Journal of Medicine* 1967;36:189-204.

INFECTIOUS AND RELATED DISORDERS

236 Neurosyphilis

Infection with the spirochete *Treponema pallidum* occurs in primary, secondary and tertiary forms. Primary syphilis typically presents with a painless chancre, and secondary syphilis with a widespread rash; following the resolution of the rash, there is a more or less lengthy "latent" interval after which tertiary syphilis may appear. Tertiary syphilis may affect a variety of organs, including the central nervous system, in which case one speaks of neurosyphilis.

Of the variety of manifestations of central nervous system involvement in neurosyphilis, four are of general interest to the psychiatrist: meningovascular syphilis, gummas, general paresis and tabes dorsalis.

Meningovascular neurosyphilis is characterized by a chronic, generally indolent basilar meningitis: both large arteries and cranial nerves which traverse the inflamed meninges may be affected, and there may be infarctions and cranial nerve palsies.

Gummas are granulomatous tumors, and are generally found in association with meningovascular neurosyphilis. They range in size from minute to quite large, and may present as any other space-occupying lesion would.

General paresis is characterized by a diffuse invasion of the brain by the spirochete, and typically results in a dementia. General paresis has a number of synonyms, including general paresis of the insane (often abbreviated as GPI), dementia paralytica, and paretic neurosyphilis.

Tabes dorsalis is characterized pathologically by involvement of the dorsal root ganglia and the posterior columns of the spinal cord, and clinically by ataxia and sensory disturbances.

The current prevalence of any form of tertiary neurosyphilis is not known with certainty. In the preantibiotic era it was apparently common, with general paresis being the most common cause of dementia. However, with the post-World War II widespread use of penicillin, the incidence fell dramatically, and at one point neurosyphilis almost vanished. Over the past decade, however, it has been undergoing a resurgence, particularly among those with AIDS.

Males are more likely to develop neurosyphilis than are females, and this has been true since the nineteenth century.

ONSET

Meningovascular neurosyphilis may present anywhere from 2 to 10 years after the primary infection. The onset is often acute, with meningeal signs, infarction in the area of distribution of a large cerebral artery, or a cranial nerve palsy. In cases, however, where the endarteritis affects multiple small vessels the patient may present with a dementia of gradual and insidious onset.

Gummas may likewise present anywhere from 2 to 10 years after the primary infection.

General paresis presents gradually anywhere from 10 to 20 years after the primary infection.

Tabes dorsalis exhibits the longest latency, and may not appear for anywhere from 10 to 30 years after the primary infection; the onset itself is typically gradual.

It must be borne in mind that the latency between the primary infection and the onset of neurosyphilis may be quite shortened in immunocompromised patients, as for example those with AIDS.

CLINICAL FEATURES

The symptomatology of meningovascular neurosyphilis varies according to whether only a few large vessels are affected by an endarteritis or numerous small ones, whether and which cranial nerves are affected by the basal meningitis, and whether an obstructive hydrocephalus occurs. When large vessels are involved, the middle cerebral and posterior cerebral arteries are often affected, and the subsequent stroke may be acute, or at times subacute, in onset, progressing over several days. The resultant symptomatology is essentially identical to that seen secondary to occlusion of the vessels by any other causes: hemianopia, hemiplegia, aphasia or apraxia, and so on. In instances where numerous small vessels are eventually occluded by the endarteritic process, the patient may present with a gradually progressive dementia that in and of itself may have no particular distinctive features. The cranial nerves most likely to be entrapped and inflamed include the third and sixth, with external ophthalmoplegia and diplopia; the fifth, with neuralgic pain; and the seventh, with a full facial paresis, which may become bilateral. The Argyll Robertson pupil is found in most cases of meningovascular neurosyphilis; here, although the pupil constricts on accommodation testing, one sees either a sluggish or no reaction to direct light.

Gummas, as noted earlier, generally occur in connection with meningovascular neurosyphilis. They tend to occur at the base of the brain or over the convexity and occasionally may be deep-seated. The symptoms are those of any space-occupying lesion.

General paresis is not necessarily associated with meningovascular neurosyphilis or the occurrence of gummas; indeed, general paresis may be the only manifestation of neurosyphilis. In the vast majority of cases, general paresis presents with a dementia that takes one of three classic forms: simple dementia, manic type of dementia, or melancholic type of dementia.

The majority of patients display the simple dementia, without prominent affective symptoms. The patient begins to neglect dress and personal hygiene. Judgment and self-restraint fail, and the patient may embark on ruinous financial or personal ventures. Hallucinations and delusions may occur, but they generally play only a minor role in the overall symptomatology. The hallucinations may be either visual or auditory. The delusions, though frequent, tend to be neither fixed nor systematized and often change concomitantly with the patient's shifting moods. Memory and concentration fail.

The manic type may be almost indistinguishable from a manic episode of bipolar disorder. The patients are euphoric and extremely energetic. Delusions of grandeur are common. They are presidents, kings, and titans of industry and often attempt to act as such exalted persons might. Life savings may be squandered overnight. This presentation, in connection with some of the symptoms of a simple dementia, is so characteristic that in the nineteenth and early twentieth century it was considered virtually pathognomonic for general paresis.

The melancholic, or depressive, type bears, as might be expected, a strong resemblance to a typical depressive episode. The patients are downcast, drained, agitated, and sleepless. They feel they have committed unpardonable sins and are to be executed. Suicide may occur.

Regardless of the typology of the dementia of general paresis, certain other signs and symptoms may be seen. Typically, however, they become apparent only after the dementia has been established. Focal or generalized seizures occur in about one half of the cases, and they tend to become more common as the dementia progresses. Speech gradually becomes slow, slurred, and monotonous; dysnomia may occur, and echolalia may occasionally be seen. Dysgraphia occurs—handwritten letters become misshapen, misspellings are common, and eventually sentences become unintelligible. Very typically, the facial musculature loses its tone and becomes flabby, giving the patient a vacant, almost stupid, facial appearance. The Argyll Robertson pupil is present in almost all patients but may not be complete. Coarse tremor is common, and, in addition to the fingers and hands, it is also apparent in the lips and tongue. Unless the patient has tabes dorsalis, the deep tendon reflexes tend to be hyperactive, and the plantar responses may be extensor.

With progression most patients with general paresis, regardless of the initial typology of the dementia, eventually come to a common end. Short-term and eventually long-term memory become profoundly deficient, and patients may confabulate wildly. The mood becomes increasingly labile, and eventually consciousness becomes profoundly clouded, with many patients sinking into a torpor. The gait becomes unsteady, and eventually a true "general paresis" occurs, with profound widespread weakness of all voluntary musculature. At the end the patient is unable to walk and becomes bedridden, existing in a vegetative state until death occurs.

The foregoing description of classical general paresis may not be entirely applicable to today's patient for two reasons. First, administration of penicillin or tetracycline in prior years for other infections may conceivably alter the clinical expression. Second, in patients with AIDS the disruption of the balance between host defense and invading spirochete may result in an atypical form of general paresis.

Tabes dorsalis is characterized by reduced vibratory sense in the lower extremities, ataxia, a positive Romberg test, urinary incontinence and erectile dysfunction. There may also be "tabetic" pains or "crises" wherein severe, lancinating, lightning-like pains occur in the lower extremities and sometimes in the abdomen.

MRI scanning in meningovascular syphilis reveals the basilar meningitis and any areas of infarction; in gummas, one sees space-occupying lesions; and in general paresis there is generalized cerebral atrophy.

Cerebrospinal fluid (CSF) pressure is usually normal; however, especially in meningovascular neurosyphilis, it may be increased. Usually a mild lymphocytic pleocytosis is present, and the total protein is usually elevated between 50 and 150 mg/dl. The IgG index is usually elevated, and oligoclonal bands may be present.

The serum Venereal Disease Research Laboratory (VDRL) test for syphilis is positive in only about 70% of cases of neurosyphilis, and the CSF VDRL is even less sensitive. The serum fluorescent treponemal antibody (FTA) test is positive in almost 100% of cases; however, the CSF FTA is less sensitive, being positive in only about 75% of patients. False positive VDRLs may occur in collagen vascular disease, such as lupus, and also in heroin addicts; generally these false positives are of low titer (e.g., less than 1:8). False positive FTAs may occur under the same circumstances but are very rare.

In practice, demented patients are often screened with a serum VDRL, which, if positive, is followed up by a serum FTA to exclude a false positive. However, given that the serum VDRL has only about a 70% sensitivity, one may want to screen all demented patients with a serum FTA. If the serum FTA is negative, then neurosyphilis is effectively ruled out. If the serum FTA is positive in a demented patient, then CSF should be obtained for cell count and differential, total protein, IgG index, oligoclonal bands and VDRL. If the CSF VDRL is positive, then the diagnosis of neurosyphilis is almost certain. If the CSF VDRL is negative, but there is evidence of infection (e.g., pleocytosis, increased protein) suggesting active disease, then it may be prudent to determine a CSF FTA, although this is controversial: even minute contamination of the CSF with blood may create a false positive CSF FTA, and hence caution must be utilized in interpreting a positive result. In the rare case where both the CSF VDRL and the CSF FTA are negative, but the clinical picture is highly suggestive of neurosyphilis and there is evidence of infection in the CSF, then one may want to treat the patient as if neurosyphilis were present, providing that no significant contraindications are evident.

Given the increasingly frequent concurrence of AIDS and syphilis, all patients with syphilis should be tested for HIV infection.

Before leaving this section on symptomatology, mention should also be made of congenital general paresis, as more cases may be seen in the decades to come. Congenitally infected children may not show the classical "Hutchinson's triad" of cataracts, sensorineuronal deafness, and "Hutchinson's teeth," wherein the central incisors are notched, widely spaced, and often tapering; indeed patients may be normal until their teenage years when an otherwise typical general paresis may gradually appear.

COURSE

Untreated, both meningovascular syphilis and general paresis are generally fatal, with death occurring in from 3 to 5 years.

COMPLICATIONS

The complications of dementia are as described in that chapter.

ETIOLOGY

The spirochete in question, *Treponema pallidum,* gains access to the central nervous system early in the course of untreated syphilis. Indeed, in up to one third of all patients with secondary syphilis, the CSF has either an elevated total protein or a pleocytosis, indicating that invasion of the nervous system has occurred. In most cases, however, host defenses are adequate to eradicate the spirochete from the central nervous system before tissue damage and symptoms occur. However, in perhaps a tenth of cases defenses fail, and neurosyphilis occurs.

In meningovascular neurosyphilis a granulomatous basilar meningitis is present. Those cranial nerves traversing the thickened meninges become inflamed and undergo degenerative changes. Likewise large and medium arteries undergo an inflammatory endarteritis, which may lead to occlusion and subsequent infarction. Obstruction of cerebrospinal fluid pathways may lead to hydrocephalus.

Gummas are granulomatous tumors and are often considered to be a "localized" form of meningovascular neurosyphilis. They may be small and miliary, or at times large and solitary, in which case they present, as noted earlier, as any other tumor might.

In general paresis, cortical atrophy occurs, more prominently in the frontal and temporal lobes. The ventricles are dilated and generally display a granular ependymitis. Spirochetes are present throughout the parenchyma; neurons are lost or degenerated, with a disruption of the normal cortical architecture. Microglia and astrocytes are present in abundance. Small penetrating vessels may show perivascular cuffing of lymphocytes and plasma cells; however, no endarteritis is present, as seen in meningovascular neurosyphilis.

Tabes dorsalis is characterized primarily by atrophy and softening of the posterior columns of the cord.

DIFFERENTIAL DIAGNOSIS

Meningovascular neurosyphilis, when presenting primarily with symptoms referable to basilar meningitis and cranial nerve palsies, may be mimicked by sarcoidosis, tuberculosis, or meningeal carcinomatosis, and the differential may depend on CSF findings.

Gummas may be mimicked by other granulomatous lesions or by neoplasms, such as a glioma.

General paresis, when presenting with mania or depression, may be mistaken for a mood disorder. The occurrence of similar episodes earlier in a patient's life, of course, would argue against the diagnosis of general paresis. The appearance of cognitive deficits out of proportion to the affective symptoms would also suggest the correct diagnosis. When general paresis presents with a simple dementia, the differential diagnosis is quite wide as discussed in the chapter on dementia. Given the similar clinical presentations, Alzheimer's disease, alcoholic dementia, lacunar dementia, and Binswanger's disease along with AIDS dementia all deserve extra consideration.

In evaluating a patient with a clinical picture consistent with neurosyphilis, one must not rely on the patient's recollection of ever having had primary or secondary syphilis: in some cases it may never have been diagnosed, and many patients are simply too ashamed to admit the diagnosis. Serologic testing is mandatory.

TREATMENT

Intravenous aqueous penicillin G should be given in a dose of 2 to 4 million units every four hours for two weeks; patients allergic to penicillin should probably undergo desensitization. It must be stressed that benzathine penicillin is not effective.

A minority of patients, after institution of antibiotic treatment, experience a transient exacerbation of symptoms accompanied by fever and other constitutional symptoms. This Jarisch-Herxheimer reaction is probably due to an inflammatory reaction to dying spirochetes.

Penicillin halts progression of meningovascular neurosyphilis; however, cranial nerve palsies and symptoms referable to ischemic infarcts persist. Likewise, in general paresis, progression is halted; however, more than a partial remission of established symptoms is not to be expected.

Gummas may respond to treatment with penicillin; the addition of prednisone may also be beneficial. Surgical removal of large gummas, however, may be required.

Cerebrospinal fluid should be reexamined at a minimum of 6 and 12 months after penicillin treatment. The pretreatment abnormalities resolve very slowly, over months or a year or more. The cell count drops first, followed by the total protein, and finally by a reduction in the CSF VDRL titer. The CSF VDRL may never become negative; however, should the titer rise, this would be an indication for treatment. Follow-up testing is especially critical in patients who are also infected with HIV, as relapse, despite otherwise adequate treatment with penicillin, is not uncommon in this group.

The serum VDRL usually becomes negative with penicillin treatment; however, some patients remain "sero-fast," with persistently low titers. The serum FTA generally remains positive for the life of the patient, despite completely adequate treatment.

Symptomatic treatment may be required either before treatment with penicillin or after, if residual symptoms persist. Antipsychotics are useful for delusions and hallucinations, antidepressants for depression, and lithium, valproate, or carbamazepine may be tried when general paresis presents with manic symptoms. Tabetic pains may respond to carbamazepine.

BIBLIOGRAPHY

Fleet WS, Watson RT, Ballinger WE. Resolution of gumma with steroid therapy. *Neurology* 1986;36:1104-1107.

Gimenez-Roldan S, Martin M. Tabetic lightning pains: high-dosage intravenous penicillin versus carbamazepine therapy. *European Neurology* 1981;20:424-428.

Gordon SM, Eaton ME, George R, et al. The response of symptomatic neurosyphilis to high-dose intravenous penicillin G in patients with human immunodeficiency virus infection. *The New England Journal of Medicine* 1994;331:1469-1473.

Holmes MD, Brant-Zawadzki MM, Simon RP. Clinical features of meningovascular syphilis. *Neurology* 1984;34:553-556.

Katz DA, Berger JR, Duncan RC. Neurosyphilis. A comparative study of the effects of infection with human immunodeficiency virus. *Archives of Neurology* 1993;50:243-249.

Merritt HH, Adams RD, Solomon HC. *Neurosyphilis,* New York, 1946, Oxford University Press.

Nordenbo AM, Sorenson PS. The incidence and clinical presentation of neurosyphilis in Greater Copenhagen 1974 through 1978. *Acta Neurologica Scandinavica* 1981;63:237-246.

Simon RP. Neurosyphilis. *Archives of Neurology* 1985;42:606-613.

Zifko U, Lindner K, Wimberger D, et al. Jarisch-Herxheimer reaction in a patient with neurosyphilis. *Journal of Neurology, Neurosurgery, and Psychiatry* 1994;57:865-867.

Mycobacterium tuberculosis is an acid-fast intracellular bacillus that in most cases is spread by droplets from persons who have cavitary pulmonary disease. In many patients a focus of infection may lie dormant in the body for years or decades, held in check by adequate host defenses until some loss of immunocompetence, as in AIDS, or some other debilitating illness, is followed by reactivation and hematogenous spread to various other organs, including the meninges or the brain, where it may cause a basilar meningitis or parenchymal tuberculomas.

The incidence of tuberculosis has risen greatly over the past two decades, primarily because of infection in intravenous drug users and in patients with HIV infection.

ONSET

The basilar meningitis is generally of subacute onset, over a matter of weeks; tuberculomas tend to present gradually.

CLINICAL FEATURES

Meningitis is characterized by delirium, often marked by intervals of partial lucidity, headache, stiff neck and fever. Tremor is common, and there may be hyponatremia secondary to a syndrome of inappropriate antidiuretic hormone secretion (SIADH). Cranial nerve palsies may occur, especially of the third, fourth, and sixth cranial nerves, and in a small minority obstructive hydrocephalus may occur, with an acute worsening of the delirium.

Infarctions, often of the basal ganglia, may occur secondary to arteritis of vessels passing through the meningeal exudate, and one may see chorea and dystonia and other focal signs.

Tuberculomas present as any other mass lesion; they may be solitary, but tend to be multiple, and may occur either above or below the tentorium. Seizures may occur.

Enhanced CT or MRI scanning demonstrates the meningitis and any tuberculoma. Unfortunately, however, it may not be possible to distinguish tuberculomas from other masses without a biopsy.

In meningitis the cerebrospinal fluid shows a pleocytosis, which initially may be polymorphonuclear but eventually becomes lymphocytic. The sugar is generally low, and protein is generally elevated. A stained smear is made from a centrifuged tube, but even after the most diligent of searches the acid-fast rods are generally not found. Culture results, though positive in over one-half of patients with tuberculous meningitis, are not available for at least a month, and hence reliance is often placed on a PCR assay for M. tuberculosis, which is generally positive.

In tuberculomas the cerebrospinal fluid is generally normal; in some cases a mild lymphocytic pleocytosis and mild elevation of total protein are present.

The purified protein derivative (PPD) test is generally, but not always, positive in meningitis and tuberculomas.

COURSE

Meningitis almost always terminates fatally in anywhere from a week up to a couple of months. In some cases tuberculomas undergo an arrest in growth and become partially calcified.

COMPLICATIONS

Complications of delirium are as described in that chapter.

ETIOLOGY

Meningitis is characterized by a thick, often basilar, exudate that may affect arteries traversing the subarachnoid space and may also obstruct the CSF outflow. The tuberculomas usually undergo typical caseation necrosis and may be minute or so large as to destroy an entire cerebral lobe.

DIFFERENTIAL DIAGNOSIS

Tuberculous meningitis must be differentiated from the basilar meningitides seen in mycotic infections, sarcoidosis, meningovascular neurosyphilis, and meningeal carcinomatosis. As noted above, the tuberculomas must be differentiated from other brain tumors.

TREATMENT

Tuberculous meningitis demands urgent treatment, and a quadruple drug regimen, such as isoniazid, rifampin, pyrazinamide and ethambutol, is often used. When isoniazid is used chronically, one must add B6 to prevent pellagra, keeping in mind that, albeit rarely, pellagra may occur despite adjunctive treatment with B6.

Tuberculomas, if solitary and accessible, may be surgically removed. In other cases, a regimen similar to that described above may be used.

The general treatment of delirium is as outlined in that chapter.

Resistant organisms are being encountered with increasing frequency, especially in patients with AIDS; treatment, even by specialists, is difficult.

BIBLIOGRAPHY

Alarcon F, Duenas G, Cevallos N, et al. Movement disorders in 30 patients with tuberculous meningitis. *Movement Disorders* 2000;15:561-569.

Davis LE, Rastogi KR, Lambert LC, et al. Tuberculous meningitis in the southwest United States: a community-based study. *Neurology* 1993;43:1775-1778.

Ishii N, Nishihara Y. Pellagra encephalopathy among tuberculosis patients: its relation to isoniazid therapy. *Journal of Neurology, Neurosurgery, and Psychiatry* 1985;48:628-634.

Kennedy DH, Fallon RJ. Tuberculous meningitis. *The Journal of American Medical Association* 1979;241:264-268.

Traub M, Colchester ACF, Kingsley DPE, et al. Tuberculosis of the central nervous system. *Quaterly Journal of Medicine* 1984;53:81-100.

Yechoor VK, Shandera WX, Rodriguez P, et al. Tuberculous meningitis among adults with and without HIV infection. Experience in an urban public hospital. *Archives of Internal Medicine* 1996;156:1710-1716.

A small proportion of patients with Lyme disease eventually develop a dementia. Classically, after being infected with *Borrelia burgdorferi* by the bite of an ixodid tick, patients experience an illness loosely organized into three stages. Stage I is characterized by erythema chronicum migrans, and stage II is characterized by cardiac involvement and/or symptoms of widespread nervous system involvement. Finally, in stage III, patients may develop an oligoarthritis or a dementia.

ONSET

The infectious tick bite tends to occur in the summer, and patients of any age may be affected. The onset of the dementia is gradual and tends to occur about 2 years after the tick bite; the range, however, is wide, from less than a year to more than a decade.

CLINICAL FEATURES

Stage I develops within days up to a month after the tick bite and is characterized by a gradually enlarging, generally ringlike erythematous rash with an indurated center, known as erythema chronicum migrans, which may or may not be accompanied by satellite lesions. It generally remits within weeks.

Stage II follows stage I within weeks or months, and may be characterized by involvement of the heart, joints or nervous system. Cardiac involvement may manifest as atrioventricular block or, less commonly, a pericarditis or myocarditis. Joint involvement is announced by a polyarthralgia. Nervous system involvement, seen in about 15% of stage II cases, is characterized by any or all of the following: meningitis, encephalitis, radiculitis, peripheral polyneuritis or mononeuritis multiplex, and a cranial neuritis, classically producing bilateral or unilateral Bell's palsy. Stage II symptoms generally remit spontaneously in a matter of months.

Stage III Lyme disease, appearing anywhere from months to many years after the fateful bite, is characterized by either an oligoarthritis or, in a minority of cases, a dementia. The dementia tends to be mild and is characterized by forgetfulness, hypersomnolence, depression and irritability, and is often accompanied by fatigue and a sensory polyneuropathy. A minority of patients may also have an expressive aphasia, long-tract signs or cerebral infarctions. MRI scanning may disclose a number of small circular areas of increased signal intensity on T2-weighted scans within the white matter, often in a periventricular distribution. Most patients with Lyme dementia have anti-Borrelia antibodies present in the serum; more than half have either antibodies or increased total protein in the cerebrospinal fluid, and in some cases a mononuclear pleocytosis may also be found.

COURSE

Lyme dementia appears to be chronic, and, in some cases, gradually progressive.

COMPLICATIONS

The complications of dementia are as described in that chapter.

ETIOLOGY

After inoculation by the bite of an ixodid tick, *Borrelia burgdorferi* spreads locally, creating the erythema chronicum migrans. Hematogenous spread then occurs to the heart, joints and nervous system, creating stage II. Stage III central nervous system involvement is characterized by both a vasculitis and by periventricular demyelinization.

DIFFERENTIAL DIAGNOSIS

Patients with Lyme dementia may or may not recall stage I or stage II. When the oligoarthritis of stage III is present in a patient with dementia, this is a strong clue; however, there are cases of Lyme dementia lacking arthritis. MRI findings may suggest multiple sclerosis.

Although the absence of anti-Borrelia serum antibodies argues strongly against the diagnosis, their presence does not carry the same strong weight, as many patients living in endemic areas are sero-positive and never have any symptoms.

TREATMENT

The general treatment of dementia is as described in that chapter. Whether or not antibiotic treatment is effective is hotly debated. If treatment is elected, patients should receive at least a four week course of intravenous ceftriaxone, keeping in mind that within the first 1 to 3 days of antibiotic treatment, a Jarisch-Herxheimer reaction may occur with constitutional symptoms and worsening of any preexisting symptoms.

BIBLIOGRAPHY

Benke T, Gasse T, Hittmair-Delazer M, et al. Lyme encephalopathy: long-term neuropsychological deficits years after acute neuroborreliosis. *Acta Neurologica Scandinavica* 1995;91:353-357.

Fallon BA, Nields JA. Lyme disease: a neuropsychiatric illness. *The American Journal of Psychiatry* 1994;151:1571-1583.

Kaiser R. Neuroborreliosis. *Journal of Neurology* 1998;245:247-255.

Klempner MS, Hu LT, Evans J, et al. Two controlled trials of antibiotic treatment in patients with persistent symptoms and a history of Lyme disease. *The New England Journal of Medicine* 2001;345:85-92.

Oschmann P, Dorndorf W, Hornig C, et al. Stages and syndromes of neuroborreliosis. *Journal of Neurology* 1998;245:262-272.

Traub J, Fernandez A, Haass A, et al. Clinical and serologic follow-up in patients with neuroborreliosis. *Neurology* 1998;51:1489-1491.

239 Whipple's Disease

Whipple's disease, also known as intestinal lipodystrophy, although generally presenting with a malabsorption syndrome and articular complaints, may occasionally involve the central nervous system. It is a rare disorder and most commonly seen in white males.

ONSET

Whipple's disease generally occurs in middle years, and symptoms appear and evolve fairly gradually.

CLINICAL FEATURES

Although cases have been reported wherein Whipple's disease presented with symptoms of central nervous system dysfunction alone, the vast majority of patients with central nervous system disease secondary to Whipple's disease have had either a malabsorption syndrome or joint involvement. The malabsorption syndrome is characterized by steatorrhea, weight loss, fever, and abdominal pain, and joint involvement usually manifests with a large joint polyarthralgia or nondeforming polyarthritis.

Central nervous system involvement may be announced by a personality change, delirium or dementia. In most instances other symptoms of central nervous system dysfunction also occur, including supranuclear ophthalmoplegia, nystagmus, ataxia, myoclonus, and seizures. Hypothalamic involvement may cause hypersomnolence, hyperphagia, changes in libido and diabetes insipidus. A minority of patients may also display a peculiar movement disorder known as oculomasticatory myoarrhythmia: here there are conjugate, pendular eye movments occurring in concert with jaw movements.

Diagnosis may be confirmed by the demonstration of PAS positive macrophages within affected tissue, as for example upon small bowel biopsy, or by PCR assay of such tissue.

CT or MRI scanning often demonstrates localized lesions consistent with the patient's focal symptomatology. The cerebrospinal fluid usually shows a moderate monocytic pleocytosis. Glucose is generally normal; protein may or may not be elevated. Occasionally PAS-positive cells may be found in the cerebrospinal fluid; however, PCR assay is more sensitive.

COURSE

Untreated, Whipple's disease is generally progressive; the appearance of central nervous system involvement is a grave sign, and some patients may slip into coma in a matter of months.

COMPLICATIONS

Complications are as described in the chapters on personality change, delirium and dementia. If malabsorption is severe, vitamin B_{12} deficiency may occur.

ETIOLOGY

Whipple's disease is caused by a bacillus, *Tropheryma whippelii*, which may be seen in macrophages.

Within the central nervous system cortical atrophy and ventricular dilatation is seen. Focal areas of inflammation are scattered throughout the cerebral cortex, subcortical gray, brainstem and cerebellar cortex, and within these areas one finds macrophages containing the bacillus.

DIFFERENTIAL DIAGNOSIS

Articular and intestinal symptoms may suggest the correct diagnosis. In those very rare cases wherein central nervous system disease occurs in their absence, the diagnosis may be in doubt pending cerebral biopsy or lumbar puncture.

TREATMENT

The general treatment of delirium, dementia or personality change is as described in those chapters.

Trimethoprim/sulfamethoxazole produces a variable degree of recovery, depending on how much structural central nervous system damage has already occurred. Treatment should be continued until PCR assay of the CSF is negative, a process that may take a year or more. Relapses may occur, and in some cases lifelong treatment may be required.

BIBLIOGRAPHY

Adams M, Rhyner PA, Day J, et al. Whipple's disease confined to the central nervous system. *Annals of Neurology* 1987;21:104-108.

Dumler JS, Baisden BL, Yardley JH, et al. Immunodetection of Tropheryma whippelii in intestinal tissues from Dr. Whipple's 1907 patient. *The New England Journal of Medicine* 2003;348:1411-1412.

Durand DV, Lecomte C, Cathebras P, et al. Whipple disease. Clinical review of 52 cases. *Medicine* 1997;76:170-184.

Gerard A, Sarrot-Reynauld F, Liozon E, et al. Neurologic presentation of Whipple disease: report of 12 cases and review of the literature. *Medicine* 2002;81:443-457.

Marth T, Raoult D. Whipple's disease. *Lancet* 2003;361:239-246.

Pollock S, Lewis PD, Kendall B. Whipple's disease confined to the nervous system. *Journal of Neurology, Neurosurgery, and Psychiatry* 1981;44:1104-1109.

Relman DA, Schmidt TM, MacDermott RD, et al. Identification of the uncultured bacillus of Whipple's disease. *The New England Journal of Medicine* 1992;327:293-301.

240 Progressive Rubella Panencephalitis

■

Progressive rubella panencephalitis represents a late complication of the congenital rubella syndrome, or, less commonly, an otherwise unremarkable case of German measles; it typically presents with a dementia and is a vanishingly rare disease.

ONSET

The onset occurs anywhere from 4 to 19 years after the original infection, and thus most cases occur either in childhood or adolescence.

CLINICAL FEATURES

School failure may be the first evidence of the dementia, which progressively worsens. Ataxia is common, and eventually pyramidal tract signs are seen. Although seizures may occur, myoclonus is generally absent.

The electroencephalogram demonstrates generalized slowing. Rarely, a burst-suppression pattern occurs. CT or MRI scanning reveals ventricular enlargement and cerebral and cerebellar cortical atrophy. The cerebrospinal fluid often shows a moderate lymphocytic pleocytosis, elevated protein, and oligoclonal bands. Serum and CSF antirubella antibody titers are elevated.

As noted, progressive rubella panencephalitis may occur in the setting of the congenital rubella syndrome, which in turn is characterized by a varying combination of mental retardation, microcephaly, deafness, cataracts, and cardiac disease.

COURSE

This is a progressive disorder, with death in about ten years.

COMPLICATIONS

The complications of dementia are as described in that chapter.

ETIOLOGY

Pathologically one sees a widespread perivascular inflammatory response, with neuronal loss and demyelinization. Although measles virus particles may be recovered from the brain, immunoglobulin deposits are also found on vessels and the precise etiology of the disease is unclear.

DIFFERENTIAL DIAGNOSIS

The appearance of new intellectual deterioration in a previously stable patient with the congenital rubella syndrome suggests the diagnosis. In patients without the congenital rubella syndrome, subacute sclerosing panencephalitis is often considered; however, the absence of myoclonus argues against this diagnosis.

TREATMENT

The general treatment of dementia is as outlined in that chapter. No specific treatment is available.

BIBLIOGRAPHY

Coyle PK, Wolinsky JS. Characterization of immune complexes in progressive rubella panencephalitis. *Annals of Neurology* 1981;9: 557-562.

Townsend JJ, Baringer JR, Wolinsky JS, et al. Progressive rubella panencephalitis. Late onset after congenital rubella. *The New England Journal of Medicine* 1975;292:990-993.

Townsend JJ, Wolinsky JS, Baringer JR. The neuropathology of progressive rubella panencephalitis of late onset. *Brain* 1976;99:81-90.

Wolinsky JS, Berg BO, Maitland CJ. Progressive rubella panencephalitis. *Archives of Neurology* 1976;33:722-723.

241 Subacute Measles Encephalitis

■

Subacute measles encephalitis, also known as measles inclusion body encephalitis, is a rare disorder, occurring generally, but not always, in immunocompromised patients who have recently had a case of measles.

ONSET

The onset is subacute, over days or a week or so.

CLINICAL FEATURES

Patients may experience delirium, myoclonus, focal signs and seizures. The seizures may be grand mal or partial, and simple partial status epilepticus has been noted.

The cerebrospinal fluid, although generally normal, may display a mild pleocytosis or a mildly elevated protein; measles antibodies may or may not be present. Brain biopsy may be required for a definitive diagnosis.

COURSE

This illness is rapidly progressive and patients become lethargic and eventually comatose; death occurs within weeks to months.

COMPLICATIONS

The complications of delirium are as described in that chapter.

ETIOLOGY

Subacute measles encephalitis appears to represent a reactivation of the measles virus, and, as noted earlier, is generally seen only in those who are immunocompromised, such as children with leukemia or patients of any age who are taking immunosuppressant drugs. The mechanism underlying those rare cases occurring in immunocompetent patients is not clear. Pathologically, there are intranuclear inclusions within neurons throughout the central nervous system; an inflammatory response is notably absent.

DIFFERENTIAL DIAGNOSIS

There are four disorders wherein measles is associated with an encephalopathy: acute measles encephalitis, post-infectious encephalitis, subacute measles encephalitis and subacute sclerosing panencephalitis. Acute measles encephalitis is distinguished by its appearance concurrent with the measles rash, and a post-measles post-infectious encephalitis by its appearance within days to weeks after resolution of the rash. Subacute measles encephalitis has a longer latency, not occurring until months after the rash has cleared, and subacute sclerosing panencephalitis has the longest latency, with its appearance delayed for years.

TREATMENT

The general treatment of delirium is as described in that chapter. There are case reports of positive responses to intravenous ribavirin.

BIBLIOGRAPHY

Agamanolis DP, Tan JS, Parker DL. Immunosuppressive measles encephalitis in a patient with a renal transplant. *Archives of Neurology* 1979;36: 686-690.

Aicardi J, Goutieres F, Arsenio-Nunes M, et al. Acute measles encephalitis in children with immunosuppression. *Pediatrics* 1977;59:232-235.

Chen RE, Ramsay DA, deVeber LL, et al. Immunosuppressive measles encephalitis. *Pediatric Neurology* 1994;10:325-327.

Croxson MC, Anderson NE, Vaughan AA, et al. Subacute measles encephalitis in an immunocompetent adult. *Journal of Clinical Neuroscience* 2002;9:600-604.

Gazzola P, Cocito L, Capello E, et al. Subacute measles encephalitis in a young man immunocompromised for ankylosing spondylitis. *Neurology* 1999;23:1074-1077.

Lyon G, Ponsot G, Lebon P. Acute measles encephalitis of the delayed type. *Annals of Neurology* 1977;2:322-327.

Wolinsky JS, Swoveland P, Johnson KP, et al. Subacute measles encephalitis complicates Hodgkin's disease in an adult. *Annals of Neurology* 1977;1:452-457.

242 Subacute Sclerosing Panencephalitis

Subacute sclerosing panencephalitis (SSPE), also known as Dawson's disease or subacute inclusion body encephalitis, results from a kind of reactivation of a prior measles infection and presents with dementia, myoclonus, and ataxia. Out of a million cases of measles, anywhere from 5 to 10 subsequent cases of SSPE may occur. The number of cases has decreased significantly since the introduction of the measles vaccination. However, in very rare instances SSPE may follow vaccination itself. Males are affected three to four times more commonly than females, and the disease appears more common in rural areas.

ONSET

Dementia is usually the first symptom, and it appears gradually and insidiously. The average age of onset is probably about 7 years; however, the range is wide, from the age of 2 up to, exceptionally, the early thirties. Most patients will have had measles before the age of 4, and the latency between the measles infection and the onset of SSPE is about 7 or 8 years.

CLINICAL FEATURES

Although the progressive evolution of symptoms may be roughly divided into three stages, overlap is not at all uncommon. In the first stage, the patient may become restless, distractible, and forgetful. Academic performance suffers, and irritability and moodiness may be present. Hallucinations have been noted, and, rarely, the first stage may be characterized by a psychosis with both hallucinations and delusions. The second stage is characterized by progression of dementia and the appearance of myoclonus and ataxia, with, in many, grand mal seizures. Abnormal involuntary movements such as chorea, athetosis, and dystonia are occasionally seen. The third stage is characterized by generalized spastic rigidity, stupor, and eventually coma.

The EEG often shows a characteristic generalized burst-suppression pattern, which may or may not be correlated with the occurrence of myoclonus. CT scanning generally reveals diffuse cortical atrophy, generalized ventricular dilatation, and scattered lucencies in the white matter, which, on MRI scanning, appear as foci of increased signal intensity on T2-weighted scans.

Measles antibody titer is increased both in serum and the cerebrospinal fluid; the increase in the cerebrospinal fluid titer, however, is disproportionately large.

The cerebrospinal fluid may have an elevated total protein, and although generally acellular, occasionally there may be a slightly elevated cell count. The IgG level, however, is greatly increased, and oligoclonal bands are typically present.

COURSE

Although the course is variable, most patients gradually pass through the stages outlined above and die within several years. In some cases, however, death may come within a few months. Conversely, in a small minority of patients, the course may stretch out to as long as 10 years and be marked by partial remissions, which, however, are almost always followed by exacerbations and, eventually, a fatal outcome.

COMPLICATIONS

The complications of dementia are as described in that chapter. The symptoms of the third stage of the disease necessitate vigorous supportive care.

ETIOLOGY

It appears that after the initial measles infection the measles virus becomes dormant, only to reactivate many years later. The measles viruses found in this disease appear defective in that they lack a normal M protein, and, rather than undergoing "budding," depend on cell fusion to spread throughout the nervous system. Pathologically, there is widespread perivascular cuffing with neuronal loss, patchy demyelinization, and gliosis. Intranuclear, and occasionally intracytoplasmic, inclusion bodies are seen, which, by electronmicroscopy, appear similar to the nucleocapsids of the measles virus, and which stain with fluorescent antimeasles antibodies.

DIFFERENTIAL DIAGNOSIS

During the first stage of SSPE the differential includes any dementia that may occur in childhood or teenage years. Both SSPE and progressive rubella panencephalitis share certain features; clinically, however, ataxia is relatively prominent in progressive rubella panencephalitis, whereas the presence of generalized seizures and prominent myoclonus favors SSPE.

In those rare cases wherein the first stage is characterized by a psychosis, early onset schizophrenia may be considered; however, the appearance of second stage symptoms immediately suggests the correct diagnosis.

TREATMENT

Although there are no blinded studies, it appears that the progression of the disease may be halted by a combination of oral isoprinosine and intraventricular interferon; recently similarly promising results have been reported with a combination of oral isoprinosine, subcutaneous interferon and oral lamivudine.

Anticonvulsants may be used for seizures and clonazepam or carbamazepine may suppress the myoclonus. Antipsychotics may be used for restlessness or hallucinations.

Eventually, institutional care is almost always required.

BIBLIOGRAPHY

Anlar B, Saatci I, Kose G, et al. MRI findings in subacute sclerosing panencephalitis. *Neurology* 1996;47:1278-1283.

Anlar B, Yalaz K, Oktem F, et al. Long-term follow-up of patients with subacute sclerosing panencephalitis treated with intraventricular alpha-interferon. *Neurology* 1997;48:526-528.

Aydin OF, Senbil N, Kuyucu N, et al. Combined treatment with subcutaneous interferon-alpha, oral isoprinosine, and lamivudine for subacute sclerosing panencephalitis. *Journal of Child Neurology* 2003;18: 104-108.

Cobb WA, Marshall J, Scaravilli F. Long survival in subacute sclerosing panencephalitis. *Journal of Neurology, Neurosurgery, and Psychiatry* 1984;47:176-183.

Dawson JR. Cellular inclusions in cerebral lesions of epidemic encephalitis. *Archives of Neurology and Psychiatry* 1934;31:685-700.

Donner M, Waltimo O, Poros J, et al. Subacute sclerosing panencephalitis as a cause of chronic dementia and relapsing brain disorder. *Journal of Neurology, Neurosurgery, and Psychiatry* 1972;35:180-185.

Duncalf CM, Kent JNG, Harbord M, et al. Subacute sclerosing panencephalitis presenting as schizophreniform psychosis. *The British Journal of Psychiatry* 1989;155:557-559.

Ozturk A, Gurses C, Bayakn B, et al. Subacute sclerosing panencephalitis: clinical and magnetic resonance imaging evaluation of 36 patients. *Journal of Child Neurology* 2002;17:25-29.

Risk WS, Haddad FS, Chemali R. Substantial spontaneous long-term improvement in subacute sclerosing panencephalitis: six cases from the Middle East and a review of the literature. *Archives of Neurology* 1978;35:495-502.

Singer C, Lange AE, Suchowersky O. Adult-onset subacute sclerosing panencephalitis: case reports and review of the literature. *Movement Disorders* 1997;12:342-353.

243 Infectious Mononucleosis

In anywhere from 0.5 to 5% of cases of infectious mononucleosis, encephalitis or other symptoms of central nervous system involvement may dominate the clinical picture.

ONSET

Mononucleosis is most common among teenagers; symptoms referable to the central nervous system may either follow or at times precede more typical symptoms of mononucleosis.

CLINICAL FEATURES

Typically, mononucleosis presents with malaise, fatigue, and headache. Fever, pharyngitis, and cervical lymphadenopathy typically ensue after several days, and may be joined by hepatomegaly and splenomegaly.

When the central nervous system is involved, the most common manifestation is an aseptic meningitis, with headache and stiff neck. Encephalitis is less common, and generally manifests with delirium; grand mal seizures may also occur, and rarely status epilepticus may be seen. Catatonia may appear, but this is very rare. Other evidence of central nervous system involvement includes ataxia, cranial nerve palsies (involving especially the facial nerve), chorea and transverse myelitis. The peripheral nervous system may also be involved and both mononeuritis multiplex and a Guillain-Barre type syndrome have been reported.

Most cases are marked by an atypical lymphocytosis, and over 90% of cases will have a positive "monospot" test. In cases where the monospot test is negative, but clinical suspicion is high, one should test for the IgM anti-viral capsid (VCA) and anti-early antigen (EA) antibody levels, as these are more sensitive. In cases of central nervous system involvement, PCR analysis of the cerebrospinal fluid may reveal Epstein-Barr viral DNA.

COURSE

Central nervous system involvement generally resolves, as do the more typical symptoms, and most patients recover within a month or so; occasionally, however, the course may be lingering, and fatigue may persist for months.

COMPLICATIONS

Fatigue may at times be debilitating. Complications of delirium are as described in that chapter.

ETIOLOGY

Mononucleosis results from infection by the Epstein-Barr virus and is typically communicated by saliva during kissing. The virus gains entry via the oropharynx, and is transported by lymphocytes to various organs, including the brain.

DIFFERENTIAL DIAGNOSIS

Prominent fatigue may suggest a depressive episode, either of a major depression or bipolar disorder. In mononucleosis, however, one fails to see depressed mood, tearfulness, guilt, and the like.

Consideration may be given to cytomegalovirus infection or to the meningeal picture seen during seroconversion in HIV infection.

Falsely positive VDRL and ANA may at times occur.

TREATMENT

Rest and adequate nutrition are generally sufficient. The general approach to delirium is as described in that chapter. Both acyclovir and corticosteroids have been advocated for encephalitis; however, there is no evidence to support their use.

BIBLIOGRAPHY

Edelstein H, Knight RT. Epstein-Barr virus causing encephalitis in an elderly woman. *Southern Medical Journal* 1989;82:1192-1193.

Ersurum S, Kalavsky SM, Watanakunakorn C. Acute cerebellar ataxia and hearing loss as initial symptoms of infectious mononucleosis. *Archives of Neurology* 1983;40:760-762.

Gautier-Smith PC. Neurological complications of glandular fever (infectious mononucleosis). *Brain* 1965;88:323-334.

Rea TD, Russo JE, Katon W, et al. Prospective study of the natural history of infectious mononucleosis caused by Epstein-Barr virus. *The Journal of the American Board of Family Practice* 2001;14:234-242.

Rubin RL. Adolescent infectious mononucleosis with psychosis. *The Journal of Clinical Psychiatry* 1978;39:773-775.

Russell J, Fisher M, Zivin JA, et al. Status epilepticus and Epstein-Barr virus encephalopathy. Diagnosis by modern serologic techniques. *Archives of Neurology* 1985;42:789-792.

Schlesinger RD, Crelinsten GL. Infectious mononucleosis dominated by neurologic symptoms and signs. *Canadian Medical Association Journal* 1977;117:652-653.

Schnell RG, Dyck PJ, Walter EJ, et al. Infectious mononucleosis: neurologic and EEG findings. *Medicine* 1966;45:51-63.

Silverstein A, Steinberg G, Nathanson M. Nervous system involvement in infectious mononucleosis. *Archives of Neurology* 1972;26:353-358.

244 Mumps Meningoencephalitis

Although the mumps virus invades the central nervous system in over one-half of all cases, clinical evidence of such invasion is seen in only a fraction: roughly 15% of patients will have an aseptic meningitis and less than 1% will have an encephalitis.

Although mumps per se is as likely to occur in males as females, central nervous system involvement is far more common in males.

ONSET

Onset is seen typically in childhood or teenage years, and generally during the winter or spring.

CLINICAL FEATURES

Mumps typically presents with fever, myalgia and malaise, followed, within one to seven days, by a parotitis; males may also develop unilateral or bilateral orchitis.

Meningitis is manifest by headache, drowsiness and a stiff neck, and generally follows the onset of parotitis by from 2 to 20 days; occasionally meningitis may precede the parotitis and, in some cases, meningitis may occur in the absence of parotitis.

Encephalitis presents with a high fever, and either delirium or stupor; seizures, ataxia and focal signs may also occur.

Acute and convalescent sera demonstrate a greater than four-fold rise in IgG and IgM antibodies. In cases of meningitis or encephalitis the CSF typically shows a lymphocytic pleocytosis, mildly elevated total protein, and either a normal glucose or, in about 10% of cases, a reduced glucose level; both the IgM and IgG indices are increased and mumps virus RNA may be detected by PCR assay.

COURSE

Overall, mumps generally runs its course within three to four weeks; meningitis and encephalitis usually resolve within a week or two. Although meningitis typically leaves no sequelae, patients with encephalitis may be left with deafness, seizures, ataxia, dementia, or, rarely, hydrocephalus secondary to aqueductal stenosis.

COMPLICATIONS

The complications of delirium are as described in that chapter.

ETIOLOGY

The invasion by the inherently neurotropic mumps virus leads to diffuse inflammation.

DIFFERENTIAL DIAGNOSIS

A mumps postinfectious encephalomyelitis may be difficult to distinguish from a mumps encephalitis on clinical grounds; MRI scanning in postinfectious cases, however, typically displays the classic white matter abnormalities, changes not seen in mumps encephalitis.

TREATMENT

The general treatment of delirium is as described in that chapter; there is no specific treatment for mumps meningitis or encephalitis.

BIBLIOGRAPHY

Bistrian B, Phillips CA, Kaye IS. Fatal mumps meningoencephalitis. *Journal of the American Medical Association* 1972;322:478-479.

Finklestein H. Meningoencephalitis in mumps. *Journal of the American Medical Association* 1938;111:17-19.

Forsberg P, Fryden A, Link H, et al. Viral IgM and IgG antibody synthesis within the central nervous system in mumps meningitis. *Acta Neurologica Scandinavica* 1986;73:372-380.

Koskiniemi M, Donner M, Pettay O. Clinical appearance and outcome in mumps encephalitis in children. *Acta Paediatrica Scandinavica* 1983;72:603-609.

Levitt LP, Rich RA, Kinde SW, et al. Central nervous system mumps: a review of 64 cases. *Neurology* 1970;20:829-834.

Poggio GP, Rodriguez C, Cisterna D, et al. Nested PCR for rapid detection of mumps virus in cerebrospinal fluid form patients with neurological diseases. *Journal of Clinical Microbiology* 2000;38:274-278.

Russell RR, Donald JC. The neurological complications of mumps. *British Medical Journal* 1958;2:27-30.

245 Arbovirus Encephalitis

Viruses transmitted by arthropods are known as arboviruses, a word derived from <u>ar</u>thropod <u>bo</u>rne. In the contiguous 48 United States there are eight endemic arboviruses known to cause encephalitis, including seven mosquito-borne viruses (eastern equine encephalitis, western equine encephalitis, Venezualan equine encephalitis, California virus encephalitis, St. Louis encephalitis, LaCrosse virus and the newest member, West Nile virus) and one tick-borne virus, Powassan virus. Most cases occur in the Summer months, when the responsible arthropods are active, and epidemics may occur. Japanese encephalitis, although not endemic in the United States, is very common in the Far East, and may be contracted by travelers.

COURSE

The onset is typically acute, with the full illness evolving over a matter of days or just a few hours.

CLINICAL FEATURES

Patients present with a delirium, fever, and, typically, meningeal signs, such as headache, stiff neck, and often photophobia. Seizures and focal signs may or may not be present, and a syndrome of inappropriate ADH secretion may occur. Although distinguishing among the various arbovirus infections on clinical grounds is difficult, St. Louis encephalitis is often marked by prominent tremor, West Nile encephalitis by a motor polyneuropathy with widespread weakness, and Japanese virus by parkinsonism.

The peripheral white blood cell count is typically elevated, often with a left shift.

Enhanced CT or MRI scanning may show focal areas of cerebritis.

The EEG typically shows generalized slowing, but focal changes may be seen.

The cerebrospinal fluid pressure may or may not be increased. Protein is generally elevated, and glucose is normal. The cell count is generally increased; early on, polymorphonuclear cells may predominate; however, over time the pleocytosis becomes lymphocytic. Specific IgM antibodies may be present, and more and more viruses may now be identified by PCR assay for viral RNA.

COURSE

The mortality rate for encephalitis secondary to arboviruses ranges from 1% or less for California virus encephalitis, up to over 50% for eastern equine encephalitis.

For those who survive, the encephalitis tends to run its course within a couple of weeks, sometimes longer. With more severe infections sequelae are not uncommon and may include dementia, personality change, seizures or a persistence of any focal signs seen during the acute illness.

COMPLICATIONS

The complications of delirium are as described in that chapter.

ETIOLOGY

Pathologically there is diffuse perivascular inflammation, which may coalesce into focal areas of cerebritis. Involved arteries may become thrombosed, with infarction of downstream tissues.

DIFFERENTIAL DIAGNOSIS

Bacterial meningoencephalitis is distinguished by a low glucose in the cerebrospinal fluid. Measles virus encephalitis is distinguished by the rash, mumps by parotitis or orchitis, and mononucleosis by cervical lymphadenopathy. Herpes simplex encephalitis is suggested by the absence of meningeal signs and by the finding, on MRI scanning, of medial temporal involvement. Given that herpes simplex virus encephalitis is treatable, this diagnosis should always be strongly considered in any case of viral encephalitis. Postinfectious encephalitis is suggested by a preceding viral infection and, on MRI scanning, prominent white matter involvement.

TREATMENT

Aggressive supportive treatment in an ICU may be required; osmotic agents may be used to lower intracranial pressure, and anticonvulsants may be given preventively.

BIBLIOGRAPHY

Baker AB, Noran HH. Western variety of equine encephalitis in man. *Archives of Neurology and Psychiatry* 1942;47:565-587.
Chaudhuri A, Kennedy PG. Diagnosis and treatment of viral encephalitis. *Postgraduate Medical Journal* 2002;78:575-583.
Klein C, Kimiagar I, Pollak L, et al. Neurological features of West Nile virus infection during the 2000 outbreak in a regional hospital in Israel. *Journal of the Neurological Sciences* 2002;200:63-66.
Lambert AJ, Martin DA, Lanciotti RS. Detection of North American eastern and western equine encephalitis viruses by nucleic acid amplification assays. *Journal of Clinical Microbiology* 2003;41:379-385.
Przelomski MM, O'Rourke E, Grady GF, et al. Eastern equine encephalitis in Massachusetts. *Neurology* 1988;38:736-739.
Smardel JE, Bailey P, Baker AB. Sequelae of the arthropod-borne encephalitides. *Neurology* 1958;8:873-896.
Tiroumourougane SV, Raghava P, Srinivasan S. Japanese viral encephalitis. *Postgraduate Medical Journal* 2002;78:205-215.
Whitley RJ, Gnann JW. Viral encephalitis: familiar infections and emerging pathogens. *Lancet* 2002;359:507-513.

246 Postinfectious and Postvaccinial Encephalomyelitis

Occurring most probably on an autoimmune basis, this disorder, also known as acute disseminated encephalomyelitis, occurs after patients have either recovered from an infection, usually viral, or have received a vaccination. Responsible viral infections include measles, chickenpox, mumps, German measles, infectious mononucleosis, scarlet fever, whooping cough and influenza; other infections associated with this disorder include mycoplasma and typhoid. Vaccinations capable of triggering the disorder include those for measles, chickenpox, mumps, influenza, rabies, typhoid and hepatitis. In some cases, no obvious cause, other than a trivial, "non-specific" viral upper respiratory illness, can be discerned.

ONSET

The latency between the infection or vaccination and the onset ranges from a few days up to three weeks and tends to be somewhat longer after vaccination. The onset itself is quite acute, with symptoms evolving over several hours or a day or so.

CLINICAL FEATURES

The symptomatology of postinfectious and postvaccinial encephalomyelitis reflects which part of the central nervous system bears the brunt of the autoimmune onslaught. Thus, with encephalitis, one sees delirium, meningeal signs, such as headache and stiff neck, seizures and various focal signs, such as hemiparesis. Although any of the cranial nerves may be involved, the optic nerve is most commonly affected, with bilateral visual loss. Cerebellar involvement produces ataxia, and cord involvement presents with a typical transverse myelitis with paraplegia.

The electroencephalogram shows generalized slowing with occasional localized seizure discharges.

CT or MRI scanning may show either large areas of diffuse white matter edema, or scattered areas of localized white matter lesions, as demonstrated in the MRI scan shown in Figure 246-1.

The cerebrospinal fluid generally displays some abnormalities. The opening pressure may be elevated but tends to be normal. Total protein is elevated. Glucose is normal, and often a modest pleocytosis, generally mononuclear, is seen. Myelin basic protein and IgG levels may be elevated, and in some cases oligoclonal bands are present.

In severe cases, which were previously known as acute hemorrhagic leukoencephalitis, a fever and an elevated peripheral white blood cell count may be present. The cerebrospinal fluid opening pressure is generally elevated, as is the total protein level.

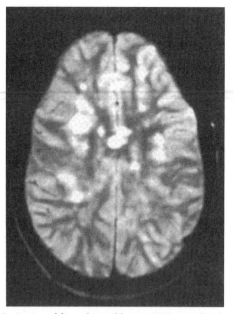

FIG. 246-1. Scattered hyperintensities on MRI scanning in postinfectious encephalitis. (From Yock DH. *Imaging of CNS disease: a CT and MR teaching file*, ed 2, St. Louis, 1991, Mosby.)

The pleocytosis is mixed, containing, in addition to monocytes, both erythrocytes and polymorphonuclear leukocytes.

COURSE

Up to 20% of cases have a fatal outcome; patients who survive tend to recover after a week or two. Although most appear to recover completely, a minority are left with some residual symptoms such as seizures, emotional lability, or dementia.

COMPLICATIONS

The complications of delirium are as described in that chapter.

ETIOLOGY

Widespread perivascular mononuclear inflammation in the white matter is present, most prominently in the centrum semiovale, cerebellum and spinal cord. Demyelinization is prominent, with relative sparing of axons and almost universal sparing of neurons. Meningeal inflammation is typically mild.

In the severe cases of acute hemorrhagic leukoencephalitis, the inflammation tends to be polymorphonuclear, with scattered petechial hemorrhages.

In all likelihood the damage is secondary to an autoimmune response directed at the central nervous system, which was precipitated by the preceding viral infection or vaccination.

DIFFERENTIAL DIAGNOSIS

When the illness occurs after vaccination or resolution of a typical viral illness, the diagnosis is relatively straightforward. In cases where the precipitating illness was so trivial as to have been forgotten, consideration must be given to an arbovirus encephalitis, herpes simplex encephalitis, and multiple sclerosis. The distinction between postinfectious encephalomyelitis and multiple sclerosis may be difficult. Certainly if the patient had had similar episodes in the past, one would favor a diagnosis of multiple sclerosis, given that postinfectious encephalomyelitis is a "monophasic" illness, and does not recur. However, if there were no such history the differential may rest on MRI findings. If the MRI scan, in addition to showing "fresh" white matter lesions, also demonstrated old, "inactive" lesions, this would favor a "multiphasic" illness, such as multiple sclerosis.

TREATMENT

The general treatment of delirium is as described in that chapter. Intravenous methylprednisolone, given via the same protocol as described in the chapter on multiple sclerosis, may at times be dramatically effective. In resistant cases, consideration may be given to intravenous immunoglobulins, plasmapheresis or immunosuppressants.

BIBLIOGRAPHY

Dolgopol VB, Greenberg M, Aronoff R. Encephalitis following smallpox vaccination. *Archives of Neurology and Psychiatry* 1955;73:216-223.

Garg RK. Acute disseminated encephalomyelitis. *Postgraduate Medical Journal* 2003;79:11-17.

Hung KL, Liao HT, Tsai ML. Postinfectious encephalomyelitis: etiologic and diagnostic trends. *Journal of Child Neurology* 2000;15:666-670.

Miller HG, Stanton JB, Gibbons JL. Parainfectious encephalomyelitis and related syndromes. *Quarterly Journal of Medicine* 1956;25:427-505.

O'Riordan JI, Gomez-Anson B, Moseley IF, et al. Long term MRI follow-up of patients with post infectious encephalomyelitis: evidence for a monophasic disease. *Journal of the Neurological Sciences* 1999;167:132-136.

Patel SP, Friedman RS. Neuropsychiatric features of acute disseminated encephalomyelitis: a review. *The Journal of Neuropsychiatry and Clinical Neurosciences* 1997;9:534-540.

Straub J, Chofflon M, Delavelle J. Early high-dose intravenous methylprednisolone in acute disseminated encephalomyelitis: a successful recovery. *Neurology* 1997;49:1145-1147.

247 Herpes Zoster Vasculopathy and Encephalitis

During chickenpox, the varicella-zoster virus infects various sensory ganglia, including the trigeminal ganglion, where it may remain latent for years or decades until, during a period of reduced immunocompetence, it reactivates, and spreads both distally and, in a small minority, proximally. With distal spread, one sees the typical zoster rash, but with proximal spread the central nervous system may be involved. In cases where the ophthalmic division of the trigeminal ganglion is involved, distal spread leads to "zoster ophthalmicus" with a rash in the ophthalmic division of the trigeminal nerve, whereas proximal spread may be followed by a vasculopathy involving the internal carotid artery or its major branches.

Another mechanism whereby the central nervous system may be affected occurs in cases of disseminated herpes zoster, wherein a viremia occurs with hematogenous seeding of the brain and a consequent vasculitis.

ONSET

The reduced immunocompetence that permits the reactivation of the varicella-zoster virus may occur with aging, during certain illnesses, such as cancer or AIDS, or during treatment with corticosteroids or immunosuppressants, and consequently a zoster vasculopathy or encephalitis may occur at any age. Most cases, however, are found in the elderly or in patients with AIDS.

CLINICAL FEATURES

Zoster is ushered in by several days of constitutional symptoms, after which the zosteriform rash appears. Figure 247-1 shows a zoster ophthalmicus, caused by a reactivation within the trigeminal ganglion and distal spread down the ophthalmic division of the trigeminal nerve.

Zoster vasculopathy may be delayed for weeks or months after the appearance of the zoster ophthalmicus. In most cases the internal carotid artery, or one of its branches, is involved and patients

may present with an ischemic infarction ipsilateral to the side where the rash was, with hemiplegia, aphasia, apraxia, or the like.

Zoster encephalitis develops more rapidly, often within days of the onset of the rash, and is characterized by delirium, which may or may not be accompanied by seizures, focal signs or meningismus. In such cases the EEG typically shows generalized slowing, and MRI scanning may reveal areas of increased signal intensity on T2-weighted scans in both the white and gray matter. The cerebrospinal fluid typically shows a lymphocytic pleocytosis with an elevated protein and normal glucose; viral DNA may be demonstrated by PCR assay.

The spinal cord may also be involved during zoster: with centripetal spread of the virus from the dorsal root ganglion to the cord, a more or less extensive myelitis occurs, producing a more or less complete transverse myelitis.

COURSE

In immunocompetent patients the encephalitis usually resolves within weeks, with only rare fatalities; in immunoincompetent patients, however, especially those with AIDS, the encephalitis may be chronic and progressive, and, in a not inconsiderable minority, fatal.

COMPLICATIONS

The complications of delirium are as described in that chapter. In cases of severe encephalitis, patients may be left with a dementia, seizures or various focal deficits.

ETIOLOGY

In cases of zoster vasculopathy, the artery may or may not undergo significant inflammation; in some cases one finds a thrombus with very little in the way of an inflammatory response. In cases of encephalitis, there is a widespread, diffuse vasculitis with surrounding cerebritis.

DIFFERENTIAL DIAGNOSIS

The diagnosis should be suspected whenever a cerebral infarction occurs in a patient with a relatively recent history of zoster ophthalmicus and whenever an encephalitis occurs in close proximity to a disseminated case of herpes zoster.

TREATMENT

The general treatment of delirium is as described in that chapter. Intravenous acyclovir, in a dose of 10 mg/kg tid for two weeks, is indicated for both the vasculopathy and the encephalitis.

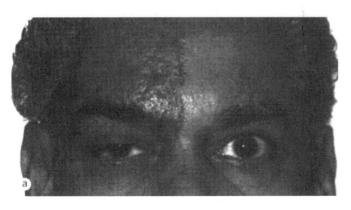

FIG. 247-1. Zoster in the ophthalmic division of the trigeminal nerve. (From Perkin GD, Hochberg FH, Miller DC. *Atlas of clinical neurology*, ed 2, London, 1993, Wolfe.)

BIBLIOGRAPHY

Applebaum E, Krebs SI, Sunshine A. Herpes zoster encephalitis. *The American Journal of Medicine* 1962;32:25-31.

Bourdette DN, Rosenberg NL, Yates FM. Herpes zoster ophthalmicus and delayed ipsilateral cerebral infarction. *Neurology* 1983;33:1428-1432.

Eidelberg D, Sotrel A, Horoupian DS, et al. Thrombotic cerebral vasculopathy associated with herpes zoster. *Annals of Neurology* 1986;19:7-14.

Gilden DH, Murray RS, Wellish M, et al. Chronic progressive varicella-zoster virus encephalitis in an AIDS patient. *Neurology* 1988;38:1150-1153.

Jemsek J, Greenberg SB, Tabor L, et al. Herpes zoster-associated encephalitis: clinicopathologic report of 12 cases and review of the literature. *Medicine* 1983;62:81-97.

MacKenzie RA, Forbes GS, Karnes WE. Angiographic findings in herpes zoster arteritis. *Annals of Neurology* 1981;10:458-464.

Peterslund NA. Herpes zoster associated encephalitis: clinical findings and acyclovir treatment. *Scandinavian Journal of Infectious Diseases* 1988;20:583-592.

Weaver S, Rosenblum MK, DeAngelis LM. Herpes varicella zoster encephalitis in immunocompromised patients. *Neurology* 1999;52:193-195.

248 Herpes Simplex Encephalitis

The encephalitis caused by herpes simplex typically begins in the temporal lobes and generally presents with a delirium.

Herpes simplex encephalitis occurs in a sporadic, nonepidemic fashion. Although, relative to the epidemic encephalitides, it is an uncommon disorder, it remains the most common cause of sporadic encephalitis in North America. It appears to be equally common among males and females.

ONSET

Although herpes simplex encephalitis can occur at any age, most cases occur in middle adult years.

The onset itself is generally subacute, spanning several days: a wide range, however, exists, from explosive onsets over several hours to very gradual ones lasting weeks or months. There may or may not be a flu-like prodrome.

CLINICAL FEATURES

The delirium may be ushered in by a change in the patient's behavior: there may be withdrawal, agitation, or, in some cases, psychosis or hypomania. With progression, however, confusion and disorientation supervene. Headache is common, as is nausea, and over 90% of patients will be febrile. Partial or grand mal seizures are common, and with progression, focal signs, such as hemiplegia or aphasia, may occur. Although a stiff neck may occur, it is not a prominent finding.

A peripheral leukocytosis may occur. The electroencephalogram, although normal early in the course, eventually shows temporal slowing, often accompanied by periodic sharp waves. CT scanning may show radiolucencies in the medial aspect of one or both temporal lobes; however, CT scanning is not sensitive and may remain normal throughout the entire illness. MRI scanning is far more sensitive, and typically shows areas of increased signal intensity in the medial aspect of one or both temporal lobes, as illustrated in Figure 248-1.

The cerebrospinal fluid typically shows an elevated protein with a normal, or occasionally reduced, glucose. Typically there is a polymorphonuclear and lymphocytic pleocytosis, and an increased number of red cells. PCR assay almost always reveals herpes simplex viral DNA.

Brain biopsy, once commonly performed to confirm the diagnosis, is rarely done now, and PCR assay of the CSF has become the "gold standard." In cases where lumbar puncture is not possible, diagnostic reliance may be placed on finding typical inferior or medial temporal lobe involvement on MRI scanning.

COURSE

The disease is fatal in a majority of patients, with progressive deterioration occurring over days or weeks. In rare instances the course may be prolonged for over a month, and even more rarely a relapsing and remitting course is seen. Among those patients who survive, only a minority recover completely: most are left with some permanent deficit.

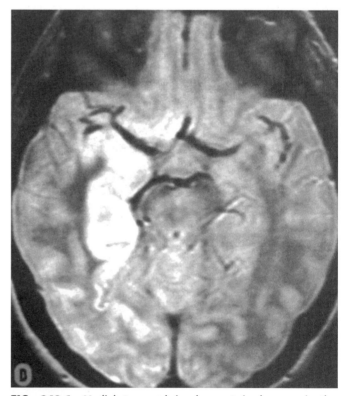

FIG. 248-1. Medial temporal involvement in herpes simplex encephalitis. (From Kuchaczyk W, ed. *MRI central nervous system*, New York, 1990, Gower.)

COMPLICATIONS

The potential deficits seen in those who survive include dementia, Korsakoff's syndrome, personality change, the Kluver-Bucy syndrome, psychosis, epilepsy and persistence of any focal signs seen during the acute illness.

ETIOLOGY

Perhaps 90% of all adults have been infected by herpes simplex type I, and it appears that the encephalitis occurs secondary to a reactivation of this virus. Pathologic material suggests strongly that the virus gains entry from the olfactory mucosa via the olfactory filia to the olfactory nerve, thence spreading to the ipsilateral, and then the contralateral, temporal lobe. Although the vast majority of cases of herpes simplex encephalitis occur secondary to infection by type I, there are documented cases of the type II virus causing an encephalitis.

Hemorrhagic necrosis, often accompanied by a substantial amount of edema, is seen in the temporal lobes, inferior frontal lobes, insula, and cingulate gyrus. Typically, one sees asymmetric involvement of the hemispheres, and uncal and subfalcal herniation are not uncommon. Chronically, in those who survive, one may see atrophy and cystic changes in the affected areas.

DIFFERENTIAL DIAGNOSIS

When the onset is gradual and marked by a psychosis or hypomania, consideration may be given to schizophrenia or bipolar disorder; however, the eventual appearance of fever, delirium, seizures or focal signs will rule these diagnoses out.

Herpes simplex encephalitis may be distinguished from arboviral encephalitis by the paucity of meningeal signs and by the presence, on MRI scanning, of medial temporal lobe involvement early on in the illness.

In instances of encephalitis where a reliable differential cannot be made between herpes simplex and other viral encephalitides, as for example when lumbar puncture is not possible and MRI findings, though suggestive of herpes, are not classic, most clinicians will make a presumptive diagnosis of herpes simplex encephalitis and treat the patient accordingly. Given that herpes simplex encephalitis is treatable, whereas the other viral encephalitides generally are not, and given the benign side-effect profile of anti-herpes treatment, such a course is justifiable.

TREATMENT

The mainstay of treatment is intravenous acyclovir, and this should be commenced as soon as there is a reasonable suspicion of herpes simplex. Should the results of CSF assay, or subsequent clinical events, necessitate a diagnostic revision, then the acyclovir may be stopped. Although most patients are adequately treated by a ten day course, relapses have been noted, and in some cases two or three weeks of treatment may be required.

The general treatment of delirium is as discussed in that chapter; antiepileptic drugs are often required, and steroids may be needed should tentorial or subfalcal herniation threaten.

BIBLIOGRAPHY

Domingues RB, Fink MC, Tsanaclis AM, et al. Diagnosis of herpes simplex encephalitis by magnetic resonance imaging and polymerase chain reaction assay of cerebrospinal fluid. *Journal of the Neurological Sciences* 1998;157:148-153.

Esiri MM. Herpes simplex encephalitis. An immunohistochemical study of the distribution of viral antigen within the brain. *Journal of the Neurological Sciences* 1982;54:209-226.

Fisher CM. Hypomanic symptoms caused by herpes simplex encephalitis. *Neurology* 1996;47:1374-1378.

Greenwood R, Bhalla A, Gordon A, et al. Behavior disturbances during recovery from herpes simplex encephalitis. *Journal of Neurology, Neurosurgery, and Psychiatry* 1983;46:809-817.

Kapur N, Barker S, Burrows EH, et al. Herpes simplex encephalitis: long-term magnetic resonance imaging and neuropsychological profile. *Journal of Neurology, Neurosurgery, and Psychiatry* 1994;57:1334-1342.

Kennedy PGE. A retrospective analysis of forty-six cases of herpes simplex encephalitis seen in Glasgow between 1962 and 1985. *Quarterly Journal of Medicine* 1988;68:533-540.

McGrath N, Anderson NE, Croxson MC, et al. Herpes simplex encephalitis treated with acyclovir: diagnosis and long term outcome. *Journal of Neurology, Neurosurgery, and Psychiatry* 1997;63:321-326.

Oommen KJ, Johnson PC, Ray CG. Herpes simplex type 2 virus encephalitis presenting as psychosis. *The American Journal of Medicine* 1982;73: 445-448.

Whitley RJ, Alford CA, Hirsch MS, et al. Vidarabine versus acyclovir therapy in herpes simplex encephalitis. *The New England Journal of Medicine* 1986;314:144-149.

Wilson LG. Viral encephalopathy mimicking functional psychosis. *The American Journal of Psychiatry* 1976;133:165-170.

Yamada S, Kameyama T, Nagaya S, et al. Relapsing herpes simplex encephalitis: pathological confirmation of viral reactivation. *Journal of Neurology, Neurosurgery, and Psychiatry* 2003;74:262-264.

249 Encephalitis Lethargica

■

Encephalitis lethargica, first described by Dr. Constantin von Economo at a meeting of the Vienna Psychiatric Society in April 1917, swept the world in an epidemic lasting from 1917 to 1928. Although there have been no further epidemics, sporadic cases still occur, and as yet the etiology remains obscure.

ONSET

The encephalitic stage is of acute or subacute onset; subsequent to its resolution, sequelae might appear immediately or after a latent interval lasting anywhere from months to decades.

CLINICAL FEATURES

The encephalitic stage is characterized by fever, headache, varying degrees of external ophthalmoplegia, and lethargy or, classically, sleep reversal. Other symptoms seen during this stage include oculogyric crises, psychosis, catatonia or euphoria. This encephalitic stage had a mortality rate approaching 25%; those who survived tended to recover in a few weeks.

Of those who survived the encephalitic stage, a significant number developed one or more sequelae. The most common was a "post-encephalitic" parkinsonism, which clinically was very similar to the parkinsonism seen in idiopathic Parkinson's disease, with the exception that the patients with post-encephalitic parkinsonism often had other abnormal movements, such as dystonia, blepharospasm, or, most importantly, oculogyric crises, as illustrated in Figure 249-1. Oculogyric crises could also occur in isolation, and it is of special interest that these crises, whether occurring with parkinsonism or in isolation, could also be accompanied by obsessions or compulsions. Some patients were also left with a dementia, and in children a syndrome similar to attention-deficit/hyperactivity disorder was noted. Some patients also developed narcoleptic and cataplectic attacks.

COURSE

For most patients the sequelae ran a chronic course.

COMPLICATIONS

The complications of secondary psychosis, catatonia, and dementia are as described in those chapters.

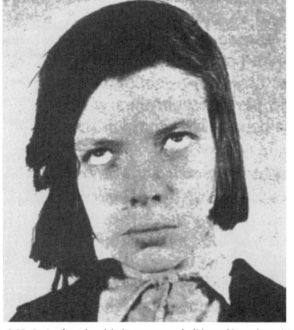

FIG. 249-1. Oculogyric crisis in postencephalitic parkinsonism. (From Roberts GW, Leigh PN, Weinberger DR. *Neuropsychiatric disorders*, Singapore, 1993, Mosby Europe.)

ETIOLOGY

Given that the epidemic of encephalitis lethargica roughly paralleled the Spanish influenza epidemic, it was assumed for many years that encephalitis lethargica represented an infection by the influenza A virus; recent PCR analysis of archival tissue samples, however, failed to disclose any influenzal RNA, and hence the nature of the etiologic agent remains obscure.

Pathologically, during the encephalitic state the mesencephalon bore the brunt of a widespread inflammation of the gray matter. Autopsy studies of those suffering from post-encephalitic parkinsonism have disclosed neuronal loss in the mesencephalic tegmentum, locus ceruleus, dorsal raphe nucleus and substantia nigra, with, in surviving neurons, neurofibrillary tangles similar to those seen in Alzheimer's disease.

DIFFERENTIAL DIAGNOSIS

Diagnosing a sporadic acute encephalitic case of encephalitis lethargica would require a high index of suspicion: the presence of ophthalmoplegia, oculogyric crises, and pronounced sleep reversal in a delirious patient, however, should raise the possibility.

Diagnosing a case of post-encephalitic parkinsonism would also require a high index of suspicion, and here the possibility should be raised by the presence of oculogyric crises, dystonia or blepharospasm.

TREATMENT

Treatment for acute encephalitic cases is supportive. Post-encephalitic parkinsonism responds to levodopa, but patients are prone to develop dyskinesias. Anticholinergics are better tolerated than levodopa, but somewhat less effective; there are no data on the effect of direct-acting dopaminergic agents.

BIBLIOGRAPHY

Buzzard EF, Greenfield JG. Lethargic encephalitis: its sequelae and morbid anatomy. *Brain* 1919;42:305-338.

Dickman MS. von Economo encephalitis. *Archives of Neurology* 2001;58:1696-1698.

Haraguchi T, Ishizu H, Terada S, et al. An autopsy case of postencephalitic parkinsonism of von Economo type: some new observations concerning neurofibrillary tangles and astrocytic tangles. *Neuropathology* 2000;20:143-148.

Howard RS, Lees AJ. Encephalitis lethargica: a report of four recent cases. *Brain* 1987;110:19-33.

Jelliffe SE. Oculogyric crises as compulsion phenomena in postencephalitis: their occurrence, phenomenology and meaning. *The Journal of Nervous and Mental Disease* 1929;69:59-68, 165-184, 278-297, 415-426, 531-551, 666-669.

Kun LN, Yian SY, Haur LS, et al. Bilateral substantia nigra changes on MRI in a patient with encephalitis lethargica. *Neurology* 1999;53:1860-1862.

McCall S, Henry JM, Reid AH, et al. Influenza RNA not detected in archival brain tissues from acute encephalitis lethargica cases or in postencephalitic Parkinson cases. *Journal of Neuropathology and Experimental Neurology* 2001;60:696-704.

Rail D, Scholtz C, Swash M. Postencephalitic parkinsonism: current experience. *Journal of Neurology, Neurosurgery, and Psychiatry* 1981;44:670-676.

von Economo C. *Encephalitis lethargica: its sequelae and treatment*, translated by Newman KO, New York, 1931, Oxford University Press.

Creutzfeldt-Jakob disease, also known as subacute spongiform encephalopathy, is characterized by a rapidly progressive dementia, typically accompanied by myoclonus and other signs of central nervous system disease. In the past Creutzfeldt-Jakob disease was felt to represent a "slow virus" infection; however, the infectious agent, now known as a "prion," is unlike any known virus or bacterium and indeed appears to be unique.

Creutzfeldt-Jakob disease is a very rare disorder, occurring at a rate of less than 5 per 1,000,000 per year. It is equally common among males and females. Eighty-five percent or more of cases occur sporadically, 15% are inherited in an autosomal dominant fashion and the remainder are iatrogenic.

In passing, it may be appropriate to point out that this disease is more properly termed Jakob-Creutzfeldt rather than Creutzfeldt-Jakob. Drs. Creutzfeldt and Jakob, two German psychiatrists, both described cases of rapidly progressive dementia, and although Dr. Creutzfeldt's description appeared first, his patient, in fact, did not have this disease. By contrast, at least two of the patients described a year later by Dr. Jakob probably did have the disease, and consequently the honor is more properly bestowed on him.

ONSET

Sporadic cases usually have an onset in the early sixties, with a wide range, from teenage years to the ninth decade. Familial cases tend to have a slightly earlier onset in the late fifties; in iatrogenic cases the latency from infection to onset ranges from 6 months to 25 years.

In about one third of cases one may see a prodrome of nonspecific symptoms such as fatigue, loss of appetite, and insomnia, all lasting a matter of weeks. The onset itself is typically gradual, spanning weeks or months; however, in a minority of cases an acute onset spanning only days may be seen.

CLINICAL FEATURES

Creutzfeldt-Jakob disease may present with dementia, personality change, psychosis, ataxia or visual symptoms, such as hemianopia or cortical blindness. Eventually, all patients become demented, and over 90% develop myoclonus, which may be stimulus-responsive. Parkinsonism may occur, as may upper and lower motor neuron signs, and a small minority may have seizures.

The electroencephalogram eventually becomes abnormal in about three quarters of cases, exhibiting periodic spike and slow wave complexes.

Routine MRI scanning is generally normal, apart from some cortical atrophy, the progression of which may be documented with serial examinations. Diffusion-weighted scanning, however, may disclose bright areas in the cortex which correspond to areas of spongiform change.

The cerebrospinal fluid is acellular with a normal glucose, but may have a slightly elevated protein. More importantly, in a majority of cases one will find an elevated 14-3-3 protein. This is an especially important test, as it is positive in only a few other conditions, such as paraneoplastic disorders (e.g., limbic encephalitis), herpes simplex encephalitis and acute cerebral infarctions.

Although brain biopsy is required for a definitive diagnosis, this is rarely performed.

COURSE

This disease progresses rapidly. A profound degree of dementia may evolve in as little as a few weeks. Most patients survive no more than 6 months; perhaps 90% are dead within a year.

COMPLICATIONS

Complications are as described in the chapter on dementia.

ETIOLOGY

Microscopically, as illustrated in Figure 250-1, there is a widespread spongiform change in the gray matter which, in turn, is accounted for by grossly swollen and vacuolated dendrites and axons. A modest degree of neuronal loss is seen, and although astrocytosis is widespread there is very little, if any, inflammation.

The responsible agent, known as a "prion," is composed of an abnormal, pathogenic, isoform of the normally occurring prion protein. This normal prion protein is a normal constituent of the neuronal cell membrane, and undergoes recycling from the exterior of the membrane into the cytoplasm where it is digested by lysozymal enzymes. This normal prion protein exists in an alpha helical conformation, and it is a change from this normal conformation to a beta-sheet conformation which transforms the normal prion protein into a pathogenic one. Once in a beta-sheet

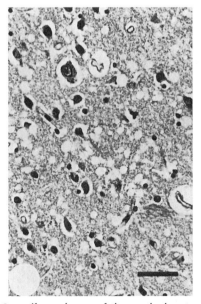

FIG. 250-1. Spongiform change of the cerebral cortex in a case of Creutzfeldt-Jakob disease. (From Vinken PJ, Bruyn GW. *Handbook of clinical neurology*, vol 56 (revised 12), New York, 1989, Elsevier.)

conformation, the pathogenic prion proteins coalesce into a large particle, known as a prion, which, being indigestible by lysozymal enzymes, accumulates within the neuron, eventually leading to the spongiform change. This fateful change in conformation from alpha-helical to beta-sheet may occur secondary to mutations in the gene for the prion protein on chromosome 20 or secondary to iatrogenic introduction of pathogenic prions into the brain, as may occur with corneal transplants, dura mater grafts, use of improperly sterilized neurosurgical instruments and injections of human growth hormone. In these cases of iatrogenic spread, it appears that the introduced pathogenic prion protein serves as a template, facilitating a change to the beta-sheet conformation. The mechanism underlying the far more common sporadic cases is not clear: some believe it represents the end result of a very slowly incubating infection, whereas others suggest it may occur secondary to a somatic mutation occurring with age.

DIFFERENTIAL DIAGNOSIS

Creutzfeldt-Jakob disease must be distinguished from three other "prion" diseases, namely "new-variant" Creutzfeldt-Jakob disease, Gerstmann-Straussler-Scheinker disease and fatal familial insomnia. "New-variant" Creutzfeldt-Jakob disease is an infectious disorder acquired by eating beef products obtained from cows suffering from bovine spongiform encephalopathy; clinically it is similar to Creutzfeldt-Jakob disease but the EEG does not show periodic complexes and the MRI scan may reveal increased signal intensity on T2-weighted scans in the pulvinar. Gerstmann-Straussler-Scheinker disease is an autosomal dominant disorder characterized by dementia and ataxia, and may be distinguished from Creutzfeldt-Jakob disease by a lack of myoclonus and EEG changes. Finally, fatal familial insomnia is also an autosomal dominant disorder and is marked, as the name suggests, by severe and intractable insomnia.

Hashimoto's encephalopathy may be difficult to distinguish on clinical grounds, as it, like Creutzfeldt-Jakob disease, may also be characterized by dementia and myoclonus: testing for antithyroid antibodies, however, will resolve the diagnostic question.

TREATMENT

The general treatment of dementia is as described in that chapter. Specific treatment for Creutzfeldt-Jakob disease is lacking.

Every effort should be made to prevent iatrogenic spread of this disease, and although there is as yet no evidence that casual contact can lead to infection, universal precautions are not unreasonable. Routine sterilization measures with formaldehyde or autoclaving are not effective, and the only way to disinfect instruments is by immersion in a 5% solution of sodium hypochlorite. Given that pins used in neurologic exams may become infectious, they should never be used twice.

BIBLIOGRAPHY

Brown P, Cathala F, Castaigne P, et al. Creutzfeldt-Jakob disease: clinical analysis of a consecutive series of 230 neuropathologically verified cases. *Annals of Neurology* 1986;20:597-602.

Brown P, Gibbs CJ, Rodgers-Johnson P, et al. Human spongiform encephalopathy: the National Institutes of Health series of 300 cases of experimentally transmitted disease. *Annals of Neurology* 1994;35: 513-529.

Brown P, Preece M, Brandel JP, et al. Iatrogenic Creutzfeldt-Jakob disease at the millennium. *Neurology* 2000;55:1075-1081.

Geschwind MD, Martindale J, Miller D, et al. Challenging the clinical utility of the 14-3-3 protein for the diagnosis of sporadic Creutzfeldt-Jakob disease. *Archives of Neurology* 2003;60:813-816.

May WW. Creutzfeldt-Jakob disease. I. Survey of the literature and clinical diagnosis. *Acta Neurologica Scandinavica* 1968;44:1-32.

Mittal S, Farmer P, Kalina P, et al. Correlation of diffusion-weighted magnetic resonance imaging with neuropathology in Creutzfeldt-Jakob disease. *Archives of Neurology* 2002;59:128-134.

Roos R, Cajdusek DC, Gibbs CJ. The clinical characteristics of transmissible Creutzfeldt-Jakob disease. *Brain* 1973;96:1-20.

Siepelt M, Zerr I, Nau R, et al. Hashimoto's encephalitis as a differential diagnosis of Creutzfeldt-Jakob disease. *Journal of Neurology, Neurosurgery, and Psychiatry* 1999;66:172-176.

Spencerf MD, Knight RS, Will RG. First hundred cases of variant Creutzfeldt-Jakob disease: retrospective case note review of early psychiatric and neurological features. *British Medical Journal* 2002; 324:1479-1482.

Will RG, Matthews WB. A retrospective study of Creutzfeldt-Jakob disease in England and Wales 1970-79. I. Clinical features. *Journal of Neurology, Neurosurgery, and Psychiatry* 1984;47:134-140.

251 New Variant Creutzfeldt-Jakob Disease

New variant Creutzfeldt-Jakob disease is a rare, infectious prion disease acquired by eating meat from cows that had bovine spongiform encephalopathy, or "mad cow disease." Of great interest to psychiatry is the fact that this new variant form of Creutzfeldt-Jakob disease typically presents with psychiatric features.

Although most cases have occurred in Great Britain, the disease has now spread to Europe and Asia, and at least one case has occurred in the United States.

ONSET

The onset is subacute and may occur anywhere from adolescence to the fifth decade.

CLINICAL FEATURES

Most patients present with psychiatric symptoms, most commonly depression. Other psychiatric features include withdrawal, agitation, insomnia or emotional lability. With time the majority of patients also develop a psychosis with hallucinations or delusions, which, in a minority, may include Schneiderian first rank symptoms. Within six months, ataxia occurs, followed by dementia and myoclonus.

The EEG does not show the periodic complexes typical of Creutzfeldt-Jakob disease. MRI scanning shows increased signal intensity on T2-weighted scans in the pulvinar in about three-quarters of all cases, and the CSF contains the 14-3-3 protein in about one-half. Tonsilar biopsy demonstrates prion proteins in the majority of cases.

COURSE

The disease is relentlessly progressive with death occurring within one-half to three years; at the end, patients are mute and akinetic, and myoclonus may be prominent.

COMPLICATIONS

The complications of secondary psychosis and of dementia are as noted in that chapter.

ETIOLOGY

As noted earlier, humans become infected by eating meat obtained from cows with bovine spongiform encephalopathy; these cows, in turn, became infected by eating feed made from the offal of sheep which had been affected by the sheep prion disease, scrapie. Of note, at least in humans, it appears that host factors are very important in determining susceptibility to infection, in that all cases of new variant Creutzfeldt-Jakob disease, to date, have occurred in patients who have the normal MM polymorphism at codon 129 of the gene for the normally occurring cellular form of the prion protein.

Pathologically, new variant Creutzfeldt-Jakob disease is quite different from classical Creutzfeldt-Jakob disease in that, in addition to widespread spongiform change, there are also widespread prion-containing plaques.

DIFFERENTIAL DIAGNOSIS

The differential is as discussed for Creutzfeldt-Jakob disease in the preceding chapter.

TREATMENT

This is also as discussed for Creutzfeldt-Jakob disease.

Strenuous efforts are underway to prevent bovine spongiform encephalopathy, and thus protect humans from acquiring new variant Creutzfeldt-Jakob disease. Given the difficulties involved in protecting the food chain, however, continual vigilance is required.

BIBLIOGRAPHY

Allroggen H, Dennis G, Abbott RJ, et al. New variant Creutzfeldt-Jakob disease: three case reports from Leicestershire. *Journal of Neurology, Neurosurgery, and Psychiatry* 2000;68:275-278.

Streichenberger N, Jordan D, Verejan I, et al. The first case of new variant Creutzfeldt-Jakob disease in France: clinical data and neuropathological changes. *Acta Neuropathologica* 2000;99:704-708.

Will RG, Ironside JW, Zeidler M, et al. A new variant Creutzfeldt-Jakob disease in the UK. *Lancet* 1996;347:921-925.

Will RG, Zeidler M, Stewart GE, et al. Diagnosis of new variant Creutzfeldt-Jakob disease. *Annals of Neurology* 2000;47:575-582.

Zeidler M, Stewart GE, Barraclough CR, et al. New variant Creutzfeldt-Jakob disease: neurological features and diagnostic tests. *Lancet* 1997; 350:903-907.

Zeidler M, Johnstone EC, Bamber RW, et al. New variant Creutzfeldt-Jakob disease: psychiatric features. *Lancet* 1997;350:908-910.

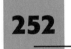 252 AIDS Dementia

Although at autopsy some 90% of patients with AIDS will have some evidence of central nervous system infection by HIV, only about one-half of patients actually develop a dementia. This AIDS dementia, or, as it is also called, AIDS dementia complex or HIV encephalopathy, is an ominous sign, for, as noted below, most patients die within a year of its onset.

The human immunodeficiency virus type I, or HIV-I, attacks a variety of cells, most importantly CD4+ T cells (the "helper" lymphocyte), and monocytes and macrophages. CD4+ T cells are gradually destroyed, and as the absolute CD4+ T cell count falls below 200 and the ratio of CD4+ T cells to CD8+ "suppressor" T cells gradually falls from its normal of 2 down to and below 1, the patient begins to develop some of the common manifestations of AIDS, such as opportunistic infections and Kaposi's sarcoma.

HIV is found in semen, vaginal fluid, breast milk, colostrum, and blood and may be spread by these fluids; transplacental spread may also occur. Although also found in saliva, urine, and tears, these fluids are unlikely to spread the virus. In the United States,

AIDS is most common among homosexual or bisexual men, particularly those who practice anal intercourse. Intravenous drug abusers who share needles and fail to sterilize their "works" constitute the next target group. Currently, in the United States the overwhelming majority of AIDS patients are male; however, as heterosexual spread grows as a common means of transmission, the sex ratio in the United States may eventually approach the 1:1 ratio found in patients in Africa, with a consequent rise in the number of affected infants.

ONSET

The onset of the dementia is typically insidious, occurring on average ten years after the initial infection.

CLINICAL FEATURES

Patients typically complain of apathy, forgetfulness, and trouble concentrating, and exhibit considerable psychomotor retardation;

some may also develop delusions and hallucinations. Ataxia and dysarthria typically appear, and pyramidal tract signs and tremor may also be seen. With progression of disease, the dementia may become quite profound, with confusion, muteness, and double incontinence. Myoclonus may eventually appear, as may seizures.

Both CT and MRI scanning generally demonstrate cortical atrophy and ventricular dilatation. Evidence of bilateral, generally symmetric white matter lesions may be seen on CT scanning but is much better demonstrated on MRI scanning as multiple, often confluent areas of increased signal intensity on T2-weighted images, as shown in Figure 252-1. Most patients also have abnormal cerebrospinal fluid, with any or all of increased protein, a mild mononuclear pleocytosis, an increased IgG index or oligoclonal bands.

The spinal cord and peripheral nerves are also commonly affected in patients with AIDS dementia. Vacuolar myelopathy typically presents with spastic paraparesis. Involvement of the peripheral nerves may present with a sensorimotor polyneuropathy (often with painful paraesthesiae) or a mononeuritis multiplex.

Although typically occurring subsequent to and in the setting of other symptoms of AIDS, this dementia may rarely be the presenting symptom of AIDS. Typically, however, the patient with an AIDS dementia also has one or more of the following: generalized lymphadenopathy, thrush, constitutional symptoms, diarrhea, cytopenia (including thrombocytopenia), Kaposi's sarcoma, shingles and opportunistic infections, such as pneumocystis carinii pneumonia. Of particular importance are those infections and neoplasms that may themselves cause a delirium or dementia, and these are discussed under Differential Diagnosis.

Antibodies to HIV-I appear between 2 and 12 weeks after the initial infection, and these are screened for with an ELISA test. Given that false positive ELISA tests may occur, positive sera are then tested with the more specific Western blot technique.

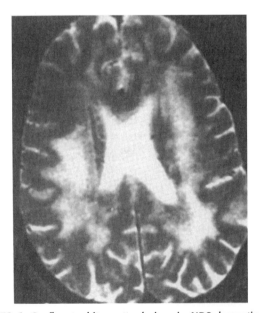

FIG. 252-1. Confluent white matter lesions in AIDS dementia. (From Stark DD, Bradely WG. *Magnetic resonance imaging*, vol 1, ed 2, St. Louis, 1992, Mosby.)

COURSE

Typically the dementia undergoes a relentless progression to a state of profound dementia and death, often within a matter of months or, less commonly, up to a year or more.

COMPLICATIONS

In addition to the complications described in the chapter on dementia, the plight of the AIDS patient is often worsened by social ostracism.

ETIOLOGY

Pathologically, there is widespread myelin pallor, with, in some cases, vacuolization. Macrophages and microglial nodules are widespread, and although there may be some neuronal loss, this is not marked. Of note, although HIV is found in microglia and macrophages, very little, if any, is found in neurons or astrocytes.

Although it is not known for certain, it is suspected that HIV gains entry into the central nervous system by a "Trojan horse" technique, wherein an infected peripheral monocyte passes through the blood-brain barrier and then transforms into a macrophage. Subsequent damage to the white matter appears to be the result of toxins released by infected microglia and macrophages.

DIFFERENTIAL DIAGNOSIS

When the dementia occurs as the presenting symptom of AIDS, the differential diagnosis is wide, as described in the chapter on dementia. Certainly, a dementia occurring in a young or middle-aged person, especially if in a high risk group, should arouse great suspicion.

When a dementia occurs in a patient known to be HIV positive, the most common cause is AIDS dementia; however, other illnesses, listed in the box on p. 425, strongly associated with AIDS, must also be considered. With regard to neurosyphilis it must be kept in mind that in patients with AIDS, treatment of secondary syphilis with benzathine penicillin may not prevent the development of tertiary syphilis. The nature of the association of AIDS and B12 deficiency is not entirely clear; however, it is a strong one, and patients with AIDS should be routinely tested for their B12 level.

AIDS dementia must also be distinguished from delirium that may occur during seroconversion: this mononucleosis-like syndrome occurs in about one-half of all patients, and typically remits spontaneously within one or two weeks. Other, not uncommon causes of delirium in AIDS include diarrhea-induced electrolyte disturbance, hypoxia secondary to pneumocystis pneumonia, intracerebral hemorrhage due to thrombocytopenia or cerebral infarction occurring secondary to herpes zoster arteritis or to emboli from a nonbacterial endocarditis.

TREATMENT

Antiretroviral treatment slows the progression of the dementia, and in some cases may be followed by significant, albeit temporary, initial clinical improvement. Given that treatment recommendations for AIDS change frequently, referral to a specialist is appropriate in all cases. Seizures may be treated with phenytoin.

The general treatment of dementia is described in that chapter. If antipsychotics are required, dose titration should be cautious,

Causes of Dementia in HIV Positive Patients

Neurosyphilis*	Mycoses*
Tuberculosis*	Toxoplasmosis*
Herpes simplex encephalitis*	Zoster vasculopathy or encephalitis*
Progressive multifocal leukoencephalopathy*	Non-Hodgkin's lymphoma (either primary or secondary)
Cytomegalovirus encephalopathy*	Kaposi's sarcoma (rare)

*See the respective chapter.

as these patients are particularly likely to develop extrapyramidal side effects. There is some evidence that selegiline, 10 mg daily, may improve memory in patients with AIDS dementia.

All patients must be counseled regarding "safe sex" including using latex condoms and nonoxynol-9 spermicide. Patients should also be informed that oral sex (including both fellatio and cunnilingus) has, albeit rarely, transmitted the virus. Addicts should be instructed to always sterilize their "works" with undiluted household bleach.

All patients must be prohibited from donating blood or any organ; breast-feeding should also be prohibited.

Vitamin B_{12} deficiency, if present, should be treated as outlined in that chapter.

BIBLIOGRAPHY

Arendt G, Hefter H, Figge C, et al. Two cases of cerebral toxoplasmosis in AIDS patients mimicking HIV-related dementia. *Journal of Neurology* 1991;238:439-442.

Bouwman FH, Skolasky RL, Hes D, et al. Variable progression of HIV-associated dementia. *Neurology* 1998;50:1814-1820.

Dana Consortium on the Therapy of HIV Dementia and Related Cognitive Disorders. A randomized, double-blind, placebo-controlled trial of deprenyl and thioctic acid in human immunodeficiency virus-associated cognitive impairment. *Neurology* 1998;50:645-651.

Dunlop O, Bjorklund B, Bruun JN, et al. Early psychomotor slowing predicts the development of HIV dementia and autopsy-verified HIV encephalitis. *Acta Neurologica Scandinavica* 2002;105:270-275.

Glass JD, Wesselingh SL, Seines OA, et al. Clinical-neuropathologic correlation in HIV-associated dementia. *Neurology* 1993;43:2230-2237.

Herzlich BC, Schiano TD. Reversal of apparent AIDS dementia complex following treatment with vitamin B12. *Journal of Internal Medicine* 1993;233:495-497.

Hriso E, Kuhn T, Masdeu JC, et al. Extrapyramidal symptoms due to dopamine-blocking agents in patients with AIDS encephalopathy. *The American Journal of Psychiatry* 1991;148:1558-1561.

Lang W, Miklossy J, Deruaz JP, et al. Neuropathology of the acquired immune deficiency syndrome (AIDS): a report of one hundred and thirty-five consecutive autopsy cases from Switzerland. *Acta Neuropathologica* 1989;77:379-390.

Maher J, Choudhri S, Halliday W, et al. AIDS dementia complex with generalized myoclonus. *Movement Disorders* 1997;12:593-597.

Navia BA, Jordon BD, Price RW. The AIDS dementia complex: I. Clinical features. *Annals of Neurology* 1986;19:517-524.

Navia BA, Cho ES, Petito CK, et al. The AIDS dementia complex: II. Neuropathology. *Annals of Neurology* 1986;19:525-535.

Zunt JR, Tu RK, Anderson DM, et al. Progressive multifocal leukoencephalopathy presenting as human immunodeficiency virus type 1 (HIV)-associated dementia. *Neurology* 1997;49:263-265.

253   Progressive Multifocal Leukoencephalopathy

Progressive multifocal leukoencephalopathy is an opportunistic infection of the central nervous system by the JC virus. Multifocal areas of demyelinization occur, producing various focal signs and, in many, eventually a dementia. In almost all cases, the patient has a condition that depressed cell-mediated immunity, most commonly AIDS, wherein progressive multifocal leukoencephalopathy is seen in from 1 to 5% of patients.

ONSET

The age of onset is determined by the age of onset of the condition responsible for the decreased cell-mediated immunity; the mode of onset is subacute, over weeks, but more rapid onsets may be seen, especially in those with AIDS.

CLINICAL FEATURES

In most cases the presentation is with a progressively worsening focal deficit, such as hemianopia, aphasia, apraxia, hemisensory loss or hemiplegia. With time, these initially unilateral deficits become bilateral, and many patients will also develop a personality change, dementia, or, rarely, a delirium. Cerebellar signs may occur, but are not common, and seizures of various types may be seen in a minority.

Diffuse or focal slowing may be seen on the electroencephalogram.

CT scanning may demonstrate nonenhancing lucencies in the white matter. MRI scanning is more sensitive, demonstrating multiple areas in the centrum semiovale of increased signal intensity on T2-weighted scans, with the same areas showing decreased signal intensity on T1-weighted scans, as illustrated in Figure 253-1. Although enhancement generally does not occur, in a minority there may be a faint degree of enhancement along the periphery of the lesions.

The cerebrospinal fluid is characteristically normal; occasionally, however, a mild elevation in total protein and, occasionally, a mild lymphocytic pleocytosis are seen. PCR assay for the JC virus, though very specific, may be falsely negative. In doubtful cases, a brain biopsy is required.

In almost all cases, patients with progressive multifocal leukoencephalopathy are immunocompromised, often by AIDS, Hodgkin's disease, other lymphomas, leukemia, and other cancers.

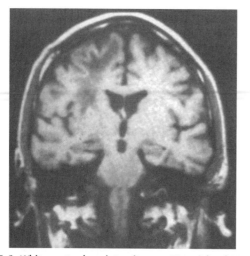

FIG. 253-1. White matter hypointensity on a T1-weighted MRI scan in progressive multifocal leukoencephalopathy. (From Yock DH. *Imaging of CNS disease: a CT and MR teaching file*, ed 2, St. Louis, 1991, Mosby.)

It has also been noted in association with tuberculosis and sarcoidosis and in patients undergoing therapeutic immunosuppression after transplantation.

COURSE

In most cases symptoms progress relentlessly, with death occurring on average within four to six months of onset. Rarely the course may stretch out for years, and even more rarely there may be spontaneous remissions.

COMPLICATIONS

Complications are as described in the chapters on personality change, dementia and delirium.

ETIOLOGY

More than 80% of the adult population of the United States has latent infection with the JC virus. In a very small minority of patients with depressed cell-mediated immunity, this infection is reactivated and the JC virus spreads to the central nervous system where it replicates in oligodendrocytes and, to a much lesser degree, astrocytes.

Oligodendrocytes are lost, and with this loss demyelination occurs, with only relative sparing of the axon itself. The multiple foci of demyelination in the white matter are generally, at least initially, asymmetrically distributed. With time, however, both hemispheres are involved, and lesions become confluent and at times cystic. Involvement of the white matter of the cerebellum, brain stem, or cord is much less common. Although generally absent, at times a mild inflammatory response may be evident.

DIFFERENTIAL DIAGNOSIS

In considering the diagnosis of progressive multifocal leukoencephalopathy in an immunocompromised patient, other opportunistic infections must be considered, such as cytomegalovirus infection and toxoplasmosis. In patients with AIDS, an AIDS dementia must also be considered.

TREATMENT

The general treatment of dementia is as described in that chapter. No specific treatment for progressive multifocal leukoencephalopathy itself is available; however, in the case of AIDS it is clear that highly active antiretroviral treatment with three or more agents prolongs survival.

BIBLIOGRAPHY

Astrom KE, Mancall EL, Richardson EP. Progressive multifocal leukoencephalopathy: a hitherto unrecognized complication of chronic lymphatic leukaemia and Hodgkin's disease. *Brain* 1958;81:93-111.

Clifford DB, Yiannoutsos C, Glicksman M, et al. HAART improves prognosis in HIV-associated progressive multifocal leukoencephalopathy. *Neurology* 1999;52:623-625.

Davies JA, Hughes JT, Oppenheimer DR. Richardson's disease (progressive multifocal leukoencephalopathy). *Quarterly Journal of Medicine* 1973;42:481-493.

Krupp LB, Lipton RB, Swerdlow ML, et al. Progressive multifocal leukoencephalopathy: clinical and demographic features. *Annals of Neurology* 1985;17:344-349.

Moulignier A, Mikol J, Pialoux G, et al. AIDS-associated progressive multifocal leukoencephalopathy revealed by new-onset seizures. *The American Journal of Medicine* 1995;99:64-68.

Richardson EP. Progressive multifocal leukoencephalopathy. *The New England Journal of Medicine* 1961;265:815-823.

von Giesen HJ, Neuen-Jacob E, Dorries K, et al. Diagnostic criteria and clinical procedures in HIV-1 association progressive multifocal leukoencephalopathy. *Journal of the Neurological Sciences* 1997; 147: 63-72.

Zunt JR, Tu RK, Anderson DM, et al. Progressive multifocal leukoencephalopathy presenting as human immunodeficiency virus type 1 (HIV)-associated dementia. *Neurology* 1997;49:263-265.

The majority of adults, and almost all patients with AIDS, show evidence of past infection with cytomegalovirus (CMV). In conditions of decreased cellular immunity, as for example after solid organ transplants and in AIDS when the CD4+ count falls to below 50 to 100 cells, the virus may reactivate and then produce, in a minority of these patients, an encephalitis. Although about one-third of patients dying of AIDS have autopsy evidence of CMV encephalitis, it is not clear what percentage of these had symptoms related to this.

ONSET

The onset of symptoms is subacute, generally over weeks.

CLINICAL FEATURES

Most patients present with a delirium, which may be accompanied by headache, apathy and hyperreflexia. In a minority of cases, the encephalitis extends to the brainstem and such patients may demonstrate ataxia, nystagmus and various cranial nerve palsies. Patients may also develop myelitis and a polyradiculopathy.

MRI scanning typically reveals increased signal intensity on T2-weighted scans in a periventricular distribution, as illustrated in Figure 254-1. Occasionally, there may be a faint degree of meningeal enhancement. In some cases, serial scans may demonstrate progressive ventricular enlargement.

Given the high rate of infection with cytomegalovirus, serologic testing is typically not helpful. The CSF may be normal or may show elevated protein and a pleocytosis, and CMV DNA may be demonstrated by PCR assay.

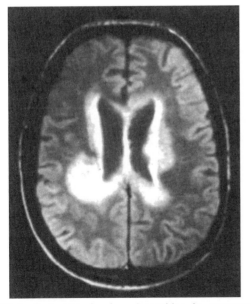

FIG. 254-1. Periventricular hyperintensities in cytomegalovirus encephalopathy. (From Yock DH. *Imaging of CNS disease: a CT and MR teaching file*, ed 2, St. Louis, 1991, Mosby.)

Cytomegalovirus infection in the immunocompromised host is not limited to the central nervous system, and the retina, esophagus, stomach, colon, liver and, most especially, the adrenal glands are typically involved.

COURSE

In patients with AIDS a CMV encephalitis carries a grave prognosis, with most patients dying within several months.

COMPLICATIONS

Complications are as described in the chapter on delirium.

ETIOLOGY

At autopsy, pronounced periventricular inflammation is present, along with scattered microglial nodules throughout the cerebrum, but most especially in the basal ganglia.

DIFFERENTIAL DIAGNOSIS

Consideration must be given to other opportunistic infections, such as progressive multifocal leukoencephalopathy, and to AIDS dementia. In cases where the encephalitis extends to the brainstem the combination of delirium, ataxia, nystagmus and ophthalmoplegia may suggest a Wernicke's encephalopathy.

TREATMENT

The treatment of the underlying cause of the immunosuppression is the primary goal. Although ganciclovir is useful for cytomegalovirus retinitis and colitis, it may not prevent the development of cytomegalovirus encephalopathy.

BIBLIOGRAPHY

Arribas JR, Storch GA, Clifford DB, et al. Cytomegalovirus encephalitis. *Annals of Internal Medicine* 1996;125:577-587.

Berman SM, Kim RC. The development of cytomegalovirus encephalitis in AIDS patients receiving ganciclovir. *The American Journal of Medicine* 1994;96:415-419.

Holland NR, Power C, Mathews VP, et al. Cytomegalovirus encephalitis in acquired immunodeficiency syndrome (AIDS). *Neurology* 1994;44: 507-514.

Torgovnik J, Arsura EL, Lala D. Cytomegalovirus ventriculoencephalitis presenting as a Wernicke's encephalopathy-like syndrome. *Neurology* 2000;55:1910-1913.

Fungal, or mycotic, infection of the central nervous system generally occurs only in the debilitated or immunocompromised host, such as in patients with AIDS, and includes candidiasis, histoplasmosis, cryptococcosis, coccidioidomycosis and aspergillosis: in patients with AIDS, candidiasis is the most common mycosis, while aspergillosis is relatively uncommon. Other, far less common, mycoses include mucormycosis, nocardiosis and blastomycosis. Generally the primary site of infection is in the respiratory tract, often the lung, and this may represent either a recent infection or reactivation of a dormant one. In either case hematogenous spread from the primary site carries the fungus to the central nervous system.

ONSET

Typically the onset is subacute.

CLINICAL FEATURES

Pathologically, there may be either multiple, scattered abscesses and granulomas, or a basilar meningitis or both. In candidiasis abscesses and granulomas predominate, whereas in histoplasmosis, cryptococcosis and coccidioidomycosis the clinical picture is often determined by a basilar meningitis; in aspergillosis abscesses and granulomas are dominant, but here one also sees evidence of mycotic aneurysms.

Abscesses and granulomas may present as mass lesions, with focal signs determined by the location of the mass.

The basilar meningitis typically presents with headache, delirium, and cranial nerve palsies; obstructive hydrocephalus may occur with a dramatic worsening of the clinical condition, and arterial involvement may lead to cerebral infarction.

CT or, more especially, MRI scanning will reveal abscesses and granulomas or the basilar meningitis. Figure 255-1 shows a

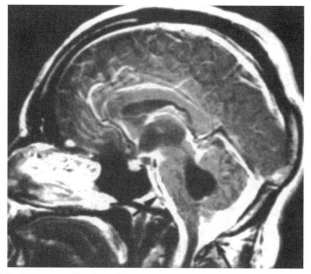

FIG. 255-1. Basilar fungal meningitis. (From Osborn AG. *Diagnostic neuroradiology,* St. Louis, 1994, Mosby.)

T1-weighted MRI scan with enhancement in a patient with coccidioidal fungal meningitis, demonstrating striking enhancement of the basilar meninges.

The CSF is generally abnormal; however, in cases where there are only abscesses or granulomas with no accompanying basilar meningitis, the CSF may be normal. When abnormal, the protein is generally increased, and the glucose may be normal or reduced. A pleocytosis is generally present and may be lymphocytic, polymorphonuclear, or mixed. In the case of cryptococcosis, the "India Ink Prep" is positive in over one-half of cases. Antigen assays may reveal evidence of cryptococcosis and coccidioidomycosis.

COURSE

Fungal meningitis tends to be progressive with a fatal outcome in from a month to a year.

COMPLICATIONS

Complications are as described in the chapter on delirium.

ETIOLOGY

Abscesses and granulomas may be single or multiple. In the case of a basilar meningitis, there is a thick exudate at the base of the brain; cranial nerves may be entrapped, and the exit foramina of the fourth ventricle may be obstructed. Vascular involvement of vessels traversing the meninges may lead to thrombosis and infarction.

DIFFERENTIAL DIAGNOSIS

In the immunocompromised host, this includes toxoplasmosis and tuberculosis. Sarcoidosis may also be considered.

TREATMENT

The general treatment of delirium is as described in that chapter. Initial treatment is usually with amphotericin B; other agents may be used in combination with the amphotericin B or as maintenance treatment.

BIBLIOGRAPHY

Davis LE. Fungal infections of the central nervous system. *Neurologic Clinics* 1999;17:761-781.

Gottfredsson M, Perfect JR. Fungal meningitis. *Seminars in Neurology* 2000;20:307-322.

Mori T, Ebe T. Analysis of central nervous system fungal infections reported in Japan between January 1979 and June 1989. *Internal Medicine* 1992;31:174-179.

Walsh TJ, Hier DB, Caplan LR. Aspergillosis of the central nervous system: clinicopathological analysis of 17 patients. *Annals of Neurology* 1985;18:574-582.

Walsh TJ, Hier DB, Caplan LR. Fungal infections of the central nervous system: comparative analysis of risk factors and clinical signs in 57 patients. *Neurology* 1985;35:1654-1657.

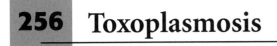

Infection by *Toxoplasma gondii* is common among birds and mammals. The cat serves as the definitive host, and oocysts excreted in cat feces may remain viable for up to a year in suitably warm and moist soil.

Human infection occurs secondary to ingesting contaminated soil or material from cat litter boxes, eating fruits or vegetables from which contaminated soil has not been washed, or eating improperly cooked meat from infected animals, such as lamb, pork, or, less commonly, beef. Infection with toxoplasma is common; over 20% of American adults display serologic evidence of past infection.

In the immunocompetent host, infection may be asymptomatic or cause a self-limited mononucleosis-like illness characterized by malaise, fever, lymphadenopathy (which tends to be cervical), and lymphocytosis. In the immunocompromised host the central nervous system is often infected, producing a variety of symptoms, including delirium. Toxoplasmosis is perhaps the most common cause of brain abscesses in patients with AIDS and is generally seen only when the CD4+ cell count falls below 200.

ONSET

The age of onset varies with the age at which immunoincompetence occurs; the mode of onset is generally subacute, over weeks.

CLINICAL FEATURES

Typically patients present with headache, fever, focal signs (such as hemianopia, hemiplegia, aphasia or abnormal movements) and delirium; seizures may occur in a minority.

CT scanning typically displays one or more ring-enhancing lesions; MRI scanning, however, is more sensitive, and may demonstrate abscesses not seen with CT.

The CSF may be normal or may display increased protein and a mild lymphoctyic pleocytosis. PCR assay is generally positive for toxoplasma DNA, and occasionally staining of the cerebrospinal fluid sediment with Wright's or Giesma's stain may reveal the organism.

Serologic studies may or may not be helpful. As noted earlier, antitoxoplasma antibodies are not uncommonly found in the general population, and in the immunocompromised host a toxoplasma infection may not provoke the classic fourfold rise in antibody titers.

Most patients will have evidence of toxoplasmal infection of other organs, such as the eye, lung or heart.

COURSE

Untreated, cerebral toxoplasmosis is generally fatal within months.

COMPLICATIONS

Complications are as described in the chapter on delirium.

ETIOLOGY

In the immunocompromised patient, toxoplasmosis may result from either a de novo infection or, more commonly, from a reactivation of some encysted toxoplasma that had lain latent since an infection earlier in the patient's life. Hematogenous seeding brings the organism to the brain, where abscess formation occurs.

In some cases, only a few large abscesses form, and these tend to occur near the junction of the cerebral cortex and the white matter or deep within the basal ganglia.

In other cases, large numbers of miliary abscesses or microscopic foci of cerebritis are scattered widely throughout the cerebrum, leptomeninges, and ependyma. Hydrocephalus may occur when aqueductal ependymitis occurs, and hypothalamic or anterior pituitary function may likewise be compromised by abscess formation.

DIFFERENTIAL DIAGNOSIS

Toxoplasmosis may be mimicked or may coexist with other opportunistic infections in the patient with AIDS, such as fungal infections, tuberculosis, and progressive multifocal leukoencephalopathy. Cerebral lymphoma may also mimic toxoplasmosis when there is a solitary lesion on neuroimaging: in such cases SPECT scanning may aid in the differential. In practice, a "diagnosis by treatment response" is often attempted in patients with suggestive clinical and MRI findings. A response within two weeks confirms the diagnosis, whereas a lack of response should prompt consideration of a brain biopsy.

TREATMENT

A combination of pyrimethamine with sulfadiazine inhibits replication of toxoplasma and leads to clinical improvement typically within about 2 weeks. The organism, however, is not eradicated, and in the immunocompromised patient chronic thrice weekly treatment is often required to prevent relapse. The general treatment of delirium is as described in that chapter.

BIBLIOGRAPHY

Arendt G, Hefter H, Figge C, et al. Two cases of cerebral toxoplasmosis in AIDS patients mimicking HIV-related dementia. *Journal of Neurology* 1991;238:439-442.

Gray F, Gherardi R, Wingate E, et al. Diffuse "encephalitic" cerebral toxoplasmosis in AIDS. Report of four cases. *Journal of Neurology* 1989;236:273-277.

Maggi P, de Mari M, De Blasi R, et al. Choreathetosis in acquired immune deficiency syndrome patients with cerebral toxoplasmosis. *Movement Disorders* 1996;11:434-436.

Navia BA, Petito CK, Gold JWM, et al. Cerebral toxoplasmosis complicating the acquired immune deficiency syndrome: clinical and neuropathological findings in 27 patients. *Annals of Neurology* 1986;19:224-238.

Porter SB, Sande MA. Toxoplasmosis of the central nervous system in the acquired immunodeficiency syndrome. *The New England Journal of Medicine* 1992;327:1643-1648.

257 Hyperglycemia

Hyperglycemia of sufficient degree to cause delirium is generally found only in one of two conditions: diabetic ketoacidosis, occurring generally as a complication of type I insulin-dependent diabetes mellitus; and the hyperglycemic hyperosmolar nonketotic syndrome occurring generally as a complication of type II non-insulin dependent diabetes mellitus.

Diabetic ketoacidosis is generally seen in the patient who fails to take insulin or whose insulin requirements, elevated by some intercurrent illness or stress, far outstrip the present dosage. The hyperglycemic hyperosmolar nonketotic syndrome, on the other hand, is usually seen in the elderly or debilitated patient with non-insulin dependent diabetes mellitus who becomes dehydrated in the course of an intercurrent illness.

ONSET

Polyuria precedes both disorders, often by a few days for diabetic ketoacidosis and for a week or more for the hyperglycemic hyperosmolar nonketotic syndrome.

CLINICAL FEATURES

In diabetic ketoacidosis the patient may experience drowsiness and delirium and at times may slip into a coma. Thirst is severe, and almost all patients have nausea, vomiting or abdominal pain, which may be severe. Kussmaul breathing is generally present, and there is typically an odor of acetone on the breath. Blood sugar is typically in the range of 300 to 700 mg/100 dL, the osmolality from 310 to 320 mOsm/L, and the BUN is only slightly elevated. Ketonemia and ketonuria are present.

In the hyperglycemic hyperosmolar nonketotic syndrome, delirium and coma may likewise occur. In addition, focal findings, such as hemiplegia or hemichorea, may occur, and perhaps a quarter of patients may have seizures, which are generally of the motor or sensory simple partial type. Abdominal complaints, Kussmaul breathing and acetone on the breath are generally absent. Clinical signs of dehydration may be severe. Blood sugar is higher, typically in the range of 600 to over 2000 mg/100 dL, the osmolality is likewise higher, often over 360 mOsm/L, and the BUN is often 80 mg/dL or above. Ketonemia and ketonuria are generally not present.

COURSE

Both disorders may be acutely life threatening. Those who survive generally recover completely.

COMPLICATIONS

Complications of delirium are as described in that chapter.

ETIOLOGY

In both disorders the mental status changes result primarily from neuronal and glial dehydration secondary to osmotic shifts of fluid from the intracellular space to the hyperosmolar extracellular space.

In the hyperglycemic, hyperosmolar, nonketotic syndrome the preexisting diabetes mellitus may be quite mild and may in fact have escaped diagnosis. In the elderly or debilitated patient, however, an intercurrent illness such as pneumonia, myocardial infarction, or stroke may cause an increase in glucose level and, by impairing the patient's ability to care for himself, cause the patient to drink less, thus leading to dehydration. Thus dehydrated, renal glucose clearance falls, and blood glucose levels rise even further.

TREATMENT

Insulin and fluid replacement form the cornerstones of treatment for both disorders. Given their lethality, hospitalization is required, often in an intensive care unit where meticulous attention to fluid and electrolyte balance may be achieved.

BIBLIOGRAPHY

Asplund K, Eriksson S, Hagg F, et al. Hyperosmolar non-ketotic coma in diabetic stroke patients. *Acta Medical Scandinavica* 1982;212:407-411.

Chiasson JL, Aris-Jilwan N, Belanger R, et al. Diagnosis and treatment of diabetic ketoacidosis and the hyperglycemic hyperosmolar state. *Canadian Medical Association Journal* 2003;168:859-866.

Delaney MF, Zisman A, Kettyle WM. Diabetic ketoacidosis and hyperglycemic hyperosmolar nonketotic syndrome. *Endocrinology and Metabolism Clinics of North America* 2000;29:683-705.

Gomez Diaz RA, Rivera Moscoso R, Ramos Rodriguez R, et al. Diabetic ketoacidosis in adults: clinical and laboratory features. *Archives of Medical Research* 1996;27:177-181.

Gonzalez-Campoy JM, Robertson RP. Diabetic ketoacidosis and hyperosmolar nonketotic state: gaining control over extreme hyperglycemic complications. *Postgraduate Medicine* 1996;99:143-152.

Khardori R, Soler NG. Hyperosmolar hyperglycemic nonketotic syndrome. Report of 22 cases and brief review. *The American Journal of Medicine* 1984;77:899-904.

Hypoglycemia may be followed by one or both of the following: autonomic symptoms, such as tremor (which occurs secondary to hyperepinephrinemia), or neuroglycopenic symptoms, such as confusion (which occurs as the central nervous system's stores of glucose are depleted). The latency between the occurrence of hypoglycemia and the onset of autonomic symptoms tends to be very brief. By contrast, cerebral stores of glucose are generally capable of sustaining cerebral activity for 30 minutes or more. Consequently, a longer latency exists between the development of hypoglycemia and the development of neuroglycopenic symptoms. Repeated episodes of severe prolonged hypoglycemia may eventually lead to a dementia.

From a clinical point of view, it is useful to distinguish between postprandial hypoglycemia, on the one hand, and fasting (or "postabsorptive") hypoglycemia, on the other. Postprandial hypoglycemia tends to occur within hours of food intake and is usually associated with autonomic symptoms, with few, if any, cerebral ones. A common example is found in the early stages of type II non-insulin dependent diabetes mellitus, when insulin secretion is prolonged past the point where most of the food has been absorbed. By contrast, fasting hypoglycemia, as the name implies, is typically seen in the "fasting" state, often in the early morning hours, or just before breakfast. Important examples include excessive dosage of insulin or the presence of an insulinoma. Here the autonomic symptoms are mild and may be absent; the cerebral ones, by contrast, are prominent.

ONSET

The onset is determined by the underlying etiology.

CLINICAL FEATURES

In general, symptoms are likely to occur when the glucose level drops below 50 mg/dL. This is not invariable, however, and some patients may have levels lower than this and not have symptoms.

Autonomic symptoms tend to come on fairly abruptly and consist of anxiety, palpitations, tremulousness, diaphoresis, and pallor. Often the patient also complains of hunger or nausea, generalized weakness, and headache. Beta-blockers may prevent autonomic symptoms, except diaphoresis, and anticholinergics may prevent this. Hence patients on these medicines may not display the typical autonomic picture.

Neuroglycopenic symptoms tend to be of more gradual onset. Some patients complain of easy fatigability or a sense of lightheadedness and depersonalization may occur. Some patients develop a delirium, which may be characterized by bizarre behavior and delusions of persecution.

Other neuroglycopenic symptoms include headache, blurry vision, and diplopia and seizures, which may be either partial or grand mal. Rarely, in cases where localized cerebral perfusion is compromised (e.g., in cerebral arteriosclerosis), the addition of hypoglycemia may be enough to produce transient localizing signs, such as aphasia or hemiplegia. Eventually, if the blood glucose continues to fall, a coma will occur.

If possible, blood should be drawn while the patient is symptomatic and tested for the following: glucose level, insulin level, and, if there is any suspicion of factitious disease or malingering, C peptide and oral antidiabetic drug levels. In cases of insulinoma, the insulin level is inappropriately high relative to the reduced glucose level, and the level of C peptide, which is derived from endogenous insulin, is also high. In cases of excessive exogenous insulin administration, however, the C peptide level is low, reflecting the exogenous source of the insulin. Oral antidiabetic agents, as they stimulate endogenous insulin production, cause an elevated C peptide, but these drugs can be detected in the blood or urine.

COURSE

The course is determined by the underlying etiology.

COMPLICATIONS

The complications of delirium are as described in that chapter.

Patients who have sustained one or more episodes of prolonged and severe hypoglycemia, with blood sugars below 20 mg/dL, may be left with dementia and ataxia.

ETIOLOGY

Postprandial hypoglycemia may occur in postgastrectomy patients, patients in the early stages of type II non-insulin dependent diabetes mellitus or on an idiopathic basis (also known as "functional" or "essential").

Important causes of fasting hypoglycemia include insulinoma, excessive use of insulin (either iatrogenic or factitious) or oral hypoglycemics, tumors, such as hepatomas or large mesenchymal tumors, and subsequent to excessive alcohol use in the fasting patient. Alcohol inhibits gluconeogenesis, and in patients who are malnourished or who have missed several meals, hypoglycemia may develop within 4 to 24 hours after a binge. Thus, while recovering from intoxication, patients may experience a deterioration in their clinical condition, which if untreated may lead to permanent brain damage.

Multiple causes of hypoglycemia exist in childhood, many of them inherited.

In patients who eventually become demented, ventricular dilatation and generalized cortical atrophy is present, with the temporal lobe and hippocampus bearing the brunt of the damage. Microscopically there is neuronal loss, which tends to be laminar but may, in severe cases, involve the entire cortical mantle.

DIFFERENTIAL DIAGNOSIS

Given that the autonomic and cerebral symptoms of hypoglycemia are relatively nonspecific, one must demonstrate Whipple's triad before attributing them to hypoglycemia. Hence one must demonstrate the following: the presence of typical symptoms, the concurrent presence of significant hypoglycemia, and the prompt relief of symptoms with correction of the hypoglycemia. Mere demonstration that hypoglycemia occurs during a 5-hour glucose tolerance test is not adequate support for a diagnosis of postprandial hypoglycemia because a substantial minority of otherwise completely normal and asymptomatic subjects demonstrate this finding. In some cases of suspected fasting hypoglycemia, one may have to admit the patient and impose a fast until symptoms appear.

Panic attacks may be confused with the episodic appearance of postprandial hypoglycemic autonomic symptoms. The self-remitting nature of the panic attack, in the absence of any glucose ingestion, is a clue to the correct diagnosis.

When neuroglycopenic symptoms present as a delirium, the differential diagnosis is very wide and is discussed in that chapter. The fact that autonomic symptoms may be very mild or even totally lacking may make the correct diagnosis even more elusive.

Alcohol-induced hypoglycemia may readily be mistaken for alcohol withdrawal or delirium tremens. Thus any withdrawing alcoholic who is unable to take glucose orally should be monitored closely for any hypoglycemia.

TREATMENT

If the patient is able to take fluids, a glass of orange juice mixed with two or three tablespoonfuls of sugar is often adequate treatment. Patients unable to take fluids may be given 50 ml of a 50% solution of glucose intravenously. Glucagon represents an alternative to intravenous glucose when intravenous administration is impractical, such as at home. The dose is 1 mg im. However, because glucagon relies on mobilizing hepatic stores of glucose, it is of little avail in those with significant liver damage. In any case,

the patient should be closely observed to see if repeat doses of glucose or glucagon are required.

In the alcoholic patient, one must give parenteral thiamine well before glucose is administered because a glucose load may precipitate Wernicke-Korsakoff syndrome.

With administration of glucose or glucagon recovery usually occurs within 10 minutes. Lack of response calls for diagnostic reevaluation.

Once hypoglycemia is corrected, treatment is directed at the underlying cause.

BIBLIOGRAPHY

Ben-Ami H, Nagachandran P, Mendelson A, et al. Drug-induced hypoglycemic coma in 102 diabetic patients. *Archives of Internal Medicine* 1999;159:281-284.

Dizon AM, Kowalyk S, Hoogwerf BJ. Neuroglycopenic and other symptoms in patients with insulinomas. *The American Journal of Medicine* 1999;106:307-310.

Fujikowa M, Okuchi K, Hiramatsu KI, et al. Specific changes in human brain after hypoglycemic injury. *Stroke* 1997;28:584-587.

Kalimo H, Olsson Y. Effects of severe hypoglycemia on the human brain: neuropathologic case reports. *Acta Neurologica Scandinavica* 1980;62: 345-356.

Malouf R, Brust JCM. Hypoglycemia: causes, neurological manifestations, and outcome. *Annals of Neurology* 1985;17:421-430.

Palardy J, Havrankova J, Lepage R, et al. Blood glucose measurements during symptomatic episodes in patients with suspected postprandial hypoglycemia. *The New England Journal of Medicine* 1989;321: 1421-1425.

Shintani S, Tsuruoka S, Shiigai T. Hypoglycemic hemiplegia: a repeat SPECT study. *Journal of Neurology, Neurosurgery, and Psychiatry* 1993;56:700-701.

259 Hypernatremia

When the serum sodium level is elevated acutely above 150 mEq/L, neuronal dysfunction occurs, the severity of which increases as the sodium concentration increases further: acute elevations of the serum sodium to 160 mEq/L are almost invariably associated with significant delirium.

ONSET

Acute elevations of serum sodium are followed by a delirium of acute onset; gradual rises in serum sodium, on the other hand, may be fairly well tolerated, and levels of 170 mEq/L or more, if gradually attained, may be associated with few, if any, symptoms.

CLINICAL FEATURES

When symptomatic, patients are confused and somnolent, and there may be irritability. Generalized weakness may occur and may be accompanied by myalgia and muscle cramping, which, in severe cases, may cause rhabdomyolysis. Partial or grand mal seizures may occur in a minority, and, rarely, chorea and myoclonus may also be seen. Eventually, with further rises of the sodium level, coma supervenes.

COURSE

Untreated severe acute hypernatremia carries a high mortality rate, ranging from 15% to 66%.

COMPLICATIONS

Complications of delirium are as described in that chapter.

ETIOLOGY

Normally, when serum sodium rises above normal, osmoreceptors in the hypothalamus stimulate both the release of arginine vasopressin (also known simply as vasopressin or as antidiuretic hormone) and thirst. Vasopressin is transported from the hypothalamus via the supraoptico-hypophyseal tract through the pituitary stalk to the posterior pituitary where it is secreted into the circulation: vasopressin stimulates the kidneys to conserve free water, in turn also rendering the urine more concentrated. Thirst, provided that patients have access to water, and are able to get to it, is followed by increased water intake. The combination of these two mechanisms fairly rapidly brings the serum sodium concentration back to normal.

Serum sodium may rise above normal for a number of reasons. In some cases, patients are subject to a "salt overload", as for example when patients take an excessive amount of "salt tablets" or are given hypertonic intravenous saline. In other cases, excessive fluid loss may lead to dehydration, as may be seen with severe diarrhea or diaphoresis, or in cases of nephrogenic diabetes insipidus. In nephrogenic diabetes insipidus, the kidneys are resistant to vasopressin, and hence free water is lost in a dilute urine despite the presence of hypernatremia and elevated serum levels of vasopressin. In general medicine, nephrogenic diabetes insipidus is most commonly seen as a side-effect to medications, most notably lithium.

Regardless of the reason for the rising sodium, significant hypernatremia in most cases simply does not occur because patients get thirsty and drink a sufficient amount of water to bring the sodium level within normal limits. It is generally only when access to water is restricted, or patients are unable to drink, that symptomatic hypernatremia occurs, as for example when patients are restrained, or too weak or confused to drink.

Determining the etiology of hypernatremia requires, in addition to a serum sodium level, simultaneous plasma and urine osmolalities and a urine sodium level. In cases of salt overload or dehydration the plasma and urine osmolalities are both increased; however, in salt overload the urine sodium is above 20 mEq/L whereas in dehydration the urine sodium is below 10 mEq/L. In cases of nephrogenic diabetes insipidus, whereas the plasma osmolality is high, the urine osmolality is either normal or low.

Before leaving this discussion of the etiology of hypernatremia, another cause must be mentioned, namely the central type of diabetes insipidus. This, relative to the other causes of hypernatremia, is a rare disorder and is characterized by a deficient release of vasopressin from the posterior pituitary, which in turn can result from either hypothalamic or pituitary disease. In hypothalamic disease osmoreceptors are damaged, with the double result of not only a lack of thirst but also a deficient production of vasopressin: possible causes include ischemic infarction (as may occur as a complication of clipping of an anterior communicating artery aneurysm), tumors, granulomas (e.g., as in sarcoidosis) and a condition known as "essential hypernatremia," wherein it appears that the hypothalamic osmoreceptor "set point" is so high that high levels of serum sodium fail to trigger it. In pituitary disease either the pituitary stalk is sectioned or the posterior pituitary is damaged: here, although thirst is preserved, vasopressin cannot be secreted into the circulation. Possible causes include head trauma, tumors or pituitary apoplexy. In cases of hypothalamic central diabetes insipidus patients become "adipsic" and, not experiencing thirst, simply do not drink despite the fact that because of deficient vasopressin production a loss of free water through the kidneys causes hypernatremia. In cases of pituitary central diabetes insipidus, thirst is preserved and, unless patients lack access to water or are too confused to drink, significant hypernatremia generally does not occur. Regardless of whether the central diabetes insipidus is of hypothalamic or pituitary origin, the plasma and urine osmolalities are similar to those seen within nephrogenic diabetes insipidus and the differential rests on the serum vasopressin level: in central diabetes insipidus it is low, whereas in nephrogenic diabetes insipidus it is high.

Hypernatremia provokes cerebral symptoms by establishing an osmotic gradient between neurons and the extracellular fluid, leading to cell shrinkage. When the hypernatremia occurs gradually, compensation occurs, and intracellular osmolality rises to approach the extracellular osmolality. However, when hypernatremia occurs rapidly or when an acute exacerbation of a chronic hypernatremia occurs, intracellular compensation cannot occur rapidly enough, and cell shrinkage occurs. In severe cases this shrinkage may be profound; intracerebral veins may be torn with widespread intracerebral hemorrhages; "bridging" veins may also rupture, and subdural hematomas may form.

DIFFERENTIAL DIAGNOSIS

Whenever delirium occurs in the elderly, especially those who, for one reason or another, have been subject to a potential overload of salt or who have become dehydrated, hypernatremia should always be one of the suspects.

TREATMENT

In severe or rapidly progressive cases, one may have to give intravenous fluids to correct the hypernatremia. In chronic cases where intracellular osmolality has undergone a compensatory rise, rapid correction of the hypernatremia creates a reversal of the osmotic gradient leading to cellular swelling and symptoms similar to those described in the chapter on hyponatremia. To be on the safe side, the sodium level should be lowered no more rapidly than 0.5 mEq/L every hour, and then only until the patient becomes asymptomatic, after which further correction may be undertaken in a more leisurely manner. Treatment is then directed at the underlying etiology; in cases of central diabetes insipidus, DDAVP may be given intranasally.

BIBLIOGRAPHY

Addleman M, Pollard A, Grossman RF. Survival after severe hypernatremia due to salt ingestion by an adult. *The American Journal of Medicine* 1985;78:176-178.

Androque HJ, Madias NE. Hypernatremia. *The New England Journal of Medicine* 2000;342:1493-1499.

Bendz H, Aurell M. Drug-induced diabetes insipidus: incidence, prevention and management. *Drug Safety* 1999;21:449-456.

Brown MA, Mullins R, Stokes GS, et al. Essential hypernatremia: disordered thirst and blood pressure control. *The Australian and New Zealand Journal of Medicine* 1985;15:751-754.

Fall PJ. Hyponatremia and hypernatremia. A systematic approach to causes and their correction. *Postgraduate Medicine* 2000;107:75-82.

Nguyen BN, Yablon SA, Chen CY. Hypodipsic hypernatremia and diabetes insipidus following anterior communicating artery aneurysm clipping: diagnostic and therapeutic challenges in the amnestic rehabilitation patient. *Brain Injury* 2001;15:975-980.

Palevsky PM, Bhagrath R, Greenberg A. Hypernatremia in hospitalized patients. *Annals of Internal Medicine* 1996;124:197-203.

Sparacio RR, Anziska B, Schutta HS. Hypernatremia and chorea. A report of two cases. *Neurology* 1976;26:46-50.

Young RS, Truax BT. Hypernatremic hemorrhagic encephalopathy. *Annals of Neurology* 1979;5:588-591.

In hyponatremia, the appearance and severity of symptoms is determined not only by the degree of hyponatremia but also by the rapidity with which it develops. For example, a rapid fall to a concentration of 120 mEq/L may cause delirium and seizures, whereas, if reached very gradually, levels of 110 mEq/L or less may be tolerated with few if any symptoms.

ONSET

The onset is determined by the underlying etiology.

CLINICAL FEATURES

The principal symptom of hyponatremia is delirium, which is often accompanied by lethargy and seizures; nausea and vomiting may also occur, as may myoclonus and asterixis. With further decreases in sodium, coma and eventually death occur.

In addition to determining the serum sodium level, one must also determine the plasma and urine osmolality and a urine sodium concentration, as explained below, under "Etiology."

COURSE

Acute symptomatic hyponatremia with sodium levels below 120 mEq/L carries a high mortality rate.

COMPLICATIONS

Complications of delirium are as described in that chapter.

ETIOLOGY

Antidiuretic hormone (ADH, also know as arginine vasopressin, or simply vasopressin) is the hormone primarily responsible for maintaining the sodium concentration within normal limits. ADH is synthesized in the hypothalamus, transported in the supraoptico-hypophyseal tract via the pituitary stalk to the posterior pituitary, and then secreted into the circulation to make its way to the kidney where it promotes the reabsorption of free water, in the process increasing the osmolality of the urine. The secretion of ADH is under the control of both osmoreceptors and baroreceptors. Osmoreceptors are present in the hypothalamus, and, in response to increasing plasma osmolality, stimulate a greater production of ADH. The baroreceptors are located in the cardiac atria, the aorta and the carotid arteries, and when pressure is low in these structures the hypothalamus is influenced via the vagus nerve and ascending fibers from the nucleus solitarius, leading again to an increased production of ADH. Normally the "osmoreceptor" mechanism is predominant; however, when pressure is very low the "baroreceptor" mechanism will override the "osmoreceptor" one, leading to an increased production of ADH despite a normal or even a decreased plasma osmolality.

Hyponatremia, in general, occurs only when either the intake of fluids is so massive as to overwhelm the kidney's ability to excrete free water or when ADH secretion is inappropriately high given the falling serum sodium concentration: this latter condition is known as the syndrome of inappropriate ADH secretion (SIADH).

Excessive ingestion of fluids is most commonly seen in what has been termed "compulsive water drinking" or "psychogenic polydipsia." Here, the serum sodium is low, the plasma osmolality is low and, critically, the urine osmolality is also low. Although compulsive water drinking may be seen in a number of conditions, and sometimes even in otherwise normal individuals, the most common associated condition is schizophrenia. A similar condition, known as "beer potomania," may be seen in heavy beer drinkers: here, the prodigious quantities of relatively solute-free beer the drinker consumes simply overwhelms the kidney's ability to excrete free water.

The syndrome of inappropriate ADH secretion is characterized by a low serum sodium accompanied by a low plasma osmolality, and, in stark distinction from compulsive water drinking, a less than maximally dilute urine. SIADH may occur due to dysfunction of the hypothalamus, ectopic secretion of ADH-like substances (e.g., as in various cancers), in states of volume contraction or decreased effective circulating volume when the baroreceptor control mechanisms override the osmoreceptors, and, finally, as a side-effect to drugs which may either stimulate ADH secretion or increase the sensitivity of the kidney to ADH.

Hypothalamic dysfunction capable of increasing ADH production may occur after cerebral infarction, subarachnoid hemorrhage, meningoencephalitis, tumors, or basilar skull fractures. Ectopic secretion of ADH-like substances may occur in bronchogenic carcinoma, oat cell carcinoma, cancer of the pancreas, duodenum, prostate, bladder or ureters, and in relation to various pulmonary disorders, including COPD, pneumonia, lung abscess and tuberculosis; positive pressure ventilation has also been associated with SIADH. In all these cases, the urinary sodium concentration is above 20 mEq/L.

Volume contraction may be seen in dehydration, and decreased effective circulating volume in congestive heart failure or cirrhosis with ascites; in both cases, as noted earlier, there is activation of the baroreceptors with consequent increased secretion of ADH despite hyponatremia. In these cases, the urinary sodium concentration is below 10 mEq/L.

Drugs capable of either stimulating ADH secretion or sensitizing the renal tubule to ADH include amitriptyline, tranylcypromine, SSRIs, venlafaxine, thioridazine, fluphenazine, thiothixene, haloperidol, risperidone, carbamazepine, oxcarbazepine, valproic acid, phenobarbital, vincristine, cyclophosphamide, amiodarone, theophylline, morphine, clofibrate, chlorpropamide and tolbutamide.

In addition to the above mechanisms, hyponatremia may also occur secondary to treatment with thiazide diuretics, in hepatic porphyria, adrenocortical insufficiency or hypothyroidism, and, of course, in cases of overdose of DDAVP, as may occur in patients treated for enuresis.

Regardless of the mechanism whereby hyponatremia occurs, the end result in the central nervous system is the same. As sodium is the principal determinant of serum osmolality, a reduction in serum sodium (with the exceptions mentioned in the section on differential diagnosis) is paralleled by a fall in serum osmolality. Should this fall be sufficiently rapid, the ability of cells to make compensatory reductions in intracellular osmolality will be overtaken and an osmotic shift of water into neurons and glia occur, leading to swelling and increased intracranial pressure. However, if the fall in serum sodium is slow, often enough time may be available for compensatory reductions in cellular osmolality so that osmotic equilibrium is maintained with no shift of water to inside the cell.

DIFFERENTIAL DIAGNOSIS

Occasionally, hyponatremia is not accompanied by hypoosmolality, and thus does not cause symptoms. Examples include the administration of mannitol and in conditions of hyperglycemia.

Spurious hyponatremia, representing a laboratory artifact, occurs when the serum sodium is measured by flame photometry in the presence of hyperproteinemia or hyperlipidemia.

TREATMENT

In the treatment of hyponatremia, efforts are directed both at the underlying etiology and toward symptomatic relief.

If patients are asymptomatic, then simple fluid restriction is generally recommended. An exception to this would be a situation wherein the sodium level has fallen very rapidly and it can be predicted that symptoms would occur soon if aggressive treatment were not undertaken. In an afebrile adult, insensible losses approximate 800 ml/day; thus fluid restriction in the range of 600 to 1200 ml/24 hours is usually adequate.

If the hyponatremia is symptomatic or judged likely to become symptomatic soon, normal saline may be given. Some authors advocate use of hypertonic saline; however, this is a risky procedure and should be reserved for life-threatening cases. The rate at which hyponatremia is corrected is determined not only by the severity of the patient's clinical situation but also with reference to whether the hyponatremia was of acute or chronic onset. In chronic hyponatremia, as noted earlier, osmotic equilibrium has often occurred. Thus if the serum sodium is corrected too rapidly, compensatory intracellular mechanisms are not able to increase intracellular osmolality fast enough and an osmotic shift of fluid from the cells into the extracellular fluid occurs, putting the patient at risk for central pontine myelinolysis. Consequently, if the hyponatremia is chronic, or if its duration is uncertain, serum sodium must be increased slowly, generally no faster than 0.4 mEq/L/hour. When it is certain that the hyponatremia is of recent origin, within the past 24 to 48 hours, then a brisker pace is an option.

The goal of acute treatment of hyponatremia is not to render the sodium level within normal limits; rather the goal is simply to make the patient safe, and this may generally be accomplished by elevating the serum sodium to 120 mEq/L. Higher levels are simply not necessary; restoration to normal sodium levels from this concentration may proceed at a much more leisurely pace.

Concurrent with symptomatic treatment, the underlying etiology must also be addressed. In cases of compulsive water drinking

in schizophrenia where other neuroleptics have failed, clozapine has been effective. In cases of SIADH where the underlying cause cannot be corrected, then demeclocycline, which has an anti-ADH effect, may be utilized. Clinical trials are underway with specific ADH receptor antagonists which appear to be better tolerated and more effective than demeclocycline.

BIBLIOGRAPHY

Ayus JC, Arieff Al. Pathogenesis and prevention of hyponatremic encephalopathy. *Endicrinology and Metabolism Clinics of North America* 1993;22:425.

Branten AJ, Wetzels JF, Weber AM, et al. Hyponatremia due to sodium valproate. *Annals of Neurology* 1998;43:265-267.

Canuso CM, Goldman MB. Clozapine restores water balance in schizophrenic patients with polydipsia-hyponatremia syndrome. *The Journal of Neuropsychiatry and Clinical Neurosciences* 1999;11:86-90.

DeWardener HE, Barlow ED. Compulsive water drinking. *Quarterly Journal of Medicine* 1958;27:567.

Gerbes AL, Gulberg V, Gines P, et al. Therapy of hyponatremia in cirrhosis with a vasopressin receptor antagonist: a randomized double-blind multicenter trial. *Gastroenterology* 2003;124:933-939.

Goldberg M. Hyponatremia and the inappropriate secretion of antidiuretic hormone. *American Journal of Medicine* 1963;35:293.

Illowsky BP, Kirch DG. Polydipsia and hyponatremia in psychiatric patients. *American Journal of Psychiatry* 1988;145:675.

Liberopoulos EN, Alexandridis GH, Christidis DS, et al. SIADH and hyponatremia with theophylline. *The Annals of Pharmacotherapy* 2002;36:1180-1182.

Liu BA, Mittmann N, Knowles SR, et al. Hyponatremia and the syndrome of inappropriate antidiuretic hormone associated with the use of selective serotonin reuptake inhibitors: a review of spontaneous reports. *Canadian Medical Association Journal* 1996;155:519-527.

Masood GR, Karki SD, Patterson WR. Hyponatremia and venlafaxine. *The Annals of Pharmacotherapy* 1998;32:49-51.

Mulloy AL, Caruana RJ. Hyponatremic emergencies. *Medical Clinics of North America* 1995;79:155.

Odeh M, Beny A, Oliven A. Severe symptomatic hyponatremia during citalopram therapy. *The American Journal of the Medical Sciences* 2002;321:159-160.

Oh MS, Kim HJ. Recommendations for treatment of symptomatic hyponatremia. *Nephron* 1995;70:143.

Patel GP, Kasiar JB. Syndrome of inappropriate antidiuretic hormone-induced hyponatremia associated with amiodarone. *Pharmacotherapy* 2002;22:649-651.

Shindel A, Tobin G, Klutke C. Hyponatremia associated with desmopressin for the treatment of nocturnal polyuria. *Urology* 2002;60:344.

Spital A. Diuretic-induced hyponatremia. *American Journal of Nephrology* 1999;19:447-452.

Swanson AG, Iseri OA. Acute encephalopathy due to water intoxication. *The New England Journal of Medicine* 1958;258:831.

Thomas A, Verbalis JG. Hyponatremia and the syndrome of inappropriate antidiuretic hormone secretion associated with drug therapy in psychiatric patients. *CNS Drugs* 1995;4:357.

Welli W. Delirium with low serum sodium. *Archives of Neurology and Psychiatry* 1956;76:559.

Whitten JR, Ruchter VL. Risperidone and hyponatremia: a case report. *Annals of Clinical Psychiatry* 1997;9:181-183.

Hypokalemia of any cause, if sufficiently severe, may cause weakness, lethargy, and, in a minority, delirium. Patients with anorexia nervosa or bulimia who use diuretics or laxatives, or who recurrently induce vomiting, represent one group at definite risk for hypokalemia.

ONSET

The age of onset is determined by the underlying etiology. Acute falls in potassium level tend to create acute symptoms. The same potassium level, however, if reached gradually, may be met by a more gradual onset of much milder symptoms.

CLINICAL FEATURES

In general, patients with potassium levels below 3 mEq/L may complain of fatigue, muscle weakness, and at times muscle cramping. As the level falls below 2.5 mEq/L, weakness becomes more pronounced and hyporeflexia may occur; lethargy and a delirium may appear. With further reduction, respiratory paralysis and death may follow. The electrocardiogram reveals a progressive reduction in the height of the T-wave, paralleled by the appearance and progressive enlargement of a U-wave. Premature atrial or ventricular contractions may occur, and ventricular fibrillation may follow.

COURSE

The course is determined by the underlying etiology.

COMPLICATIONS

Complications of delirium are as described in that chapter.

ETIOLOGY

Inadequate intake of potassium may occur in patients with anorexia nervosa or those on starvation diets. Excessive loss may occur with recurrent vomiting, gastric suction, or diarrhea, as may be seen with laxative abuse or with a villous adenoma.

Hypokalemia may be seen in Cushing's syndrome (including that due to high dose corticosteroid treatment), hyperaldosteronism, during treatment with mineralocorticoids (e.g., fludrocortisone), or with chronic licorice chewing.

Various drugs may have hypokalemia as a side effect, and of these the most important are the loop and thiazide diuretics. Others include acetazolamide, insulin, beta-adrenergic agonists, theophylline, penicillin (and its derivatives), gentamycin and amphotericin B. Toluene inhalation may also cause hypokalemia.

Other conditions associated with hypokalemia include hypomagnesemia, treatment of vitamin B_{12} deficiency with B_{12}, hypokalemic periodic paralysis, clay-eating, and Gitelman's syndrome, a rare inherited disorder of adults characterized by hypokalemia, hypomagnesemia and hypocalcemia.

Hypokalemia may also occur in agitated patients, as for example those with an exacerbation of schizophrenia.

DIFFERENTIAL DIAGNOSIS

The delirium of hypokalemia may be mimicked by some of the other metabolic encephalopathies, and given that differentiating among them on clinical grounds is difficult, it is customary in evaluating a patient with a suspected metabolic encephalopathy to obtain not only a potassium level but also levels of sodium, calcium, magnesium, and glucose.

TREATMENT

If the patient is symptomatic or shows electrocardiographic changes, potassium supplementation is indicated. Oral treatment is preferable and may be accomplished with potassium chloride liquid (10%) in a total daily dose of 30 to 60 mEq, given in divided doses. For alcoholics the effervescent tablets should be used because the elixir contains alcohol. When patients cannot tolerate the taste of the liquid, micro-encapsulated potassium, available in 8 and 10 mEq sizes, may be used. In life-threatening situations intravenous potassium may be given in quarter-normal saline solutions containing no more than 40 mEq/L of potassium, administered at a rate no faster than 10 mEq/hour: in such cases, potassium levels must be monitored closely, sometimes on an hourly basis, to avoid hyperkalemia.

As noted earlier, when hypokalemia is of gradual onset and chronic, there may be no symptoms: indeed, levels as low as 1.6 mEq/L have been well-tolerated by some patients with anorexia nervosa. In such cases, a conservative approach to replenishment is indicated.

BIBLIOGRAPHY

Barakat AJ, Rennert OM. Gitelman's syndrome (familial hypokalemia-hypomagnesemia). *Journal of Nephrology* 2001;14:43-47.

Bonne OB, Bloch M, Berry EM. Adaptation to severe chronic hypokalemia in anorexia nervosa: a plea for conservative management. *The International Journal of Eating Disorders* 1993;13:125-128.

Greenfeld D, Mickley D, Quinlan DM, et al. Hypokalemia in outpatients with eating disorders. *The American Journal of Psychiatry* 1995;152:60-63.

Hatta K, Takahashi T, Nakamura H, et al. Hypokalemia and agitation in acute psychotic patients. *Psychiatry Research* 1999;86:85-88.

Kim GH, Han JS. Therapeutic approach to hypokalemia. *Nephron* 2002; 92(Suppl 1):28-32.

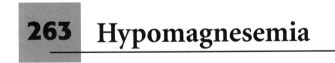

262 Hypermagnesemia

Hypermagnesemia is a relatively rare condition that, among multiple other signs and symptoms, may also cause delirium. It generally results from ingestion of magnesium containing medicines, and although typically occurring only in those with a greater or lesser degree of renal failure, it may also occur in those with normal renal function.

ONSET

Most patients are elderly, and the onset is generally subacute, over days.

CLINICAL FEATURES

As the serum magnesium level rises over 5 mEq/L, lethargy, signs of generalized weakness and delirium appear, and the deep tendon reflexes become depressed. As the magnesium level rises toward 15 mEq/L these symptoms worsen, blood pressure drops, respiratory depression begins and various cardiac abnormalities appear, including bradycardia, conduction delays, occasional U waves, and ventricular tachyarrythmias; eventually coma and either respiratory or cardiac arrest occur.

Magnesium suppresses parathyroid hormone release, and hypocalcemia often accompanies hypermagnesemia.

COURSE

The course of this disorder is determined by the underlying cause.

COMPLICATIONS

Complications of delirium are as described in that chapter.

ETIOLOGY

Various over-the-counter medications contain magnesium, including laxatives (milk of magnesia), antacids (magnesium hydroxide) and Epsom salts (magnesium sulfate), which are occasionally used as gargles. As magnesium is excreted primarily by the kidneys, renal failure puts patients taking such medications at risk for the accumulation of magnesium; however, it should be kept in mind that constipation, by allowing for a greater absorption of magnesium, may also increase the risk.

DIFFERENTIAL DIAGNOSIS

Hypermagnesemia may be difficult to distinguish from hypokalemia on clinical grounds; in general, whenever a patient is suspected of having a metabolic encephalopathy, it is prudent to obtain not only a magnesium level, but also levels of potassium, sodium, glucose, BUN and ammonia.

TREATMENT

Typically, eliminating the excess intake of magnesium is all that is required. In emergency situations, however, calcium, which antagonizes magnesium, may be given intravenously over about one-half hour as 10 to 20 ml of a 10% solution of calcium gluconate. In addition, if renal failure is not a significant factor, intravenous furosemide combined with half-normal sailine may also hasten excretion of magnesium. When renal failure renders furosemide ineffective, hemodialysis may be used.

BIBLIOGRAPHY

Birrer RB, Shallash AJ, Totten V. Hypermagnesemia-induced fatality following epsom salt gargles. *The Journal of Emergency Medicine* 2002;22:185-188.

Choist IN, Steinberg SF, Tropper PJ, et al. The influence of hypermagnesemia on serum calcium and parathyroid hormone levels in human subjects. *The New England Journal of Medicine* 1984;1310:1221-1225.

Clark BA, Brown RS. Unsuspected morbid hypermagnesemia in elderly patients. *American Journal of Nephrology* 1992;12:336-343.

McLaughlin SA, McKinney PE. Antacid-induced hypermagnesemia in a patient with normal renal function and bowel obstruction. *The Annals of Pharmacotherapy* 1998;32:312-315.

Qureshi T, Melonakos TK. Acute hypermagnesemia after laxative use. *Annals of Emergency Medicine* 1996;28:552-555.

263 Hypomagnesemia

Magnesium is obtained primarily from the chlorophyll of green vegetables; other sources include fish and meat. Roughly 25 mEq, or 300 mg, is required on a daily basis for the average adult. The bioavailability of ingested magnesium is a little less than 40%, and absorption takes place primarily in the proximal small bowel, with excretion via the kidney.

Magnesium is required for the proper functioning of numerous enzymes; it also is required for the release of parathyroid hormone from the parathyroid glands. The most common cause of hypomagnesemia is alcoholism. Frequently, in addition to hypomagnesemia, one also finds other electrolyte changes and vitamin deficiencies.

ONSET

The onset of symptoms is typically gradual. Weeks or a month or more may be required before hypomagnesemia develops in those on a diet low in magnesium.

CLINICAL FEATURES

Symptoms typically begin when the serum magnesium level drops to 1 mEq/L or lower. Patients may become apathetic and irritable, and may complain of fatigue and generalized weakness. With further reductions, a delirium may occur with confusion, disorientation, and at times hallucinations; myoclonus, fasciculations and grand mal seizures may also occur.

Various arrhythmias, including ventricular fibrillation, may occur, and patients show an enhanced sensitivity to digitalis preparations.

As noted earlier, hypomagnesemia causes deficient parathyroid hormone release, and hypocalcemic tetany may occur. Hypokalemia is also frequently present.

COURSE

The course of this disorder is determined by the course of the underlying etiology.

COMPLICATIONS

Complications of delirium are as described in that chapter.

ETIOLOGY

The most common cause, as noted above, is alcoholism. Other conditions associated with a decreased intake or absorption of magnesium include anorexia nervosa, prolonged intravenous feeding without magnesium supplementation, various malabsorption syndromes, such as pancreatic insufficiency or sprue, and prolonged vomiting, naso-gastric suctioning or diarrhea. Multiple medications may lower magnesium levels, and of all these the most common culprits are diuretics, especially thiazide diuretics; others include gentamycin, pentamidine, amphotericin B, cyclosporine, cisplatin and foscarnet.

DIFFERENTIAL DIAGNOSIS

Unless magnesium levels are checked, one might mistake the clinical features for hypocalcemia.

TREATMENT

Magnesium for parenteral use is supplied as magnesium sulfate: a 10% solution (0.812 mEq/ml) is available for intravenous use, and a 50% solution (4.06 mEq/ml) for intramuscular use.

In emergency situations, such as when convulsions or serious arrhythmias occur, one may add 20 cc of a 10% solution to 80 cc of D5W and then infuse the resulting 100 cc over approximately 10 minutes. This will deliver 16.2 mEq, which is usually sufficient to bring patients out of mortal danger.

In urgent, but non-emergency situations, the 10% solution may be utilized to make final concentrations of anywhere from 8.1 to 48.6 mEq/1000cc to be infused over 24 hours. Magnesium sulfate may also be given intramuscularly, and although injections are often painful, some authors believe this is a safer route. The 50% solution is used for intramuscular administration and anywhere from 2 ml (8.12 mEq) to 4 ml (16.2 mEq) may be given intramuscularly every six hours.

Regardless of whether magnesium is given intravenously or intramuscularly, the dose must be lower if renal failure is present. Furthermore, magnesium levels must be monitored, either directly, by obtaining serum magnesium concentrations, or indirectly, by serially checking deep tendon reflexes, keeping in mind that depressed deep tendon reflexes are an indicator of hypermagnesemia.

In cases where ongoing magnesium loss cannot be stopped, oral supplementation may be accomplished by giving magnesium gluconate or magnesium oxide.

BIBLIOGRAPHY

Barton CH, Vaziri ND, Martin DC, et al. Hypomagnesemia and renal magnesium wasting in renal transplant recipients receiving cyclosporine. *The American Journal of Medicine* 1987;83:693-699.

Hall RCW, Joffe JR. Hypomagnesemia: physical and psychiatric symptoms. *Journal of the American Medical Association* 1973;224:1749-1751.

Martin BJ, Milligan K. Diuretic-associated hypomagnesemia in the elderly. *Archives of Internal Medicine* 1987;147:1768-1771.

Palla B, Litt IF. Medical complications of eating disorders in adolescents. *Pediatrics* 1988;81:613-623.

Shils ME. Experimental human magnesium depletion. *Medicine* 1969;48:61-85.

Whang R. Magnesium deficiency: pathogenesis, prevalence and clinical implications. *The American Journal of Medicine* 1987;82(Suppl 3):24-29.

Hypercalcemia, as may be seen in certain malignancies or in hyperparathyroidism, may, among other symptoms, cause a delirium.

ONSET

The onset, as determined by the underlying disease, may range from acute to one that is insidious and gradual, extending over many years.

CLINICAL FEATURES

The normal range for total serum calcium is from 8.9 to 10.1 mg/dL, and symptoms generally do not appear until the level rises above 12; at this point there may be apathy, fatigue, depression and irritability, along with nausea, vomiting, constipation and colicky abdominal pain. Patients may also complain of headache and there may be proximal muscle weakness and decreased deep tendon reflexes. At levels between 14 and 16 mg/dL, delirium may appear, and, rarely, either grand mal or partial seizures. Higher levels bring somnolence and eventually coma, and death may ensue at levels of over 18 mg/dL.

It must be kept in mind that there is only a very rough correlation between total serum calcium levels and symptomatology. Calcium is bound to albumin, and as it is the free, ionized calcium that is important, a "normal" total serum calcium in the presence of hypoalbuminemia may be associated with symptoms.

The ECG typically shows a shortened QT interval, and the electroencephalogram typically shows generalized slowing.

In long-standing cases, one may see nephrocalcinosis, nephrolithiasis, and, possibly, an increased incidence of peptic ulcer disease. An association with pancreatitis also exists.

COURSE

The course is determined by the underlying disease. In some cases of hyperparathyroidism, the course may extend for many years.

COMPLICATIONS

Complications of delirium are as described in that chapter.

ETIOLOGY

Most cases of clinically significant hypercalcemia are caused by either hyperparathyroidism or malignant disease, and severe elevations of calcium are generally associated with malignancies.

Granulomatous disease, as may occur in sarcoidosis, is also an important cause, as is vitamin D intoxication, and, in children, prolonged immobilization.

Hypercalcemia may occur secondary to various other conditions; however, it is rarely severe enough to cause symptoms. These conditions include thiazide diuretics, lithium, the milk-alkali syndrome; hyperthyroidism or hypothyroidism; and adrenocortical insufficiency.

DIFFERENTIAL DIAGNOSIS

Other metabolic encephalopathies may mimic hypercalcemia, and thus a "screen," including sodium, potassium, glucose, calcium, BUN and ammonia, is generally in order.

TREATMENT

Mild or asymptomatic hypercalcemia may be approached by treating the underlying disease.

Hypercalcemia at levels of 13 mg/dL or above, or those above 12 mg/dL that are associated with symptoms, requires urgent symptomatic treatment in addition to treatment of the underlying disease. Once any volume deficit has been corrected, patients may be diuresed with intravenous normal saline, with potassium supplements as needed, and furosemide, with a goal of producing a urinary output of approximately 3 liters/day. Once the level has fallen and patients are no longer symptomatic, oral treatment with furosemide, sodium chloride tablets, and a high fluid intake generally is satisfactory pending more definitive treatment. Throughout acute treatment, the patient should be kept ambulatory to prevent the hypercalcemic effect of immobilization.

BIBLIOGRAPHY

Edelson GW, Kleerekoper M. Hypercalcemic crisis. *The Medical Clinics of North America* 1995;79:79-92.

Karpati G, Frame B. Neuropsychiatric disorders in primary hyperparathyroidism: clinical analysis with review of the literature. *Archives of Neurology* 1964;10:387-397.

Reinfrank RF. Primary hyperparathyroidism with depression. *Archives of Internal Medicine* 1961;108:162-166.

Watson LC, Marx CE. New onset of neuropsychiatric symptoms in the elderly: possible primary hyperparathyroidism. *Psychosomatics* 2002;43:413-417.

Weizman A, Eldar M, Schoenfeld Y, et al. Hypercalcemia-induced psychopathology in malignant disease. *The British Journal of Psychiatry* 1979;135:363-366.

Regardless of the cause, hypocalcemia, if of sufficient degree, may cause mood changes or delirium. In addition, chronic hypocalcemia, if secondary to hypoparathyroidism, may be followed by cerebral and cerebellar calcification and a dementia or a movement disorder.

ONSET

The age and mode of onset is determined by the underlying etiology; subacute onsets may be seen after parathyroidectomy, whereas very gradual onsets may be seen in idiopathic hypoparathyroidism.

CLINICAL FEATURES

The degree of hypocalcemia required to cause symptoms varies with the acuteness of the fall in serum calcium level: rapid falls to only 8 mg/dL may produce very obvious symptoms, whereas a gradual fall to 7 mg/dL may be asymptomatic; at 6 mg/dL, however, symptoms almost always occur no matter how gradual the fall.

Mood changes may consist of depression, irritability and, especially, anxiety. Should a delirium occur, it may be marked by prominent hallucinations and delusions. Other symptoms include muscle cramping, especially in the back and legs, widespread parasthesiae, affecting the toes, fingers and face, and tetany, which may range in severity from mild carpal spasm (Figure 265-1) to opisthotonotic posturing, and may also manifest as laryngospasm. Seizures, either grand mal, or, less commonly, partial, are not uncommon and may or may not be accompanied by tetany; rarely, status epilepticus may occur secondary to hypocalcemia.

"Latent" tetany may be unmasked by either Chvostek's sign (twitching of the mouth upon tapping the seventh cranial nerve just anterior to the tragus) or Trousseau's sign (carpal spasm upon inflating a blood pressure cuff on the forearm well above systolic pressure for up to three minutes).

The QT interval is prolonged in hypocalcemia and is a reliable guide to its severity.

When chronic hypocalcemia occurs secondary to hypoparathyroidism, calcification may occur. CT or MRI scanning may display calcification in the basal ganglia (Figure 265-2), cerebellum, and occasionally in the cerebral cortex. Although these calcifications are at times asymptomatic and represent only incidental findings, they may cause Fahr's syndrome, characterized by a dementia or abnormal movements, including varied combinations of parkinsonism, chorea, dystonia, or ataxia. Calcification may also occur in the lens with cataract formation.

COURSE

The course is determined by the underlying etiology. The relatively common condition of postthyroidectomy hypoparathyroidism may be either transient and self-limiting, or, occasionally, chronic.

COMPLICATIONS

Complications of delirium or dementia are as described in those chapters.

ETIOLOGY

The most important causes of hypocalcemia are hypoparathyroidism, vitamin D deficiency, renal failure, hypomagnesemia, acute pancreatitis, malnutrition, pregnancy and lactation; certain medications, as for example foscarnet, may also cause hypocalcemia.

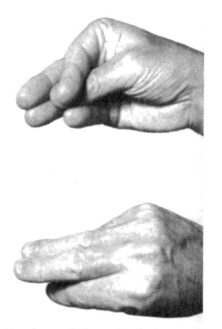

FIG. 265-1. Carpal spasm in hypocalcemia. (From Hall R, Evered DC. *Color atlas of endocrinology,* ed 2, London, 1990, Wolfe.)

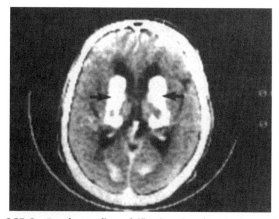

FIG. 265-2. Basal ganglia calcification in chronic hypocalcemia secondary to hypoparathyroidism. (From Hall R, Evered DC. *Color atlas of endocrinology,* ed 2, London, 1990, Wolfe.)

DIFFERENTIAL DIAGNOSIS

In general, the free, or ionized, calcium level parallels that of the total serum calcium. An exception occurs in hypoalbuminemia, wherein although total calcium is reduced, the ionized calcium remains normal and no symptoms are evident. Conversely, in any condition accompanied by alkalosis, such as in hyperventilation, although the total calcium remains within normal limits, the ionized calcium level falls and may produce extreme symptoms, such as tetany.

TREATMENT

Acute symptoms, such as delirium, tetany, or seizures, are treated with 10 to 20 ml of a 10% solution of calcium gluconate given slowly intravenously over about 10 to 20 minutes: although this generally is effective, repeat doses may be required every two or three hours. In the case of patients taking a digitalis preparation, continuous ECG monitoring is required during the infusion. Treatment is then directed at the underlying condition. Chronic oral therapy with calcium, generally with vitamin D, may be required.

Although delirious or demented patients may require treatment with antipsychotics these agents must be used cautiously, as these patients are prone to extrapyramidal side effects: either second generation agents or low-potency first-generation agents are preferred.

BIBLIOGRAPHY

Cheek JC, Riggs JE, Lilly RL. Extensive brain calcification and progressive dysarthria and dysphagia associated with chronic hypoparathyroidism. *Archives of Neurology* 1990;47:1038-1039.

Eraut D. Idiopathic hypoparathyroidism presenting as dementia. *British Medical Journal* 1974;1:429-430.

Kline CA, Esekogwu VI, Henderson SO, et al. Non-convulsive status epilepticus in a patient with hypocalcemia. *The Journal of Emergency Medicine* 1998;16:715-718.

Lawlor BA. Hypocalcemia, hypoparathyroidism, and organic anxiety syndrome. *The Journal of Clinical Psychiatry* 1988;49:317-318.

Reber PM, Heath H. Hypocalcemic emergencies. *The Medical Clinics of North America* 1995;79:93-106.

Slyter H. Idiopathic hypoparathyroidism presenting as dementia. *Neurology* 1979;29:393-394.

Tambyah PA, Ong BKC, Lee KO. Reversible parkinsonism and asymptomatic hypocalcemia with basal ganglia calcification from hypoparathyroidism 26 years after thyroid surgery. *The American Journal of Medicine* 1993;94:444-445.

Tohme JF, Bilezikian JP. Hypocalcemic emergencies. *Endocrinology and Metabolism Clinics of North America* 1993;22:363.

266 Uremic Encephalopathy

In severe renal failure, patients may develop a delirium, a condition known as uremic encephalopathy.

ONSET

The age of onset is determined by the underlying etiology, and the mode of onset, whether acute or insidious, reflects the rapidity with which the kidneys fail.

CLINICAL FEATURES

Patients complain of fatigue and difficulty concentrating, and they may present with a certain lassitude and appear less than fully alert. With progression, a delirium, often marked by visual hallucinations, appears, and is typically accompanied by asterixis and dysarthria.

With further progression, stupor supervenes, often accompanied by multifocal myoclonus, diffuse muscle twitching, and, in a minority, grand mal seizures; coma and death may follow.

In chronic renal failure one may also see a polyneuropathy. Initially this presents with a sensory component which often manifests with prominent dysesthesiae and restlessness, similar to that seen in the restless legs syndrome; over time a motor component appears which may progress, in severe cases, to quadriparesis.

The severity of delirium correlates positively not only with a rise in the BUN but also with the rapidity of that rise. For example, whereas in acute renal failure most patients with a BUN over 100 mg/dL would have some symptoms, in chronic renal failure of gradual onset, patients may tolerate levels of 200 mg/dL or higher with few if any symptoms.

The EEG typically shows generalized slowing. MRI scans may reveal cortical atrophy, and in some cases T2-weighted scans may reveal increased signal intensity both cortically and subcortically, findings which reverse with successful treatment.

COURSE

Typically, the symptomatology of the encephalopathy fluctuates from day to day, and even hour to hour; its overall course parallels that of the underlying renal disease.

COMPLICATIONS

The complications of delirium are as described in that chapter.

ETIOLOGY

Although there is a rough correlation between the rise in BUN and the severity of the delirium, the BUN, itself, is not responsible for the encephalopathy. In all likelihood the delirium results from an "auto-intoxication" by other substances normally excreted by the kidneys.

DIFFERENTIAL DIAGNOSIS

Certain diseases capable not only of causing renal failure but also of directly affecting the brain must be considered, including polyarteritis nodosa, systemic lupus erythematosus and malignant hypertension, with an associated hypertensive encephalopathy.

Both hypocalcemia and hypokalemia are common in renal failure, and may make independent contributions to the delirium seen in renal failure.

Certain drugs (most notably lithium), normally excreted by the kidneys, may accumulate in renal failure, causing a delirium in their own right.

TREATMENT

If the underlying cause of the renal failure is untreatable and spontaneous improvement is not expected, then uremic encephalopathy is an indication for dialysis. With dialysis, delirium typically clears promptly, within a day or two.

If antipsychotics are required, treatment is initiated with very low doses and titrated up very slowly. Lithium is generally contraindicated in renal failure; if an alternative to lithium is required, carbamazepine or valproate may be more safely used.

BIBLIOGRAPHY

Chadwick D, French AT. Uremic myoclonus: an example of reticular reflex myoclonus? *Journal of Neurology, Neurosurgery, and Psychiatry* 1979; 42:52-55.
Fraser CL, Arieff AA. Nervous system complications in uremia. *Annals of Internal Medicine* 1988;109:143-149.
Moe SM, Sprague SM. Uremic encephalopathy. *Clinical Nephrology* 1994;42:251-256.
Okada Y, Yoshikawa K, Matsue H, et al. Reversible MRI and CT findings in uremic encephalopathy. *Neuroradiology* 1991;33:524-526.
Raskin NH, Fishman RA. Neurologic disorders in renal failure. *The New England Journal of Medicine* 1976;294:143-148,204-210.
Schmidt M, Sitter T, Lederer SR, et al. Reversible MRI changes in a patient with uremic encephalopathy. *Journal of Nephrology* 2001;14:424-427.

267 Dialysis Dysequilibrium Syndrome

Perhaps 5% of patients undergoing hemodialysis will develop a transient delirium during or shortly after a dialysis run, and this is most likely to occur early on in treatment or with rapid dialysis.

ONSET

The delirium typically occurs several hours after the start of a dialysis run; rarely it may be delayed for up to 24 hours.

CLINICAL FEATURES

The delirium is typically accompanied by headache, nausea and muscle cramping, and seizures may occur; rarely one may see focal signs, papilledema or exophthalmos. The EEG typically reveals generalized slowing.

COURSE

The delirium remits spontaneously, generally within hours, or at the most a few days.

COMPLICATIONS

Complications are as described in the chapter on delirium.

ETIOLOGY

In all likelihood this syndrome results from cerebral edema occurring secondary to an extracellular to intracellular osmotic shift of water.

DIFFERENTIAL DIAGNOSIS

The principal differentials for delirium occurring during or shortly after dialysis include subdural hematoma and intracerebral hemorrhage.

TREATMENT

Symptomatic treatment is as described in the chapter on delirium. Future episodes may be prevented by scrupulous attention to fluid and electrolyte balance during dialysis runs and by slowing the dialysis run itself.

BIBLIOGRAPHY

Fraser CL, Arieff AI. Nervous system complications in uremia. *Annals of Internal Medicine* 1988;109:143-149.
Leonard A, Shapiro FL. Subdural hematoma in regularly hemodialyzed patients. *Annals of Internal Medicine* 1975;82:650-658.
Mawdsley C. Neurological complications of hemodialysis. *Proceedings of the Royal Society of Medicine* 1972;65:871-873.
Peterson H, Swanson AC. Acute encephalopathy occurring during hemodialysis. *Archives of Internal Medicine* 1964;113:877-880.
Raskin NH, Fishman RA. Neurologic disorders in renal failure. *The New England Journal of Medicine* 1976;294:143-148, 204-210.
Walters RJ, Fox NC, Crum WR, et al. Haemodialysis and cerebral oedema. *Nephron* 2001;87:143-147.

With significant shunting of portal blood past the liver and directly into the systemic circulation, as may be seen in hepatitis, cirrhosis or after surgical creation of a shunt, toxins normally removed by the liver reach the brain. When this toxic insult is relatively brief, the result is a potentially fully reversible delirium, known as hepatic encephalopathy or portal systemic encephalopathy. When the toxic insult is severe and repetitive or prolonged, however, irreversible brain damage may occur causing a permanent condition, known as acquired hepatocerebral degeneration.

ONSET

The onset of hepatic encephalopathy may be either acute or gradual, depending on the rapidity with which the underlying disease develops. For example, acute viral hepatitis may cause a delirium of fulminant onset; on the other hand, a slowly developing alcoholic cirrhosis may present with a delirium of very insidious onset.

The onset of acquired hepatocerebral degeneration is usually gradual, often punctuated by a series of intercurrent episodes of hepatic encephalopathy.

CLINICAL FEATURES

In hepatic encephalopathy the initial symptoms often consist of impaired judgment and difficulty with abstract thinking, perhaps also with some mild, evanescent confusion. With progression, the mood may change, often in the direction of euphoria; indeed in rare cases definite manic symptoms may be seen. Eventually a delirium appears which is often accompanied by drowsiness, sleep reversal, asterixis, myoclonus and constructional apraxia; a small minority may have seizures or focal signs, such as hemiparesis. Fetor hepaticus, a characteristic sickly sweet odor to the breath, may also be noted. With progression, stupor and coma eventually supervene, and are accompanied by rigidity and bilateral Babinski signs.

The EEG in hepatic encephalopathy initially shows generalized slowing; however, with progression triphasic delta waves often appear. Epileptiform abnormalities may be seen in a small minority of patients.

Although the blood ammonia level is elevated in almost all cases, the degree of its elevation is not a reliable guide to the severity of the encephalopathy; indeed, although quite rare, a normal ammonia level has been seen in some patients who progress to coma.

Acquired hepatocerebral degeneration is characterized by dementia and/or a sometimes complex movement disorder with elements of parkinsonism, dystonia, tremor, chorea and ataxia. MRI scanning may reveal, on T1-weighted images, an increased signal intensity in the globus pallidus.

COURSE

The mortality rate in hepatic encephalopathy rises with the severity of the encephalopathy to the point where most patients who progress to coma have a fatal outcome. Generally, patients who survive experience a full recovery; however, depending on the underlying liver disease and the presence or absence of precipitating factors, recurrences may occur.

Acquired hepatocerebral degeneration is, in the natural course of events, irreversible and, with repeated intercurrent bouts of hepatic encephalopathy, progressively worsens.

COMPLICATIONS

The complications of delirium and of dementia are as described in their respective chapters.

ETIOLOGY

As noted in the introduction, both hepatic encephalopathy and acquired hepatocerebral degeneration are the result of the action of toxins found in portal blood on the brain. Although the identity of the toxin or toxins has not been clarified, various candidates have been proposed, including ammonia, mercaptans, various aromatic amino acids, short-chain fatty acids and gamma-aminobutyric acid.

The most common causes of portal-systemic shunting are alcoholic cirrhosis and viral hepatitis. In many cases, the onset of any particular episode of encephalopathy may be traced to an event which increased the nitrogenous load in the gut beyond the detoxifying capacity of whatever hepatic tissue remained. Examples include high protein meals, blood, as for example from bleeding esophageal varices or peptic ulcers, and constipation. Other precipitants include diuretics, hypokalemia, azotemia, anesthesia, surgery, various infections, and exposure to alcohol or to sedative hypnotics.

Pathologic changes in hepatic encephalopathy are limited to a partial breakdown of the blood-brain barrier and an increased number of Alzheimer-type II astrocytes. In fatal cases cerebral edema is found.

The etiology of acquired hepatocerebral degeneration, although clearly tied to repeated episodes of hepatic encephalopathy, is not clearly understood; there is some evidence for an accumulation of manganese. Pathologically, there is widespread spongiform change throughout the cerebral cortex and basal ganglia.

DIFFERENTIAL DIAGNOSIS

Especially in alcoholics, hepatic encephalopathy must be distinguished from delirium tremens, hypoglycemia, Wernicke's encephalopathy, and subdural hematoma.

Acquired hepatocerebral degeneration is distinguished from alcoholic dementia by the presence of abnormal involuntary movements, and from Wilson's disease by the normal copper and ceruloplasmin levels.

TREATMENT

Hepatic encephalopathy is treated by attending to the underlying cause and any precipitating factors, and also by reducing the protein load in the gut. Patients are placed on a 20 g low-protein diet; lactulose is given in a dose of 30 to 45 ml hourly until the patient begins to have bowel movements; the dose is then adjusted to produce three or four soft stools per day (usually achieved with 30 to 45 ml of lactulose three to four times a day). In severe cases, neomycin, from 4 to 8 g daily in divided doses, may be given. As improvement occurs, however, neomycin is generally discontinued to prevent ototoxicity or nephrotoxicity. In contrast to other deliria, antipsychotics and, especially, benzodiazepines are generally contraindicated because they may exacerbate clinical symptoms; however, if restraints fail to control an agitated patient, haloperidol may be used, keeping in mind that lower doses are required. Some patients may experience symptomatic improvement with intravenous flumazenil; however, this should generally be reserved for emergent situations.

When hepatic failure is chronic, repeat episodes of hepatic encephalopathy may be prevented by avoiding precipitating factors, instituting modest protein restriction of about 60 gm/day, and administering sufficient lactulose (usually 30 to 40 ml/d) to ensure at least two soft bowel movements per day.

Acquired hepatocerebral degeneration may show significant improvement with liver transplantation.

BIBLIOGRAPHY

Burkhard PR, Delavelle J, Du Pasquier R, et al. Chronic parkinsonism associated with cirrhosis: a distinct subset of acquired hepatocerebral degeneration. *Archives of Neurology* 2003;60:521-528.

Cadranel JF, Lebiez E, Di Martino V, et al. Focal neurological signs in hepatic encephalopathy in cirrhotic patients: an underestimated entity. *The American Journal of Gastroenterology* 2001;96:515-518.

Ficker DM, Westmoreland BF, Sharbrough FW. Epileptiform abnormalities in hepatic encephalopathy. *Journal of Clinical Neurophysiology* 1997;14:230-234.

Finlayson MH, Superville B. Distribution of cerebral lesions in acquired hepatocerebral degeneration. *Brain* 1981;104:79-95.

Fraser CL, Arieff AI. Hepatic encephalopathy. *The New England Journal of Medicine* 1985;313:865-873.

Hernandez-Avila CA, Shoemaker WJ, Ortega-Soto HA. Plasma concentrations of endogenous benzodiazepine-receptor ligands in patients with hepatic encephalopathy: a comparative study. *Journal of Psychiatry & Neuroscience* 1998;23:217-222.

Jog MS, Lange AE. Chronic acquired hepatocerebral degeneration: case reports and new insights. *Movement Disorders* 1995;10:714-722.

Krieger D, Drieger S, Jansen O, et al. Manganese and chronic hepatic encephalopathy. *Lancet* 1995;346:274.

Laccetti M, Manes G, Uomo G, et al. Flumazenil in the treatment of acute hepatic encephalopathy in cirrhotic patients: a double-blind randomized placebo controlled study. *Digestive and Liver Disease* 2000;32:335-338.

Read AE, Laidlaw J, Sherlock S. Neuropsychiatric complications of portocaval anastomosis. *Lancet* 1961;1:961-964.

Summerskill WHJ, Davidson EA, Sherlock S, et al. The neuropsychiatric syndrome associated with hepatic cirrhosis and an extensive portal collateral circulation. *Quarterly Journal of Medicine* 1956;25:245-266.

Victor M, Adams RD, Cole M. The acquired "non-Wilsonian" type of chronic hepatocerebral degeneration. *Medicine* 1965;44:345-396.

269 Fahr's Syndrome

Fahr's syndrome is characterized by the occurrence of a movement disorder or dementia secondary to calcification of the basal ganglia. As noted under etiology, below, this may occur either secondary to some other disorder, as for example hypoparathyroidism, or on an idiopathic basis, in which case one speaks of Fahr's disease.

Fahr's syndrome is probably a rare disorder.

ONSET

Regardless of whether the presentation is with a movement disorder or a dementia, the onset is generally insidious in the early or middle adult years.

CLINICAL FEATURES

The movement disorder is generally a parkinsonism; choreoathetosis or dystonia may also be seen. Less commonly, there may be dysarthria and ataxia.

The dementia is characterized by poor memory, poor concentration and overall slowness of thought.

Rarely, one may see depression, psychosis or obsessions and compulsions.

CT scanning reveals symmetric calcification of the basal ganglia, and, in severe cases, the thalamus, dentate nuclei of the cerebellum and the gray-white junction in the cerebral and cerebellar cortices.

In cases occurring secondary to hypoparathyroidism, hypocalcemia may cause seizures.

Serum calcium, phosphorous and parathyroid hormone levels may or may not be abnormal, depending on the underlying cause.

COURSE

The course is one of very slow progression, and in cases presenting with dementia, many years may pass before a movement disorder occurs.

COMPLICATIONS

The complications of dementia are as described in that chapter.

ETIOLOGY

Microscopically, calcification is seen in the same areas imaged on CT scanning.

Fahr's syndrome may occur secondary to hypoparathyroidism (either idiopathic or surgical), pseudo-hypoparathyroidism or pseudo-pseudo-hypoparathyroidism. Idiopathic cases, that is to say cases of Fahr's disease, may occur sporadically or be inherited in an autosomal dominant fashion: in one such family, linkage was established to chromosome 14q.

DIFFERENTIAL DIAGNOSIS

The most important aspect of differential diagnosis is to keep in mind that asymptomatic basal ganglia calcification is a common finding, being noted incidentally on up to 0.6% of CT scans. Consequently, the diagnosis of Fahr's syndrome should not be made simply on the basis of a finding of calcification on CT scanning, but must be reserved for cases where this calcification is accompanied by a typical clinical picture. Should the clinical picture be atypical, then one would have to consider the possibility that the patient had another disorder which just happened to be accompanied by calcification of the basal ganglia.

TREATMENT

In secondary cases, treatment is directed at the underlying cause; Fahr's disease, as yet, has no specific treatment.

The general treatment of dementia is as outlined in that chapter; if antipsychotics are used care must be taken to not aggravate any parkinsonism. The parkinsonism may or may not respond to levodopa.

BIBLIOGRAPHY

Chabot B, Roulland C, Dolifus S. Schizophrenia and familial idiopathic basal ganglia calcification: a case report. *Psychological Medicine* 2001;31:741-747.

Geschwind DH, Loginov M, Stern JM. Identification of a locus on chromosome 14q for idiopathic basal ganglia calcification (Fahr disease). *American Journal of Human Genetics* 1999;65:764-772.

Koller WC, Cochran JW, Klawans HL. Calcification of the basal ganglia: computerized tomography and clinical correlation. *Neurology* 1979; 29:328-333.

Lopez-Villegas D, Kulisevsky J, Deus J, et al. Neuropsychological alterations in patients with computed tomography-detected basal ganglia calcification. *Archives of Neurology* 1996;53:251-256.

Trautner RJ, Cummings JL, Read SL, et al. Idiopathic basal ganglia calcification and organic mood disorder. *The American Journal of Psychiatry* 1988;145:350-353.

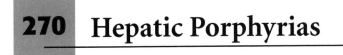

270 Hepatic Porphyrias

Of the hepatic porphyrias, four can cause delirium. Three of these are inherited in an autosomal dominant fashion, namely acute intermittent porphyria, variegate porphyria, and hereditary coproporphyria, whereas the fourth, ALA dehydratase deficiency, is an autosomal recessive disorder. Acute intermittent porphyria is found worldwide and may have an incidence as high as 5 to 10 per 100,000. Variegate porphyria is rare in the United States but relatively common in Sweden and among whites in South Africa. Hereditary coproporphyria appears to be quite rare. ALA dehydratase deficiency is extraordinarily rare, with only a handful of cases reported worldwide, and is not considered further here. Acute intermittent porphyria is more common among females than males.

From a clinical viewpoint, these three hepatic porphyrias are essentially the same, with the exception that both variegate porphyria and hereditary coproporphyria may cause a photosensitive rash, a finding not seen in acute intermittent porphyria.

Of some historical interest is the fact that the periodic "madness" of King George III represented attacks of hepatic porphyria.

ONSET

These disorders are episodic illnesses with the first attack usually appearing in adolescence or young adulthood. The episodes themselves tend to come on acutely and are often precipitated by one of the many drugs noted under Etiology or by infection, menstruation, or pregnancy.

CLINICAL FEATURES

Up to half of all attacks are characterized by a delirium which is often marked by lability, hallucinations and delusions of persecution; in severe cases stupor or coma may occur. Rarely, rather than a delirium, the attack may present with a psychosis with auditory hallucinations and delusions.

Almost all patients experience abdominal pain during an attack, which is usually accompanied by nausea, vomiting, and constipation, or, occasionally, diarrhea.

Most patients also experience a polyneuropathy, which is primarily motor. This may progress rapidly to a quadriplegia, and respiratory failure may occur.

Seizures occur in a minority of patients; rarely, status epilepticus may occur.

Cranial nerve palsies occur rarely, presenting most commonly with ophthalmoplegia or facial palsy, which may be bilateral.

Hyponatremia may occur in a small number of patients and may be severe, with sodium values below 100 mEq/L. This apparently is secondary to a combination of inappropriate ADH secretion and either intestinal or renal sodium loss.

Hypertension and tachycardia both occur in a majority of patients.

Patients with variegate porphyria or hereditary coproporphyria may or may not have a photosensitive rash, which may or may not be contemporaneous with the other symptoms described above.

During an attack a 24-hour urine sample generally reveals elevated porphobilinogen and aminolevulinic acid in all three of these forms of porphyria. Both variegate porphyria and hereditary coproporphyria also generally display elevated urinary coproporphyrin. Distinguishing between variegate and hereditary coproporphyria requires a 24-hour stool collection for coproporphyrin and protoporphyrin. In variegate porphyria, protoporphyrin is greater than coproporphyrin; in hereditary coproporphyria the converse is true. In between attacks these abnormalities may or may not be demonstrable.

During an attack of acute intermittent porphyria, MRI scanning may reveal multiple areas of increased signal intensity in the cerebrum.

COURSE

The duration of individual attacks ranges from a few days up to several weeks. Although most patients recover, death may occur secondary to respiratory failure or cardiac arrhythmias. As noted earlier, repeated attacks are prone to occur.

COMPLICATIONS

Complications are as described in the chapter on delirium.

ETIOLOGY

Acute intermittent, variegate, and hereditary coproporphyria each result from mutations in the genes for different enzymes in the biosynthetic pathway for heme: porphobilinogen deaminase (also known as hydroxymethylbilane synthase) on chromosome 11 in acute intermittent porphyria, protoporyphyrinogen oxidase on chromosome 1 in variegate porphyria, and coproporphyrinogen oxidase on chromosome 3 in hereditary coproporphyria. Although, as mentioned earlier, these are autosomal dominant conditions, these enzymatic deficiencies generally do not become symptomatic until the heme biosynthetic pathway is stressed by a specific precipitating factor; consequently many individuals with the mutation remain asymptomatic carriers.

Precipitants for attacks of hepatic porphyria include infection, menstruation, pregnancy, fasting (or merely a carbohydrate-restricted diet), or any one of a large number of drugs, including barbiturates, meprobamate, methyprylon, ethanol, ergot preparations, progesterone preparations, danazol, phenytoin, valproate, carbamazepine, nortriptyline, methyldopa, glutethimide, chlorpropamide, chloroquine, griseofulvin, and sulfonamides. Importantly, the following drugs appear to be safe: propranolol, chlorpromazine, trifluoperazine, diphenhydramine, diazepam, gabapentin, aspirin and acetaminophen.

The mechanism whereby the delirium is produced is not clear. One theory holds that aminolevulinic acid is an agonist at gamma-aminobutyric acid (GABA) receptor sites, creating a hypergabaergic state. At autopsy some brains have shown small areas of focal ischemia; however, these may be secondary to the hypertension seen during the attack.

DIFFERENTIAL DIAGNOSIS

The combination of delirium and abdominal pain is highly suggestive; the addition of a primarily motor polyneuropathy or seizures is quite distinctive.

Polyarteritis nodosa may produce a similar picture: here, however, one generally finds a pronounced leukocytosis and also proteinuria and an elevated ESR.

TREATMENT

Acute attacks may be treated with a high carbohydrate diet, or, if the patient is NPO, intravenous glucose in a total daily dose of approximately 300 gm. Although in mild cases these dietary changes may be sufficient, most cases will require treatment with intravenous hematin, which effectively suppresses the heme biosynthetic pathway. Hematin treatment is generally followed by a resolution of all symptoms within a matter of four days, with the exception of the motor polyneuropathy which may take months or even a year to resolve.

Various measures may also be employed on a symptomatic basis including chlorpromazine, in doses of from 25 to 50 mg every 4 to 6 hours, which may not only control the delirium but may also reduce abdominal pain. Meperidine may be used for persistent abdominal pain, and propranolol, in daily doses ranging from 20 to 200 mg, may relieve hypertension and tachycardia. Chloral hydrate may be used for sleep, gabapentin for seizures and diazepam for status epilepticus.

Prevention is accomplished by avoiding the drugs listed above, maintaining a high carbohydrate diet and by vigorously treating infections. When attacks are associated with menstruation, leutenizing hormone releasing hormone may prevent attacks. When attacks persist despite these measures, prophylactic hematin may be considered.

BIBLIOGRAPHY

Becker DM, Kramer S. The neurological manifestations of porphyria: a review. *Medicine* 1977;56:411-423.

Goldberg A. Acute intermittent porphyria. *Quarterly Journal of Medicine* 1959;28:183-209.

Hierons R. Changes in the nervous system in acute porphyria. *Brain* 1957;80:176-192.

King PH, Bragdon AC. MRI reveals multiple reversible cerebral lesions in an attack of acute intermittent porphyria. *Neurology* 1991;41:1300-1302.

McAlpine I, Hunter R. The "insanity" of King George III: a classic case of porphyria. *British Medical Journal* 1966;1:65-71.

Menawat AS, Panwar RB, Kochar DK, et al. Propranolol in acute intermittent porphyria. *Postgraduate Medical Journal* 1979;55:546-547.

Muhlbauer JE, Pathak MA, Tishler PV, et al. Variegate porphyria in New England. *The Journal of the American Medical Association* 1982;247:3095-3102.

Suarez JI, Cohen ML, Larkin J, et al. Acute intermittent porphyria: clinico-pathologic correlation. Report of a case and review of the literature. *Neurology* 1997;48:1678-1683.

Tatum WO, Zachariah SB. Gabapentin treatment of seizures in acute intermittent porphyria. *Neurology* 1995;45:1216-1217.

Respiratory failure is characterized by hypoxemia and, if hypoventilation is present (as is often the case), hypercapnia. Both hypoxemia and hypercapnia, either individually or in combination, may cause delirium. Furthermore, severe hypoxemia may be followed by a post-anoxic dementia.

ONSET

The onset of delirium parallels the onset of the respiratory failure and may range from acute, as for example when a patient with compensated COPD is over-sedated or develops an aspiration pneumonia, to gradual, as may occur in cases of very slowly progressive COPD.

CLINICAL FEATURES

In hypoxemia, symptoms typically appear by the time Pao_2 reaches 50 mm Hg. Inattentiveness, insomnia, and drowsiness appear; fatigue may occur, and patients typically show a delayed reaction time and have difficulty completing any complex motor tasks. Eventually a delirium occurs that may be accompanied by agitation, delusions, and hallucinations. Cyanosis is not a helpful sign, as many clinicians are unable to recognize its presence until the Pao_2 falls below 50. Levels below 30 typically produce coma and lower levels may cause neuronal death, and, as noted earlier, survivors may be left with a post-anoxic dementia.

In hypercapnia of acute onset, symptoms tend to appear as the arterial $Paco_2$ approaches 70 mm Hg. By contrast, in gradually progressive cases adaptation occurs, and some patients may remain asymptomatic despite a $Paco_2$ of 90 mm Hg or above. Apprehension and lethargy may be seen and headache is particularly common. Eventually, as the $Paco_2$ rises a delirium occurs during which delusions and hallucinations may appear. Typically, these delirious patients appear intoxicated, a finding that prompted the older term "CO_2 narcosis." Asterixis and myoclonus may occur, and there may be bilateral extensor plantar responses and, rarely, seizures; occasionally papilledema may be found. Eventually, with progressive rises, coma supervenes.

COURSE

The course is determined by the underlying etiology.

COMPLICATIONS

Complications of delirium and of dementia are as described in those chapters.

ETIOLOGY

Common causes of respiratory failure include chronic obstructive pulmonary disease, asthma, pneumonia, pulmonary edema, the Pickwickian syndrome, myasthenia gravis, the Guillain-Barre syndrome and amyotrophic lateral sclerosis.

DIFFERENTIAL DIAGNOSIS

Delirium secondary to respiratory failure is generally readily recognized as such, given the more or less obvious respiratory distress of the patient. Often, however, a delirium in patients with respiratory failure will be multifactorial, with contributions from fever, sepsis, electrolyte imbalances and various medications.

TREATMENT

Treatment is directed not only at the underlying etiology but also toward ensuring adequate oxygenation. Oxygen, however, must be administered with extreme caution to those with chronic hypercapnia. In these cases adaptation has rendered hypercapnia an ineffective respiratory stimulant, and patients breathe on "hypoxic drive" alone. Too much oxygen, by removing this drive, may plunge the patient into acute life-threatening respiratory failure.

The general treatment of delirium is as discussed in that chapter. Great caution must be exercised in the use of any medications that might sedate patients, including benzodiazepines and most antipsychotics.

BIBLIOGRAPHY

Grant I, Heaton RK, McSweeney AJ, et al. Brain dysfunction in COPD. *Chest* 1980;77(Suppl 2):308-309.

Grant I, Heaton RK, McSweeney AJ, et al. Neuropsychologic findings in hypoxemic chronic obstructive pulmonary disease. *Archives of Internal Medicine* 1982;142:1470-1476.

Grant I, Prigatano GP, Heaton RK, et al. Progressive neuropsychiatric impairment and hypoxia. Relationship in chronic obstructive pulmonary disease. *Archives of General Psychiatry* 1987;44:999-1006.

Meissner HH, Franklin C. Extreme hypercapnia in a fully alert patient. *Chest* 1992;102:1298-1299.

Mouallem M, Wolf I. Olanzapine-induced respiratory failure. *The American Journal of Geriatric Psychiatry* 2001;9:304-305.

272 Tricyclic Antidepressants

All tricyclic antidepressants share a common three-ringed structure, from the middle ring of which arises a carbon side chain, which, in turn, has a nitrogen atom at its end. The tricyclics are usefully divided into two groups according to the number of methyl groups attached to this nitrogen atom. The tertiary amines have two methyl groups and include amitriptyline, imipramine, trimipramine and doxepin. The secondary amines have only one methyl group and include nortriptyline, desipramine, protriptyline, and maprotiline. Clomipramine and amoxapine, although tricyclics, are treated in separate chapters because of the unique therapeutic effect and side effect profile of clomipramine and, in the case of amoxapine, because of the antipsychotic activity of one of its metabolites.

The mechanism whereby the tricyclics induce their antidepressant effect is not clear. All of these agents block, to varying degrees, the reuptake of both serotonin and norepinephrine from the synaptic cleft: the tertiary amines are primarily serotoninergic, whereas the secondary amines (and maprotilene) are primarily noradrenergic. Initially, this reuptake blockade was felt to be the mechanism; however, as this blockade occurs immediately, and the antidepressant effect takes weeks to appear, attention has now shifted to the long-term compensatory changes that occur with prolonged treatment. Specifically, all these agents downregulate, to varying degrees, post-synaptic serotonin receptors, post-synaptic beta receptors and both post- and presynaptic alpha receptors. The fact that the time course for these downregulatory changes and the time course for the antidepressant effects are similar suggests strongly that the two are mechanistically linked, and research is currently exploring this possibility.

The most important indications for the tricyclics are as follows: a depressive episode of major depression or bipolar disorder or schizoaffective disorder; dysthymia; a "postpsychotic" depression of schizophrenia; premenstrual syndrome; posttraumatic stress disorder; panic disorder; generalized anxiety disorder; bulimia; various secondary depressions (e.g., the depression of Parkinson's disease); and migraine prophylaxis. Other indications include enuresis, separation anxiety disorder, attention-deficit/hyperactivity and nicotine dependence. Protriptyline has been used in the obstructive form of sleep apnea, and various tricyclics may relieve the cataplexy seen in narcolepsy. Interestingly, tricyclics such as nortriptyline may reduce the pathologic crying and laughter seen in pseudobulbar palsy.

A very important indication for tricyclic antidepressants is any chronically painful condition that has failed to respond to routine medical or surgical management. One must bear in mind that these agents are effective regardless of whether the patient has any depressive symptoms; their analgesic effect is independent of any antidepressant effect. Both amitriptyline and nortriptyline have been used; low doses (e.g., 75 mg of amitriptyline) may be effective; however, at times, full antidepressant doses may be required. Should the response to an antidepressant be less than robust, an antipsychotic may be added. Traditionally, fluphenazine in doses of 2.5 to 5 mg/day has been used and may convert a "nonresponder" to a "responder." Blood levels of the tricyclic should be obtained before and after starting the antipsychotic because its introduction may be followed by a rise in the blood level and a dosage reduction may be required.

Guidelines for selecting which tricyclic to use for a specific indication in a specific given patient are discussed under Therapeutic Usage. At this point, one should know that in most cases tertiary tricyclics have relatively prominent serotoninergic activity, whereas those with a secondary amine structure are relatively more adrenergic. In general, patients with psychomotor agitation tend to do better, at least initially, with tertiary amines, whereas those with psychomotor retardation may initially do better with the secondary amines.

PHARMACOKINETICS

All of the tricyclics are well absorbed after oral administration; all reach peak blood levels within 2 to 8 hours, and all are strongly protein bound. Metabolism occurs in the liver by either demethylation of the side ring or by hydroxylation of the ring structure itself: demethylation is primarily via cytochrome P450 2D6, whereas hydroxylation occurs via several cytochrome P450 enzymes, including 3A4, 1A2 and 2C19. There is an extraordinarily wide inter-patient variability in the activity of these enzymes, and, on the same dose, up to 40-fold variations may be seen in blood level.

Estimates as to half-life vary considerably among studies. For clinical purposes, however, the following rough guidelines are useful: 6 to 36 hours for amitriptyline, doxepin, imipramine, and desipramine; 1 to 2 days for nortriptyline and maprotiline; and 3 days for protriptyline. It must also be borne in mind that a small minority of patients, perhaps 10% or less of Caucasians, are "slow hydroxylaters," and such patients may have very high blood levels on relatively modest doses.

Amitriptyline has as its major metabolite nortriptyline, which in turn is hydroxylated to 10-hydroxynortriptyline, which is pharmacologically active. Similarly, imipramine has as its major metabolite desipramine, which in turn is hydroxylated to 2-hydroxydesipramine, which is also pharmacologically active.

Doxepin has as its major metabolite desmethyldoxepin, again a pharmacologically active compound.

SIDE EFFECTS

Sedation is prominent with amitriptyline, trimipramine, doxepin, and with imipramine to a somewhat lesser extent. Mild degrees of sedation may be seen with nortriptyline and maprotiline. Desipramine and protriptyline may have slight or no sedative effects or may at times have a mild stimulant effect.

Anticholinergic side effects, to varying degrees, may occur with all tricyclics. They include dry mouth, blurry vision, constipation, and urinary hesitancy. At times urinary retention may occur, and although this is more common in the setting of prostatic hypertrophy, it may at times be seen in men with normal prostates, and may even occasionally occur in women, especially those with a concurrent lower urinary tract infection. Anticholinergic effects are very prominent with amitriptyline and protriptyline, somewhat less common with imipramine, doxepin, desipramine, and nortriptyline, and less still with maprotiline.

Weight gain can be a very troubling side effect, especially because patients often require long-term treatment. Amitriptyline, doxepin, and, to a somewhat lesser extent, imipramine are the main offenders. Although some patients may gain only a few pounds, others may suffer a gain of 10 to 20 or more pounds. With maprotiline and nortriptyline, weight gain is slight or absent, and with desipramine some patients may actually lose a small amount of weight.

Other, not uncommon side effects include fine tremor, flushing and increased perspiration, allergic rashes, and sexual side effects including ejaculatory dysfunction, delayed ejaculation, painful ejaculation, anorgasmia, decreased libido, and decreased lubrication. Speech blockage occasionally occurs but is rarely spontaneously reported by patients.

Cardiovascular effects are often a major concern, particularly in the elderly or those with heart disease. Orthostatic hypotension is common with amitriptyline, doxepin and imipramine; less common with desipramine, protriptyline, and maprotiline; and least common with nortriptyline. Elderly patients, in particular, must be watched closely for the resulting orthostatic dizziness to prevent falls and fractured hips.

All tricyclics slow cardiac conduction, with resultant prolongation of the PR interval, QRS duration, and corrected QT interval. In otherwise healthy patients these prolongations are insignificant; however, complications may develop in cardiac patients. Second or higher degree AV block may occur, as may bundle branch blocks. All the tricyclics have a quinidine-like effect. Thus in some cases they may be antiarrhythmic, and this is often the case with therapeutic blood levels. However, as the blood level rises above 500 ng/ml (or at even lower levels in those with heart disease), ventricular arrhythmias may occur.

Cardiac contractility may or may not be depressed.

Benign ECG changes may be seen with all the tricyclics and consist of flattening or inversion of the T-wave.

All tricyclics lower the seizure threshold; however, this is clinically significant only in the case of maprotiline, clomipramine and amoxapine: in the case of maprotiline, the risk of seizures rises at doses of only 75 mg and becomes significant at doses of over 200 mg daily.

Rare side effects include hyponatremia secondary to SIADH, agranulocytosis, jaundice, and what has been termed "behavioral toxicity," with poor memory, confusion, or agitation. Such "behavioral toxicity" is unusual at total tricyclic levels below 450 ng/ml.

One must keep in mind that the tricyclics may precipitate mania in patients with bipolar disorder or schizoaffective disorder, bipolar type, and may also exacerbate the symptoms of schizophrenia.

All tricyclics are excreted in the breast milk; however, the amount found in the infant is generally negligible. Whether tricyclics are teratogenic is not known.

DRUG-DRUG INTERACTIONS

A variety of drugs, by inhibiting hepatic microsomal enzymes, may cause increased tricyclic blood levels. Most of the SSRIs, by inhibiting the CYP2D6 enzyme, impair the demethylation and hydroxylation of tricyclics: in this regard, the SSRIs may be ranked with regard to their potency as CYP2D6 inhibitors, with fluoxetine and paroxetine being most potent, followed by sertraline and finally citalopram and escitalopram, which have very little effect on CYP2D6; fluvoxamine has essentially none. Fluvoxamine, on the other hand, does inhibit the cytochrome P450 enzymes 3A4, 1A2 and 2C19, and thereby impairs hydroxylation, thus increasing tricyclic levels. Other drugs capable of increasing tricyclic blood levels include methylphenidate, amphetamine, antipsychotics, cimetidine, methadone, and, to a lesser degree, oral contraceptives. The elevation seen with fluoxetine, paroxetine, or methylphenidate may be 100% or more; those seen with antipsychotics are substantially less.

Other drugs, by inducing hepatic enzymes, may cause a reduction of tricyclic levels. These include barbiturates, carbamazepine and tobacco smoke, and, to a small degree, phenytoin.

Tricyclics may inhibit the metabolism of phenytoin, leading to elevated phenytoin levels.

Tricyclics and alpha-2 autoreceptor agonists may have mutually antagonistic pharmacodynamic effects. The antihypertensives clonidine and guanabenz both produce their hypotensive effect by stimulating alpha-2 receptors; tricyclics block this effect, and blood pressure control may be lost.

Tricyclics may block the uptake of guanethidine into the presynaptic neuron, thus blocking its hypotensive effect.

Additive effects may occur between the tricyclics and other "quinidine-like" drugs, such as class I antiarrhythmics quinidine, disopyramide, and procainamide. If a tricyclic is used concurrently with a class I antiarrhythmic, the dose of the antiarrhythmic may have to be reduced to retain the antiarrhythmic effect and to prevent precipitating an arrhythmia.

As discussed in detail in the chapter on monoamine oxidase inhibitors (MAOIs), tricyclics should not be added to a preexisting regimen of an MAOI. In treatment-resistant patients, however, an MAOI may be cautiously added to a tricyclic without incurring a significantly increased risk of a hypertensive crisis.

The combination of sedative tricyclics with hypnotics, sedatives, or alcohol produces further central nervous system depression. Likewise, the addition of an anticholinergic tricyclic to low-potency first generation antipsychotics or to anticholinergics such as atropine, scopolamine, benztropine and so forth, produces an augmented anticholinergic effect.

OVERDOSAGE

Overdosage of from 1 to 2 grams, or total tricyclic levels of over 1000 nanogram/ml, are generally associated with serious symptoms. An anticholinergic delirium is common, as described in that chapter. Coma may ensue, and seizures, which are more common with maprotiline, may occur.

Hypotension and respiratory depression may be seen.

Cardiac effects are common. As might be expected, cardiac conduction is slowed; indeed, in patients with normal conduction systems, a QRS duration of over 0.1 second is highly suggestive of a serious overdose. Tachycardia is common, and arrhythmias may occur, especially when the QRS duration rises above 0.16 seconds: these include ventricular tachycardia and torsades de pointes.

Patients should be admitted to an intensive care unit and undergo cardiac monitoring for at least a day. If the patient is seen within 8 hours of the overdose, gastric lavage and activated charcoal are used; as enterohepatic recirculation occurs, prolonged administration of activated charcoal through a nasogastric tube may be helpful. Intubation and respiratory support may be required, and antiarrythmics may be required: in this regard, class I antiarrhythmics are contraindicated.

Seizures may be treated with intravenous lorazepam; phenytoin may or may not prevent them.

Although physostigmine, as described in the chapter on anticholinergic delirium, may dramatically reverse delirium or coma, it has little or no effect on arrhythmias and may precipitate seizures.

THERAPEUTIC USAGE

Amitriptyline is available in 10, 25, 50, 75, 100 and 150 mg tablets, imipramine in 10, 25 and 50 mg tablets, trimipramine in 25, 50 and 100 mg capsules, doxepin in 10, 25, 50, 75, 100 and 150 mg capsules, nortriptyline in 10, 25, 50 and 75 mg capsules, desipramine in 10, 25, 50, 75 and 150 mg tablets, protriptyline in 5 and 10 mg capsules, and maprotiline in 25, 50 and 75 mg tablets.

In selecting a tricyclic for the treatment of a depressive episode, dysthymia, postpsychotic depression, or premenstrual syndrome, one is guided by the following: the effect of anticipated side effects in any particular patient; the kind of psychomotor change present, if any; and a history of past response to a tricyclic. As noted earlier, the various tricyclics vary widely in their ability to produce certain side effects such as sedation, anticholinergic effects, weight gain, and orthostatic hypotension. In general, the tricyclic with the most favorable side effect profile is nortriptyline; desipramine runs a close second. Side effects with amitriptyline, imipramine, and doxepin are considerable. The long half-life of protriptyline makes it difficult to use, and the risk of seizures with maprotiline argues for caution in its use.

As mentioned in the introduction, some patients with psychomotor agitation seem to do better with a tertiary amine, and in such cases doxepin is a good choice. Conversely, those with prominent psychomotor retardation may do better with a secondary amine, such as nortriptyline or desipramine. This guideline, however, is not hard and fast; even extraordinarily agitated patients may eventually do well with a secondary amine such as nortriptyline.

A history of a past good response to a certain tricyclic is a good predictor of a current response. Concern about side effects, however, may prevail over this guideline. For example, if a patient gained 60 pounds while on amitriptyline in the past, switching to its secondary amine metabolite, nortriptyline, for current treatment may be prudent.

Patients should be clearly informed that, in general, once an optimum dose is reached, at least 1 or 2 weeks must elapse before any significant benefit can be seen. They must also be encouraged to endure any side effects that immediately occur and wait until a therapeutic response appears before deciding whether the side effects are "worth it." It must also be emphatically stated that the tricyclics only "work" if taken regularly; using them on a "PRN" basis does not help.

Once a particular tricyclic is chosen, the average "optimum" dose is noted, and, in general, the patient is started on one quarter to one third of the optimum dose, with increases of similar increments every 3 to 5 days until either the optimum is reached or limiting side effects occur. This incremental increase in dosage may be hastened in hospitalized patients who are closely monitored. Average "optimum" doses are as follows: 150 to 200 mg for amitriptyline, imipramine, trimipramine, desipramine, and doxepin; 50 to 75 mg for nortriptyline; 20 to 60 mg for protriptyline; and 150 mg for maprotiline. As noted in the section on side effects, when using maprotiline, increasing the dose in smaller increments and at longer intervals may be prudent. In any case 225 mg is the recommended maximum for this medicine.

Giving tricyclics in divided doses is rarely necessary; in almost all cases a single bedtime dose is satisfactory. An exception to this rule may occur if stimulation occurs with either desipramine or protriptyline; in such cases the dose may be divided or, in most cases, simply given once a day in the morning. Another exception would be when a bedtime dose produces limiting side effects, whereas divided doses render the side effects tolerable.

Much has been written about "therapeutic" blood levels for the tricyclics. Unfortunately, with the exception of nortriptyline, the data regarding the existence or lack of a curvilinear dose-response curve (i.e., a "therapeutic window") are conflicting. Of all the tricyclics, only nortriptyline has been shown to have a "therapeutic window." Levels of nortriptyline below 50 ng/ml and levels above 150 ng/ml are both associated with a poor response; hence the dosage should be adjusted to achieve a blood level of about 100 ng/ml.

For the rest of the tricyclics, only a rough estimate can be given for a minimum blood level below which a therapeutic response is unlikely. If the total tricyclic level is below the range of 100 to 200 ng/ml, the likelihood of a response is reduced. For the tertiary amines, amitriptyline, imipramine, trimipramine and doxepin, this "total" tricyclic level equals the level of the tertiary amine and of its pharmacologically active desmethylated metabolite: nortriptyline, desipramine, and desmethyldoxepin, respectively. As yet, an upper limit, or therapeutic window, has not been reliably demonstrated for tricyclics other than nortriptyline.

After an average "optimum" dose has been reached, only in the case of nortriptyline should one routinely obtain a blood level. In the case of all other tricyclics, a blood level is optional; however, in doubtful or questionable cases, obtain a level to make sure that the patient is not such a "rapid metabolizer" that the level is below 100 ng/ml. One may also want to obtain a level when concerned about possible cardiotoxicity, and in such cases a simultaneous ECG should also be obtained and compared with a pre-treatment ECG. Blood levels are obtained after at least 4 or 5 half-lives have elapsed and are drawn between 8 and 12 hours after the bedtime dose.

In cases where side effects preclude the attainment of an average "optimum" dose, one may want to check a blood level before switching to another agent. Some patients are slow metabolizers and may have relatively high blood levels on "low" doses. For example, in an occasional patient, a dose of 75 mg of doxepin may yield a total tricyclic level of over 150 ng/ml. In cases where the blood level is low, yet side effects are prominent, treating the side effect directly may be possible, thus allowing for a dose increase. Constipation may be countered by psyllium, blurry vision by reading glasses, and dry mouth with sugar-free lemon drops. Furthermore, all anticholinergic side effects, if necessary, may be treated with bethanechol at a dosage of about 10 mg t.i.d. Daytime sedation may be relieved by giving all or most of the dose at bedtime. Fine tremor may be relieved by propranolol. However, in cases where side effects preclude a dose increase and the blood level is low, continuing the drug makes no sense, and the patient should be switched to an agent with a more favorable side effect profile.

After an "optimum" dose has been achieved and the blood level, if obtained, is appropriate, one must wait at least 1 to 2 weeks to assess whether or not an initial response has occurred. It must be borne in mind that, for many patients, 6 weeks are required to see a significant response at any given dose; indeed, in a not inconsiderable minority, 3 or 4 months may be required before a complete response is seen. Patients should be informed that, after an initial response, one or more setbacks are to be expected before an enduring robust response is seen.

In cases where only a partial response is seen, despite treatment at an adequate blood level for an adequate duration, provided that no limiting side effects are seen, one may gradually increase the dose of the tricyclic (with the exception of nortriptyline) until limiting side effects do occur. At times, doses of 500 or 600 mg of doxepin, imipramine, or desipramine may be not only well tolerated but also required. When such "high dose" treatment is used, the patient should be carefully monitored clinically and with blood levels and simultaneous ECGs. Blood levels of 450 ng/ml or more are not necessarily a contraindication to continued treatment provided that the patient is closely monitored and free of cardiac disease, that the cardiac conduction time is not unduly slowed, and that one sees no evidence of "behavioral toxicity," as described above. Where the cardiac status of the patient is in question, cardiologic consultation is appropriate.

For depressive episodes of major depression, bipolar disorder or schizoaffective disorder, and for dysthymia, any of the tricyclics may be used. For other indications, however, certain specific tricyclics may have certain advantages, as discussed in the respective chapters.

When tricyclics are discontinued, it is important to taper the dose over three or four days in order to avoid the syndrome of "cholinergic rebound" as described in that chapter.

BIBLIOGRAPHY

Bigger JT, Giardina EG, Perel JM, et al. Cardiac antiarrhythmic effect of imipramine hydrochloride. *The New England Journal of Medicine* 1977;296:206-208.

Boehnert MT, Lovejoy FH. Value of the QRS duration versus the serum drug level in predicting seizures and ventricular arrhythmias after an acute overdose of heterocyclic antidepressants. *The New England Journal of Medicine* 1985;313:474-479.

Boyce P, Judd F. The place for the tricyclic antidepressants in the treatment of depression. *The Australian and New Zealand Journal of Psychiatry* 1999;33:323-327.

Garner EM, Kelly MW, Thompson DF. Tricyclic antidepressant withdrawal syndrome. *The Annals of Pharmacotherapy* 1993;27:1068-1072.

Giardina EGB, Barnard T, Johnson L, et al. The antiarrhythmic effect of nortriptyline in cardiac patients with ventricular premature depolarizations. *Journal of the American College of Cardiology* 1986;7: 1363-1369.

Glausser J. Tricyclic antidepressant poisoning. *Cleveland Clinic Journal of Medicine* 2000;67:704-706, 709-713, 717-719.

Jabbari B, Bryan GE, Marsh EE, et al. Incidence of seizures with heterocyclic and tetracyclic antidepressants. *Archives of Neurology* 1985;42: 480-481.

Max MB, Lynch SA, Muir J, et al. Effects of desipramine, amitriptyline, and fluoxetine on pain in diabetic neuropathy. *The New England Journal of Medicine* 1992;326:1250-1256.

Meador-Woodruff JH, Akil M, Wisner-Carlson R, et al. Behavioral and cognitive toxicity related to elevated plasma heterocyclic antidepressant levels. *Journal of Clinical Psychopharmacology* 1988;8:28-32.

Perry JP, Zeilman C, Arndt S. Tricyclic antidepressant concentrations in plasma: an estimate of their sensitivity as a predictor of response. *Journal of Clinical Psychopharmacology* 1994;14:230-240.

Preskom SH, Jerkovich GS. Central nervous system toxicity of heterocyclic antidepressants: phenomenology, course, risk factors, and role of therapeutic drug monitoring. *Journal of Clinical Psychopharmacology* 1990;10:88-95.

Schatzberg AF, Cole JO, Blumer DP. Speech blockage: a heterocyclic side effect. *The American Journal of Psychiatry* 1978;135:600-601.

273 Clomipramine

Clomipramine is a tricyclic antidepressant that is structurally identical to imipramine except for the addition of a chlorine atom on one of the rings, an addition which confers a stronger serotoninergic activity on this compound. Like the other tricyclics, it is effective in the treatment of depression and panic disorder; however, unlike the other tricyclics, it is also effective in the treatment of obsessive-compulsive disorder. It is also effective for body dysmorphic disorder, trichotillomania, developmental stuttering, cataplexy (as seen in narcolepsy), premature ejaculation, and for self-injurious behaviors associated with mental retardation.

PHARMACOKINETICS

Clomipramine is well absorbed and then undergoes a significant first-pass effect. Peak blood levels are obtained in about 2 to 6 hours, and 95% or more is protein bound. Clomipramine is metabolized in the liver to desmethylclomipramine, which is strongly noradrenergic and which has antidepressant but not antiobsessive activity.

The metabolism of both clomipramine and desmethylclomipramine is capacity limited. At doses of 150 mg or less, the half-life of clomipramine ranges from 20 to 40 hours, and that of desmethylclomipramine from 54 up to 77 hours. At doses higher than 150 mg, however, the half-lives and steady state concentrations of both clomipramine and its metabolite increase, at times several-fold.

SIDE EFFECTS

Sedation and anticholinergic side effects such as dry mouth, blurry vision, and constipation are common. Urinary hesitancy or retention may occur. Dizziness, nausea and vomiting, tremor, and increased sweating may be seen.

Erectile dysfunction, retarded ejaculation and anorgasmia are common and distressing, as is weight gain.

Transient mild evaluations of SGOT and SGPT have occurred. Rarely, serious, even fatal, hepatotoxicity has occurred.

On the electrocardiogram, ST segment and T wave changes may occur; the QT interval may be lengthened, and occasionally premature ventricular contractions may be seen.

As with all antidepressants, clomipramine may also precipitate mania in bipolar patients.

Seizures are more common with clomipramine than with all other tricyclic antidepressants, with the exception of maprotiline. The overall incidence at doses of 250 mg or less appears to be about 0.5%; with higher doses the incidence rises to over 1.5%.

The teratogenicity of clomipramine is not known; it is excreted in breast milk.

DRUG-DRUG INTERACTIONS

Haloperidol increases clomipramine levels. By analogy with other tricyclics, one should anticipate that fluoxetine, paroxetine, sertraline and methylphenidate will also increase clomipramine levels. Fluvoxamine increases clomipramine levels; conversely, clomipramine increases fluvoxamine levels. Heavy smoking decreases clomipramine levels. Clomipramine elevates phenobarbital and modafinil levels. The combination of clomipramine with a monoamine oxidase inhibitor may produce hyperpyrexia, seizures, and death. By analogy with other tricyclics, mutual antagonism may be anticipated between clomipramine and alpha-2 blockers, such as clonidine.

OVERDOSAGE

Overdoses may produce stupor, coma, respiratory depression, hypotension, severe anticholinergic symptoms, seizures, arrhythmias, and fever.

Treatment is supportive with cardiac monitoring and any necessary respiratory support. Admission to an intensive care unit is indicated. Fluids, pressor agents, such as dopamine, and a cooling blanket may be required.

THERAPEUTIC USAGE

Clomipramine is available in 25, 50 and 75 mg tablets.

For depression or for obsessive-compulsive disorder, treatment is begun with 25 or 50 mg, and the dose is increased in 50 mg increments weekly, up to 150 mg. For panic disorder begin with 25 mg and increase in 25 mg increments. During the initial titration, the total daily dose may be divided and given three times daily to reduce the risk of nausea or vomiting. Once the titration is done, however, most patients may be switched to either a twice daily or all-at-bedtime schedule. If patients have not shown a response after waiting at least a month, the dose may be gradually increased, but generally no higher than 250 mg. Given the nonlinear kinetics noted above, however, dose increases above 150 mg should be done in increments of 25 mg and the total clomipramine plus desmethylclomipramine level should be monitored: levels above 150 nanogram/ml are associated with a response.

BIBLIOGRAPHY

Balant-Gorgia AE, Gex-Fabry M, Balant LP. Clinical pharmacokinetics of clomipramine. *Clinical Pharmacokinetics* 1991;20:447-462.

Kuss HJ, Jungkunz G. Non-linear pharmacokinetics of clomipramine after infusion and oral administration in patients. *Progress in Neuro-psychopharmacology & Biological Psychiatry* 1986;10:739-748.

McTavish D, Benfield P. Clomipramine: an overview of its pharmacological properties and a review of its therapeutic use in obsessive compulsive disorder and panic disorder. *Drugs* 1990;39:136-153.

Panerai AE, Monza G, Movilia P, et al. A randomized, within-patient, cross-over, placebo-controlled trial on the efficacy and tolerability of the tricyclic antidepressants clomipramine and nortriptyline in central pain. *Acta Neurologica Scandinavica* 1990;82:34-38.

Schacter M, Parkes JD. Fluvoxamine and clomipramine in the treatment of cataplexy. *Journal of Neurology, Neurosurgery, and Psychiatry* 1980;43:171-174.

274 Amoxapine

Amoxapine, though classed as a tricyclic antidepressant, has certain unique, and unfavorable, properties. Amoxapine is a derivative of the antipsychotic loxapine, and two of amoxapine's metabolites, 8-hydroxyamoxapine and 7-hydroxyamoxapine, possess antipsychotic properties themselves.

Amoxapine may be used for treatment of depression, and its antidepressant activity is contingent on its ability to blockade norepinephrine reuptake and, to a lesser extent, serotonin reuptake.

Given its antipsychotic activity and significant side effects, as noted below, there appears to be little justification for its use: some authors have advocated it for the treatment of depression with psychotic features, but in this regard it is no more effective than a combination of a better-tolerated tricyclic with an antipsychotic, and, unlike combination treatment where one can stop the antipsychotic when recovery occurs, there is no way to "stop" the antipsychotic activity of amoxapine except by stopping the drug entirely.

PHARMACOKINETICS

Amoxapine reaches peak blood levels in about $1\frac{1}{2}$ hours, and about 90% is protein bound. Amoxapine itself is almost completely metabolized in the liver, with a half-life of about 8 hours; its two metabolites with antipsychotic activity, 8-hydroxyamoxapine and 7-hydroxyamoxapine, have half-lives of 30 and 8 hours, respectively.

SIDE EFFECTS

The most common side effects are sedation and anticholinergic side effects such as dry mouth, constipation, and blurry vision. Postural dizziness may occur.

Amoxapine lowers the seizure threshold and in high doses may cause seizures.

Side effects seen with antipsychotics are also seen with amoxapine, including parkinsonism, the neuroleptic malignant syndrome, tardive dyskinesia and hyperprolactinemia.

Although in comparison with tricyclics such as imipramine and amitriptyline, amoxapine is relatively noncardiotoxic, atrial flutter has been reported.

Whether amoxapine is teratogenic is not known; it is excreted in the breast milk.

DRUG-DRUG INTERACTIONS

Amoxapine may potentiate sedative or anticholinergic side effects of other drugs, and, as with other tricyclics, the combination of amoxapine with an MAOI may cause a hypertensive crisis.

OVERDOSAGE

Amoxapine has a higher mortality rate in overdose than other tricyclics, due, in large measure, to the frequency of grand mal seizures; renal failure may also occur. Cardiotoxicity is not a major feature of overdose, and, in contrast to overdose with standard tricyclics, the width of the QRS complex is not a reliable guide to the severity of amoxapine overdose.

Patients should be admitted to an ICU, and treatment may proceed as described in the chapter on tricyclics, with particular attention to renal function.

THERAPEUTIC USAGE

Amoxapine is available in 25, 50, 100 and 150 mg tablets.

In otherwise healthy adults, treatment is begun at 100 to 150 mg daily, increasing by 50 mg every few days until either limiting side effects occur or a dose of 300 mg is reached. If no response to 300 mg is seen after several weeks, and if the patient has no risk factors for seizures, the dose may be gradually increased up to a maximum of 600 mg.

At total daily doses below 300 mg, the dose may be either divided or given all at bedtime; at doses over 300 mg, divided doses are recommended, with the largest single dose being no more than 300 mg.

BIBLIOGRAPHY

Anton RF, Burch EA. Amoxapine versus amitriptyline combined with perphenazine in the treatment of psychotic depression. *The American Journal of Psychiatry* 1990;147:1203-1208.

Calvo B, Garcia MJ, Pedraz JL, et al. Pharmacokinetics of amoxapine and its active metabolites. *International Journal of Clinical Pharmacology, Therapy, and Toxicology* 1985;23:180-185.

Giannini AJ, Price WA. Amoxapine-induced seizures: case reports. *The Journal of Clinical Psychiatry* 1984;45:385-389.

Jennings AE, Levy AS, Harrington JT. Amoxapine-associated acute renal failure. *Archives of Internal Medicine* 1983;143:1525-1527.

Litovitz TL, Troutman WG. Amoxapine overdose: seizures and fatalities. *Journal of the American Medical Association* 1983;250:1069-1071.

Taylor NE, Schwartz HI. Neuroleptic malignant syndrome following amoxapine overdose. *The Journal of Nervous and Mental Disease* 1988;176:249-251.

Thornton JE, Stahl SM. Case report of tardive dyskinesia and parkinsonism associated with amoxapine therapy. *The American Journal of Psychiatry* 1984;141:704-705.

275 Selective Serotonin Reuptake Inhibitors

The selective serotonin reuptake inhibitors (SSRIs), fluoxetine, paroxetine, sertraline, citalopram, escitalopram and fluvoxamine, are all remarkably versatile and safe medicines that almost exclusively affect serotonin transmission by blocking reuptake of serotonin by presynaptic neurons. This chapter deals with fluoxetine, paroxetine, sertraline, citalopram and escitalopram; as fluvoxamine differs substantially from these five SSRIs, especially with regard to drug-drug interactions and pharmacokinetics, it is dealt with separately in the next chapter.

It should be noted that escitalopram is another name for the *S*-isomer of citalopram: citalopram exists as a racemic mixture of *R*-citalopram and *S*-citalopram, and *S*-citalopram is the more active of the two, and probably, in fact, accounts for much of the therapeutic effect of racemic citalopram.

The principal indications for an SSRI are a depressive episode of major depression, bipolar disorder or schizoaffective disorder, premenstrual dysphoric disorder, postpsychotic depression, post-partum depression, secondary depressions (as may be seen in Alzheimer's disease and multi-infarct dementia), panic disorder, obsessive-compulsive disorder, posttraumatic stress disorder, generalized anxiety disorder, social phobia, premature ejaculation, body dysmorphic disorder and bulimia. Although in the case of some of these indications (e.g., depressive episodes) each one of these SSRIs has been shown to be effective, this is not universally the case, and for some indications only one or a few of the SSRIs have support from double-blinded studies. Consequently, although it may well be the case that, in terms of efficacy, the SSRIs are all generally equivalent, the reader is directed to the respective chapters for each indication to find out which of these SSRIs have the best support for that specific indication.

PHARMACOKINETICS

All of these five SSRIs are all well absorbed after oral administration, and peak blood levels are obtained within 1 to 8 hours. Fluoxetine, paroxetine and sertraline each undergo over 95% protein binding, whereas for citalopram and escitalopram the figure is about 50%. All five SSRIs undergo extensive hepatic metabolism, but only in the case of fluoxetine is there an active metabolite of any significance. Fluoxetine, which is sequestered in the lungs, has a half-life of about 2 or 3 days, and its active metabolite, norfluoxetine, has a much longer half-life of from 7 to 10 days. The other four SSRIs have half-lives of from 1 to 1½ days.

SIDE EFFECTS

All these SSRIs may produce nausea, vomiting, diarrhea, and anorexia. Weight loss may occur, but this is generally seen only in those who were overweight prior to treatment; exceptions to this rule, however, do occur, especially among the elderly, who may, even though of normal weight prior to treatment, lose substantial amounts. Uncommonly patients may gain weight. Sexual dysfunction is seen in almost one-half of patients, and may consist of decreased libido, erectile dysfunction, delayed ejaculation or anorgasmia; of these five SSRIs, paroxetine may be most likely to cause these effects. Anxiety, tremor, and insomnia may occur; conversely, some patients may experience sedation or an urge to take a nap, an urge which generally coincides with peak blood levels. A minority of patients may experience an akathisia that may at times be severe and may be associated with an increase in any preexisting agitation or suicidal ideation; such symptoms are promptly relieved by propranolol, used as described in that chapter. Dystonia or parkinsonism may also occur, but these are generally mild; in patients with preexisting Parkinson's disease, the SSRIs may also increase the parkinsonism seen in this condition. A slight reduction in heart rate may also be present; rarely a bradyarrhythmia may occur. In bipolar patients mania may be precipitated. In a small minority, there may be an increase in liver enzymes and, although this is generally benign and transient, fatal hepatotoxicity has occurred. SSRIs also increase the risk of gastrointestinal bleeding, and this is especially the case when used with NSAIDs or aspirin. Occasionally a syndrome of inappropriate antidiuretic hormone (SIADH) secretion may occur with hyponatremia. Rarely, a systemic vasculitis may be precipitated by an SSRI.

All the SSRIs are excreted in the breast milk.

None of these SSRIs have been associated with major malformations in infants; however, there may be an increased risk of miscarriage with fluoxetine.

Fluoxetine, rarely, may be associated with a systemic vasculitis, which may be fatal.

DRUG-DRUG INTERACTIONS

Although all of these SSRIs inhibit cytochrome P450 2D6 (CYP2D6), their potency in this regard varies widely: fluoxetine and paroxetine are most potent; sertraline has only modest effects in this regard; and both citalopram and escitalopram have negligible effect. Of the many drugs metabolized by CYP2D6 whose blood levels may be increased with inhibition of CYP2D6, the most important are the tricyclic antidepressants whose levels may be increased into toxic ranges by fluoxetine or paroxetine.

SSRIs, especially fluoxetine and paroxetine, may increase warfarin levels, thus increasing the risk of bleeding; phenytoin and metoprolol levels may also be increased.

Concurrent use of an SSRI with a monoamine oxidase inhibitor (MAOI) is contraindicated because it may cause a "serotonin syndrome" with confusion, myoclonus, agitation, hyperthermia, long-tract signs, and possibly death. If a patient is initially taking an MAOI, at least 2 weeks should elapse after discontinuing the MAOI before starting the SSRI to allow for a regeneration of monoamine oxidase. If the patient was initially taking the SSRI, at least 2 weeks should elapse between discontinuing paroxetine or sertraline and starting the MAOI; in the case of fluoxetine, given its longer half-life and the long half-life of its active metabolite nor-fluoxetine, generally 7 weeks should pass before starting the MAOI.

In some cases the addition of cyproheptadine to an SSRI in depressed patients may be followed by a relapse of depressive symptoms.

OVERDOSAGE

All of these five SSRIs are remarkably safe in overdose: nausea, vomiting, and agitation are generally the only symptoms; rarely, seizures may occur.

Activated charcoal and gastric lavage may be used, and lorazepam may be used for seizures.

THERAPEUTIC USAGE

Fluoxetine is available in a 10 mg tablet and in 10 and 20 mg capsules, and in a 90 mg capsule designed for once weekly use; paroxetine in 10, 20, 30, and 40 mg tablets and in a "controlled release" preparation of 12.5, 25 and 37.5 mg; sertraline in 25, 50 and 100 mg tablets; citalopram in 10, 20 and 40 mg tablets; and escitalopram in 10 and 20 mg tablets. All of these SSRIs, with the exception of escitalopram, are also available in liquid form.

All of these five SSRIs may each be given in a single daily dose either at bedtime or in the morning, depending on patient convenience and on whether any sedation or insomnia occurs as side effects.

For a depressive episode, dose ranges are 20 to 80 mg for fluoxetine, 10 to 50 mg for paroxetine, 50 to 200 mg for sertraline, 10 to 40 mg for citalopram and 5 to 20 mg for escitalopram. Dosing ranges for other indications are outlined in the respective chapters.

BIBLIOGRAPHY

Beasley CM, Masica DM, Heiligenstein JH, et al. Possible monoamine oxidase inhibitor-serotonin uptake inhibitor interaction. *Journal of Clinical Psychopharmacology* 1993;13:312-320.

DeVane CL. Pharmacokinetics of the selective serotonin reuptake inhibitors. *The Journal of Clinical Psychiatry* 1992;53(suppl):13-20.

Feder R. Reversal of antidepressant activity of fluoxetine by cyproheptadine in three patients. *The Journal of Clinical Psychiatry* 1991;52:163-164.

Feighner JP, Boyer WF, Tyler DL, et al. Adverse consequences of fluoxetine-MAOI combination therapy. *The Journal of Clinical Psychiatry* 1990;51:222-225.

Jimenez-Jimenez FJ, Tejeiro J, Martinez-Junquera G, et al. Parkinsonism exacerbated by paroxetine. *Neurology* 1994;44:2406.

Lane RM. Pharmacokinetic drug interaction potential of selective serotonin reuptake inhibitors. *International Clinical Psychopharmacology* 1996;11(Suppl 5):31-61.

Leo RJ. Movement disorders associated with the serotonin selective reuptake inhibitors. *The Journal of Clinical Psychiatry* 1996;57:449-454.

Montejo-Gonzalez AL, Llorca G, et al. SSRI-induced sexual dysfunction: fluoxetine, paroxetine, sertraline, and fluvoxamine in a prospective, multicenter, and descriptive clinical study of 344 patients. *Journal of Sex & Marital Therapy* 1997;23:176-194.

Rothschild AJ, Locke CA. Reexposure to fluoxetine after serious suicide attempts by three patients: the role of akathisia. *The Journal of Clinical Psychiatry* 1991;52:491-493.

van Harten J. Clinical pharmacokinetics of selective serotonin reuptake inhibitors. *Clinical Pharmacokinetics* 1993;24:203-220.

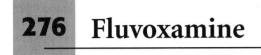

276 Fluvoxamine

Fluvoxamine is a selective serotonin reuptake inhibitor (SSRI) that, like the other SSRIs (fluoxetine, paroxetine, sertraline, citalopram and escitalopram), inhibits reuptake of serotonin by presynaptic neurons. As noted in the preceding chapter on selective serotonin reuptake inhibitors, however, it is treated separately here given its significant differences from the other SSRIs, particularly with regard to pharmacokinetics and drug-drug interactions. Fluvoxamine is indicated for obsessive-compulsive disorder and is also useful in the treatment of a depressive episode of major depression, panic disorder, and social phobia of the generalized type.

PHARMACOKINETICS

Fluvoxamine is well absorbed from the gastrointestinal tract, but because of a first-pass effect it has a bioavailability of only about 50%. Peak blood levels are obtained in 2 to 8 hours, with about 80% protein binding. Extensive hepatic metabolism occurs, with at least 11 different metabolites, none of which are known to have any significant pharmacologic activity. The half-life at steady state ranges from 15 hours to 20 hours.

Fluvoxamine exhibits nonlinear kinetics, with disproportionately higher blood levels with multiple or increasing doses. For unclear reasons, females tend to have higher blood levels than males.

SIDE EFFECTS

A minority of patients may experience somnolence, insomnia, nausea, nervousness, agitation, headache, diarrhea, constipation, dry mouth, dizziness, delayed ejaculation, impotence, decreased libido, or anorgasmia; rarely hyponatremia secondary to SIADH may occur.

Fluvoxamine is excreted in the breast milk. Its teratogenic potential in humans is not known.

DRUG-DRUG INTERACTIONS

Unlike paroxetine and fluoxetine, fluvoxamine only minimally inhibits the cytochrome P450 2D6 enzyme system. However, alone among the SSRIs, fluvoxamine inhibits the cytochrome P450 1A2, 2C9, and 3A4 enzymes with significant consequences.

Cytochrome P450 1A2 is partially responsible for demethylating the tertiary amine tricyclics; thus levels of imipramine, trimipramine, clomipramine, amitriptyline, and maprotiline are all increased. Cytochrome P450 1A2 is also partially responsible for metabolizing warfarin, caffeine, theophylline, propranolol, and metoprolol, with each of these agents undergoing significant elevations in blood level.

P450 3A4 has substantial responsibility for metabolizing cyclosporine and all of the benzodiazepines (with the exception of lorazepam, temazepam and oxazepam), with all these agents undergoing a significant increase in blood level.

Fluvoxamine also increases diazepam and desmethyldiazepam, methadone, clozapine, carbamazepine, phenytoin and mirtazapine levels.

Fluvoxamine levels may be increased by haloperidol and by clomipramine.

The combination of fluvoxamine and lithium has been reported to cause somnolence and seizures, and the combination of fluvoxamine and risperidone was reported to induce a syndrome similar to the neuroleptic malignant syndrome.

The combination of fluvoxamine and an MAOI would probably predispose to a serotonin syndrome; at least 2 weeks should separate the administration of these agents.

OVERDOSAGE

In addition to an exacerbation in side effects noted above, overdose of fluvoxamine may also cause tachycardia, bradycardia, hypotension, coma, and convulsions; deaths have occurred secondary to fluvoxamine overdose alone.

Treatment is supportive; gastric lavage and activated charcoal may be used; lorazepam, and not diazepam, should be used for seizures.

THERAPEUTIC USAGE

Fluvoxamine is available in 25, 50 and 100 mg capsules.

Treatment is initiated at 50 mg/day and increased in 50 mg increments every 4 to 7 days to a maximum of 300 mg. Doses over 100 mg are divided, with the larger fraction generally being given at bedtime. In the elderly, debilitated, or those with impaired hepatic function, doses should be decreased and the intervals between increments increased.

Should concurrent treatment with a benzodiazepine be required, lorazepam, oxazepam, or temazepam should be used because their metabolism is not inhibited by fluvoxamine. Similarly, if a beta-blocker is required, atenolol may be safely used.

BIBLIOGRAPHY

Anttila AK, Rasanen L, Leinonen EV. Fluvoxamine augmentation increases serum mirtazapine concentration three- to fourfold. *The Annals of Pharmacotherapy* 2001;35:1221-1223.

Liu BA, Mittmann N, Knowles SR, et al. Hyponatremia and the syndrome of inappropriate secretion of antidiuretic hormone associated with the use of selective serotonin reuptake inhibitors: a review of spontaneous reports. *Canadian Medical Association Journal* 1996;155:519-527.

Lu ML, Lane HY, Chen KP, et al. Fluvoxamine reduces the clozapine dosage needed in refractory schizophrenic patients. *The Journal of Clinical Psychiatry* 2000;61:594-599.

Mamiya K, Kojima K, Yukawa E, et al. Phenytoin intoxication induced by fluvoxamine. *Therapeutic Drug Monitoring* 2001;23:75-77.

Perucca E, Gatti G, Spina E. Clinical pharmacokinetics of fluvoxamine. *Drugs* 1994;27:175-190.

Reeves RR, Mark JE, Beddingfield JJ. Neurotoxic syndrome associated with risperidone and fluvoxamine. *The Annals of Pharmacotherapy* 2002; 36:440-443.

van Harten J. Overview of the pharmacokinetics of fluvoxamine. *Clinical Pharmacokinetics* 1995;29(Suppl 1):1-9.

277 Venlafaxine

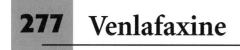

Venlafaxine blocks the reuptake of serotonin at all dosages, and, in addition, blocks the reuptake of norepinephrine at higher doses; it has little or no effect on cholinergic or histaminergic transmission and does not block postsynaptic alpha-1 receptors. Venlafaxine is indicated for major depression, generalized anxiety disorder and social phobia of the generalized type; other uses include cataplexy (as seen in narcolepsy), painful neuropathy and, curiously, in the treatment of hot flashes in males undergoing anti-androgen therapy, and in post-menopausal females.

PHARMACOKINETICS

Venlafaxine is well absorbed, and although food may delay absorption, it does not reduce it. Peak levels occur in from 1.5 to 2.5 hours for the immediate release preparation and in from 5 to 6 hours for the extended release preparation. Protein binding is only about 25%. Venlafaxine has a half-life of from 3.5 to 5 hours and is extensively metabolized in the liver, with only about 5% being excreted unchanged in the urine.

One of venlafaxine's major metabolites, O-desmethylvenlafaxine, is active, has a half-life of about 11 hours, and is partially metabolized in the liver, with about 30% excreted unchanged in the urine.

SIDE EFFECTS

A minority of patients may experience nausea, sweating, dizziness, somnolence, insomnia, tremor, anxiety, anorexia (generally with only slight weight loss), or sexual dysfunction.

Some patients may experience an increase in supine diastolic blood pressure, averaging about 7 mm Hg; this effect is dose related, and at higher doses may be 15 mm Hg or more above baseline in about 5% of patients. Some patients may also experience a rise in resting heart rate of about three beats/minute.

Rarely, seizures may occur.

In those with a bipolar disorder, mania may be precipitated.

There is a case report of the serotonin syndrome occurring secondary to monotherapy with venlafaxine.

Venlafaxine is excreted in breast milk; it is not known if it is teratogenic.

DRUG-DRUG INTERACTIONS

Venlafaxine is a relatively weak inhibitor of P450 2D6; nevertheless blood levels of drugs dependent on this enzyme, such as tricyclics, may be increased.

Both diphenhydramine and cimetidine increase venlafaxine blood level; however, in the case of cimetidine this is generally minimal.

The serotonin syndrome can occur with a combination of venlafaxine and an MAOI and this combination should not be used. Although the serotonin syndrome has also been reported with the combination of venlafaxine and lithium, this is rare, and this combination may be used and either phenelzine or lithium.

OVERDOSAGE

Although venlafaxine is not as toxic as a tricyclic in overdose, it is not benign, and there may be seizures, sedation and a prolongation of the QT interval. Gastric lavage and activated charcoal may be administered, along with supportive care.

THERAPEUTIC USAGE

Venlafaxine is supplied in immediate release tablets of 25, 37.5, 50, 75 and 100 mg, and as an extended release preparation available in 37.5, 75 and 150 mg strengths.

For depression, venlafaxine treatment is initiated at 37.5 or 75 mg total per day and then increased in 75 mg/d increments no more rapidly than every four days. Most patients respond to total daily doses of from 150 to 225 mg; however, in some, often more severe cases, doses up to 375 mg may be required. If the immediate release preparation is used, the total daily dose should be divided into a twice or thrice daily schedule; the extended release preparation, however, may be given once daily, either in the morning or at bedtime.

Doses should be decreased and the interval between doses increased in those with significant hepatic or renal failure.

A minority of patients who have taken venlafaxine for 6 or more weeks will, upon abrupt discontinuation of the drug, develop a syndrome characterized by headache, nervousness, electric shock-like sensations, dizziness, and nausea. Thus in patients treated for this duration, the dose of venlafaxine should be tapered gradually, over perhaps 2 weeks.

If patients are switched from an MAOI to venlafaxine, 14 days should be allowed to pass so that a new "crop" of monoamine oxidase may be generated; conversely, if patients are switched from venlafaxine to an MAOI, about 7 days should be allowed to pass to allow enough time for all the venlafaxine to "wash out."

BIBLIOGRAPHY

Harvey AT, Rudolph RL, Preskorn SH. Evidence of the dual mechanism of action of venlafaxine. *Archives of General Psychiatry* 2000;57:503-509.

Lessard E, Yessine MA, Hamelin BA, et al. Diphenhydramine alters the disposition of venlafaxine through inhibition of CYP2D6 activity in humans. *Journal of Clinical Psychopharmacology* 2001;21:175-184.

Loprinzi CL, Pisansky TM, Fonsecca R, et al. Pilot evaluation of venlafaxine hydrochloride for the therapy of hot flushes in cancer survivors. *Journal of Clinical Oncology* 1998;16:2377-2381.

Morton WA, Sonne SC, Verga MA. Venlafaxine: a structurally unique and novel antidepressant. *The Annals of Pharmacotherapy* 1995;29:387-395.

Pan JJ, Shen WW. Serotonin syndrome induced by low-dose venlafaxine. *The Annals of Pharmacotherapy* 2003;37:209-211.

Reeves RR, Mack JE, Beddingfield JJ. Shock-like sensations during venlafaxine withdrawal. *Pharmacotherapy* 2003;23:678-681.

Sindrup SH, Bach FW, Madsen C, et al. Venlafaxine versus imipramine in painful polyneuropathy: a randomized, controlled trial. *Neurology* 2003;60:1284-1289.

Thase ME. Effects of venlafaxine on blood pressure: a meta-analysis of original data from 3744 depressed patients. *The Journal of Clinical Psychiatry* 1998;59:502-508.

Whyte IM, Dawson AH, Buckley NA. Relative toxicity of venlafaxine and selective serotonin reuptake inhibitors in overdose compared to tricyclic antidepressants. *Quarterly Journal of Medicine* 2003;96:369-374.

278 Duloxetine

Duloxetine, like venlafaxine, is a selective serotonin-norepinephrine reuptake inhibitor. It is scheduled to be released in the United States soon, and is indicated for the treatment of major depression. It may also be useful in the treatment of stress urinary incontinence.

PHARMACOKINETICS

Duloxetine reaches peak blood levels in about five hours, and has a half life ranging from 9 to 19 hours. Extensive hepatic metabolism occurs, involving, in part, CYP2D6, and both of its main metabolites are pharmacologically active.

SIDE EFFECTS

Nausea, vomiting, anorexia, diarrhea or constipation, somnolence, dizziness and insomnia may occur. Trivial increases in blood pressure and pulse have been noted, and a slight weight loss may occur.

It is not known if duloxetine is excreted in the breast milk or if it is teratogenic.

DRUG-DRUG INTERACTIONS

There is very limited experience in this area. Duloxetine levels are increased by the CYP2D6 inhibitor paroxetine, and it is reasonable to expect that other 2D6 inhibitors will have the same effect. Duloxetine itself appears to inhibit CYP2D6 and increases desipramine levels: it is also reasonable to expect that other drugs metabolized by 2D6 will also be affected.

Duloxetine should not be used with MAOIs, nor within two weeks of the discontinuation of an MAOI.

OVERDOSAGE

There is no published information regarding this.

THERAPEUTIC USAGE

Duloxetine will probably be available in 20 mg capsules.

Based on currently published work, treatment of depression may be initiated at a total daily dose of 20 to 40 mg and increased in weekly increments of 40 mg to a maximum dose of 120 mg: most patients with depression appear to respond to doses between 60 and 80 mg. The total daily dose may be given once daily or in two divided doses.

BIBLIOGRAPHY

Detke MJ, Lu Y, Goldstein DJ, et al. Duloxetine, 60 mg once daily, for major depressive disorder: a randomized double-blind placebo-controlled trial. *The Journal of Clinical Psychiatry* 2002;63:308-315.

Detke MJ, Lu Y, Goldstein DJ, et al. Duloxetine 60 mg once daily dosing versus placebo in the acute treatment of major depression. *Journal of Psychiatric Research* 2002;36:383-390.

Goldstein DJ, Mallinckrodt C, Lu Y, et al. Duloxetine in the treatment of major depressive disorder: a double-blind clinical trial. *The Journal of Clinical Psychiatry* 2002;63:225-231.

Karps KD, Caveanaugh JE, Lakoski JM. Duloxetine pharmacology: profile of a dual monamine modulator. *CNS Drug Reviews* 2002;8:361-376.

Sharma A, Goldberg MJ, Cerimele BJ. Pharmacokinetics and safety of duloxetine, a dual-serotonin and norepinephrine reuptake inhibitor. *Journal of Clinical Pharmacology* 2000;40:161-171.

Skinner MH, Kuan HY, Pan A, et al. Duloxetine is both an inhibitor and a substrate of cytochrome P4502D6 in healthy volunteers. *Clinical Pharmacology and Therapeutics* 2003;73:170-177.

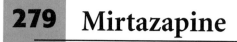

Mirtazapine is a structurally unique antidepressant which, by virtue of its antagonism at presynaptic alpha-2 autoreceptors and heteroreceptors, and at post-synaptic 5-HT2 and 5-HT3 receptors, has prominent effects on both noradrenergic and serotoninergic transmission. Mirtazapine is also a potent antagonist at H1 receptors, and this may account for the sedation and weight gain seen during its use. Antagonism also occurs at peripheral post-synaptic alpha-1 receptors, and this may account for the side effect of dizziness. Anticholinergic effects also occur, but are relatively modest.

Mirtazapine is indicated for the treatment of major depression.

PHARMACOKINETICS

Mirtazapine has a bioavailability of about 50% and reaches peak blood levels in about two hours. About 85% is protein-bound, and the half life ranges from 20 to 40 hours. Metabolism is via hepatic cytochrome P450 enzymes 2D6, 1A2 and 3A4, and one of its metabolites, though active, is only about 10 or 20% as potent as the parent compound.

SIDE EFFECTS

The main side effects are sedation, dizziness, increased appetite and weight gain. Dry mouth and constipation may occur, but generally only to a minimal degree, and both cholesterol and triglyceride levels may be increased.

Transaminase levels may increase in a small minority of patients, but revert to normal whether or not the drug is discontinued.

When given to patients with Parkinson's disease, mirtazapine may precipitate REM sleep behavior disorder.

It is not known if mirtazapine is teratogenic, nor is it clear whether it is excreted in breast milk or not.

In terms of side effects, one of the great advantages of mirtazapine is the low incidence of sexual dysfunction.

DRUG-DRUG INTERACTIONS

Both phenytoin and carbamazepine, by inducing enzymes, reduce mirtazapine levels.

Fluvoxamine may increase mirtazapine levels several-fold.

Cimetidine, by increasing bioavailability, may increase blood levels without altering the half-life of mirtazapine.

Concurrent use of mirtazapine and an MAOI may cause the serotonin syndrome.

Clonidine exerts its therapeutic effect by stimulating presynaptic alpha-2 autoreceptors, and, as might be predicted, the addition of mirtazapine may negate the antihypertensive effect of clonidine.

The addition of mirtazapine to levodopa was noted in one case report to cause a psychosis.

Mirtazapine itself does not inhibit cytochrome P450 enzymes, and has little effect on the metabolism of other drugs.

OVERDOSAGE

Mirtazapine is generally safe in overdose; gastric lavage and supportive care are generally sufficient.

THERAPEUTIC USAGE

Mirtazapine is available in 15, 30 and 45 mg tablets and also in orally disintegrating tablets in the same strengths.

Mirtazapine is generally given once daily, at bedtime, and in otherwise healthy adults treatment is initiated at 15 mg and increased in 15 mg increments every week or two until limiting side effects occur or a maximum dose of 60 mg is reached: most patients respond to doses between 15 and 45 mg. For hospitalized patients, a more rapid titration may be undertaken.

The dose should be reduced in the elderly or those with significant hepatic or renal failure.

BIBLIOGRAPHY

Abo-Zena RA, Bobek MB, Dweik RA. Hypertensive urgency induced by an interaction of mirtazapine and clonidine. *Pharmacotherapy* 2000; 20:476-478.

Anttila AK, Rasanen L, Leinonen EV. Fluvoxamine augmentation increases serum mirtazapine concentrations three- to four-fold. *The Annals of Pharmacotherapy* 2001;35:1221-1223.

Bremner JD, Wingard P, Walshe TA. Safety of mirtazapine in overdose. *The Journal of Clinical Psychiatry* 1998;59:233-235.

Normann C, Hesslinger B, Frauenknecht S, et al. Psychosis during chronic levodopa therapy triggered by the new antidepressive drug mirtazapine. *Pharmacopsychiatry* 1997;30:263-265.

Onofrj M, Luciano AL, Thomas A, et al. Mirtazapine induces REM sleep behavior disorder (RBD) in parkinsonism. *Neurology* 2003;60: 113-115.

Sitsen JM, Maris FA, Timmer CJ. Concomitant use of mirtazapine and cimetidine: a drug-drug interaction study in healthy male subjects. *European Journal of Clinical Pharmacology* 2000;56:389-394.

Spaans E, van den Heuvel MW, Schnabel PG, et al. Concomitant use of mirtazapine and phenytoin: a drug-drug interaction study in healthy male subjects. *European Journal of Clinical Pharmacology* 2002;58: 423-429.

Timmer CJ, Sitsen JM, Delbressine LP. Clinical pharmacokinetics of mirtazapine. *Clinical Pharmacokinetics* 2000;38:461-474.

Nefazodone is structurally similar to trazodone, and appears to exert its antidepressant effect by virtue of blocking the reuptake of serotonin and norepinephrine by presynaptic neurons and by blocking postsynaptic serotonin ($5HT_2$) receptors. Although nefazodone also blocks alpha-1 receptors, it has no significant activity at alpha-2, acetylcholine, beta-adrenergic or dopaminergic receptors.

Nefazodone is indicated for the treatment of depressive episodes of major depression; of note, nefazodone, in contrast with many other antidepressants, does not, in depressed patients, delay the onset of REM sleep, nor does it suppress REM sleep; in normals, nefazodone has little effect on any sleep parameter. Nefazodone is rarely used, given its hepatotoxicity, as noted below.

PHARMACOKINETICS

Nefazodone undergoes extensive first-pass metabolism, with a bioavailability of only about 20%. Peak blood levels are obtained in from 1 to 2 hours, and about 99% is protein bound. Nefazodone is extensively metabolized in the liver, with a half-life ranging from 2 to 4 hours. Of nefazodone's multiple metabolites, three have been identified: hydroxynefazodone, a triazole-dione metabolite, and meta-chlorophenylpiperazine (mCPP). Hydroxynefazodone is pharmacologically very similar to nefazodone and has a half-life from $1^1/_2$ to 4 hours. The triazole-dione metabolite is less well characterized pharmacologically, but does appear to block $5HT_2$ receptors; it has a half-life of about 18 hours. mCPP is a mixed agonist-antagonist at $5HT_2$ receptors and has a half-life of 4 to 8 hours.

Food both delays the time to peak for nefazodone and decreases its bioavailability by about 20%.

Both nefazodone and hydroxynefazodone display nonlinear kinetics with multiple dosing, and this is probably due to a saturation of the first-pass effect. With multiple dosing, both the half-lives and the peak blood levels increase. In practice, steady state blood levels are not reached for 3 to 5 days.

SIDE EFFECTS

Nausea, sedation, dry mouth, blurry vision, postural dizziness, constipation, confusion, visual scotomata, visual "trailing," insomnia, agitation, and tremor may all occur and there is a case report of clitoral priapism.

Sinus bradycardia may occur, as may orthostatic hypotension.

The most serious side effect of nefazodone is hepatotoxicity: this appears to be idiosyncratic, and, although rare, has been fatal. Most cases appear to occur within the first half year of treatment.

Nefazodone is excreted in the breast milk; whether it is teratogenic in humans is not known.

DRUG-DRUG INTERACTIONS

Nefazodone inhibits cytochrome P450 3A4 and increases blood levels of all of the benzodiazepines, with the exception of lorazepam, temazepam and oxazepam, each of which undergoes direct glucuronidation.

Nefazodone increases digoxin, carbamazepine and haloperidol levels.

A serotonin syndrome has been reported secondary to a combination of nefazodone and paroxetine.

OVERDOSAGE

Overdosage with nefazodone is generally benign; some patients may have no symptoms at all whereas others may experience nausea, vomiting, or sedation.

Treatment is supportive; gastric lavage may be performed.

THERAPEUTIC USAGE

Nefazodone is available in 50, 100, 150, 200 and 250 mg tablets.

Treatment is generally initiated at 200 mg/day, and the dose may be increased in increments of from 100 to 200 mg at an interval of approximately every 7 days, to a maximum of 600 mg. Most patients respond at doses between 300 and 600 mg daily. In the elderly, debilitated, or those with some hepatic failure, the initial dose and any subsequent incremental doses should be lower, and the intervals between dose increments longer. In all cases, the total daily dose should be given on a divided, b.i.d. schedule.

Liver function tests should be ordered before instituting treatment and performed periodically during the first six months, and patients should be monitored for any symptoms suggestive of hepatic injury.

BIBLIOGRAPHY

Benson BE, Mathiason M, Dahl B, et al. Toxicities and outcomes associated with nefazodone poisoning: an analysis of 1,338 exposures. *The American Journal of Emergency Medicine* 2000;18:587-592.

Brodie-Meijer CC, Diemont WL, Buijs PJ. Nefazodone-induced clitoral priapism. *International Clinical Psychopharmacology* 1999;14: 257-258.

Dockens RC, Greene DS, Barbhaiya RH. Assessment of pharmacokinetic and pharmacodynamic drug interactions between nefazodone and digoxin in healthy volunteers. *Journal of Clinical Pharmacology* 1996; 36:160-167.

Greene DS, Barbhaiya RH. Clinical pharmacokinetics of nefazodone. *Clinical Pharmacokinetics* 1997;33:260-275.

John L, Perreault MM, Tao T, et al. Serotonin syndrome associated with nefazodone and paroxetine. *Annals of Emergency Medicine* 1997;29: 287-289.

Kaul S, Shukla UA, Barbhaiya RH. Nonlinear pharmacokinetics of nefazodone after escalating single and multiple oral doses. *Journal of Clinical Pharmacology* 1995;35:830-839.

Kroboth PD, Folan MM, Lush RM, et al. Coadministration of nefazodone and benzodiazepines: I. Pharmacodynamic assessment. *Journal of Clinical Pharmacology* 1995;15:306-319.

Rush AJ, Armitage R, Gillin JC, et al. Comparative effects of nefazodone and fluoxetine on sleep in outpatients with major depressive disorder. *Biological Psychiatry* 1998;44:3-14.

Stewart DE. Hepatic adverse reactions associated with nefazodone. *Canadian Journal of Psychiatry* 2002;47:375-377.

Vogal G, Cohen J, Mullis D, et al. Nefazodone and REM sleep: how do antidepressant drugs decrease REM sleep? *Sleep* 1998;21:70-77.

The mechanism of action of trazodone is not clear but probably involves both blockade of reuptake of serotonin by presynaptic receptors and antagonism at postsynaptic serotonin receptors. It does not block reuptake of norepinephrine.

Trazodone does not block postsynaptic cholinergic receptors; however, it does block postsynaptic alpha-1 receptors, and this action may account for some of its side effects.

Trazodone is effective for depressive episodes of major depression, generalized anxiety disorder, bulimia and also for agitation or aggressiveness seen in dementia. Trazodone is also an effective hypnotic which increases slow-wave sleep but neither suppresses REM sleep nor prolongs REM latency.

PHARMACOKINETICS

Trazodone is well absorbed after oral administration and has a bioavailability of about 80%. In fasting subjects the time to peak concentration is about 1 hour. In the presence of food, absorption is delayed with peak blood levels occurring in about 2 hours; however, the total amount absorbed is actually slightly greater. Protein binding is over 90% and trazodone is almost completely metabolized in the liver with a half-life of about 6 hours. An active metabolite, m-chlorophenylpiperazine, is a mixed agonist-antagonist at postsynaptic serotonin receptors and, as noted, can increase symptoms in patients with obsessive-compulsive disorder.

SIDE EFFECTS

Sedation and postural dizziness are especially common and may be so severe as to preclude full dosing. Other relatively common side effects include nausea, headache, dry mouth, and blurred vision. Some patients may also complain of difficulty with concentration and irritability.

Although trazodone has negligible effect on cardiac conduction, it may, rarely, produce ventricular ectopy. Sinus bradycardia has also been noted.

Priapism has been noted in males, and there is one case report of clitoral priapism; increased libido has also been noted in females.

Rare side effects include palinopsia, parkinsonism and hepatic injury.

The teratogenicity of trazodone is not clear; it is excreted in the breast milk.

DRUG-DRUG INTERACTIONS

The antihypertensive effects of methyldopa and clonidine may be reduced.

Trazodone may increase levels of digoxin and phenytoin, and there are reports suggesting an increase in warfarin levels.

Ritonavir may increase trazodone levels and carbamazepine may decrease them.

The serotonin syndrome has been reported with combinations of trazodone and buspirone, paroxetine or an MAOI.

OVERDOSAGE

Overdose may be followed by vomiting, coma, respiratory depression, seizures, priapism, complete A-V block and ventricular tachycardia.

THERAPEUTIC USAGE

Trazodone is available in 50, 100 and 150 mg tablets.

The most common reason for using trazodone currently is insomnia, and here doses of from 50 to 100 mg hs are generally effective. If trazodone is used for depression, then, in otherwise healthy depressed adults, treatment is begun at 100 or 150 mg daily, increasing by 50 to 100 mg every 3 or 4 days, until a dose between 400 and 600 mg is arrived at or unacceptable side effects occur. A more rapid dosage escalation may be used in hospitalized patients. Doses much less than 400 mg are generally not likely to be effective, and should sedation occur at lower doses, as is often the case, another antidepressant should probably be used. Although the short half-life suggests using divided doses, most patients, in fact, do just as well taking the entire daily dose all at bedtime. No established therapeutic range for trazodone blood levels is available.

Males should be warned that prolonged erections may be a precursor to priapism and should be instructed to contact their physician immediately should this occur.

BIBLIOGRAPHY

Dorn JM. A case of phenytoin toxicity possibly precipitated by trazodone. *The Journal of Clinical Psychiatry* 1986;47:89-90.

Fernandes NF, Martin RR, Schenker S. Trazodone-induced hepatotoxicity: a case report with comments on drug-induced hepatotoxicity. *The American Journal of Gastroenterology* 2000;95:532-535.

Fukunishi I, Kitaoka T, Shirai T, et al. A hemodialysis patient with trazodone-induced parkinsonism. *Nephron* 2002;90:222-223.

Gartrell N. Increased libido in women receiving trazodone. *The American Journal of Psychiatry* 1986;143:781-782.

Greenblatt DJ, von Moltke LL, Harmatz JS, et al. Short-term exposure to low-dose ritonavir impairs clearance and enhances adverse effects of trazodone. *Journal of Clinical Pharmacology* 2003;43:414-422.

Hughes MS, Lessell S. Trazodone-induced palinopsia. *Archives of Ophthalmology* 1990;108:399-400.

Nierenberg AA, Adler LA, Peselow E, et al. Trazodone for antidepressant-associated insomnia. *The American Journal of Psychiatry* 1994;151:1069-1072.

Otani K, Ishida M, Kaneko S, et al. Effects of carbamazepine on plasma concentrations of trazodone and its active metabolite, m-chlorophenylpiperazine. *Therapeutic Drug Monitoring* 1996;18:164-167.

Pescatori ES, Engelman JC, Davis G, et al. Priapism of the clitoris: a case report following trazodone use. *The Journal of Urology* 1993;149:1557-1559.

Small NL, Giomanna KA. Interaction between warfarin and trazodone. *The Annals of Pharmacotherapy* 2000;34:734-736.

Sultzer DL, Gray KF, Gunay I, et al. Does behavioral improvement with haloperidol or trazodone treatment depend on psychosis or mood symptoms in patients with dementia? *Journal of the American Geriatrics Society* 2001;49:1294-1300.

Warner MD, Peabody CA, Whiteford HA, et al. Trazodone and priapism. *The Journal of Clinical Psychiatry* 1987;48:244-245.

Yamadera H, Nakamura S, Suzuki H, et al. Effects of trazodone hydrochloride and imipramine on polysomnography in healthy subjects. *Psychiatry and Clinical Neurosciences* 1998;52:439-443.

282 Bupropion

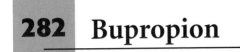

The mechanism of action of bupropion is not clear. Originally bupropion was thought to have a relatively selective effect on dopamine transmission, with little effect on other neurotransmitters. Recent work, however, suggests a role for one of bupropion's metabolites, hydroxybupropion, especially as it affects norepinephrine transmission. A relatively negligible effect is noted on serotonin, acetylcholine, or histamine metabolism. Bupropion is indicated for depression, primarily those depressions marked by psychomotor retardation and hypersomnia. Bupropion is also effective in attention deficit disorder with hyperactivity and in the treatment of nicotine dependence. Unlike most other antidepressants, it is not effective in panic disorder. Of interest, bupropion was recently shown to also be effective in the treatment of painful polyneuropathies.

PHARMACOKINETICS

Peak blood levels are obtained within 2 hours for the immediate release preparation, within 3 hours for the sustained release preparation, and within 5 hours for the extended release preparation; over 80% is protein bound. Bupropion is almost completely metabolized in the liver; less than 1% is excreted unchanged in the urine; its half-life ranges from 6 to 24 hours, averaging about 12 hours. Three metabolites, hydroxybupropion, threohydrobupropion, and erythrohydrobupropion, are all metabolically active; each has a longer half-life than the parent compound, and their steady state blood levels are anywhere from several up to 10 times higher than that of bupropion itself. Wide interpatient variability in blood levels of both bupropion and its active metabolites is evident, with twofold to fivefold differences being found among patients on the same dose. Interestingly, high levels of the active metabolites have been associated with a negative therapeutic effect.

SIDE EFFECTS

Anxiety, agitation, and insomnia are troubling and relatively common. Nausea, vomiting, dry mouth, constipation, and dizziness may also occur. Supine blood pressure may rise slightly, and in some patients an orthostatic fall in blood pressure may occur which, however, in most cases is not clinically significant. Left ventricular function and cardiac conduction appear unaffected, and arrhythmias do not appear to occur. Both weight loss and weight gain can occur; however, in most cases bupropion is weight-neutral. Sexual dysfunction is less frequent with bupropion than with most other antidepressants, with the possible exceptions of nefazodone and mirtazapine, which also have a lesser effect on sexual functioning. In bipolar patients, bupropion may precipitate mania; however, it may be somewhat less likely to do this than other antidepressants.

Bupropion may cause seizures. For the immediate-release preparation the overall incidence appears to be about 0.4% and for the sustained release preparation it is about 0.1%; the risk, however, increases at doses over 450 mg/day. Rapid or large dosage increases also appear to increase the risk. Other risk factors include current or prior bulimic episodes, either as part of bulimia or anorexia nervosa; a prior history of seizures; a history of head trauma; any other potentially epileptogenic lesion; and withdrawal from alcohol or sedative-hypnotics. Although most seizures tend to occur within days or a week after initiating treatment or increasing the dose, this is not always the case, and weeks may pass before a seizure occurs.

Other, rare, side effects include psychosis, delirium and dystonia.

The teratogenicity of bupropion is not known; it is excreted in breast milk.

DRUG-DRUG INTERACTIONS

Bupropion inhibits CYP P450 2D6 and may elevate tricyclic blood levels.

Bupropion, in one case report, caused a decline in cyclosporine levels.

Carbamazepine grossly reduces the levels of bupropion, threohydrobupropion, and erythrohydrobupropion, and increases the level of hydroxybupropion.

The use of bupropion with other dopaminergic agents, such as levodopa, amantadine, bromocriptine, pergolide, and methylphenidate, should be done with great caution, as dyskinesias and confusion have been reported with such combinations.

OVERDOSAGE

Overdose may cause tachycardia, hypertension, nausea and vomiting and, in up to one-third of patients, seizures; agitation, stupor or coma may also occur.

Treatment is primarily supportive. Gastric lavage may be performed if the patient is seen early enough, and activated charcoal should be administered; lorazepam may be used for seizures.

THERAPEUTIC USAGE

Bupropion is available in immediate release tablets containing 75 and 100 mg, in sustained release tablets containing 100, 150 or 200 mg, and in extended release tablets of 150 and 300 mg.

For depression, if the immediate release preparation is used, treatment is initiated at 100 mg twice daily and increased to 100 mg three times daily no sooner than 4 days later. If no response is seen within a month, the dose may be increased to 150 mg t.i.d. If the sustained release preparation is used, begin at 150 mg once daily, in the morning, and, after 4 or more days, increase the dose to 150 mg b.i.d.; if no response is seen within a month, the dose may be increased to 200 mg b.i.d. In general, the last dose of the day should be given in the late afternoon or early evening in order to reduce the risk of insomnia. If the extended release preparation is used, begin at 150 mg in the morning, and, after 4 or more days, increase the dose to 350 mg in the morning; if no response is seen in a month, the dose may be increased to 450 mg in the morning.

Doses of bupropion above 450 mg are not recommended, given the increased risk of seizures; furthermore, patients with a history of bulimic episodes should not be prescribed bupropion. Doses should also be reduced in the elderly or those with hepatic disease.

BIBLIOGRAPHY

Balit CR, Lynch CN, Isbister GK. Bupropion poisoning: a case series. *The Medical Journal of Australia* 2003;178:61-63.

Dager SR, Heritch AJ. A case of bupropion-associated delirium. *The Journal of Clinical Psychiatry* 1990;51:307-308.

Detweiller MB, Harpold GJ. Bupropion-induced acute dystonia. *The Annals of Pharmacotherapy* 2002;36:251-254.

Golden RN, James SP, Sherer MA, et al. Psychoses associated with bupropion treatment. *The American Journal of Psychiatry* 1985;142: 1459-1462.

Horne RL, Ferguson JM, Pope HG, et al. Treatment of bulimia with bupropion: a multicenter controlled trial. *The Journal of Clinical Psychiatry* 1988;49:262-266.

Johnston JA, Lineberry CG, Ascher AJ, et al. A 102-center prospective study of seizures in association with bupropion. *The Journal of Clinical Psychiatry* 1991;52:450-456.

Ketter TA, Jenkins JB, Schroeder DH, et al. Carbamazepine but not valproate induces bupropion metabolism. *Journal of Clinical Psychopharmacology* 1995;15:327-333.

Lai AA, Schroeder DH. Clinical pharmacokinetics of bupropion: a review. *The Journal of Clinical Psychiatry* 1983;44(suppl 5):82-85.

Laizure SC, DeVane CL, Stewart JT, et al. Pharmacokinetics of bupropion and its major basic metabolites in normal subjects after a single dose. *Clinical Pharmacology and Therapeutics* 1985;38:586-589.

Lewis BR, Aoun SL, Bernstein GA, et al. Pharmacokinetic interactions between cyclosporine and bupropion or methylphenidate. *Journal of Child and Adolescent Psychopharmacology* 2001;11:193-198.

Semenchuk MR, Sherman S, Davis B. Double-blind, randomized trial of bupropion SR for the treatment of neuropathic pain. *Neurology* 2001; 13:1583-1588.

283 Monoamine Oxidase Inhibitors

Currently, three monoamine oxidase inhibitors (MAOIs) are available in the United States: phenelzine, selegiline (formerly known as deprenyl) and tranylcypromine. Each of these drugs exerts its therapeutic effect primarily by inhibiting the enzyme monoamine oxidase.

Monoamine oxidase exists in two separate molecular forms: monoamine oxidase type A and monoamine oxidase type B. For each form, Table 283-1 lists its primary location and preferential substrate.

Monoamine oxidase type A provides protection against tyramine, which is a naturally occurring indirect sympathomimetic found in many foods and drinks (a list of which is found under Side Effects). Once absorbed from the gut, a percentage of tyramine is destroyed by monoamine oxidase type A in the gut wall, and that which escapes into the portal venous blood is then destroyed by monoamine oxidase type A in the liver. When monoamine oxidase type A is irreversibly inhibited, the stage is set for a catastrophic reaction.

With inhibition of monoamine oxidase type A, norepinephrine, found in presynaptic neurons, is not degraded and its concentration in the presynaptic neuron rises. Furthermore, now that the monoamine oxidase type A in the gut and liver is inhibited, tyramine has relatively free access to the systemic circulation and subsequently reaches the brain in high concentration. Making contact with presynaptic neurons in the brain, tyramine triggers the release of large stored amounts of norepinephrine, causing, among other things, a profound and potentially lethal rise in blood pressure. This resultant "hypertensive crisis" was originally called the "cheese reaction" as it was initially noted in a patient taking an MAOI who had eaten some aged cheese, a food high in tyramine.

The MAOIs available in the United States are classified as either selective or nonselective, depending on whether they selectively inhibit just one of the two types of monoamine oxidase or nonselectively inhibit both. Both phenelzine and tranylcypromine are nonselective. Selegiline, on the other hand, is selective, but only relatively so: at doses of 10 mg or less it inhibits monoamine oxidase type B with very little effect on type A; at doses of 20 or 30 mg, however, it also inhibits type A and thus becomes nonselective.

Antidepressant effectiveness, as might be expected, depends on inhibition of monoamine oxidase type A; only by increasing levels of norepinephrine and serotonin are depressive symptoms relieved. Consequently, whereas the nonselective MAOIs phenelzine and tranylcypromine have some antidepressant effect at any dose, the selective MAOI, selegiline, lacks antidepressant effectiveness at doses of 10 mg or less because at those doses it inhibits only monoamine oxidase type B.

This selectivity of selegiline at low doses, however, has been used to advantage in the treatment of Parkinson's disease. Because selegiline, at doses of 10 mg, leaves monoamine oxidase type A

■**TABLE 283-1.** Locations and Preferential

SUBSTRATES OF MAO ISOFORMS		
	Location	**Preferential Substrate**
Isoform		
MAO-A	Gastrointestinal tract, liver, brain	Norepinephrine, serotonin, tyramine
MAO-B	Brain	Dopamine

untouched, the body is still protected from tyramine, and thus patients taking low doses of selegiline may eat whatever they like and not risk the "hypertensive crisis." The ability of low-dose selegiline to inhibit monoamine oxidase type B, however, increases the supply of dopamine in presynaptic neurons, and this is one of the mechanisms whereby selegiline is beneficial for patients with Parkinson's disease.

Phenelzine is useful in the following disorders: atypical depression, panic disorder, social phobia of the generalized type, and posttraumatic stress disorder. Phenelzine is also helpful in the treatment of a depressive episode of major depression, and some studies indicate that it is as useful here as are tricyclic antidepressants. Bulimia, narcolepsy, and migraine and cluster headache also constitute indications; however, in each of these cases phenelzine is generally a second choice to other available agents. This is particularly true for patients with bulimia, who may have considerable difficulty adhering to the strict tyramine-free "MAOI diet" described in the section on side effects.

Selegiline, in a high dose of 30 or more mg, is effective in depression, and in a dose of 20 mg in narcolepsy; low dose selegiline is indicated for the treatment of Parkinson's disease, Alzheimer's disease and AIDS dementia.

Tranylcypromine is effective in depression (where it may be superior to phenelzine for the treatment of psychomotorically retarded patients) and attention-deficit/hyperactivity disorder. Tranylcypromine is unique among the nonselective MAOIs in that it is structurally similar to amphetamine and may have a slight stimulant effect. Indeed, albeit rarely, some patients have come to abuse tranylcypromine at very high doses, precisely for this amphetamine-like effect, and in fact have become addicted to it.

The nonselective MAOIs are out of clinical favor. The MAOI diet is very difficult to follow, and the number of potentially fatal drug-drug interactions is impressive, thus prompting clinicians and patients to look to newer and safer antidepressants, such as the selective serotonin reuptake inhibitors. Phenelzine, however, may be uniquely effective in atypical depression and generalized social phobia, and thus it has enjoyed something of a small renaissance. In addition, both phenelzine and tranylcypromine constitute valuable alternative treatments when standard antidepressants either fail or are otherwise contraindicated.

PHARMACOKINETICS

Each of these three MAOIs reach peak blood levels in from 1/2 to 4 hours and all are metabolized in the liver: for phenelzine, metabolites include phenylacetic acid and parahydroxyphenylacetic acid; for selegiline, L-amphetamine and L-methamphetamine; and for tranylcypromine, D-amphetamine.

Although the half-life of the MAOI itself is short, the inhibition of monoamine oxidase produced by the MAOI is prolonged. The available MAOIs bind irreversibly to monoamine oxidase, and it generally takes about 2 weeks for a new "crop" of monoamine oxidase to appear. Thus, even after an MAOI is discontinued, the actual inhibition of monoamine oxidase persists.

SIDE EFFECTS

The most common side effects of the MAOIs are orthostatic hypotension and dizziness, which may not become clinically apparent until several weeks have passed. Other side effects include dry mouth, blurry vision, constipation, decreased libido, anorgasmia, retarded ejaculation, and erectile dysfunction.

Phenelzine may cause weight gain and, rarely, may also be associated with pyridoxine deficiency and a peripheral neuropathy. Other rare side effects include delirium and myoclonus.

Tranylcypromine is less likely to cause weight gain; however, it may cause insomnia if given late in the day and may also cause restlessness or agitation.

Rarely, phenelzine may cause hepatotoxicity; this is even less common with tranylcypromine.

The most feared side effect of the nonselective MAOIs (and of selegiline in doses over 10 mg) is the hypertensive crisis. As noted earlier, this occurs when patients with inhibited monoamine oxidase type A ingest tyramine. Clinically the hypertensive crisis presents with the following: a severe throbbing headache, often beginning occipitally and radiating frontally; tachycardia and palpitations; hypertension; nausea; diaphoresis; and photophobia. Fever may occur, and, rarely, intracranial hemorrhage.

The list of foods that contain tyramine is formidable. Those with relatively large amounts are listed in the box on this page.

Hypertensive crises may also occur secondary to drug-drug interactions as described below.

The teratogenicity of the MAOIs is not known. Tranylcypromine is excreted in the breast milk; whether the other MAOIs are excreted in breast milk is not known.

DRUG-DRUG INTERACTIONS

A large number of drugs, if given to a patient whose monoamine oxidase type A is inhibited, may cause a hypertensive crisis. These include indirect sympathomimetic agents, such as pseudoephedrine, ephedrine, and the like; stimulants such as amphetamine, dextroamphetamine, methylphenidate, and cocaine; the anorectics diethylpropion and phentermine; and certain antihypertensives such as reserpine, alpha-methyldopa and guanethidine. The pressor response to such direct acting sympathomimetics as epinephrine and isoproterenol may also be increased.

The tricyclic antidepressants and amoxapine, if added to an MAOI, may precipitate a hypertensive crisis (however, as noted in the section on therapeutic usage, it is generally safe if the sequence is reversed and the MAOI is added to the tricyclic). Similar reactions may occur if carbamazepine or cyclobenzaprine, both chemically similar to the tricyclics, are added to an MAOI.

Interestingly, if a switch is made immediately from one MAOI to another, a hypertensive crisis may occur; consequently, if such a switch is desired, one should wait at least two weeks before starting the second agent.

Tyramine-Containing Foods

Aged cheeses
Sour cream
Yogurt
Pickled herring
Sausage
Aged or "cured" meats
Liver
Red wines
Certain beers
Concentrated yeast
Ripe avocados
Broad bean pods

The serotonin syndrome may occur secondary to the combination of an MAOI and an SSRI, a tricyclic, venlafaxine, meperidine or dextromethorphan.

MAOIs may potentiate the hypoglycemic effect of sulfonylureas.

Certain of the antimigraine "triptans" are metabolized by MAO-A and should not be used in patients taking phenelzine or tranylcypromine or selegiline (in doses of over 10 mg): these include sumatriptan, rizatriptan and zolmitriptan. The other available triptans, naratriptan, almotriptan and frovatriptan, are all metabolized by the cytochrome P450 system and thus may be safely taken with an MAOI.

In assessing possible drug-drug interactions, one should keep in mind that inhibition of monoamine oxidase actively persists for at least 2 weeks after discontinuation of the MAOI, during which time the patient is still vulnerable to an interaction.

OVERDOSAGE

Symptoms of overdose, which may not be apparent for up to 12 hours, include agitation, delirium, fever, convulsions, increased or decreased blood pressure, and coma.

Gastric lavage may be helpful, even up to several hours after overdose. Treatment is generally supportive; cooling blankets may be required. Pressor agents must be used with extreme caution. Acidification of the urine and diuresis may speed elimination of the drug.

THERAPEUTIC USAGE

Phenelzine is available in 15 mg tablets, tranylcypromine in 10 mg tablets, and selegiline in 5 mg capsules.

For depression, phenelzine is begun at 15 mg twice daily and increased every few days in 15 or 30 mg increments up to a minimum of 60 mg; some patients may require doses of 90 mg for a therapeutic effect. Eventually, many patients may be managed on a once daily dose at bedtime. Tranylcypromine is begun at 10 mg twice daily, with the last dose no later than midday. The dose is increased every few days up to 30 or 40 mg; some patients may require doses as high as 60 mg. Nighttime dosing is not practical, as insomnia may occur with tranylcypromine. When selegiline is used for depression, begin at 5 mg twice daily, with the second dose no later than midday, and increase every few days in 10 mg increments up to 30 mg total.

Doses may have to be reduced in the elderly, with longer intervals between each successive dose increase. Once an optimum dose of an MAOI is reached, several weeks may be required to see a clinical effect. The patient should be given a list of all forbidden foods and drugs and instructed to inform all physicians that he is taking an MAOI. Furthermore, the patient should be informed that he must abstain from these foods and drugs for at least 2 weeks following discontinuation of the MAOI. In any case, the nonselective MAOIs should not be prescribed to unreliable patients or to those with a pheochromocytoma or those with illness, such as asthma, which may require the use of sympathomimetics.

In general, MAOIs should not be abruptly discontinued. They are very effective REM suppressants, and after abrupt discontinuation a severe "REM rebound" may occur with insomnia, agitation, and hallucinations.

Should a hypertensive crisis occur, treatment may be initiated with nitroprusside, phentolamine, or nifedipine. Some physicians give patients a small supply of 10 mg tablets of nifedipine to be crushed and taken orally for use in case of a suspected hypertensive crisis.

For Parkinson's disease, selegiline may be given at a dose of 5 mg in the morning and 5 mg at midday. When selegiline is added to L-dopa, peak dose dyskinesias may appear several days later, necessitating a reduction by about 10% to 30% of the dose of levodopa.

BIBLIOGRAPHY

Briggs NC, Jefferson JW, Koenecke FH. Tranylcypromine addiction: a case report and review. *The Journal of Clinical Psychiatry* 1990;51:426-429.

Halle MT, Dilsaver SC. Tranylcypromine withdrawal phenomena. *Journal of Psychiatry & Neuroscience* 1993;18:49-50.

Liskin B, Roose SP, Walsh BT, et al. Acute psychosis following phenelzine discontinuation. *Journal of Clinical Psychopharmacology* 1985;5:46-47.

Mahmood I. Clinical pharmacokinetics and pharmacodynamics of selegiline. An update. *Clinical Pharmacokinetics* 1997;33:91-102.

Mann JJ, Aarons SF, Wilner PJ, et al. A controlled study of the antidepressant efficacy and side effects of (-)-deprenyl. A selective monoamine oxidase inhibitor. *Archives of General Psychiatry* 1989;46:45-50.

Robinson DS, Nies A, Ravaris CL, et al. Clinical pharmacology of phenelzine. *Archives of General Psychiatry* 1978;35:629-635.

Shulman KI, Walker SE, MacKenzie S, et al. Dietary restriction, tyramine, and the use of monoamine oxidase inhibitors. *Journal of Clinical Psychopharmacology* 1989;9:397-402.

Stewart JW, Harrison W, Quitkin F, et al. Phenelzine-induced pyridoxine deficiency. *Journal of Clinical Psychopharmacology* 1984;4:225-226.

White PD. Myoclonus and episodic delirium associated with phenelzine: a case report. *The Journal of Clinical Psychiatry* 1987;48:340-341.

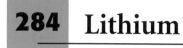

284 Lithium

Although lithium has seen medicinal use since the first half of the nineteenth century, the modern era of lithium did not begin until the publication of John Cade's 1949 paper documenting its effectiveness in the treatment of mania. Lithium subsequently became the acknowledged treatment for bipolar disorder, and, although newer agents have come into use, it still remains the standard against which all bipolar treatments must be measured.

In addition to its use in bipolar disorder, lithium is useful for cyclothymia, hyperthymia, and those cases of schizoaffective disorder wherein manic episodes occur. It is also useful in postpartum psychosis, especially when accompanied by manic-like symptoms. Although depressive episodes occurring in a bipolar disorder may respond to lithium alone, those occurring as part of a major depression generally do not. Nevertheless, lithium does have a place in certain cases of major depression, namely as an augmenting agent in cases resistant to treatment with either tricyclics or SSRIs and as prophylactic treatment in cases where, for one reason or other, the patient is unable to tolerate long-term treatment with an antidepressant. One of the great advantages of lithium in the long term treatment of mood disorders is a reduction in the risk of suicide and suicide attempts, an effect that argues strongly for its use.

Violent behavior, especially if impulsive, may be reduced by lithium. Similarly, in patients with conduct disorder who display considerable impulsivity, lithium may likewise be useful. Preliminary work also suggests an effectiveness of lithium in attention-deficit/hyperactivity.

Lithium relieves or prevents mania secondary to steroids and is useful for the prevention of both cluster and migraine headaches. Occasionally, lithium is used in the treatment of neutropenia and, rarely, hyperthyroidism.

Although lithium is advocated by some for the treatment of schizophrenia, the evidence for this indication is less than robust. Indeed some patients with hebephrenic schizophrenia deteriorate if given lithium.

Although the mechanism or mechanisms whereby lithium exerts its manifold effects on the central nervous system is unknown, some theories have been advanced, with varying degrees of experimental support. Lithium does substitute for sodium and could thereby profoundly affect the generation of neuronal action potentials. Lithium also affects the functioning of G proteins, thus potentially altering transmembrane signal transduction. Finally, the functioning of both the adenylate cyclase and phosphoinositide second-messenger systems is altered, again with potentially significant effects of signal transduction.

PHARMACOKINETICS

Lithium is completely absorbed, and, with immediate-release preparations, peak blood levels are obtained within 1 to 2 hours; with the slow- or controlled-release preparations, the peak is delayed until 4 or 4 1/2 hours. Lithium is neither protein bound nor does it undergo any metabolism. The "lithium ratio," or ratio of intracellular to extracellular lithium concentration, as measured using red blood cells, is about 0.4; however, this ratio can vary widely among patients, with "high" blood lithium levels actually coexisting with low intracellular levels and vice versa. About 95% of lithium is excreted through the kidney; the rest is eliminated in sweat and feces.

Lithium is freely filtered at the glomerulus. In the proximal tubule, it competes with sodium for reabsorption, and when sodium levels are normal, about 80% of lithium is reabsorbed. Whereas mild degrees of hypernatremia cause a slight reduction in the amount of lithium reabsorbed and a consequent insignificant fall in blood lithium levels, hyponatremia may cause profound changes. In hyponatremia, a substantially greater amount of lithium is reabsorbed, and lithium levels may rise high enough to produce toxicity.

In otherwise healthy adults, the half-life of lithium is from 18 to 24 hours; thus, anywhere from 4 to 6 days is required before steady state blood levels are obtained. With age, creatinine clearance normally decreases, and in those 60 and over, the half-life of lithium may correspondingly rise to about 36 hours. Similarly, should renal failure occur, the half-life of lithium also increases.

SIDE EFFECTS

The most troubling side effects of lithium are weight gain, hypothyroidism, nephrogenic diabetes insipidus, a fine tremor, hair loss, acne, slight incoordination, and a certain hard to describe, yet definite, lassitude.

Weight gain occurs in over half the patients; in some it is slight, only a few pounds. In others, however, gains of 20 to 40 pounds or more may occur. The mechanism of weight gain is not known. It does not appear to be caused by water retention or by a greatly increased appetite.

Thyroid hormone release from the thyroid gland is reduced with lithium treatment. In perhaps a third of patients, the resulting fall in thyroid hormone levels is sufficient to provoke a rise in TSH levels. In most cases such rises are transitory and return to normal with continued treatment; however, in about 4% of patients, despite high TSH levels, thyroid hormone levels fall below the statistical normal. Such cases are more likely to occur in females and in those with antimicrosomal antibodies. A goiter may or may not occur. Apart from its direct clinical consequences, any degree of hypothyroidism, even if manifest only by an elevated TSH, is extremely significant, as it may blunt the response to lithium, antidepressants, and carbamazepine.

Polyuria and polydipsia, secondary to the nephrogenic effects of lithium, occur in from one-third to one-half of patients; only a minority of these patients, however, find these symptoms troublesome. Although in the vast majority of cases polyuria and polydipsia clear upon discontinuation of lithium, it appears that in a small minority of cases these symptoms will persist, suggesting some permanent renal dysfunction.

Of more concern than polyuria, however, is the vexed question of whether lithium can cause renal failure. Lithium does, in a small minority of patients, cause an interstitial renal fibrosis, and has also been associated with specific lesions of the renal tubule; furthermore there are well-documented cases of lithium-induced nephrotic syndrome and distal renal tubular acidosis. Despite these findings, however, it remains unclear whether lithium does, indeed, cause chronic renal failure. Although long-term treatment with lithium is associated, in a minority, with increasing creatinine levels, it is not clear whether this association is causal or not: renal function declines normally with age, and age brings with it an increased vulnerability to various renal diseases.

A mild fine tremor of the hands occurs in somewhat less than half the patients. In most cases, this is of no concern, and indeed many patients are unaware of it. It should be clearly differentiated from the coarse tremor that may be seen in lithium overdose, as described below.

Telogen hair loss may very gradually occur in a small minority. Patients complain that their hair is thinner and more brittle; it may be found in great quantities on the pillow or in combs and brushes.

Acne may occur in a minority of patients. Most have a history of acne; however, in some it may occur de novo. In some cases it is quite mild; in others, cystic acne may occur. Another cutaneous side effect is psoriasis. In most of these cases, as with acne, the patient has a history of psoriasis; rarely, it may also occur de novo.

Incoordination may be seen in a minority of patients. This is generally quite slight and must be distinguished from the gross ataxia seen with overdose. Most patients are unaware of it; however, tennis players, dancers, and the like may complain of it.

Lassitude occurs in a substantial minority of patients and is often bitterly complained of. Patients may bemoan their lack of creativity, energy, sparkle, or enthusiasm.

Nausea and loosening of bowel movements may also occur and must be distinguished from the vomiting and diarrhea seen with overdose.

Other, much less common side effects of lithium include ankle edema, mild cogwheel rigidity, insignificant degrees of hypermagnesemia, very rare cases of pseudotumor cerebri, downbeat nystagmus or peripheral polyneuropathy, and benign flattening or inversion of T waves. Lithium may also cause an increase in parathyroid hormone levels, and although this generally results only in an insignificant elevation of serum calcium, there are rare instances of lithium-induced parathyroid adenomas requiring surgical correction. Lithium may also occasionally cause sinus node dysfunction. Occasionally, one may also see a modest, benign increase in circulating neutrophils. Lithium may cause generalized EEG slowing; occasionally petit mal and, much less frequently, complex partial seizures may be aggravated. Exacerbation of myasthenia gravis with lithium treatment has been reported.

Although lithium is teratogenic during the first trimester, previous estimates of the incidence of major malformations, especially Ebstein's anomaly, appear to have been inaccurately high. Lithium treatment during pregnancy may also cause fetal goiter and hypothyroidism. Lithium is excreted in the breast milk.

DRUG-DRUG INTERACTIONS

Both thiazide diuretics and, to a lesser extent, ACE inhibitors may cause an increased lithium level. Most nonsteroidal antiinflammatory agents, including the cox-2 inhibitors, increase lithium levels; a notable exception is sulindac. Aspirin does not elevate lithium levels. Metronidazole may also increase lithium levels. Theophylline may decrease lithium levels. As carbamazepine may cause a tertiary hypothyroidism with a reduced TSH, it may "mask" the tell-tale rise of TSH that signals a lithium-induced hypothyroidism. The combination of fluvoxamine and lithium has been reported to cause sedation and possibly seizures, and there are rare reports of the serotonin syndrome with the combination of lithium and SSRIs, clomipramine or venlafaxine.

The possibility that the combined use of haloperidol and lithium may cause severe neurotoxicity has caused much concern. A careful review of such cases, however, suggests strongly that some of these patients were actually overdosed with lithium and would have become toxic whether they had been treated with concurrent haloperidol or not. In fact the combination of lithium and haloperidol is commonly used and appears to be quite safe.

Lithium may potentiate the action of neuromuscular blocking agents such as succinylcholine or curare.

The combination of lithium and iodide salts increases the risk of hypothyroidism.

OVERDOSAGE

Lithium levels between 2 and 2.5 mEq/L often cause the following: nausea, vomiting, diarrhea; coarse tremor; dysarthria, ataxia, and nystagmus; and delirium or stupor. With increasing lithium level, coma, seizures, arrhythmias, hypotension, and death may occur. In those who survive a severe degree of intoxication, permanent brain damage, most particularly affecting the cerebellum, may occur.

Gastric lavage should be performed if the patient is seen early, and general supportive measures should be instituted. The goal of treatment is to reduce the lithium level, and, although the effect is debated, some authorities recommend forced diuresis with furosemide and isotonic saline. In any case, hemodialysis should be instituted in cases of severe toxicity or in cases where the lithium level has risen above 2.5 mEq/L and neurological manifestations are present.

THERAPEUTIC USAGE

Lithium is available in the United States as the carbonate in immediate release tablets of 300 mg and immediate release capsules of 150, 300 and 600 mg; a liquid preparation, lithium citrate, is also available which contains an amount of lithium equivalent to that found in a 300 mg tablet or capsule. Lithium is also available in a "slow-release" 300 mg tablet and a "controlled release" 450 mg tablet.

In otherwise healthy adults with normal renal function, treatment may be initiated with a total daily dose of 900 to 1200 mg of lithium carbonate, which is divided in anywhere from 2 to 3 doses. Lower doses are indicated in the following situations: renal failure, dehydration, debilitating illness, old age, and use of diuretics or of the other medicines cited earlier that may elevate lithium levels. Special caution is required in the elderly, and indeed in some elderly patients, therapeutic levels of lithium may be obtained on just 150 mg total per day. Higher doses are suggested when the patient is large or overweight or in cases of acute or delirious mania. The patient is observed for any signs of overdosage, and the dose is lowered accordingly should they occur. After the patient has taken the same daily dose for at least 4 days, a lithium level is obtained.

Controversy exists over what constitutes a "therapeutic" lithium level for the acutely ill manic patient. The level itself is standardized to be drawn 12 hours after a previous dose, and this is generally most conveniently done in the early morning after a bedtime dose the night before. Most authorities recommend a level somewhere between 0.8 and 1.2 mEq/L. However, good clinical judgment must prevail. Keeping in mind that the lithium ratio varies among patients, one should be content with a "low" lithium level if higher levels cause toxicity. In such cases the lithium ratio may be quite high, and whereas the blood level is "low," the more clinically important intracellular level may be quite "therapeutic." Conversely, and perhaps even more important, if a patient is not responding to a level that is at the "high end" of the therapeutic "range" and is not having side effects, one may cautiously increase the dose.

After the first lithium level is obtained, subsequent dosage adjustments are made every 4 days or so depending on the clinical response, side effects, and subsequent lithium levels. As noted earlier, some patients do well with very low doses: conversely, some patients, for example young, large manic patients, may require Herculean doses, up to 2700 or 3000 mg of lithium carbonate per day.

Once an optimum dose has been reached, one must then endure the notorious "lag period" for lithium until an antimanic response is seen, often 7 to 10 days. As noted in the chapter on bipolar disorder, most patients with mania require temporary treatment with antipsychotics or benzodiazepines during this time. Often, when the mania does go into remission, one observes a rise in the lithium level, despite the fact that the dose has been held constant. Typically the rise is small and of no clinical significance; however, at times it may be enough to cause toxicity and require a dose decrease.

When initiating treatment for less urgent indications, such as a patient with bipolar disorder who is currently mildly depressed, one may proceed at a more leisurely pace, starting with lower doses and perhaps allowing a week between each lithium level and subsequent dose adjustment.

Once the acute illness has been controlled by lithium and depending on the course of the disorder, one may wish to initiate a preventive phase of treatment. Although there is debate as to what constitutes an adequate level for preventive purposes, a level anywhere from 0.6 to 1.0 mEq/L is generally recommended. If a decision is made to discontinue lithium, the dose should be tapered gradually, over a minimum of 2 to 4 weeks, as more rapid discontinuation may be associated with a higher risk of subsequent relapse.

At this point one may also wish to consider once-daily dosing, in order to increase compliance. Although some clinicians who choose this option will switch from an immediate to a slow- or controlled-release preparation, keeping the total daily dose in milligrams the same, it is also possible to give the entire daily dose once daily using an immediate-release preparation, and most patients are able to tolerate this without an increase in side effects.

Laboratory monitoring is critical when using lithium. Before treatment is initiated, one should generally obtain the following: thyroid function tests, including TSH; serum electrolytes, BUN, creatinine; urinalysis. With the exception of the white blood cell count, these tests should be repeated once every 3 to 12 months or as indicated by the clinical situation. In the elderly or those suspected of sinus node disease, one may also wish to obtain an electrocardiogram.

Patients should be warned about possible drug-drug interactions and they should also be advised to call should they develop an illness characterized by diarrhea or vomiting, which could lead to sodium loss and elevated lithium levels. Reduced salt diets may have the same effect, and should these be necessary the lithium level should be closely monitored. In the past, patients were warned also to avoid excessive sweating because it was feared that this might lead to elevated lithium levels. In fact, however, provided that neither heat exhaustion, heat stroke, nor dehydration occurs, one has little cause for concern. Indeed, as lithium is excreted in greater concentration in sweat than is sodium, lithium levels may actually fall during vigorous, sweaty exercise.

Given that many patients end up taking lithium chronically, particular attention must be paid to side effects. Persistent evidence of hypothyroidism is an indication for treatment with levothyroxine, and the patient should be maintained on a dose of levothyroxine that normalizes both the free T4 (or free thyroxine index) and the TSH for at least as long as the lithium is taken.

Polyuria and polydipsia are sometimes mitigated by taking the entire daily dose of lithium at bedtime using a timed-release preparation. Should nephrogenic diabetes insipidus continue to be a problem, one may add amiloride or a thiazide diuretic, and this often alleviates the problem. Naturally, if a diuretic is added, the dose of lithium generally has to be reduced to prevent a rise in lithium level and toxicity.

Tremor may be treated with a beta-blocker, such as propranolol, nadolol, or atenolol, provided that no contraindications are evident, as discussed in the chapter on propranolol; the dosage range for propranolol is from 60 to 240 mg daily. Primidone is also effective.

Acne, if mild, may respond to benzoyl peroxide, perhaps with tetracycline or erythromycin. When severe, however, it often does not respond and may necessitate discontinuation of the lithium. Psoriasis, likewise, may or may not respond to conventional treatments.

Nausea may be minimized by taking lithium with a meal; mild loosening of bowel movements may be treated by reducing dietary fiber content or by using loperamide.

Weight gain may or may not respond to diet and exercise; it is sometimes the limiting side effect. Hair loss, likewise, if distressing, indicates alternative treatment. Certainly, if either weight gain or hair loss occurs, one should first rule out hypothyroidism.

BIBLIOGRAPHY

Batlle DC, von Riotte AB, Gaviria M, et al. Amelioration of polyuria by amiloride in patients receiving long-term lithium therapy. *The New England Journal of Medicine* 1985;312:408-414.

Bocchetta A, Mossa P, Velluzzi F, et al. Ten-year follow-up of thyroid function in lithium patients. *Journal of Clinical Psychopharmacology* 2001;21:594-598.

Cade JFJ. Lithium salts in the treatment of psychotic excitement. *The Medical Journal of Australia* 1949;36:349-352.

Chan HH, Wing Y, Su R, et al. A control study of the cutaneous side effects of chronic lithium therapy. *Journal of Affective Disorders* 2000;57: 107-113.

Finley PR, O'Brien JG, Coleman RW. Lithium and angiotensin-converting enzyme inhibitors: evaluation of a potential interaction. *Journal of Clinical Psychopharmacology* 1996;16:68-71.

Gitlin M. Lithium and the kidney: an updated review. *Drug Safety* 1999;20:231-243.

Jefferson JW. Lithium carbonate-induced hypothyroidism: its many faces. *Journal of the American Medical Association* 1979;242:271-272.

Jefferson JW, Greist JH, Ackerman DL, et al. *Lithium encyclopedia for clinical practice*, 2/e, Washington, DC, 1987, American Psychiatric Press.

Lenox RH, Hahn CG. Overview of the mechanism of action of lithium in the brain: fifty-year update. *The Journal of Clinical Psychiatry* 2000; 61(Suppl 9):5-15.

Meckler G, Woggon B. A case of serotonin syndrome caused by venlafaxine and lithium. *Pharmacopsychiatry* 1997;30:272-273.

Meltzer E, Steinlauf S. The clinical manifestations of lithium intoxication. *The Israel Medical Association Journal* 2002;4:265-267.

Perlis RH, Sachs GS, Lafer B, et al. Effect of abrupt change from standard to low serum levels of lithium: a reanalysis of double-blind lithium maintenance data. *The American Journal of Psychiatry* 2002;159: 115-119.

Carbamazepine, related structurally to the tricyclic antidepressants, is useful for the treatment of mania in bipolar disorder, and may also occasionally be useful in the treatment of bipolar depression. It is one of the first line drugs for partial seizures, whether simple or complex, and for generalized tonic-clonic seizures. It is also effective in the treatment of alcohol withdrawal and benzodiazepine withdrawal, and for agitation in dementia; uncontrolled studies also suggest a usefulness in intermittent explosive disorder. Despite this broad range of therapeutic effectiveness, carbamazepine is falling out of favor, in large part due to its many side effects and to the multitude of its clinically significant drug-drug interactions.

PHARMACOKINETICS

Carbamazepine is variably absorbed; bioavailability is generally over 70%, but this may be reduced if it is taken with food. Peak blood levels occur anywhere from 4 to 8 hours later; however, in a minority of cases, the peak may not be achieved for up to 26 hours. About 75% is protein bound. Carbamazepine is metabolized in the liver, primarily by the CYP 3A4 enzyme; its main metabolite, the 10-11 epoxide, is active, and indeed may account for many of the side effects seen with carbamazepine treatment; the epoxide's half-life is about 6 hours. With chronic, repeated dosing, carbamazepine induces its own metabolism, and this process of autoinduction may take a month to become complete. Half-life at the initiation of treatment ranges from 18 to 65 hours; when autoinduction is completed, however, the range falls to 2 to 26 hours.

SIDE EFFECTS

Sedation, ataxia, dizziness and diplopia are common and may be mitigated by increasing the dose slowly. Nausea and vomiting may occur, and patients may complain of dry mouth, blurry vision, and constipation.

A mild leukopenia, which usually partially resolves in a few months with continued treatment, occurs in up to 10% of patients. A very small minority of patients, however, may develop an agranulocytosis or an aplastic anemia. Periodic blood counts are prudent; however, since an agranulocytosis may develop abruptly, patients should be instructed to report the occurrence of fever, sore throat, or severe fatigue. Thrombocytopenia occurs rarely during the first few weeks and may manifest with petechiae.

Rashes, which may be serious in a small minority, may occur in perhaps a tenth of all patients, typically within the first 2 weeks of treatment.

A transient, mild elevation of liver enzymes occurs in about 5% to 10% of patients. Hyponatremia is not rare and may be treated with demeclocycline at a dose of 600 mg.

A reduction in free thyroxine levels is not uncommon and may be accompanied by either an increase or a decrease in TSH levels. The clinical significance of these changes is not clear.

Carbamazepine, rarely, may increase seizure frequency, especially in cases of petit mal epilepsy.

Carbamazepine reduces folate levels, with an accompanying increase in homocysteine levels: the clinical significance of this is uncertain.

Carbamazepine is teratogenic and is excreted in the breast milk.

DRUG-DRUG INTERACTIONS

Carbamazepine reduces the blood levels of a large number of medications, including phenytoin, primidone, phenobarbital, valproic acid, lamotrigene, topiramate, tiagabine, tricyclic antidepressants, trazodone, haloperidol, risperidone (and 9-hydroxyrisperidone), clozapine, clonazepam, alprazolam, warfarin, theophylline, doxycycline, indinavir, cyclosporin, and oral birth control pills: in the case of oral birth control pills, dose increases may be required to maintain contraception.

Carbamazepine levels are increased by concurrent use of medications such as fluoxetine, fluvoxamine, risperidone, erythromycin, clarithromycin, metronidazole, ketoconazole, fluconazole, isoniazid, acetazolamide, allopurinol, propoxyphene, cimetidine, omeprazole, verapamil and diltiazem.

The level of the 10,11-epoxide metabolite is increased by both valproic acid and quetiapine, without any change in the level of carbamazepine itself.

Clonidine apparently antagonizes the anticonvulsant effect of carbamazepine.

Given carbamazepine's structural resemblance to the tricyclic antidepressants, caution should be used if it is combined with a monoamine oxidase inhibitor.

OVERDOSAGE

Overdose may lead to coma, seizure activity, and respiratory depression. As blood levels slowly fall, patients awaken into a delirium that may be accompanied by hallucinations and chorea. With further recovery, patients become more alert but may display cerebellar signs. When patients clear, they may soon after experience a relapse due to absorption of drugs that may have been trapped in the anticholinergic-paralyzed bowel. Cardiac conduction defects and arrhythmias may occur. Treatment involves repeated gastric lavage and the use of activated charcoal. Hemoperfusion may also be effective.

THERAPEUTIC USAGE

Carbamazepine is available in immediate release 100 and 200 mg tablets, and in extended release 100, 200 and 400 mg tablets and 200 and 300 mg capsules.

In the non-urgent treatment of adults with depression or epilepsy, treatment is initiated in a total daily dosage ranging from 100 to 400 mg, increasing in similar increments every week until reaching one of the following end points: unacceptable side effects, a maximum of 2000 mg, or a therapeutic effect, with most patients responding to between 600 and 1200 mg; one of the extended release preparations should be used and the total daily dose should be divided into a twice-daily regimen. There is debate as to whether or not one should initiate treatment in small increments or proceed more rapidly, beginning with 400 mg increments: clearly, the slower one goes the better tolerated the medicine will be; however, some clinical situations may preclude such a leisurely approach.

In urgent situations, as for example in the treatment of mania or alcohol withdrawal, a much more rapid escalation is desirable, and, interestingly, patients in such heightened clinical conditions often tolerate such rapid escalations with little discomfort: total daily dose of 600 to 1000 mg may be appropriate on the first day of treatment.

Before treatment, a baseline determination is made of the CBC, liver enzymes, sodium level, free thyroxine, and TSH, and these are repeated periodically as indicated.

In the treatment of epileptic conditions, therapeutic levels for carbamazepine range from 4 to 12 µg/ml. Although this range is also used for treatment of mania, prospective studies to verify this are lacking. Blood levels should be checked after initial titration and also after autoinduction has had a chance to occur, with the understanding that, in almost all cases, dose increases will be required to maintain a therapeutic effect.

BIBLIOGRAPHY

Albani F, Riva R, Baruzzi A. Carbamazepine clinical pharmacology: a review. *Pharmacopsychiatry* 1995;28:235-244.

Arroyo S, Sander JW. Carbamazepine in comparative trials: pharmacokinetic characteristics too often forgotten. *Neurology* 1999;53:1170-1174.

Fitzgerald BJ, Okos AJ. Elevation of carbamazepine-10,11 epoxide by quetiapine. *Pharmacotherapy* 2002;22:1500-1503.

Furukori H, Otani K, Yasui N, et al. Effect of carbamazepine on the single dose pharmacokinetics of alprazolam. *Neruopsychopharmacology* 1998;18:364-369.

Gansaeuer M, Alsaadi TM. Carbamazepine-induced seizures: a case report and review of the literature. *Clinical Electroencephalography* 2002;33:174-177.

Hesslinger B, Normann C, Langosch JM, et al. Effects of carbamazepine and valproate on haloperidol plasma levels and on psychopathologic outcome in schizophrenic patients. *Journal of Clinical Psychopharmacology* 1999;19:310-315.

Mula M, Monaco F. Carbamazepine-risperidone interactions in patients with epilepsy. *Clinical Neuropharmacology* 2002;25:97-100.

Ono S, Mihara K, Suzuki A, et al. Significant pharmacokinetic interactions between risperidone and carbamazepine: its relationship with CYP2D6 genotypes. *Psychopharmacology* 2002;162:50-54.

Spina E, Pisani F, Perucca E. Clinically significant pharmacokinetic drug interactions with carbamazepine. An update. *Clinical Pharmacokinetics* 1996;31:198-214.

286 Oxcarbazepine

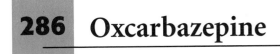

Oxcarbazepine is a keto-analog of carbamazepine which was developed in the hope of creating a compound with similar efficacy but fewer side effects and drug-drug interactions: this hope has been fulfilled. While the mechanism of action of oxcarbazepine is suspected to be similar to that of carbamazepine, namely blockade of voltage-gated sodium channels, this has not as yet been unequivocally demonstrated.

Oxcarbazepine is indicated for the treatment of partial seizures with or without secondary generalization, either as monotherapy or as an "add on" drug to other antiepileptic agents. Controlled trials have demonstrated that, as monotherapy, it is equivalent in efficacy to carbamazepine, phenytoin and valproate, and overall better tolerated than either carbamazepine or phenytoin. Oxcarbazepine is also used for trigeminal neuralgia.

Whether or not oxcarbazepine will prove as effective as carbamazepine in the treatment of bipolar disorder, alcohol withdrawal, agitation in dementia, and impulsive aggression has not as yet been determined: preliminary work with oxcarbazepine in mania, however, is favorable.

PHARMACOKINETICS

Oxcarbazepine has a bioavailability approaching 100%, reaches peak blood levels in from 4 to 5 hours and is about 50% protein-bound. Oxcarbazepine is rapidly metabolized via hepatic enzymes, with a half life of only about two hours, to its 10-monohydroxy-derivative (MHD), which is primarily responsible for oxcarbazepine's

pharmacologic effects. MHD is about 40% protein-bound and has a half life of about nine hours: about 25% is excreted unchanged in the urine, and about 50% undergoes hepatic glucuronidation.

SIDE EFFECTS

Overall, oxcarbazepine is well-tolerated: sedation, fatigue, dizziness, ataxia, diplopia and headache have been noted in a minority of patients.

Hyponatremia is more frequent with oxcarbazepine than with carbamazepine, and although it is generally mild, hyponatremic coma has been recorded with oxcarbazepine treatment. The hyponatremia with oxcarbazepine is not due to inappropriate ADH secretion, and may occur secondary to sensitization of the renal tubule cells to circulating ADH.

Mild reduction in free thyroxine levels may occur in a minority, without concurrent elevations in TSH levels.

Mild, transient elevations of hepatic transaminases may occur in a minority.

Rash may appear; however, this is less common than in the case of carbamazepine: of patients who did experience a rash secondary to carbamazepine, about 25% will have a rash when switched to oxcarbazepine.

Oxcarbazepine is found in breast milk; although its teratogenic potential is not known, its structural similarity to carbamazepine suggests that it has significant potential in this regard.

DRUG-DRUG INTERACTIONS

Oxcarbazepine has relatively little effect on the P450 enzyme system, with the exception of the P450 3A4 and 3A5 enzymes, which do undergo induction. Estrogen and progestin levels may be reduced in patients taking oral contraceptives, with a subsequent loss of effectiveness.

Oxcarbazepine may increase phenytoin levels.

MHD levels may fall with concurrent use of phenytoin, carbamazepine, valproate and verapamil.

Importantly, when patients are switched from carbamazepine to oxcarbazepine and enzyme induction is gradually reduced, blood levels of certain concurrently used drugs may undergo significant increases, as has been shown with haloperidol and clozapine.

OVERDOSAGE

Oxcarbazepine is relatively safe in overdose; gastric lavage, activated charcoal and supportive care are generally sufficient.

THERAPEUTIC USAGE

Oxcarbazepine is supplied in 150, 300 and 600 mg tablets and as a 300 mg/5ml suspension.

In adults with normal renal function, oxcarbazepine is given in two equal divided doses, beginning at a total daily dose of 600 mg, and increasing in increments of 600 mg/day every week (when being used as an "add on" to other antiepileptic drugs) or every two to four days (when used as monotherapy). In the treatment of epilepsy, the dosage range is from 600 to 3000 mg: when used as an "add on," most patients do best at 1200 mg, and when used as monotherapy, at 2400 mg.

MHD blood levels may be used as rough guides for dosage adjustments: in epilepsy, therapeutic responses have been associated with levels of from 10 to 25 microgram/ml.

In the elderly or those with moderate renal failure (i.e., creatinine clearance of from 10 to 30 ml) dosages should be cut by one-half, with longer intervals between incremental increases. The dosage adjustments required for severe renal failure are not as yet clear.

BIBLIOGRAPHY

Baruzzi A, Albani F, Riva R. Oxcarbazepine: pharmacokinetic interactions and their clinical relevance. *Epilepsia* 1994;35(Suppl 3):14-19.

Bill PA, Vigonius U, Pohlmann H, et al. A double-blind controlled trial of oxcarbazepine versus phenytoin in adults with previously untreated epilepsy. *Epilepsy Research* 1997;27:195-204.

Christe W, Kramer G, Vigonius U, et al. A double-blind controlled trial: oxcarbazepine versus sodium valproate in adults with newly diagnosed epilepsy. *Epilepsy Research* 1997;26:451-460.

Dam M, Ekberg R, Loyning V, et al. A double-blind study comparing oxcarbazepine and carbamazepine in patients with newly diagnosed, previously untreated epilepsy. *Epilepsy Research* 1989;3:70-76.

Dickinson RG, Hooper WD, Dunstan PR, et al. First dose and steady-state pharmacokinetics of oxcarbazepine and its 10-hydroxy metabolite. *European Journal of Clinical Pharmacology* 1989;37:69-74.

Hellewell JS. Oxcarbazepine (Trileptal) in the treatment of bipolar disorders: a review of efficacy and tolerability. *Journal of Affective Disorders* 2002;72(Suppl 1):23-34.

Isojarvi JI, Turkka J, Pakarinen AJ, et al. Thryoid function in men taking carbamazepine, oxcarbazepine, or valproate for epilepsy. *Epilepsia* 2001;42:930-934.

Lloyd P, Flesch G, Dieterle W. Clinical pharmacology and pharmacokinetics of oxcarbazepine. *Epilepsia* 1994;35(Suppl 3):10-13.

Raitasuo V, Lehtovarra R, Huttunen MO. Effect of switching carbamazepine to oxcarbazepine on the plasma levels of neuroleptics. A case report. *Psychopharmacology* 1994;116:115-116.

Rouan MC, Lecaillon JB, Godbillon J, et al. The effect of renal impairment on the pharmacokinetics of oxcarbazepine and its metabolites. *European Journal of Clinical Pharmacology* 1994;47:161-167.

Sachdeo R, Beydoun A, Schacter S, et al. Oxcarbazepine (Trileptal) as monotherapy in patients with partial seizures. *Neurology* 2001;57:864-871.

Sachdeo RC, Wasserstein A, Mesenbrink PJ, et al. Effects of oxcarbazepine on sodium concentration and water handling. *Annals of Neurology* 2002;51:613-620.

Tecoma ES. Oxcarbazepine. *Epilepsia* 1999;40(Suppl 5):37-46.

287 Valproate

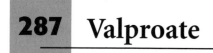

Valproate is an anion derived from either valproic acid or sodium valproate; oral preparations available for use in the United States include valproic acid and divalproex, which is a coordination compound of valproic acid and sodium valproate. Valproate's original use was in epilepsy, and it is indicated as monotherapy or adjunctive therapy in the treatment of partial seizures with or without secondary generalization, primary generalized grand mal epilepsy and petit mal epilepsy. It is also indicated for treatment of mania in bipolar disorder, and is useful for the treatment of the alcohol withdrawal syndrome. Preliminary work suggests it may be used adjunctively with antipsychotics in the treatment of acute exacerbations of schizophrenia and for agitation in traumatic brain injury.

Other uses include migraine, where it is used prophylactically, posthypoxic intention myoclonus and painful diabetic polyneuropathy.

PHARMACOKINETICS

Absorption of valproate is nearly complete; food may delay, but does not reduce, the total amount of valproate absorbed. Valproate levels peak in about 2 hours after administration of valproic acid, and within 3 to 8 hours after divalproex is taken. Protein binding is on the average 90%; however, this figure varies, becoming progressively less as the valproate concentration rises. Valproate is subject to almost complete metabolism in the liver, and one of its major metabolites, 2-propyl-pentenoic acid, is almost twice as potent as valproate itself.

The half-life of valproate is about 14 or 15 hours, but ranges from 6 to 17 hours.

SIDE EFFECTS

Nausea, vomiting, abdominal cramping, diarrhea, or constipation may occur, and gastrointestinal side effects are a not uncommon limiting factor; importantly, these are less common with the enteric-coated divalproex. Sedation may likewise be troublesome. Occasionally patients may develop a fine tremor: ataxia may also at times be seen, and rarely there may be chorea. Weight gain and hair loss may occur with chronic use. Acute pancreatitis, which may be fatal, is a rare side effect, which may be more common in the mentally retarded than in those of normal intelligence. Thrombocytopenia and thrombasthenia may occur, with petechiae and easy bruisability.

A mild increase in liver enzymes (SGOT, SGPT, and LDH) may occur within the first few months of treatment in up to almost one half of all patients, but is of no clinical significance. Rarely, however, a potentially fatal hepatotoxicity may occur. In this situation, patients complain of the acute onset of nausea, vomiting, weakness, and lethargy, which, interestingly, may not be preceded by the mild elevation of liver enzymes just mentioned. Hepatotoxicity, if it does occur, generally presents within about 2 months of the start of treatment; the range of onset, however, is wide, from only a few days up to 6 months. It appears to occur for the most part among very young children who are taking multiple anticonvulsants. Preexisting hepatic disease may also increase the risks. Should hepatotoxicity occur, consideration may be given to intravenous or oral carnitine as a treatment.

Hyperammonemia may occur, and may be accompanied by delirium, stupor or coma. Of interest, this may or may not be accompanied by a rise in hepatic enzymes, and appears to be more likely in patients with one of the inherited diseases of urea metabolism, such as ornithine transcarbamylase deficiency.

Rarely, valproate may cause cortical atrophy and dementia; importantly, this syndrome is of insidious onset and may not occur until the patient has been taking valproate for two or more years. Parkinsonism may also occur, either in conjunction with a dementia or independently. Both the dementia and the parkinsonism often resolve or improve with discontinuation of valproate; however, many months or a year or more may be required for full recovery.

Valproate is teratogenic and is excreted in breast milk.

DRUG-DRUG INTERACTIONS

The combination of valproate with several other antiepileptic drugs may have significant effects. Valproate combined with phenobarbital causes a reduced valproate and grossly increased phenobarbital level. Valproate and lamotrigine together lead to a reduction in valproate level and up to a doubling of the lamotrigine level. Valproate with carbamazepine leads to a reduced valproate level and an increase in the level of the 10,11-epoxide of carbamazepine. Finally, if valproate is combined with phenytoin, although the total phenytoin level may decrease, the level of free phenytoin increases.

Valproate levels may be increased by amitriptyline, fluoxetine and guanfacine.

Valproate may increase levels of amitriptyline, clomipramine and zidovudine.

Aspirin displaces valproate from plasma proteins, and the elevated free fraction has occasionally led to toxicity. The added thrombasthenic effect of aspirin to that of valproate may lead to an increased risk of bleeding. Valproate may displace diazepam from plasma proteins, with possibly increased sedation.

The concurrent use of clonazepam and valproate in patients with absence seizures may precipitate absence status.

OVERDOSAGE

Valproate overdose, if severe, may cause coma and death. In addition to supportive measures, gastric lavage and activated charcoal, naloxone may be given to reverse the coma; in patients with epilepsy, however, this may precipitate seizures. Hemodialysis may be effective.

It must be borne in mind that if divalproex is taken in overdose, peak levels may not occur for up to eight hours: such patients must be monitored clinically and with blood levels until the peak has been passed.

THERAPEUTIC USAGE

As noted earlier, valproate may be obtained either from valproic acid or sodium valproate, and several preparations are available. Valproic acid is available in 250 mg capsules or in a syrup containing the equivalent of 250 mg of valproic acid in 5 cc. Valproic acid and sodium valproate are also combined in a coordination compound known as divalproex, which contains equimolar amounts of valproic acid and sodium valproate: divalproex is available in 125, 250 and 500 mg tablets and in a "sprinkle" capsule containing 125 mg; there is also an extended release form of divalproex, available in a 500 mg tablet for once daily dosing. Sodium valproate is available for intravenous use in a solution containing 100 mg of sodium valproate per 1 cc.

Given the greater gastrointestinal side effects of valproic acid, divalproex is the preferred form. In non-urgent situations, treatment may be initiated at a total daily dose of about 15 mg/kg/day and is increased in weekly increments of from 5 to 10 mg/kg/day until a desired effect, limiting side effects, or a maximum dose of about 60 mg/kg/day is reached. In general, a trough blood level of between 50 and 100 μg/ml is desirable. In urgent situations, such as acute mania, a more rapid titration schedule may be employed, starting with a loading dose of 20 mg/kg/day, with dosage adjustments made on a daily basis to achieve a serum level between 50 and 100 mg/ml; typically, doses of approximately 2000 mg/day are required. The total daily dose is generally given in two or three divided doses, and once patients are stable a twice-daily schedule may be used or patients may be directly switched to the "extended release" form of divalproex, thus allowing once-daily dosage.

A baseline determination should be made of liver enzymes and platelet count. These tests should then be repeated as clinically indicated. During the first 6 months of treatment, one may decide to monitor these values on a regular basis. However, as noted earlier, hepatotoxicity may occur abruptly and may or may not be foreshadowed by mild elevations in liver enzymes.

BIBLIOGRAPHY

Armon C, Shin C, Miller P, et al. Reversible parkinsonism and cognitive impairment with chronic valproate use. *Neurology* 1996;47:626-635.
Bohan TP, Helton E, McDonald I, et al. Effect of L-carnitine treatment for valproate-induced hepatotoxicity. *Neurology* 2001;56:1405-1409.

Chatham Showalter PE, Kimmel DN. Agitated symptom response to divalproex following acute brain injury. *The Journal of Neuropsychiatry and Clinical Neurosciences* 2000;12:195-197.

DeToledo JC, Haddad H, Ramsay RE. Status epilepticus associated with the combination of valproic acid and clomipramine. *Therapeutic Drug Monitoring* 1997;19:71-73.

Feil D, Chuang K, Sultzer DL. Valproate-induced hyperammonemia as a cause of altered mental status. *American Journal of Geriatric Psychiatry* 2002;10:476-478.

Gunal DI, Guleryuz M, Bingol CA. Reversible valproate-induced choreiform movements. *Seizure* 2002;11:205-206.

Oechsner M, Steen C, Tturenburg HJ, et al. Hyperammonaemic encephalopathy after initiation of valproate therapy in unrecognized ornithine transcarbamylase deficiency. *Journal of Neurology, Neurosurgery, and Psychiatry* 1998;64:680-682.

Onofrj M, Thomas A, Paci C. Reversible parkinsonism induced by prolonged treatment with valproate. *Journal of Neurology* 1998;245:794-796.

Papazian O, Canizales E, Alfonso I, et al. Reversible dementia and apparent brain atrophy during valproate therapy. *Annals of Neurology* 1995; 38:687-691.

Perucca E. Pharmacological and therapeutic properties of valproate: a summary after 35 years of clinical experience. *CNS Drugs* 2002;16: 695-714.

Wassef AA, Dott SG, Harris A, et al. Randomized, placebo-controlled pilot study of divalproex sodium in the treatment of acute exacerbations of chronic schizophrenia. *Journal of Clinical Psychopharmacology* 2000;20:357-361.

Wong SL, Cavanaugh J, Shi H, et al. Effects of divalproex sodium on amitriptyline and nortriptyline pharmacokinetics. *Clinical Pharmacology and Therapeutics* 1996;60:48-53.

288   Lamotrigine

Lamotrigine is indicated for monotherapy of partial seizures with or without secondary generalization, and in this regard is generally equivalent to gabapentin, phenytoin and carbamazepine, and is overall better tolerated than either phenytoin or carbamazepine. It is also effective in the treatment of petit mal epilepsy and primary grand mal epilepsy.

Of great interest to psychiatry, lamotrigine is also effective as maintenance treatment in bipolar disorder. Here, it is most effective in preventing recurrence of depression.

Lamotrigine appears to exert its therapeutic effect in epilepsy by virtue of a use-dependent blockade of sodium channels, leading to a reduction in the amount of glutamate release from presynaptic neurons.

PHARMACOKINETICS

The bioavailability of lamotrigine is almost 100%, and peak levels are reached within 1 to 3 hours, with protein binding of about 55%. Hepatic metabolism is extensive, and primarily involves glucuronidation; there are no active metabolites.

SIDE EFFECTS

Lamotrigine is generally well-tolerated; a minority of patients may experience a degree of sedation, dizziness, ataxia, blurred vision, nausea or vomiting. The most problematic side effect of lamotrigine is a rash which may occur in anywhere from 3 to 10% of patients, and may range in severity from benign to life-threatening.

There are case reports of patients developing tics secondary to lamotrigine, and one case report of blepharospasm.

DRUG-DRUG INTERACTIONS

Lamotrigine levels are reduced by phenobarbital, primidone, phenytoin, carbamazepine, oral contraceptives and rifampicin.

Lamotrigine levels are increased, in a dose-dependent manner, by valproate. There is also an anecdotal report of sertraline increasing lamotrigine levels.

Lamotrigine may increase the level of the 10,11-epoxide of carbamazepine, although this is controversial.

OVERDOSAGE

Overdosage is manifest by stupor which may progress to coma and death. Gastric lavage, activated charcoal and vigorous supportive care are indicated; hemodialysis is of little benefit.

THERAPEUTIC USAGE

Lamotrigine is available in 25, 100, 150 and 200 mg scored tablets.

Given that the likelihood of a rash increases in proportion to the rapidity with which the dose of lamotrigine is escalated, treatment is generally initiated gradually.

In cases where the patient is already taking an enzyme-inducing drug, such as phenobarbital, primidone, phenytoin or carbamazepine, treatment is begun at a total daily dose of 50 mg for two weeks, then 100 mg for the next two weeks, and then increased in 100 mg/d increments every week until limiting side effects occur or there is a response: most patients with epilepsy respond to doses between 200 and 500 mg/day, and for bipolar disorder the dosage range is from 200 to 400 mg. When added to an enzyme-inducer, lamotrigine is given in two divided doses.

In cases where the patient is already taking valproate, treatment is begun at a total daily dose of 25 mg given every other day for two weeks, then increased to 25 mg daily for the next two weeks, with subsequent incremental increases of 25-50 mg/d every week or two thereafter until limiting side effects occur or there is a response: most patients concurrently taking valproate respond to lamotrigine in doses of from 100 to 200 mg daily. When added to valproate, the total daily dose of lamotrigine may be given once daily.

When lamotrigine is used as monotherapy, treatment is commenced at 25 mg given every other day for two weeks, then increased to 25 mg daily for the next two weeks, with subsequent incremental increases of 25-50 mg/d every week or two thereafter until limiting side effects occur or there is a response: most patients under monotherapy require doses between 200 and 400 mg, given in two divided doses.

In the elderly or those with hepatic failure, the dose must be decreased and the intervals between dose escalations should be increased.

BIBLIOGRAPHY

Bowden CL, Calabrese JR, Sachs G, et al. A placebo-controlled 18-month trial of lamotrigine and lithium maintenance treatment in recently manic or hypomanic patients with bipolar I disorder. *Archives of General Psychiatry* 2003;60:392-400.

Brodie MJ, Chadwick DW, Anhut H, et al. Gabapentin versus lamotrigine monotherapy: a double-blind comparison in newly diagnosed epilepsy. *Epilepsia* 2002;43:993-1000.

Calabrese JR, Bowden CL, Sachs GS, et al. A double-blind placebo-controlled study of lamotrigine monotherapy in outpatients with bipolar I depression. *The Journal of Clinical Psychiatry* 1999;60:79-88.

Frank LM, Enlow T, Holmes GL, et al. Lamictal (lamotrigine) monotherapy for typical absence seizures in children. *Epilepsia* 1999;40:973-979.

Kaufman KR, George R. Lamotrigine toxicity secondary to sertraline. *Seizure* 1998;7:163-165.

Marcellin P, de Bony F, Garret C, et al. Influence of cirrhosis on lamotrigine pharmacokinetics. *British Journal of Clinical Pharmacology* 2001;51: 410-414.

Rambeck B, Wolf P. Lamotrigine clinical pharmacokinetics. *Clinical Pharmacokinetics* 1993;25:433-443.

Sabers A, Buchholt JM, Uldall P, et al. Lamotrigine plasma levels reduced by oral contraceptives. *Epilepsy Research* 2001;47:151-154.

Sotero de Menezes MA, Rho JM, Murphy P, et al. Lamotrigine-induced tic disorder: report of five pediatric cases. *Epilepsia* 2000;41:862-867.

Steiner TJ, Dellaportas CI, Findley LJ, et al. Lamotrigine monotherapy in newly diagnosed untreated epilepsy: a double-blind comparison with phenytoin. *Epilepsia* 1999;40:601-607.

Verma A, Miller P, Carwile ST, et al. Lamotrigine-induced blepharospasm. *Pharmacotherapy* 1999;19:877-880.

289 Gabapentin

Although gabapentin is a structural analog of GABA, it does not, in fact, function as a GABA agonist, and its mechanism of action remains unknown. It is useful as monotherapy for partial seizures with or without secondary generalization, and in this regard is comparable to lamotrigine. It is also useful for social phobia of the generalized type, restless legs syndrome, nocturnal myoclonus, post-herpetic neuralgia and painful diabetic polyneuropathy; it may also have a place in the treatment of essential tremor, orthostatic tremor and in migraine prophylaxis. Importantly, although unblinded studies suggested efficacy in the treatment of bipolar disorder, two double-blinded studies have not borne this out.

PHARMACOKINETICS

Gabapentin is absorbed in the proximal small bowel by the L-amino acid transporter system. This system is saturable within the therapeutic dosage range of gabapentin: although bioavailability is about 60% at doses of 900 mg, it falls to roughly 35% at a dose of 3600 mg. Peak blood levels are reached in from two to three hours, and protein binding is negligible. Gabapentin is not metabolized, and is excreted unchanged in the urine with a half life of from 5 to 7 hours.

SIDE EFFECTS

Sedation, dizziness and ataxia are most common, but these are generally mild and transient. At high doses, some weight gain may occur. Overall gabapentin is remarkably well tolerated.

There are two case reports of hypomania occurring as a side effect of gabapentin.

Gabapentin is excreted in breast milk; its teratogenic potential is not known.

DRUG-DRUG INTERACTIONS

Gabapentin may increase felbamate levels.

Concomitant use of antacids may reduce gabapentin absorption by about 20%.

OVERDOSAGE

Somnolence and lethargy may occur; general supportive care is generally sufficient.

THERAPEUTIC USAGE

Gabapentin is available in 100, 300 and 400 mg capsules, as 600 and 800 mg tablets, and as a 250 mg/5 mL oral solution.

Early work with gabapentin employed a slow titration, beginning at 300 mg; however, it is now clear that most patients tolerate a dose of 900 to 1200 mg on the first day, with daily increases in similar increments until symptoms are controlled, unacceptable side effects occur or a maximum total daily dose of 3600 mg is reached. Given gabapentin's short half life, this total daily dose should generally be divided into three equal doses. Although increasing the total daily dose above 3600 generally does not substantially increase the blood level of gabapentin, there are exceptions to this rule, and some patients may require doses as high as 4800. In general, total daily doses of from 900 to 2400 mg are sufficient for the indications noted above. The dose should be reduced in renal failure: for creatinine clearances of from 30 to 60 mL/min, the dose is reduced by about 60%, and may be given in two divided doses; at 15 to 30 mL/min, the dose is reduced by about 80% and may be given once daily; and at a creatinine clearance below 15 mL/min, the dose should be reduced by about 90%, and may be given once daily. Dosage reductions should also be made for the elderly.

BIBLIOGRAPHY

Berry DJ, Beran RG, Plunkeft MJ, et al. The absorption of gabapentin following high dose escalation. *Seizure* 2003;12:28-36.

Beydoun A, Uthman BM, Sackellares JC. Gabapentin: pharmacokinetics, efficacy, and safety. *Clinical Neuropharmacology* 1995;18:469-481.

Brodie MJ, Chadwick DW, Anhut H, et al. Gabapentin versus lamotrigine monotherapy: a double-blind comparison in newly diagnosed epilepsy. *Epilepsia* 2002;43:993-1000.

Fisher RS, Sachdeo RC, Pellock J, et al. Rapid initiation of gabapentin: a randomized, controlled trial. *Neurology* 2001;56:743-748.

Frye MA, Ketter TA, Kimbrell TA, et al. A placebo-controlled study of lamotrigine and gabapentin monotherapy in refractory mood disorders. *Journal of Clinical Psychopharmacology* 2000;20:607-614.

Garcia-Borreguero D, Larrosa O, de la Llave Y, et al. Treatment of restless legs syndrome with gabapentin: a double-blind, cross-over study. *Neurology* 2002;59:1573-1579.

Morello CM, Leckband SG, Stoner CP, et al. Randomized, double-blind study comparing the efficacy of gabapentin with amitriptyline on diabetic peripheral neuropathy pain. *Archives of Internal Medicine* 1999;159:1931-1937.

Pande AC, Crockatt JG, Janney CA, et al. Gabapentin in bipolar disorder: a placebo-controlled trial of adjunctive therapy. *Bipolar Disorders* 2000;2:249-255.

Rice AS, Maton S. Gabapentin in postherpetic neuralgia: a randomized, double blind, placebo controlled study. *Pain* 2001;94:215-224.

Trinka E, Niedermuller U, Thaler C, et al. Gabapentin-induced mood changes with hypomanic features in adults. *Seizure* 2000;9:505-508.

290   Topiramate

Topiramate is useful as monotherapy for the treatment of partial seizures with or without secondary generalization, and in this regard is of comparable efficacy with either carbamazepine or valproate. Topiramate also reduces the frequency of binging in binge-eating disorder, and a case series report suggested that it may also be effective in the treatment of bulimia nervosa. As noted below, one of topiramate's side effects is weight loss, and in one open study this was turned to good advantage in the successful treatment of weight gain occurring secondary to treatment with SSRIs. Multiple open studies have suggested that topiramate may be effective in the acute treatment of mania in bipolar disorder; however, unpublished studies have not borne this out. One single-blind study suggested that it is comparable to bupropion in the treatment of bipolar depression. Topiramate, in one double-blinded study of alcoholism, reduced drinking days and the amount drunk per day. Finally, topiramate is also effective in the treatment of essential tremor and in the prevention of migraine.

Although it is clear that topiramate blocks sodium channels and enhances chloride flux at GABA receptor sites, the precise mechanism responsible for its therapeutic effects is not clear.

PHARMACOKINETICS

The bioavailability of topiramate is about 75%, and peak levels are reached in about two hours; protein binding is almost negligible, at about 15%. Somewhat more than 70% of topiramate is excreted unchanged in the urine and the rest is metabolized in the liver to inactive metabolites; the half life ranges from 15 to 24 hours.

SIDE EFFECTS

Sedation, fatigue, poor concentration and ataxia may occur, and are generally related not only to dose but also to the rapidity with which the dose is increased. Other side effects related to rapid dose titration include psychosis, mood changes, irritability, aggression, agitation and anxiety.

Word-finding difficulties occur in roughly 7% of patients, regardless of the rapidity of dose escalation.

Weight loss, as noted earlier, may occur during the first year of therapy, and this may be quite significant.

Topiramate is a carbonic anhydrase inhibitor, and a metabolic acidosis may occur which, rarely, may lead to hyperventilation. Paresthesiae may also occur, but are generally mild and transient.

Hypohidrosis and elevated temperature may occur, but are rare.

Acute narrow-angle glaucoma is a rare, but dreaded, side effect.

DRUG-DRUG INTERACTIONS

Topiramate levels are reduced by phenytoin and carbamazepine.

Topiramate may cause an increase in phenytoin level.

Topiramate may reduce ethinyl estradiol levels in patients taking oral contraceptives; however, this is dose-dependent, with little effect until the dose is above 200 mg.

OVERDOSAGE

Stupor may occur. Gastric lavage is indicated, but activated charcoal may not be effective. Hemodialysis removes topiramate, but this is rarely required and supportive care is generally sufficient.

THERAPEUTIC USAGE

Topiramate is available in 25, 100 and 200 mg tablets.

Treatment is generally initiated at 25 to 50 mg per day and increased in similar increments every week until limiting side effects occur or a maximum dose of 500 mg, with the total daily dose being divided into two doses. A more rapid titration schedule may be considered, but, as noted above, this is not as well tolerated: patients may be started at 100 mg/day with the dose increased in 100 to 200 mg increments every week.

In the treatment of epilepsy, a dose of 400 mg is recommended; however, some patients do well at lower doses. For the other indications, the dose ranges from 100 to 200 mg.

When topiramate is added to a regimen containing either phenytoin or carbamazepine and the original drug is then discontinued, it may be necessary to subsequently lower the dose of topiramate to avoid toxicity.

Dosage should also be reduced in cases of hepatic or renal failure.

BIBLIOGRAPHY

Bourgeois BF. Drug interaction profile of topiramate. *Epilepsia* 1996;37(Suppl 2):14-17.

Connor GS. A double-blind placebo-controlled trial of topiramate for essential tremor. *Neurology* 2002;59:132-134.

McIntyre RS, Mancini DA, McCann S, et al. Topiramate versus bupropion SR when added to mood stabilizer therapy for the depressive phase of bipolar disorder: a preliminary single-blind study. *Bipolar Disorders* 2002;4:207-213.

Mula M, Trimble MR, Lhatoo SD, et al. Topiramate and psychiatric adverse events in patients with epilepsy. *Epilepsia* 2003;44:659-663.

Mula M, Trimble MR, Thompson P, et al. Topiramate and word-finding difficulties in patients with epilepsy. *Neurology* 2003;60:1104-1107.

Privitera MD, Broide MJ, Mattson RH, et al. Topiramate, carbamazepine and valproate monotherapy: double-blind comparison in newly diagnosed epilepsy. *Acta Neurologica Scandinavica* 2003;107:165-175.

Storey JR, Calder CS, Hart DE, et al. Topiramate in migraine prevention: a double-blind, placebo-controlled study. *Headache* 2001;41:968-975.

Suppes T. Review of the use of topiramate for treatment of bipolar disorders. *Journal of Clinical Psychopharmacology* 2002;22:599-609.

Van Ameringen M, Mancini C, Pipe B, et al. Topiramate treatment for SSRI-induced wieght gain in anxiety disorders. *The Journal of Clinical Psychiatry* 2002;63:981-984.

291 First Generation Antipsychotics

The first generation antipsychotics are a large group of drugs whose principal indication is the treatment of schizophrenia. These drugs are also at times referred to as neuroleptics, and were, in the past, termed "major tranquilizers," but this term has fortunately been abandoned.

The antipsychotics may be divided into two broad groups, namely the "first generation" or "typical" antipsychotics and the more recent "second generation" or "atypical" antipsychotics. The various first generation antipsychotics are listed in the box on p. 476; the second generation antipsychotics include clozapine, risperidone, olanzapine, ziprasidone, quetiapine and aripiprazole. The distinction between the first and the second generation antipsychotics is based on differences in receptor activity, side effects and overall efficacy. With regard to receptor activity, the first generation drugs are primarily dopamine receptor blockers; by contrast the second generation antipsychotics, though also possessing dopamine blocking activity, exert prominent inhibitory effects at serotonin receptors. With regard to side effects, most of the second generation drugs are, by and large, better tolerated than the first generation ones. There are, however, some notable exceptions here, especially with regard to clozapine and, possibly, olanzapine. With regard to efficacy in schizophrenia, it is clear that clozapine, risperidone and olanzapine are superior to the first generation agents; whether or not the other second generation drugs share this superiority has not as yet been demonstrated in double-blinded studies.

This chapter deals with the first generation antipsychotics; each of the second generation antipsychotics is dealt with separately in its own chapter. Before proceeding to the first generation antipsychotics, however, it may be appropriate to say a few words as to why these agents are still used. One very important reason is the incredible wealth of experience we have with these agents: there are very few surprises here, whereas, as noted in the chapters on second generation agents, unanticipated, and at times serious, side effects are now coming to light, such as significant weight gain, hyperlipidemia and diabetes. Another reason is the availability of long-acting decanoate preparations of haloperidol and fluphenazine;

however, this advantage may soon pale should the long-acting form of risperidone become available. Finally, there is the matter of price: many patients do quite well on a first generation agent and would gain little, except a sometimes huge expense, if treated with a second generation agent.

The first generation antipsychotics come from several different chemical classes: phenothiazines (divided into aliphatic, piperidine, and piperazine subgroups), thioxanthenes, butyrophenones, dibenzoxazepines, and dihydroindolones. These classes are listed in the box on p. 476, where they are also designated as low- or high-potency antipsychotics, a useful distinction.

Although all of the foregoing antipsychotics are equally effective, on the average, in the treatment of schizophrenia, haloperidol is by far the most widely used of the first generation antipsychotics, and this is true not only for schizophrenia but for most of the other indications noted below. An additional first generation antipsychotic, pimozide, is sufficiently unique, especially with regard to side effects, that it is treated in its own chapter.

First generation antipsychotics are useful for the treatment of schizophrenia; schizoaffective disorder; delusional disorder; alcohol hallucinosis and alcoholic paranoia; mania; postpartum psychosis; dementia and delirium; borderline, paranoid and schizotypal personality disorders; Tourette's syndrome; psychosis occurring secondary to intoxication with cocaine, stimulants, phencyclidine, cannabis or anabolic steroids; occasionally in delirium tremens; occasionally in a depressive episode with psychotic features; autism; conduct disorder when characterized by aggression and impulsivity; mental retardation when complicated by stereotypies or aggression and impulsivity; developmental stuttering; chorea (e.g., Huntington's disease or Sydenham's chorea); ballism; porphyria; and as an adjunct to tricyclic antidepressants for chronic pain syndrome.

As noted earlier, on the average, all the antipsychotics considered in this chapter are equally effective in the treatment of schizophrenia and most of the other disorders just mentioned. Thus choosing among them is often based on their anticipated side effects. This task, in turn, is made easier if one groups the antipsychotics as

Antipsychotics

■

Phenothiazines
    Aliphatic
        Chlorpromazine*
    Piperidine
        Thioridazine*
        Mesoridazine*
    Piperazine
        Perphenazine†
        Trifluoperazine†
        Fluphenazine†
Thioxanthines
    Thiothixene†
Butyrophenone
    Haloperidol†
Dibenzoxazepine
    Loxapine‡
Dihydroindolone
    Molindone‡

*Low-potency drug.
†High-potency drug.
‡High-potency drug, although some consider these "medium-potency" drugs.

either "low potency" or "high potency," with reference to the average dose required for a therapeutic effect. The low-potency drugs require relatively large doses and are more likely to produce sedation, hypotension, and anticholinergic effects; they are less likely, however, to produce extrapyramidal side effects. The high-potency drugs, by contrast, require relatively small doses and are less likely to produce sedation, hypotension, and anticholinergic effects and more likely to produce extrapyramidal side effects.

Some authors consider loxapine and molindone to be in a separate group, namely a "medium-potency" group, because their tendency to produce side effects of all types is somewhere between the low- and high-potency drugs. In practice, however, both loxapine and molindone are more similar to the traditional high-potency drugs and are usefully included in that subgroup.

Two high-potency antipsychotics, fluphenazine and haloperidol, are also available in a long-acting injectable form. In each case the parent molecule is esterified with a decanoate moiety, producing fluphenazine decanoate and haloperidol decanoate, respectively.

The antipsychotics produce their therapeutic effect, at least initially, by competitively blockading postsynaptic dopamine receptors. Of the three principal dopaminergic pathways, blockade in the nigrostriatal system results in extrapyramidal effects, and blockade in the mesolimbic and mesocortical systems is responsible for the therapeutic effect in schizophrenia and most of the other indications.

PHARMACOKINETICS

Bioavailability ranges from 20 to 70%, and is consistently higher with liquid preparations than with tablets. Protein binding ranges from 90 to 99%, and peak levels are obtained within 1 to 4 hours. The interpatient variability in blood levels given the same oral dose may be quite high, as much as tenfold or more in the case of chlorpromazine. Metabolism is via hepatic enzymes, and the half-lives range from 8 to 36 hours, averaging from 18 to 24. Most of these antipsychotics have active metabolites: chlorpromazine may have more than 50, and in the case of thioridazine one of its active metabolites is the commercially available mesoridazine. In the case

of haloperidol, there may be no active metabolites; "reduced" haloperidol may or may not be active in and of itself; in any case, it can undergo "reverse" metabolism back to the parent compound, haloperidol.

Given the limited bioavailability of most antipsychotics, intramuscular administration of doses equivalent to oral doses result in higher blood levels, sometimes twofold or threefold higher, or even more.

SIDE EFFECTS

As noted earlier, although all the first generation antipsychotics can cause sedation, hypotension, and anticholinergic effects, the low-potency drugs are more likely to do so. Hypotension is often postural and may lead to light-headedness or syncope. Anticholinergic effects include dry mouth, blurry vision, constipation, urinary hesitancy or retention, tachycardia, and, given a high enough dose, an anticholinergic delirium, as described in that chapter.

The acute extrapyramidal side effects, which are more common with high-potency agents, include parkinsonism, bradykinesia and bradyphrenia, akathisia, dystonia, oculogyric crisis, and a difficult to describe yet very definite and unpleasant sense of dysphoria.

Parkinsonism may manifest with any or all of the following: a pill-rolling tremor, masked facies, excessive salivation, a stooped flexion posture, festination, and cogwheel rigidity. Bradyphrenia and bradykinesia, although also part of the parkinsonian syndrome, often occur in isolation and thus deserve special note. Although not stiff or rigid, patients move slowly (as if in molasses), and they complain that their thoughts come slowly, if at all. Often this bradyphrenia and bradykinesia is mistaken for a psychomotorically retarded depression. Antipsychotic-induced parkinsonism appears within days to several weeks after initiation of treatment or a substantial increase in dose and persists until the dose is lowered or effective antiparkinsonian treatment is initiated.

Akathisia, classically, manifests as a restless inability to sit or lie still. Patients typically complain of a restlessness "in the legs" that is worse when they lie or sit down, and is partially relieved by getting up and perhaps pacing around. At times, such an akathisia may be mistaken for agitation. In addition to such motoric restlessness, many patients also complain of a restlessness or racing of their thoughts. Occasionally, akathisia may manifest only as such cognitive restlessness, and when it does, great diagnostic confusion may arise. Patients may appear more psychotic; their speech may be more disorganized and their behavior more fragmented. At times, such patients with cognitive akathisia may, rather than appear restless, become withdrawn, almost mute, and only when they evidence a dramatic response to propranolol or benztropine is the correct diagnosis confirmed. Lacking a correct diagnosis, such patients may be treated with ever-escalating doses of antipsychotics, with an ever-increasing worsening of their clinical status. Akathisia, whether motoric or cognitive or both, is typically of gradual onset, anywhere from 1 to 8 weeks after initiation of treatment or substantial dose increase. Like parkinsonism, akathisia is chronic and persists until either the dose is lowered or treatment with propranolol or an anticholinergic, antiparkinsonian drug is begun.

Dystonic manifestations, in order of decreasing frequency, include torticollis, thick tongue (which may present as dysarthria), dystonic posturing of the upper or, less frequently, lower extremities, torsion dystonia involving the trunk and extremities, and, rarely, opisthotonic posturing. Very rarely, laryngeal dystonia may occur, and in such cases aspiration has occurred. Oculogyric crises, although properly considered an extraocular dystonia, are sufficiently singular in appearance that they deserve special note. These relatively common dystonias typically present with involuntary upward deviation of both eyes. Patients often complain that they cannot "look down" and they may fall down stairs. Although all dystonias may involve some discomfort, the oculogyric crisis at times may be actually painful. Dystonias tend to occur earlier than parkinsonism or akathisia, typically within days, and rather than being chronic, they tend to be episodic. In most cases, if nothing is done, the dystonia remits spontaneously, often within hours. Most patients, however, are unwilling to wait and welcome the dramatic relief with benztropine or diphenhydramine.

The last of the acute extrapyramidal side effects to consider lacks an agreed upon name—"antipsychotic-induced dysphoria" is probably as good as any other. Patients may complain that they feel unwell or not themselves. Some, less articulate than others, may simply say that they do not like the medicine, that it does not "agree" with them. This antipsychotic-induced dysphoria may occur within days and tends to be chronic. One should inquire of patients whether their medicine "agrees" with them, because this dysphoria may respond to benztropine or propranolol.

Weight gain is another important side effect of first generation antipsychotics, and although more common with low-potency drugs, it is also frequently seen with high-potency ones. Molindone appears to be an exception, with little or no associated weight gain.

All of the antipsychotics reliably cause an elevation of prolactin levels, with possible associated breast enlargement and galactorrhea. Such elevated prolactin levels do not appear associated with an increased risk of breast cancer. Antipsychotics may also cause menstrual irregularities or amenorrhea. False positive urine pregnancy tests may also occur; however, false positive serum pregnancy tests are very rare.

The seizure threshold may be reduced, especially by low-potency agents. Epilepsy, however, is not a contraindication to antipsychotic treatment. In such cases, adequate seizure control may be obtained by generally increasing the dose of the antiepileptic drug.

First generation antipsychotics, particularly low-potency antipsychotics, may predispose to heat stroke. This probably results from a combination of factors, including decreased sweating (an anticholinergic effect) and a tendency toward poikilothermia, which is most marked with low-potency drugs.

ECG changes are most common with low-potency agents and include prolonged corrected QT interval, depressed ST segments, depressed or inverted T-waves, and, occasionally, the appearance of a U-wave. Thioridazine, which (unique among these antipsychotics) appears to have calcium channel blocking activity, seems most likely to produce these changes. Occasionally, severe ventricular arrhythmias may occur, and the incidence of sudden cardiac death is higher for thioridazine than for the other first generation agents. Rarely, one may see a clinically significant degree of suppression of cardiac contractility.

Disturbances in sexual functioning are common with antipsychotics and are more likely with low-potency agents. They include erectile dysfunction, delayed ejaculation, anorgasmia, and decreased libido. Retrograde ejaculation may occur, and this is particularly common with thioridazine, occurring in perhaps half of the men who take it. Painful ejaculation may also occur.

Thioridazine may also cause a distressing nasal stuffiness and congestion.

Photosensitivity, which is more common with low-potency drugs, may occur and may lead to severe sunburn. In patients treated for long periods with high doses of chlorpromazine or thioridazine, one may also, very rarely, see a slate-blue pigmentation, more prominent on exposed surfaces.

Thioridazine may rarely cause a pigmentary retinopathy. This usually occurs with chronic treatment at high doses of 1 g or more daily. Doses of 800 mg or less are considered safe.

All the antipsychotics, with chronic treatment, may cause particulate deposits in the cornea or lens. These are rare and generally detectable only with slit lamp examination and are rarely symptomatic.

Another rare side effect of the antipsychotics is hyponatremia secondary to SIADH.

Allergic manifestations may occur and include rashes, jaundice, and agranulocytosis. Rashes tend to occur early in treatment, cholestatic jaundice within the first month, and agranulocytosis at any time in treatment. All of these allergic manifestations are uncommon or rare and tend to occur more frequently with the low-potency drugs.

Tardive dyskinesia and the neuroleptic malignant syndrome are discussed in their respective chapters.

The teratogenicity of the antipsychotics is not known, but it is believed to be quite low. In all likelihood all of them are excreted in the breast milk.

DRUG-DRUG INTERACTIONS

Most, but not all, first generation antipsychotics inhibit CYP2D6 enzymes and thus may cause a significant rise in tricyclic antidepressant blood levels. Haloperidol may increase fluvoxamine levels, and in turn carbamazepine may reduce haloperidol levels. The effectiveness of L-dopa or dopamine agonists such as bromocriptine or pergolide is reduced by antipsychotics.

Other interactions of questionable clinical significance include reduced antipsychotic levels due to antacids, anticholinergics, or phenobarbital; increased antipsychotic levels due to propranolol; and reduced levels of valproic acid and oral anticoagulants with concurrent administration of antipsychotics.

OVERDOSAGE

Taken alone in overdose, antipsychotics are generally not lethal. In severe cases, coma and hypotension may occur. Convulsions may occur; arrhythmias may also occur and are more common with thioridazine.

Gastric lavage and activated charcoal are generally indicated. No attempt should be made to induce emesis. Hypotension may be treated with fluids; if pressor agents are required, epinephrine and isoproterenol should be avoided because they may aggravate the hypotension.

THERAPEUTIC USAGE

The various available preparations of the first generation antipsychotics are listed in Table 291-1.

The treatment of schizophrenia, schizoaffective disorder, paranoia, alcohol hallucinosis, and alcoholic paranoia with antipsychotics may be initiated as follows. The choice among antipsychotics is based on the following factors: personal or family history of past response, anticipated need for long-acting decanoate preparations, and the effect of anticipated side effects in any particular patient.

■TABLE 291-1. First Generation Preparations

	Strength, mg	Liquid Preparation	Injectable
chlorpromazine	10, 25, 50, 100, 200	100 mg/mL	Y
thioridazine	10, 25, 50, 100, 200	N	N
mesoridazine	10, 25, 50, 100	25 mg/mL	N
perphenazine	2, 4, 8, 16	16 mg/5 mL	Y
trifluoperazine	1, 2, 5, 10	10 mg/mL	Y
fluphenazine	1, 2.5, 5, 10	2.5 mg/5 mL	Y
thiothixene	1, 2, 5, 10, 20	5 mg/mL	Y
haloperidol	0.5, 1, 2, 5, 10, 20	2 mg/mL	Y
loxapine	5, 10, 25, 50	25 mg/mL	Y
molindone	5, 10, 25, 50, 100	20 mg/mL	N

Presuming that one gets no compelling history of a good previous response and that one does not anticipate a problem with compliance that would suggest using a decanoate, then the choice is based on side effects. In broad terms, therefore, one must choose between either a low-potency agent or a high-potency agent. For example, patients who must remain alert or who could not tolerate hypotension or anticholinergic effects should probably not be given a low-potency drug. Conversely, those who might not tolerate extrapyramidal side effects should probably not be offered a high-potency drug. In cases where one has no clear-cut contraindications to either low- or high-potency drugs, one generally does best to choose a high-potency drug. Extrapyramidal side effects, should they appear, are generally treatable, whereas sedation, hypotension, and anticholinergic effects are less amenable to treatment and may necessitate lowering the dose with a possible loss of effectiveness.

If the choice is to use one of the high-potency drugs either haloperidol or fluphenazine should be chosen because they allow for an easy transition to use of a decanoate form, should that be required in the future, as it often is: of these two agents, haloperidol is by far the most commonly used. If, however, the choice is to use a low-potency drug, chlorpromazine should be chosen.

Once an agent is chosen, the patient is started on an "average" dose. For high-potency drugs this should be roughly in the range of 5 to 15 mg; for low-potency drugs the range is roughly anywhere from 100 to 300 mg. For loxapine and molindone the range is from 50 to 100 mg. Large body size and extremely severe symptoms suggest a dose in the upper end of the range; whereas small size, debilitation, old age, hepatic insufficiency, and concern over possible side effects suggest using a dose on the lower end of the range. Indeed, in some frail elderly patients doses of 0.5 or 1 mg of a high-potency drug may be preferred. In most cases giving the entire daily dose at bedtime is appropriate; an exception might be when some degree of sedation is desired during the day. When intramuscular dosing is required, given the generally low bioavailability of oral antipsychotics, one can use a dose equivalent to anywhere from 50% to 75% of the oral dose.

In general, one should wait 3 to 5 days before increasing the dose, as a significant response is rarely seen before then; indeed, one may have to wait 6 to 8 weeks to see a full response to any given dose. An exception would be when severe agitation is present, and in such cases the protocol for rapid treatment, as outlined in that chapter, may be followed.

The goal is to use the lowest possible dose consistent with an optimum remission of symptoms. Earlier practices of using high doses (e.g., 60 to 100 mg of haloperidol or 2 to 3 g of chlorpromazine) for initial treatment have been largely abandoned because they fail to produce better results than the lower doses outlined above and produce very troubling degrees of side effects.

Sedation, anticholinergic effects, hypotension, and extrapyramidal side effects are all dose related, and, if they do occur to a troubling degree, may be lessened by reducing the dose. Furthermore, even with continued treatment at the same dose, sedation and anticholinergic effects tend to lessen over days or weeks. When dose reduction is not practical, the following treatments for side effects may be considered. For sedation, one should attempt to give most of, if not the entire, daily dose at bedtime; caffeine may also help during the day. Hypotensive patients should be cautioned to rise slowly; support stockings, though often impractical, may help. Dry mouth may be relieved by sucking sugar-free hard candy, blurry vision by using reading glasses, constipation by using psyllium and as-needed laxatives, and urinary hesitancy by using bethanechol.

Extrapyramidal side effects are generally amenable to treatment. Parkinsonism may be treated with an anticholinergic, as described in that chapter. In general, the effective dose of the anticholinergic should be continued until the antipsychotic dose is decreased, at which time a complementary decrease in the dose of the anticholinergic may be attempted.

Akathisia is best treated with propranolol, which is clearly superior to anticholinergics in this case; average daily doses range from 60 to 240 mg. As with parkinsonism, treatment is chronic, with the dose adjusted after antipsychotic doses are changed. If propranolol is ineffective or not tolerated, consideration may be given to cyproheptadine in doses of approximately 8 mg bid.

Dystonias respond very well to intramuscular injection of 2 mg of benztropine or intravenous injection of 50 mg of diphenhydramine. After the first dystonia has occurred, most clinicians start a prophylactic dose of benztropine to prevent a recurrence.

Treatment of the antipsychotic-induced dysphoria is not as yet clearly worked out. Some patients appear to respond to benztropine, and others may respond to propranolol.

Certain other side effects are also amenable to treatment. Patients taking low-potency drugs should be instructed to use a sunscreen to prevent photosensitive sunburn and should be cautioned to avoid activity that might predispose to heat stroke. The treatment of sexual side effects is not as yet clearly worked out; a cautious trial of sildenafil may be considered for erectile dysfunction, with due regard to potentially additive hypotensive effects. Gynecomastia may be treated with amantadine.

If side effects preclude treatment with an "average" dose, then another antipsychotic, statistically less likely to cause the side effects in question, should be used.

Presuming that the patient is taking an "average" dose, a trial of that antipsychotic should be of "adequate" duration before assessing the drug's effectiveness. In most cases an initial response is seen within the first week; however, a full response to any given dose may take 6 to 8 weeks.

The usefulness of blood levels is a controversial subject. The existence of multiple active metabolites for most antipsychotics (with the notable exception of haloperidol) makes correlation between clinical response and levels of the parent compound very difficult. With this caveat in mind, it may be noted that therapeutic responses have been noted for chlorpromazine levels between 30 and 100 nanogram/mL, for fluphenazine between 0.2 and 2 nanogram/mL, and for haloperidol between 2 and 15 nanogram/mL. It is not clear whether the upper figure in each case represents the high end of a true "therapeutic window," or rather is a level at which unacceptable side effects, including antipsychotic-induced dysphoria, occurs.

If a given antipsychotic at "average" dose produces little or no clinical response after a trial of adequate duration, one may either increase the dose or switch to a different antipsychotic. In general, provided that side effects are not limiting, a reasonable "high dose" upper limit for a low-potency drug is about 1 to 2 g, and for a high-potency drug it is anywhere from 30 to 50 mg (for loxapine and molindone, the figure would be about 200 mg). If the decision is made to switch to a different antipsychotic, then one from a different class should be chosen. Thus if the patient fails to respond to a phenothiazine, it would be appropriate to switch to a thioxanthene or to a butyrophenone. No evidence indicates that a combination of two or more first generation antipsychotics works any better than a single agent, and such "polypharmacy" is to be avoided.

When patients with schizophrenia fail to respond to the strategy just outlined, some authors advocate "megadose" treatment. Thus patients have been treated with chlorpromazine in doses of over 3 g, or with haloperidol in doses of 100 mg or more. Although it appears that some previously unresponsive patients may do better with such "megadoses," the response is unpredictable, and the side effects may be intolerable.

Compliance is often a problem and, in such cases, consideration should be given to utilizing a decanoate preparation. Either fluphenazine or haloperidol may be used, as it appears that, by and large, they are equally effective. Regardless of which decanoate preparation is chosen, one should demonstrate first by using oral preparations that the patient is neither allergic to it nor prone to suffer disabling side effects. Some authors also recommend demonstrating first that the patient will respond to the oral agent; however, in many cases of noncompliant outpatients, this is simply not possible precisely because of the noncompliance. In choosing an initial dose, attempting to extrapolate from an oral dosage to a dose of the decanoate is not practical. Many authors have attempted to provide formulae for the conversion from oral to decanoate dosage, but in practice such conversion formulas simply are not reliable. Fluphenazine decanoate is generally given every 2 weeks, and the initial dose generally ranges between 12.75 and 50 mg. Haloperidol decanoate is given generally every 4 weeks, and the initial dosage range is from 100 to 300 mg.

Deciding whether to use a dose on the higher or lower end of the range is based on the same guidelines outlined earlier for oral preparations. For the elderly or others likely to be intolerant of otherwise "average" doses, an initial dose of 5 mg of fluphenazine decanoate or 50 mg of haloperidol decanoate might be preferable. Dosage adjustments are made generally every 2 weeks for fluphenazine and every 4 weeks for haloperidol

decanoate, based on clinical response. One should continue the oral preparation for a few days after the first injection of the decanoate because it takes at least that long to see an initial response to a decanoate. Subsequently, oral preparations may be available on a "prn" basis, and the need for such prn doses may be taken as an indication to increase the decanoate dose at the time of the next injection. Although definite exceptions exist, in general doses of over 150 mg of fluphenazine decanoate or 500 mg of haloperidol decanoate are unlikely to provide further benefit. In some cases, one may see a falling off of clinical effectiveness before the end of the "average" interval between injections, and in such cases shorter dosage intervals are required (e.g., perhaps 1 week for fluphenazine decanoate or 2 to 3 weeks for haloperidol decanoate). Conversely, in some patients who are doing well, one may be able to lengthen the interval, sometimes up to 4 weeks for fluphenazine or even 8 weeks for haloperidol.

In assessing the effectiveness of any given decanoate dosage, one must keep in mind that "steady state" blood levels will not be obtained until after 4 or 5 dosage intervals have passed. Thus in practice, if possible, when adjusting "maintenance" doses of the decanoate, one should allow at least 4 dosage intervals to pass before making an assessment. In cases where patients have done well for extended periods of time, gradual dosage reductions are indicated. For fluphenazine decanoate, the minimum dose is 5 mg, and for haloperidol decanoate, 50 mg probably constitutes a minimum dose.

By and large, as between fluphenazine and haloperidol, the decanoate of haloperidol is preferable. Fewer injections and fewer clinic visits are required, and this greatly increases compliance. The decanoates are greatly underutilized; they clearly prevent relapses and are a boon to most patients who take them.

The treatment of mania, as discussed in that chapter, often involves initially using an antipsychotic until the "lag period" between initiation of treatment with an antimanic agent passes and a therapeutic effect occurs. In general, the protocol for rapid pharmacologic treatment of agitation, as outlined in that chapter, may be followed.

For the other indications listed in the introduction, in general the same principles as described for schizophrenia may be used. Lower doses, however, are often indicated in borderline personality disorder, Tourette's syndrome, and chronic pain syndrome. For porphyria, relatively low doses of chlorpromazine are recommended. When discontinuing a low-potency drug, one should taper the dose over 3 to 4 days to prevent a cholinergic rebound. This should also be done if one is switching from a low-potency drug to a high-potency one.

BIBLIOGRAPHY

Adler LA, Angrist B, Peselow E, et al. Efficacy of propranolol in neuroleptic-induced akathisia. *Journal of Clinical Psychopharmacology* 1985;5:164-166.

Compton MT, Miller AH. Antipsychotic-induced hyperprolactinemia and sexual dysfunction. *Psychopharmacology Bulletin* 2002;36:143-164.

Gardos G, Cole JO. Weight reduction in schizophrenia by molindone. *The American Journal of Psychiatry* 1977;134:302-304.

Reilley JG, Ayis SA, Ferrier IN, et al. Thioridazine and sudden unexplained death in psychiatric inpatients. *The British Journal of Psychiatry* 2002;180:515-522.

Remington GJ, Adams ME. Depot neuroleptic therapy: clinical considerations. *Canadian Journal of Psychiatry* 1995;40(Suppl 1):5-11.

Tonda ME, Guthrie SK. Treatment of acute neuroleptic-induced movement disorders. *Pharmacotherapy* 1994;14:543-560.

VanPutten T, May PRA. "Akinetic depression" in schizophrenia. *Archives of General Psychiatry* 1978;35:1101-1107.

Wiles DH, McCreadie RG, Whitehead A. Pharmacokinetics of haloperidol and fluphenazine decanoates in chronic schizophrenia. *Psychopharmacology* 1990;101:274-281.

Wirshing WC. Movement disorders associated with neuroleptic treatment. *The Journal of Clinical Psychiatry* 2001;62(Suppl 21):15-18.

Yeung PK, Hubbard JW, Korchinski ED, et al. Pharmacokinetics of chlorpromazine and key metabolites. *European Journal of Clinical Pharmacology* 1993;45:563-569.

292 Pimozide

Although pimozide is a first generation antipsychotic, it is treated here separately in light of its side effects and drug interactions.

Pimozide is at best a second choice agent for schizophrenia and Tourette's syndrome.

PHARMACOKINETICS

Bioavailability is between 50 and 60%, with peak levels reached within 6 to 8 hours; protein binding is 99% and the half life averages 55 hours with a very wide range (15 to 168 hours). Metabolism is primarily via CYP3A and there is a greater than tenfold variability in blood levels given the same oral dose. It is not known whether pimozide's metabolites are active or not.

SIDE EFFECTS

With regard to autonomic and extrapyramidal side effects, pimozide is similar to the "high-potency" first generation antipsychotics described in that chapter. Thus extrapyramidal side effects are relatively common, whereas sedation, blurry vision, dry mouth, and constipation occur with less frequency. Erectile dysfunction apparently is not rare with pimozide.

When given to children, pimozide may cause a syndrome similar to that seen in separation anxiety disorder, or, as it is also known, "school phobia."

Pimozide reduces the seizure threshold, and seizures have been reported at doses of over 20 mg.

The most troubling side effect of pimozide is its tendency to prolong the QT interval and to cause ventricular arrhythmias, such as torsade de pointes.

The teratogenicity of pimozide is not known, nor is it known whether it is excreted in breast milk.

DRUG-DRUG INTERACTIONS

Clarithromycin increases pimozide levels and the combination has been associated with torsade de pointes and death; similar reactions may be anticipated with other macrolide antibiotics, such as erythromycin and zithromycin. Both ketoconazole and itraconazole also increase pimozide levels.

There is a case report of severe bradycardia seen with the combination of pimozide and fluoxetine.

The QT lengthening effect of pimozide may be augmented by other drugs capable of the same effect, such as tricyclics, ziprasidone, quinidine, procainamide, disopyramide, bretylium, and amiodarone.

OVERDOSAGE

Stupor, coma, depressed respirations, hypotension, and ventricular arrhythmias, such as torsade, may occur.

Continuous ECG monitoring is required; fluids and pressor agents may be required, but epinephrine should not be used.

THERAPEUTIC USAGE

Pimozide is available in 1 and 2 mg tablets.

For Tourette's syndrome, the starting dose is 1 mg, and this may be increased in 1 mg increments every week until a satisfactory response, limiting side-effects or a maximum dose is reached, generally considered to be about 10 mg: most patients respond to a dose of 3 or 4 mg.

For schizophrenia most patients respond to a dose of from 4 to 8 mg, with a maximum of 20 mg.

An ECG should be obtained before treatment and as indicated thereafter.

BIBLIOGRAPHY

Bloch M, Tager S, Braun A, et al. Pimozide-induced depression in men who stutter. *The Journal of Clinical Psychiatry* 1997;58:433-436.

Flockhart DA, Drici MD, Kerbusch T, et al. Studies on the mechanism of a fatal clarithromycin-pimozide interaction in a patient with Tourette syndrome. *Journal of Clinical Psychopharmacology* 2000;20:317-324.

Krahenbuhi S, Sauter B, Kupferschmidt H, et al. Case report: reversible QT prolongation with torsades de pointes in a patient with pimozide intoxication. *The American Journal of the Medical Sciences* 1995;309:315-316.

Lechin F, van der Dijs B, Lechin ME, et al. Pimozide therapy for trigeminal neuralgia. *Archives of Neurology* 1989;46:960-963.

Linet LS. Tourette syndrome, pimozide, and school phobia: the neuroleptic separation anxiety syndrome. *The American Journal of Psychiatry* 1985;142:613-615.

Sallee FR, Pollock BG, Stiller RL, et al. Pharmacokinetics of pimozide in adults and children with Tourette's syndrome. *Journal of Clinical Pharmacology* 1987;27:776-781.

Clozapine is a second generation antipsychotic whose primary indication is treatment resistant schizophrenia, where it is superior to all other antipsychotics, both of the first and second generations. In addition to being effective against "positive" symptoms of schizophrenia, it also, in contrast to most other antipsychotics, has a robust effect on "negative" symptoms. Unfortunately, however, clozapine, as detailed under Side Effects, carries a substantial burden of side effects, including agranulocytosis, and consequently it should be reserved for patients with schizophrenia who fail to respond to adequate trials of at least two other antipsychotics (one of which should probably be either risperidone or olanzapine), or who are intolerant of the side effects of other, safer antipsychotics.

Clozapine is also being used for treatment resistant schizoaffective disorder and treatment resistant bipolar mania, but here too, as in the case of schizophrenia, it should not be used until aggressive trials with safer agents have been unsuccessful.

Another use for clozapine is Parkinson's disease complicated by psychosis. Here, clozapine reduces the psychosis but does not, in contrast to other antipsychotics, increase the parkinsonism; indeed, in many cases motor symptoms such as tremor improve with clozapine.

Clozapine's unique therapeutic effect is probably related to its strong binding to serotonin receptors; although it also binds to dopamine receptors, it has a preference for D4 receptors, with relatively little affinity for the D2 receptors in the basal ganglia, a fact that may account for its general lack of extrapyramidal side effects.

PHARMACOKINETICS

The bioavailability of clozapine is about 50%, and peak levels are reached in from 1 to 4 hours, with over 95% protein binding. Metabolism is via hepatic enzymes and the half life averages about 12 hours, with a wide range, from 4 to 66 hours. Clozapine does have active metabolites, the most prominent of which are desmethylclozapine and clozapine N-oxide.

SIDE EFFECTS

Agranulocytosis, or a granulocyte count of less than 500, occurs in about 1.3% of patients. Most cases have occurred 6 to 18 weeks after the initiation of treatment; nevertheless, cases have occurred both during the first month and after long-term chronic use. Granulocytopenia may occur abruptly, within days, and the first evidence of it may be a sore throat, lethargy, fever, "the flu," or some other infection. It appears that agranulocytosis is more common among those of Ashkenazi Jewish descent, particularly those with the HLA-B38 phenotype.

Sedation is very common, and although it tends to wane with continued treatment, it may be severe. Constipation may occur, and weight gain is common and may be substantial. There are some data suggesting a causal relationship between clozapine treatment and both diabetes mellitus and hyperlipidemia; however, this association is not as yet firm. Patients may report nausea and vomiting, headache, dry mouth, increased sweating and vivid dreams. Urinary frequency and urgency, urinary retention, and erectile dysfunction may occur and there are rare reports of priapism. Nocturnal incontinence occurs in a minority, and may be very troubling. This side effect generally responds to ephedrine in a total daily dose of 150 mg.

Unique among the antipsychotics, clozapine also causes excessive salivation, and this may occur in the absence of a parkinsonian syndrome. Some patients complain that their pillows are drenched with saliva when they awaken in the morning. When this is troubling, it may be treated with low doses of benztropine, trihexyphenidyl or clonidine.

In a minority of patients, obsessions and compulsions may occur de novo, and any obsessions or compulsions present before treatment with clozapine may be aggravated; furthermore, a small minority will also develop generalized social anxiety, similar to that seen in social phobia of the generalized type.

Postural hypotension and dizziness may occur. Interestingly, one may also see a sustained nonpostural tachycardia, with the elevation in heart rate being dose dependent and ranging from 10 to 25 beats per minute. Venous thromboembolism and pulmonary embolism have been reported, as has myocarditis. The myocarditis, which may be fatal, tends to appear within the first six weeks of treatment and presents with a "flu-like" illness with chest discomfort, fever, tachycardia and congestive heart failure. This myocarditis is probably autoimmune in nature, and its occurrence demands admission and treatment with steroids.

Grand mal seizures may occur in 1% to 5% of patients taking clozapine, and the risk appears higher in those with preexisting epilepsy, CNS lesions and with higher doses. Other side effects include myoclonus and the neuroleptic malignant syndrome (NMS). The neuroleptic malignant syndrome seen secondary to clozapine is somewhat atypical, in that it tends to present with delirium, diaphoresis and tachycardia, with relatively little in the way of rigidity and tremor. Finally, there are rare reports of tardive dyskinesia secondary to clozapine.

Some 10% to 15% of patients become mildly febrile within the first few weeks of treatment. The temperature generally rises only 3 or 4 degrees Fahrenheit and resolves spontaneously within 3 to 8 days. The differential diagnosis of such a temperature, however, would include not only granulocytopenia but also the neuroleptic malignant syndrome.

Transient, benign eosinophilia may occur during the third through the fifth weeks of treatment. Occasionally, transient salivary gland enlargement may occur, which may be either bilateral or unilateral.

In contrast to other antipsychotics, prolactin levels are either not elevated or only very mildly and transiently.

The teratogenicity of clozapine is not known. It is excreted in breast milk.

DRUG-DRUG INTERACTIONS

Clozapine levels are significantly increased by fluvoxamine and fluoxetine; the data regarding elevations secondary to paroxetine and sertraline are contradictory, but it does appear that citalopram has no effect on clozapine levels. Clozapine levels are also increased by erythromycin, ciprofloxacin, ketoconazole, cimetidine and valproate.

Clozapine levels are decreased by phenytoin, valproate and carbamazepine.

Smoking decreases clozapine levels, and with admission or discharge from non-smoking facilities one may expect significant changes in blood levels.

Clozapine should not be used with any other medication, such as carbamazepine, which may have a myelosuppressive effect.

There are rare reports of apnea occurring secondary to a combination of clozapine and a benzodiazepine, and likewise rare reports of delirium with the combination of clozapine and either lorazepam or clonazepam.

OVERDOSAGE

Stupor, coma, hypotension, respiratory depression, and seizures may occur. Tachycardia, other arrhythmias, and heart block may also be seen.

Epinephrine should not be used for hypotension, and neither procainamide nor quinidine should be used for arrhythmias.

THERAPEUTIC USAGE

Clozapine is available in 25 and 100 mg tablets.

Pretreatment and weekly white blood cell counts and differentials are obtained for the first six months, and then biweekly thereafter for the duration of treatment. If treatment is discontinued in the first six months, then weekly CBCs should be obtained for 4 weeks, and if discontinuation is after 6 months, then the CBC should be obtained at twice weekly intervals for a month. In the event that the white blood cell count falls below 3500, or the granulocyte count below 1500, one proceeds as outlined in Table 293-1. In the event the granulocyte count falls below 1000, the patient should be admitted and undergo appropriate isolation and antibiotic treatment. These patients should probably never receive clozapine again. If the patient survives, the white cell count generally returns to normal within 2 to 4 weeks after clozapine is discontinued; granulocyte colony-stimulating factor may hasten recovery.

Treatment is initiated at 25 or 50 mg/day, increasing by 25 or 50 mg increments every day until the patient experiences unacceptable side effects or a dose between 300 and 450 mg is obtained. During this initial titration, the total daily dose is given in three divided doses; subsequently, a twice daily regimen may be appropriate. Subsequent dose increases may be made in 50 and 100 mg increments on a weekly basis up to a maximum of 900 mg. Most patients with schizophrenia, however, appear to respond to doses

between 300 and 600 mg. Blood levels are sometimes useful here, as it appears that a clozapine level below 350 nanogram/mL is unlikely to be effective.

It appears that if a response is going to occur at any given dose, that it begins within eight weeks of the initiation of that dose. Consequently, if a patient on an optimum tolerated dose has shown no improvement after eight weeks of treatment, it is probably appropriate to taper and discontinue the clozapine, rather than subject the patient to the risk of agranulocytosis. Although a partial response is to be expected by eight weeks, a full response may not be seen for up to three months; once a full response has occurred, the dose often may be reduced, often to 300 mg, without loss of therapeutic effect.

When clozapine is used in Parkinson's disease, lower doses are generally satisfactory, in the range of 6.25 to 50 mg.

If seizures occur, clozapine may be stopped, or, if the clinical response warrants, it may be continued at a lower dose. Some patients have been successfully treated with a combination of clozapine and valproate.

If clozapine is to be discontinued this should be done gradually, as abrupt discontinuations in patients with schizophrenia have been associated with severe and rapid recurrences of psychosis; this withdrawal phenomenon has also been noted with the transition from brand name clozapine to a generic preparation. In addition to psychosis, rapid discontinuation of clozapine may also be followed by abnormal movements, such as dystonia. If a rapid discontinuation is required, it appears that the withdrawal psychosis may be prevented by immediately starting another second generation antipsychotic such as olanzapine.

In the case of Parkinson's disease, rapid withdrawal has been followed by a syndrome similar to the serotonin syndrome, with stupor, myoclonus, tremor, rigidity and hyperreflexia. It appears that this syndrome may be successfully treated with cyproheptadine, as described in the chapter on the serotonin syndrome.

BIBLIOGRAPHY

Ahmed S, Chengappa KN, Naidu VR, et al. Clozapine withdrawal-emergent dystonias and dyskinesias: a case series. *The Journal of Clinical Psychiatry* 1998;59:472-477.

Bak TH, Bauere M, Schaub RT, et al. Myoclonus in patients treated with clozapine: a case series. *The Journal of Clinical Psychiatry* 1995;56: 418-422.

Baker RW, Chengappa KN, Baird JW. Emergence of obsessive compulsive symptoms during treatment with clozapine. *The Journal of Clinical Psychiatry* 1992;53:439-442.

Banov MD, Tohen M, Friedberg J. High risk of eosinophilia in women treated with clozapine. *The Journal of Clinical Psychiatry* 1993;54:466-469.

Barnas C, Zwiersina H, Hummer M, et al. Granulocyte-macrophage colony-stimulating factor (GM-CSF) treatment of clozapine-induced agranulocytosis: a case report. *The Journal of Clinical Psychiatry* 1992;53:245-247.

Centorrino F, Baldessarini RJ, Frankenburg FR, et al. Serum levels of clozapine and norclozapine in patients treated with selective serotonin reuptake inhibitors. *The American Journal of Psychiatry* 1996;153:820-826.

Cohen LG, Chesley S, Eugenio L, et al. Erythromycin-induced clozapine toxic reaction. *Archives of Internal Medicine* 1996;156:675-677.

Cohen S, Chiles J, MacNaughton A. Weight gain associated with clozapine. *The American Journal of Psychiatry* 1990;147:503-504.

Conley RR, Carpenter WT, Tamminga CA. Time to clozapine response in a standardized trial. *The American Journal of Psychiatry* 1997;154: 1243-1247.

Dave M. Clozapine-related tardive dyskinesia. *Biological Psychiatry* 1994;35:886-887.

■**TABLE 293-1.** White Cell Monitoring for Clozapine

White Cell Count		Granulocyte Count	Frequency	Action
>3500	and	>1500	Weekly	Continue clozapine
<3500	and	>1500	Twice weekly	Continue clozapine
<3000	or	<1000	Twice weekly	Discontinue clozapine and restart only when WBC >3500
<2000	or	<1000	Daily	Discontinue clozapine and admit; do not restart clozapine

Fuller MA, Borovicka MC, Jaskiw GE, et al. Clozapine-induced urinary incontinence: incidence and treatment with ephedrine. *The Journal of Clinical Psychiatry* 1996;57:514-518.

Hagg S, Spigset O, Soderstrom TG. Association of venous thromboembolism and clozapine. *Lancet* 2000;355:1155-1156.

Hagg S, Spigset O, Bate A, et al. Myocarditis related to clozapine treatment. *Journal of Clinical Psychopharmacology* 2001;21:382-388.

Hummer M, Kurz M, Kurzthaler I, et al. Hepatotoxicity of clozapine. *Journal of Clinical Psychopharmacology* 1997;17:314-317.

Jackson CW, Markowitz JS, Brewerton TD. Delirium associated with clozapine and benzodiazepine combinations. *Annals of Clinical Psychiatry* 1995;7:139-141.

Jann MW, Grimsley SR, Gray EC, et al. Pharmacokinetics and pharmacodynamics of clozapine. *Clinical Pharmacokinetics* 1993;24:161-176.

Karagianis JL, Phillips LC, Hogan KP, et al. Clozapine-induced neuroleptic malignant syndrome: two new cases and a review of the literature. *The Annals of Pharmacotherapy* 1999;33:623-630.

Kluznik JC, Walbek NH, Farnsworth MG, et al. Clinical effects of a randomized switch from Clozaril to generic clozapine. *The Journal of Clinical Psychiatry* 2001;62(Suppl 5):14-17.

Koller E, Schneider B, Bennett K, et al. Clozapine-associated diabetes. *The American Journal of Medicine* 2001;111:716-723.

Kronig MH, Munne RA, Szymanski S, et al. Plasma clozapine levels and clinical response for treatment-refractory schizophrenic patients. *The American Journal of Psychiatry* 1995;152:179-182.

Lieberman JA, Yunis J, Egea E, et al. HLA-B38, DR4, DQw3 and clozapine-induced agranulocytosis in Jewish patients with schizophrenia. *Archives of General Psychiatry* 1990;47:945-948.

Lund BC, Perry PJ, Brooks JM, et al. Clozapine use in patients with schizophrenia and the risk of diabetes, hyperlipidemia, and hypertension: a claims-based approach. *Archives of General Psychiatry* 2001;58:1172-1176.

Miller DD. Effect of phenytoin on plasma clozapine concentrations in two patients. *The Journal of Clinical Psychiatry* 1991;52:23-25.

Pacia SV, Devinsky O. Clozapine-related seizures. *Neurology* 1994;44:2247-2249.

Pallanti S, Quercioli L, Rossi A, et al. The emergence of social phobia during clozapine treatment and its response to fluoxetine augmentation. *The Journal of Clinical Psychiatry* 1999;60:819-823.

Parkonson Study Group. Low-dose clozapine for the treatment of drug-induced psychosis in Parkinson's disease. *The New England Journal of Medicine* 1999;340:757-763.

Raaska K, Neuvonen PJ. Ciprofloxacin increases serum clozapine and N-desmethylclozapine: a study in patients with schizophrenia. *European Journal of Clinical Psychopharmacology* 2000;56:585-589.

Spina E, Avenoso A, Facciola G, et al. Effect of fluoxetine on the plasma concentrations of clozapine and its major metabolites in patients with schizophrenia. *International Clinical Psychopharmacology* 1998;13:141-145.

Spina E, Avenoso A, Salemi M, et al. Plasma concentrations of clozapine and its major metabolites during combined treatment with paroxetine or sertraline. *Pharmacopsychiatry* 2000;33:213-217.

Spivak B, Adlersberg S, Rosen L, et al. Trihexyphenidyl treatment of clozapine-induced hypersalivation. *International Clinical Psychopharmacology* 1997;12:213-215.

Szymanski S, Libermann JA, Picou D, et al. A case report of cimetidine-induced clozapine toxicity. *The Journal of Clinical Psychiatry* 1991;52:21-22.

Taylor D, Ellison Z, Ementon Shaw L, et al. Co-administration of citalopram and clozapine: effect on plasma clozapine levels. *International Clinical Psychopharmacology* 1998;13:19-21.

Than JC, Dickson RA. Clozapine-induced fevers and 1-year clozapine discontinuation rate. *The Journal of Clinical Psychiatry* 2002;63:880-884.

Tollefson GD, Deliva MA, Mattler CA, et al. Controlled, double-blind investigation of the clozapine discontinuation symptoms with conversion to either olanzapine or placebo. The Collaborative Crossover Study Group. *Journal of Clinical Psychopharmacology* 1999;19:435-443.

Wetzel H, Anghelescu I, Szegedi A, et al. Pharmacokinetic interactions of clozapine with selective serotonin reuptake inhibitors: differential effects of fluvoxamine and paroxetine in a prospective study. *Journal of Clinical Psychopharmacology* 1998;18:2-9.

Zesiewicz TA, Borra S, Hauser RA. Clozapine withdrawal symptoms in a Parkinson's disease patient. *Movement Disorders* 2002;17:1365-1367.

294 Risperidone

Risperidone is a second generation antipsychotic that is superior to the first generation agents for the treatment of schizophrenia, being effective not only against the positive but also the negative symptoms of that disorder. Although, like first generation antipsychotics, risperidone blocks post-synaptic D2 dopamine receptors, it also, and unlike the first generation agents, exerts a prominent blockade against 5-HT2 serotonin receptors, which probably accounts for its superior efficacy. Risperidone also blocks post-synaptic histamine and alpha-2 receptors, and these actions probably account for many of its side effects.

In addition to its use in schizophrenia, risperidone is also effective in bipolar disorder (for the acute treatment of mania), schizoaffective disorder, delusional disorder, paranoid and schizotypal personality disorders, conduct disorder (when accompanied by aggressivity), autism, mental retardation (when accompanied by aggressivity and impulsivity), developmental stuttering, Tourette's syndrome, Huntington's disease and dementia. Risperidone has also been used for psychosis in Parkinson's disease; however, as pointed out further on, this must be done with caution.

PHARMACOKINETICS

Risperidone is well absorbed from the gastrointestinal tract, with a bioavailability of about 70%, and peak blood levels are generally reached in about one hour. Risperidone is normally metabolized in the liver by the CYP 2D6 enzyme to 9-hydroxyrisperidone, which is as pharmacologically active as risperidone itself; 9-hydroxyrisperidone is then excreted, for the most part unchanged, in the urine. Protein binding for risperidone is about 90%, and for 9-hydroxyrisperidone, about 75%.

In patients with normal CYP 2D6 activity, the half life of risperidone is about 3 hours; however, in "poor metabolizers," who have deficient CYP 2D6 activity, the half life rises to about 21 hours. Regardless of metabolizer status, the half life of 9-hydroxyrisperidone is the same, about 22 hours.

Initially, slow metabolizers were thought to be subject to an increased drug effect; however, this does not appear to be the case. As noted above, the antipsychotic activity of risperidone is a reflection of the sum of the blood levels of risperidone and 9-hydroxyrisperidone.

In the case of slow metabolizers, the increased level of risperidone is offset by the decreased level of 9-hydroxyrisperidone, with the result that the sum of these two levels in the slow metabolizer is roughly equivalent to their sum in those with normal cytochrome P450 2D6 activity. In addition, as the prolonged half-life of risperidone in slow metabolizers is roughly equivalent to the half-life of 9-hydroxyrisperidone, there is likewise no significant change in time to steady state of the total antipsychotic activity.

SIDE EFFECTS

If risperidone is started at a "full" dose, there is a significant risk of sedation and orthostatic hypotension, with dizziness and, possibly, falls. A gradual titration, however, generally avoids these problems.

Other side effects include sedation, difficulty with concentration, anxiety, insomnia, nausea, abdominal pain, or constipation. Nasal congestion may be seen, and some patients may experience mild weight gain, decreased libido, erectile dysfunction, and ejaculatory delay or anorgasmia. Prolactin levels are elevated in both males and females, and may be associated with galactorrhea. In a minority of patients, the corrected QT interval may be prolonged.

Extrapyramidal side effects, such as akathisia, parkinsonism, and dystonia, are uncommon with risperidone, provided that the dose is below 6 mg, whereas at doses much above this, risperidone appears as likely to produce these side effects as are first generation high-potency antipsychotics, such as haloperidol. In the case of patients with Parkinson's disease, however, it appears that risperidone carries a higher risk of exacerbating the parkinsonism, and in some cases delirium may occur. Rarely, risperidone may cause tardive dyskinesia or the neuroleptic malignant syndrome. There are also rare reports of obsessions or compulsions occurring secondary to risperidone.

Risperidone is excreted in breast milk; its teratogenic potential in humans in not known.

DRUG-DRUG INTERACTIONS

Both fluoxetine and paroxetine increase risperidone levels, without any significant effect on 9-hydroxyrisperidone levels.

Carbamazepine reduces both risperidone and 9-hydroxyrisperidone levels; in turn, risperidone increases the carbamazepine level.

Risperidone augments the hypotensive effect of prazosin.

OVERDOSAGE

Overdosage may cause sedation, dystonia, hypotension, tachycardia and, with prolongation of the corrected QT interval, arrhythmias; seizures have also been reported. Cardiac monitoring should be performed, and arrhythmias should not be treated with agents that might further prolong the QT interval. Hypotension may be treated with fluids; epinephrine and dopamine should not be given.

THERAPEUTIC USAGE

Risperidone is available in 0.25, 0.5, 1, 2, 3 and 4 mg tablets and as a 1 mg/mL liquid. A long-acting intramuscular preparation has been developed, and should be available by the time this book is published.

For schizophrenia or schizoaffective disorder, doses between 2 and 4 mg daily are generally adequate, and for the acute treatment of mania, 2 to 6 mg. Although some patients may require higher doses, it must be borne in mind that doses much above 6 mg are associated with an incidence of extrapyramidal side effects similar to that seen with high potency first generation antipsychotics, such as haloperidol. If non-compliance becomes problematic, the long acting form may be given in a dose of 25 to 50 mg IM every two weeks.

To reduce the risk of postural hypotension, treatment may be initiated at 0.5 to 1 mg twice daily, and increasing in 1 or 2 mg increments every day until the target dose is reached. It should be noted, however, that otherwise healthy adults generally tolerate starting at 2 or 3 mg on the first day. Once the optimum dose has been reached, most patients may be switched to once daily dosage, at bedtime.

In the elderly or debilitated, or those with significant hepatic or renal failure, lower doses are appropriate, with longer intervals between dose increases.

Although a therapeutic response in schizophrenia may be seen in the first 2 weeks of treatment, a full response to any given dose may not occur until 8 or more weeks have passed.

For the other indications, lower doses are generally satisfactory, such as 0.25 to 2 mg for schizotypal personality disorder, 1 to 3 mg for autism, and 1 to 2 mg for dementia: in the case of dementia, low doses are preferable, as these patients may be particularly liable to side effects. If risperidone is used for psychosis in Parkinson's disease low doses are again preferable, given that higher doses are associated with an exacerbation of parkinsonism and, in some cases, delirium.

BIBLIOGRAPHY

Acri AA, Henretig FM. Effects of risperidone in overdose. *The American Journal of Emergency Medicine* 1998;16:498-501.

Alevizos B, Lykouras L, Servas IM, et al. Risperidone-induced obsessive-compulsive symptoms: a series of six cases. *Journal of Clinical Psychopharmacology* 2002;22:461-467.

Bajjoka I, Patel T, O'Sullivan T. Risperidone-induced neuroleptic malignant syndrome. *Annals of Emergency Medicine* 1997;30:698-700.

Fontaine CS, Hynan LS, Koch K, et al. A double-blind comparison of olanzapine versus risperidone in the acute treatment of dementia-related behavioral disturbances in extended care facilities. *The Journal of Clinical Psychiatry* 2003;64:726-730.

Huang ML, Van Peer A, Woestenborghs R, et al. Pharmacokinetics of the novel antipsychotic agent risperidone and the prolactin response in healthy subjects. *Clinical Pharmacology and Therapeutics* 1993;54:257-268.

Kane JM, Eerdekens M, Lindenmayer JP, et al. Long-acting injectable risperidone: efficacy and safety of the first long-acting atypical antipsychotic. *The American Journal of Psychiatry* 2003;160:1125-1132.

Kleinberg DL, Davis JM, de Coster R, et al. Prolactin levels and adverse events in patients treated with risperidone. *Journal of Clinical Psychopharmacology* 1999;19:57-61.

Koenigsberg HW, Reynolds D, Goodman M, et al. Risperidone in the treatment of schizotypal personality disorder. *The Journal of Clinical Psychiatry* 2003;64:628-634.

Kumar S, Malone DM. Risperidone implicated in the onset of tardive dyskinesia in a young woman. *Postgraduate Medical Journal* 2000;76:316-317.

Leopald NA. Risperidone treatment of drug-related psychosis in patients with parkinsonism. *Movement Disorders* 2000;15:301-304.

Merlo MC, Hofer H, Gekle W, et al. Risperidone, 2 mg/day vs. 4 mg/day, in first-episode, acutely psychotic patients: treatment efficacy and effects on fine motor functioning. *The Journal of Clinical Psychiatry* 2002;63:885-891.

Mula M, Monaco F. Carbamazepine-risperidone interactions in patients with epilepsy. *Clinical Neuropharmacology* 2002;25:97-100.

Ono S, Mihara K, Suzuki A, et al. Significant pharmacokinetic interaction between risperidone and carbamazepine: its relationship with CYP2D6 genotypes. *Psychopharmacology* 2002;162:50-54.

Rich SS, Friedman JH, Ott BR. Risperidone versus clozapine in the treatment of psychosis in six patients with Parkinson's disease and other akinetic-rigid syndromes. *The Journal of Clinical Psychiatry* 1995;56:556-559.

Scordo MG, Spina E, Facciola G, et al. Cytochrome P450 2D6 genotype and steady state plasma levels of risperidone and 9-hydroxyrisperidone. *Psychopharmacology* 1999;147:300-305.

Spina E, Avenoso A, Facciola G, et al. Plasma concentrations of risperidone and 9-hydroxyrisperidone during combined treatment with paroxetine. *Therapeutic Drug Monitoring* 2001;23:223-227.

Spina E, Avenoso A, Scordo MG, et al. Inhibition of risperidone metabolism by fluoxetine in patients with schizophrenia: a clinically relevant pharmacokinetic drug interaction. *Journal of Clinical Psychopharmacology* 2002;22:419-423.

295 Olanzapine

Olanzapine is a second generation antipsychotic that is more effective than the first generation agents in the treatment of schizophrenia. Other uses include schizoaffective disorder, bipolar disorder and agitation in dementia.

Olanzapine is thought to exert its therapeutic effect by virtue of a blockade of postsynaptic 5-HT2 and dopamine D2 receptors. Both H1 and muscarinic receptors are also blocked, accounting, in part, for some of olanzapine's side effects.

PHARMACOKINETICS

Olanzapine has a bioavailability of about 60%, reaches peak blood levels in about 6 hours, and undergoes 93% protein binding. Extensive hepatic metabolism occurs, without any active metabolites being produced, and the half life ranges from 21 to 54 hours.

SIDE EFFECTS

Sedation and dizziness are the most common side effects: these are dose-related, and tend to subside with continued treatment. Dry mouth and constipation may also occur.

Weight gain occurs in a majority of patients, and tends to be significant, averaging about 15 pounds.

The incidence of diabetes mellitus is increased in patients taking olanzapine, and this increase is independent of any weight gain; new onset diabetic ketoacidosis has occurred, and there have been fatalities.

The incidence of hyperlipidemia is also increased.

Elevated liver transaminases may occur in a small minority; these are generally transient and tend to resolve while treatment is ongoing.

Akathisia, parkinsonism and dystonia may occur but these are far less frequent than with first generation agents.

There are rare case reports of olanzapine-induced neuroleptic malignant syndrome and tardive dyskinesia.

Olanzapine is excreted in the breast milk; its teratogenic potential is not known.

DRUG-DRUG INTERACTIONS

Olanzapine levels are increased by fluvoxamine and ritonavir.

Olanzapine levels are decreased by carbamazepine, phenytoin and cigarette smoking.

OVERDOSAGE

Olanzapine is generally safe in overdose: stupor may occur, but gastric lavage, activated charcoal and supportive care generally suffice.

THERAPEUTIC USAGE

Olanzapine is available in 2.5, 5, 10, 15 and 20 mg tablets and in orally disintegrating tablets of 5, 10, 15 and 20 mg strength.

In otherwise healthy adults, treatment is begun at 10 mg, once daily at bedtime: most patients respond to doses between 10 and 30 mg. The use of intramuscular olanzapine is discussed in the chapter on Rapid Pharmacologic Treatment of Agitation.

In the elderly the dose should be reduced, and it is generally appropriate to begin at a 2.5 mg dose and observe the patient for from days to a week before increasing the dose.

BIBLIOGRAPHY

Gunal DI, Onultan O, Afsar N, et al. Tardive dystonia associated with olanzapine therapy. *Neurological Sciences* 2001;22:331-332.

Hall KL, Taylor WH, Ware MR. Neuroleptic malignant syndrome due to olanzapine. *Psychopharmacology Bulletin* 2001;35:49-54.

Hiemke C, Peled A, Jabarin M, et al. Fluvoxamine augmentation of olanzapine in chronic schizophrenia: pharmacokinetic interactions and clinical effects. *Journal of Clinical Psychopharmacology* 2002;22: 502-506.

Koro CE, Fedder DO, L'Italien GJ, et al. An assessment of the independent effects of olanzapine and risperidone exposure on the risk of hyperlipidemia in schizophrenic patients. *Archives of General Psychiatry* 2002;59:1021-1026.

Koro CE, Fedder DO, L'Italien GJ, et al. Assessment of independent effect of olanzapine and risperidone on risk of diabetes among patients with schizophrenia: population based nested case-control study. *British Medical Journal* 2002;325:243.

Meatherall R, Younes J. Fatality from olanzapine induced hyperglycemia. *Journal of Forensic Sciences* 2002;47:893-896.

Penzak SR, Hon YY, Lawhorn WD, et al. Influence of ritonavir on olanzapine pharmacokinetics in healthy volunteers. *Journal of Clinical Psychopharmacology* 2002;22:366-370.

Ziprasidone is a second generation antipsychotic indicated for the treatment of schizophrenia and schizoaffective disorder. Although ziprasidone is clearly superior to placebo for these disorders, it is not as yet clear whether it is superior in efficacy to the first generation agents. Ziprasidone is also useful for acute mania, and preliminary work also supports efficacy in Tourette's syndrome.

Ziprasidone is an antagonist at 5HT2A and 5HT2D receptors, and at dopamine D2 receptors; it also functions as an agonist at 5HT1A receptors. Unlike other antipsychotics, ziprasidone also inhibits reuptake of both serotonin and norepinephrine by presynaptic neurons, and in this regard is of comparable potency to the tricyclic antidepressant imipramine.

PHARMACOKINETICS

Ziprasidone is highly lipid soluble, and its pharmacokinetics are strongly influenced by whether it is taken fasting or with meals. Bioavailability fasting is about 30%, and with food about 60%. Peak levels in the fasting state are obtained in 2 to 6 hours, but in the fed state in from 6 to 8 hours. The half life when taken fasting is about 7 hours, but when taken with food is roughly 5 hours. Ziprasidone undergoes extensive hepatic metabolism and there are no active metabolites; protein binding is high, over 99%.

SIDE EFFECTS

Ziprasidone is generally very well tolerated; nausea, constipation, abdominal pain and lightheadedness are seen in a minority. Unlike the case with other antipsychotics, there is little associated weight gain with ziprasidone, and, in contrast with some of the other second generation agents, ziprasidone, rather than increasing lipid levels, actually reduces them. Extrapyramidal side effects, such as akathisia, parkinsonism or dystonia, are very uncommon with ziprasidone.

There are rare reports of ziprasidone precipitating mania in patients with bipolar disorder.

Ziprasidone does increase the corrected QT interval (QTc), but only to a modest degree, and not as much as is seen with the first generation agent thioridazine. Initially, there was concern about the possibility of ventricular arrhythmias, such as torsade de pointes, because of this, but as yet these fears have not materialized.

DRUG-DRUG INTERACTIONS

Ziprasidone levels are decreased by carbamazepine and increased by ketoconazole.

An additive effect on the QTc would be expected with other medications capable of prolonging this interval, such as quinidine and quinidine-like drugs.

OVERDOSAGE

Ziprasidone appears safe in overdose. Gastric lavage, activated charcoal and supportive care are generally sufficient. Due to the possibility of a significantly prolonged QTc in overdose, periodic EKGs are appropriate, with cardiac monitoring if the QTc becomes prolonged beyond 500 msec.

THERAPEUTIC USAGE

Ziprasidone is available in 20, 40, 60 and 80 mg capsules and as an injection.

When given with meals, treatment is initiated at 20 mg bid, increasing in similar increments every two or three days until a response is seen, limiting side effects occur, or a maximum dose of 120 mg bid: most patients do best at a dose of from 60 to 80 mg bid.

When given in a fasting state, the dose should be increased by from 50% to 100%.

Regardless of whether patients elect to take their ziprasidone with or without meals, it is critical that they stick to their schedule in order to avoid widely fluctuating blood levels.

Given concerns over unduly prolonged corrected QT intervals, it is important to avoid conditions that may prolong the interval (e.g., hypokalemia, hypomagnesemia) or medications that themselves may prolong the QTc, such as class IA antiarrhythmics (quinidine, procainamide, disopyramide), class III antiarrhythmics (bretyllium, sotalol, amiodarone, ibutilide), macrolide antibiotics, tricyclics and first generation antipsychotics (esp. thioridazine and pimozide). In doubtful cases, it may be appropriate to obtain a baseline EKG followed by a repeat EKG once the patient has been treated.

Doses should be reduced in the elderly or in those with hepatic failure.

BIBLIOGRAPHY

Baldassano CF, Ballas C, Datto SM, et al. Ziprasidone-associated mania: a case series and review of the mechanism. *Bipolar Disorders* 2003;5: 72-75.

Gunasekara NS, Spencer CM, Keating GM. Ziprasidone: a review of its use in schizophrenia and schizoaffective disorder. *Drugs* 2002;62: 1217-1251.

Hamelin BA, Allard S, Laplante L, et al. The effect of timing of a standard meal on the pharmacokinetics of the novel atypical antipsychotic ziprasidone. *Pharmacotherapy* 1998;18:9-15.

Keck PE, Versiani M, Potkin S, et al. Ziprasidone in the treatment of acute bipolar mania: a three-week, placebo-controlled, double-blind, randomized trial. *The American Journal of Psychiatry* 2003;160: 741-748.

Kingsbury SJ, Fayek M, Trufasiu D, et al. The apparent effects of ziprasidone on plasma lipids and glucose. *The Journal of Clinical Psychiatry* 2001;62:347-349.

Miceli JJ, Anziano RJ, Robarge L, et al. The effect of carbamazepine on the steady-state pharmacokinetics of ziprasidone in healthy volunteers. *British Journal of Clinical Pharmacology* 2000;49(Suppl 1):56-70.

Miceli JJ, Smith M, Robarge L, et al. The effects of ketoconazole on ziprasidone pharamacokinetics—a placebo-controlled crossover study in healthy volunteers. *British Journal of Clinical Pharmacology* 2000; 49(Suppl 1):71-76.

Schmidt AW, Lebel LA, Howard HR, et al. Ziprasidone: a novel antipsychotic agent with a unique receptor binding profile. *European Journal of Pharmacology* 2001;425:197-201.

Taylor D. Ziprasidone in the management of schizophrenia: the QT interval issue in context. *CNS Drugs* 2003;17:423-430.

Quetiapine is a second generation antipsychotic indicated for schizophrenia: although it is better tolerated than first generation agents, it has not as yet been shown to be superior to either haloperidol or chlorpromazine. It has also been shown to be useful for acute mania. Open studies support its use in dementia, delirium, psychosis seen in diffuse Lewy body disease, and dopaminergic-induced psychosis in Parkinson's disease, where it appears to be as effective as clozapine. Unlike clozapine, however, quetiapine can increase the parkinsonism seen in both these conditions, albeit to a mild degree.

Quetiapine has broad pharmacologic activity, binding to 5HT1A, 5HT2, dopamine D1 and D2, H1 and both alpha-1 and alpha-2 receptors.

PHARMACOKINETICS

The bioavailability of quetiapine is not known; peak blood levels are reached within one to two hours, and protein binding occurs at 83%. The half life is about six hours, and there is extensive hepatic metabolism with at least 11 metabolites, two of which possess minimal activity.

SIDE EFFECTS

Somnolence and postural dizziness are most common, but tend to subside with continued treatment; dry mouth and constipation may also occur. A mild weight gain may occur, and in about 5% there is a transient rise in transaminases.

Extrapyramidal side effects, such as parkinsonism or akathisia, are very uncommon except in patients with an underlying parkinsonian condition, such as Parkinson's disease.

Very rarely, quetiapine may cause the neuroleptic malignant syndrome.

Free thyroxine levels may undergo a mild reduction, and in a very small percentage this may be accompanied by an elevated TSH.

Administration of quetiapine to beagles in preclinical work resulted in cataract formation. This has not as yet been observed in humans.

Quetiapine is excreted in the breast milk; its teratogenic potential is not known.

DRUG-DRUG INTERACTIONS

Quetiapine levels are reduced by thioridazine, carbamazepine and phenytoin, and in the case of phenytoin the reduction is five-fold.

Quetiapine levels are increased by ketoconazole.

Quetiapine increases the level of carbamazepine's 10,11-epoxide metabolite.

OVERDOSAGE

Sedation, dizziness and tachycardia may occur, and the corrected QT interval may be prolonged. In severe overdoses, coma may occur, and this may develop very rapidly.

Treatment is with gastric lavage, activated charcoal and supportive care.

THERAPEUTIC USAGE

Quetiapine is available in 25, 100, 200 and 300 mg tablets.

For schizophrenia, treatment in otherwise healthy adults may be initiated at a total daily dose of 100 mg, increasing in similar increments every day until unacceptable side effects occur or a dose of from 400 to 500 mg is reached: although most patients respond to this dose, higher doses, up to 800 mg, may be required in some cases. The total daily dose should be divided into two doses: although some patients respond to once daily dosing, a considerable minority will not.

For dementia, delirium and psychosis in parkinsonian conditions, titration should start at a lower dose and proceed more gradually: most patients are optimally treated at doses of from 25 to 150 mg.

Doses should generally be reduced in the elderly and in those with significant hepatic failure.

BIBLIOGRAPHY

Arvanitis LA, Miller BG. Multiple fixed doses of "Seroquel" (quetiapine) in patients with acute exacerbation of schizophrenia: a comparison with haloperidol and placebo. *Biological Psychiatry* 1997;42:233-246.

Copolov DL, Link CG, Kowalcyk B. A multicentre, double-blind, randomized comparison of quetiapine (ICI 204,636, "Seroquel") and haloperidol in schizophrenia. *Psychological Medicine* 2000;30:95-105.

DeVane CL, Nemeroff CG. Clinical pharmacokinetics of quetiapine: an atypical antipsychotic. *Clinical Pharmacokinetics* 2001;40:509-522.

Fernandez HH, Trieschman ME, Burke MA, et al. Quetiapine for psychosis in Parkinson's disease versus dementia with Lewy bodies. *The Journal of Clinical Psychiatry* 2002;63:513-515.

Fitzgerald BJ, Okos AJ. Elevation of carbamazepine-10,11-epoxide by quetiapine. *Pharmacotherapy* 2002;22:1500-1503.

Hatch CD, Lund BC, Perry PJ. Failed challenge with quetiapine after neuroleptic malignant syndrome with conventional antipsychotics. *Pharmacotherapy* 2001;21:1003-1006.

Hustey FM. Acute quetiapine poisoning. *The Journal of Emergency Medicine* 1999;17:995-997.

Kim KY, Bader GM, Kotlyar V, et al. Treatment of delirium in older adults with quetiapine. *Journal of Geriatric Psychiatry and Neurology* 2003; 16:29-31.

Morgante L, Epifanio A, Spina E, et al. Quetiapine versus clozapine: a preliminary report of comparative effects on dopaminergic psychosis in patients with Parkinson's disease. *Neurological Sciences* 2002; 23(Suppl 2):89-90.

Peuskens J, Link CG. A comparison of quetiapine and chlorpromazine in the treatment of schizophrenia. *Acta Psychiatrica Scandinavica* 1997;96:265-273.

Wong YW, Yeh C, Thyrum PT. The effects of concomitant phenytoin administration on the steady-state pharmacokinetics of quetiapine. *Journal of Clinical Psychopharmacology* 2001;21:89-93.

Aripiprazole is a second generation antipsychotic indicated for schizophrenia: although it is better tolerated than first generation agents, aripiprazole has not as yet been demonstrated to be therapeutically superior to haloperidol. Aripiprazole is also useful in the treatment of acute mania and in the treatment of schizoaffective disorder.

Aripiprazole functions as a partial agonist at dopamine D2 receptors, where it displays some interesting properties: whereas in hypodopaminergic states it functions as a D2 agonist, in hyperdopaminergic states it is an antagonist. Aripiprazole is also a partial agonist at 5HT1A receptors and an antagonist at 5HT2A receptors.

PHARMACOKINETICS

The bioavailability of aripiprazole is 83% and peak levels are reached in from 3 to 5 hours, with over 99% protein binding. Metabolism occurs in the liver, primarily via cytochrome P450 2D6 and 3A4 enzymes: the major metabolite, dehydro-aripiprazole, is roughly as active as the parent compound. The half life of aripiprazole is 75 hours and of dehydro-aripiprazole, 94 hours.

SIDE EFFECTS

Headache, sedation, insomnia and postural dizziness may be seen in a small minority; extrapyramidal side effects, such as akathisia, are very uncommon.

Prolactin levels are not increased, and there is little if any weight gain or prolongation of the corrected QT interval.

DRUG-DRUG INTERACTIONS

Aripiprazole levels are increased by inhibitors of CYP2D6, such as quinidine, fluoxetine and paroxetine, and by inhibitors of CYP3A4, such as ketoconazole.

Aripiprazole levels are decreased by inducers of CYP3A4, such as carbamazepine.

OVERDOSAGE

Sedation and vomiting may occur. Gastric lavage, activated charcoal and routine supportive care are generally adequate.

THERAPEUTIC USAGE

Aripiprazole is available in 5, 10, 15, 20 and 30 mg tablets.

The total daily dose should be given once daily, either in the morning or at bedtime; most patients respond to a dose of 15 mg.

When a CYP2D6 or CYP3A4 inhibitor is used, the dose should be reduced by roughly one-half. Conversely, if carbamazepine is used, the dose should be increased, roughly two-fold.

BIBLIOGRAPHY

Bowles TM, Levin GM. Aripiprazole: a new atypical antipsychotic drug. *The Annals of Pharmacotherapy* 2003;37:687-694.

Burris KD, Molski TF, Xu C, et al. Aripiprazole, a novel antipsychotic, is a high-affinity partial agonist at human D2 receptors. *The Journal of Pharmacology and Experimental Therapeutics* 2002;302:381-389.

Kane JM, Carson WH, Saha AR, et al. Efficacy and safety of aripiprazole and haloperidol versus placebo in patients with schizophrenia and schizoaffective disorder. *The Journal of Clinical Psychiatry* 2002; 63:763-771.

Keck PE, Marcus R, Tourkodimitris S, et al. A placebo-controlled, double-blind study of the efficacy and safety of aripiprazole in patients with acute bipolar mania. *The Journal of Clinical Psychiatry* 2003;160: 1651-1658.

McGavin JK, Goa KL. Aripiprazole. *CNS Drugs* 2002;16:779-786.

Pigott TA, Carson WH, Saha AR, et al. Aripiprazole for the prevention of relapse in stabilized patients with chronic schizophrenia: a placebo-controlled 26-week study. *The Journal of Clinical Psychiatry* 2003; 64:1048-1056.

Biperiden, procyclidine, trihexyphenidyl and benztropine are all antimuscarinic anticholinergic agents that are especially useful in the treatment of antipsychotic-induced extrapyramidal side effects such as dystonia, oculogyric crisis, akinesia, and parkinsonism. Although also useful for akathisia, propranolol is the preferred treatment for this extrapyramidal side effect.

These agents are also useful in the treatment of the tremor of Parkinson's disease, the postencephalitic parkinsonism of von Economo's disease, torsion dystonia, some focal dystonias, and also in tardive dystonia, a variant of tardive dyskinesia. Rarely,

these agents may be abused; this appears most likely with trihexyphenidyl.

PHARMACOKINETICS

Relatively little is known of the pharmacokinetics of these agents. The time to peak blood levels after oral ingestion is under 2 hours for biperiden, procyclidine, and trihexyphenidyl; the figure for benztropine is not known. The half-life for biperiden is under 24 hours, for procyclidine under 12 hours, and for trihexyphenidyl about

4 hours. The half-life for benztropine is not known, but it is suspected to be relatively long.

SIDE EFFECTS

The most common side effects are dry mouth, blurry vision with mydriasis, and constipation. Occasionally a degree of anhidrosis may occur, and the resultant decreased heat loss ability may predispose to heat stroke. Pulmonary secretions may become dried and difficult to clear. Occasionally, urinary hesitancy may occur and in men with prostatism this may progress to urinary retention. Rarely, retention may also occur in women, especially those with a concurrent urinary tract infection.

In those so predisposed, the anticholinergic may precipitate acute narrow angle glaucoma.

An important side effect is memory loss. This is most noticeable in those whose memory is already impaired, as in patients with a parkinsonian dementia, but may also be detected, albeit to a slight degree, in otherwise healthy young patients, such as those being treated for schizophrenia.

The teratogenicity of these drugs is not known, nor is it known whether they are excreted in breast milk.

DRUG-DRUG INTERACTIONS

Additive effects may occur when any of these agents are combined with other drugs with anticholinergic effects, such as tricyclic anti-depressants, low-potency antipsychotics, and the like. The addition of amantadine may also potentiate anticholinergic effects.

OVERDOSAGE

The consequences and treatment of overdose are as described in the chapter on anticholinergic delirium.

THERAPEUTIC USAGE

Biperiden is available in 2 mg tablets, procyclidine in 5 mg tablets, trihexyphenidyl in 2 mg tablets and as a 2 mg/5 ml oral elixir, and benztropine in 0.5, 1 and 2 mg tablets and, for either intramuscu-lar or intravenous injection, as a 1 mg/ml solution.

In psychiatric practice, benztropine is the most commonly used of these agents. Once or twice daily dosing may be used, with the total daily dose ranging from 0.5 to 6 mg. In emergency situations, 1 or 2 mg may be given intramuscularly; intravenous use does not appear to provide a quicker response.

Biperiden may be given once or twice daily, with doses ranging from 2 up to 16 mg/day. Procyclidine is given in two or three divided doses, with the total daily dose ranging from 10 to 30 mg. Trihexyphenidyl is likewise given in two or three divided doses, with the total daily dose ranging from 2 to 20 mg.

When any of these agents has been used chronically, it is impor-tant to not discontinue it abruptly but to taper the dose over several days in order to avoid a cholinergic rebound, as described in that chapter.

Overall, there appears to be little in the way of clinical differences in these agents, and it is reasonable to pick one and become thoroughly familiar with it; benztropine is a good choice. In any case the initial dose is chosen with due regard to severity of symptoms, age, and the effect on the patient of any anticipated side effects. The dose may then be adjusted as indicated.

BIBLIOGRAPHY

Burke RE, Fahn S. Pharmacokinetics of trihexyphenidyl after short-term and long-term administration to dystonic patients. *Annals of Neurology* 1985;18:35-40.
Burke RE, Fahn S, Marsden CD. Torsion dystonia: a double-blind, prospective trial of high-dosage trihexyphenidyl. *Neurology* 1986;36:160-164.
Friedman JH, Koller WC, Lannon MC, et al. Benztropine versus clozapine for the treatment of tremor in Parkinson's disease. *Neurology* 1997;48:1077-1088.
Gelenberg AJ, Van Putten T, Lavori PW, et al. Anticholinergic effects on memory: benztropine versus amantadine. *Journal of Clinical Psychopharmacology* 1989;9:180-185.
Zemishlany Z, Aizenberg D, Weiner Z, et al. Trihexyphenidyl (Artane) abuse in schizophrenic patients. *International Clinical Psychopharmacology* 1996;11:199-202.

300 Cholinesterase Inhibitors

There are currently four acetylcholinesterase inhibitors available in the United States, including donepezil, galantamine, rivastigmine and tacrine. Tacrine, alone among these cholinesterase inhibitors, is associated with significant hepatotoxicity, and, given that it has no advantages over the other three, it should probably not be used, and is not covered further here.

The primary indication for donepezil, galantamine and rivastigmine is Alzheimer's disease; other uses include vascular dementia, Parkinson's disease and diffuse Lewy body disease. In all these conditions, the principal effect of the cholinesterase inhibitor is improved memory, cognition and global functioning; furthermore, in the case of Parkinson's disease and diffuse Lewy body disease, there is also a distinct reduction in associated hallucinations and delusions, without any deterioration in motor status.

All three agents are effective in mild to moderate Alzheimer's disease, and donepezil has also demonstrated effectiveness in moderate to severe disease. Galantamine has been demonstrated to be effective in vascular dementia, donepezil in Parkinson's disease and rivastigmine in diffuse Lewy body disease.

All three of these agents, by inhibiting central nervous system acetylcholinesterase, increase cholinergic tone, thereby exerting their therapeutic effect. In addition, galantamine, alone among the cholinesterase inhibitors, also allosterically modifies the post-synaptic nicotinic acetylcholine receptor complex, rendering it more sensitive to stimulation by acetylcholine.

Donepezil and galantamine are both reversible inhibitors of acetylcholinesterase; rivastigmine is considered "pseudo-irreversible" in that although it does bind irreversibly to acetylcholinesterase, it is also, albeit very gradually, cleaved and metabolized by that same enzyme.

PHARMACOKINETICS

There are substantial differences in pharmacokinetics among these three agents, as illustrated in Table 300-1. From a practical, clinical point of view, the most important differences here are in half life and metabolic pathway. As noted below, whereas donepezil, given its long half life, may be given once daily, the other two must be given in divided doses. Further, as noted under drug-drug interactions, the dependence of donepezil and galantamine on the CYP 2D6 and 3A4 enzymes renders them susceptible to significant interactions.

SIDE EFFECTS

The most common side effects are anorexia, nausea, vomiting, diarrhea, fatigue and insomnia. Bradycardia may appear, as may A-V heart block; dizziness and, uncommonly, syncope have occurred.

Bronchial secretions are increased, and patients with significant asthma or COPD may experience a worsening of their condition. Acid gastric secretions also increase, and this may place some patients, particularly those taking aspirin or NSAIDs, at risk for gastrointestinal bleeding.

DRUG-DRUG INTERACTIONS

All three of these agents may augment the effect of succinylcholine and antagonize the effect of anticholinergic drugs.

Because donepezil and galantamine are metabolized by the CYP 3A4 and 2D6 enzymes, increased levels would be anticipated with concurrent use of drugs such as ketoconazole, fluvoxamine, fluoxetine, paroxetine and quinidine, and indeed this has been demonstrated in the case of galantamine. Although such demonstrations are lacking for donepezil, it is prudent to assume that they do exist.

OVERDOSAGE

Overdose may produce a cholinergic crisis, with vomiting, diarrhea, diaphoresis, bradycardia, respiratory depression, weakness and convulsions.

■**TABLE 300-1.** Pharmacokinetic Profiles of Cholinesterase Inhibitors

	Donepezil	Galantamine	Rivastigmine
Bioavailability	?*	90%	40%
Time to peak	3-4 h	1 h	1 h
Protein binding	96%	18%	40%
Half life	70 h	7 h	1.5 h
Metabolic pathway	CYP 2D6 CYP 3A4	CYP 2D6 CYP 3A4	acetylcholinesterase**

*Although the absolute bioavailability of donepezil is not known, the oral bioavailability is almost 100% relative to intravenous administration.
**Metabolism of rivastigmine by acetylcholinesterase is non-linear at doses above 6 mg (i.e., a doubling of the dose from 6 to 12 mg of rivastigmine results in more than a three-fold increase in the AUC).

In addition to intense supportive care, atropine is given intravenously in a dose of from 0.5 to 2 mg, with repeat doses as needed.

THERAPEUTIC USAGE

Donepezil is available in 5 and 10 mg tablets. Treatment is initiated at 5 mg once daily, either in the morning or evening, and then, if tolerated, increased to 10 mg after four to six weeks: although there is some benefit at 5 mg, 10 mg, overall, is more effective.

Galantamine is available in 4, 8 and 12 mg tablets and as a 4 mg/ml oral solution. Treatment is begun at a total daily dose of 8 mg and increased in similar increments every four weeks until either limiting side effects occur or a maximum total daily dose of 32 mg is reached: most patients require at least 16 mg to benefit, and doses of from 24 to 32 mg appear most effective. In all cases, the total daily dose is divided into two equal doses.

Rivastigmine is available in 1.5, 3, 4.5 and 6 mg capsules and as a 2 mg/ml oral solution. Treatment is initiated at a total daily dose of 3 mg and increased in similar increments every two weeks until either limiting side effects occur or a maximum dose of 12 mg is reached: doses of from 6 to 12 mg are generally required for a therapeutic effect. As with galantamine, the total daily dose is divided into two equal doses.

For donepezil and galantamine, the dose must be reduced in cases of hepatic failure. For rivastigmine, given that it is not dependent on hepatic enzymes for its metabolic degradation, no adjustment is necessary.

The implications of "missing" doses for a few days varies widely among these agents. In the case of galantamine and rivastigmine, both of which have short half lives, a few days without treatment allows for up-regulation of acetylcholine receptors, and in such a case, reinstitution of treatment at the previously tolerated dose will generally result in severe cholinergic side effects; consequently, with these agents, reinstitution of treatment must be by gradual titration. With donepezil, however, given its very long half life, one can generally restart treatment at 10 mg without any adverse effects.

Switching between cholinesterase inhibitors must also be approached with different strategies, depending on which cholinesterase is already in place. For example, when patients are already on donepezil, one cannot simply stop donepezil and switch more or less directly to a full replacement dose of either galantamine or rivastigmine without grossly increasing cholinergic tone. Given donepezil's long half life, either galantamine or rivastigmine would have to be titrated up slowly, over roughly two weeks time. Conversely, when switching from either galantamine or rivastigmine to donepezil, however, one may generally begin with donepezil at 5 mg the next day, and, if tolerated, up to 10 mg the day following that.

BIBLIOGRAPHY

Aarsland D, Laake K, Larsen JP, et al. Donepezil for cognitive impairment in Parkinson's disease: a randomized controlled study. *Journal of Neurology, Neurosurgery, and Psychiatry* 2002;72:708-712.

Erkinjuntti T, Kurz A, Gautier S, et al. Efficacy of galantamine in probable vascular dementia and Alzheimer's disease combined with cerebro-vascular disease: a randomized trial. *Lancet* 2002;359:1283-1290.

Feldman H, Gautier S, Hecker J, et al. A 24-week, double-blind study of donepezil in moderate to severe Alzheimer's disease. *Neurology* 2001;57:13-20.

Hossain M, Jhee SS, Shiovitz T, et al. Estimation of the absolute bioavailability of rivastigmine in patients with mild to moderate dementia of the Alzheimer's type. *Clinical Pharmacokinetics* 2002;41:225-234.

Lillienfeld S. Galantamine—a novel cholinergic drug with a unique dual mode of action for the treatment on patients with Alzheimer's disease. *CNS Drug Reviews* 2002;8:159-176.

McKeith I, Del Ser T, Spano R, et al. Efficacy of rivastigmine in dementia with Lewy bodies: a randomized, double-blind, placebo-controlled international study. *Lancet* 2000;356:2031-2036.

Maelicke A, Samochoki M, Jostock R, et al. Allosteric sensitization of nicotinic receptors by galantamine, a new treatment strategy for Alzheimer's disease. *Biological Psychiatry* 2001;49:279-288.

Rockwood K, Mintzer J, Truyen L, et al. Effects of a flexible galantamine dose in Alzheimer's disease: a randomized, controlled trial. *Journal of Neurology, Neurosurgery, and Psychiatry* 2001;71:589-595.

Rosier M, Anand R, Cicin-Sain A, et al. Efficacy and safety of rivastigmine in patients with Alzheimer's disease: international randomized controlled trial. *British Medical Journal* 1999;318:633-638.

Tiseo PJ, Rogers SL, Friedhoff LT. Pharmacokinetic and pharmacodynamic profile of donepezil HCL following evening administration. *British Journal of Clinical Pharmacology* 1998;46(Suppl 1):13-18.

301 Amantadine

Amantadine blocks NMDA glutamate receptors and also increases dopaminergic tone, not only by blocking reuptake of dopamine from the synaptic cleft but also by facilitating release of dopamine from the presynaptic membrane. The drug has minimal anticholinergic effect, generally evident only when high doses are used.

Amantadine is indicated for the treatment of antipsychotic-induced extrapyramidal side effects, where it may be as effective as are the anticholinergic drugs, such as benztropine. Amantadine is effective against levodopa-induced dyskinesias seen in Parkinson's disease and also against the parkinsonian motor symptoms themselves; however, its effect here is modest at best when compared to levodopa. Huntington's disease constitutes another indication; however, as pointed out below, relatively high doses must be utilized before a reduction in chorea is seen. Other indications; include cocaine withdrawal, fatigue seen in multiple sclerosis, and hyperprolactinemia and gynecomastia occurring as a side effect to antipsychotics. Amantadine may also enhance cognitive recovery in patients with traumatic brain injuries.

PHARMACOKINETICS

Amantadine is well absorbed after oral administration and has a bioavailability of anywhere from 50% to 90%. Peak blood levels are obtained in 1 to 4 hours and about 70% is protein bound. Only about 10% of amantadine is metabolized in the liver, with the rest being excreted unchanged in the urine. In patients with normal renal function the half life is about 16 hours; in those with severe renal failure, this may be prolonged to up to 34 days. Hemodialysis removes 5% or less of amantadine in each run, and in patients on chronic hemodialysis, the half life of amantadine is about 8 days.

SIDE EFFECTS

In general, side effects are more common and more severe at doses over 200 mg/day. Perhaps the most common side effects are difficulty in concentration, lightheadedness, lethargy, and insomnia. Less frequent are depression, irritability, nausea, dry mouth, blurry vision, difficulty with urination, confusion, and visual hallucinations. Infrequent side effects include dysarthria and ataxia, and there are rare reports of peripheral neuropathy, delusions and mania. Rarely, congestive heart failure may occur, and likewise, rarely, epileptic patients may experience an increased frequency of seizures. Not uncommonly, livedo reticularis may develop in patients, especially females, who take amantadine for a month or more.

Amantadine may be teratogenic; it is excreted in the breast milk.

DRUG-DRUG INTERACTIONS

Combination treatment with either anticholinergics or levodopa is more likely to produce confusion and hallucinations.

Amantadine levels have been increased by quinidine, trimethoprim/sulfamethoxazole and hydrochlorthiazide/triamterene.

OVERDOSAGE

In addition to an intensification of the side effects noted above, torsade de pointes and ventricular fibrillation may occur.

Gastric lavage should be considered in cases of recent overdose, and patients should be monitored for arrhythmias. Acidification of the urine hastens excretion and should be considered. Hemodialysis, as noted earlier, is relatively ineffective, but in some cases repeated hemodialysis has been used to good effect.

THERAPEUTIC USAGE

Amantadine is available in a 100 mg tablet and a 50 mg/5 ml syrup.

In patients with normal renal function, the dosage range is from 100 to 400 mg total per day, generally in two divided doses, with most patients responding to 200 or 300 mg; an exception to this is Huntington's disease, where it appears that doses of 400 mg are required. In patients with impaired renal function or the elderly, the dose should be reduced.

Amantadine should not be abruptly discontinued, as this may be followed by a delirium or the neuroleptic malignant syndrome. Although these consequences are rare, they are clearly severe, and prudence dictates tapering the dose over a few days or more.

BIBLIOGRAPHY

Factor SA, Molho ES, Brown DL. Acute delirium after withdrawal of amantadine in Parkinson's disease. *Neurology* 1998;50:1456-1458.

Horadam VW, Sharp JG, Smilack JD, et al. Pharmacokinetics of amantadine hydrochloride in subjects with normal and impaired renal function. *Annals of Internal Medicine* 1981;94:454-458.

Ing TS, Mahurkar SD, Dunea G, et al. Removal of amantadine hydrochloride by dialysis in patients with renal insufficiency. *Canadian Medical Association Journal* 1976;115:515.

Krupp LB, Coyle PK, Doscher C, et al. Fatigue therapy in multiple sclerosis: results of a double-blind, randomized, parallel trial of amantadine, pemoline, and placebo. *Neurology* 1995;45:1956-1961.

McNamara P, Durso R. Reversible jealousy (Othello syndrome) associated with amantadine. *Journal of Geriatric Psychiatry and Neurology* 1991; 4:157-159.

Metman LV, Del Dotto P, LePoole K, et al. Amantadine for levodopa-induced dyskinesias: a 1-year follow-up study. *Archives of Neurology* 1999;56:1383-1386.

Meythaler JM, Brunner RC, Johnson A, et al. Amantadine to improve neurorecovery in traumatic brain-injury-associated diffuse axonal injury: a pilot double-blind randomized trial. *The Journal of Head Trauma Rehabilitation* 2002;17:300-313.

Postma JU, Van Tilburg W. Visual hallucinations and delirium during treatment with amantadine. *Journal of the American Geriatrics Society* 1975;23:212-215.

Rego MD, Giller EL. Mania secondary to amantadine treatment of neuroleptic-induced hyperprolactinemia. *The Journal of Clinical Psychiatry* 1989;50:143-144.

Sartori M, Pratt CM, Young JB. Torsade de pointe. Malignant cardiac arrhythmia induced by amantadine poisoning. *The American Journal of Medicine* 1984;77:388-391.

Siever LJ. The effect of amantadine on prolactin levels and galactorrhea on neuroleptic-treated patients. *Journal of Clinical Psychopharmacology* 1981;1:2-7.

Simpson DM, Davis GC. Case report of neuroleptic malignant syndrome associated with withdrawal from amantadine. *The American Journal of Psychiatry* 1984;141:796-797.

Speeg KV, Leighton JA, Maldonado AL. Toxic delirium in a patient taking amantadine and trimethoprim-sulfamethoxazole. *The American Journal of the Medical Sciences* 1989;298:410-412.

Verhagen Metman L, Morris MJ, Farmer C, et al. Huntington's disease: a randomized, controlled trial using the NMDA-antagonist amantadine. *Neurology* 2002;59:694-699.

Wilson TW, Rajput AH. Amantadine-Dyazide interaction. *Canadian Medical Association Journal* 1983;129:974-975.

302 Propranolol

Propranolol is a nonselective beta-blocker with equal affinity for beta-1 and beta-2 receptors, and is available in both immediate- and sustained-release preparations. It is an immensely versatile medicine, being useful for the treatment of acute antipsychotic-induced akathisia, tardive akathisia, social phobia of the circumscribed type, intermittent explosive disorder, violence (when impulsive), alcohol or benzodiazepine withdrawal, medication-induced tremor (e.g., lithium), hyperthyroidism, essential tremor, and in the prophylaxis of migraine. Of all these conditions, the most robust indication is akathisia; for the rest propranolol is generally used only as a second line medication or adjunctively.

PHARMACOKINETICS

Propranolol is well absorbed after oral administration but because of an extensive first-pass effect bioavailability is about 25% for the immediate-release preparation and only about 15% for the sustained-release preparation. Peak blood levels are obtained in from 1 to 1½ hours with the immediate-release preparation and in about 6 hours with the sustained-release preparation. About 90% is protein-bound. Propranolol is metabolized almost completely in the liver, with less than 0.5% being excreted unchanged in the urine. The half-life of the immediate release preparation is about 4 hours and of the sustained-release preparation about 10 hours. It should be kept in mind that there is an up to 20-fold interpatient variability of blood level on any given dose.

SIDE EFFECTS

Propranolol may cause both bronchospasm and vasospasm and is thus generally contraindicated in asthma, COPD, vasospastic angina, and Raynaud's phenomenon.

Bradycardia occurs routinely, and preexisting sinus bradycardia constitutes a relative contraindication. Atrioventricular conduction time is prolonged; thus those with second or third degree AV block should generally not receive the drug, not should patients with Wolff-Parkinson-White syndrome who are in atrial flutter or fibrillation. Congestive heart failure may be aggravated due to propranolol's negative inotropic effect. Hypotension may occur and may cause dizziness, especially in patients with preexisting hypotension. Fatigue is common; depression may also occur but does not appear to be as common as was once feared. Vivid dreams may be complained of, and hallucinations and confusion have been reported. Erectile dysfunction may occur.

DRUG-DRUG INTERACTIONS

Aluminum hydroxide (as found in certain antacids), colestipol and cholestyramine may all reduce absorption.

Propranolol levels are decreased by nicotine, phenobarbital, phenytoin and rifampin.

Propranolol levels are increased by fluvoxamine, cimetidine, thioridazine and chlorpromazine (in the case of fluvoxamine this increase may be up to fivefold). Further, in the case of chlorpromazine, the concurrent use of chlorpromazine and propranolol is followed by increased chlorpromazine levels.

Propranolol has an additive effect with other antihypertensive medications.

The teratogenicity of propranolol is not known; it is excreted in breast milk.

OVERDOSAGE

Overdosage may produce delirium, bradycardia, hypotension, congestive failure, and bronchospasm. Atropine is used for bradycardia, epinephrine for hypotension, digoxin for congestive failure, and aminophylline and isoproterenol for bronchospasm.

THERAPEUTIC USAGE

Propranolol is available as an immediate-release preparation in 10, 20, 40 and 80 mg tablets and as an oral solution containing 20, 40 or 80 mg per 5cc. A sustained-release preparation is available as 60, 80, 120 and 160 mg capsules.

The dose ranges for each of the indications noted earlier are contained in the respective chapters; for essential tremor and for migraine prophylaxis it is from 60 to 240 mg. In general, it is prudent to begin with an immediate-release preparation at a starting total daily dose ranging from 20 to 40 mg, dividing this total into at least two doses. Increases may then be made in similar increments every day or two until an adequate therapeutic effect is obtained, the upper limit of the dose range is reached or intolerable side effects occur. Once an optimum dose has been found it is appropriate in most cases (with the notable exception of the circumscribed subtype of social phobia) to switch to a sustained-release preparation which may be given once daily. In switching to a sustained-release preparation, it is often necessary, given the increased first-pass effect, to increase the total daily dose by from 30 to 50%.

In patients with hypertension or coronary artery disease, propranolol should not be abruptly discontinued, as angina or infarction or rebound hypertension may occur. The dose may be safely tapered over a 2-week period.

BIBLIOGRAPHY

Bailly D, Servant D, Blandin N, et al. Effects of beta-blocking drugs in alcohol withdrawal: a double-blind comparative study with propranolol and diazepam. *Biomedicine & Pharmacotherapy* 1992;46:419-424.

Gelenberg AJ, Jefferson JW. Lithium tremor. *The Journal of Clinical Psychiatry* 1995;56:283-287.

Gironell A, Kulisevsky J, Barbanoj M, et al. A randomized placebo-controlled comparative trial of gabapentin and propranolol in essential tremor. *Archives of Neurology* 1990;56:475-480.

Hartley LR, Ungapen S, Davie I, et al. The effect of beta adrenergic blocking drugs on speakers' performance and memory. *The British Journal of Psychiatry* 1983;142:512-517.

Henderson JM, Portmann L, Van Melle G, et al. Propranolol as an adjunct therapy for hyperthyroid tremor. *European Neurology* 1997;37:182-185.

Jenkins SC, Maruta T. Therapeutic use of propranolol for intermittent explosive disorder. *Mayo Clinic Proceedings* 1987;62:204-214.

Kramer MS, Gorkin R, DiJohnson C. Treatment of neuroleptic-induced akathisia with propranolol: a controlled replication study. *Hillside Journal of Clinical Psychiatry* 1989;11:107-119.

Lapierre YD. Control of lithium tremor with propranolol. *Canadian Medical Association Journal* 1976;114:619-620.

Mattes JA. Comparative effectiveness of carbamazepine and propranolol for rage outbursts. *The Journal of Neuropsychiatry and Clinical Neurosciences* 1990;2:159-164.

Meilbach RC, Dunner D, Wilson LG, et al. Comparative efficacy of propranolol, chlordiazepoxide, and placebo in the treatment of anxiety: a double-blind trial. *The Journal of Clinical Psychiatry* 1987;48:355-358.

Nace GS, Wood AJ. Pharmacokinetics of long acting propranolol. Implications for therapeutic use. *Clinical Pharmacokinetics* 1987;13:51-64.

Ravaris CL, Friedman MJ, Hauri PJ, et al. A controlled study of alprazolam and propranolol in panic-disordered and agoraphobic outpatients. *Journal of Clinical Psychopharmacology* 1991;11:344-350.

Silver JM, Yudofsky SC, Slater JA, et al. Propranolol treatment of chronically hospitalized aggressive patients. *The Journal of Neuropsychiatry and Clinical Neurosciences* 1999;11:328-335.

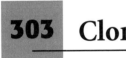

303 Clonidine

The primary mechanism of action of clonidine appears to be stimulation of presynaptic alpha-2 receptors within the central nervous system, leading to an overall decrease in sympathetic tone. At supratherapeutic doses, however, clonidine may stimulate vascular alpha-2 receptors, leading to vasoconstriction.

Clonidine is useful for attention deficit disorder/hyperactivity, Tourette's syndrome, autism, opioid withdrawal, tardive dyskinesia and the restless legs syndrome.

PHARMACOKINETICS

Oral clonidine has a bioavailability of 95% and peak blood levels are obtained in about 3 hours, with a range of 1 to 5 hours; about 20% is protein bound. Roughly 50% is metabolized in the liver and 50% is excreted unchanged in the urine; the half-life averages about 12 hours, with a range from 6 to 24 hours. In renal failure, the half-life increases to as high as 40 hours.

SIDE EFFECTS

Sedation, dry mouth, and hypotension with dizziness are not uncommon. Erectile dysfunction may occur, and depression has been reported. Clonidine is excreted in breast milk; it is not known if it has teratogenic effect.

DRUG-DRUG INTERACTIONS

Desipramine, and probably other tricyclics as well, blocks the interaction between clonidine and the presynaptic alpha-2 receptor, with a loss of clonidine's therapeutic effect.

Agents capable of decreasing blood pressure, notably other antihypertensives and trazodone, potentiate clonidine's hypotensive effect.

OVERDOSAGE

Overdosage, if sufficiently severe, may initially cause a dramatic surge in blood pressure; as the level of clonidine falls, however, the blood pressure falls and patients develop stupor or coma, respiratory depression, bradycardia, miosis and decreased deep tendon reflexes; seizures may also occur.

If seen early enough, gastric lavage and activated charcoal are indicated. In cases where blood pressure becomes dangerously high, nitroprusside may be given. When blood pressure falls, fluids are indicated, and, if this is not sufficient, dopamine; bradycardia may be treated with atropine.

THERAPEUTIC USAGE

Clonidine is available in 0.1, 0.2 and 0.3 mg tablets and in a transdermal delivery system, applied once weekly, which may deliver, on a daily basis, 0.1, 0.2 or 0.3 mg.

The recommended approach for each of the disorders mentioned earlier is described in the appropriate chapter; overall the dose must be reduced in the elderly or in those with significant hepatic or renal failure. Those taking clonidine chronically may benefit by using transdermal patches rather than tablets.

After chronic use, clonidine tablets must be gradually tapered over 3 to 7 days to prevent a withdrawal syndrome. In a minority of patients, abrupt discontinuation is followed within 18 to 36 hours by tremulousness, anxiety, diaphoresis, tachycardia, and hypertension. This syndrome is worse if the patient is concurrently taking a beta-blocker; hence, in patients taking both a beta-blocker and clonidine, the beta-blocker should be gradually tapered and discontinued first, followed then by tapering of the clonidine.

In addition to this "sympathetic" rebound, patients with Tourette's syndrome, if abruptly withdrawn from clonidine, may experience a dramatic increase in tics which, even with reinstitution of treatment, may take months to resolve.

It appears that a withdrawal syndrome is less likely when the transdermal system is used, as the blood level falls gradually, over days, after the patch is removed.

BIBLIOGRAPHY

Anavekar SN, Howes LG, Jarrott B, et al. Pharmacokinetics and antihypertensive effects of low dose clonidine during chronic therapy. *Journal of Clinical Pharmacokinetics* 1989;29:321-326.

Briant RH, Reid JL, Dollery CT. Interaction between clonidine and desipramine in man. *British Medical Journal* 1973;1:522-523.

Domino LE, Domino SE, Stockstill MS. Relationship between plasma concentrations of clonidine and mean arterial pressure during an accidental clonidine overdose. *British Journal of Clinical Pharmacology* 1986;21:71-74.

Fankhauser MP, Karumanchi VC, German ML, et al. A double-blind, placebo-controlled study of the efficacy of transdermal clonidine in autism. *The Journal of Clinical Psychiatry* 1992;53:77-82.

Fauler J, Verner L. The pharmacokinetics of clonidine in high dosage. *European Journal of Clinical Pharmacology* 1993;45:165-167.

Frye CB, Vance MA. Hypertensive crisis and myocardial infarction following massive clonidine overdose. *The Annals of Pharmacotherapy* 2000; 34:611-615.

Jasinski DR, Johnson RE, Kocher DR. Clonidine in morphine withdrawal: differential effects on signs and symptoms. *Archives of General Psychiatry* 1985;42:1063-1066.

Leckman JF, Ort S, Caruso KA, et al. Rebound phenomena in Tourette's syndrome after abrupt withdrawal of clonidine. Behavioral, cardiovascular, and nuerochemical effects. *Archives of General Psychiatry* 1986;43:1168-1176.

Leckman JF, Hardin MT, Riddle MA, et al. Clonidine treatment of Gilles de la Tourette's syndrome. *Archives of General Psychiatry* 1991;48:324-328.

Singer HS, Brown J, Quaskey S, et al. The treatment of attention-deficit hyperactivity disorder in Tourette's syndrome: a double-blind, placebo-controlled study with clonidine and desipramine. *Pediatrics* 1995;95: 74-81.

304 Guanfacine

Guanfacine, like clonidine, stimulates pre-synaptic alpha-2 receptors, with an overall decrease in sympathetic tone, and, also like clonidine, is effective in attention-deficit hyperactivity disorder and Tourette's syndrome. Overall, it is better tolerated than clonidine, and easier to use.

PHARMACOKINETICS

Guanfacine has a bioavailability of about 80% and is about 70% protein bound. The half-life ranges from 12 to 24 hours, and about 70% is metabolized in the liver with the remainder being excreted unchanged in the urine.

SIDE EFFECTS

Side effects are similar to those seen with clonidine, but less severe, and include sedation, dry mouth, hypotension and dizziness.

There is a case series of pediatric patients, all with family histories of bipolar disorder, who became manic when given guanfacine.

DRUG-DRUG INTERACTIONS

Although not documented, it is reasonable to assume that desipramine, and other tricyclics, would block guanfacine's stimulation of alpha-2 receptors, just as they do in the case of clonidine.

Guanfacine appears to increase valproate levels.

Other agents capable of reducing blood pressure would have an additive effect with guanfacine.

OVERDOSAGE

Hypotension and stupor may occur, with respiratory depression, miosis and bradycardia.

Gastric lavage and activated charcoal should be given. Hypotension may be controlled with fluids or dopamine, and bradycardia may be treated with atropine.

THERAPEUTIC USAGE

Guanfacine is available in 1 and 2 mg tablets.

Treatment is initiated at a total daily dose of 1 mg and increased in similar increments every three to seven days until a response is seen, limiting side effects occur or a maximum dose of 4 mg is reached. Although once-daily dosing may be attempted, in many cases dividing the dose into two doses is required to maintain control throughout the day.

Dosage adjustments are not required in renal failure.

Abrupt discontinuation of guanfacine may be followed by a sympathetic rebound, but this is generally less severe than that seen with clonidine. There may be agitation, tremor, headache, tachycardia, hypertension and diaphoresis.

BIBLIOGRAPHY

Ambrosini PJ, Sheikh RM. Increased plasma valproate concentrations when coadministered with guanfacine. *Journal of Child and Adolescent Psychopharmacology* 1998;8:143-147.

Carchman SH, Crowe JT, Wright GJ. The bioavailability and pharmaco-kinetics of guanfacine after oral and intravenous administration to healthy volunteers. *Journal of Clinical Pharmacology* 1987;27: 762-767.

Horrigan JP, Barnhill LJ. Guanfacine and secondary mania in children. *Journal of Affective Disorders* 1999;54:309-314.

Kirch W, Kohler H, Braun W, et al. The influence of renal function on plasma concentration, urinary excretion and antihypertensive effect of guanfacine. *Clinical Pharmacokinetics* 1980;5:476-483.

Scahill L, Chappell PB, Kin YS, et al. A placebo-controlled study of guanfacine in the treatment of children with tic disorders and attention deficit hyperactivity disorder. *The American Journal of Psychiatry* 2001;158:1067-1074.

Taylor FB, Russo J. Comparing guanfacine and dextroamphetamine for the treatment of adult attention-deficit/hyperactivity disorder. *Journal of Clinical Psychopharmacology* 2001;21:223-228.

Yamadera H, Ferber G, Matejcek M, et al. Electroencephalographic and psychometric assessment of the CNS effects of single doses of guanfacine hydrochloride (Estulic) and clonidine (Catapres). *Neuropsychobiology* 1985;14:97-107.

305 Buspirone

Buspirone, an azapirone, is a full agonist at presynaptic 5-HT$_{1A}$ receptors and a partial agonist at post-synaptic 5-HT$_{1A}$ receptors; it also binds to both pre- and post-synaptic dopamine D2 receptors, and in this regard its predominant effect is an antagonism at the presynaptic receptor. One of buspirone's major active metabolites, 1-pyramidinylpiperazine, also has antagonistic activity at both presynaptic and postsynaptic alpha-2 receptors.

Buspirone is indicated for generalized anxiety disorder; it may also be of modest use in cases of ataxia secondary to cerebellar cortical atrophy.

PHARMACOKINETICS

Buspirone is well absorbed after oral administration but is subject to an extensive first-pass effect, with bioavailability of only about 4%. Peak blood levels are obtained in 40 to 90 minutes, and about 95% is protein bound. Metabolism occurs in the liver via CYP3A4, and less than 0.1% is excreted as the parent compound in the urine. The half-life ranges from 2 to 11 hours, with an average of about 6 hours.

SIDE EFFECTS

Sedation, headache, dizziness, nausea and diarrhea may be seen, and a small minority of patients may complain of a sense of restlessness similar to an akathisia. Prolactin levels are generally increased.

There are rare case reports of abnormal movements occurring within hours to weeks of initiation of treatment, including myoclonus, tremor, an exacerbation of preexisting parkinsonism, and dystonia; in one case the dystonia persisted despite discontinuation of the drug.

DRUG-DRUG INTERACTIONS

Buspirone levels may be increased, in some cases several-fold, by CYP3A4 inhibitors such as erythromycin, ketoconazole, itracona-zole, verapamil, diltiazem, nefazodone and fluvoxamine. Grapefruit juice also increases buspirone levels.

Buspirone levels may be decreased by CYP3A4 inducers, such as rifampin.

Combination with an MAOI may lead to hypertension.

There is a case report of a serotonin syndrome occurring secondary to the combination of fluoxetine and buspirone.

OVERDOSAGE

Buspirone appears to be remarkably safe in overdose, producing for the most part only an exaggeration of the side effects noted earlier. Although no deaths have occurred secondary to buspirone alone, there is one case report of a grand mal seizure occurring after an overdose.

THERAPEUTIC USAGE

Buspirone is supplied in 5, 7.5, 10, 15 and 30 mg tablets.

Treatment is generally initiated at a total daily dose of 15 mg, increasing in 5 or 10 mg increments every 2 to 4 days to the desired dose, which, in the case of generalized anxiety disorder, ranges from 15 to 60 mg, with the total daily dose generally given in three divided doses. Importantly, unlike benzodiazepines, buspirone is slow acting, and several weeks may be required to see the full therapeutic effect. Furthermore, there is no cross-tolerance with the benzodiazepines; consequently, if the patient who has chronically taken a benzodiazepine is to be switched to buspirone, the benzodiazepine must be gradually tapered to prevent withdrawal symptoms.

BIBLIOGRAPHY

Catalano G, Catalano MC, Hanley PF. Seizures associated with buspirone overdose: case report and literature review. *Clinical Neuropharmacology* 1998;21:347-350.

Hammerstead JP, Carter J, Nutt JG, et al. Buspirone in Parkinson's disease. *Clinical Neuropharmacology* 1986;9:556-560.

Lamberg TS, Kivisto KT, Laitila J, et al. The effect of fluvoxamine on the pharmacokinetics and pharmacodynamics of buspirone. *European Journal of Clinical Pharmacology* 1998;54:761-766.

LeWitt PA, Walters A, Hening W, et al. Persistent movement disorders induced by buspirone. *Movement Disorders* 1993;8:331-334.

Liegghio NE, Yeragani VK, Moore NC. Buspirone-induced jitteriness in three patients with panic disorder and one patient with generalized anxiety disorder. *The Journal of Clinical Psychiatry* 1988;49:165-166.

Lilja JJ, Kivisto KT, Backman JT, et al. Grapefruit juice substantially increases plasma concentrations of buspirone. *Clinical Pharmacology and Therapeutics* 1998;64:655-660.

Mahmood I, Sahajwalla C. Clinical pharmacokinetics and pharmacodynamics of buspirone, an anxiolytic drug. *Clinical Pharmacokinetics* 1999;36:277-287.

Manos GH. Possible serotonin syndrome associated with buspirone added to fluoxetine. *The Annals of Pharmacotherapy* 2000;34:871-874.

Meltzer HY, Maes M. Effects of buspirone on plasma prolactin and cortisol levels in major depressed and normal subjects. *Biological Psychiatry* 1994;35:316-323.

Ritchie EC, Bridenbaugh RH, Jabbari B. Acute generalized myoclonus following buspirone administration. *The Journal of Clinical Psychiatry* 1988;49:242-243.

Salazar DE, Frackiewicz EF, Dockens R, et al. Pharmacokinetics and tolerability of buspirone during oral administration to children and adolescents with anxiety disorder and normal healthy adults. *Journal of Clinical Pharmacology* 2001;41:1351-1358.

Strauss A. Oral dyskinesia associated with buspirone use in an elderly woman. *The Journal of Clinical Psychiatry* 1988;49:322-323.

Trouillas P, Xie J, Adeleine P, et al. Buspirone, a 5-hydroxytryptamine 1A agonist, is active in cerebellar ataxia. Results of a double-blind drug placebo study in patients with cerebellar cortical atrophy. *Archives of Neurology* 1997;54:749-752.

306 Benzodiazepines

Each of the benzodiazepines exerts its clinical effect by virtue of enhancing the postsynaptic effectiveness of the naturally occurring inhibitory neurotransmitter gamma-aminobutyric acid (GABA). When GABA binds to the beta subunit of the postsynaptic GABA$_A$-benzodiazepine chloride ionophore receptor complex, the chloride channel is opened and an influx of chloride ions into the postsynaptic neuron occurs, thus hyperpolarizing the neuron and rendering it relatively refractory to any stimulatory influences.

Benzodiazepines bind to the alpha subunit of the same ionophore receptor complex. Subsequent to this binding, the configuration of the complex changes, with a greater influx of chloride whenever GABA binds to the beta subunit.

Benzodiazepines are used for generalized anxiety disorder, panic disorder, social phobia of the generalized subtype, recurrent nightmares, somnambulism, nocturnal myoclonus, the restless legs syndrome, alcohol withdrawal (and, of course, benzodiazepine withdrawal) and agitation. Both lorazepam and diazepam are also used in the treatment of status epilepticus.

Perhaps the most common reason why benzodiazepines are prescribed is to relieve anxiety, regardless of cause, or to relieve insomnia, again regardless of cause. Benzodiazepines reduce sleep latency, and although they prolong total sleep time, they actually reduce the amount of slow-wave sleep. The duration of REM episodes is decreased, but their number is increased.

Unfortunately, when a patient complains of anxiety or insomnia, a prescription for a benzodiazepine is often given without first pursuing a diagnostic workup. Thus many patients with dysthymia, depressive episodes, and many other disorders go undiagnosed and fail to receive appropriate treatment. Indeed, if careful diagnostic inquiry is pursued, one rarely finds a patient complaining of anxiety or of insomnia for whom a benzodiazepine is the unequivocal drug of first choice.

With the exception of alprazolam and clonazepam, which are each discussed in their respective chapters, the individual benzodiazepines are introduced below.

PHARMACOKINETICS

In general, benzodiazepines are well absorbed and reach peak blood levels within one-half to two hours; they are all extensively protein bound, most over 90%.

All of the benzodiazepines undergo metabolism in the liver: some proceed directly to glucuronidation, whereas others are first metabolized to active metabolites, which themselves subsequently undergo glucuronidation. It is customary to divide the various benzodiazepines into those with a short (S) half life, less than 6 hours, those with an intermediate (I) half life from 6 to 24 hours, and those with a long (L) half life of over 24 hours. Lorazepam (I), temazepam (I) and oxazepam (I) lack active metabolites and undergo direct glucuronidation. Diazepam (L) is metabolized to desmethyldiazepam (L) (which is not commercially available), which in turn is metabolized to oxazepam. Clorazepate (S) is unusual in that it is a "pro-drug" which is converted in the acidic gastric juices to desmethyldiazepam (L), which is then absorbed. Chlordiazepoxide (I) has several active metabolites, eventually being converted to desmethyldiazepam (L). Flurazepam (S) has an active metabolite (L) which is then glucuronidated. Estazolam (I) also has an active metabolite (S) which is glucuronidated. Finally, triazolam (S) also has an active metabolite (S) which is also glucuronidated.

In prescribing a benzodiazepine, it is clearly important to keep in mind whether it has an active metabolite before estimating its duration of effect. For example, given that lorazepam, temazepam and oxazepam all lack active metabolites, their intermediate half-lives allow a rough approximation of the duration of their clinical effect. In the case of diazepam, clorazepate, chlordiazepoxide, and flurazepam, however, the presence of active metabolites with long half-lives predicts a duration of effect far longer than that suggested by the half-life of the parent compound. Estazolam and triazolam both have active metabolites, but in these two instances the metabolites have short half-lives, and do not add much to the duration of effect of the parent compound.

Certain important clinical guidelines may be derived from the foregoing. First, since in hepatic failure intermediary metabolism is slowed, whereas glucuronidation generally is not, it makes sense to use lorazepam, temazepam or oxazepam in patients with any significant degree of hepatic failure. Second, little, if any, pharmacologic rationale exists for prescribing the pro-drug clorazepate, as one would accomplish essentially the same purpose by prescribing diazepam. Third, one must be prepared for drug accumulation when drugs with long or intermediate half-lives or metabolites with similar half-lives are used.

SIDE EFFECTS

All of the benzodiazepines are capable of causing tolerance, and withdrawal symptoms may occur even at "therapeutic" doses if taken long enough; indeed, in some cases neuroadaptation may occur in less than a month. The most common withdrawal symptom is "rebound insomnia"; other withdrawal symptoms are as described in the chapter on sedative, hypnotic, or anxiolytic related disorders. Withdrawal symptoms are both more common and more rapidly appearing with short half-life agents. Agents with long half-lives or those with active metabolites with long half-lives may undergo a "self-tapering" process: the blood levels decline so slowly that the withdrawal symptoms are delayed and remain mild or subclinical.

The most common acute side effects are sedation, lightheadedness, and slowed reaction time. These can be dangerous when agents with long half-lives or active metabolites with long half-lives are given as hypnotics. Blood levels the next day may be sufficiently high so as to render the patient incapable of safely driving or of using machinery. If the dose is too high, ataxia may occur, and, particularly in the elderly, one may see falls with fractures and subdural hematomas.

Short-term memory is impaired, and if the dose is high enough, anterograde amnesia may occur, producing a blackout. This may be more likely with triazolam than with the other benzodiazepines.

With the possible exception of alprazolam (discussed in the next chapter), all the benzodiazepines appear capable of worsening depressive symptoms in patients with a depressive episode, dysthymia, and the like. Benzodiazepines may also disinhibit patients leading to increased hostility. This appears to be least likely with oxazepam.

Benzodiazepines readily cross the placenta, and neonates may experience respiratory depression and may go into withdrawal. Although controversial, it also appears that chronic use during pregnancy may cause a syndrome similar to the fetal alcohol syndrome. Finally, benzodiazepines do appear in the breast milk.

DRUG-DRUG INTERACTIONS

The combination of a benzodiazepine with another drug with sedative effects, such as alcohol, may lead to increased sedation, unsteadiness, and the like.

In general, lorazepam, temazepam and oxazepam, as they all undergo immediate glucuronidation, are free of drug-drug interactions. The remainder, or their metabolites, however, undergo a significant increase in blood level when the following drugs are administered: erythromycin, clarithromycin, ritonavir, isoniazid, itraconazole, ketoconazole, nefazodone and fluvoxamine; grapefruit juice also increases these blood levels. The remainder also undergo a decrease in blood level when rifampin or carbamazepine are given; smoking also reduces blood levels.

For unclear reasons, benzodiazepines increase digoxin levels.

OVERDOSAGE

Overdoses with benzodiazepines alone are rarely fatal. In a mild case, ataxia and drowsiness may be seen; in severe cases coma with some degree of hypotension and respiratory depression may occur.

Gastric lavage and activated charcoal are generally appropriate; in severe cases one may consider giving flumazenil, as described in that chapter.

THERAPEUTIC USAGE

Lorazepam is available in 0.5, 1 and 2 mg scored tablets and for injection, temazepam in 15 and 30 mg capsules, oxazepam in 10, 15 and 30 mg capsules, diazepam in scored 2, 5 and 10 mg tablets and for injection, clorazepate in 3.75, 7.5 and 15 mg tablets, chlordiazepoxide in 5, 10 and 25 mg capsules and for injection, flurazepam in 15 and 30 mg capsules, estazolam in 1 and 2 mg tablets, and triazolam in 0.125 and 0.25 mg tablets.

The decision as to which benzodiazepine to use is based largely on the potential for drug-drug interactions and on pharmacokinetics. Agents which undergo direct glucuronidation have far fewer potential drug-drug interactions, and in this regard are therefore preferable. With regard to pharmacokinetics, an argument may be made for the directly glucuronidated agents on two counts. First, as noted earlier, they are relatively safe to use in cases of hepatic failure, whereas the remaining agents will all have prolonged half lives in this condition. Second, given that the half lives of these directly glucuronidated compounds are all in the intermediate range of 6 to 24 hours, there is less risk of drug accumulation and increased side effects. On the other hand, the intermediate half life of these glucuronidated agents make withdrawal symptoms more likely in cases of chronic treatment, whereas, by contrast, those agents with long half lives, or with long half life metabolites, are much less likely to be associated with withdrawal symptoms as their slowly falling blood levels in effect create a "self-taper."

On balance, and all other things being equal, it appears prudent to use one of the directly glucuronidated agents, and of these three, lorazepam enjoys the widest popularity, perhaps in large part due to its availability in an injectable form. In cases, however, where one wishes a longer duration of effect, one of the other agents should be chosen, and of them either diazepam or chlordiazepoxide is a reasonable choice.

For insomnia, lorazepam may be given in a dose of 1 or 2 mg hs. For daytime anxiolysis, lorazepam may be given in a total daily dose of 1 to 4 mg, diazepam in a dose of 15-25 mg or chlordiazepoxide in a dose of 25 to 75 mg, with the total daily dose being divided into two or three doses; in all cases, one should start with a low dose and build up gradually, always aiming for the lowest effective dose. The use of benzodiazepines for other indications is discussed in the respective chapters.

If a benzodiazepine is to be given parenterally, lorazepam is the first choice, as it is available for intravenous use and is well-absorbed after intramuscular administration. Diazepam, although available for intravenous use, is erratically absorbed after intramuscular use; chlordiazepoxide is also erratically absorbed after intramuscular administration and is not safe if given intravenously.

In all cases, doses must be reduced in the elderly, the very young, or debilitated patients.

BIBLIOGRAPHY

Busto U, Sellers EN, Naranjo CA, et al. Withdrawal reaction after long-term therapeutic use of benzodiazepines. *The New England Journal of Medicine* 1986;315:854-859.

Dietch JT, Jennings RK. Aggressive dyscontrol in patients treated with benzodiazepines. *The Journal of Clinical Psychiatry* 1988;49:184-188.

Laegrid L, Olegard R, Walstrom J, et al. Teratogenic effects of benzodiazepine use during pregnancy. *The Journal of Pediatrics* 1989;114: 126-131.

Mohler H, Fritschy JM, Rudolph U. A new benzodiazepine pharmacology. *The Journal of Pharmacology and Experimental Therapeutics* 2002; 300:2-8.

Rickels K, DeMartinis N, Rynn M, et al. Pharmacologic strategies for discontinuing benzodiazepine treatment. *Journal of Clinical Psychopharmacology* 1999;19(Suppl 2):12-16.

Sand P, Kavvadias D, Feineis D, et al. Naturally occurring benzodiazepines: current status of research and clinical implications. *European Archives of Psychiatry and Clinical Neuroscience* 2000;250:194-202.

Tanaka E. Clinically significant pharmacokinetic drug interactions with benzodiazepines. *Journal of Clinical Pharmacy and Therapeutics* 1999; 24:347-355.

307 Alprazolam

Alprazolam is an intermediate half-life benzodiazepine which is useful in the treatment of generalized anxiety disorder, panic disorder, premenstrual syndrome and essential tremor. Furthermore, and in distinction from other benzodiazepines, there are some studies supporting its effectiveness in the treatment of major depression: in this regard, however, alprazolam is not commonly used.

PHARMACOKINETICS

Alprazolam is available in both an immediate release and an extended release preparation. In both cases the bioavailability is about 90%; peak levels are obtained in from 1 to 2 hours for the immediate release preparation and in about 6 hours for the sustained release preparation. Protein binding is about 80%. Metabolism is via the liver, and although there are active metabolites these are found in extremely low concentration. The half life is about 12 hours in otherwise healthy adults; in the elderly it may be prolonged 4 hours, in hepatic failure 8 hours, and in the obese up to 10 hours.

SIDE EFFECTS

The side effects seen with alprazolam are generally similar to those reported for other benzodiazepines in the preceding chapter. In addition to these, alprazolam may be more likely to cause disinhibition with hostility, especially in patients with borderline personality disorder. There are also rare reports of alprazolam inducing mania, and one report of stuttering occurring secondary to alprazolam.

Although controversial, it appears that alprazolam may also be more likely to cause neuroadaptation than the other benzodiazepines, and thus more likely to cause a withdrawal syndrome (as described in the chapter on sedative, hypnotic, or anxiolytic related disorders); indeed there are case reports of grand mal seizures and delirium occurring within a day after abrupt discontinuation of relatively short-term (e.g., 10 weeks) therapeutic use of alprazolam.

Consequently, it is very important to taper the dose of alprazolam, generally at a rate no faster than 10% of the total daily dose every 3 or 4 days; indeed, in some cases patients are unable to tolerate a rate as slow as 10% per week.

Alprazolam is probably present in the breast milk and it is assumed that, like other benzodiazepines, it is teratogenic.

DRUG-DRUG INTERACTIONS

Alprazolam levels are increased by fluvoxamine, nefazodone, and, to a lesser extent, by fluoxetine; levels are also increased by ketoconazole, itraconazole, cimetidine and propoxyphene.

Alprazolam levels are decreased by carbamazepine, phenytoin, rifampin and theophylline.

Alprazolam may increase digoxin levels; however, this is significant only in the elderly. Imipramine and desipramine levels may also be increased; however, this generally is of little clinical significance.

Additive sedative effects typically occur when alprazolam is combined with alcohol or with other drugs with sedative effects.

OVERDOSAGE

The principal manifestations of alprazolam overdose are stupor, coma, and hypotension. In addition to general supportive treatment, gastric lavage and activated charcoal should be considered; fluid and pressor agents may be required for hypotension, and intubation may be necessary. Flumazenil may be considered; however, in patients who have taken alprazolam for more than a few weeks, this carries the risk of precipitating a seizure.

THERAPEUTIC USAGE

Alprazolam is available in immediate release scored tablets of 0.25, 0.5, 1 and 2 mg strength, and in extended release tablets of 0.5, 1, 2 and 3 mg.

In otherwise healthy adults, treatment is initiated in a total daily dose of 0.75 to 1.5 mg, with the dose increased in 1 mg or less increments about every 4 days or more until either a response is seen or limiting side effects occur: most patients require doses between 2 and 4 mg. When the immediate release preparation is used the total daily dose should be divided into at least three doses in order to prevent the emergence of withdrawal symptoms; in the case of the extended release preparation the entire daily dose may generally be given once a day in the morning.

In the elderly, those with significant liver disease, or the obese, smaller doses and longer intervals between incremental dose increases should be used.

BIBLIOGRAPHY

Abernathy DR, Greenblatt DJ, Divoll M, et al. Interaction of cimetidine with the triazolobenzodiazepines alprazolam and triazolam. Psychopharmacology 1983;80:275-278.

Abernathy DR, Greenblatt DJ, Divoll M, et al. The influence of obesity on the pharmacokinetics of oral alprazolam and triazolam. Clinical Pharmacokinetics 1984;9:177-183.

Abernathy DR, Greenblatt DJ, Morse DS, et al. Interaction of propoxyphene with diazepam, alprazolam and lorazepam. British Journal of Clinical Pharmacology 1985;19:51-57.

Busto UE, Kaplan HL, Wright CE, et al. A comparative pharmacokinetic and dynamic evaluation of alprazolam sustained-release, bromazepam, and lorazepam. Journal of Clinical Psychopharmacology 2000;20:628-635.

Elliott RL, Thomas BJ. A case report of alprazolam-induced stuttering. Journal of Clinical Psychopharmacology 1985;5:159-160.

Fleishaker JC, Hulst LK. A pharmacokinetic and pharmacodynamic evaluation of the combined administration of alprazolam and fluvoxamine. European Journal of Clinical Pharmacology 1994;46:35-39.

Gardner DL, Cowdry RW. Alprazolam-induced dyscontrol in borderline personality disorder. The American Journal of Psychiatry 1985;142:98-100.

Goodman WK, Charney DS. A case of alprazolam, but not lorazepam, inducing manic symptoms. The Journal of Clinical Psychiatry 1987;48:117-118.

Gunal DI, Afsar N, Bekiroglu N, et al. New alternative agents in essential tremor therapy: double-blind placebo-controlled study of alprazolam and acetazolamide. Neurological Sciences 2000;21:315-317.

Guven H, Tuncok Y, Guneri S, et al. Age-related digoxin-alprazolam interaction. Clinical Pharmacology and Therapeutics 1993;54:42-44.

Juergens SM, Morse RM. Alprazolam dependence in seven patients. The American Journal of Psychiatry 1988:145:625-627.

Levy AB. Delirium and seizures due to abrupt alprazolam withdrawal: case report. The Journal of Clinical Psychiatry 1984;45:38-39.

Rosenbaum JF, Woods SW, Groves JE, et al. Emergence of hostility during alprazolam treatment. The American Journal of Psychiatry 1984;141:792-793.

Yuan R, Flockhart DA, Balian JD. Pharmacokinetic and pharmacodynamic consequences of metabolism-based drug interactions with alprazolam, midazolam, and triazolam. Journal of Clinical Pharmacology 1999;39:1109-1125.

308 Clonazepam

Clonazepam is a long half-life benzodiazepine which, in addition to being effective in panic disorder, social phobia and generalized anxiety disorder, is also effective for treatment of nocturnal myoclonus, restless legs syndrome, intention myoclonus (as may be seen in post-anoxic states) and hyperekplexia or "startle disease"; it also plays a secondary role in Tourette's syndrome, treatment of petit mal, myoclonic and primary grand mal seizures and partial seizures of either the simple or complex type. Unfortunately, in about one-third of cases where it is used for seizure control, tolerance to the antiepileptic effect of clonazepam develops within a matter of months.

PHARMACOKINETICS

The bioavailability of clonazepam ranges from 80 to 98% and peak levels are reached within 1 to 4 hours with about 85% protein binding. Clonazepam is extensively metabolized in the liver and its metabolites have little or no pharmacologic activity; the half life ranges from 20 to 80 hours.

SIDE EFFECTS

The most common side effects are drowsiness and ataxia, which may subside over time with continued treatment. Unlike other benzodiazepines, clonazepam may also produce increased salivation. Disinhibition may occur, and thus caution should be used in prescribing to patients who are having trouble controlling their anger or impulses. Clonazepam shares with other benzodiazepines the risk of producing neuroadaptation, with withdrawal symptoms after abrupt discontinuation.

Clonazepam is excreted in the breast milk and is suspected of being teratogenic.

DRUG-DRUG INTERACTIONS

Clonazepam levels are decreased by phenytoin, carbamazepine and phenobarbital.

Clonazepam levels are increased by cimetidine.

Concurrent use of clonazepam and valproate in epileptic patients has been followed by status epilepticus, and concurrent use with other sedating drugs will have an additive effect.

OVERDOSAGE

Coma and respiratory depression may occur in overdose. Supportive treatment is indicated, and intubation may be required. In severe cases one may consider using flumazenil, as described in that chapter, with due regard for the risks of precipitating seizures, or, in those with epilepsy, status epilepticus.

THERAPEUTIC USAGE

Clonazepam is available in 0.5, 1 and 2 mg tablets.

For panic disorder, social phobia or generalized anxiety disorder treatment is initiated at a total daily dose of from 0.5 to 1 mg, which is then increased in 1 to 2 mg increments every week until satisfactory control, limiting side effects or a maximum dose of about 6 mg is reached; most patients respond to a dose of from 1 to 4 mg. In general, the total daily dose may be divided into two doses to mitigate side effects.

For nocturnal myoclonus, a dose of 0.5 to 1.5 mg at bedtime is generally adequate.

For seizure control, adults may be started at a dose of 1 to 2 mg daily, increasing in 0.5 to 1 mg increments every few days until control is established, limiting side effects occur or a maximum dose of 20 mg is reached; most adults respond to total daily doses of from 3 to 6 mg. Dividing the dose early on may mitigate side effects.

After chronic use, clonazepam should be slowly tapered, at a rate of perhaps 1 mg/week, in order to avoid a withdrawal syndrome or an exacerbation of the symptoms that were being treated.

BIBLIOGRAPHY

Binder RL. Three case reports of behavioral disinhibition with clonazepam. *General Hospital Psychiatry* 1987;9:151-153.

Chataway J, Fowler A, Thompson PJ, et al. Discontinuation of clonazepam in patients with active epilepsy. *Seizure* 1993;2:295-300.

Crevoisier C, Delisle MC, Joseph I, et al. Comparative single-dose pharmacokinetics of clonazepam following intravenous, intramuscular and oral administration to healthy volunteers. *European Neurology* 2003;49: 173-177.

Goldberb MA, Dorman JD. Intention myoclonus: successful treatment with clonazepam. *Neurology* 1976;26:24-26.

Lai AA, Levy RH, Cutler RE. Time-course of interaction between carbamazepine and clonazepam in normal man. *Clinical Pharmacology and Therapeutics* 1978;24:316-323.

Mikkelson B, Birket-Smith E, Holm P, et al. A controlled trial of clonazepam (Ro 5-4023, Rivitrol (R)) in the treatment of focal epilepsy and secondary generalized grand mal epilepsy. *Acta Neurologica Scandinavica* 1975;60:55-61.

Mikkelson B, Birket-Smith E, Bradt S, et al. Clonazepam in the treatment of epilepsy. A controlled clinical trial in simple absences, bilateral massive epileptic myoclonus, and atonic seizures. *Archives of Neurology* 1976;33:322-325.

Mikkelson B, Berggreen P, Joensen P, et al. Clonazepam (Rivitrol) and carbamazepine (Tegretol) in psychomotor epilepsy: a randomized multicenter trial. *Epilepsia* 1981;22:415-420.

Nanda RN, Johnson RH, Keogh HJ, et al. Treatment of epilepsy with clonazepam and its effect on other anticonvulsants. *Journal of Neurology, Neurosurgery, and Psychiatry* 1977;40:538-543.

Ryan SG, Sherman SL, Terry JC, et al. Startle disease, or hyperekplexia: response to clonazepam and assignment of the gene (5THE) to chromosome 5q by linkage analysis. *Annals of Neurology* 1992;31:663-668.

Sjo O, Hvidberg EF, Naestoft J, et al. Pharmacokinetics and side-effects of clonazepam and its 7-amino-metabolite in man. *European Journal of Clinical Pharmacology* 1975;8:249-254.

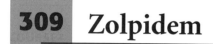

309 Zolpidem

Although structurally dissimilar to benzodiazepines, zolpidem shares certain agonist properties with them. As noted in the chapter on benzodiazepines, the post-synaptic GABA-A-benzodiazepine receptor complex consists of subunits, including the beta subunit, which naturally occurring GABA binds to, and the alpha subunit. This alpha subunit has subtypes, including BZ-1 (also known as omega-1) and BZ-2 (also known as omega-2). Zolpidem is an agonist preferentially at the BZ-1 subtype, whereas the benzodiazepines act as agonists at both the BZ-1 and BZ-2 subtypes.

Zolpidem is indicated for the short term treatment of insomnia.

PHARMACOKINETICS

Zolpidem has a bioavailability of about 70%, reaches peak concentrations in from one to two hours and undergoes 92% protein binding. Metabolism is via hepatic enzymes, including CYP 3A4, and the half life is about 2.5 hours; there are no active metabolites.

SIDE EFFECTS

In general, zolpidem is remarkably well tolerated: a small minority may be troubled by morning sedation, headache, dizziness or nausea.

Although abuse and dependence are less likely than with benzodiazepines, they have occurred, and there are reports of a withdrawal syndrome similar to that seen with benzodiazepines and, rarely, of withdrawal seizures.

There is a case report of a blackout with zolpidem, similar phenomenologically to an alcoholic blackout.

Zolpidem is excreted in the breast milk, albeit in very small amounts. The teratogenic potential of zolpidem is not known.

DRUG-DRUG INTERACTIONS

Zolpidem levels may be increased by ketoconazole (and, to a lesser extent, itraconazole) and by sertraline.

Zolpidem levels are decreased by rifampin.

Combination of zolpidem with other agents with sedative properties will have an additive effect.

OVERDOSAGE

Drowsiness is seen, and with severe overdoses there may be coma and respiratory depression.

Treatment is with gastric lavage, activated charcoal and supportive measures; flumazenil is also effective.

THERAPEUTIC USAGE

Zolpidem is available in 5 and 10 mg tablets. The average dose for otherwise healthy adults is 10 mg at bedtime; in the elderly, frail, or those with hepatic failure, the dose should be reduced.

BIBLIOGRAPHY

Aragona M. Abuse, dependence, and epileptic seizures after zolpidem withdrawal: review and case report. *Clinical Neuropharmacology* 2000; 23:281-283.

Canady BR. Amnesia possibly associated with zolpidem administration. *Pharmacotherapy* 1996;16:687-689.

Garnier R, Guerault E, Muzard D, et al. Acute zolpidem poisoning—analysis of 344 cases. *Journal of Toxicology, Clinical Toxicology* 1994;32:391-404.

Greenblatt DJ, von Moltke LL, Harmatz JS, et al. Kinetic and dynamic interaction study of zolpidem with ketoconazole, itraconazole, and fluconazole. *Clinical Pharmacology and Therapeutics* 1998;64:661-671.

Liappas IA, Malitas PN, Dimopoulos NP, et al. Zolpidem dependence case series: possible neurobiological mechanisms and clinical management. *Journal of Psychopharmacology* 2003;17:131-135.

Nowell PD, Mazumdar S, Buysse DJ, et al. Benzodiazepines and zolpidem for chronic insomnia: a meta-analysis of treatment efficacy. *The Journal of the American Medical Association* 1997;278:2170-2177.

Salva P, Costa J. Clinical pharmacokinetics and pharmacodynamics of zolpidem. Therapeutic implications. *Clinical Pharmacokinetics* 1995;29:142-153.

Villikka K, Kivisto KT, Luurila H, et al. Rifampin reduces plasma concentrations and effects of zolpidem. *Clinical Pharmacology and Therapeutics* 1997;62:629-634.

310 Zaleplon

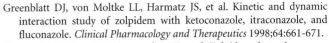

Zaleplon's mechanism of action is essentially the same as that described in the preceding chapter for zolpidem. The main difference between these two hypnotics is in half life, which is very short in the case of zaleplon.

Zaleplon is indicated for the short term treatment of insomnia. Because of its short half life, zaleplon, unlike all other hypnotics, can safely be taken by patients in the middle of the night should they awaken and have trouble getting back to sleep. When patients present with such a complaint, however, it is very important to rule out a depressive illness as the cause of the middle insomnia.

Although zaleplon is very effective in reducing sleep latency, its half life is so short that it does not reduce the number of awakenings, nor does it increase total sleep time.

PHARMACOKINETICS

Zaleplon has a bioavailability of about 30%, reaches peak levels in about one hour and undergoes 60% protein binding. The half life is roughly one hour, and metabolism is via hepatic enzymes, primarily aldehyde oxidase, with a minor contribution by CYP 3A4: there are no active metabolites.

SIDE EFFECTS

Zaleplon is remarkably well tolerated; a small minority may be troubled by headache.

The potential for abuse appears very low for zaleplon.

Zaleplon is excreted in the breast milk in very small amounts; its teratogenic potential is not known.

DRUG-DRUG INTERACTIONS

Zaleplon levels are reduced by rifampin, and increased by cimetidine.

Concurrent use of other sedating agents will have an additive effect.

OVERDOSAGE

Drowsiness is seen with overdose.

Gastric lavage and activated charcoal are appropriate, along with general supportive measures. Flumazenil may be considered in extreme cases.

THERAPEUTIC USAGE

Zaleplon is available in 5 and 10 mg capsules. The average dose for an otherwise healthy adult is 10 mg; the dose should be reduced in the elderly, frail, or those with hepatic failure.

Given zaleplon's rapid onset of action, it should not be taken until just before patients are ready to get into bed.

BIBLIOGRAPHY

Dooley M, Plosker GL. Zaleplon: a review of its use in the treatment of insomnia. *Drugs* 2000;60:413-445.

Drover D, Lemmens H, Naidu S, et al. Pharmacokinetics, pharmacodynamics, and relative pharmacokinetic/pharmacodynamic profiles of zaleplon and zolpidem. *Clinical Therapeutics* 2000;22:1443-1461.

Elie R, Ruther E, Farr I, et al. Sleep latency is shortened during 4 weeks of treatment with zaleplon, a novel nonbenzodiazepine hypnotic. *The Journal of Clinical Psychiatry* 1999;60:536-544.

Fry J, Scharf M, Mangano R, et al. Zaleplon improves sleep without producing rebound effects in outpatients with insomnia. *International Clinical Psychopharmacology* 2000;15:141-152.

Verster JC, Volkerts ER, Schreuder AH, et al. Residual effects of middle-of-the-night administration of zaleplon and zolpidem on driving ability, mental functions, and psychomotor performance. *Journal of Clinical Psychopharmacology* 2002;22:576-583.

311 Diphenhydramine

Diphenhydramine is an antihistamine H1 blocker that also has anticholinergic effects. It is commonly used as an hypnotic, and is also dramatically effective in the emergent treatment of antipsychotic-induced dystonias.

PHARMACOKINETICS

Diphenhydramine has a bioavailability of about 70%, reaches a peak blood level in from 2 to 3 hours, and undergoes about 80% protein binding. It is metabolized in the liver and has a half life of about 9 hours in otherwise healthy adults.

SIDE EFFECTS

Sedation and dizziness are common, and anticholinergic side effects, such as dry mouth, blurry vision, constipation and urinary hesitation or retention, may occur. Other side effects include nausea, dizziness and tinnitus. Bronchial secretions may be thickened and due caution must be used in patients with COPD or pneumonia; vaginal lubrication may also be reduced. Acute narrow-angle glaucoma may be exacerbated and, rarely, in adults, one may see a "paradoxic" reaction with agitation and restlessness.

In the elderly, diphenhydramine not uncommonly is a primary or contributory cause of delirium.

DRUG-DRUG INTERACTIONS

Diphenhydramine appears to inhibit CYP2D6 activity and, in extensive metabolizers, the addition of diphenhydramine prolongs the half lives of both venlafaxine and metoprolol.

Concomitant use of other sedatives or of anticholinergic agents will increase the respective side effects seen with diphenhydramine.

It is not known if diphenhydramine appears in the breast milk or if it is teratogenic.

OVERDOSAGE

Diphenhydramine, as it is available without a prescription, is not uncommonly used during suicide attempts. In mild cases one may see only an exaggeration of the familiar sedative and anticholinergic side effects. In moderate cases, however, delirium, often with visual hallucinations, and agitation may appear and the QRS complex may become quite widened. In severe cases seizures and coma may appear and respiratory depression and circulatory collapse may lead to death.

Treatment should include gastric lavage and activated charcoal along with vigorous supportive measures.

THERAPEUTIC USAGE

Diphenhydramine is available in 25 mg capsules, 50 mg tablets, 12.5 mg chewable tablets, in an elixir containing 12.5 mg/5 ml, and for injection.

For insomnia, diphenhydramine is given in a dose of from 50 to 100 mg. In some cases the sedative effect may wane after several days of regular use; however, this effect may be restored with several days of abstinence.

For dystonia diphenhydramine may be given intravenously, slowly, in a dose of from 25 to 50 mg.

BIBLIOGRAPHY

Agostini JV, Leo-Summers LS, Inouye SK. Cognitive and other adverse effects of diphenhydramine use in hospitalized older patients. *Archives of Internal Medicine* 2001;24:2091-2097.

Blyden GT, Greenblatt DJ, Scavone JM, et al. Pharmacokinetics of diphenhydramine and a demethylated metabolite following intravenous and oral administration. *Journal of Clinical Pharmacology* 1985;26:529-533.

Cheng KL, Dwyer PN, Amsden GW. Paradoxic excitation with diphenhydramine in an adult. *Pharmacotherapy* 1997;17:1311-1314.

Hamelin BA, Bouayad A, Mehot J, et al. Significant interaction between the nonprescription antihistamine diphenhydramine and the CYP2D6 substrate metoprolol in healthy men with high or low CYP2D6 activity. *Clinical Pharmacology and Therapeutics* 2000;67:466-477.

Kudo Y, Kurihara M. Clinical evaluation of diphenhydramine hydrochloride for the treatment of insomnia in psychiatric patients: a double-blind study. *Journal of Clinical Pharmacology* 1990;30: 1041-1048.

Lessard E, Yessine MA, Hamelin BA, et al. Diphenhydramine alters the disposition of venlafaxine through inhibition of CYP2D6 activity in humans. *Journal of Clinical Psychopharmacology* 2001;21:175-184.

Radovanovic D, Meier PJ, Guirguis M, et al. Dose-dependent toxicity of diphenhydramine overdose. *Human & Experimental Toxicology* 2000;19:489-495.

Sharma AN, Hexdall AH, Chang EK, et al. Diphenhydramine-induced wide complex dysrhythmia responds to treatment with sodium bicarbonate. *The American Journal of Emergency Medicine* 2003;21: 212-215.

Simons KJ, Watson WT, Martin TJ, et al. Diphenhydramine: pharmacokinetics and pharmacodynamics in elderly patients, young adults, and children. *Journal of Clinical Pharmacology* 1990;30:665-671.

Hydroxyzine is an antihistamine which blocks H1 receptors and also has some anticholinergic effects. It is commonly used as an hypnotic and occasionally in the short term treatment of anxiety.

PHARMACOKINETICS

Hydroxyzine is well absorbed and reaches peak blood levels in about 2 hours. Metabolism occurs in the liver, and hydroxyzine has a half life of about 20 hours; there is an active metabolite, ceterizine, which has a half life of about 25 hours.

SIDE EFFECTS

Sedation and anticholinergic effects may occur; however, the anticholinergic effects do not appear as pronounced as those seen with diphenhydramine. There is a case report of priapism occurring secondary to hydroxyzine.

DRUG-DRUG INTERACTIONS

Cimetidine increases hydroxyzine levels.

Concurrent use with other sedating agents will have an additive effect.

OVERDOSAGE

Taken in overdose, hydroxyzine may produce stupor, and an anticholinergic delirium.

Treatment should include gastric lavage, activated charcoal, and supportive measures.

THERAPEUTIC USAGE

Hydroxyzine is available in 10, 25, 50 and 100 mg capsules, as a syrup containing 10 mg/5 ml, and for injection.

For anxiolysis, 50 to 75 mg total per day is generally sufficient, with the total dose divided into two or three doses. For insomnia, the bedtime dose ranges from 25 to 100 mg.

BIBLIOGRAPHY

Llorca PM, Spadone C, Sol O, et al. Efficacy and safety of hydroxyzine in the treatment of generalized anxiety disorder: a 3-month double-blind study. *The Journal of Clinical Psychiatry* 2002;63:1020-1027.

Simons FE, Simons KJ, Frith EM. The pharmacokinetics and antihistaminic of the H1 receptor antagonist hydroxyzine. *The Journal of Allergy and Clinical Immunology* 1984;73:69-75.

Simons FE, Sussman GL, Simons KJ. Effect of the H2-receptor antagonist cimetidine on the pharmacokinetics and pharmacodynamics of the H1-receptor antagonists hydroxyzine and cetirizine in patients with chronic urticaria. *The Journal of Allergy and Clinical Immunology* 1995;95:685-693.

Simons KJ, Watson WT, Chen XY, et al. Pharacokinetic and pharmacodynamic studies of the H1-receptor antagonist hydroxyzine in the elderly. *Clinical Pharmacology and Therapeutics* 1989;45:9-14.

Thavundayil JX, Hambalek R, Kin NM, et al. Prolonged penile erections induced by hydroxyzine: possible mechanism of action. *Neuropsychobiology* 1994;30:4-6.

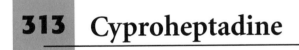

Cyproheptadine is an H1 antihistamine and a 5HT2A serotonin blocker; it also has some anticholinergic activity.

Cyproheptadine is useful for the serotonin syndrome, nightmares (as may appear in posttraumatic stress disorder), as an adjunct in the treatment of anorexia nervosa of the classical restrictor subtype, antipsychotic-induced akathisia and SSRI-induced inhibited orgasm.

PHARMACOKINETICS

Little is known of cyproheptadine's pharmacokinetics. It appears to have a rapid onset of action, and its clinical effects tend to persist for from four to six hours. It is clear that metabolism occurs in the liver, and there do not appear to be any active metabolites.

SIDE EFFECTS

Sedation, dry mouth, blurry vision, constipation and weight gain may occur.

DRUG-DRUG INTERACTIONS

There is an additive effect when cyproheptadine is administered with any agents with antihistaminergic, antiserotoninergic or anticholinergic properties.

There are scattered case reports of cyproheptadine negating the therapeutic effects of SSRIs in patients with depression or bulimia.

OVERDOSAGE

Sedation, agitation, and an anticholinergic delirium (as described in that chapter) may occur.

Treatment is by gastric lavage, activated charcoal and supportive measures; when anticholinergic effects are prominent, treatment may proceed as described in the chapter on anticholinergic delirium.

THERAPEUTIC USAGE

Cyproheptadine is available in a 4 mg scored tablet.

Treatment of the serotonin syndrome, posttraumatic stress disorder and anorexia nervosa are as described in those chapters. For antipsychotic-induced akathisia, the average total daily dose is 16 mg, which should be divided into at least two doses. In the case of SSRI-induced inhibited orgasm, anywhere from 4 to 12 mg may be taken about one to two hours before sexual activity.

BIBLIOGRAPHY

Aizenberg D, Zemishlany Z, Weizman A. Cyproheptadine treatment of sexual dysfunction induced by serotonin reuptake inhibitors. *Clinical Neuropharmacology* 1995;18:320-324.

Feder R. Reversal of antidepressant activity of fluoxetine by cyproheptadine in three patients. *The Journal of Clinical Psychiatry* 1991;52: 163-164.

Fischel T, Hermesh H, Aizenberg D, et al. Cyproheptadine versus propranolol for the treatment of acute neuroleptic-induced akathisia: a comparative double-blind study. *Journal of Clinical Psychopharmacology* 2001;21:612-615.

Goldbloom DS, Kennedy SH. Adverse interaction of fluoxetine and cyproheptadine in two patients with bulimia nervosa. *The Journal of Clinical Psychiatry* 1991;52:261-262.

Silverstone T, Schuyler D. The effect of cyproheptadine on hunger, caloric intake and body weight in man. *Psychopharmacologia* 1975;40: 335-340.

314   Amphetamine

■

Amphetamine is a racemic mixture of dextroamphetamine and levoamphetamine, and of these two stereoisomers, dextroamphetamine may be up to three or four times more potent. Pharmacologically, amphetamine is an indirect sympathomimetic, facilitating release of both norepinephrine and dopamine from presynaptic neurons. Dextroamphetamine is commercially available; levoamphetamine is not used by itself, but is marketed along with dextroamphetamine in a combination product, as noted below.

Amphetamine is useful for attention-deficit/hyperactivity disorder. It has also been used in narcolepsy; however, here other agents are preferable. Dextroamphetamine has also been used in the treatment of debilitating fatigue or apathy in general medical patients. Although somewhat controversial, there are also studies demonstrating that dextroamphetamine, when administered shortly after ischemic cerebral infarction and in combination with physical and speech therapy, may facilitate recovery from hemiplegia and aphasia.

Dextroamphetamine, as noted below, is liable to abuse, and thus must be prescribed with great caution.

PHARMACOKINETICS

Dextroamphetamine is available in both immediate-release and extended-release forms.

Dextroamphetamine is well absorbed, and peak levels are reached within 2 to 3 hours with the immediate-release preparation and in about 8 hours with the extended-release form. A little under one-half is excreted unchanged in the urine, with the rest being metabolized to inactive metabolites in the liver. Urinary excretion of amphetamine is dependent on urinary pH: when the urine is acidified the percent excreted increases, and when alkalinized, it decreases. Consequently, the half-life of amphetamine is strongly influenced by urinary pH: whereas the average half-life is about 10 hours, it is reduced to 8 with acidification and increased up to 30 hours with alkalinization.

SIDE EFFECTS

If the dose is excessive, intoxication, as described in the chapter on amphetamine (or amphetamine-like)-related disorders, will occur. At therapeutic doses, blood pressure may be increased; heart rate may be either reflexively slowed or more often increased as a direct result of dextroamphetamine's sympathomimetic effect; palpitations may occur. Anorexia and weight loss may occur; patients may report either constipation or diarrhea. Whether or not dextroamphetamine retards linear growth in children, and, if it does, whether this has any effect on eventual adult stature, is unclear. It may exacerbate symptoms of Tourette's syndrome and of schizophrenia; mania may be precipitated or worsened in patients with bipolar disorder.

Dextroamphetamine is excreted in breast milk. It is suspected of being a teratogen; infants born of women taking amphetamines may go into withdrawal.

DRUG-DRUG INTERACTIONS

As noted earlier, agents that either acidify or alkalinize the urine respectively either shorten or prolong the half-life. The antihypertensive effects of alpha-methyldopa and of guanethidine are blunted by dextroamphetamine. Dextroamphetamine may elevate tricyclic blood levels. The combination of dextroamphetamine and a monoamine oxidase inhibitor may provoke a hypertensive crisis.

OVERDOSAGE

The consequences of overdose are as described in the chapter on amphetamine (or amphetamine-like)-related disorders. Gastric lavage and activated charcoal are indicated, and the urine should be acidified with ammonium chloride in a dose of 500 mg q4h. Chlorpromazine, in a dose of 50 to 100 mg orally or intramuscularly every hour or so, combats the agitation and often also lowers the blood pressure; when blood pressure is dangerously high, sodium nitroprusside may be used. Seizures may be treated with lorazepam and arrhythmias with propranolol.

THERAPEUTIC USAGE

Dextroamphetamine is available as immediate release tablets in 5, 10 and 15 mg strengths and in extended release capsules of 5, 10 and 15 mg. A combination of dextroamphetamine and levoamphetamine salts is available, containing equal amounts of dextroamphetamine sulfate, dextroamphetamine saccharate, amphetamine aspartate and amphetamine sulfate: this is supplied in immediate release 5, 7.5, 10, 12.5, 15, 20 and 30 mg tablets and in extended release capsules of 5, 10, 15, 20, 25 and 30 mg.

The use of amphetamine in attention-deficit/hyperactivity disorder is discussed in that chapter. In the case of narcolepsy, if other agents fail, immediate release dextroamphetamine may be started in a total daily dose of 10 or 20 mg daily, with the total daily dose increased in 10 mg increments every week until one arrives at satisfactory daytime alertness, limiting side effects, or a maximum dose of about 60 mg. The total daily dose should be divided into at least two doses, once in the morning and once in the early afternoon. Once an optimum regimen with the immediate release preparation has been determined, a trial using the extended release preparation, with the total daily dose being given in the morning, may be attempted.

In those with general medical illnesses, the dose is tailored to patients' overall clinical condition, with special reference to renal status; generally, low doses are used, with careful upward titration.

If dextroamphetamine is used to aid in the rehabilitation of stroke patients, low doses, of 5 or 10 mg, are also recommended. Further, especially in this setting, careful attention must be paid to any elevations of blood pressure or heart rate.

BIBLIOGRAPHY

Angrist B, Corwin J, Bartlik B, et al. Early pharmacokinetic and clinical effects of oral D-amphetamine in normal subjects. *Biological Psychiatry* 1987;22:1357-1368.

Arnold LE, Huestis RD, Smeltzer DJ, et al. Levoamphetamine vs dextroamphetamine in minimal brain dysfunction. Replication, time response, and differential effect by diagnostic group and family rating. *Archives of General Psychiatry* 1976;33:292-301.

Martinsson L, Wahlgren NG. Safety of dexamphetamine in acute ischemic stroke: a randomized, double-blind, controlled dose-escalation trial. *Stroke* 2003;34:475-481.

Sonde L, Nordstrom M, Nilsson CG, et al. A double-blind placebo-controlled study of the effects of amphetamine and physiotherapy after stroke. *Cerebrovascular Diseases* 2001;12:253-257.

Walker-Batson D, Smith P, Curtis S, et al. Amphetamine paired with physical therapy accelerates motor recovery after stroke. Further evidence. *Stroke* 1995;26:2254-2259.

Walker-Batson D, Curtis S, Natarajan R, et al. A double-blind, placebo-controlled study of the use of amphetamine in the treatment of aphasia. *Stroke* 2001;32:2093-2098.

315 Methylphenidate

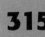

Methylphenidate is an indirect-acting sympathomimetic which, though facilitating release of both dopamine and norepinephrine from presynaptic neurons, preferentially affects dopaminergic tone.

Methylphenidate is indicated in attention-defict/hyperactivity disorder and narcolepsy. It also appears effective in the treatment of post-stroke depression, and in depression occurring in AIDS and in the elderly with general medical problems: in these disorders, however, standard antidepressants are also effective and the only clear-cut advantage of methylphenidate is the rapidity with which symptoms are relieved. Methylphenidate is also effective in hastening the overall recovery of patients admitted to rehabilitation units after stroke.

Other, less well-substantiated indications include apathy (as may be seen in those with serious and long-lasting general medical illnesses), cognitive slowing (as may be seen in AIDS, traumatic brain injury or in cancer patients) and opioid-induced somnolence (as may be seen in terminally ill cancer patients). In the case of apathy in the elderly with general medical illnesses who have stopped eating and taken to bed, methylphenidate may be life-saving.

Importantly, in the case of major depression occurring in otherwise healthy adults, however, methylphenidate does not appear generally effective: nevertheless, there are case reports of patients resistant to antidepressants who have responded to methylphenidate.

PHARMACOKINETICS

Methylphenidate is available in both immediate and slow release forms. With both forms, bioavailability is around 20%, and protein binding is on the order of 15%. With the immediate release form peak concentrations are reached in about 2 hours and the half life ranges from 2 to 6 hours. For the slow release form, the peak is reached in from 3 to 8 hours, and the half life is prolonged to from 3 to 6 hours. Metabolism is by the liver, and over 80% is converted into an inactive metabolite, ritalinic acid.

SIDE EFFECTS

Methylphenidate may cause a loss of appetite and weight loss. If taken too late in the day, it may also cause insomnia. Occasionally, one may see palpitations or a rise in blood pressure. Methylphenidate may exacerbate the symptoms of schizophrenia and may also, albeit rarely, cause chorea. Although methylphenidate may also cause or exacerbate tics, it is not contraindicated in the treatment of concurrent attention-deficit/hyperactivity disorder and Tourette's syndrome, for in such situations the benefits of methylphenidate outweigh the risks. Children chronically treated with methylphenidate may exhibit growth retardation. However, provided methylphenidate is discontinued well before epiphyseal closure, most patients "catch up" and obtain a normal adult stature. As methylphenidate is liable to abuse, as described in the chapter on amphetamine (or amphetamine-like)-related disorders, it should not be prescribed to alcoholics, drug addicts, or those who are judged to be at risk for the misuse of these substances.

DRUG-DRUG INTERACTIONS

Methylphenidate may increase blood levels of tricyclic antidepressants, phenylbutazone, phenobarbital, phenytoin, and warfarin. Of these interactions, the elevation of tricyclic levels is perhaps the most important, as increases of 100% or more may occur. The concurrent administration of methylphenidate and a monoamine oxidase inhibitor may cause a hypertensive crisis. Methylphenidate decreases the antihypertensive effect of guanethidine.

OVERDOSAGE

The effects of overdose are as described in the chapter on amphetamine (or amphetamine-like)-related disorders. Treatment, as described there, includes chlorpromazine, which may be given intramuscularly or as an oral concentrate, in a dose of 50 to 100 mg every hour, which usually controls not only agitation but also lowers blood pressure. Should blood pressure not be controlled by chlorpromazine, nitroprusside may be used. Seizures are treated with lorazepam and arrhythmias with propranolol.

THERAPEUTIC USAGE

Immediate release methylphenidate is available in 5, 10 and 20 mg tablets. Slow release forms are available as tablets containing 10, 18, 20, 27, 36 and 54 mg and as a capsule containing 20 mg. It should be noted that the various slow release forms display modest differences in the time required to reach peak levels and in half lives.

The use of methylphenidate in attention-deficit/hyperactivity disorder and narcolepsy is as discussed in those chapters. For the other indications, methylphenidate should generally be given in divided doses, once in the early morning and once in the early afternoon, beginning with a total daily dose of 5 to 10 mg and increasing in similar increments every day or two until a good response, limiting side effects or a maximum dose of 60 mg is reached. In the frail, the elderly, or those with debilitating general medical illnesses, low total daily doses, on the order of 10 to 20 mg, are often quite effective. The response to any given dose is often rapid, within one to two days.

BIBLIOGRAPHY

Challman TD, Lipsky JJ. Methylphenidate: its pharmacology and uses. *Mayo Clinic Proceedings* 2000;75:711-721.

Denckla MB, Bemporad JR, MacKay MC. Tics following methylphenidate administration. A report of 20 cases. *The Journal of the American Medical Association* 1976;235:1349-1351.

Fernandez F, Levy JK, Samley HR, et al. Effects of methylphenidate in HIV-related depression: a comparative trial with desipramine. *International Journal of Psychiatry in Medicine* 1995;25:53-67.

Grade C, Redford B, Chrostowski J, et al. Methylphenidate in early poststroke recovery: a double-blind, placebo-controlled study. *Archives of Physical Medicine and Rehabilitation* 1998;79:1047-1050.

Hinken CH, Castellon SA, Hardy DJ, et al. Methylphenidate improves HIV-1-associated cognitive slowing. *The Journal of Neuropsychiatry and Clinical Neurosciences* 2001;13:48-54.

Lazarus LW, Moburg PJ, Langsley PR, et al. Methylphenidate and nortriptyline in the treatment of poststroke depression: a retrospective comparison. *Archives of Physical Medicine and Rehabilitation* 1994;75: 403-406.

Levy DL, Smith M, Robinson D, et al. Methylphenidate increases thought disorder in recent onset schizophrenics, but not in normal controls. *Biological Psychiatry* 1993;34:507-514.

Plenger PM, Dixon CE, Castillo RM, et al. Subacute methylphenidate treatment for moderate to moderately severe traumatic brain injury: a preliminary double-blind placebo-controlled study. *Archives of Physical Medicine and Rehabilitation* 1996;77:536-540.

Plutchik L, Snyder S, Drooker M, et al. Methylphenidate in post liver transplant patients. *Psychosomatics* 1998;39:118-123.

Rottenhausler HB, Ehrentraut S, von Degenfeld G, et al. Treatment of depression with methylphenidate in patients difficult to wean from mechanical ventilation in the intensive care unit. *The Journal of Clinical Psychiatry* 2000;61:750-757.

Rozans M, Dreisbach A, Lertorra JJ, et al. Palliative use of methylphenidate in patients with cancer: a review. *Journal of Clinical Oncology* 2002;20: 335-339.

Wallace AE, Kofoed LL, West AN. Double-blind, placebo-controlled trial of methylphenidate in older, depressed, medically ill patients. *The American Journal of Psychiatry* 1995;152:929-931.

Weiner WJ, Nausieda PA, Klawans HL. Methylphenidate-induced chorea: case report and pharmacologic implications. *Neurology* 1978;28: 1041-1044.

316 Atomoxetine

Atomoxetine is indicated for the treatment of attention-deficit/hyperactivity disorder in both children and adults, and exerts its pharmacologic effect primarily via blockade of norepinephrine reuptake by presynaptic neurons.

PHARMACOKINETICS

Atomoxetine is metabolized primarily by CYP2D6, and its pharmacokinetics are quite different in extensive metabolizers (EM) versus the 7% of the Caucasian population that are poor metabolizers (PM).

Bioavailability in EMs is about 60%, and in PMs about 90%; in both EMs and PMs, peak levels are reached within one to two hours and protein binding is about 98%. The half life in EMs is about 5 hours, and in PMs it rises to about 21 hours: this increased half life in PMs is accompanied by a five-fold increase in peak blood levels.

SIDE EFFECTS

Nausea is common, but apart from this, atomoxetine is generally well tolerated: mild increases in pulse and blood pressure may occur, and appetite is generally reduced with a modest weight loss.

Rarely, urinary retention may occur.

To date, it appears that atomoxetine's liability to abuse is very low.

It is not known whether atomoxetine is excreted in the breast milk, nor is it known if it is teratogenic in humans.

DRUG-DRUG INTERACTIONS

CYP2D6 inhibitors such as fluoxetine, paroxetine, sertraline and quinidine effectively turn an EM into a PM, with pharmacokinetic consequences as noted above and an exaggeration of side effects.

The combination of albuterol and atomoxetine has been reported to cause marked tachycardia and hypertension.

Atomoxetine should not be used in combination with an MAOI or within two weeks of the discontinuation of an MAOI, as the theoretical risk of a hypertensive crisis is high.

OVERDOSAGE

There is limited information regarding overdosage with atomoxetine. Gastric lavage, activated charcoal and general supportive measures are prudent.

THERAPEUTIC USAGE

Atomoxetine is available in 10, 18, 25, 40 and 60 mg capsules.

For patients weighing under 70 kg, treatment is initiated at a total daily dose of approximately 0.5 mg/kg, and then, after three days, increased to approximately 1.2 mg/kg; if there is no response after two weeks, the dose may be increased to a maximum of 1.8 mg/kg. For patients weighing more than 70 kg, one may begin at 40 mg/d, increasing after three days to 80 mg/d, with an option to increase to 100 mg after two weeks if there is no response.

In poor metabolizers the dose should be 25% or less than that just noted, and the intervals between dosage increases should be roughly four times as long.

In most patients, once daily dosing in the morning is adequate; in cases where there is a falling-off of clinical effect in the late afternoon or evening, consideration may be given to dividing the dose into an early morning and early afternoon schedule.

In hepatic failure the dose should be only 25% to 50% of that noted above.

BIBLIOGRAPHY

Belle DJ, Ernest CS, Sauer JM, et al. Effect of potent CYP2D6 inhibition by paroxetine on atomoxetine. *Journal of Clinical Pharmacology* 2002;42: 1219-1227.

Chalon SA, Desager JP, Desante KA, et al. Effect of hepatic impairment on the pharmacokinetics of atomoxetine and its metabolites. *Clinical Pharmacology and Therapeutics* 2003;73:178-191.

Farid NA, Bergstrom RF, Ziege EA, et al. Single-dose and steady-state pharmacokinetics of tomoxetine in normal subjects. *Journal of Clinical Pharmacology* 1985;25:296-301.

Heil SH, Holmes HW, Bickel WK, et al. Comparison of the subjective, physiological, and psychomotor effects of atomoxetine and methylphenidate in light drug users. *Drug and Alcohol Dependence* 2002;57:149-156.

Sauer JM, Ponsler GD, Mattiuz EL, et al. Disposition and metabolic fate of atomoxetine hydrochloride: the role of CYP2D6 in human disposition and metabolism. *Drug Metabolism and Disposition* 2003;31: 98-107.

Witcher JW, Long A, Smith B, et al. Atomoxetine pharmacokinetics in children and adolescents with attention deficit hyperactivity disorder. *Journal of Child and Adolescent Psychopharmacology* 2003;13:53-63.

317 Modafinil

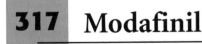

The primary indication for modafinil is excessive daytime sleepiness in narcolepsy; similar alerting effects are found in myotonic dystrophy and, to a modest degree, in Parkinson's disease. Modafinil is also effective in attention-deficit/hyperactivity disorder, and has been used to relieve drowsiness in individuals who have been sleep deprived; however, in this latter regard it was no more effective than caffeine.

Modafinil's mechanism of action is not clear, and may involve either blockade of reuptake of dopamine by presynaptic neurons or stimulation at postsynaptic alpha-1 receptors.

PHARMACOKINETICS

The absolute bioavailability of modafinil is not known. Peak blood levels are reached in from two to four hours, and protein binding occurs at about 60%. The half life ranges from 11 to 15 hours, and about 90% of modafinil is metabolized in the liver to inactive metabolites.

SIDE EFFECTS

Modafinil is generally well-tolerated: a small minority may experience headache, nausea, anxiety or insomnia.

In patients with left ventricular hypertrophy or mitral valve prolapse, there may be palpitations, chest pain and ischemic changes on the EKG.

Although modafinil can produce a euphoriant effect, to date the potential for abuse seems very low.

DRUG-DRUG INTERACTIONS

Modafinil may reduce levels of ethinyl estradiol, and the effectiveness of oral contraceptives may be reduced.

In one case report, modafinil increased clomipramine levels.

OVERDOSAGE

Agitation is the principal manifestation of overdose. Gastric lavage, activated charcoal and supportive care, with periodic EKG monitoring, is appropriate.

THERAPEUTIC USAGE

Modafinil is available in 100 mg and scored 200 mg tablets.

Most patients respond to 200 mg daily, given in the morning; occasionally 300 or 400 mg may be required to obtain a full effect.

The dose should be reduced by about one-half in those with hepatic failure or in the elderly.

BIBLIOGRAPHY

Adler CH, Caviness JN, Hentz JG, et al. Randomized trial of modafinil for treating subjective sleepiness in patients with Parkinson's disease. *Movement Disorders* 2003;18:287-293.

Grozinger M, Hartter S, Hiemke C, et al. Interaction of modafinil and clomipramine as comedication in a narcoleptic patient. *Clinical Neuropharmacology* 1998;21:127-129.

MacDonald JR, Hill JD, Tarnopolsky MA. Modafinil reduces excessive somnolence and enhances mood in patients with myotonic dystrophy. *Neurology* 2002;59:1876-1880.

Robertson P, Hellriegel ET. Clinical pharmacokinetic profile of modafinil. *Clinical Pharmacokinetics* 2003;42:123-137.

Taylor FB, Russo J. Efficacy of modafinil compared to dextroamphetamine for the treatment of attention deficit hyperactivity disorder in adults. *Journal of Child and Adolescent Psychopharmacology* 2000;10:311-320.

Wesensten NJ, Belenky G, Kautz MA, et al. Maintaining alertness and performance during sleep deprivation: modafinil versus caffeine. *Psychopharmacology* 2002;159:238-247.

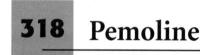

318 Pemoline

Pemoline is an indirect-acting sympathomimetic which facilitates release of both norepinephrine and dopamine from presynaptic neurons, with a preferential effect on dopaminergic tone. It is effective in attention-deficit/hyperactivity disorder, narcolepsy, and, although controversial, perhaps also in multiple sclerosis-related fatigue. Given, however, its potential for hepatotoxicity and the availability of alternative treatments that are of equal or superior efficacy, pemoline should be held in reserve.

PHARMACOKINETICS

Pemoline is well absorbed after oral administration, reaches peak blood levels in from 2 to 4 hours and undergoes about 50% protein binding. One-half the dose is metabolized in the liver to inactive metabolites and the rest is excreted unchanged in the urine; the half-life ranges from 5 to 12 hours.

SIDE EFFECTS

Insomnia, irritability and anorexia are the most common side effects. Choreiform movements, facial grimacing, tics and oculogyric crises may occur, and the tics seen in Tourette's syndrome may be exacerbated. Hallucinations or psychosis may rarely occur, and the seizure threshold is reduced. Among children, expected gain in height and weight may initially be slowed; however, within a year or two of treatment discontinuation, most adolescents "catch up."

Severe hepatic failure, resulting in death, or necessitating liver transplantation, though rare, occurs with greater frequency in patients treated with pemoline than with other stimulants; most cases have occurred only after six months of treatment.

It is not known whether pemoline is teratogenic or not, nor whether it is excreted in breast milk.

DRUG-DRUG INTERACTIONS

Pemoline appears to be compatible with most other drugs.

OVERDOSAGE

After overdose one may see delirium, agitation, abnormal involuntary movements, hallucinations, seizures, tachycardia, hypertension, and fever.

Gastric lavage and activated charcoal are generally in order. In addition to supportive measures, chlorpromazine, 50 to 100 mg via oral solution or intramuscularly every hour, may be given.

THERAPEUTIC USAGE

Pemoline is available in 18.75, 37.5 and 75 mg tablets.

For otherwise healthy children and adults, dosage starts at 37.5 mg and increases in 18.75 or 37.5 mg increments on a weekly basis until an average effective dose is reached or limiting side effects occur: for hyperactivity and for the fatigue seen in multiple sclerosis, the effective dose ranges from 56.25 to 75 mg; for narcolepsy the range is from 56.25 mg to 150 mg. The total daily dose may generally be taken once daily in the morning; however, if there is a "wearing off" of effect by late afternoon, the total daily dose may be divided into two doses, with the first in the early morning and the second in the early afternoon. Although most patients respond promptly, in a minority up to several weeks may be required to see the full effect of any given dose. Liver enzymes should be monitored periodically throughout treatment; conservatively on a biweekly basis.

Although pemoline is less liable to abuse than amphetamine or methylphenidate, physicians must still be on guard against diversion of prescriptions to illicit use.

BIBLIOGRAPHY

Bachman DS. Pemoline-induced Tourette's disorder: a case report. *The American Journal of Psychiatry* 1981;138:1116-1117.

Friedmann N, Thomas J, Carr R, et al. Effect on growth in pemoline-treated children with attention deficit disorder. *American Journal of Diseases of Children* 1981;135:329-332.

Krupp LB, Coyle PK, Doscher C, et al. Fatigue therapy in multiple sclerosis: results of a double-blind, randomized, parallel trial of amantadine, pemoline, and placebo. *Neurology* 1995;45:1956-1961.

Marotta PJ, Roberts EA. Pemoline hepatotoxicity in children. *The Journal of Pediatrics* 1998;132:894-897.

Mitler MM, Shafor R, Hajdukovich R, et al. Treatment of narcolepsy: objective studies on methylphenidate, pemoline and protriptyline. *Sleep* 1986;9:260-264.

Nakamura H, Blumer JL, Reed MD. Pemoline ingestion in children: a report of five cases and review of the literature. *Journal of Clinical Pharmacology* 2002;42:275-282.

Nausieda PA, Koller WC, Weiner WJ, et al. Pemoline-induced chorea. *Neurology* 1981;31:356-360.

Safer DJ, Zito JM, Gardner JE. Pemoline hepatotoxicity and postmarketing surveillance. *Journal of the American Academy of Child and Adolescent Psychiatry* 2001;40:622-629.

Sallee FR, Stiller RL, Perel JM, et al. Pemoline-induced abnormal involuntary movements. *Journal of Clinical Psychopharmacology* 1989;9:125-129.

Weinshenker BG, Penman M, Bass B, et al. A double-blind, randomized, crossover trial of pemoline in fatigue associated with multiple sclerosis. *Neurology* 1992;42:1468-1471.

319 Sildenafil

Sildenafil is a phosphodiesterase-5 inhibitor which is effective in the treatment of erectile dysfunction, female sexual arousal disorder, premature ejaculation and SSRI-induced sexual dysfunction. Notably, in the case of erectile dysfunction, sildenafil is effective not only in primary, or psychogenic, dysfunction, but also in secondary, or organic, cases.

Under normal conditions, penile erection occurs when sexual stimulation leads to parasympathetically-mediated release of nitrous oxide into the corpus cavernosum; nitrous oxide, in turn, activates guanylate cyclase leading to an increased production of cyclic guanosine monophosphate. Cyclic guanosine monophosphate is a vasodilator which in turn allows for increased blood flow into the corpus cavernosum, producing an erection. Phosphodiesterase-5 is the enzyme responsible for the degradation of cyclic guanosine monophosphate, and when this enzyme is inhibited by sildenafil the concentration of guanosine monophosphate remains high, allowing for increased blood flow into the corpus callosum.

PHARMACOKINETICS

Sildenafil has a bioavailability of about 40%, reaches peak levels in about one hour, and undergoes 96% protein binding. Metabolism is via the hepatic enzymes, primarily CYP3A4, with a minor contribution from CYP2C9. Of more than a half dozen metabolites, one, N-desmethylsildenafil, is active. Both sildenafil and N-desmethylsildenafil have a half life of about four hours.

SIDE EFFECTS

Headache, facial flushing, nasal congestion, heartburn and a change in color perception, with most objects acquiring a blue-green tint, may occur.

A modest fall in blood pressure may occur in normal individuals. In patients with significant autonomic failure, as may be seen in multiple system atrophy, the hypotensive effect of sildenafil may be grossly exaggerated.

In patients with migraine, sildenafil fairly reliably induces migraine headaches.

There are reports of fatal cardiovascular and cerebrovascular events associated with sildenafil, including myocardial infarction, sudden cardiac death, transient ischemic attacks and cerebrovascular accidents. In most cases patients had significant risk factors for these events, and overall, provided patients are not taking nitrates, sildenafil is a very safe medicine.

There are rare reports of priapism secondary to sildenafil, and this may be more likely in the presence of conditions, such as sickle cell anemia, which predispose to priapism.

DRUG-DRUG INTERACTIONS

Organic nitrates undergo conversion to nitrous oxide, and, in the setting of inhibition of phosphodiesterase by sildenafil, the stage is set for a disastrous, and potentially life-threatening, fall in blood pressure, and sildenafil must not be taken by patients who are using or who have recently used these agents.

Drugs such as erythromycin, ketoconazole, itraconazole, cimetidine, saquinavir and ritonavir all increase sildenafil levels.

OVERDOSAGE

An exaggeration of the side effects noted above occurs with overdose, and routine supportive measures are generally sufficient.

THERAPEUTIC USAGE

Sildenafil is available in 25, 50 and 100 mg tablets.

Sildenafil should be taken about one hour before anticipated sexual activity. The average dose is 50 mg, with a range of 25 to 100 mg. The dose should be halved in the elderly or those with hepatic failure.

BIBLIOGRAPHY

Arruda-Olson AM, Mahoney DW, Nehra A, et al. Cardiovascular effects of sildenafil during exercise in men with known of probable coronary artery disease: a randomized crossover trial. *The Journal of the American Medical Association* 2002;287:719-725.

Hussain IF, Brady CM, Swinn MJ, et al. Treatment of erectile dysfunction with sildenafil citrate (Viagra) in parkinsonism due to Parkinson's disease or multiple system atrophy with observations on orthostatic hypotension. *Journal of Neurology, Neurosurgery, and Psychiatry* 2001; 71:371-374.

Kruuse C, Thomson LL, Birk S, et al. Migraine can be induced by sildenafil without changes in middle cerebral artery diameter. *Brain* 2003;126: 241-247.

Moreira SG, Brannigan RE, Sptiz A, et al. Side-effect profile of sildenafil citrate (Viagra) in clinical practice. *Urology* 2000;56:474-476.

Muirhead GJ, Wulff MB, Fielding A, et al. Pharmacokinetic interactions between sildenafil and saquinavir/ritonavir. *British Journal of Clinical Pharmacology* 2000;50:99-107.

Muirhead GJ, Rance DJ, Walker DW, et al. Comparative pharmacokinetics and metabolism of single-dose oral and intravenous sildenafil. *British Journal of Pharmacology* 2002;53(Suppl 1):13-20.

Muirhead GJ, Faulkner S, Harness JA, et al. The effects of steady-state erythromycin and azithromycin on the pharmacokinetics of sildenafil in healthy volunteers. *British Journal of Clinical Pharmacology* 2002; 53(Suppl 1):37-43.

Nurnberg HG, Hensley PL, Gelenberg AJ, et al. Treatment of antidepressant-associated sexual dysfunction with sildenafil: a randomized controlled trial. *The Journal of the American Medical Association* 2003;289:56-64.

Wilner K, Laboy L, LeBel M. The effects of cimetidine and antacid on the pharmacokinetic profile of sildenafil citrate in healthy male volunteers. *British Journal of Clinical Pharmacology* 2002;53(Suppl 1):31-36.

320 Yohimbine

■

Yohimbine is a selective presynaptic alpha-2 receptor blocking agent that reliably increases the firing rate of the locus ceruleus and increases sympathetic tone.

Yohimbine may be effective in some cases of erectile dysfunction, but is generally a second choice after other agents, such as sildenafil.

PHARMACOKINETICS

The bioavailability of yohimbine ranges widely from 10 to 90%. Yohimbine is almost completely metabolized in the liver, with a half-life of from 1 to 2 hours; two active metabolites exist, 10-hydroxy-yohimbine and 11-hydroxy-yohimbine.

SIDE EFFECTS

Yohimbine may cause anxiety, especially at higher doses, and especially in patients with panic disorder; tremor, tachycardia and elevations of both systolic and diastolic pressure may also occur. There are rare reports of mania and of SIADH occurring secondary to yohimbine.

It is not known whether yohimbine is excreted in breast milk or whether it is teratogenic.

DRUG-DRUG INTERACTIONS

Yohimbine and clonidine are mutually antagonistic. Given yohimbine's pharmacology, one could expect that combination use with tricyclic antidepressants or monoamine oxidase inhibitors would be followed by excessive sympathetic activity.

OVERDOSAGE

A gross exaggeration of side effects is seen, and supportive treatment is generally satisfactory.

THERAPEUTIC USAGE

Yohimbine is available in 5.4 mg scored tablets.

In cases of primary erectile dysfunction where other medical treatments, e.g. sildenafil, are ineffective or not tolerated, yohimbine may be considered. Treatment should begin at a dose of 2.7 mg tid, and increased gradually: when used by itself, the average effective dose is 10.8 mg tid (given the wide range of bioavailability, however, if the average dose is ineffective or poorly tolerated it is reasonable to try different doses). There is also a recent study which demonstrated an effect from a dose of 5.4 mg tid when combined with trazodone, 50 mg once daily.

BIBLIOGRAPHY

Albus M, Zahn TP, Breier A. Anxiogenic properties of yohimbine. I. Behavioral, physiological and biochemical measures. *European Archives of Psychiatry and Clinical Neuroscience* 1992;241:337-344.

Friesen K, Palatnick W, Tenenbein M. Benign course after massive ingestion of yohimbine. *The Journal of Emergency Medicine* 1993; 11:287-288.

Guthrie SK, Hariharan M, Grunhaus LJ. Yohimbine bioavailability in humans. *European Journal of Clinical Pharmacology* 1990;39:409-411.

Kunelius P, Hakkinen J, Lukkarinen O. Is high-dose yohimbine hydrochloride effective in the treatment of mixed-type impotence? A prospective, randomized, controlled double-blind crossover study. *Urology* 1997;49:441-444.

LeCorre P, Dollo G, Chevanne F, et al. Biopharmaceutics and metabolism of yohimbine in humans. *European Journal of Pharmaceutical Sciences* 1999;9:79-84.

Montorsi F, Strambi LF, Guazzoni G, et al. Effect of yohimbine-trazodone on psychogenic impotence: a randomized, double-blind, placebo-controlled study. *Urology* 1994;44:732-736.

Owen JA, Nakatsu SL, Fenemore J, et al. The pharmacokinetics of yohimbine in man. *European Journal of Clinical Pharmacology* 1987; 32:577-582.

Price LH, Charney DS, Heninger GR. Three cases of manic symptoms following yohimbine administration. *The American Journal of Psychiatry* 1984;141:1267-1268.

321 Flumazenil

Flumazenil competitively antagonizes the interaction of benzodiazepines with the postsynaptic ionophore GABA receptor complex and as such is useful for reducing the stupor or coma seen with benzodiazepines taken in overdose. Flumazenil itself is essentially devoid of agonist or reverse agonist properties and as such generally has no effect if given to a normal subject who has not taken a benzodiazepine. Interestingly, however, flumazenil is an effective panicogen and, if given to a benzodiazepine-naive patient with panic disorder, generally induces a panic attack.

In treating patients who have overdosed with a benzodiazepine, one must determine whether prior use of the drug was sufficient to cause neuroadaptation. If neuroadaptation has occurred, the administration of flumazenil may provoke seizures. Additionally, one should also determine whether the overdose was mixed and if so whether proconvulsant drugs, such as tricyclics, bupropion or theophylline, were also taken, as in such cases the likelihood of seizures is even higher.

Flumazenil is also indicated for the reversal of benzodiazepine-induced anesthesia and may be useful in the symptomatic treatment of hepatic encephalopathy.

Flumazenil may also be useful in reversing alcohol-induced coma; however, here high doses, on the order of 2 to 5 mg, may be required. As in the treatment of benzodiazepine overdose, here also one must be wary of precipitating seizures.

PHARMACOKINETICS

After intravenous administration, flumazenil is almost completely metabolized in the liver to inactive metabolites, with the half-life averaging a little less than 60 minutes. About 50% is protein bound.

SIDE EFFECTS

In benzodiazepine-naive subjects, flumazenil may produce nausea, vomiting, headache, diaphoresis, dizziness, and agitation. Patients may have pain at the injection site. Rarely, complete heart block may occur.

DRUG-DRUG INTERACTIONS

Apart from interacting with benzodiazepines, no significant drug-drug interactions occur.

OVERDOSAGE

No consequences to overdose are known in benzodiazepine-naive subjects.

THERAPEUTIC USAGE

Flumazenil is available for injection in a 0.1mg/ml solution.

Treatment of benzodiazepine overdose is accomplished with sequential bolus injections, with each bolus being given over 30 seconds into a freely running intravenous line. In patients who have overdosed on benzodiazepines alone and who are not likely to go into withdrawal, the initial bolus is 0.2 mg; an interval of 60 seconds is then allowed to pass from the ending of that bolus to the next, which contains 0.3 mg. After another 60-second interval, 0.5 mg is given, and then 0.5 mg boluses may be repeated at 60-second intervals until the patient either awakens or a total of 3 mg is given. Most patients respond to 3 mg or less. Occasionally the sequential bolus administration may have to be continued up to a total of 5 mg. A lack of response to 5 mg effectively rules out a benzodiazepine as the major cause of coma.

In patients who are at risk for going into withdrawal or in those who have overdosed on a tricyclic or other proconvulsant drug, the administration of flumazenil should be done cautiously by either reducing the size of the bolus (to no more than 0.1 mg) or increasing the interval between boluses (up to 5 minutes) or both. If seizures do occur, large doses of benzodiazepines or phenobarbital may be required.

Once the patient has awakened sufficiently, repeat doses of anywhere from 0.1 to 1 mg may be required every 20 to 60 minutes until the offending benzodiazepine taken in overdose has "washed out."

Treatment of hepatic encephalopathy is less consistently effective than that of benzodiazepine overdose, and may be attempted using the same bolus approach as just described. Given, however, that the half-life of flumazenil is prolonged in hepatic failure, the intervals between repeat doses is generally much longer.

BIBLIOGRAPHY

Barbaro G, Di Lorenzo G, Soldini M, et al. Flumazenil for hepatic encephalopathy grade III and IVa in patients with cirrhosis: an Italian multicenter double-blind, placebo-controlled, cross-over study. *Hepatology* 1998;28:374-378.

Laccetti M, Manes G, Uomo G, et al. Flumazenil in the treatment of acute hepatic encephalopathy in cirrhotic patients: a double blind randomized placebo controlled study. *Digestive and Liver Disease* 2000;32:335-338.

Mintner MZ, Stoller KB, Griffiths RR. A controlled study of flumazenil-precipitated withdrawal in chronic low-dose benzodiazepine users. *Psychopharmacology* 1999;147:200-209.

Spivey WH. Flumazenil and seizures: analysis of 43 cases. *Clinical Therapeutics* 1992;14:292-305.

Weinbroum A, Rucick V, Sorkine P, et al. Use of flumazenil in the treatment of drug overdose: a double-blind and open clinical study in 110 patients. *Critical Care Medicine* 1996;24:199-206.

Naloxone is essentially a pure opioid antagonist whose primary use is the reversal of opioid-induced sedation, coma or respiratory depression. There are also case reports suggesting its utility in overdosage with valproate and with dextromethorphan.

PHARMACOKINETICS

Naloxone is generally given intravenously: although subcutaneous and intramuscular routes may also be utilized, the onset of action is much slower. After intravenous administration effects are seen within one to two minutes. Naloxone is almost completely metabolized in the liver, primarily by direct glucuronidation, and has a half life ranging from 30 minutes to 1 1/2 hours.

SIDE EFFECTS

In opioid-naive patients, naloxone has virtually no effect at all. In those addicted to opioids, however, even small doses may precipitate a severe withdrawal syndrome, with prominent agitation, hypertension, tachycardia, and, in some, ventricular arrhythmias. Very rarely, naloxone may cause acute pulmonary edema.

DRUG-DRUG INTERACTIONS

Essentially no drug-drug interactions are known, except with opioids.

OVERDOSAGE

No effect from overdose appears likely.

THERAPEUTIC USAGE

Naloxone is available for injection in various concentrations: 0.02 mg/mL, 0.4 mg/mL and 1 mg/mL.

To reverse respiratory depression in an overdose, give anywhere from 0.4 to 2 mg intravenously every 3 to 5 minutes until the patient is out of danger. As the duration of effect is anywhere from 15 minutes to an hour or more, repeat doses generally are required until the offending opioid has "washed out." If a total of 10 mg fails to bring any improvement, the diagnosis of opioid overdose should be questioned.

In patients who are addicted to opioids, smaller doses (e.g., 0.1 to 0.4 mg) should be considered, as patients who are precipitated into opioid withdrawal may be combative. In such cases it may be prudent to apply restraints before administering naloxone.

BIBLIOGRAPHY

Alberto G, Erickson T, Popiel R, et al. Central nervous system manifestations of a valproic acid overdose responsive to naloxone. *Annals of Emergency Medicine* 1989;18:889-891.

Barsan WG, Seger D, Danzl DF, et al. Duration of antagonistic effects of nalmefene and naloxone in opiate-induced sedation for emergency department procedures. *The American Journal of Emergency Medicine* 1989;7:155-161.

Gaddis GM, Watson WA. Naloxone-associated patient violence: an overlooked toxicity? *The Annals of Pharmacotherapy* 1992;26:196-198.

Kanof PD, Handelsman L, Aronson MJ, et al. Clinical characteristics of naloxone-precipitated withdrawal in human opioid-dependent subjects. *The Journal of Pharmacology and Experimental Therapeutics* 1992;260:363-366.

Olsen KS. Naloxone administration and laryngospasm followed by pulmonary edema. *Intensive Care Medicine* 1990;16:340-341.

Schneider SM, Michelson EA, Boucek CD, et al. Dextromethorphan poisoning reversed by naloxone. *The American Journal of Emergency Medicine* 1991;9:237-238.

Watson WA, Steele MT, Muelleman RL, et al. Opioid toxicity recurrence after an initial response to naloxone. *Journal of Toxicology and Human Toxicology* 1998;36:11-17.

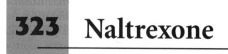

323 Naltrexone

Naltrexone is a competitive inhibitor at post-synaptic opioid receptors, and is essentially devoid of any agonist properties.

Naltrexone plays a modest role in the overall treatment of opioid dependence and in alcoholism. In opioid dependence, naltrexone blocks the euphoria of opioids, and in alcoholism it appears to both reduce craving and blunt the intoxication. Naltrexone is generally useful only in highly motivated patients. Poorly motivated patients are rarely compliant; most either refuse

to take it or stop it after perhaps a few weeks, and then again resume using opioids or drinking.

Naltrexone may also have a minor place in the treatment of bulimia nervosa and pathological gambling; there is also the possibility of effectiveness in kleptomania and in reducing self-injurious behavior in patients with borderline personality disorder.

In children with autism, naltrexone may reduce irritability, but is otherwise without effect. It should not be given to patients with Rett's syndrome as it may worsen that disorder.

PHARMACOKINETICS

Naltrexone undergoes considerable first-pass hepatic metabolism, and the bioavailability is about 60%. Peak blood levels are obtained in about 1 hour, and about 20% is protein bound. The half-life of naltrexone is about 10 hours; about 95% is metabolized in the liver, in part to a weak opioid antagonist, 6-beta naltrexone, that has a half-life of about 13 hours.

SIDE EFFECTS

A significant number of patients experience some fatigue, dysphoria, nausea and headache; these side effects tend to clear gradually with continued use over 1 or 2 months.

Naltrexone exhibits dose-related hepatotoxicity. At typical therapeutic doses, one sees little or no evidence of hepatic injury; however, at doses of 300 mg, significant elevations of liver transaminases may occur.

DRUG-DRUG INTERACTIONS

Naltrexone blocks the activity not only of opioid analgesics but also of opioid antitussives and antidiarrheal agents. Patients facing elective surgery where opioid analgesia may be required should discontinue naltrexone at least three days ahead of time.

OVERDOSAGE

Experience with naltrexone overdose is very rare; should this occur, close monitoring and general supportive care are prudent.

THERAPEUTIC USAGE

Naltrexone is available in 50 mg scored tablets.

In the treatment of opioid dependence, naltrexone is typically withheld until one has determined with certainty that the patient has been free of opioids for at least a week. As urine drug tests, although helpful, are not completely reliable, it is often appropriate to give a naloxone challenge before starting naltrexone to be sure that the naltrexone does not precipitate withdrawal symptoms. Naloxone is given in a dose of 0.2 mg intravenously, and if no symptoms of withdrawal are seen after 30 seconds, another 0.6 mg is given. If the patient remains completely free of withdrawal symptoms for the next 20 minutes, he may be given his first dose of naltrexone, at 25 mg, followed an hour later by another 25 mg. Possible subsequent dosage schedules include the following: 50 mg every morning 7 days a week; 50 mg every morning Monday through Thursday and 150 mg on Friday morning; or 100 mg on Monday and Wednesday mornings, and 150 mg on Friday morning.

In the treatment of alcoholism, naltrexone is given in a dose of 50 mg daily. Importantly, should alcoholics have a "slip" while taking naltrexone they should be encouraged to persevere with treatment.

The optimum duration of naltrexone treatment in these addictions is not clear: documentation of benefit much beyond several months is slim. However, in highly motivated patients who appear unable to maintain abstinence without naltrexone, a case for chronic treatment could be made. Regardless of the duration of treatment it is clear that pharmacologic treatment of opioid or alcohol dependence is of little benefit unless given in the context of a comprehensive treatment program.

For children with autism, the recommended dose is roughly 1 mg/kg/d.

Dosage requirements for other indications have not been well worked out, but probably fall in the range of 50 to 250 mg daily.

Naltrexone should not be given to patients with hepatic failure or those with active hepatic inflammation, as indicated by transaminase levels elevated three-fold or more above normal. All patients should have baseline liver function tests, which should be repeated monthly for three months, then every three to six months thereafter: more frequent testing may be appropriate when the dose is above 50 mg.

Finally, opioid addicts should be warned that, although very high doses of opioids may overcome naltrexone blockade and produce some euphoria, such high doses may very well also cause respiratory depression and death.

BIBLIOGRAPHY

Gonzalez JP, Brogden RN. Naltrexone: a review of its pharmacodynamic and pharmacokinetic properties and therapeutic efficacy in the management of opioid dependence. *Drugs* 1988;35:192-213.

Grant JE, Kim SW. An open-label study of naltrexone in the treatment of kleptomania. *The Journal of Clinical Psychiatry* 2002;63:349-356.

Griengel H, Sendera A, Dantendorfer K. Naltrexone as a treatment of self-injurious behavior—a case report. *Acta Psychiatrica Scandinavica* 2001;103:234-236.

Guardia J, Case C, Arias F, et al. A double-blind, placebo-controlled study of naltrexone in the treatment of alcohol-dependence disorder: results from a multicenter clinical trial. *Alcoholism, Clinical and Experimental Research* 2002;26:1381-1387.

Kim SW, Grant JE, Adson DE, et al. Double-blind naltrexone and placebo comparison study in the treatment of pathological gambling. *Biological Psychiatry* 2001;49:914-921.

McCaul ME, Wand GS, Eissenberg T, et al. Naltrexone alters subjective and psychomotor responses to alcohol in heavy drinking subjects. *Neuropsychopharmacology* 2000;22:480-492.

Marrazzi MA, Bacon JP, Kinzie J, et al. Naltrexone use in the treatment of anorexia nervosa and bulimia nervosa. *International Clinical Psychopharmacology* 1995;10:163-172.

Percy AK, Glaze DG, Schultz RJ, et al. Rett syndrome: controlled study of an oral opiate antagonist, naltrexone. *Annals of Neurology* 1994; 35:464-470.

Willensem-Swinkels SH, Buitelaar JK, van Engeland H. The effects of chronic naltrexone treatment in young autistic children: a double-blind, placebo-controlled crossover study. *Biological Psychiatry* 1996;39:1023-1031.

Disulfiram is indicated as an adjunct in the treatment of alcoholism. It is generally useful only for patients committed to sobriety who, despite active attendance at Alcoholics Anonymous, continue to drink. Disulfiram is effective by virtue of an irreversible inhibition of acetaldehyde dehydrogenase. Ethanol is initially metabolized by alcohol dehydrogenase to acetaldehyde, a highly toxic substance that, however, is immediately removed through conversion to acetic acid by acetaldehyde dehydrogenase. When acetaldehyde dehydrogenase is inhibited and the patient takes a drink, acetaldehyde levels rise to 5 to 10 times the concentration that would normally occur, thus producing the extremely unpleasant "acetaldehyde syndrome." This syndrome, which occurs within 5 to 10 minutes of taking a drink, is characterized initially by scarlet red facial flushing, which quickly spreads and is joined by throbbing headache, diaphoresis, vomiting, chest pain, palpitations, dyspnea, dizziness, and vertigo. When a large amount of alcohol has been taken, these symptoms may be joined by delirium and convulsions, severe hypotension that may lead to shock, acute congestive heart failure, myocardial infarction, respiratory depression, coma and death. The syndrome generally lasts anywhere from 30 minutes to several hours, depending on how much alcohol was taken. The patient then often feels exhausted and falls asleep for several hours.

The fear of such a reaction may keep patients from taking a drink until, eventually, their involvement with Alcoholics Anonymous provides them with the protection required to abstain from the next drink. Patients who are not committed to sobriety get little benefit from disulfiram; they either stop it so that they can drink again or simply drink while taking it, perhaps protecting themselves somewhat from the acetaldehyde syndrome by taking some diphenhydramine before they drink.

PHARMACOKINETICS

Disulfiram has about 80% bioavailability and reaches peak blood levels within 1 to 2 hours. It is metabolized in the liver to several active and inactive metabolites. Of the active metabolites, diethylthiomethylcarbonate is most important, as it, probably rather than disulfiram itself, is responsible for the irreversible inhibition of aldehyde dehydrogenase. Of the inactive metabolites, carbon disulfide is probably responsible for most of the neurologic side effects of disulfiram. Disulfiram has a long half-life; well over a week is required for its full metabolism.

SIDE EFFECTS

Although disulfiram is generally very well tolerated, a small minority of patients may experience side effects such as sedation, fatigue, headache, dizziness, tremor, restlessness, and impotence. Most of these side effects tend to lessen with continued treatment. Acneiform rashes may occur, as may a metallic taste. Rarely, a potentially fatal hepatitis may occur, typically within the first 2 months. Rare neurologic side effects may also occur, including a peripheral neuropathy, dystonia, parkinsonism and a dementia, which, though typically having an onset in the first few months of treatment, may not appear until after many years of treatment. Patients with schizophrenia may experience an exacerbation of their psychotic symptoms. Whether disulfiram is teratogenic or whether it is excreted in breast milk is not known.

DRUG-DRUG INTERACTIONS

Inhibition of hepatic enzymes by disulfiram may lead to elevated blood levels of certain tricyclic antidepressants (e.g., imipramine and desipramine), certain benzodiazepines (e.g., diazepam and chlordiazepoxide), phenobarbital, phenytoin, theophylline, rifampin, INH, and warfarin, and dosage adjustments may be necessary. Concurrent use of disulfiram and INH in particular may be followed by ataxia and a delirium. The combination of metronidazole and disulfiram may also cause a delirium.

OVERDOSAGE

Overdoses of disulfiram are rare. Severe encephalopathy and quadriplegia may ensue.

THERAPEUTIC USAGE

Disulfiram is available in 250 mg tablets.

As noted earlier, disulfiram is indicated only for patients who are committed to sobriety and who are attending Alcoholics Anonymous. In general, several months of treatment may be required before the patient is firmly enough established in Alcoholics Anonymous to be able to remain sober without disulfiram. Some patients may go on to take disulfiram on a "prn" basis, such as when traveling or entering into other situations where the temptation to drink might be acutely increased.

Treatment is generally initiated at 500 mg/day, with the dose decreased to 250 mg daily after 1 or 2 weeks. Generally, patients should be instructed to take the disulfiram first thing upon arising, as that is when the desire to stay sober is often strongest. However, when sedation is pronounced, half the dose may be taken at bedtime. Disulfiram should be used only with great caution in patients with heart disease or those with untreated hypothyroidism. In any case, treatment should not be started until the patient's blood alcohol level is zero.

Patients should be warned that even extremely small amounts of alcohol may provoke the acetaldehyde syndrome. Liquid medicines that contain alcohol (e.g., certain "cough" or "cold" preparations), vinegars, certain sauces, cologne, perfumes, and aftershave lotions must all be avoided. Furthermore, given the irreversible inhibition of aldehyde dehydrogenase and the time required for a new "crop" of the enzyme to be synthesized, patients should be made aware that an acetaldehyde syndrome may still occur within 14 days following discontinuation of disulfiram.

In the past the patient taking disulfiram was customarily given a drink to initiate the acetaldehyde syndrome. Provided, however, that the patient is given a graphic description of the syndrome, such a "test dose" procedure is not necessary. Additionally, some patients would not have a reaction during the test dose.

Should an acetaldehyde reaction occur, observation and supportive care are usually sufficient. Should the syndrome be severe, the following measures may be helpful: intravenous diphenhydramine; intravenous vitamin C; and carbogen (a mixture of 95% oxygen and 5% carbon dioxide) inhalation. If shock occurs, the usual treatment measures are instituted.

Liver function should probably be checked every 2 weeks for the first 2 months to guard against the rare occurrence of hepatitis, and perhaps every few months after that.

BIBLIOGRAPHY

Bergouignan FX, Vital C, Henry P, et al. Disulfiram neuropathy. *Journal of Neurology* 1988;235:382-383.

Borrett D, Ashby P, Bilbao J, et al. Reversible, late-onset disulfiram-induced neuropathy and encephalopathy. *Annals of Neurology* 1985;17:396-399.

Chick J, Gough K, Falkowski W, et al. Disulfiram treatment of alcoholism. *The British Journal of Psychiatry* 1992;161:84-89.

Christensen JK, Ronsted P, Vaag UH. Side effects after disulfiram. Comparison of disulfiram and placebo in a double-blind multicentre study. *Acta Psychiatrica Scandinavica* 1984;69:265-273.

Forns X, Caballeria J, Bruguera M, et al. Disulfiram-induced hepatitis. Report of four cases and review of the literature. *Journal of Hepatology* 1994;21:853-857.

Fuller RK, Branchey L, Brightwell DR, et al. Disulfiram treatment of alcoholism: a Veterans Administration cooperative study. *The Journal of the American Medical Association* 1986;256:1449-1455.

Krauss JK, Mohadjer M, Wakhloo AK. Dystonia and akinesia due to pallidoputaminal lesions after disulfiram intoxication. *Movement Disorders* 1991;6:166-170.

Laplane D, Attal N, Sauron B, et al. Lesions of basal ganglia due to disulfiram neurotoxicity. *Journal of Neurology, Neurosurgery, and Psychiatry* 1992;55:925-929.

Park CW, Riggio S. Disulfiram-ethanol induced delirium. *The Annals of Pharmacotherapy* 2001;35:32-35.

Wright C, Vafier JA, Lake CR. Disulfiram-induced fulminating hepatitis: guidelines for liver-panel monitoring. *The Journal of Clinical Psychiatry* 1988;49:430-434.

Zorzon M, Mase G, Biasutti E, et al. Acute encephalopathy and polyneuropathy after disulfiram intoxication. *Alcohol* 1995;30:629-631.

325 Rapid Pharmacologic Treatment of Agitation

When agitation becomes severe enough to constitute a danger to the patient or to others, rapid pharmacologic treatment should be considered. This is also called "rapid tranquilization," and although this term has much to recommend itself, it appears to have fallen into disfavor.

The most commonly used drugs for rapid pharmacologic treatment of agitation are antipsychotics (e.g., haloperidol, risperidone, olanzapine, ziprasidone and chlorpromazine) and the benzodiazepine, lorazepam. The reader is referred to the respective chapters for a discussion of the pharmacology of each of these agents.

INDICATIONS

The most common indications for rapid treatment are mania, an acute exacerbation of schizophrenia or schizoaffective disorder, or delirium. Intoxications with cocaine, stimulants, phencyclidine or hallucinogens may also be associated with considerable agitation. Occasionally, certain patients with a borderline, histrionic, paranoid, or antisocial personality disorder may also become severely agitated and require rapid pharmacologic treatment.

However, rapid pharmacologic treatment is indicated only for severe agitation and should not be used when patients are readily manageable by other means. Although this may seem self-evident, errors have been made in the past. For example, some patients admitted for schizophrenia have been rapidly treated with high doses of antipsychotics despite being only "quietly" psychotic and of no immediate danger to themselves or others. Although such an approach was rationalized by invoking the idea of a "loading" dose, using 60 mg of haloperidol in such patients provides no more benefit than using 5 to 10 mg, but does, however, cause more extrapyramidal side effects.

CHOICE OF DRUG

The choice of which drug to use is determined, in large part, by the underlying cause of the agitation.

For patients with mania or acute exacerbations of schizophrenia or schizoaffective disorder, any one of the antipsychotics is probably superior to lorazepam used alone, and, in the cases of haloperidol and risperidone, the addition of lorazepam creates a combination superior to either of these antipsychotics used alone. Whether or not the addition of lorazepam to olanzapine, ziprasidone or chlorpromazine creates a combination of superior efficacy to any of these agents alone has not as yet been determined. In choosing among these options, it must also be borne in mind that neither risperidone nor olanzapine, unlike all the other agents, are available in an intramuscular form. On balance, when rapid control is absolutely required in a patient unwilling to take oral medications, the combination of haloperidol and lorazepam is probably best; in cases where the need is not as urgent, and patients are willing to take oral medications, then the combination of risperidone and lorazepam is preferable, given risperidone's overall better tolerability as compared to haloperidol. Some clinicians prefer using olanzapine, either by itself or with lorazepam; however, as noted earlier, it is not as yet clear how effective olanzapine is, either with or without lorazepam, in comparison with the combination of haloperidol or risperidone and lorazepam. Some clinicians also prefer ziprasidone; however, experience with ziprasidone in this clinical situation, relative to the other agents, is limited. Chlorpromazine, once a standard, is now rarely used: it should, however, not be forgotten as its sedative effects may be extremely welcome in a severely agitated patient.

In the case of delirium, there is, remarkably, only one double-blinded study, and that compared haloperidol, chlorpromazine and lorazepam in AIDS patients who had developed delirium. In this study, both haloperidol and chlorpromazine were roughly equivalent, and both were superior to lorazepam, which was poorly tolerated. On balance, given that haloperidol is generally better tolerated than chlorpromazine, it is reasonable to use haloperidol in this clinical situation. Many clinicians, despite the lack of double-blinded supportive evidence, will use second generation agents, such as risperidone, in this situation, reasoning that it is in general more effective than haloperidol in other clinical situations and is also, by and large, better tolerated.

When agitation occurs secondary to intoxication with cocaine, other stimulants or phencyclidine, haloperidol is recommended; in the case of hallucinogens, however, lorazepam should be used.

In the case of agitation occurring in the context of a personality disorder, there are few solid guidelines; in practice a combination of lorazepam with either haloperidol or risperidone is often used.

TECHNIQUE

In the case of mania, schizophrenia or schizoaffective disorder, for otherwise healthy adults, haloperidol 5 to 10 mg IM and lorazepam 2 mg IM may be given every hour until an end point of clinical effectiveness or limiting side effects, or a maximum dose of 60 mg of haloperidol or 12 mg of lorazepam. The combination of haloperidol and lorazepam may also be given orally, in the same doses, but with the intervals stretched out to two hours. Risperidone and lorazepam may be given orally, in doses of 2 mg of each given every two hours, until one of the foregoing end points is reached or a maximum dose of 12 mg of either agent. Olanzapine may be given in a dose of 10 mg PO every two hours, until one of the end points or a maximum dose of 40 mg. Ziprasidone has been given in IM doses of 10 mg every 2 hours or 20 mg every 4 hours up to one of the end points or a maximum dose of 40 mg. Chlorpromazine may be given in a dose of 50 to 100 mg IM every hour or PO every two hours until one of the end points or a maximum dose of 1000 mg. In all instances where the antipsychotic is given orally, the concentrate or liquid form should generally be used.

For delirium, guidelines for rapid treatment are discussed in that chapter. As noted earlier, many clinicians will substitute risperidone for haloperidol, in a milligram to milligram ratio of roughly 1:4.

For intoxications with cocaine, other stimulants or phencyclidine, haloperidol may be given by itself in a schedule similar to that described above for mania, schizophrenia or schizoaffective disorder; for intoxication with hallucinogens, lorazepam may be used alone, again in a schedule as described above.

For agitation in a personality disorder, treatment may proceed as for mania, schizophrenia or schizoaffective disorder.

Haloperidol may also be given intravenously. This may be preferable in delirious patients who already have an IV in place and who balk at intramuscular injection. High-dose intravenous haloperidol has been associated with torsades de pointes, however, and this practice should be reserved for situations where other approaches have failed.

Once satisfactory control is achieved, the patient is placed on a regular dose of the effective drug or drugs, given orally in divided doses, with the total daily oral dose approximately equal to the amount required to initially control the agitation. An order is also left providing for "as-needed" extra doses. Every subsequent day, the oral dose is then further increased by an amount approximately equal to the total required in extra doses over the preceding

24 hours. This process is continued on a daily basis until either satisfactory control or limiting side effects occur.

In general, the patient is then maintained on this oral dose until the agitation that prompted rapid treatment has either remitted spontaneously or has been brought under control by other means. For example, in a manic patient, treatment is continued for a week or two until lithium, valproate, or carbamazepine has become effective. Or in schizophrenia, for example, once the agitation has been controlled, one generally waits a similar period of time until a true antipsychotic effect from an antipsychotic can be obtained, at which point lorazepam, if it had been used, may be tapered, after which it may also be possible to reduce the dose of the antipsychotic. In the case of delirium or intoxication, one waits out the natural course, and in the case of personality disorders, one waits until psychosocial measures have effected some further stability in the patient's life.

Certain caveats are in order regarding this technique. In the case of elderly or debilitated patients, or those with significant general medical conditions, doses should be lower, often much lower, and the interval between doses should generally be extended; furthermore, in hepatic failure the dose of the antipsychotic must also be lowered. Finally, good clinical judgment must come into play, and clinicians should monitor patients carefully during rapid treatment and be prepared to alter their technique as the clinical condition warrants.

CONCLUSIONS

Rapid pharmacologic treatment of agitation, properly and prudently performed, is a safe procedure that may spare the patient needless suffering and at times may even be lifesaving. The need for restraints and seclusion may be obviated, and in some cases hospitalization may be averted. Cardiac patients in the intensive care unit whose agitation threatens to precipitate a lethal arrhythmia or another myocardial infarction may be brought out of danger with timely institution of rapid treatment.

BIBLIOGRAPHY

Baker RW, Kinon BJ, Maguire GA, et al. Effectiveness of rapid initial dose escalation of up to 40 mg per day of oral olanzapine in acute agitation. *Journal of Clinical Psychopharmacology* 2003;23:342-348.

Battaglia J, Moss S, Rush J, et al. Haloperidol, lorazepam, or both for psychotic agitation? A multicenter, prospective, double-blind, emergency department study. *The American Journal of Emergency Medicine* 1997;15:335-340.

Bienick SA, Ownby RL, Penalver A, et al. A double-blind study of lorazepam versus the combination of haloperidol and lorazepam in managing agitation. *Pharmacotherapy* 1998;18:57-62.

Breier A, Meehan K, Birkett M, et al. A double-blind, placebo-controlled dose-response comparison of intramuscular olanzapine and haloperidol in the treatment of acute agitation in schizophrenia. *Archives of General Psychiatry* 2002;59:441-448.

Breitbart W, Marotta R, Platt MM, et al. A double-blind trial of haloperidol, chlorpromazine, and lorazepam in the treatment of delirium in hospitalized AIDS patients. *The American Journal of Psychiatry* 1996;153:231-237.

Currier GW, Simpson GM. Risperidone liquid concentrate and oral lorazepam versus intramuscular haloperidol and intramuscular lorazepam for treatment of psychotic agitation. *The Journal of Clinical Psychiatry* 2001;62:153-157.

Daniel DG, Potkin SG, Reeves KR, et al. Intramuscular (IM) ziprasidone 20 mg is effective in reducing acute agitation associated with psychosis: a double-blind, randomized trial. *Psychopharmacology* 2001;155:128-134.

Dubin WR, Waxman HM, Weiss KJ, et al. Rapid tranquilization: the efficacy of oral concentrate. *The Journal of Clinical Psychiatry* 1985;46: 475-478.

Lenox RH, Newhouse PA, Creelman WL, et al. Adjunctive treatment of manic agitation with lorazepam versus haloperidol: a double-blind study. *The Journal of Clinical Psychiatry* 1992;53:47-52.

Lesem MD, Zajecka JM, Swift RH, et al. Intramuscular ziprasidone, 2 mg versus 10 mg, in the short-term management of agitated psychotic patients. *The Journal of Clinical Psychiatry* 2001;62:12-18.

Meehan K, Zhang F, David S, et al. A double-blind, randomized comparison of the efficacy and safety of intramuscular injections of olanzapine, lorazepam, or placebo in treating acutely agitated patients diagnosed with bipolar mania. *Journal of Clinical Psychopharmacology* 2001; 21:389-397.

Meehan KM, Wang H, David SR, et al. Comparison of rapidly acting intramuscular olanzapine, lorazepam, and placebo: a double-blind, randomized study in acutely agitated patients with dementia. *Neuropsychopharmacology* 2002;26:494-504.

Neborsky R, Janowsky D, Munson E, et al. Rapid treatment of acute psychotic symptoms with high- and low-dose haloperidol. Behavioral considerations. *Archives of General Psychiatry* 1981;38:195-199.

Riker RR, Fraser GL, Cox PM. Continuous infusion of haloperidol controls agitation in critically ill patients. *Critical Care Medicine* 1994;22: 433-440.

Salzman C, Solomon D, Miyawaki E, et al. Parenteral lorazepam versus parenteral haloperidol for the control of psychotic disruptive behavior. *The Journal of Clinical Psychiatry* 1991;52:177-180.

Wright P, Birkett M, David SR, et al. Double-blind, placebo-controlled comparison of intramuscular olanzapine and intramuscular haloperidol in the treatment of acute agitation in schizophrenia. *The American Journal of Psychiatry* 2001;158:1149-1151.

326 Electroconvulsive Treatment

Electroconvulsive treatment (ECT) remains the most effective treatment for depressive episodes of either a major depression or bipolar disorder. However, given the necessity for a hospital stay and the widespread, yet wholly undeserved, public disapproval of its use, ECT is generally not performed except in emergency situations or until other treatments have failed or have caused unacceptable side effects.

In addition to being effective in depression, ECT is also effective in the treatment of a manic episode of bipolar disorder, depressive or manic episodes of schizoaffective disorder, catatonic schizophrenia (either the excited or stuporous type), post partum psychosis, and acute exacerbations of paranoid or undifferentiated schizophrenia, especially when accompanied by perplexity and prominent affective symptoms. Interestingly, as discussed in the chapter on Parkinson's disease, ECT is also effective for the motor symptoms of Parkinson's disease, regardless of whether depressive symptoms are present. This indication appears little known, and ECT is grossly underused in patients with end-stage Parkinson's disease unresponsive to medical management. Some cases of tardive dyskinesia may also improve. ECT has also been used for phencyclidine delirium and for delirium tremens; however, other treatments for these two disorders are almost always satisfactory and easier to use.

Although most clinicians reserve ECT for patients who have failed a trial of drug treatment, in certain situations one should probably proceed directly to ECT. Examples include depressed patients at immediate risk of death by suicide, debilitated and malnourished patients who might not survive long enough to experience an adequate trial of an antidepressant, and patients whose general medical condition prohibits the use of antidepressants.

The mechanism of action of ECT is unknown. Clearly, the generalized electrical seizure is necessary for a therapeutic effect; tonic and clonic motor activity may be completely prevented by succinylcholine without any loss of effect. Furthermore, the application of an electrical stimulus is likewise not necessary, since seizures induced by camphor injection or flurothyl (Indoklon) inhalation are just as effective. Despite extensive research, however, the mechanism whereby a series of generalized electrical seizures relieves depression remains unclear.

PREPARATION

In addition to a thorough history and physical, with special attention to handedness, all patients should have an electrocardiogram, a chem survey and a CBC. Other testing may include a lumbosacral spine film when pathology of the vertebral column is suspected,

and an MRI or CT scan of the head when significant intracranial pathology, such as a tumor, infarction or vascular malformation, is suspected.

Tricyclic antidepressants, which may predispose to arrhythmias, should be discontinued. Lithium should probably also be discontinued, since it may predispose to greater post-ECT confusion. Patients requiring antipsychotics may continue taking them.

Theophylline lowers the seizure threshold, and a theophylline level must be checked and appropriate adjustments made. Benzodiazepines may increase the seizure threshold, and, if possible, should be discontinued. Patients requiring benzodiazepines, or those requiring anticonvulsants, may continue with these medications; however, a greater electrical stimulus is required to induce a seizure.

As patients with hypertension are liable to severe rises in blood pressure during the ECT, one should optimize antihypertensive regimens before treatment.

As succinylcholine causes a rise in intraocular pressure, any patient with glaucoma should be under optimum treatment before receiving ECT.

Debilitated or malnourished patients should be carefully checked for any electrolyte imbalances, and these should be corrected before treatment. Loose teeth should probably be extracted, since they may break off and be aspirated when the electrical stimulus causes a vigorous contraction of the masseter muscle. One must bear in mind that the masseters are responding to direct electrical current and contract no matter how much succinylcholine is given.

The effects of succinylcholine may be prolonged by several factors. Succinylcholine is metabolized by plasma cholinesterase, and if cholinesterase levels are low, the half-life of succinylcholine will be prolonged. In about 1 in 2500 patients, one sees an inherited deficiency of cholinesterase; furthermore, cholinesterase levels are reduced during pregnancy and in the presence of hepatic insufficiency. Whenever doubt arises, a plasma cholinesterase level may be obtained.

Anticholinesterase agents, such as echothiophate or isofluorophate, also prolong succinylcholine's half-life. Cimetidine may also prolong the effects of succinylcholine. Hypokalemia, hypocalcemia, loop diuretics, and aminoglycosides all increase the response to succinylcholine.

TECHNIQUE

Treatment is scheduled for early in the morning. The night before, the scalp is thoroughly cleansed, and the application of hair or skin lotions or creams is forbidden. The patient is kept NPO after midnight, and on the morning of treatment uses the commode and is dressed in a loosely fitting hospital gown.

In the treatment room, a pulse oximeter and ECG and EEG monitors are attached, and a blood pressure cuff is placed on the arm ipsilateral to the nondominant hemisphere. Intravenous access is secured in the arm ipsilateral to the dominant hemisphere.

The clinician must decide what charge to administer during the stimulation and whether to use bilateral or nondominant unilateral electrode placement. Although electrical charge may be expressed as the actual mC delivered, it is conventional to grade the charge with reference to the patient's seizure threshold (the determination of which is discussed later): a "low" charge is about 50% over threshold, a "moderate" charge 150% above threshold, and a "high" charge is from 400% to 500% above threshold. The charge itself may be delivered either via bilateral electrode placement or unilateral nondominant placement. As noted below, transient amnesia is a common side effect of ECT, and the severity of this is related both to charge and electrode placement: bilateral placement at low, moderate or high charge creates the most amnesia, followed by nondominant high charge, nondominant moderate charge and nondominant low charge. The effectiveness of treatment also varies with charge and electrode placement: bilateral placement at moderate or high charge is probably most effective, but nondominant placement at high charge comes a close second. Nondominant placement at moderate charge is less effective than either of the foregoing, and nondominant placement at low charge is least effective. With these considerations in mind, most clinicians will begin with nondominant electrode placement at moderate charge.

If unilateral nondominant placement is elected, the first electrode is placed over the nondominant hemisphere about 1 inch superior to the midpoint of a line between the external canthus and the tragus, and the other is about 1 inch directly lateral to the vertex. If bilateral placement is used, both electrodes are placed, one on each side, about 1 inch superior to the midpoint of the line between the external canthus and the tragus. It is critical not to place an electrode over an opening in the skull, such as a burr hole, or over a steel plate. A generous amount of electrode gel is placed where the electrode will be placed; care is taken to ensure that, with unilateral placement, one does not allow a superficial conductive pathway between the electrodes.

An anticholinergic may both reduce respiratory tract secretions and bradycardia seen during ictus, and many clinicians administer them routinely. Given, however, that they may also predispose to greater tachycardia during the seizure, other clinicians prefer to utilize them only on a case by case basis. Glycopyrrolate, 0.2 to 0.4 mg, is preferred, but atropine in a dose of 0.6 to 1.0 mg may also be used. Both are given intravenously.

Anesthesia is induced with methohexital intravenously in a dose of 0.75 to 1.0 mg/kg.

The patient is oxygenated with 100% oxygen, administered through a face mask under positive pressure from this point until after spontaneous respirations have fully returned, the only exception being from when the bite block is placed until after cessation of any ictal motor activity that might interfere with respirations.

The blood pressure cuff on the arm ipsilateral to the nondominant hemisphere is immediately inflated above systolic pressure, and succinylcholine is then given intravenously in a dose of approximately 1 mg/kg. When complete relaxation is required, such as for recent fractures, higher doses may be given. Fasciculations appear within 60 seconds, starting in facial musculature and proceeding down the trunk and arm, finally to the feet. Their disappearance indicates that relaxation is completed. Patients with myotonia congenita or with myotonic muscular dystrophy may show a pronounced response to succinylcholine.

A bite block is inserted, the jaw is gently held shut, and the stimulus is applied.

Selection of the proper stimulus is of great importance. Different ECT devices allow for the setting of different parameters, and the clinician should become familiar with the device available at the hospital. If more than one device is available, the one that delivers a brief pulse should be used rather than a device delivering a sine wave current. Although both are equally effective, the sine wave device generally results in greater postictal confusion. As noted earlier, it is appropriate to determine the seizure threshold, and this may be accomplished by beginning with what would, in most patients, be a "sub-threshold" dose of perhaps 50 mC, and then increasing this in similar increments every 30 seconds until either a generalized seizure occurs or two further attempts at higher dose have failed to produce a seizure: if this latter end-point is reached, then the machine should be set to provide a maximum charge in order to ensure that the patient has a seizure before the anesthetic wears off. In such a case, during the second treatment session one may begin the titration at approximately the dose reached on the third stimulation and titrate from there. Once the seizure threshold has been determined, then the charge for subsequent treatments may be set with reference to this threshold: if nondominant leads are used, then a "moderate" charge of roughly 150% of the threshold is generally in order.

Before proceeding further, it must be noted that this titration procedure, though favored by many, is not without controversy. It has been pointed out that subconvulsive stimulations, though not producing a seizure, may however induce a vagal discharge and a consequent bradycardia which, as it is not relieved by the sympathetic discharge seen during a seizure, may be quite prolonged, thus placing some patients, particularly those with cardiac disease, at risk. With this consideration in mind, combined with the fact that the highest charge produces the greatest clinical effect, some clinicians argue against titration at all and recommend simply beginning with a "fixed" high charge (of from 350 to 500 mC) delivered via nondominantly placed leads. The resolution of this controversy awaits further study: in the meantime it may be prudent to reserve the "titration" method for those without significant cardiac disease and to consider the "fixed" high charge method for those at risk if prolonged bradycardia occurred.

Regardless of what charge is employed initially and how leads are placed, it is critical to produce a generalized seizure that lasts at least 30 seconds, as briefer seizures are unlikely to be therapeutically effective. If after the stimulus is given there is no seizure or if the seizure is of inadequate duration, then the stimulus intensity should be substantially increased and a second stimulus immediately given. Importantly, in determining whether or not a seizure has occurred, one must not confuse the masseter contraction, which is directly caused by the local stimulation, with actual tonic activity.

Two methods are available whereby seizure duration may be monitored, namely by direct observation of tonic and clonic activity in the cuffed arm and by observing the EEG monitor. As the electrical seizure generally outlasts the motor manifestations, the EEG monitor has the advantage of providing a more accurate record of seizure duration. However, as the single lead channel EEG available with most devices does not always distinguish between a localized seizure and a generalized one, the cuff method has the advantage of indisputably signaling a generalized seizure when nondominant unilateral electrode placement is used: provided that the cuff is placed ipsilateral to the electrodes, motor activity in the cuffed arm indicates that the ictal discharge has crossed the midline into the dominant hemisphere. In practice, both methods are used.

During the seizure, blood pressure and cardiac rate and rhythm are monitored. Typically, within seconds, a vagally-mediated bradycardia occurs which, in more than one-half of patients, is accompanied by a brief period of asystole, lasting up to five seconds. Subsequently, a sympathetically-mediated tachycardia and hypertension ensue and persist for the remainder of the seizure: during this time, ventricular premature beats may occur, sometimes in a trigeminal or bigeminal pattern; rarely, ventricular tachycardia may occur. At the end of the seizure, a transient bradycardia may again be seen. As noted earlier, bradycardia may be prevented by pretreating with glycopyrrolate; supplementary doses may be required. Occasionally, premature beats require the administration of an antiarrhythmic. If the blood pressure rises alarmingly high, a beta-blocker, such as labetolol, may be given. Optimum control of hypertension before beginning treatment often prevents this from happening; in some cases pre-treatment with nifedipine may also be helpful.

Seizures lasting much longer than 60 seconds are not any more therapeutic than those in the range of 30 to 60 seconds. Seizures lasting longer than 2 to 3 minutes should be terminated, either with intravenous lorazepam, 1 to 2 mg, or another dose of methohexital. Importantly, one must distinguish between the expected post-ictal delirium and the rare occurrence of ECT-induced complex partial status epilepticus. In doubtful cases, the EEG is helpful, as it will reveal generalized slowing in the case of a post-ictal delirium and rhythmic activity in the case of status.

Subsequent to the seizure and after spontaneous respiration has fully reappeared, the patient is placed in a postoperative position and closely observed for at least the next 30 minutes. Vomiting occasionally occurs and may be treated with prochloperazine, 5 mg IV.

Although upon awakening some patients are immediately clear, the majority experience a delirium of variable severity, lasting from 15 minutes up to several hours or more. Longer and more severe deliria are associated with bilateral placement, greater stimulus charge, longer seizures, greater number of treatments, and with having treatments too closely spaced together. Upon return to the ward, phone calls and visitors should generally be prohibited until the sensorium is clear. A small minority, perhaps 5%, of those who become delirious become violently agitated. Such patients may be treated with 5 to 10 mg of diazepam or 1 to 2 mg of lorazepam intravenously.

COURSE

Treatments are generally given three times a week, and in most cases from six to twelve treatments are required for a full therapeutic effect. The use of multiple monitored ECT, that is the induction of several seizures during one period of anesthesia, does not appear to hasten response, but does appear to cause considerably more confusion.

In general, an initial response is seen after the first three or four treatments. If no response is seen with nondominant electrode placement at moderate charge at this point, then one should utilize a high charge; if a high charge is already being used then one should switch to bilateral lead placement, utilizing either a moderate or high charge. If, despite an adequate seizure duration of 30 to 60 seconds with bilateral high dose stimulation, no response is seen after 12 treatments, then a subsequent response is unlikely, and the patient should be thoroughly reassessed.

Most patients show a full response after 6 to 10 treatments. Many clinicians then administer one or two "extra" treatments to "cement" the response. Although no reliable experimental data are available to support this practice, the general clinical opinion favors it.

During the course of treatment, typically one finds it necessary to progressively increase the charge to ensure a seizure of adequate duration. Should increasing the charge be ineffective, or should the maximum charge allowed by the machine be reached, one may prolong seizures by the intravenous administration of caffeine about 5 minutes before application of the stimulus in a dose of from 250 to 1000 mg. Should this be ineffective one may consider utilizing a different anesthetic.

In rare instances one may have to terminate a course of treatment before achieving a full response. This may occur when unacceptable cardiovascular complications occur. Most commonly, however, treatments are prematurely terminated because the postictal confusion persists at a severe level without significant diminution by the time the next treatment is due.

RELATIVE CONTRAINDICATIONS

During the seizure a rise in intracranial pressure occurs which, if coupled with an edematous lesion, may lead to uncal or transtentorial herniation. Examples include certain tumors, abscesses, recent (within four to six weeks) infarction, and hemorrhage. The presence of a tumor, however, is not an absolute contraindication. Indeed, with slow-growing lesions, such as a meningioma, that have no associated edema, little or no risk at all is present. The same, of course, holds true for an old infarction. In borderline cases, where a small degree of edema is present, the use of prednisone or dexamethasone may reduce the edema to the point where treatment is safe.

The paroxysmal rise in blood pressure during the seizure may be dangerous in patients with any of the following lesions: cerebral arteriovenous malformations, cerebral aneurysms, aortic or carotid aneurysm, and recent (within four to six weeks) myocardial infarction. Aggressive antihypertensive treatment may be required.

Although patients with arrhythmias or those predisposed to them (such as a patient with a recent myocardial infarction) are at an increased risk for arrhythmias during the seizure and may require aggressive antiarrhythmic treatment, overall the cardiovascular risk from ECT is low.

Pregnancy is not a contraindication to ECT; indeed ECT may be safer for the fetus than are antidepressants and is certainly safer than first trimester use of lithium, valproate, or carbamazepine.

Patients with ongoing upper or lower motor neuron disease, or those with significant crush injuries or severe burns, may experience hyperkalemia with succinylcholine treatment that may be severe enough to cause cardiac arrest. In these clinical situations other muscle relaxants should be used.

ADVERSE EFFECTS

ECT per se is generally a safe treatment; the mortality rate is no higher than for any other procedure requiring anesthesia. Before the introduction of muscle relaxants such as succinylcholine, fractures of the long bones were not uncommon; with adequate relaxation, however, fractures as a complication of ECT are almost unheard of.

An anterograde amnesia exists for the period of time when the patient is to any degree delirious postictally; a small amount of retrograde amnesia for events occurring just before the treatment may also be seen. As the delirium following a long course of treatments may persist, for several months, albeit to a progressively less severe degree, the period of amnesia may be relatively long. By 6 months post-treatment, however, one cannot detect any difficulty in acquiring new information. However, when these patients look back they may be unable to recall most events occurring from just before treatment up to a week or so after the last treatment; subsequent events that occurred over the next month or two are recalled in a spotty fashion, and events subsequent to that are recalled as well as any events that occurred before treatment began.

Paradoxically, in bipolar depressed patients, ECT may cause mania. Thus in treating a bipolar depressed patient, the first hint of mania is an indication to either discontinue treatment and observe the patient or to proceed only with great caution.

Rarely, a treatment will be followed by a postictal psychosis: here, following resolution of the post-ictal delirium, patients may develop delusions and hallucinations. This generally resolves spontaneously; however, if it is problematic it may be treated with a brief course of haloperidol.

POSTTREATMENT MANAGEMENT

As is the case with antidepressants and other medications used in the mood disorders, ECT is purely a symptomatic treatment—it does not alter the long-term course of the illness being treated. The beneficial effects of ECT endure for about two or three months and sometimes less. Consequently, if in the natural course of events the underlying illness has not gone into remission, when ECT "wears off" the patient will re-experience symptoms. Consequently, in instances where the underlying illness is expected to last longer than several months (and this is the case with almost all the indications for ECT, except for phencyclidine delirium or delirium tremens), one can begin continuation drug treatment as described in the respective chapters for these illnesses. Thus for the patient with a major depression, one may consider a single antidepressant (e.g., paroxetine) or a combination of nortriptyline and lithium; for the patient with a bipolar disorder, lithium, valproate, carbamazepine or lamotrigine; and for patients with schizophrenia, an antipsychotic.

When aggressive drug treatment fails to forestall a relapse, one may consider "maintenance ECT." Here, after a successful course of treatments, the patient receives single treatments weekly for about two months, after which the frequency of treatments may be gradually reduced, as tolerated, down to one per month. In most cases it is possible to discontinue maintenance ECT after patients have been free of depressive symptoms for from 6 to 12 months. Importantly, during maintenance ECT there will be some ongoing, albeit perhaps subtle, anterograde amnesia and this will require some modification of the patient's affairs.

BIBLIOGRAPHY

Andersen K, Balldin J, Gottfries CG, et al. A double-blind evaluation of electroconvulsive therapy in Parkinson's disease with "on-off" phenomena. *Acta Neurologica Scandinavica* 1987;76:191-199.

Burd J, Kettl P. Incidence of asystole in electroconvulsive therapy in elderly patients. *The American Journal of Geriatric Psychiatry* 1998;6:203-211.

Chung KF, Wong SJ. Stimulus dose titration for electroconvulsive therapy. *Psychiatry and Clinical Neurosciences* 2001;55:105-110.

Coffey CE, Figiel GS, Weiner RD, et al. Caffeine augmentation of ECT. *The American Journal of Psychiatry* 1990;147:579-585.

Coffey CE, Locke J, Weiner RD, et al. Seizure threshold in electroconvulsive therapy (ECT) II. The anticonvulsant effect of ECT. *Biological Psychiatry* 1995;37:777-788.

Delva NJ, Brunet D, Hawken ER, et al. Electrical dose and seizure threshold: relations to clinical outcome and cognitive effects in bifrontal, bitemporal, and right unilateral ECT. *The Journal of ECT* 2000;16: 361-369.

Griesemer DA, Kellner CH, Beale MD, et al. Electroconvulsive therapy for treatment of intractable seizures. Initial findings in two children. *Neurology* 1997;49:1389-1392.

Hansen-Grant S, Tandon R, Maixner D, et al. Subclinical status epilepticus following ECT. *Convulsive Therapy* 1995;11:134-138.

Janakiramaiah N, Motreja S, Gangadhar BN, et al. Once vs three times weekly ECT in melancholia: a randomized controlled trial. *Acta Psychiatrica Scandinavica* 1998;98:316-320.

Jha AK, Stein GS, Fenwick P. Negative interaction between lithium and electroconvulsive therapy—a case-control study. *The British Journal of Psychiatry* 1996;168:241-243.

Larsen JR, Hein L, Stromgren LS. Ventricular tachycardia with ECT. *The Journal of ECT* 1998;14:109-114.

McCall WV, Reboussin DM, Weiner RD, et al. Titrated moderately suprathreshold vs fixed high-dose right unilateral electroconvulsive therapy: acute antidepressant and cognitive effects. *Archives of General Psychiatry* 2000;57:438-444.

Mayur PM, Gangadhar BN, Janakiramaiah N, et al. Motor seizure monitoring during electroconvulsive therapy. *The British Journal of Psychiatry* 1999;174:270-272.

Patkar AA, Hill KP, Weinstein SP, et al. ECT in the presence of brain tumor and increased intracranial pressure: evaluation and reduction of risk. *The Journal of ECT* 2000;16:189-197.

Penney JF, Dinwiddie SH, Zorumski CF, et al. Concurrent and close temporal administration of lithium and ECT. *Convulsive Therapy* 1990;6:139-145.

Rabheru K, Persad E. A review of continuation and maintenance electroconvulsive therapy. *Canadian Journal of Psychiatry* 1997;42:476-484.

Sackheim HA, Prudic J, Devanand DP, et al. A prospective, randomized, double-blind comparison of bilateral and right unilateral electroconvulsive therapy at different stimulus intensities. *Archives of General Psychiatry* 2000;57:425-434.

Salaris S, Szuba MP, Traber K. ECT and intracranial vascular masses. *The Journal of ECT* 2000;16:198-203.

Squire LR, Chace PM. Memory functions six to nine months after electroconvulsive therapy. *Archives of General Psychiatry* 1975;32:1557-1564.

Stromgren LS. ECT in acute delirium and related clinical states. *Convulsive Therapy* 1997;13:10-17.

Swartz CM, Manly DT. Efficiency of the stimulus characteristics of ECT. *The American Journal of Psychiatry* 2000;157:1504-1506.

Tew JD, Mulsant BH, Haskett RF, et al. A randomized comparison of high-charge right unilateral electroconvulsive therapy and bilateral electroconvulsive therapy in older depressed patients who failed to respond to 5 to 8 moderate-charge unilateral treatments. *The Journal of Clinical Psychiatry* 2002;63:1102-1105.

Troller JN, Sachdev PS. Electroconvulsive treatment of neuroleptic malignant syndrome: a review and report of cases. *The Australian and New Zealand Journal of Psychiatry* 1999;33:650-659.

UK ECT Review Group. Efficacy and safety of electroconvulsive therapy in depressive disorders: a systematic review and meta-analysis. *Lancet* 2003;361:799-808.

Wengel SP, Burke WJ, Pfeiffer RF, et al. Maintenance electroconvulsive therapy for intractable Parkinson's disease. *The American Journal of Geriatric Psychiatry* 1998;6:263-269.

Zwil AS, Pemerantz A. Transient postictal psychosis associated with a course of ECT. *Convulsive Therapy* 1997;13:32-36.

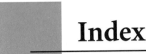

Index

Note: *vs.* denotes differential diagnosis.

A

abnormal movements, in tardive dyskinesia 267, 268
abscess, brain *see* brain abscess
absence seizures 309
abstract thought, deficiency/defects 10
  dementia 284
abulia 2
  frontal lobe syndrome 299, 300
abuse, drug/substance *see* alcohol abuse; drug abuse; substance abuse
acceleration-deceleration injuries 375
ACE inhibitors, drug interactions, lithium 466
acetaldehyde syndrome 514
acetazolamide, sleep apnea 222
Achilles tendon enlargement 338, 339
acne, as side effect, lithium 465
acquired hepatocerebral degeneration 443–444
activity disturbances 1–3
acute anxiety neurosis *see* panic disorder
acute confusional state *see* delirium
acute disseminated encephalomyelitis 364
acute intermittent porphyria 445
acute measles encephalitis 411
acute organic brain syndrome *see* delirium
acute stress disorder 172
acute toxic psychosis *see* delirium
acyclovir, herpes zoster vasculopathy/encephalitis 417
addiction 62
  symptomatology, impulsivity 2
  see also drug abuse; substance abuse
Addison's disease 392
adolescents
  antisocial personality disorder 251, 252
  attention-deficit/hyperactivity disorder 44
  borderline personality disorder 254
  disorders first diagnosed in 12–51
  hair pulling 245
  thrill-seeking 242
adrenal adenomas, Cushing's syndrome 391
adrenal carcinomas, Cushing's syndrome 391
adrenocortical insufficiency 392–393
  Addison's disease 392
  adrenocorticotropic hormone (ACTH) 392
  AIDS 393
  diabetes mellitus 393
  differential diagnosis 393
  Hashimoto's thyroiditis 393
  hypoparathyroidism 393
  pernicious anemia 393
  vitamin B_{12} deficiency 402
  vitiligo 393
adrenocorticotropic hormone (ACTH)
  adrenocortical insufficiency 392
  Cushing's syndrome 390
adrenoleukodystrophy 339–340
  differential diagnosis 340, 342
  therapy 340
    Lorenzo's oil 340
adults, attention-deficit/hyperactivity disorder 44
aerosol spray propellant abuse 71–72
affect
  blunting of affect 6, 118
  definition 4
  disturbances of 6
  flat affect 6, 118
  inappropriate affect 6
  labile affect 5–6

aggressiveness
  intermittent explosive disorder 240
  see also violence
agitation 2
  in Alzheimer's disease 316
  therapy
    benzodiazepines 496
    chlorpromazine 515
    first generation antipsychotics 515
    haloperidol 515, 516
    lorazepam 515, 516
    olanzapine 515
    risperidone 515, 516
    ziprasidone 515
agoraphobia 11, 162–163
  social phobia *vs.* 166
agranulocytosis
  clozapine causing 481
  tricyclic antidepressants 449
AIDS
  adrenocortical insufficiency 393
  fungal (mycotic) infections 428
  neurosyphilis 404
  primary nervous system lymphoma 380
AIDS dementia 423–425
  cytomegalovirus encephalitis *vs.* 427
  general paresis *vs.* 406
  neurosyphilis *vs.* 424
  vitamin B_{12} deficiency *vs.* 424
airway obstruction, obstructive sleep apnea 221, 222
akathisia 123
  antipsychotics causing 123, 476, 492
    treatment 478, 492
  restless legs syndrome *vs.* 224
  tardive dyskinesia *vs.* 270
akinesia
  secondary to antipsychotics 295
  therapy, anticholinergics 488
akinetic mutism 10
  stuporous catatonia *vs.* 293
albuterol, atomexetine interaction 507
alcohol, rubbing 111
alcohol abuse 85–88
  alcoholism *vs.* 85, 86
  posttraumatic stress disorder 171, 172
  secondary psychosis 290
alcohol dependence *see* alcoholism
alcohol hallucinosis 101–102, 475, 477
alcohol intoxication 89–90
  blackouts 90–91
    dissociative amnesia *vs.* 185
    transient global amnesia *vs.* 359
  blood alcohol level (BAL) 89
  pathological intoxication 91–92
  violence association 279
alcohol tolerance 86
alcohol withdrawal 86, 92–94
  delirium *see* delirium tremens (alcohol withdrawal delirium)
  hyperthyroidism *vs.* 387
  hypoglycemia *vs.* 432
  major depressive disorder *vs.* 138
  seizures 94–95
  therapy
    benzodiazepines 496
    propanolol 492
alcoholic cerebellar degeneration 104–105
  spinocerebellar ataxia *vs.* 334

alcoholic cirrhosis, hepatic encephalopathy 443
alcoholic dementia 100
  acquired hepatocerebral degeneration *vs.* 443
  Alzheimer's disease *vs.* 317
  general paresis *vs.* 406
alcoholic myopathy 105–106
alcoholic paranoia 102–103, 248
  delusional disorder *vs.* 130
  therapy, first generation antipsychotics 475, 477
alcoholic polyneuropathy 103–104
Alcoholics Anonymous 87–88, 252
alcohol-induced depression 86
alcohol-induced persisting amnestic disorder *see* Korsakoff's syndrome
alcohol-induced persisting dementia *see* alcoholic dementia
alcohol-induced psychotic disorder with delusions *see* alcoholic paranoia
alcohol-induced psychotic disorder with hallucinations 101–102, 473, 477
alcoholism 84–87
  alcohol abuse *vs.* 85, 86
  antisocial personality disorder *vs.* 252
  conduct disorder and 46
  delirium tremens 282
  fetal alcohol syndrome and 14–15
  gastritis 111
  head trauma 111
  hepatic injury 111–112
  hypoglycemia 112
  hypomagnesemia 437
  isopropyl (isopropanol) alcohol intoxication 111
  ketoacidosis 112
  major depressive disorder *vs.* 138
  Marchiafava–Bignami disease 107–108
  methanol intoxication 109–110
  pancreatitis 112
  posttraumatic stress disorder 171, 172
  smoking and 74, 109
  suicide risk 276
  symptomatology, impulsivity 2
  therapy 87–88
    disulfiram 514
    naltrexone 512, 513
  tobacco–alcohol amblyopia 109
  Wernicke's encephalopathy 97–98
ALD gene, adrenoleukodystrophy 340
alien hand syndrome 301, 304–305, 325
allergic reactions, first generation antipsychotics 477
alpha-2 autoreceptor agonists, drug interactions 449
alpha-2 autoreceptor blockers
  attention-deficit/hyperactivity disorder 45
  Tourette's syndrome 50
  see also clonidine; guanfacine
alpha-methyldopa, drug interactions 463, 504
alprazolam 498–499
  drug interactions 498
  essential tremor 498
  generalized anxiety disorder 174, 498
  major depressive disorder 140
  panic disorders 161, 498
  premenstrual syndrome 145, 498
  therapeutic use 498
alprostadil, erectile dysfunction therapy 195
"alternative psychosis" *see* psychosis of forced normalization
aluminium poisoning 399